KU-467-592

The ESC Textbook of
Cardiovascular Imaging

European Society of Cardiology publications

The ESC Textbook of Cardiovascular Medicine (Second Edition)
Edited by A. John Camm, Thomas F. Lüscher, and Patrick W. Serruys

The EAE Textbook of Echocardiography
Editor-in-Chief: Leda Galiuto, with Co-editors: Luigi Badano, Kevin Fox, Rosa Sicari, and José Luis Zamorano

The ESC Textbook of Intensive and Acute Cardiovascular Care (Second Edition)
Edited by Marco Tubaro, Pascal Vranckx, Susanna Price, and Christiaan Vrints

The ESC Textbook of Cardiovascular Imaging (Second Edition)
Edited by José Luis Zamorano, Jeroen Bax, Juhani Knuuti, Patrizio Lancellotti, Luigi Badano, and Udo Sechtem

Forthcoming
The EHRA Book of Pacemaker, ICD, and CRT Troubleshooting: Case-based learning with multiple choice questions
Edited by Harran Burri, Carsten Israel, and Jean-Claude Deharo

The ESC Textbook of Preventive Cardiology
Edited by Stephan Gielen, Guy De Backer, Massimo Piepoli, and David Wood

The EACVI Echo Handbook
Edited by Patrizio Lancellotti and Bernard Cosyns

The ESC Handbook of Preventive Cardiology: Putting prevention into practice
Edited by Catriona Jennings, Ian Graham, and Stephan Gielen

The ESC Textbook of
Cardiovascular Imaging

SECOND EDITION

Edited by

José Luis Zamorano

Jeroen Bax

Juhani Knuuti

Udo Sechtem

Patrizio Lancellotti

Luigi Badano

OXFORD

UNIVERSITY PRESS

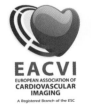

OXFORD
UNIVERSITY PRESS

Great Clarendon Street, Oxford, OX2 6DP,
United Kingdom

Oxford University Press is a department of the University of Oxford.
It furthers the University's objective of excellence in research, scholarship,
and education by publishing worldwide. Oxford is a registered trade mark of
Oxford University Press in the UK and in certain other countries

© European Society of Cardiology 2015

The moral rights of the author have been asserted

First Edition published in 2010
Second Edition published in 2015

Impression: 1

All rights reserved. No part of this publication may be reproduced, stored in
a retrieval system, or transmitted, in any form or by any means, without the
prior permission in writing of Oxford University Press, or as expressly permitted
by law, by licence or under terms agreed with the appropriate reprographics
rights organization. Enquiries concerning reproduction outside the scope of the
above should be sent to the Rights Department, Oxford University Press, at the
address above

You must not circulate this work in any other form
and you must impose this same condition on any acquirer

Published in the United States of America by Oxford University Press
198 Madison Avenue, New York, NY 10016, United States of America

British Library Cataloguing in Publication Data
Data available

Library of Congress Control Number: 2014959477

ISBN 978–0–19–870334–1

Printed in Italy by L.E.G.O. S.p.A.

Oxford University Press makes no representation, express or implied, that the
drug dosages in this book are correct. Readers must therefore always check
the product information and clinical procedures with the most up-to-date
published product information and data sheets provided by the manufacturers
and the most recent codes of conduct and safety regulations. The authors and
the publishers do not accept responsibility or legal liability for any errors in the
text or for the misuse or misapplication of material in this work. Except where
otherwise stated, drug dosages and recommendations are for the non-pregnant
adult who is not breast-feeding

Links to third party websites are provided by Oxford in good faith and
for information only. Oxford disclaims any responsibility for the materials
contained in any third party website referenced in this work.

Contents

Abbreviations

(video icon)	video	EE	embolic events
(cross reference icon)	cross reference	EF	ejection fraction
(online material icon)	additional online material	EMI	electromagnetic interference
(website icon)	website	EOA	effective orifice area
$^{13}NH_3$	^{13}N-labelled ammonia	ERNV	equilibrium radionuclide ventriculography
^{201}Tl	thallium-201	EROA	effective regurgitant orifice area
^{82}Rb	^{82}Rubidium	ESV	end-systolic volume
^{99m}Tc	technetium-99m	FBP	filtered back-projection
AAA	abdominal aortic aneurysms	FDG	fluorodeoxyglucose
ACS	acute coronary syndromes	FFA	free fatty acid
AF	atrial fibrillation	FFR	fractional flow reserve
AMI	acute myocardial infarction	FOV	field of view
ARVC/D	arrhythmogenic right ventricular cardiomyopathy/dysplasia	GFR	glomerular filtration rate
		GSD	glycogen storage diseases
AS	aortic stenosis	GSO:Ce	cerium-doped gadolinium oxyorthosilicate
ASD	atrial septal defect	$H_2{}^{15}O$	^{15}O-labelled water
AV	aortic valve	HCM	hypertrophic cardiomyopathy
AVA	aortic valve area	HFREF	heart failure patients with reduced ejection fraction
BMIPP	beta-methyl-p-iodophenyl-pentadecanoic acid		
BNP	brain natriuretic peptide	HLA	horizontal long axis
b-SSFP	balanced steady-state free precession	HM	hibernating myocardium
CAD	coronary artery disease	HMR	heart to mediastinum ratio
CDRIE	cardiac devices-related infective endocarditis	ICA	invasive coronary angiography
CFR	coronary flow reserve	ICD	implantable cardioverter-defibrillators
CHF	congestive heart failure	ICE	intra-cardiac echocardiography
CIED	cardiac implantable electric device	IE	infective endocarditis
CMR	cardiac magnetic resonance	IOD	internal orifice diameter
CP	constrictive pericarditis	IR	inversion–recovery
CRT	cardiac resynchronization therapy	IRA	infarct-related artery
CSA	cross-sectional area	IVRT	isovolumic relaxation time
CT	computed tomography	LA	left auricle
CTCA	computed tomography coronary angiography	LAA	left atrial appendage
CVF	collagen volume fraction	LBBB	left bundle branch block
CZT	cadmium-zinc-telluride	LC	lumped constant
DI	Doppler imaging	LGE	late gadolinium enhancement
DSE	dobutamine stress echocardiography	LOR	line-of-response
DTI	Doppler tissue imaging	LSO	lutetium oxyorthosilicate
ECMO	extracorporeal membrane oxygenation	LV	left ventricular
ECV	extracellular volume	LVEF	left ventricular ejection fraction
EDV	end-diastolic volume	LVOT	left ventricular outflow tract

LYSO	lutetium-yttrium		RT3D	real-time three-dimensional
MACE	major adverse cardiac events		RV	right ventricle
MBF	myocardial blood flow		RVOT	right ventricular outflow tract
MCE	myocardial contrast echocardiography		RWMA	regional wall motion abnormalities
MDCT	multi-detector computed tomography		SAM	systolic anterior motion
MI	myocardial infarction		SAR	specific absorption rate
MIBG	metaiodobenzylguanidine		SARF	severe acute respiratory failure
MIP	maximum intensity projections		SCD	sudden cardiac death
MPI or	myocardial performance index		sECG	stress electrocardiogram
Tei-index			SENC	strain-encoded cardiac magnetic resonance
MPR	multi-planar reconstructions		ShMOLLI	Shortened Modified Look-Locker Inversion
MPR	multi-planar reformatting			recovery
MPRI	myocardial perfusion reserve index		SIS	segment involvement score
MPS	myocardial perfusion scintigraphy		SNR	signal-to-noise ratio
MR	mitral regurgitation		Sp	specificity
MR	mitral regurgitation		SPECT	single photon emission computed tomography
MRI	magnetic resonance imaging		SSA	senile systemic amyloidosis
MS	mitral stenosis		SSFP	steady-state free precession
MSCT	multi-slice computed tomography		STE	speckle-tracking echocardiography
MV	mitral valve		STEMI	ST-elevation myocardial infarction
MVA	mitral valve area		SV	stroke volume
MVO_2	myocardial oxygen consumption		TA	tricuspid annulus
MVR	mitral valve replacement		TAC	time–activity curves
MVS	mitral valve stenosis		TAVI	trans-catheter aortic valve implantation
NMR	nuclear magnetic resonance		TCFA	thin-cap fibroatheroma
OSEM	ordered-subsets expectation maximization		TEE	transoesophageal
PAH	pulmonary artery hypertension		TEI	transmural extent of infarction
PAU	penetrating aortic ulcer		TGA	transposition of the great arteries
PCI	percutaneous coronary interventions		TOE	transoesophageal echocardiography
PET	positron emission tomography		TOF	time of flight
PFO	patent foramen ovale		TOF	tetralogy of Fallot
PH	pulmonary hypertension		TR	tricuspid regurgitation
PICE	percutaneous intra-pericardial cardiac echo		TS	tricuspid stenosis
PMBV	percutaneous mitral balloon valvuloplasty		TTE	transthoracic echocardiography
PMC	percutaneous mitral commissurotomy		TTR	transthyretin
PPVR	percutaneous pulmonary valve replacement		TV	tricuspid valve
PSF	point spread function		TVIR	trans-catheter valve-in-ring implantation
PSIR	phase-sensitive inversion recovery		UCA	ultrasound contrast agent
PS	pulmonic stenosis		USPIO	ultra-small superparamagnetic particles of iron
PSS	post-systolic shortening			oxides
PVIE	prosthetic valve infective endocarditis		VCAM-1	vascular cell adhesion molecule-1
PVR	paravalvular regurgitation		VCG	vector cardiogram
QCA	quantitative coronary angiography		VD	myocardial contrast volume of distribution
RAP	right atrial pressure		VHD	valvular heart disease
RCMP	restrictive cardiomyopathy		VLA	vertical long axis
RF	radiofrequency		VSDs	ventricular septal defects
RNA	radionuclide angiography			

Contributors

Stephan Achenbach
Department of Cardiology, University of Erlangen, Germany

Teresa Arcadi
Department of Radiology, Giovanni XXIII Hospital, Monastier, Italy

Luigi P. Badano
Department of Cardiac, Thoracic and Vascular sciences, University of Padova, School of Medicine, Padova, Italy

Jeroen J. Bax
Department of Cardiology, Leiden University Medical Center, Leiden, The Netherlands

Helmut Baumgartner
Director, Division of Adult Congenital and Valvular Heart Disease, Department of Cardiovascular Medicine, University Hospital Muenster, Professor of Cardiology/Adult Congenital Heart Disease, University of Muenster, Germany

Harald Becher
Heart and Stroke Foundation for Cardiovascular Research, University of Alberta; Mazankowski Heart Institute, Edmonton, Canada

Frank M. Bengel
Department of Nuclear Medicine, Hannover Medical School, Hannover, Germany

Ruxandra Beyer
TBC

Jan Bogaert
Department of Radiology, Gasthuisberg University Hospital, Leuven, Belgium

Eric Brochet
Cardiology Department, Hospital Bichat, Paris, France

Oliver Bruder
Associate Professor of Medicine, Director Department of Cardiology and Angiology, Contilia Heart and Vascular Center, Elisabeth Hospital Essen, Germany

Thomas Buck
Associate Professor of Medicine and Cardiology, Director Department of Cardiology, Klinikum Westfalen, Dortmund, Germany

Peter Buser
Professor of Cardiology, Vice-Chairman Department of Cardiology, University Hospital Basel, Switzerland

Filippo Cademartiri
Department of Radiology, Erasmus Medical Center, Rotterdam, The Netherlands; Department of Radiology, Giovanni XXIII Hospital, Monastier, Italy

Paolo G. Camici
Vita-Salute University and San Raffaele Scientific Institute, Milan, Italy

Jean-Luc Canivet
Department of General Intensive Care, University Hospital Centre, University of Liege, Domaine Universitaire du Sart-Tilman, Liege, Belgium

Giovanni La Canna
Echocardiography Unit, San Raffaele Scientific Institute, Milan, Italy

Gaby Captur
Biomedical Research Centre, University College London, UK

John-Paul Carpenter
Cardiovascular Magnetic Resonance Unit, Royal Brompton Hospital, London

Ignasi Carrió
Professor of Nuclear Medicine, Universitat Autònoma de Barcelona; Director, Nuclear Medicine Department, Hospital de la Santa Creu i Sant Pau, Sant Antoni M. Claret, Barcelona, Spain

Orlando Catalano
Department of Radiology, SDN Foundation IRCCS, Naples, Italy

Zhong Chen
BHF Clinical Research Fellow in Cardiovascular Imaging

Sofia Churzidse
University Clinic of Cardiology, University Duisburg-Essen, Germany

Paolo Colonna
Cardiology Department, Policlinico University Hospital, Bari, Italy

Nuno Cortez Dias
Cardiology Fellow, Department of Cardiology, University Hospital Santa Maria, Lisbon University, Portugal

Genevieve Derumeaux
Hôpital Louis Pradel, Lyon, France

Johan De Sutter
University Gent, Belgium and Department of Cardiology, AZ Maria Middelares Hospital, Gent, Belgium

Victoria Delgado
Department of Cardiology, Leiden University Medical Center, Leiden, The Netherlands

Erwan Donal
Cardiologie, CHU Rennes et LTSI, France

Raluca E. Dulgheru
Department of Cardiology, CHU Sart Tilman, Liège, Belgium

Perry Elliott
Professor of Cardiology, University College London, UK

Raimund Erbel
Professor of Medicine/Cardiology, European Cardiologist, Department of Cardiology, West-German Heart Center, University Duisburg-Essen, Germany

Arturo Evangelista
Director of Cardiac Imaging, Servei de Cardiología, Hospital Universitari Vall d'Hebron, Spain

Covadonga Fernández-Golfín
University Hospital Ramón y Cajal, Madrid, Spain

Frank A. Flachskampf
Uppsala Universitet, Akademiska Sjukhuset, Sweden

Albert Flotats
Associate Professor of Nuclear Medicine, Universitat Autònoma de Barcelona, Spain; Consultant, Nuclear Medicine Department, Hospital de la Santa Creu i Sant Pau, Sant Antoni M. Claret, Barcelona, Spain

Mark K. Friedberg
The Hospital for Sick Children, The University of Toronto, Toronto, Canada

Jérôme Garot
Director of Cardiovascular Magnetic Resonance, Hôpital Privé Jacques Cartier, Institut Cardiovasculaire Paris Sud (ICPS), Générale de Santé, France

Bernhard L. Gerber
Department of Cardiology, Cliniques Universitaires St. Luc UCL, Brussels, Belgium

Tjeerd Germans
Department of Cardiology, VU University Medical Center, Amsterdam, The Netherlands

Silvia Gianstefani
Locum Consultant Cardiologist and Lead of Echocardiography, Croydon University Hospital, London, UK

Carmen Ginghina
University of Medicine and Pharmacy 'Carol Davila', Euroecolab, Emergency Institute of Cardiovascular Diseases 'Prof. C. C. Iliescu', Bucharest, Romania

Alexandra Gonçalves
Cardiology Department, University of Porto Medical School/ Centro Hospitalar S. João, Porto, Portugal

Maria Magdalena Gurzun
University of Medicine and Pharmacy 'Carol Davila', Euroecolab, Emergency Institute of Cardiovascular Diseases 'Prof. C. C. Iliescu', Bucharest, Romania

Gilbert Habib
Hôpital Timone, Cardiology Department, Marseille

Andreas Hagendorff
Head of the Laboratory of Echocardiography, Department of Cardiology-Angiology, University of Leipzig, Germany

James Harrison
BHF Clinical Research Fellow in Cardiovascular Imaging

Rainer Hoffmann
Medical Clinic I, University Aachen, Germany

Michael Horacek
University Clinic of Cardiology, University Duisburg-Essen, Germany

Alexander Janosi
University Clinic of Cardiology, University Duisburg-Essen, Germany

Majo Joseph
Department of Cardiovascular Medicine (JBS, MJ), Flinders University, Flinders Medical Centre, Adelaide, Australia

Hagen Kälsch
University Clinic of Cardiology, University Duisburg-Essen, Germany

Theodoros Karamitsos
The Oxford Centre for Clinical Magnetic Resonance Research (TK, SN), University of Oxford, Oxford, UK

Philipp A. Kaufmann
Stv. Klinikdirektor Nuklearmedizin, Leiter Kardiale Bildgebung NUK/CT/MRI, UniversitätsSpital Zürich, Switzerland

Philip Kilner
CMR Unit, Royal Brompton Hospital, London, UK

Juhani Knuuti
Turku University Hospital and University of Turku, Finland

Gabriel Krestin
Department of Radiology, Erasmus Medical Center, Rotterdam, The Netherlands

Patrizio Lancellotti
GVM Care and Research, Italy

Paul Leeson
Professor of Cardiovascular Medicine and Director Oxford Cardiovascular Clinical Research Facility, University of Oxford, UK

Massimo Lombardi
Medical Director UOC Cardiovascular MR at CNR, Institute of Clinical Physiology/G. Monasterio Foundation, Pisa, Italy

Erica Maffei
Department of Radiology, Giovanni XXIII Hospital, Monastier, Italy

Julien Magne
Research Associate, Cardiology Department, CHU Limoges, France

Heiko Mahrholdt
Department of Cardiology, Robert Bosch Krankenhaus, Stuttgart, Germany

David Maintz
Director Department of Radiology, University of Cologne, Germany

Luc Mertens
The Hospital for Sick Children, The University of Toronto, Toronto, Canada

Mark J. Monaghan
Director of Non-Invasive Cardiology and Associate Medical Director, King's College Hospital, London, UK

Denisa Muraru
Department of Cardiac, Thoracic, and Vascular Sciences, University of Padova, School of Medicine, Padova, Italy

Eike Nagel
Division of Cardiovascular Imaging, Goethe University Frankfurt, Germany

Danilo Neglia
Director Multimodality Cardiovascular Imaging Program at CNR, Institute of Clinical Physiology/G. Monasterio Foundation, Pisa, Italy

Stefan Neubauer
The Oxford Centre for Clinical Magnetic Resonance Research (TK, SN), University of Oxford, Oxford, UK

Ed Nicol
Department of Radiology, Royal Brompton Hospital, London; Department of Cardiology, John Radcliffe Hospital, Oxford, UK

Petros Nihoyannopoulos
Professor of Cardiology, Imperial College London; Hammersmith Hospital, London, UK

Stefan Orwat
Division of Adult Congenital and Valvular Heart Disease, Department of Cardiovascular Medicine, University Hospital Muenster, Germany

Dudley J. Pennell
Professor of Cardiology, National Heart and Lung Institute, Imperial College; Director NIHR Cardiovascular Biomedical Research Unit; Director, Cardiovascular Magnetic Resonance Unit, Head, Non-Invasive Cardiology, Royal Brompton Hospital, UK

Pasquale Perrone-Filardi
Department of Internal Medicine, Cardiovascular and Immunological Sciences, Federico II University, Naples, Italy

Luc A. Pierard
Department of Cardiology, CHU Sart Tilman, Liège, Belgium

Fausto J. Pinto
Professor of Cardiology, Department of Cardiology, University Hospital Santa Maria, Lisbon University, Portugal

Sven Plein
Professor of Cardiology, BHF Senior Clinical Research Fellow, University of Leeds, UK

Björn Plicht
Senior Cardiologist, Assistant Director Department of Cardiology, Klinikum Westfalen, Dortmund, Germany

Bogdan A. Popescu
University of Medicine and Pharmacy 'Carol Davila', Euroecolab, Emergency Institute of Cardiovascular Diseases 'Prof. C. C. Iliescu', Bucharest, Romania

Sanjay K. Prasad
Royal Brompton NHS Foundation Trust and Imperial College, London, UK

Susanna Price
Consultant Cardiologist and Intensivist, Royal Brompton Hospital, London, UK

Frank Rademakers
Department of Cardiology, University Hospitals Leuven, Leuven, Belgium

Reza Razavi
Head of Division, Imaging Sciences and Biomedical Engineering, Division of Imaging Sciences and Biomedical Engineering, King's College London, UK

Ornella Rimoldi
IBFM, Consiglio Nazionale delle Ricerch, Segrate, Italy

Luis M. Rincón
Cardiology Department, Ramón y Cajal University Hospital, Spain

Daniel Rodriguez Munoz
Department of Cardiology, University Hospital Ramón y Cajal, Madrid, Spain

Raphael Rosenhek
Director Heart Valve Clinic, Division of Cardiology, Medical University of Vienna, Austria

Michael Rubens
Department of Radiology, Royal Brompton Hospital, London, UK

Thomas Schlosser
Institute of Diagnostic and Therapeutic Radiology, University Clinic Essen, University Duisburg-Essen, Germany

Axel Schmermund
Professor of Internal Medicine and Cardiology, Cardioangiologisches Centrum Bethanien, Germany

Juerg Schwitter
Division of Cardiology and Director Cardiac MR Center, University Hospital Lausanne, Switzerland

Udo Sechtem
Division of Cardiology, Robert-Bosch-Krankenhaus, Stuttgart, Germany

Joseph B. Selvanayagam
Department of Cardiovascular Medicine (JBS, MJ), Flinders University, Flinders Medical Centre, Adelaide, Australia

Roxy Senior
Consultant Cardiologist and Director of Echocardiography, Royal Brompton Hospital; Cardiovascular Biomedical Research Unit, Imperial College, London, UK

Benoy N. Shah
Consultant Cardiologist, University Hospital Southampton, Southampton, UK

Marta Sitges
Cardiology Department, Hospital Clinic, University of Barcelona, Spain

Rosa Sicari
CNR Institute of Clinical Physiology

Manav Sohal
St. Jude Clinical Research Fellow in Cardiovascular Imaging

James Stirrup
Clinical Research Fellow, Nuclear Cardiology and Cardiac CT, National Heart and Lung Institute, Imperial College, London, UK

Franck Thuny
Hôpital Timone, Cardiology Department, Marseille, France

S. Richard Underwood
Professor of Cardiac Imaging, National Heart and Lung Institute, Imperial College, Royal Brompton Hospital, London, UK

Albert C. van Rossum
Professor of Cardiology, Chairman of the Department of Cardiology, VU University Medical Center, Amsterdam, The Netherlands

David Vancraeynest
Cardiovascular Department, Division of Cardiology, Cliniques Universitaires St-Luc, Université Catholique de Louvain, Belgium

Jean-Louis J. Vanoverschelde
Cardiovascular Department, Division of Cardiology, Cliniques Universitaires St-Luc, Université Catholique de Louvain, Belgium

Jens-Uwe Voigt
TBC

Jeremy Wright
Department of Radiology, Gasthuisberg University Hospital, Leuven, Belgium; Greenslopes Private Hospital, Brisbane, Australia

Ali Yilmaz
Department of Cardiology and Angiology, University Hospital Münster, Germany

José L. Zamorano
Head of Cardiology, University Hospital Ramón y Cajal, Madrid, Spain

SECTION I

Technical aspects of imaging

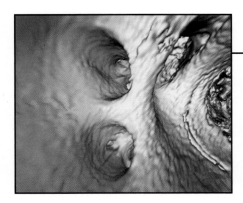

CHAPTER 1

Conventional echocardiography—basic principles

Andreas Hagendorff

Contents

Introduction

Echocardiography is an imaging technique that enables accurate assessment of cardiac structures and cardiac function. Conventional echocardiography involves different modalities—especially the M-mode, the 2D and colour Doppler, as well as the pulsed wave and continuous wave Doppler. The M-mode illustrates the reflections of a single sound beam plotted against time. 2D echocardiography enables the documentation of views, which represent characteristic sectional planes of the moving heart during one heart cycle. Colour Doppler echocardiography adds the information of blood flow to the 2D cineloop. Pulsed wave Doppler is the acquisition of a local blood flow spectrum of a defined region represented by the dimension of the sample volume, whereas continuous wave Doppler displays the blood flow spectrum of all measured blood flow velocities along a straight line sound beam from its beginning to the end. The handling of the transducer has to be target-oriented, stable with respect to the imaging targets, and coordinated with respect to angle differences between the defined views to use all these modalities correctly to get optimal image quality of the cineloops and spectra. Thus, the focus of this chapter will be a mainly practically oriented description of scanning technique in transthoracic and transoesophageal echocardiography.

The echocardiographic documentation requires ultrasound machines, which fulfil the international laboratory standards in echocardiography. Thus, the equipment has to be minimally capable to enable broadband 2D imaging, M-mode imaging, pulsed and continuous wave Doppler, as well as colour-coded imaging, pulsed tissue Doppler imaging, and complete digital storage capability. In addition, the ultrasound system has to have all technical possibilities for transoesophageal, contrast, and stress echocardiography. An ECG recording should generally be performed in order to be able to capture complete heart cycles according to the ECG trigger. This chapter is written in accordance with the current international guidelines and recommendations [1–8].

Principles of transthoracic echocardiography—practical aspects

The main principle of echocardiographic scanning is an exact or best possible manual control of the region of interest during the technical procedure. This principle includes the ability to move a certain cardiac structure within the scan sector from the left to the right and vice versa without losing the cardiac structures of the selected sectional plane.

In addition, this aspect is documented by the ability to rotate the transducer exactly about 60 or 90° without losing the defined cardiac structure in the centre of the primary scan sector before rotating. In other words, the visualization of cardiac structures in the centre of the scan sector has to be combined with the technical skill of the investigator to change only one plane within the spatial coordinates to achieve accurate characterization and documentation of the target cardiac structure. Thus, the easy message of transthoracic echocardiography is scanning by tilting without flipping and rotating, by flipping without tilting and rotating, as well as by rotating without tilting and flipping. This sounds easy, but it requires a stable transducer position next to the skin of the patient, an absolutely stable guiding of the transducer, and a stereotactic manual control of the transducer.

Regarding these aspects it is surprising that the finger position of holding a transducer has almost never been described in lectures and books about echocardiography, whereas in every book about musical instruments instructions of hand and finger positions, and illustrations of fingering charts are given.

In transthoracic echocardiography there is a complex interaction between the eyes, the brain and the hand muscles to coordinate looking to a monitor to detect incongruities between the actual view and defined views and to correct them by manual manoeuvres to get the standardized views. Thus, it is like 'seeing' the heart with your hands. A basic position of the transducer in the hand is necessary to get the orientation for the scan procedure for an easy, but controlled change of a sectional plane. This implies that a defined holding of the transducer is always linked to a defined hand position which has to be linked with a defined view. In echocardiography in adult patients, the echocardiographic investigation normally starts with the left parasternal approach. It is obvious that the basic holding of the transducer should be linked to the long-axis view of the left ventricle. In consequence, all possible long-axis views that can be acquired between the position of the left parasternal and the apical approach should be linked to this defined hand-holding of the transducer. If you change your basic position of holding the transducer during the scanning procedure of the same sectional plane, the imagination and association of the individual coordinates of the heart within the thorax will be lost by the investigator, which means that he will become disoriented or blind during scanning.

It has to be mentioned and emphasized, that scanning is possible with the right as well as with the left hand. The argument for a correct scanning technique is always the acquisition of standardized images with high image quality. Thus, echocardiographic scanning can be performed as the investigator is, or has been, taught how to do it. The author of this chapter, however, scans with the right hand. Thus, the images of how to hold the transducer and adjust the finger positions are shown for right-hand scanners.

To get a stable position for the transducer holding, all fingers are generally lifted and not extended. The pulps of the fourth and fifth fingers conveniently lie on the small edge of the transducer without any muscle tension (⊃ Fig. 1.1a). The pulp of the thumb is conveniently placed on the notch of the transducer without any muscle tension (⊃ Fig. 1.1b). This convenient relaxed transducer holding has to be conceptionally combined with the basic

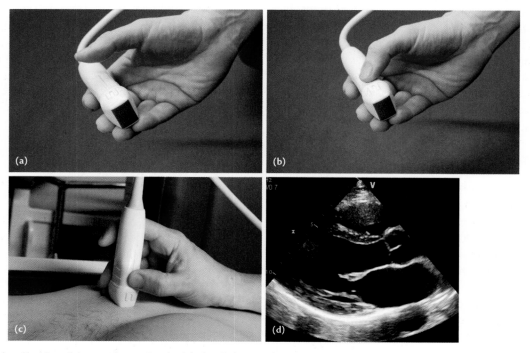

Fig. 1.1 Correct relaxed holding of the transducer using the right hand. The transducer lies on the fourth and fifth finger without any muscle tension (a), the pulp of the thumb only has contact to the notch of the transducer (b). The pulps of the fourth and fifth finger have contact to the skin (c) and the feeling of this transducer holding is combined with the parasternal log axis view (d).

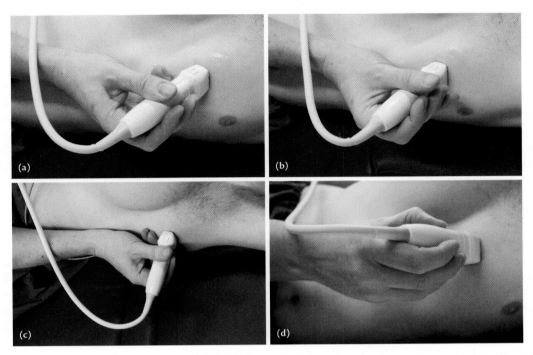

Fig. 1.2 Examples of inconveniently holding the transducer. In (a) the fourth and fifth finger are between the transducer and the skin like writing with a pencil. No stable contact to the skin results in non-stabilization of the transducer. In (b) the holding is like encompassing a horizontal bar. Thus, rotation of the transducer is not performed by the hand—it has to be done by the shoulder and/or cubital joint. In (c) the thumb is too extended and the pulp of the thumb is not at the notch causing a blind feeling when moving or rotating the transducer. In addition, the mistake in Fig. 1.2a is also seen. In (d) no finger has contact to the skin. Thus, every trembling of the hand is bridged to the transducer and consequently to the images on the monitor. It is also not possible to get a basis for a defined flipping, tilting and rotation, because the starting position is not stable.

position of the transducer in the parasternal long-axis view of the heart (⮞ Fig. 1.1c, d). The loss of the feeling for the notch and extended or tensed fingers in the starting position will induce discomfort and restrict the degrees of freedom for the movement of the transducer. Thus, wrong transducer holdings (⮞ Fig. 1.2a–d) will lead to disorientation and difficulties in fine-tuning for adjusting correct standardized views. An often observed mistake is not to fix the fourth and fifth finger on the skin of the patient, leading to an unstable transducer position. With tilting over the small edge using the transducer holding of this starting position in the long-axis view, the mitral valve, for example, can be moved from the right to the left and vice versa without losing the long-axis view.

A clockwise rotation of the transducer from the starting position is easy (⮞ Fig. 1.3a), because there is free space to turn the thumb clockwise by bending backwards the fourth and fifth fingers (⮞ Fig. 1.3b, c). A 90° rotation is easily possible and thus, you will get the feeling of rotating exactly 90° clockwise at the left parasternal window to visualize a correct short-axis view (⮞ Fig. 1.3d).

After acquisition of the necessary parasternal short-axis views the transducer is rotated counterclockwise back to the correct long-axis view. The correct position of the apical window and the correct apical long-axis view can be achieved by sliding down from the parasternal window to the apex without losing the sectional plane of the long-axis view (⮞ Fig. 1.4). At the end of this

movement the right hand can support itself against the thorax with the complete auricular finger (⮞ Figs 1.5a,b). Fingers placed between the transducer and the thorax in this position will disturb or inhibit the correct documentation of apical standard views by positioning the transducer too perpendicular to the body surface inducing a right twisted position of the heart within the scan sector and/or foreshortening views. Without tilting and flipping the correct apical long-axis view, a clockwise rotation of exactly 60° can be performed (⮞ Fig. 1.5c) to visualize a correct 2-chamber view (⮞ Fig. 1.5d).

Combining a defined transducer holding always with the long-axis view and getting the stable feeling for this combination are the prerequisites for target-controlled scanning and the accurate assessment of cardiac structures. It is obvious that minimal manipulations of the transducer position can be easily performed and stably fixed using the correct scanning technique. Thus, a correct scanning technique is the prerequisite for images with at least best possible image quality.

The aim of a sufficient transthoracic, and also transoesophageal, echocardiographic investigation should be an almost reproducible standardized documentation, which enables an accurate diagnostic analysis for correct decision-making. A standardization of the documentation enables a comparison between current and previous findings to detect changes, improvements or deterioration of the cardiac state in follow-ups. Furthermore, the more standardization is present, the more

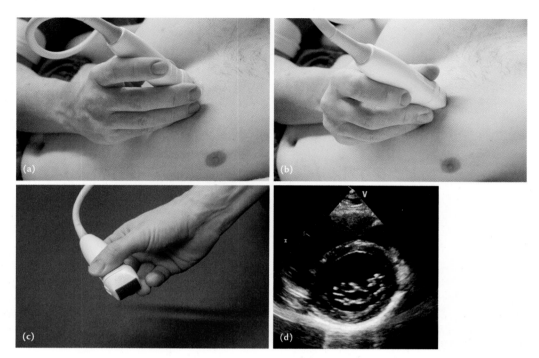

Fig. 1.3 Starting with the correct holding of the transducer for displaying the parasternal long-axis view (a) the transducer is exactly rotated 90° clockwise (b), after this movement the pulp of the thumb is at the broad side of the transducer at the top and the third finger is at the broad side of the transducer at the bottom (b), while the fourth and fifth finger are retracted (c), but they have still contact to the skin. This holding is linked with all parasternal short-axis views (d).

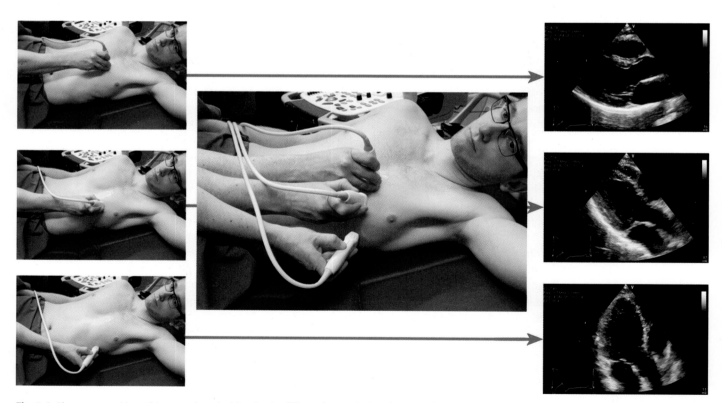

Fig. 1.4 Photo composition of the transducer holding for the different long-axis views between the standardized parasternal approach and the standardized apical approach. On the left side the different holdings at the correct parasternal position, at a position between the parasternal and apical position, as well as at the correct apical position are shown. In the centre the photomontage of all transducer holdings is shown documenting the plane of all long-axis views. On the right side the corresponding views are shown.

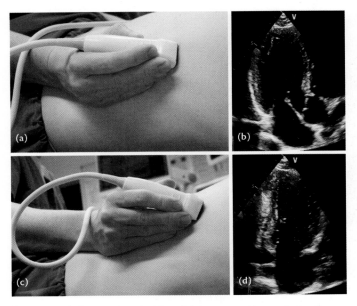

Fig. 1.5 With the transducer holding of the parasternal long-axis view the hand is slid down to the apical long-axis view (a). At the position of the apical long-axis view the fourth and fifth finger still remain on the skin. In addition, the complete ulnar area of the fifth finger is placed in position against the thorax for scanning from the apical approach (a). This transducer holding is linked with the apical long-axis view (b). A clockwise rotation of 60° without tilting and flipping has to be done (c) to get the correct apical 2-chamber view (d).

intra- and inter-observer variability is reduced. The basis for the correct configuration of an echocardiographic data acquisition and examination—including data acquisition, data documentation, data storage, interpretation and reporting of the results—as well as the correct measurements and calculations of numerical values in echocardiography is provided by already published national and international guidelines and position papers.

Standardized data acquisition in transthoracic echocardiography

Left parasternal and apical scanning should normally be performed in left lateral position of the patient.

The transthoracic echocardiographic examination should start with the correct documentation of the conventional two-dimensional left parasternal long-axis view of the left ventricle (⮕ Fig. 1.6a–b). This sectional plane is characterized by the centre of the mitral valve, the centre of the aortic valve, as well as by the 'imaginary' cardiac apex, which cannot be visualized from the parasternal approach due to the superposition of the left lung. The following anatomical structures are visualized by the parasternal long-axis view. In the nearfield of the transducer, the first myocardial structure is the free right ventricular

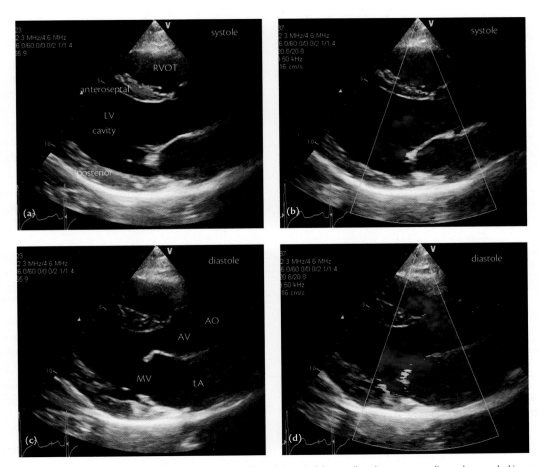

Fig. 1.6 Standardized grey-scale parasternal long-axis view during systole (a) and diastole (c), as well as the corresponding colour-coded images during systole (b) and diastole (d). Additional comments in the text.

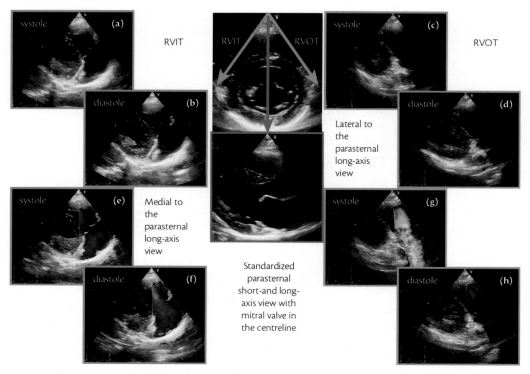

Fig. 1.7 Illustration for display of the right ventricular inflow tract and right ventricular outflow tract. Starting from the standardized parasternal long-axis view (red arrow and red surrounding), the right ventricular inflow tract is displayed by medial tilting (green arrow and green surrounding) of the sectional plane (a-systole, b-diastole), the right ventricular outflow tract by lateral tilting (blue arrow and blue surrounding) of the sectional plane (c-systole, d-diastole). The corresponding colour-coded views are displayed in e-h. Additional comments in the text.

wall—normally parts of the right ventricular outflow tract. The left ventricular cavity in the longitudinal section is surrounded by the midbasal anteroseptal and posterior regions of the left ventricle. The mitral valve is sliced in the centre of the valve plane nearly perpendicularly to the commissure. The aortic valve is also sliced in the centre of the valve in longitudinal direction. The aortic root and the proximal part of the ascending aorta are longitudinally intersected. Behind the aortic root the left atrium is longitudinally intersected. The posterior left ventricular wall is bordered by the posterior epicardium and the diaphragm. The far field of the parasternal long-axis view should include the cross-section of the descending aorta behind the left atrium. A standardized left parasternal long-axis view can be verified by the following display of the heart within the sector. The mitral valve has to be centred in the scanning sector. Then, the ventral boundary of the mid anteroseptal region of the left ventricle on the left side has to be in line with the ventral boundary of the ascending aorta on the right side of the sector. Furthermore, the check of the correct longitudinal parasternal long-axis view should include the ascending aorta visualized as a tube and not as an oblique section, the central valve separation of the mitral and aortic valves, as well as the missing of papillary muscles. If papillary muscles are sliced, the sectional plane is not in the centre of the left cavity, which corresponds to a non-standardized view. For qualitative assessment of flow phenomena at the mitral

and aortic valves, as well as for the detection of perimembranous ventricular septal defects, a colour-coded 2D cineloop of the left parasternal long-axis view can be added to the documentation (⮑ Fig. 1.6c–d).

With respect to the documentation of the right heart, tilting the transducer to the sternal regions enables the visualization of the right ventricular inflow tract with a longitudinal sectional plane through the tricuspid valve (⮑ Fig. 1.7a–b). Tilting the long-axis view to the lateral regions of the heart enables the visualization of the right ventricular outflow tract with the longitudinal sectional plane through the pulmonary valve (⮑ Fig. 1.7c–d). These views should also be documented using colour-coded 2D cineloops (⮑ Fig. 1.7e–h).

The 90° clockwise rotation of the transducer from the transducer position of the correctly set parasternal long-axis view will lead to sectional short-axis views of the heart. The correct transducer position to display standardized parasternal short-axis views using conventional transthoracic echocardiography is documented by a M-mode sweep (⮑ Fig. 1.8a). Parasternal short-axis views should be documented with respect to an accurate definition of the plane according to cardiac structures, which enables a high reproducibility of each view. Short-axis views are defined by the accurate cross-section through the left ventricular attachment of the papillary muscles (⮑ Fig.1.8b), through the papillary muscles (⮑ Fig. 1.8c), through the chord

through the LV attachment of the papillary muscles | through the papillary muscles | through the chord heads as well as the chord strands | through the mitral valve | through the inter-atrial septum and the left ventricular outflow tract | through the aortic valve

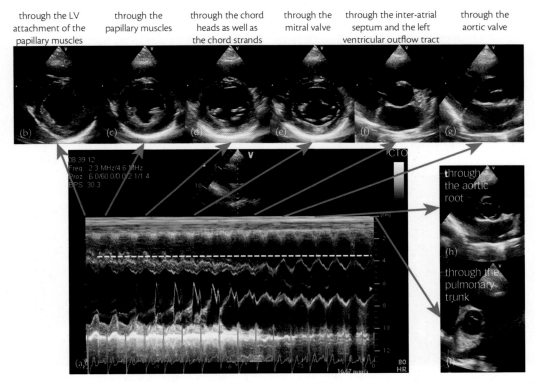

Fig. 1.8 Display of a standardized M-mode sweep (a). The correct transducer position is documented by the M-mode sweep by a horizontal line between the ventral border of the anteroseptal septum and the ventral border of the aortic root (dotted line). Short-axis views are defined by the accurate cross-section through the left ventricular attachment of the papillary muscles (b), through the papillary muscles (c), through the chord heads as well as the chord strands (d), through the mitral valve (e), through the inter-atrial septum and the left ventricular outflow tract (f), through the aortic valve (g), the aortic root and the proximal ascending aorta (h), as well as by a nearly longitudinal plane through the pulmonary trunk and the bifurcation of the pulmonary arteries (i). The red arrows show the position of the respective short-axis view in a M-mode sweep. Additional comments in the text.

heads, as well as the chord strands (➲ Fig. 1.8d), through the mitral valve (➲ Fig. 1.8e), through the inter-atrial septum and the left ventricular outflow tract (➲ Fig. 1.8f), through the aortic valve (➲ Fig.1.8g), the aortic root and the proximal ascending aorta (➲ Fig. 1.8h), as well as by a nearly longitudinal plane through the pulmonary trunk and the bifurcation of the pulmonary arteries (➲ Fig. 1.8i). The acquisition of a correct M-mode sweep is performed within 6–12 cardiac cycles using the cursor in the centre line of all parasternal short-axis views by scanning through the left ventricle over the long axis of the left ventricle by tilting the transducer starting from the short-axis view between the papillary muscles up to the cranial short-axis view of the centrally intersected aortic valve and ascending aorta (➲ Fig. 1.8a). By deriving M-modes and M-mode sweeps in the short axis, it can always be checked whether the left heart is sliced exactly in its centre line or only a secant view of the left ventricle is documented. This fact favours the acquisition of M-modes using short-axis views instead of a long-axis view. The correct transducer position is documented in the M-mode sweep by a horizontal line between the border of the ventral septum and the border of the ventral ascending aorta. The alternative to document the correct transducer position in the long-axis view simultaneously to the short-axis views is only possible by

biplane scanning. The problem of isolated short-axis views is the fact that the transducer position is too much lateral or caudal, which causes an oval conformation of the ventricular wall at the level of the left ventricle. The consequence for measurements of left ventricular dimensions and wall thicknesses is that the left ventricular cavity is measured too large and the ventricular wall is measured too thick (➲ Fig. 1.9).

For training aspects and to document manual skills of target-oriented scanning, the correct acquisition of the M-mode sweep should be integrated into the educational process like a driver's license for echocardiography. For clinical practice the correct M-mode sweep represents a characteristic profile of the individual human heart.

According to European recommendations, however, it is not mandatory to acquire the M-mode sweep. The standard documentation includes only parasternal short-axis views at the mid-papillary level, at the mitral valve level and at the aortic level. In all parasternal short-axis views the centre of the left ventricle or the aortic valve should be in the middle of the scanning sector. Near the transducer the parasternal short-axis view at the mid-papillary level (➲ Fig. 1.10a–d) shows the free right ventricular wall, the right ventricular cavity, all mid-segments of the left ventricular wall (near the transducer: anteroseptal—0°;

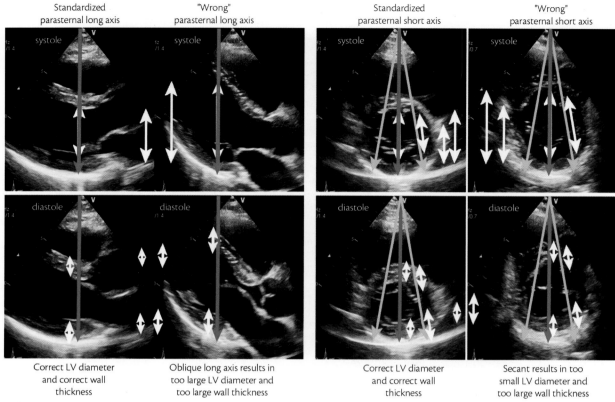

Standardized parasternal long axis · "Wrong" parasternal long axis · Standardized parasternal short axis · "Wrong" parasternal short axis

Correct LV diameter and correct wall thickness | Oblique long axis results in too large LV diameter and too large wall thickness | Correct LV diameter and correct wall thickness | Secant results in too small LV diameter and too large wall thickness

Fig. 1.9 Illustration of potential errors of measurements for left ventricular dimensions and wall thicknesses due to non-standardization. If the parasternal transducer position is too caudal and/or too lateral, the aortic root drops down on the right side of the sector. This induces too large dimensions of the left ventricular cavity and of the wall thickness (left side—differences are displayed by the white arrows). Measurements using long-axis views can be performed using secant-like sectional planes which induce too small dimensions of the left ventricular cavity and too large dimensions of the wall thickness (right side—differences are displayed by the white arrows). Additional comments in the text.

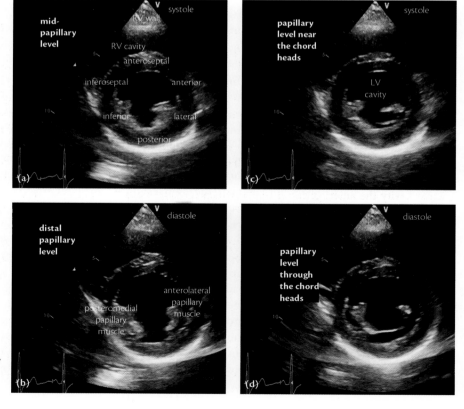

Fig. 1.10 The standardized parasternal short-axis view at the mid-papillary level. Additional comments in the text.

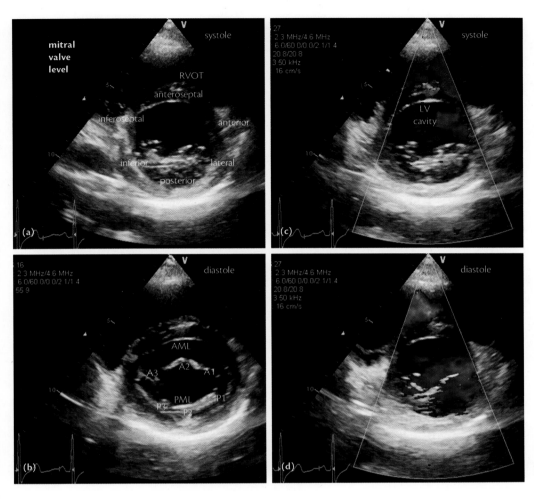

Fig. 1.11 The standardized parasternal short-axis view at the mitral valve level. Additional comments in the text.

then clockwise: anterior—60°; lateral—120°; posterior—180°; inferior—240°; inferoseptal—300°), the left ventricular cavity, the anterolateral transversal mid-papillary muscle between 60° and 90° at the inner wall of the left ventricle and the posteromedial transversal mid-papillary muscle between 210° and 240° at the inner wall of the left ventricle. The parasternal short-axis view at the mitral valve level (⊃ Fig. 1.11a–d) shows the free wall of the right ventricular outflow tract, the cavity of the right ventricular outflow tract, all basal segments of the left ventricular wall and the left ventricular cavity, near the transducer in the left ventricular cavity the anterior mitral leaflet, which is anatomically one leaflet but can be described by three portions (the A1-scallop near the anterolateral left ventricular wall, the A2-scallop in the centre of the anterior mitral leaflet, the A3-scallops near the posteromedial left ventricular wall) and far from the transducer in the left ventricular cavity the posterior mitral leaflet, which is divided anatomically into three scallops (the P1-scallop near the anterolateral left ventricular wall, the P2-scallop in the centre of the posterior mitral leaflet, the P3-scallops near the posteromedial left ventricular wall). The parasternal short-axis view at the aortic valve level (⊃ Fig. 1.12a–d) is characterized by the following cardiac structures. The basal free wall of the right ventricular outflow tract is near the transducer. The right ventricular cavity

is bounded on the left side of the sector by the tricuspid valve and on the right side by the pulmonary valve. The aortic valve is in the centre of the sector behind the right ventricle. During diastole the right coronary cusp is ventrally located, the left coronary cusp is between 60° and 180°, and the non-coronary cusp is between 180° and 300°. Close to the commissure between the right and the left coronary cusp at the aortic valve annulus, the dorsal cusp of the longitudinally intersected pulmonary valve is located. Close to the commissure between the right and the non-coronary cusp at the aortic valve annulus, the septal leaflet of the tricuspid valve is located. At the far side of the aortic valve, the left atrium is shown. Close to the aortic valve annulus, near to the non-coronary cusp, the perpendicular intersected inter-atrial septum is located. Between the aortic valve and the left atrium, the fibrotic aorticomitral junction is located. Between the inter-atrial septum and the tricuspid valve is the right atrium.

It has to be mentioned that all parasternal short-axis views display the cardiac structures mirror-inverted.

The colour-coded short-axis views through the mitral and aortic valve are additionally suitable for qualitative analysis of the location of mitral valve regurgitation and semiquantification of aortic valve regurgitation by analysing the regurgitant orifice during diastole.

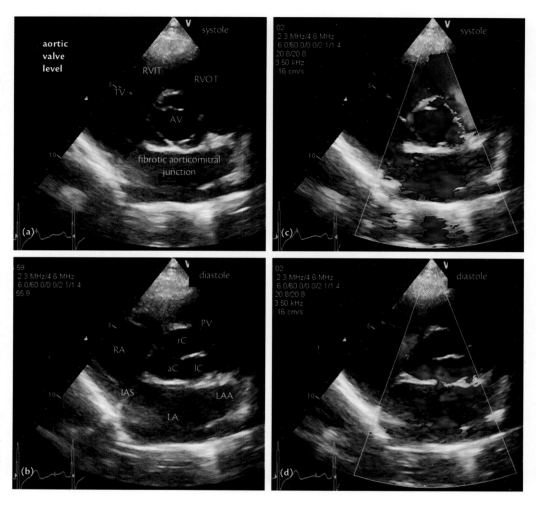

Fig. 1.12 The standardized parasternal short-axis view at the aortic valve level. Additional comments in the text.

From the parasternal approach, colour-coded and pulsed spectral Doppler imaging of the right ventricular outflow tract or the pulmonary valve should be generally added to a standard documentation in order to calculate the cardiac output of the right heart and to estimate the pulmonary pressure by acceleration time and the morphology of the flow profile, retrospectively (➲ Fig. 1.13a–e). If pulmonary regurgitation is present, and right heart or pulmonary diseases are suspected, a continuous wave Doppler spectrum through the pulmonary valve should be documented to estimate end-diastolic and mean pulmonary pressure by the end-diastolic and maximal velocities of the regurgitant flow.

The locating of the transducer directly at the cardiac apex is essential for the documentation of the correct apical sectional planes. This is possible by guiding the transducer to the correct apical position by sliding in caudolateral direction on the skin of the patient from the correct transducer position of a standardized parasternal long-axis view to the correct transducer position of a standardized apical long-axis view (➲ Fig. 1.14). The apical long-axis view is characterized by the same cardiac structures as the parasternal long-axis view (➲ Fig. 1.14). The standardized apical long-axis view is additionally characterized by the tip of the cardiac apex, which is directly below the transducer surface and the

centre of the mitral valve in the centreline of the scanning sector. The centred display of the left ventricle is essential for the correct documentation of the apical 2- and 4-chamber view by rotation of the transducer without tilting and flipping at the correct apical transducer position. If the centreline of the left ventricle is not centred in the sector of the apical long-axis view, rotation of the transducer obviously will produce foreshortening views of other sectional planes of the left ventricle.

Oblique apical views in normal hearts and failing standardization can be checked by the configuration of the apical shape of the left ventricular cavity. In normal hearts with a normal electrocardiogram, the apex of the left cavity shows a peaked, 'gothic' configuration (early 'gothic' in the 4-chamber view, mid 'gothic' in the long-axis view and late 'gothic' in the 2-chamber view). In normal hearts a 'romanic' configuration is obtained due to foreshortening views.

Due to guiding to the apical transducer position by sliding down from the parasternal long-axis view to the apical long-axis view, the apical transthoracic echocardiographic examination should start with the two-dimensional imaging of the left ventricle in the apical long-axis view (➲ Fig. 1.14a–b). The apical long-axis view of the left ventricle is normally perpendicular to the commissure of the mitral valve. Thus, the long-axis view shows

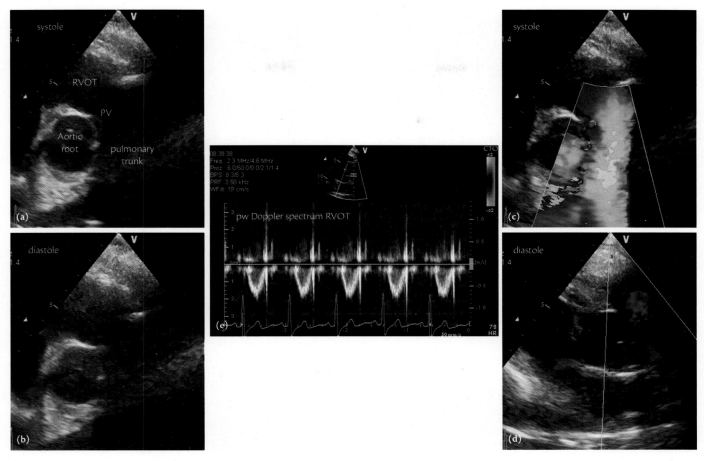

Fig. 1.13 The standardized parasternal short-axis view through the pulmonary valve and the pulmonary trunk at systole (a) and diastole (b). The corresponding colour-coded views are displayed in (c) and (d). In (e) the pulsed wave Doppler spectrum of the right ventricular outflow tract is shown. Additional comments in the text.

the functional division of the left ventricle into the complete in-flow chamber during diastole at fully opened mitral valve and the movement of the anterior mitral leaflet close to the anterior septal wall, as well as into the complete outflow chamber during systole by complete closure of the mitral valve. Monoplane planimetry of the left ventricle is performed using the apical long-axis view for estimation of global left-ventricular function by determination of the ejection fraction. The apical long-axis view is also used for visual analysis of regional wall motion in the posterior and anteroseptal regions, as well as for morphological evaluation of the mid scallops of the mitral valve (A2-/P2-scallop).

The 2D-view is followed by the colour-coded apical long-axis view (⊃ Fig. 1.14c–d) to assess mitral and aortic valve function qualitatively. Because the long-axis view shows best the blood flow direction into and out of the left ventricle, determinations of proximal jet width or vena contracta, as well as proximal isovelocity surface areas in the presence of turbulent flow at the mitral and aortic valve can usually be well performed in this sectional plane—especially for central mitral and aortic lesions. According to guidelines, jet morphology and jet size of mitral and aortic regurgitation is not recommended anymore

for assessing the severity of mitral and aortic regurgitation. The derivations of the pulsed wave Doppler spectra of the inflow and outflow tract of the left ventricle should be performed in the apical long-axis view due to the clear positioning of the sample volumes (⊃ Fig. 1.14e–f). The sample volume of the pulsed wave Doppler spectrum at the mitral valve for characterizing left ventricular inflow should be positioned in the region of the transition of the mitral leaflets to the chord strands (about 10–15 mm towards the ventricle from the mitral valve plane) in the centre of the flow direction into the left ventricle. High-quality pulsed wave Doppler spectra are depicted by bright contours at the maximum velocities. The sample volume of the pulsed wave Doppler spectrum at the left ventricular outflow tract has to be positioned in front of the aortic valve (about 5–10 mm towards the left ventricle from the aortic valve plane).

The pulsed wave Doppler spectrum of the left ventricular inflow is necessary for characterization of diastolic function by the E/A ratio, as well as for calculation of E/E′; the pulsed wave Doppler spectrum of the left ventricular outflow tract is mandatory for calculation of cardiac output or shunt volumes in case of communication defects, as well as for calculation of aortic stenotic valve area according to the continuity equation.

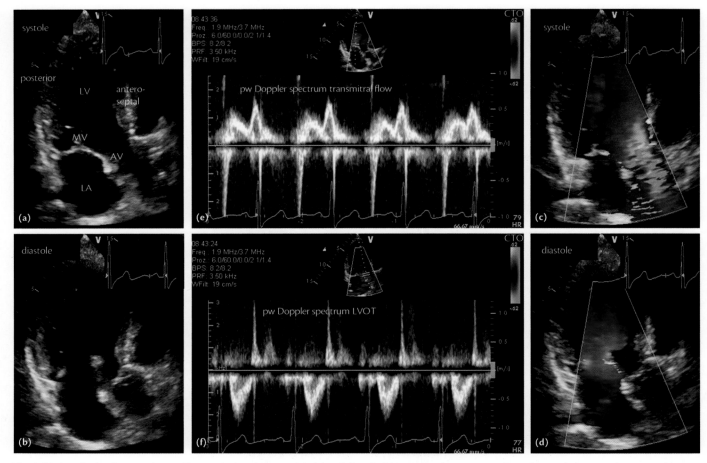

Fig. 1.14 Standardized grey-scale apical long-axis view during systole (a) and diastole (b), as well as the corresponding colour-coded images during systole (c) and diastole (d). The pulsed wave Doppler spectrum of the left ventricular inflow through the mitral valve (e) and of the left ventricular outflow tract (f) is displayed in the middle of the illustration. Additional comments in the text.

In the presence of turbulences at the mitral and aortic valves, the standard documentation should be completed by continuous wave Doppler spectra over the mitral and the aortic valves. The continuous wave Doppler spectrum over the mitral valve is necessary for determination of the velocity time integral in the presence of mitral valve stenosis for determination of mean and maximum pressure gradients, the determination of the stenotic and regurgitant velocities, as well as for calculation of the parameter dp/dt for estimation of global left ventricular function. The continuous wave Doppler spectrum over the aortic valve is necessary for estimating aortic stenosis severity by determining the mean and maximum pressure gradients and for calculation of aortic stenotic valve area according to the continuity equation. For semiquantification of aortic regurgitation, the pressure half-time method is used at the deceleration border of the regurgitant velocities.

By an approximately 60° clockwise rotation of the transducer, starting from the standardized apical long-axis view, the correct apical 2-chamber view is obtained (➲ Fig. 1.15a–b). The sectional plane of the apical 2-chamber view is characterized by the left ventricular cavity tip, the inferior left ventricular wall at the left side of the cavity, the anterior left ventricular wall at the right side of the

cavity, the centre of the mitral valve in its commissural plane, the cross-sectional coronary sinus in the region of the inferior mitral ring, the left atrium and the left atrial auricle cranial to the mitral ring and the opening of the upper left pulmonary vein cranial to the left atrial auricle. Near the anterior region the P1-scallop of the mitral valve is depicted, near the inferior region the P3-scallop. In the centre of the mitral valve the A2-scallop is normally seen. The apical 2-chamber view is used for visual assessment of global and regional left ventricular function in the inferior and anterior regions of the left ventricular wall and for the morphological evaluation of the mitral valve. The colour-coded 2-chamber view is suitable for characterization of the defect localization in mitral valve regurgitation (➲Fig. 1.15c–d).

After modifying the hand position of the transducer to enable a further approximately 60° clockwise rotation of the transducer, this isolated rotation will be performed from the correctly set apical 2-chamber view to get the standardized apical 4-chamber view (➲ Fig. 1.16a–b). The correct apical 4-chamber view is characterized by the left ventricular cavity tip, the inferoseptal left ventricular wall at the left side of the cavity, the lateral left ventricular wall at the right side of the cavity, the centre of the mitral valve (A2-scallop, P2-scallop near to the P1-scallop), the inter-ventricular

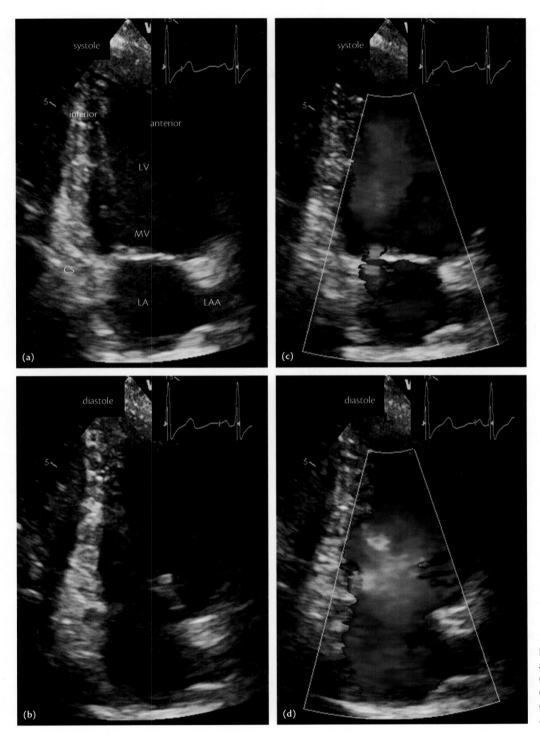

Fig. 1.15 Standardized grey-scale apical 2-chamber view during systole (a) and diastole (b), as well as the corresponding colour-coded images during systole (c) and diastole (d). Additional comments in the text.

and inter-atrial septum, the cardiac crux, the septal and the anterior leaflet of the tricuspid valve, the inflow tract of the right ventricle, the free right ventricular wall and the left and right atrium. It is essential that the origin of the anterior mitral leaflet and the septal leaflet of the tricuspid valve is almost at the same point near the cardiac crux. The standardized 4-chamber view does not show parts of the left ventricular outflow tract or the longitudinal sectional plane of the coronary sinus. The apical 4-chamber view is used for visual assessment of global and regional left ventricular function in the inferoseptal and lateral regions of the left ventricular wall and for the morphological evaluation of the central mitral valve.

Using the 2- and 4-chamber views, quantitative assessment of left ventricular function is performed by left ventricular volume analysis and determination of left ventricular ejection fraction using the Simpson's rule. It is recommended to check the

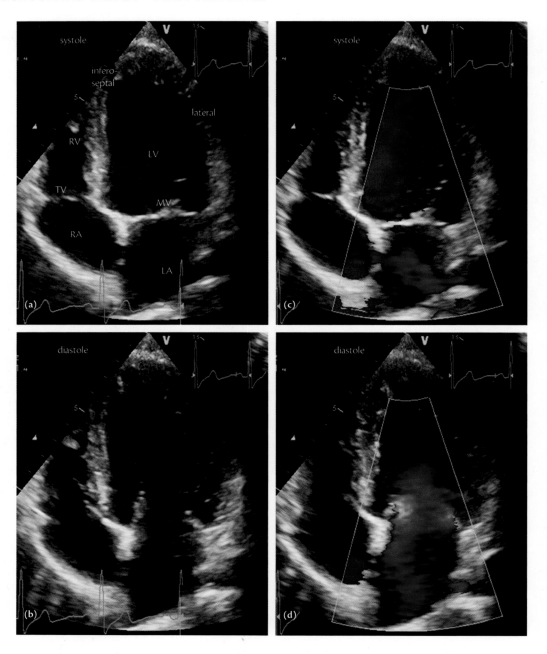

Fig. 1.16 Standardized grey-scale apical 4-chamber view during systole (a) and diastole (b), as well as the corresponding colour-coded images during systole (c) and diastole (d). Additional comments in the text.

longitudinal length of the ventricle at end-diastole in both views before starting planimetry. If, for example, the longitudinal length of the 4-chamber view is more shortened than 10 mm in comparison to the 2-chamber view, it is obvious that the 4-chamber view has to be foreshortened.

The colour-coded 4-chamber view (⊃ Fig. 1.16c–d) is necessary for characterization of the defect localization in mitral valve regurgitation and for semiquantification of the tricuspid valve regurgitation by its vena contracta (⊃ Fig. 1.17a–c; Fig. 1.17d–f). For complete semiquantification of tricuspid valve regurgitation its vena contracta has to be additionally measured in the apical right ventricular inflow tract view derived by tilting the apical long-axis view to the medial regions (⊃ Fig. 1.17g–i). In the presence of turbulences at the tricuspid valve, the continuous wave

Doppler spectra over the tricuspid valve have to be documented. The continuous wave Doppler spectrum over the tricuspid valve is necessary for estimating the right ventricular systolic pressure according to the simplified Bernoulli equation, which corresponds to the systolic pulmonary pressure if no pulmonary stenosis is present. Furthermore, the maximum velocity of tricuspid valve regurgitation is necessary for estimation of the pulmonary valvular resistance.

The 4-chamber view is also used for the acquisition of the pulsed tissue Doppler spectra for the calculation of E/E′. The sample volume is positioned at the basal inferoseptal and lateral myocardium near the mitral annulus (⊃ Fig. 1.18a–d). E′ for calculation of the E/E′-ratio is the mean E′ of both values determined at the basal inferoseptal and lateral left ventricular wall. The 4-chamber view is also used

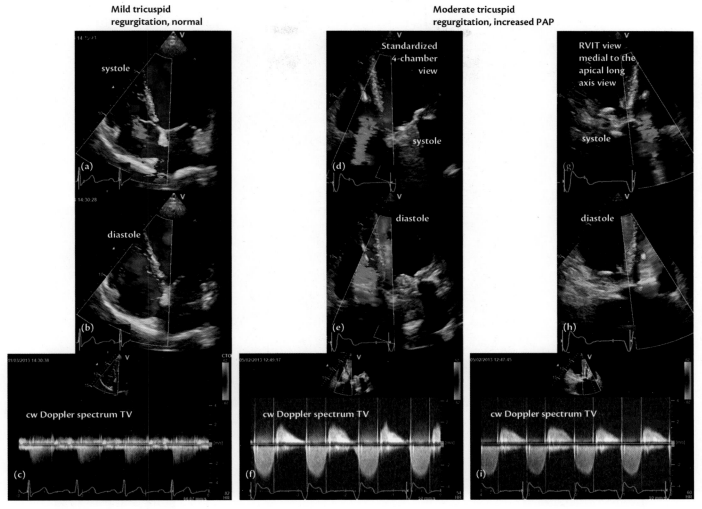

Fig. 1.17 The colour-coded 4-chamber view for qualitative and semiquantitative analysis of tricuspid valve regurgitation during systole (a) and diastole (b). The continuous wave Doppler spectrum of tricuspid valve regurgitation is given in (c). For semiquantification of moderate and severe tricuspid valve regurgitation two views are necessary. In an example of a combined tricuspid valve disease the colour-coded 4-chamber view is displayed during systole (d) and diastole (e), as well as the view of the right ventricular inflow tract by medial tilting from the apical long-axis view during systole (g) and diastole (h). In both views the vena contracta of a tricuspid valve regurgitation has to be determined for semiquantification during systole. The corresponding continuous wave Doppler spectra of the tricuspid valve regurgitation are given in (f) and (i). Additional comments in the text.

for grey scale and colour-coded imaging of the upper right pulmonary vein for documentation of the pulsed wave Doppler spectrum of the pulmonary vein flow for analysis of diastolic function. The sample volume has to be positioned into the left atrium 10–15 mm ahead of the entry of the pulmonary vein. The pulsed wave Doppler spectrum has to be acquired in low pulse repetition frequency mode to prevent overlapping of the signals of the flow through the mitral valve and the signals of the pulmonary vein (⮕ Fig. 1.19a–e).

For the documentation of the anterolateral and posteromedial commissure of the mitral valve, two further oblique views of the apical 4-chamber view have to be adjusted (⮕ Fig. 1.20). The documentation of the P3/A3 scallops of the mitral valve (= posteromedial commissure) is performed by tilting the transducer to the dorsal region of the left ventricle, which will show the dorsal mitral annulus with the target structure of a longitudinal section of the coronary sinus (⮕ Fig. 1.20a–d). The documentation of

the P1/A1 scallops of the mitral valve (= anterolateral commissure) is possible by tilting the transducer to the ventral region of the left ventricle, which will show the 5-chamber view (⮕ Fig. 1.20e–h). In the 5-chamber view the left ventricular outflow tract and parts of the aortic valve are visualized. The 5-chamber view is an oblique view through the left ventricle, which shows the anteroseptal and anterolateral basal segments of the left ventricular wall and the inferoseptal and lateral apical segments of the left ventricle. The target structure of the 5-chamber view is the left ventricular outflow tract. Both views should also be documented using colour-coded Doppler to analyse the localization of mitral valve regurgitation.

Subcostal and suprasternal scanning should be performed with the patient in strict supine position.

Subcostal scanning should start with the subcostal 4-chamber view, which is easily adjusted by holding the transducer with the

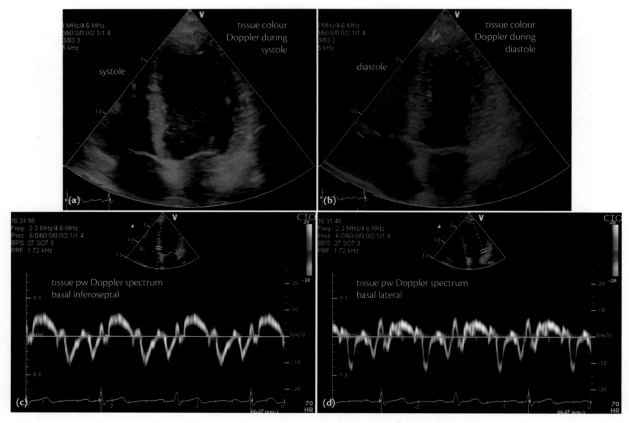

Fig. 1.18 Illustration of a colour-coded tissue Doppler 4-chamber view during systole (a) and diastole (b) and the corresponding tissue pulsed wave Doppler spectra at the basal septal (c) and lateral (d) myocardium near the mitral annulus. Additional comments in the text.

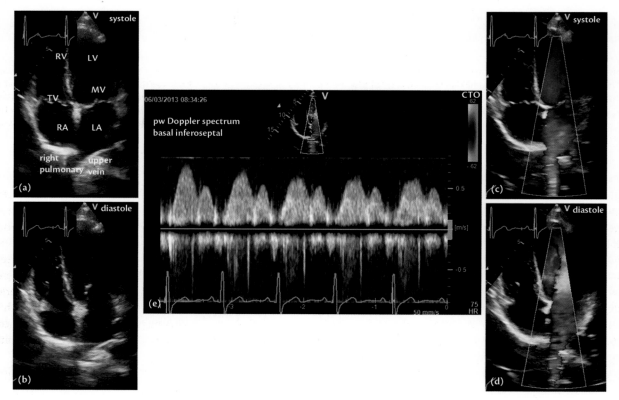

Fig. 1.19 Illustration of a deep grey scale 4-chamber view during systole (a) and diastole (b) and the corresponding colour-coded 4-chamber view during systole (c) and diastole (d). The pulsed wave Doppler spectrum of the flow in the right upper pulmonary vein is displayed in (e). Additional comments in the text.

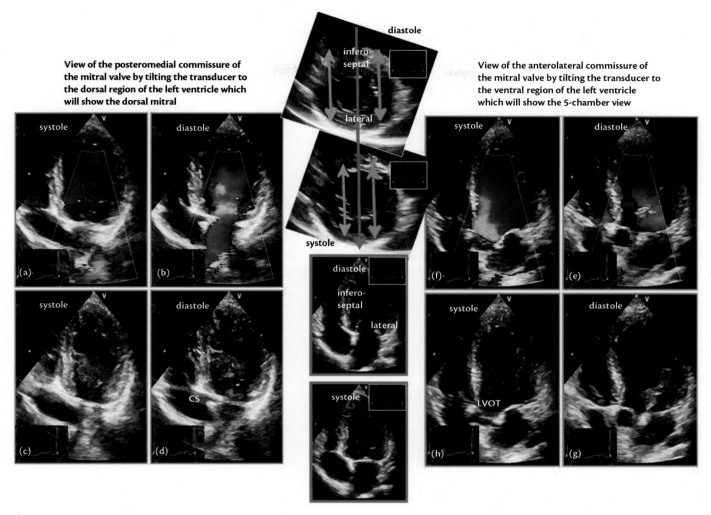

Fig. 1.20 Illustration for analysis of mitral valve regurgitation affecting the commissures. In the middle of the illustration the standardized 4-chamber view is displayed during diastole and during systole (red surrounding) and its sectional plane is displayed in a parasternal short-axis view (red arrow). For analysis of the posteromedial commissure the transducer has to be tilted to the dorsal region of the left ventricle showing a longitudinal section through the coronary sinus. The illustration shows the corresponding colour-coded images during systole (a) and diastole (b), as well as the grey scale images during systole (c) and diastole (d). For analysis of the anterolateral commissure the transducer has to be tilted to the ventral region of the left ventricle showing the left ventricular outflow tract. The illustration shows the corresponding colour-coded images during systole (e) and diastole (f), as well as the grey scale images during systole (g) and diastole (h). Additional comments in the text.

orientation of the notch in the same direction as in the apical 4-chamber view during inspiration of the patient (➲ Fig. 1.21a–b). The subcostal 4-chamber view shows the same cardiac structures as the apical 4-chamber view. A counter-clockwise rotation shows the subcostal short-axis views. The perpendicular view to the inter-atrial septum in the subcostal short-axis view of the aortic valve is suitable for the detection of inter-atrial communication defects by colour-coded Doppler imaging (➲ Fig. 1.21c–f). Subcostal short-axis views of the mitral valve and the left ventricle at mid-papillary level can replace the parasternal short-axis views for analysis of the heart if the parasternal window is not sufficient (➲ Fig. 1.22a–h). The right ventricular inflow and outflow tract, as well as the pulmonary trunk and the pulmonary bifurcation can be well visualized by the subcostal approach. Due to the excellent Doppler angle, Doppler spectra through the pulmonary valve

can be achieved in this view (➲ Fig. 1.23a–e). By counter-clockwise rotation from the subcostal 4-chamber view the longitudinal section of the inferior caval vein should be documented for estimation of the preload of the right ventricle (➲ Fig. 1.24a–b). In the presence of normal right atrial pressure, the central venous pressure is normal, which can be documented by pulsatile wall movement and a complete breath-dependent inspiratory collapse of the inferior caval vein. The right atrial pressure is increased in patients with cardiac stasis on the right side, documented by partial collapse or a complete loss of collapse of the inferior caval vein during deep inspiration.

For the analysis of the aortic arch the suprasternal long-axis view of the aortic arch has to be documented by grey scale 2D cineloop, as well as by colour-coded Doppler (➲ Fig. 1.25a–b). The transducer should be positioned with the axis directed to the

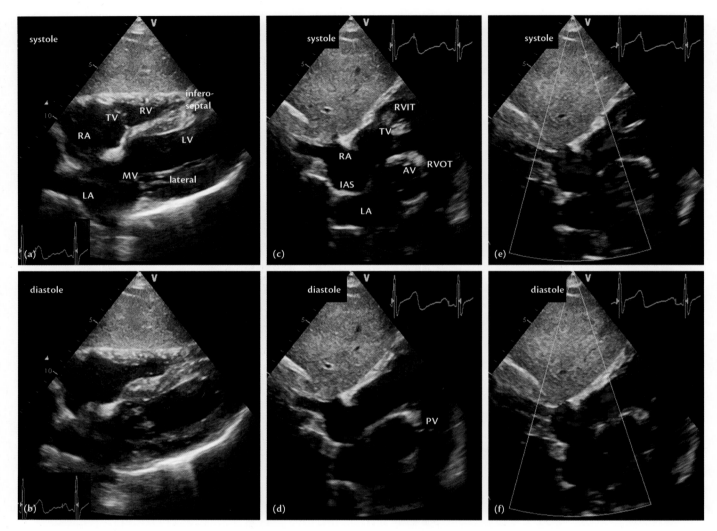

Fig. 1.21 Standardized grey-scale apical 4-chamber view during systole (a) and diastole (b). Standardized subcostal short-axis view at the aortic valve level during systole (c) and diastole (d), as well as the corresponding colour-coded images during systole (e) and diastole (f). Additional comments in the text.

centre of the left ventricle and with the notch oriented to the left shoulder. The correct view should individually be adjusted to the topography of the aortic arch. The suprasternal documentation of the aortic arch is necessary for detection of aortic pathologies—especially for the transthoracic detection of aortic dissection. Thus, it is mandatory to perform suprasternal scanning of the aortic arch in patients with aortic valve diseases and assumed aortic pathologies, as well as in the emergency scenario.

Principles of transoesophageal echocardiography—practical aspects

A transthoracic echocardiography should be generally performed prior to a transoesophageal echocardiography, if it is possible. The main reason for the transthoracic pre-examination in adult patients is the fact that multiple cineloops and Doppler spectra can be achieved and documented in a high and often better image quality in the transthoracic than in the transoesophageal

approach. This mainly concerns the short-axis views of the left ventricle and the mitral valve, which often will be visualized by oblique views in the transgastric documentation and the Doppler spectra of the left heart, which will not show optimal Doppler angulations in the transoesophageal echocardiography. This is very important for all calculations using Doppler parameters. If these parameters are falsified by incorrect Doppler angulations, calculation of pressure gradients, stroke volumes, shunt volumes and stenotic areas using the Bernoulli or continuity equation will be wrong. Therefore it is obvious that a sufficient transthoracic echocardiography prior to the transoesophageal investigation can significantly shorten the procedure time of transoesophageal echocardiography.

For transoesophageal echocardiography some prerequisites have to be fulfilled. The preparation of the patient for the procedure includes an ECG, blood pressure and oxygen saturation monitoring, a venous line for sedation, contrast administration, drug administration in the event of complications, the availability of emergency and resuscitation equipment, as well as a suction

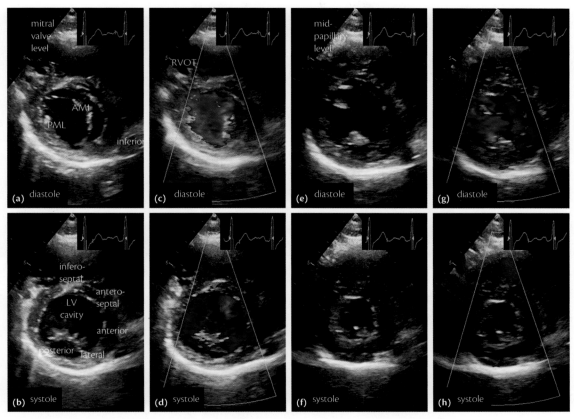

Fig. 1.22 Standardized subcostal short-axis view at the mitral valve level during diastole (a) and systole (b), as well as the corresponding colour-coded images during diastole (c) and systole (d). Standardized subcostal short-axis view at the mid-papillary level during diastole (e) and systole (f), as well as the corresponding colour-coded images during diastole (g) and systole (h). Additional comments in the text.

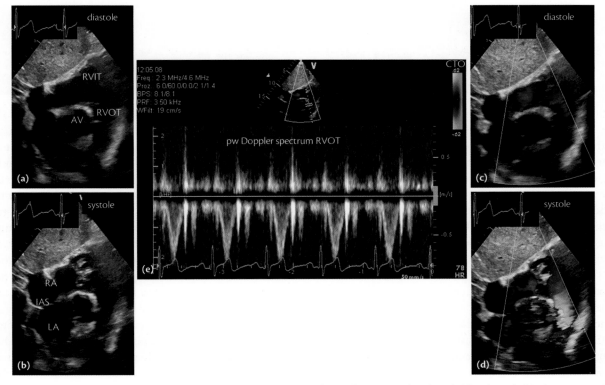

Fig. 1.23 The standardized subcostal short-axis view through the pulmonary valve and the pulmonary trunk at diastole (a) and systole (b). The corresponding colour-coded views are displayed in (c) and (d). In (e) the pulsed wave Doppler spectrum of the right ventricular outflow tract is shown. Additional comments in the text.

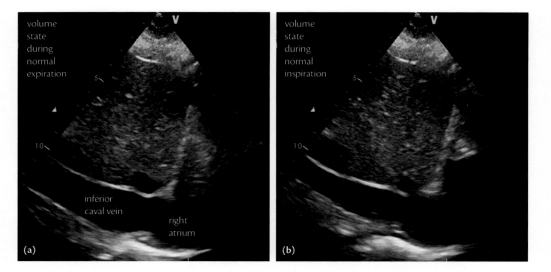

Fig. 1.24 The subcostal longitudinal view of the inferior caval vein during expiration (a) and inspiration (b). Additional comments in the text.

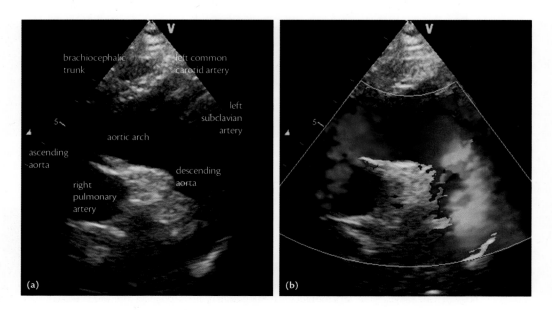

Fig. 1.25 The suprasternal view of the aortic arch using grey scale mode (a) and colour-coded imaging (b). Additional comments in the text.

system. The patient should have an empty stomach, dental fixtures should be removed and a bite guard should be used to protect the shaft of the probe. A local oropharyngeal anaesthesia with lidocaine spray is often sufficient for intubation of the oesophagus. If additional sedation is needed, intravenous administration of midazolam (0.075 mg/kg) can be added in stable patients. It is obvious that lower sedation doses should be used in patients with severe heart failure or in patients with other compromising diseases. The transoesophageal echocardiography is normally performed in the left lateral position. During intubation of the probe, the tip of the probe has to be unlocked, regarding flexion and extension, to avoid injury to the oesophageal wall. After the examination the probe has to be disinfected as well as inspected for damage according to the international guidelines.

The insertion of the probe is the most uncomfortable moment for the awake or slightly sedated patient. Assistance during the intubation is helpful to enable the most convenient mode of introduction

of the probe (⇒ Figs 1.26–1.27). The user-operated actuator should be held by the assistant directly above the patient in the vertical direction with the shaft leading downwards (⇒ Fig. 1.26a–b). Then, the shaft is touched by the operator with the right hand at the distal shaft near the movable tip (⇒ Fig. 1.26b–c). The distal ending of the unlocked probe is curved and adapted to the curvature of the oropharynx (⇒ Fig. 1.26c). The left hand of the operator is free for manipulating the tip of the probe during introduction to the oral cavity. The advantage of this setting is that by pushing the probe forward into the oesophagus, the tip, as well as the shaft, of the probe will follow the natural course of the upper pharyngeal isthmus without inducing unnecessary forces to the wall of the pharynx and the upper oesophagus. The fingers of the left hand will guide the tip of the probe. If the bite guard has to be positioned between the teeth during insertion, the second finger should be laid across the tongue. Then, the probe can be fixed to the back of the pharynx, but positioned at the ridge in the middle of the tongue for

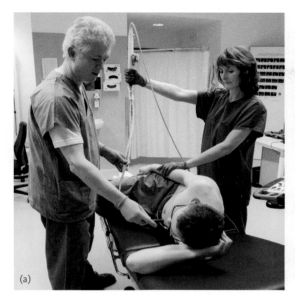
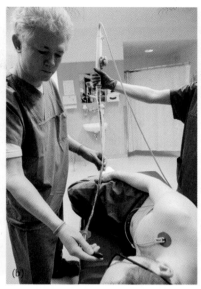
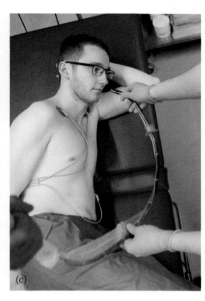

Fig. 1.26 Holding of the actuator and the shaft of the transoesophageal probe at the beginning of the investigation. An assistant during the intubation is helpful to enable the most convenient mode of introduction of the probe (a). The user-operated actuator should be held by the assistant directly above the patient in a vertical direction with the shaft leading downwards (a). The shaft is touched by the operator with the right hand at the distal shaft near the movable tip (b). The distal ending of the unlocked probe is curved to adapt to the curvature of the oropharynx (c). Additional comments in the text.

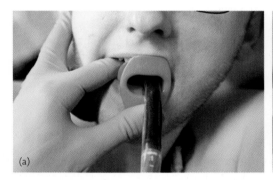
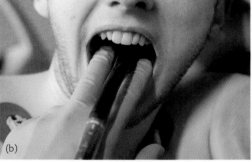

Fig. 1.27 Directly before introducing the probe the left hand of the operator is free for manipulating the tip of the probe during introduction to the oral cavity. The fingers of the left hand will guide the tip of the probe. If the bite guard has to be positioned between the teeth during insertion, the second finger should be laid across the tongue (a). Then, the probe can be fixed to the back of the pharynx, but positioned at the ridge in the middle of the tongue with the best possibility to introduce into the proximal oesophagus. If the patient can tolerate the introduction procedure without the bite guard, the second and third fingers can be used for introduction of the probe to fix the probe at the ridge in the middle of the tongue (b). Additional comments in the text.

the best possibility of introduction into the proximal oesophagus (➲ Fig. 1.27a). If the patient tolerates the introduction procedure without the bite guard, the second and third finger can be used for introduction of the probe to fix the probe at the ridge in the middle of the tongue (➲ Fig. 1.27b). The bite guard, which during this manoeuvre was at the shaft of the probe, should be positioned between the teeth after insertion of the probe.

Standardized data acquisition in transoesophageal echocardiography

The sequence of the transoesophageal image acquisition and documentation depends on the individual situation. If there is no time

limit due to emergency, cardiac or respiratory failure, cough or vomiting, agitation or high temperature, the transoesophageal investigation can be performed according to anatomical issues starting with the transgastric views followed by the oesophageal views with retraction of the probe. If there is a time limit, the investigation should focus on the target lesion and additional important findings. In conventional settings with high-quality transthoracic pre-investigations and sufficient acquisition of all necessary Doppler spectra by the transthoracic approach, documentation of the transgastric views can normally be spared with respect to the patient's comfort. Important medical indications for a transoesophageal echocardiography are the accurate visualization of cardiac structures, which cannot be analysed by transthoracic echocardiography, and the clarification of issues which were the cause for the transoesophageal procedure. Then, depending on the patient's tolerance and further circumstances, the transoesophageal study should be performed completely, if it is possible.

Most of the transoesophageal cardiac views are characterized by the left atrium nearest to the transducer. All standard views should be documented as 2D grey-scale cineloops, as well as colour-coded 2D cineloops, to document flow phenomena at the valves or other special cardiac structures. Due to the higher frequencies used in transoesophageal echocardiography, the spatial resolution is normally better than in transthoracic echocardiography. The small layers of the oesophageal and left atrial wall result in an almost direct proximity to the heart. Thus, transoesophageal echocardiography is normally performed in the fundamental mode due to the absence of tissue interferences of the ultrasound.

The transoesophageal study should normally start in the transverse position (0°) with a 5-chamber view or an oblique foreshortened 4-chamber view in the lower transoesophageal approach (⊃ Fig. 1.28a–d). With a minimal deeper insertion of the probe, the longitudinal section of the coronary sinus can be visualized (⊃ Fig. 1.28e–h). The standardized 4-chamber view is obtained by a rotation of the plane of about 0°–40° (⊃ Fig. 1.29a–b), straightening the tip of the probe and retracting the probe to the midoesophageal window to get the apex into the centre of the scanning sector. The transoesophageal 2-chamber view is shown by rotating the plane a further 60° without any movement of the tip and/or the shaft (60°–100°) (⊃ Fig. 1.29c–d). Then, the left ventricular apex is still in the centreline of the scanning sector. The transoesophageal long-axis view is obtained by further plane rotation of about 60° (120°–160°) (⊃ Fig. 1.29e–f). The angle distance between the views is like in transthoracic echocardiography—60°

if the left ventricular apex is in the centre of the scanning sector. If this is not possible and the left ventricular apex is rotating from the right side of the sector in the 4-chamber view to the left side of the sector in the long-axis view, which occurs if the correct position in the upper oesophagus cannot be achieved, the angle differences between the planes of the left ventricle will change. This is the reason why the 2-chamber view in transoesophageal echocardiography often seems to be perpendicular to the long-axis view. The normal 60°-angle difference between the standardized views of the left ventricle can be documented by the triplane approach, which will show exactly the standardized views with 60°-angle difference if the left ventricular apex is centred in the scanning sector (⊃ Fig. 1.29g–h).

An oblique 2-chamber view, which is obtained by deflecting the tip of the probe, normally enables the documentation of a longitudinal section of the left atrial appendage and the upper left pulmonary vein (⊃ Fig. 1.30a–e). This view is used for acquisition of the pulsed wave Doppler spectra of the velocities of the left atrial appendage and the pulmonary venous inflow. The Doppler spectrum of the velocities of left atrial appendage is necessary for risk estimation of thromboembolic events and the Doppler spectrum of the pulmonary vein is necessary for analysis of diastolic function, as well as for estimation of the severity of mitral valve regurgitation. The left atrial appendage should be visualized at least in a second plane perpendicular to this view to detect possible thrombus formations. Using conventional echocardiography, the left atrial appendage has to be positioned in the centre of the sector by deflecting the probe (⊃ Fig. 1.31a–c). Using multidimensional probes, this second plane can be achieved by the biplane scanning mode.

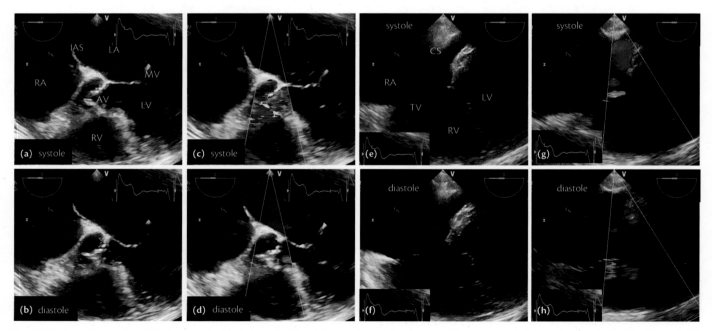

Fig. 1.28 The mid-oesophageal 5-chamber view during systole (a) and diastole (b) and the corresponding colour-coded views during systole (c) and diastole (d). A slight deeper insertion of the probe at 0° displays the inflow of the coronary sinus. The following views of the right atrium and the right ventricular inflow tract are displayed in grey scale mode during systole (e) and diastole (f) and in colour-coded mode during systole (g) and diastole (h). Additional comments in the text.

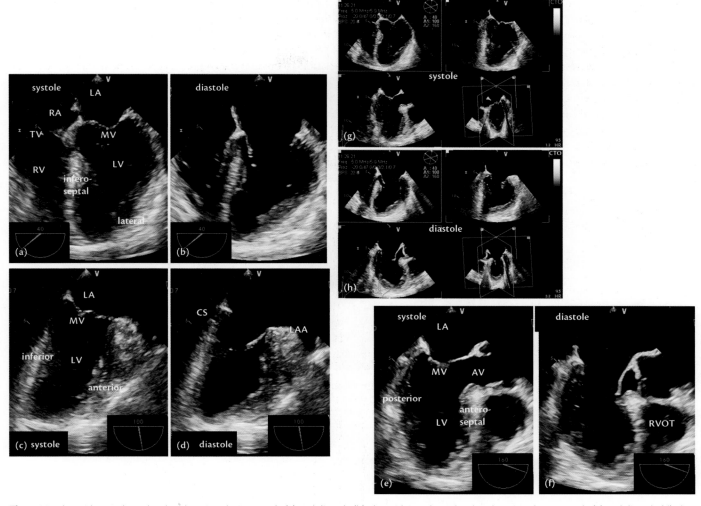

Fig. 1.29 The mid-oesophageal 4-chamber view during systole (a) and diastole (b), the midoesophageal 2-chamber view during systole (c) and diastole (d), the mid-oesophageal long-axis view during systole (e) and diastole (f) and the simultaneous triplane views during systole (g) and diastole (h) to document that angle differences between mid-oesophageal standardized views with the left ventricular apex near the centreline of the sector are about 60° like the transthoracic views. Additional comments in the text.

The aortic short-axis view is also obtained by further flexion of the tip of the probe taking the 2-chamber view as the starting view. In addition to the morphological analysis of the aortic valve, the aortic short-axis view (⊃ Figs 1.31d and 1.32a) also shows the region of the oval fossa to detect a patent foramen ovale, which is located at the connection of the inter-atrial septum with the aortic valve annulus. With rotation from 50°–75° to 120°–135° the longitudinal intersected channel of the patent foramen ovale can be visualized (⊃ Fig. 1.31d–f). In addition, colour-coded Doppler can be used or contrast can be administrated to document a communication defect. An additional long-axis view of the aortic valve (120°–135°) should be documented from the most upper oesophageal approach to display the best possible view of the ascending aorta (⊃ Fig. 1.32b). The perpendicular short-axis view of the ascending aorta (again 60°–75°) displays the cross-sected ascending aorta, as well as the bifurcation and origin of the right pulmonary artery (⊃ Fig. 1.32c–d). With a clockwise rotation of the probe shaft, the cross-sected superior caval vein is behind the

right upper pulmonary vein (⊃ Fig. 1.32e–f). This view is necessary for the detection of upper sinus venosus atrial defects.

By rotating the shaft of the transoesophageal probe clockwise from the aortic long-axis view, the bicaval view can be achieved (⊃ Fig. 1.33a–b). The bicaval view of the right atrium displays the left atrium at the top followed by the inter-atrial septum, which is longitudinally intersected and is seen as a nearly horizontal structure. Distal to the inter-atrial septum the right atrium is displayed. Located on the right side of the sector the orifice of the superior caval vein and the right atrial appendage can be documented, on the left side of the sector the orifice of the inferior caval vein enters the right atrium.

The transgastric views will be achieved after positioning the tip of the probe in the upper stomach. For the transgastric approach harmonic imaging is often superior to fundamental imaging due to the larger near field and the longer distance between the transducer and the cardiac structures. The investigation starts with a short-axis view of the left ventricle at the

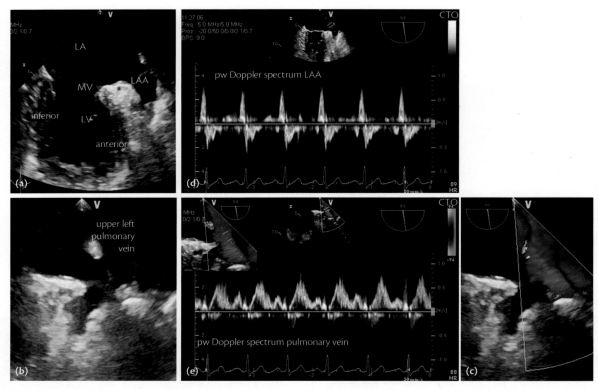

Fig. 1.30 Oblique mid oesophageal 2-chamber view (a) for visualization of the left atrial appendage (LAA) and the upper left pulmonary vein. The upper left pulmonary vein is displayed at the right side of the sector by positioning of the left atrial appendage in the centre of the sector (b). Colour-coded imaging of the pulmonary vein (c) facilitates the positioning of the sample volume for flow measurements. In the middle of the figure the pulsed wave Doppler spectra of the flow in the left atrial appendage with sinus rhythm (e) and in the upper left pulmonary vein (e) are displayed. Additional comments in the text.

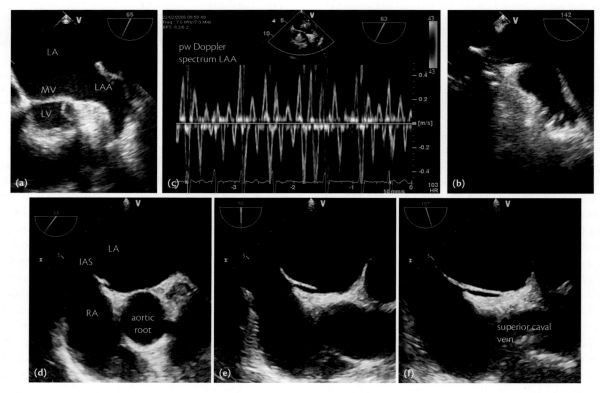

Fig. 1.31 Biplane documentation of a normal left atrial appendage (a, b) and the corresponding pulsed wave Doppler spectrum during atrial fibrillation (c). Documentation of the oval fossa in a short-axis view at the aortic root level (d). By rotation of the plane to 90° (e) and 107° (f) the channel between the septum primum and secundum is displayed. Additional comments in the text.

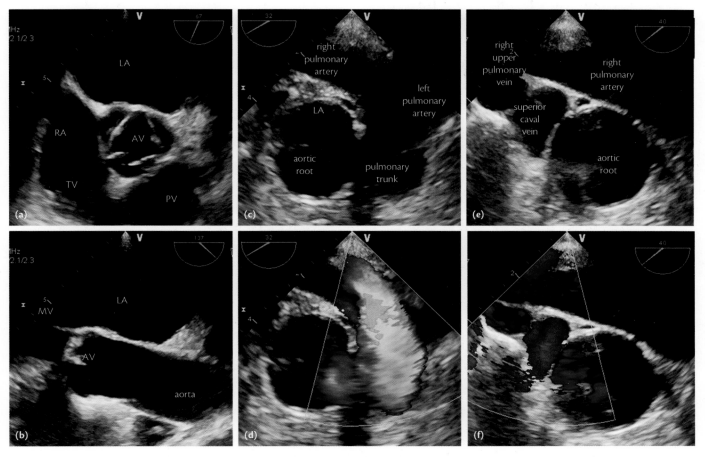

Fig. 1.32 Mid-transoesophageal short-axis view of the aortic valve (a). Upper transoesophageal long-axis view of the ascending aorta (b). Upper transoesophageal views of the ascending aorta and pulmonary artery, as well as the superior caval vein. The short-axis view of the aortic root and the pulmonary bifurcation is displayed in grey scale (c) and colour-coded mode (d). The short-axis view of the superior caval vein and the upper right pulmonary vein is displayed in grey scale (e) and colour-coded mode (f). Additional comments in the text.

mid-papillary level (0°) (⊃ Fig. 1.33c–d). If the left ventricle is displayed centrally in the sector, the perpendicular view shows the transgastric left ventricular 2-chamber view (90°) with the apex on the left side and the mitral valve on the right side (⊃ Fig. 1.33e–f). The inferior wall is in the near field, the anterior wall in the far field. The transgastric long-axis view can be displayed by further rotation of the probe to 100°–130° and a minor clockwise rotation of the shaft, which displays the aortic valve on the right side of the sector in the far field (⊃ Fig. 1.34a–f). The inflow tract of the right ventricle is also visualized by the perpendicular view (90°) to the left ventricular short-axis view (0°) after centring the right ventricle in the sector before rotating (⊃ Fig. 1.35a–d). The transgastric right ventricular longitudinal view displays the right ventricular apex on the left side and the right atrium and the tricuspid valve on the right side of the sector. A further rotation of the probe to 110°–140° and a minor rotation of the shaft enables the visualization of the inflow and outflow tracts of the right ventricle. The outflow tract and the pulmonary valve are nearly centred in the far field in this view.

The transgastric short-axis view of the mitral valve is a technically difficult view. Often only an oblique view of the mitral valve can be displayed. The short-axis view of the mitral valve is

achieved by slightly withdrawing the probe at 0°–20° from the mid-papillary short-axis view and simultaneous anteflexion of the probe. In this view the anterior mitral leaflet is on the left side of the sector and the posterior leaflet on the right side of the sector. The posteromedial commissure (A3/P3) is in the near field, the anterolateral commissure (A1/P1) in the far field (⊃ Fig. 1.36a–d).

A second possibility to visualize the left ventricular outflow tract is by deep intubation into the gastric fundus with consecutive anteflexion of the tip of the probe. Using this approach, the deep transgastric long-axis view at about 0° and the deep transgastric 5-chamber view can be achieved at about 120°–140° (⊃ Fig. 1.37a–f). The deep transgastric long-axis view displays the right ventricular outflow tract on the left side of the sector, the left ventricle on the right side of the sector in the near field, and the aortic valve centrally in the far field. Sometimes the transversely intersected aortic root and proximal ascending aorta are visualized.

After the documentation of the cardiac structures and the ascending aorta at the end of the transoesophageal investigation, the probe is turned into the opposite direction to the heart by rotating the shaft about 90°. Starting in the deep oesophagus at the diaphragm, the descending aorta is scanned using short-axis views (0°) during withdrawal of the probe to the upper oesophagus.

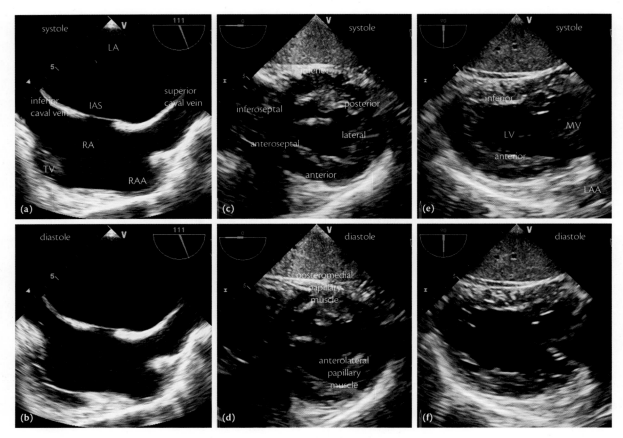

Fig. 1.33 Mid-transoesophageal bicaval view during systole (a) and diastole (b). Transgastric short-axis view at the mid-papillary level during systole (c) and diastole (d). Transgastric 2-chamber view during systole (e) and diastole (f). Additional comments in the text.

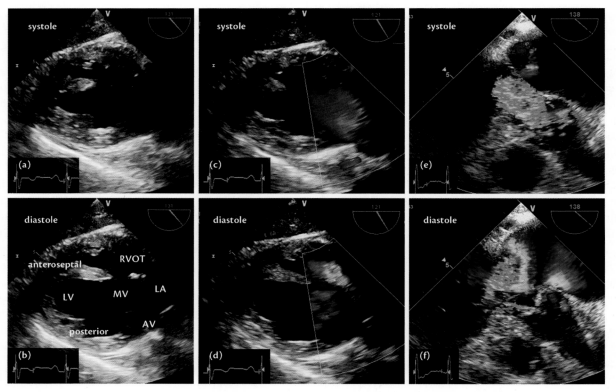

Fig. 1.34 Transgastric long-axis view during systole (a) and diastole (b), as well as the corresponding colour-coded views (c, d). The transgastric colour-coded long-axis view in a patient with hypertrophic cardiomyopathy with increased systolic (e) and diastolic flow (f). Additional comments in the text.

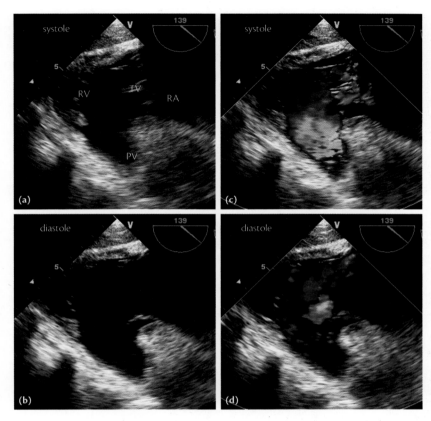

Fig. 1.35 Transgastric right ventricular inflow and outflow tract during systole (a) and diastole (b) and the corresponding colour-coded views (c, d). Additional comments in the text.

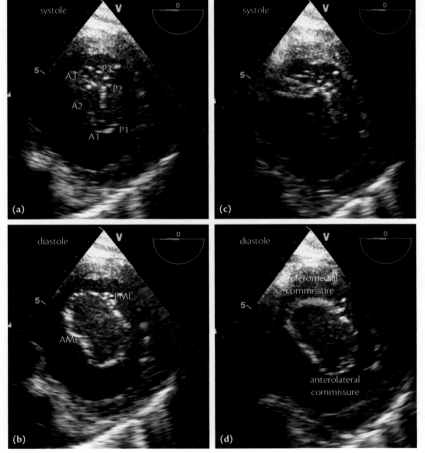

Fig. 1.36 Transgastric short-axis views at the mitral valve level. Two slightly different sectional planes of the mitral valve are displayed during systole (a, c) and diastole (b, d). Additional comments in the text.

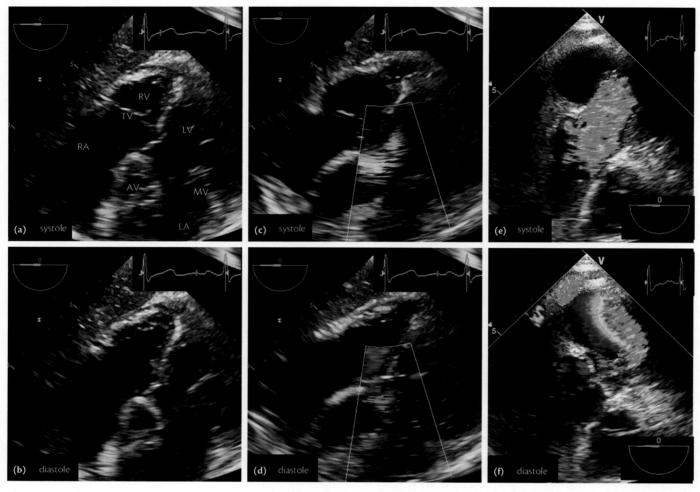

Fig. 1.37 Deep transgastric long-axis view during systole (a) and diastole (b) and the corresponding colour-coded views (c, d). Further colour-coded views of a patient with hypertrophic cardiomyopathy are displayed during systole (e) and diastole (f). Additional comments in the text.

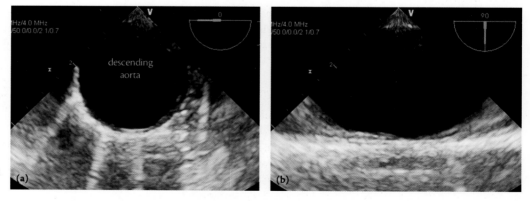

Fig. 1.38 Mid-oesophageal short-axis view (a) and long-axis view (b) of the descending aorta. Additional comments in the text.

In the region of the separation of the left subclavian artery, the probe has to be rotated (10°–60°) to display the descending aorta in short-axis views (➲ Fig. 1.38a–b). The aortic arch is displayed in a short-axis view after rotation of about 90°. Scanning of the descending aorta is necessary for the detection of plaque ruptures and other aortic pathologies. If pathological findings are present, additional long-axis views of the descending aorta should be documented.

Standard values in transthoracic and transoesophageal echocardiography

M-mode measurements

M-mode measurements in conventional echocardiography are mainly performed for analysis of left ventricular dimensions and wall thicknesses, as well as aortic root and left atrial dimensions.

For wall thickness measurements to calculate left ventricular mass according to the Penn-convention and for left ventricular diameter measurements for calculation of the left ventricular ejection fraction according to the Teichholz equation, the myocardial borders will be labelled inner-edge-to-inner-edge without endo- and epicardium at the maximum peak of the R-wave of the electrocardiogram. In contrast, according to the American Society of Echocardiography convention, measurements of the left ventricular wall will be performed leading-edge-to-leading-edge at the beginning of the QRS complex. In Europe the measurements are normally performed inner-edge-to-inner-edge. Measurements were performed at a ventricular level between the transition of the papillary muscles to the chords.

Left atrial diameter is measured at the time point of early diastole behind the aortic root. Aortic root diameter is measured inner-edge-to-inner-edge during mid-systole at the time interval of aortic valve separation.

Right ventricular diameter is measured in the M-mode at the mitral valve level during end-diastole.

Two-dimensional measurements

Two-dimensional measurements of left atrial and left ventricular volumes and function are performed by planimetry of both cavities in the standardized apical 2- and 4-chamber view during diastole and systole using Simpson's rule.

Right atrial and ventricular size is conventionally determined by the longitudinal and transverse diameter of the right atrium and the right ventricular inflow tract in the standardized apical 4-chamber view. Right ventricular function is estimated by planimetry of the right ventricular inflow tract in the standardized apical 4-chamber view during diastole and systole for determination of right ventricular fractional area change.

The diameter of the left ventricular outflow tract is normally measured in a standardized parasternal long-axis view due to a better spatial resolution than in the apical long-axis view.

Inferior caval vein diameter is measured in the subcostal longitudinal view during expiration and inspiration.

Pulsed spectral Doppler measurements

Pulsed spectral Doppler measurements are performed using the spectra of the mitral valve inflow and the left ventricular outflow tract. In normal hearts the dimension of the left ventricular outflow tract is almost the same as the dimension of the aortic valve annulus. For the left ventricular inflow, maximum velocities of the E- and A-wave, the E/A-ratio and the deceleration time of the E-wave are measured.

For estimation of diastolic function, the pulsed wave Doppler spectrum of the pulmonary vein flow is analysed for determination of the retrograde maximum A-wave velocity and the A-wave duration.

Continuous wave Doppler measurements

Continuous wave Doppler measurements are performed in all spectra documenting turbulences. This is especially important in valve pathologies. In normal hearts only the continuous wave Doppler spectrum of a mild tricuspid regurgitation is used for estimation of systolic pulmonary pressure. The maximum and mean velocities, as well as maximum and mean gradients calculated by the velocity time integrals, will be measured for the mitral valve inflow and left ventricular outflow tract or the flow through the aortic valve using the continuous wave Doppler spectra, if velocities are increased.

Pulsed spectral tissue Doppler measurements

Pulsed spectral tissue Doppler measurements are performed in the inferoseptal and lateral region of the mitral valve annulus to determine the velocity of E′ and the E/E′-ratio.

Standard values for these measurements are given in ⊃ Table 1.1.

The standard digital acquisition for transthoracic and transoesophageal echocardiography is given in Table ⊃ 1.2.

Table 1.1 Echocardiographic parameters and standard values used to quantify cardiac dimensions and function

Echocardiographic parameter	Standard value
Left ventricular wall thickness (M-mode/2D)	6–11 mm
Left ventricular end-diastolic diameter (M-mode/2D)	39–59 mm 22–32 mm/m^2 25–33 mm/m
Right ventricular wall thickness (M-mode/2D)	< 5 mm
Right ventricular diameter (M-mode/2D)	< 25 mm
Left ventricular end-diastolic volume (2D)	56–155 ml 35–75 ml/m^2
Left ventricular end-systolic volume (2D)	19–58 ml 12–30 ml/m^2
Left ventricular ejection fraction (2D)	> 55%
Left ventricular outflow tract diameter	18–31 mm
Right ventricular outflow tract and aortic annulus diameter	17–23 mm
Right ventricular base-to apex-length	71–79 mm
Basal right ventricular diameter	20–28 mm
Right ventricular diastolic area	11–28 cm^2
Right ventricular fractional area change	32–60%
Left atrial diameter (M-mode/2D)	27–40 mm 15–23 mm/m^2
Left atrial volume (atrial end-diastole) (2D)	22–58 ml < 34 ml/m^2
Aortic root diameter (M-mode/2D)	< 39 mm
Right atrial minor axis diameter (2D)	29–45 mm 17–25 mm/m^2
Inferior caval vein diameter (2D)	< 17 mm
E/A-ratio	> 1
Deceleration time	< 200 ms
A wave velocity of the pulmonary vein	< 35 cm/s
A wave duration	< 120 ms
E′-wave velocity	> 8 cm/s
E/E′-ratio	< 8

Table 1.2 Standard digital acquisition for transthoracic and transoesophageal echocardiography. The mandatory documentation is labelled in bold. 2D - two-dimensional; pw - pulsed wave Doppler; cw - continuous wave Doppler; IAS - inter-atrial septum; TTE - transthoracic echocardiography.

View	Data type
Parasternal long-axis view of the left ventricle (2D/colour-coded)	**Cineloop**
Parasternal long-axis view at the mid-papillary level (2D/M-mode)	**Cineloop**
Parasternal long-axis view at the mitral valve level (2D/colour-coded)	**Cineloop**
Parasternal long-axis view at the aortic valve level (2D/colour-coded/M-mode)	**Cineloop**
M-mode sweep	M-Mode
Parasternal right ventricular inflow tract (2D/colour-coded)	Cineloop
Parasternal right ventricular outflow tract (2D/colour-coded)	Cineloop
Right ventricular outflow tract velocities (pw Doppler)	**pw Doppler**
Apical long-axis view (2D/colour-coded, optional tissue colour-coded)	**Cineloop**
Transmitral velocities (pw Doppler/in the presence of turbulences—cw Doppler)	**pw Doppler cw Doppler**
Left ventricular outflow tract velocities (pw Doppler)	**pw Doppler**
Transaortic velocities (in the presence of turbulences—cw Doppler)	**cw Doppler**
Apical 2-chamber view (2D/colour-coded, optional tissue colour-coded)	**Cineloop**
Apical 4-chamber view (2D/colour-coded, optional tissue colour-coded)	**Cineloop**
Tricuspid valve regurgitant velocities (cw Doppler)	**cw Doppler**
Tissue pulsed wave Doppler velocities (inferoseptal, lateral—4-chamber view)	**pw Doppler**
Right pulmonary vein velocities	pw Doppler
Subcostal 4-chamber view—IAS (2D/colour-coded)	Cineloop
Subcostal short-axis view at the mitral valve level (2D/colour-coded)	Cineloop
Subcostal short-axis view at the aortic valve level (2D/colour-coded)	Cineloop
Subcostal longitudinal view of the inferior caval vein during breathing (2D)	**Cineloop**
Suprasternal view of the aortic arch (2D/colour-coded)	**Cineloop**
Mid-transoesophageal 4-chamber view (2D/colour-coded)	**Cineloop**
Mid-transoesophageal 2-chamber view (2D/colour-coded)	**Cineloop**
Mid-transoesophageal long-axis view (2D/colour-coded)	**Cineloop**
Mid-transoesophageal short-axis view at the aortic valve level (2D/colour-coded)	**Cineloop**
Mid-transoesophageal view of the left atrial appendage (2D/colour-coded) and its perpendicular view	**Cineloop**
Left atrial appendage velocities (pw Doppler)	**pw Doppler**
Left upper pulmonary vein velocities (pw Doppler)	pw Doppler
Mid-oesophageal bicaval view (2D)	**Cineloop**
Upper oesophageal aortic short-axis view	**Cineloop**
Upper oesophageal superior caval vein axis view	Cineloop
Upper oesophageal aortic long-axis view	Cineloop
Mid-oesophageal short-axis view of the descending aorta (2D)	**Cineloop**
Mid-oesophageal long-axis view of the descending aorta (2D)	**Cineloop**
Transgastric short-axis view at the mid-papillary level (2D) if TTE not possible	**Cineloop**
Transgastric 2-chamber view (2D/colour-coded) if TTE not possible	**Cineloop**
Transgastric long-axis view (2D/colour-coded) if TTE not possible	**Cineloop**
Transgastric view of the right ventricular inflow and outflow tract (2D/colour-coded) if TTE not possible	Cineloop
Transgastric short-axis view at the mitral valve level (2D/colour-coded) if TTE not possible	Cineloop
Deep transgastric 5-chamber view (2D/colour-coded) if TTE not possible	Cineloop
Deep transgastric long-axis view (2D/colour-coded) if TTE not possible	Cineloop
Transmitral velocities in the deep transgastric 5-chamber view (pw Doppler/in the presence of turbulences—cw Doppler) if TTE not possible	**pw Doppler cw Doppler**
Left ventricular outflow tract velocities in the transgastric long-axis view (pw Doppler) if TTE not possible	**pw Doppler**
Transaortic velocities in the transgastric long-axis view (in the presence of turbulences—cw Doppler) if TTE not possible	cw Doppler

Acknowledgements

The photos and the photo composition are performed by Stefan Straube, Public Relations Department, University Hospital AöR Leipzig, Germany.

All persons on the photos have given consent to be published.

References

1. Flachskampf FA, Decoodt P, Fraser AG, et al. Recommendations for performing transoesophageal echocardiography. *Eur J Echocardiography* 2001; 2: 8–21.
2. Lang R, Bierig M, Devereux R, et al. Recommendations for chamber quantification. *Eur J Echocardiography* 2006; 7: 79–108.
3. Nihoyannopoulos P, Fox K, Fraser A, et al. EAE laboratory standards and accreditation. *Eur J Echocardiography* 2007; 8:80–87.
4. Evangelista A, Flachskampf F, Lancellotti P, et al. European Association of Echocardiography recommendations for standardization of performance, digital storage and reporting of echocardiographic studies. *Eur J Echocardiography* 2008; 9:438–48.
5. Hagendorff A. Transthoracic echocardiography in adult patients—a proposal for documenting a standardized investigation. *Eur J Ultrasound* 2008; 29: 2–31.
6. Nagueh SF, Appleton CP, Gillebert TC, et al. Recommendations for the evaluation of left ventricular diastolic function by echocardiography. *Eur J Echocardiography* 2009; 10: 165–93.
7. Flachskampf FA, Badano L, Daniel WG, et al. Recommendations for transoesophageal echocardiography: update 2010. *Eur J Echocardiography* 2010; 11: 557–76.

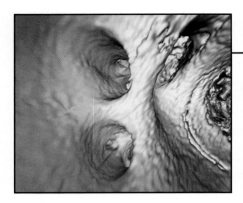

CHAPTER 2

Nuclear cardiology (PET and SPECT)—basic principles

Frank M. Bengel, Ornella Rimoldi, and
Paolo G. Camici

Contents

Introduction

Radionuclide imaging of the heart is well established for the clinical diagnostic and prognostic workup of coronary artery disease. Myocardial perfusion single photon emission computed tomography (SPECT) has been the mainstay of cardiovascular radionuclide applications for decades and its usefulness is supported by a very large body of evidence [1]. Positron emission tomography (PET) is an advanced radionuclide technique that has also been available for decades. In contrast to SPECT, PET has long been considered mainly a research tool due to its methodological complexity. But owing to several recent developments, cardiac PET is now increasingly penetrating the clinical arena [2].

Nuclear cardiology techniques are considered robust, accurate, and reliable for clinical imaging of heart disease. Yet, in a continuous effort to minimize radiation burden and maximize comfort for patients on the one hand, while maximizing the available information for the referring physician on the other hand, nuclear imaging technology is progressing towards higher sensitivity and resolution [3], and novel, highly specific radiotracers are being introduced [4]. While the techniques will continue to play a key role for the assessment of myocardial perfusion, function, and viability, on-going novel developments are indicators of a steady evolution of nuclear cardiology towards characterization of molecular events at the tissue level. In the competitive environment of cardiovascular imaging, it is therefore expected that radionuclide imaging will take a central role in the implementation of molecular imaging techniques for more specific, personalized, preventive, and therapeutic decision-making.

This chapter will outline the basic aspects of SPECT and PET as the two key nuclear cardiology techniques. Technical aspects of image acquisition will be discussed first. A brief overview on current application of radionuclide imaging procedures will then be given, and the chapter will be concluded by an outlook on novel developments of camera and tracer methodology.

Technical aspects: physics and data analysis

SPECT

Myocardial SPECT imaging has typically been performed using a multi-detector gamma camera system, which rotates around the chest to obtain tomographic images of single emitted photons (⊃ Fig. 2.1). Collimators are being used to balance detection sensitivity

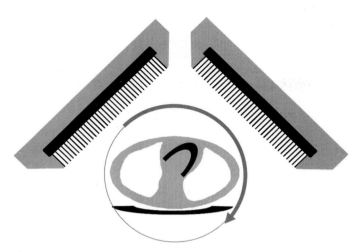

Fig. 2.1 Configuration of a SPECT system. Two gamma camera detector heads, equipped with collimators, rotate in a semicircular fashion around the chest and create images in multiple positions ('step-and-shoot').

which correct for loss of resolution at increasing distance from the detector (resolution recovery). These algorithms improve sensitivity and allow for reduction of injected activity without loss of image quality [3]. The resulting tomographic datasets are re-orientated along the left ventricular short and long axes to facilitate review of myocardial tracer distribution and comparison of rest and stress studies (⊃ Fig. 2.2a). Software tools have been developed that employ contour detection algorithms and circumferential profiles to create polar maps from the tomographic images [6–9]. These polar maps are a two-dimensional display of the three-dimensional tracer distribution throughout the myocardium, which facilitate comparison of patient data with normal databases, as well as semi-quantitative analysis of defect sizes (⊃ Fig. 2.2b).

Electrocardiographic (ECG) gating

ECG-gated acquisition of perfusion SPECT studies has become a standard procedure, which has two major advantages over non-gated acquisition. First, ECG-gating allows quantitative measurement of left ventricular (LV) ejection fraction (EF) and volumes, as well as regional evaluation of LV wall motion [10]. Second, ECG-gating may improve the diagnostic accuracy of perfusion imaging in the event of attenuation artefacts [11]. Such artefacts may appear as apparently irreversible perfusion defects, but normal regional wall motion prevents a wrong interpretation as scar tissue.

It should be noted that functional gated SPECT acquired after stress shows the LV at rest, although sometimes, transient wall motion abnormality and possibly dilated LV and reduced EF (myocardial stunning) may persist and be observed during the acquisition phase, up to 90 min or even later after the resolution of ischaemia [12].

For ECG-gating, the patient should have a fairly regular heart rhythm. The cardiac cycle is usually divided into 8, and sometimes

and optimize spatial resolution. For imaging, the patient is typically positioned supine on the table, although prone positioning has been shown to be useful for reducing attenuation artefacts [5].

During acquisition, the system creates 'raw' data, which consist of multiple planar projection images at different angles. As for any other tomographic acquisition, the raw data must be transformed into tomographic images for subsequent analysis and interpretation. This process, known as reconstruction, produces an image that reflects, as closely as possible, the tracer's distribution in the organ/tissue of interest at the time of acquisition. This is achieved using either standard filtered back-projection (FBP) or novel iterative reconstruction algorithms. The process of reconstruction is then followed by filtering to reduce image noise. Of note, novel reconstruction algorithms have been introduced recently,

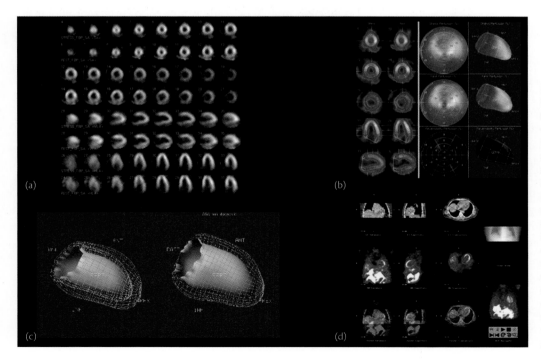

Fig. 2.2 State-of-the-art myocardial SPECT imaging. (a) Display of matched stress (rows 1, 3, 5, 7) and rest (rows 2, 4, 6, 8) tomographic images, re-angulated along the short and long axes of the left ventricle for visual analysis. (b) Creation of two- (middle column), and three-dimensional polar maps (right column) using software-assisted detection of myocardial contours (left column), for semiquantitative analysis of perfusion defects. (c) Three-dimensional display of endocardial contours throughout the cardiac cycle from gated SPECT acquisition, for visual and quantitative analysis of left ventricular function. (d) Creation of density maps from transmission images, for attenuation correction of SPECT data.

into 12 or 16 gates (time bins). Based on relative timing after the R-wave, counts in each projection image are then accumulated for each of the gates. For reproducible functional analysis, software products are available that generate semi-automatically three-dimensional (3D) myocardial contours throughout the cardiac cycle. Volumetric data from the contours can then be used for 3D display and calculation of quantitative global parameters (⊃ Fig. 2.2c).

Attenuation correction

Attenuation of radiation in the body can lead to a non-uniform reduction in the apparent activity in the myocardium and to the introduction of artefacts in the images. Additionally, scatter of radiation both within the body and in the detector degrades image contrast and potentially affects the accurate quantification of activity and relative distribution of perfusion. Finally, resolution decreases with distance from the collimator face, which can alter the apparent distribution of activity in the myocardium.

Among those factors, attenuation is considered to have the most significant effect. The amount of attenuation in a clinical study depends on the type of tissue (soft tissue, bone, or lung), the energy of the radiation, and the thickness of the body. Hence, compensation for soft-tissue attenuation requires exact knowledge of the attenuation characteristics for each patient. While many schemes for the generation of the attenuation characteristics have been reported [13], nowadays the attenuation map of a patient is usually generated by transmission imaging, using the X-ray CT in hybrid systems (⊃ Fig. 2.2d). Software and hardware methods used in these systems vary significantly from one vendor to another, but it has been documented for several systems that attenuation correction improves image quality and image interpretation [14–16]. Importantly, failure to incorporate effects of scatter into the attenuation compensation technique will result in introduction of artefacts, so that a combination of attenuation and scatter correction is necessary.

Systematic data analysis

For adequate interpretation of myocardial perfusion images, a systematic visual review of raw data and reconstructed images on a computer screen is warranted [17]. The system of reviewing comprises several reviewing levels. First, raw projection data are reviewed to identify motion artefacts and assess tracer distribution in organs other than the heart. Next, re-orientated tomographic images are reviewed without and, if available, with attenuation/scatter compensation and gated cine data. Then, software-derived semiquantitative data are reviewed and used in order to strengthen the visual impression of tomographic image readout. Finally, the impression of the image readout is integrated with stress performance and with clinical data and should be reported in a standardized format.

PET

There are multiple methodological differences between conventional SPECT and PET. Most importantly, PET scanners have a different geometry and a different detection principle.

Multiple corrective algorithms are routinely applied to yield images of absolutely quantitative tracer distribution within the body. Second, much shorter lived positron emitting radioisotopes are being utilized, which increase flexibility of imaging protocols and biologic targets, but at the same time increase complexity and limit availability of the methodology.

Acquisition

The goal of PET scanning is to produce a three-dimensional image volume that is an accurate map of the distribution of tracer in the body. To allow absolute quantification, a series of such volumes is normally generated over a time to describe the time–activity curves (TAC) and investigate the kinetics of tracer uptake and release from different tissues and blood.

Annihilation

Positron-emitting radioisotopes are generated by cyclotrons, which accelerate protons or deuterons interacting with target atoms to produce 'proton-rich' radioisotopes. During decay, a proton converts to a neutron and a positron is emitted. Under the influence of surrounding atomic electrons, the positron is slowed down until interaction with an electron results in the annihilation of both particles and two photons are emitted (each with energy of 511 keV) in practically opposite directions (⊃ Fig. 2.3). Compared to radionuclides emitting single gamma-ray photons, the emission of pairs of 511 keV annihilation photons gives PET imaging higher detection efficiency, better uniformity of spatial resolution and easier correction for attenuation (scattering) of photons in tissue (⊃ Fig. 2.4).

Attenuation

In PET, the probability to detect a coincidence along a line, meaning none of the two photons forming the coincidence have interacted with the matter, is independent of the position of annihilation along the detected line-of-response (LOR). This property is different from SPECT and is utilized to correct for photon attenuation in a robust manner.

Coincidence detection

If photons interact with the detectors' ring within a specified time period, known as the coincidence window, then an event is recorded and is termed a prompt coincidence. True coincidences, formed by the two photons detected within the coincidence window

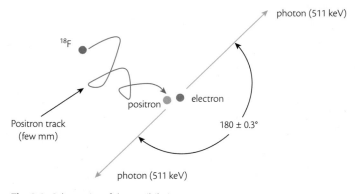

Fig. 2.3 Schematics of the annihilation process.

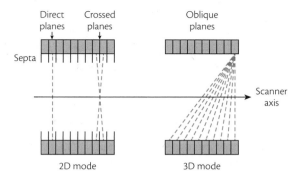

Fig. 2.6 Comparison of the two acquisition modes permitted by some PET systems. In 2D mode, because of the use of lead septa reducing the transaxial acceptance angle, the device only detects photons in the direct or crossed planes, whereas in 3D mode, all the planes, direct or oblique, can be recorded.

Data correction

To exploit the potential of PET to provide quantitative data, a number of corrections need to be carried out:

Normalization

The geometry of a PET system introduces variation in the detection sensitivity. Normalization corrects for this by measuring the count rate for each line of response using a source with predefined radioactivity.

Dead time

The response time of a detector system is finite. Dead time is the period when a detector is unable to record an event [18, 19]. This might be because of the electronics' delay or if more than one photon strikes a detector within its resolving time and is rejected. New lutetium oxyorthosilicate (LSO), lutetium-yttrium (LYSO), and cerium-doped gadolinium oxyorthosilicate (GSO:Ce) crystals have higher light output and shorter decay constants, which result in improved spatial resolution and reduction of random coincidences affecting the counting rate capabilities of the system.

Attenuation

In the past, an external positron-emitting source has been used to measure the attenuating factor before administration of radioactivity [20–22]. This process results in an image representing the distribution of the density of the patient's organs. With the advent of hybrid PET-CT, a CT scan provides a substitute for the conventional PET transmission scan [23]. Hybrid systems are equipped

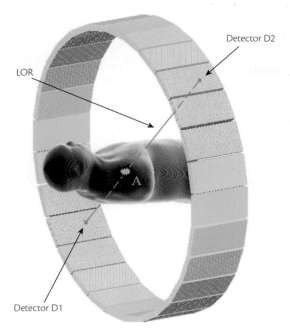

Fig. 2.4 Representation of the detection of the two emitted photons. Two photons arise from annihilation at point A and impinge on detectors D1 and D2. A circular ring of individual detectors is shown here but the same principles apply for other position-sensitive systems, such as rings of planar detectors or rotating gamma cameras. Imposing a coincidence condition on the detection process, such that an event is only recorded when signals are produced from both detectors simultaneously, effects an automatic electronic collimation and enables the annihilation to be localized to the line D1–D2, conventionally termed a line-of-response (LOR). The width of the LOR is the intrinsic spatial resolution of the detectors. It can also readily be seen that the resolution will be quite constant along the LOR.

without having undergone any interaction with matter need to be separated from scattered and random coincidences (⊃ Fig. 2.5).

3D Imaging

⊃ Figure 2.6 shows an axial section through a multi-ring PET tomograph. The 3D mode makes maximum use of the detectors available within all rings, as well as the same ring allowing the use of lower doses of radioactivity. This seems the obvious solution, but registration of scattered and random coincidences complicates the situation and often leads to a retreat from 3D acquisition to a more conservative 2D mode. In the latter, tungsten annuli called Septa are placed between detector rings.

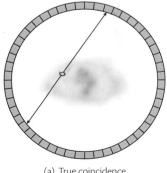
(a). True coincidence

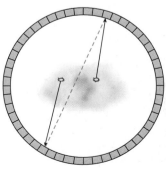
(b). Random coincidence

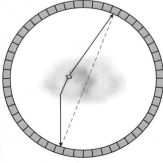
(c). Scattered coincidence

Fig. 2.5 Representation of the different types of coincidences.

with fast, multi-slice CT components, allowing the correction of soft-tissue attenuation artefact with a brief CT scan before or after emission imaging [24–26]. The duration of the CT scan is much less than the PET transmission scan, around 20 seconds, hence, a problem to overcome is movement of the patient (cardiac, respiratory, other voluntary and involuntary movements), resulting in misalignment of CT and PET.

Scattered coincidences

Some correction methods employ mathematical modelling (using, for example, data from point sources in scattering media) to deconvolute scattered events from the total signal [27]. In the chest, however, scatter distribution is complex due to the range of tissue densities. An alternative but more challenging approach is that of calculation of scattered photon distribution from raw-image data, a process that can be repeated iteratively until satisfactory accuracy is achieved [28]. Iterative reconstruction methods (ordered-subsets expectation maximization (OSEM)) are now used to reconstruct the data acquired with high resolution tomographs showing promising results, which should be translated into clinical practice in a short while [29].

Random coincidences

In cardiac scanning the correction for, and treatment of, random coincidence events is very important. The most commonly used method estimates randoms using a delayed coincidence circuit [30], which is employed with a temporal delay so that no true coincidences will be registered. Randoms are then estimated and can be subtracted on-line from the prompt events or stored separately for later processing.

Motion

A very important consequence of the high timing resolution made possible by the data acquisition in list mode is that it makes effective motion correction possible. ECG-gating is a standard procedure for use with PET and studies have also been carried out into respiratory gating, making feasible the monitoring of, and the correction for, both cardiac and respiratory movements of the patient [26, 31, 32].

Partial volume

Despite the technological developments in PET, basic physical characteristics mean that its spatial resolution is limited and the signal in a particular region will be 'diluted' due to the presence of surrounding tissues—there will be a 'spillover' of radioactivity between adjacent structures. The same is true for SPECT, which usually has an approximately 2-fold lower spatial resolution compared to PET. Combination of transmission and emission data has been used to correct for this effect in the myocardium and PET and CT or MRI images have been combined to enable corrections [33].

Time of flight (TOF)

The electronics of the detectors are linked so that the detection events that occur within a certain time window (5–15 ns depending on the crystal material) are assumed to have come from the same annihilation, i.e. coincident. In TOF, electronics are capable

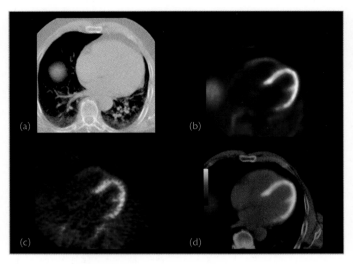

Fig. 2.7 Example of a cardiac 3D PET image with $^{13}NH_3$. (a) CT transmission image. (b) High statistic PET data reconstructed—3D OSEM point spread function (PSF) and time of flight (TOF), spatial resolution FWHM (full width at half maximum) 2 mm. (c) Low statistic PET data reconstruction for comparison–3D Filter Back projection, Hanning filter spatial resolution FWHM 4.3 mm. (d) Co-registration of PET and CT images, motion corrected. Note the lower noise, the higher contrast and the better definition of the myocardial wall in the PET images reconstructed with the iterative 3D-OSEM algorithm also accounting for the PET system, PSF and TOF.
Courtesy of Dr L. Gianolli and Dr V. Bettinardi, Nuclear Medicine Department, Ospedale San Raffaele, Milan.

of measuring the real-time interval between (1 ns) detection along the coincidence ray between the two detectors. This allows TOF scanners to localize more accurately the origin of annihilation. An example of the improvement of the image quality in 3D with a TOF scanner is shown in ⊃ Fig. 2.7.

Current imaging procedures and applications

SPECT

SPECT is widely used for the clinical workup of suspected or known coronary artery disease (CAD). Its diagnostic and prognostic usefulness is supported by a large body of evidence [1]. Most importantly, SPECT-derived information is utilized as a gatekeeper to invasive procedures and as a guide for further clinical decision-making. Assessment of myocardial perfusion and function are the two major clinical applications [17, 34].

Myocardial perfusion

For perfusion imaging, two technetium-99m (^{99m}Tc) labelled radiopharmaceuticals (sestamibi and tetrofosmin) are commonly employed, while use of the longer-lived tracer thallium-201 (^{201}Tl) is discouraged due to resulting higher radiation exposure.

The higher energy of ^{99m}Tc generally leads to better quality images (because of less attenuation and scatter) compared to ^{201}Tl. Moreover, the short half-life permits much higher activities to be administered, giving good counting statistics (⊃ Fig. 2.8),

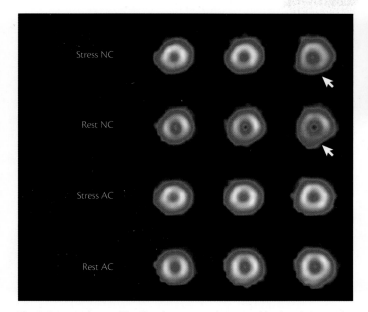

Fig. 2.8 Non-corrected (NC) and attenuation corrected (AC) mid-ventricular short-axis myocardial perfusion SPECT images using 99mTc-sestamibi in an individual with suspected coronary artery disease. Note inferior wall defect in NC images (arrows), which resolves after AC, indicating presence of artefact rather than disease.

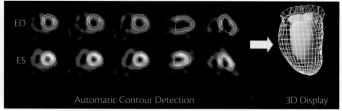

Fig. 2.9 Gated myocardial perfusion SPECT. Automated contour detection (left) is employed for creation of three-dimensional displays (right) to review wall motion, volumes and ejection fraction. ED, enddiastolic frame; ES, end-systolic frame.

while still resulting in lower radioactivity doses compared to 201Tl. However, tracer kinetic properties are somewhat inferior when compared to 201Tl [35]. Uptake and extraction of both 99mTc-labelled tracers as a function of myocardial perfusion is less avid, and reaches a plateau at higher flow.

99mTc -sestamibi is a cationic complex, which diffuses passively through the capillary and cell membrane, although less readily than 201Tl, resulting in lower immediate extraction. Within the cell it is trapped in the mitochondria. Retention is based on intact mitochondria, reflecting viable myocytes [36, 37]. Tetrofosmin is also cleared rapidly from the blood and its myocardial uptake is similar to that of sestamibi. Hepatic clearance is slightly more rapid than in the case of sestamibi [38, 39]. Two-day, same-day stress–rest or same-day rest–stress imaging protocols have been established [40, 41].

SPECT imaging usually begins 30–60 min after injection to allow for hepatobiliary clearance. Longer delays are required for resting images and for stress with vasodilators alone because of the risk of higher subdiaphragmatic activity. For improved assessment of myocardial viability, resting injections can be given following nitrate administration to avoid underestimation in areas with reduced resting perfusion [42].

Ventricular function

Assessment of LV function and volumes is not only important for the assessment of prognosis in CAD. Addition of gating has also been shown to improve diagnostic and prognostic accuracy of myocardial perfusion SPECT [11, 43]. Additionally, assessment of the function of the right ventricle (RV) is recognized to be important in some diseases such as arrhythmogenic RV and pulmonary hypertension. Finally, determination with equilibrium

radionuclide ventriculography of LV-EF is recognized as one of the methods-of-choice for monitoring of cardiotoxicity of cytotoxic anti-cancer drugs [44].

Functional radionuclide cardiac studies include several techniques, and ECG-gating with R-wave triggering is a key point in these methods.

First-pass radionuclide ventriculography comprises a short sequence of cardiac cycles acquired during the transit of a bolus of any radionuclide through the heart. It can be performed at rest and during stress [45], provides high target-to-background ratio with temporal separation of the RV and LV, but imaging is possible in only one projection and tomographic SPECT images cannot be obtained [34].

Equilibrium radionuclide ventriculography is performed after 99mTc-labelling of red blood cells using different techniques [34]. It provides high-quality planar images and may even be performed as a SPECT study for accurate separation of RV and LV and for accurate assessment of regional wall motion [46].

Finally, as mentioned, SPECT (and PET) perfusion studies can be acquired in ECG-gated mode in order to obtain parameters of LV function on top of myocardial perfusion [47] (◗ Fig. 2.9).

PET

In contrast to SPECT, which is the clinical mainstay for the diagnostic workup of CAD by nuclear imaging techniques, PET offers deeper insights into myocardial patho-physiology and biology. Although PET has the potential to probe a number of complex functions (including genes), the current clinical applications of PET imaging in cardiology can be divided into three main categories: studies of regional myocardial blood flow, metabolism, and pharmacology.

Myocardial blood flow (MBF)

Mainly three tracers are used for the measurement of MBF using PET: 15O-labelled water ($H_2$15O) [48, 49], 13N-labelled ammonia (13NH3) [50, 51], and the cationic potassium analogue 82Rubidium (82Rb) [52]. Recently an 18F-labelled PET perfusion tracer 18F-BMS747158-02 (flurpiridaz) has been validated in animals [53] and humans [54, 55]. This novel tracer is an analogue of the insecticide pyridaben that binds the mitochondrial complex I of the electron transport chain with high affinity and shows good uptake in the heart. 18F-BMS747158-02 has a relatively long $t_{1/2}$ (110 min), good image quality high extraction at first pass

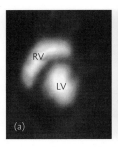
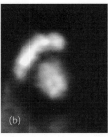
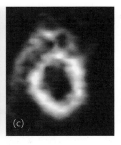

Fig. 2.10 Short-axis images obtained from one representative study showing the blood pool (a) measured with $C^{15}O$, which labels the erythrocytes through the formation of carboxyhaemoglobin, and the distribution of $H_2^{15}O$ separated in a blood (b) and myocardial tissue (c) component. (b) and (c) are both calculated by means of factor analysis. RV = right ventricle; LV = left ventricle. This research was originally published in *J Nucl Med*. 2002 Aug;43(8):1031-40. © by the Society of Nuclear Medicine and Molecular Imaging, Inc.

(3.1% of injected dose per gram), at present the comparison with ^{99m}Tc SPECT appears favourable in a phase 2 evaluation study [55]; larger studies are warranted to weigh the real potential of ^{18}F-flurpiridaz to enter clinical practice.

^{82}Rb is produced by a strontium-82/^{82}Rb generator that generally requires replacement once a month. The high positron energy of ^{82}Rb results in a relatively inferior image quality and reduced spatial resolution due to its long positron track (4 mm). Kinetic models [56–58] have been proposed for quantification of MBF using ^{82}Rb [59]; these are limited by the dependence of the myocardial extraction of this tracer on the prevailing flow rate and myocardial metabolic state [60]. Nevertheless, in the past few years both semiquantitive [61] and fully quantitative measurements [62] of myocardial perfusion with ^{82}Rb have been proven to be feasible on a large scale. An incremental prognostic value of quantitative ^{82}Rb PET for cardiac and all-cause death has been shown in patients with known or suspected CAD.

For $H_2^{15}O$ and $^{13}NH_3$, tracer kinetic models have been successfully validated in animals against the radiolabelled microsphere method over a wide flow range [48, 49, 51, 63, 64]. The values of MBF determined in normal human volunteers using both tracers either at rest or during pharmacologically induced coronary vasodilatation are similar [48, 51]. Recent advances in image processing [64] enhanced the quality of myocardial $H_2^{15}O$ images

(⊃ Fig. 2.10) to match the quality of $^{13}NH_3$ images. Both tracers have short physical half-lives (2 and 10 min, respectively), which allow repeated measurements of MBF in the same session [65].

The major regulatory site of tissue perfusion is at the level of arterioles of less than 300 μm diameter (i.e. the microcirculation). Information on this section of the coronary circulation in humans *in vivo* can only be obtained indirectly by measuring parameters such as MBF and coronary flow reserve (CFR), i.e. the ratio of maximal MBF following pharmacologically induced coronary vasodilatation to resting MBF (⊃ Figs 2.11 and 2.12).

The use of PET has highlighted the effects of age [48, 51, 66], gender [67], and sympathetic tone [68] on MBF. The accuracy of PET has been used to detect impairments of MBF in asymptomatic subjects with cardiovascular risk factors [69, 70], in the relatives of patients with CAD, in whom coronary arteriography is not justifiable on the basis of family history alone [71], and in diabetic patients without symptoms of cardiac disease [72].

In patients with CAD, the measurement of CFR is useful for assessment of the functional significance of coronary stenoses [73]. Myocardial perfusion imaging and CFR have a predictive value of long-term prognosis in patients with suspected myocardial ischaemia. In patients with normal perfusion, abnormal CFR is independently associated with a higher annual event rate over 3 years compared with normal CFR [74]. Hybrid multislice CT systems can provide comprehensive assessment of cardiac and coronary morphology in addition to the assessment of inducible ischaemia [62] in suspected coronary artery disease [75].

In addition, PET is particularly effective in those circumstances where the CFR is diffusely (and not regionally) blunted, e.g. in patients with hypertrophic or dilated cardiomyopathy. The improved spatial resolution of the latest generation of 3D PET scanners [76] has allowed the quantification of the transmural distribution of myocardial blood flow in patients with LV hypertrophy secondary to aortic stenosis demonstrating a more significant reduction of subendocardial CFR, which was directly related to the reduction of the aortic valve area [77].

Myocardial metabolism

In the post-absorptive state, the heart relies mainly on oxidation of free fatty acid (FFA) as its main source of high-energy phosphates,

Fig. 2.11 (a) Blood (arterial and venous) and (b) tissue time activity curves (TAC) measured from the dynamic scan sequence obtained after injection of $H_2^{15}O$. The arterial and venous TAC were obtained from regions of interest (ROI) drawn in the right and left ventricles, while the tissue TAC was obtained from an ROI placed in left ventricular myocardium. These data are then used to compute myocardial blood flow in ml/min/g.

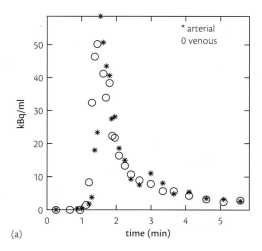
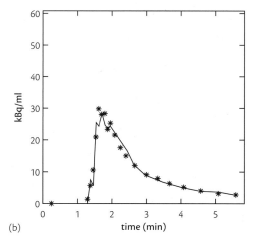

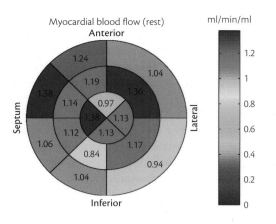

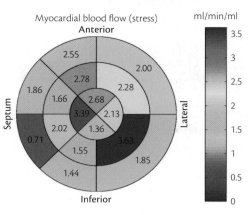

Fig. 2.12 Polar maps of myocardial blood flow measured with $H_2{}^{15}O$ at rest and during adenosine stress in a patient with significant disease of the left anterior descending and right coronary arteries.

while glucose uptake and oxidation are low. In the fed state, glucose uptake is high and accounts for virtually all of the concurrent oxygen uptake [78]. The factors that regulate myocardial substrate utilization are complex and depend, in addition to substrate concentration, upon the action of different hormones. Insulin, which stimulates myocardial glucose uptake and utilization, also inhibits adipose tissue lipolysis, so that during hyperinsulinaemia the circulating levels of FFA are low [78]. On the other hand, catecholamines decrease rather than increase glycolysis in the heart, together with a greatly increased uptake and oxidation of FFA [78]. Myocardial utilization of carbohydrates is also affected by cardiac workload, with oxidation of carbohydrates accounting for more than 50% of energy produced during conditions of maximal stress [79]. Finally, glucose utilization is increased during conditions of reduced oxygen supply; under these circumstances exogenous glucose uptake and glycogen breakdown are increased, glycolysis is stimulated, and ATP can be produced from the anaerobic catabolism of glucose with the concomitant formation of lactate [78].

In order to assess this metabolic pathway under normoxic and ischaemic conditions, PET imaging has been performed after intravenous administration of the natural FFA palmitate labelled with ^{11}C (^{11}C-palmitate) [80]. Furthermore, ^{11}C-labelled acetate has been advocated as a tracer of tricarboxylic acid cycle activity [81] and used as an indirect marker of myocardial oxygen consumption (MVO_2) by PET in both experimental animals [82, 83] and humans [84–86].

The utilization of exogenous glucose by the myocardium can be assessed using PET with ^{18}F-2-fluoro-2-deoxyglucose (FDG) [87]. FDG is transported into the myocyte by the same trans-sarcolemmal carriers (GLUT-1, GLUT-4) as glucose and is then phosphorylated to FDG-6-phosphate by hexokinase. This is essentially a unidirectional reaction, as no glucose-6-phosphatase (the enzyme that hydrolyses FDG-6-phosphate back to free FDG and free phosphate) has yet been identified in cardiac muscle [87]. Thus, measurement of the myocardial uptake of FDG is proportional to the overall rate of trans-sarcolemmal transport and hexokinase-phosphorylation of exogenous circulating glucose by

heart muscle, but it does not provide information about the further intracellular disposal of glucose.

A number of kinetic modelling approaches have been used for the quantification of glucose utilization rates using FDG [88]. The major limitation of these approaches is that quantification of glucose metabolism requires the knowledge of the lumped constant (LC), a factor that relates the kinetic behaviour of FDG to naturally occurring glucose in terms of the relative affinity of each molecule for the trans-sarcolemmal transporter and for hexokinase. The value of the LC in humans under different physiologic and pathophysiologic conditions is not known, thus making true *in vivo* quantification of myocardial metabolic rates of glucose very difficult [89]. Nevertheless, the quantification of the uptake of FDG under standardized dietary conditions, such as during insulin clamp [90] allows comparison of absolute values from different individuals.

Non-invasive metabolic imaging of ischaemia basically relies on two simple observations. first, the uptake of glucose by the myocardium is increased by hypoxia and mild to moderate ischaemia, but decreased by very severe ischaemia. Second, during both mild and severe ischaemia the extraction, uptake, and oxidation of FFA are reduced. Hence the uptake of an appropriately labelled FFA is seen to be decreased in the ischaemic myocardium [91].

Myocardial pharmacology

Different tracers have been used to study presynaptic sympathetic terminals: ^{18}F-labelled fluorometaraminol [92, 93], ^{11}C-labelled hydroxyephedrine (^{11}C-HED) [94], and ^{11}C-labelled epinephrine [95], which compete with endogenous noradrenaline for the transport into the presynaptic nerve terminal.

A benzylguanidine analogue that acts as substrate for the noradrenaline transporter LMI1195 (*N*-[3-Bromo-4-(3-[18F] fluoro-propoxy)-benzyl]-guanidine) has been recently tested in experimental animals, interestingly it incorporates ^{18}F thus achieving a longer half-life [96].

Several beta-blocker drugs have been labelled with ^{11}C to act as radioligands for the study of postsynaptic ß-adrenoceptor [97]. ^{11}C-(S)-CGP 12177 is a non-selective ß-adrenoceptor antagonist, which is particularly suited for PET studies due to its high affinity and low lipophilicity, thus enabling the functional receptor pool on the cell surface to be studied [98]. Studies in patients have demonstrated diffuse downregulation of ß-adrenoceptor density in hypertrophic cardiomyopathy [99, 100] and in congestive heart failure [101–103].

In addition to studies of the sympathetic nervous system, the density and affinity constants of myocardial muscarinic receptors can be evaluated non-invasively with 11C-MQNB (methylquinuclidinyl benzilate), a specific hydrophilic antagonist, in both experimental animals [104] and in humans [105, 106]. In patients with congestive heart failure, mean receptor concentration (Bmax) was significantly higher compared with normal subjects [105], a clear indication that congestive heart failure is associated with an upregulation of myocardial muscarinic receptors paralleling the downregulation of ß-adrenoceptors.

Recent trends
Novel dedicated SPECT cameras

Economic pressure, competition from alternative modalities, and an increasing awareness of patient radiation exposure have triggered a rapid development of novel cardiac SPECT technology in recent years. The goal is to establish systems with higher sensitivity and resolution, and with the potential to provide faster acquisition protocols or imaging with lower radiation dose. Those goals have been achieved by various measures. On the one hand, several manufacturers have integrated novel semiconductor detector materials, such as cadmium-zinc-telluride (CZT), together with innovative collimators, into dedicated cardiac scanners [107]. On the other hand, new collimators and reconstruction algorithms have led to increased speed and accuracy of conventional gamma cameras [108]. Imaging times now can be reduced to as much as 10% of that of previous standard protocols, and/or injected activity can be reduced. This is achieved without loss of diagnostic accuracy. These novel developments are still in an early phase of clinical implementation. Yet, first multi-centre trials have shown that test results using ultra-fast acquisition protocols are at least of equal quality when compared to standard gamma camera acquisitions [109]. The potential of these novel systems for a profound change of the clinical practice of radionuclide myocardial perfusion imaging is obvious. Some of these new systems are

even suited for dynamic applications, which may facilitate measurements of CFR. It is expected that SPECT nuclear cardiology procedures with these novel techniques will be faster and more accurate, while radiotracer dose and thus radiation exposure can be reduced (Fig. 2.13).

Reduction of radiation dose

The success and high frequency of non-invasive testing in coronary artery disease have contributed to an increasingly critical perception of radiation exposure from nuclear cardiology [110]. Given the growing emphasis of radiation-induced risk, cardiovascular imaging must adapt and be a forerunner in addressing concerns. Methodological advances in myocardial perfusion SPECT and PET have enabled a significant reduction of radiation exposure, while at the same time allowing for maximization of information content of a single test.

Increased gamma camera sensitivity through resolution recovery reconstruction algorithms, new solid state detector materials, and novel camera designs allow for a significant reduction of injected radiotracer dose, which in turn reduces radiation exposure to the patient proportionally [111]. When combining such novel technology with a stress-only imaging approach, where the stress study is performed first and rest studies are only acquired if stress perfusion is abnormal, then the average injected dose per patient can be reduced to less than 20% of previous standard protocols.

Likewise, PET as an advanced methodology that uses shorter lived radiotracers, and thus results in lower radiation exposure when compared to SPECT, is increasingly available for clinical application. A switch from SPECT to PET is resulting in reduced radiation exposure by itself, but on top of that, PET scanners have also improved. Today, PET-scanner sensitivity is maximized by 3D acquisition, extended field of view, and novel reconstruction algorithms correcting for loss of resolution at the edge of the field of view [112]. Like in SPECT, these technical innovations allow for reduction of injected dose without loss of image quality and thus enable reduction of radiation exposure.

PET MR

Magnetic resonance imaging (MRI) appears to have a great potential for replacing CT in hybrid tomographs in cardiac indications,

Fig. 2.13 (a) Configuration of a new, dedicated cardiac SPECT system. Small solid-state detectors are focused on the heart and positioned in a semicircle, enabling imaging of multiple projections without camera motion. (b) Representative tomographic images and polar maps of a healthy subject imaged on a novel dedicated fast camera system equipped with cadmium-zinc-telluride (CZT) detectors (top, 3 min acquisition time), compared to regular SPECT of the same patient (bottom, 20 min acquisition).

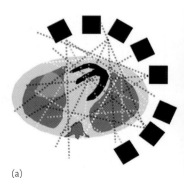
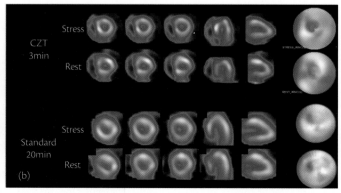

where MRI may have certain benefits over CT such as superior soft tissue contrast and lack of radiation exposure when compared to CT as the adjunct to PET in a hybrid device. Technical challenges exist because phototubes are sensitive even to low magnetic field [113], and new approaches are required for a MRI-based attenuation correction [114]. The integration of MBF or 18-FDG PET measurement with structural and functional MR parameters, such as the contractile response on dobutamine or the transmural extension of late gadolinium enhancement, might help to improve the prediction of recovery of dysfunctional segments after revascularization [115].

Molecular imaging

The tracer principle—the attachment of a radioisotope to a biomolecule in order to follow its distribution throughout the body—is attractive not only for imaging of physiologic mechanisms such as perfusion or contractile function. It is especially suitable for non-invasive detection of biologic processes at the level of tissue and cells [4, 116–118]. Myocardial metabolism and sympathetic innervation have emerged as the first applications of clinical biologic/molecular cardiac radionuclide imaging. The FDA-approved glucose analogue F-18 fluorodeoxyglucose (FDG) is not only used for myocardial viability assessment, but has more recently proven to be versatile and has been successfully utilized for imaging of atherosclerotic plaque and post-infarct inflammation, and labelling of stem cells for tracking after transplantation. Another FDG application may be ischaemic memory imaging, where, more recently, fatty acid analogues such as I-123 BMIPP have also been introduced [4, 116]. For innervation imaging, the integrity of presynaptic sympathetic nerve terminals is measured using catecholamine analogues such as the recently FDA-approved I-123 metaiodobenzylguanidine (MIBG), or several available PET compounds [119]. Risk stratification in heart failure has emerged as a promising application for innervation imaging, where the degree of impaired innervation may provide more accurate information than conventional markers. Additionally, a broad spectrum of other tracers for specific biologic targets in the cardiovascular system is being evaluated on the preclinical level. These targets include various receptors, the renin–angiotensin system, integrins, matrix metalloproteinases, cell death, reporter genes, and transplanted stem cells [4, 116, 118]. The goal is a visualization of key mechanisms involved in subjects of ongoing basic cardiovascular science, including early disease development and novel therapeutic interventions. It is expected that molecular imaging, early disease detection, and molecular therapy will progress hand in hand from the preclinical to the clinical level in the future. Radionuclides are likely to play a key role in this paradigm.

Conclusion

Radionuclide imaging techniques are well established for imaging of myocardial function, perfusion, viability, and biologic mechanisms. While SPECT is the clinical workhorse for the workup of CAD, PET is an advanced technique that is utilized to obtain quantitative, more specific insights into disease mechanisms. Advances in imaging methodology aim at more rapid, more accurate acquisition and radiation dose reduction. Additionally, the advent of various molecular-targeted probes is expected to result in novel clinical applications of nuclear cardiology in the future.

References

1. Marcassa C, Bax JJ, Bengel F, Hesse B, Petersen CL, Reyes E, et al. Clinical value, cost-effectiveness, and safety of myocardial perfusion scintigraphy: a position statement. *Eur Heart J* 2008; 29(4): 557–63.
2. Le Guludec D, Lautamaki R, Knuuti J, Bax JJ, Bengel FM. Present and future of clinical cardiovascular PET imaging in Europe-a position statement by the European Council of Nuclear Cardiology (ECNC). *Eur J Nucl Med Mol Imaging* 2008; 35: 1709–24.
3. Garcia EV. Physical attributes, limitations, and future potential for PET and SPECT. *J Nucl Cardiol* 2012; 19 Suppl 1: S19–29. Epub 2011/12/ 14.
4. Higuchi T, Bengel FM. Cardiovascular nuclear imaging: from perfusion to molecular function: non-invasive imaging. *Heart* 2008; 94(6): 809–16.
5. Segall GM, Davis MJ. Prone versus supine thallium myocardial SPECT: a method to decrease artefactual inferior wall defects. *J Nucl Med* 1989; 30(4): 548–55.
6. Ficaro EP, Lee BC, Kritzman JN, Corbett JR. Corridor4DM: the Michigan method for quantitative nuclear cardiology. *J Nucl Cardiol* 2007; 14(4): 455–65.
7. Klein JL, Garcia EV, DePuey EG, Campbell J, Taylor AT, Pettigrew RI, et al. Reversibility bull's-eye: a new polar bull's-eye map to quantify reversibility of stress-induced SPECT thallium-201 myocardial perfusion defects. *J Nucl Med* 1990; 31(7): 1240–6.
8. Nekolla SG, Miethaner C, Nguyen N, Ziegler SI, Schwaiger M. Reproducibility of polar map generation and assessment of defect severity and extent assessment in myocardial perfusion imaging using positron emission tomography. *Eur J Nucl Med* 1998; 25(9): 1313–21.
9. Slomka PJ, Nishina H, Berman DS, Akincioglu C, Abidov A, Friedman JD, et al. Automated quantification of myocardial perfusion SPECT using simplified normal limits. *J Nucl Cardiol* 2005; 12(1): 66–77.
10. Germano G, Kiat H, Kavanagh PB, Moriel M, Mazzanti M, Su HT, et al. Automatic quantification of ejection fraction from gated myocardial perfusion SPECT. *J Nucl Med* 1995; 36(11): 2138–47.
11. Choi JY, Lee KH, Kim SJ, Kim SE, Kim BT, Lee SH, et al. Gating provides improved accuracy for differentiating artefacts from true lesions in equivocal fixed defects on technetium 99m tetrofosmin perfusion SPECT. *J Nucl Cardiol* 1998; 5(4): 395–401.
12. Johnson LL, Verdesca SA, Aude WY, Xavier RC, Nott LT, Campanella MW, et al. Postischaemic stunning can affect left ventricular ejection fraction and regional wall motion on post-stress gated sestamibi tomograms. *J Am Coll Cardiol* 1997; 30(7): 1641–8.
13. Corbett JR, Ficaro EP. Clinical review of attenuation-corrected cardiac SPECT. *J Nucl Cardiol.* 1999; 6(1 Pt 1): 54–68.
14. Bateman TM, Cullom SJ. Attenuation correction single-photon emission computed tomography myocardial perfusion imaging. *Semin Nucl Med* 2005; 35(1): 37–51.

15. Hendel RC, Berman DS, Cullom SJ, Follansbee W, Heller GV, Kiat H, et al. Multicenter clinical trial to evaluate the efficacy of correction for photon attenuation and scatter in SPECT myocardial perfusion imaging. *Circulation* 1999; 99(21): 2742–9.

16. Tonge CM, Manoharan M, Lawson RS, Shields RA, Prescott MC. Attenuation correction of myocardial SPECT studies using low resolution computed tomography images. *Nucl Med Commun* 2005; 26(3): 231–7.

17. Hesse B, Tagil K, Cuocolo A, Anagnostopoulos C, Bardies M, Bax J, et al. EANM/ESC procedural guidelines for myocardial perfusion imaging in nuclear cardiology. *Eur J Nucl Med Mol Imaging* 2005; 32(7): 855–97.

18. Cranley K, Millar R, Bell T. Correction for deadtime losses in a gamma camera data analysis system. *Eur J Nucl Med* 1980; 5: 377–82.

19. Daube-Witherspoon ME, Carson RE. Unified deadtime correction model for PET. IEEE *Trans Med Imag* 1991; 10(3): 267–75.

20. deKemp RA, Nahmias C. Attenuation correction in PET using single photon transmission measurement. *Med Phys* 1994; 21(6): 771–8.

21. Karp JS, Muehllehner G, Qu H, Yan XH. Singles transmission in volume-imaging PET with a 137Cs source. *Phys Med Biol* 1995; 40(5): 929–44.

22. Yu SK, Nahmias C. Single-photon transmission measurements in positron tomography using 137Cs. *Phys Med Biol* 1995; 40(7): 1255–66.

23. Burger C, Goerres G, Schoenes S, Buck A, Lonn AH, Von Schulthess GK. PET attenuation coefficients from CT images: experimental evaluation of the transformation of CT into PET 511-keV attenuation coefficients. *Eur J Nucl Med Mol Imaging* 2002; 29(7): 922–7.

24. Goetze S, Brown TL, Lavely WC, Zhang Z, Bengel FM. Attenuation correction in myocardial perfusion SPECT/CT: effects of misregistration and value of reregistration. *J Nucl Med* 2007; 48(7): 1090–5.

25. Lautamaki R, Brown TL, Merrill J, Bengel FM. CT-based attenuation correction in (82)Rb-myocardial perfusion PET-CT: incidence of misalignment and effect on regional tracer distribution. *Eur J Nucl Med Mol Imaging.* 2008; 35(2): 305–10.

26. Fayad HJ, Lamare F, Le Rest CC, Bettinardi V, Visvikis D. Generation of 4-dimensional CT images based on 4-dimensional PET-derived motion fields. *J Nucl Med* 2013; 54(4): 631–8. Epub 2013/03/ 09.

27. Ollinger JM. A model-based scatter correction for fully 3D PET. *Phys Med Biol* 1996; 41(1): 153–76.

28. Watson CC, Newport D, Casey ME. The Effect of Energy Threshold on Image Variance in Fully 3D PET. In: *Three-dimensional Image Reconstruction in Radiology and Nuclear Medicine.* In: Grangeat P, Amans JL, editors. Dordrecht, Kluwer Academic; 1996, pp. 255–68.

29. van Velden FH, Kloet RW, van Berckel BN, Lammertsma AA, Boellaard R. Accuracy of 3-dimensional reconstruction algorithms for the high-resolution research tomograph. *J Nucl Med* 2009; 50(1): 72–80. Epub 2008/12/19.

30. Dyson NA. The annihilation coincidence method of localizing positron-emitting isotopes, and a comparison with parallel counting. *Phys Med Biol* 1960; 4: 376–90.

31. Dawood M, Kösters T, Fieseler M, Büther F, Jiang X, Wübbeling F, Schäfers KP. Motion correction in respiratory gated cardiac PET/CT using multi-scale optical flow. *Med Image Comput Comput Assist Interv.* 2008;11(Pt 2):155–62.

32. Lamare F, Teras M, Kokki T, Fayad H, Knuuti J, Visvikis D. Correction of respiratory motion in dual gated PET cardiac imaging. *J Nucl Med* 2008; 49 (Suppl 1): 389P.

33. Boussion N, Hatt M, Lamare F, Rest CC, Visvikis D. Contrast enhancement in emission tomography by way of synergistic PET/CT image combination. *Computer Methods & Programs in Biomedicine* 2008; 90(3): 191–201.

34. Hesse B, Lindhardt TB, Acampa W, Anagnostopoulos C, Ballinger J, Bax JJ, et al. EANM/ESC guidelines for radionuclide imaging of cardiac function. *Eur J Nucl Med Mol Imaging* 2008; 35(4): 851–85.

35. Takahashi N, Reinhardt CP, Marcel R, Leppo JA. Myocardial uptake of 99mTc-tetrofosmin, sestamibi, and 201Tl in a model of acute coronary reperfusion. *Circulation* 1996; 94(10): 2605–13.

36. Beanlands RS, Dawood F, Wen WH, McLaughlin PR, Butany J, D'Amati G, et al. Are the kinetics of technetium-99m methoxyisobutyl isonitrile affected by cell metabolism and viability? *Circulation* 1990; 82(5): 1802–14.

37. Meerdink DJ, Leppo JA. Comparison of hypoxia and ouabain effects on the myocardial uptake kinetics of technetium-99m hexakis 2-methoxyisobutyl isonitrile and thallium-201. *J Nucl Med* 1989; 30(9): 1500–6.

38. Jain D, Wackers FJ, Mattera J, McMahon M, Sinusas AJ, Zaret BL. Biokinetics of technetium-99m-tetrofosmin: myocardial perfusion imaging agent: implications for a one-day imaging protocol. *J Nucl Med* 1993; 34(8): 1254–9.

39. Munch G, Neverve J, Matsunari I, Schroter G, Schwaiger M. Myocardial technetium-99m-tetrofosmin and technetium-99m-sestamibi kinetics in normal subjects and patients with coronary artery disease. *J Nucl Med* 1997; 38(3): 428–32.

40. Berman DS, Kiat HS, Van Train KF, Germano G, Maddahi J, Friedman JD. Myocardial perfusion imaging with technetium-99m-sestamibi: comparative analysis of available imaging protocols. *J Nucl Med* 1994; 35(4): 681–8.

41. Heo J, Kegel J, Iskandrian AS, Cave V, Iskandrian BB. Comparison of same-day protocols using technetium-99m-sestamibi myocardial imaging. *J Nucl Med* 1992; 33(2): 186–91.

42. Sciagra R, Bisi G, Santoro GM, Rossi V, Fazzini PF. Nitrate versus rest myocardial scintigraphy with technetium 99m-sestamibi: relationship of tracer uptake to regional left ventricular function and its significance in the detection of viable hibernating myocardium. *Am J Card Imaging* 1995; 9(3): 157–66.

43. Sharir T, Germano G, Kang X, Lewin HC, Miranda R, Cohen I, et al. Prediction of myocardial infarction versus cardiac death by gated myocardial perfusion SPECT: risk stratification by the amount of stress-induced ischaemia and the poststress ejection fraction. *J Nucl Med* 2001; 42(6): 831–7.

44. Klocke FJ, Baird MG, Lorell BH, Bateman TM, Messer JV, Berman DS, et al. ACC/AHA/ASNC guidelines for the clinical use of cardiac radionuclide imaging—executive summary: a report of the American College of Cardiology/American Heart Association Task Force on Practice Guidelines (ACC/AHA/ASNC Committee to Revise the 1995 Guidelines for the Clinical Use of Cardiac Radionuclide Imaging). *Circulation* 2003; 108(11): 1404–18.

45. Nichols K, DePuey EG, Gooneratne N, Salensky H, Friedman M, Cochoff S. First-pass ventricular ejection fraction using a single-crystal nuclear camera. *J Nucl Med* 1994; 35(8): 1292–300.

46. Daou D, Van Kriekinge SD, Coaguila C, Lebtahi R, Fourme T, Sitbon O, et al. Automatic quantification of right ventricular function with gated blood pool SPECT. *J Nucl Cardiol.* 2004; 11(3): 293–304.

47. Germano G, Berman DS. On the accuracy and reproducibility of quantitative gated myocardial perfusion SPECT. *J Nucl Med* 1999; 40(5): 810–3.

48. Araujo LI, Lammertsma AA, Rhodes CG, McFalls EO, Iida H, Rechavia E, et al. Non-invasive quantification of regional myocardial blood flow in coronary artery disease with oxygen-15-labelled carbon dioxide inhalation and positron emission tomography. *Circulation* 1991; 83(3): 875–85.

49. Bergmann SR, Herrero P, Markham J, Weinheimer CJ, Walsh MN. Non-invasive quantitation of myocardial blood flow in human subjects with oxygen-15-labelled water and positron emission tomography. *J Am Coll Cardiol* 1989; 14(3): 639–52.

50. Schelbert HR, Phelps ME, Hoffman EJ, Huang SC, Selin CE, Kuhl DE. Regional myocardial perfusion assessed with N-13 labelled ammonia

and positron emission computerized axial tomography. *Am J Cardiol* 1979; 43(2): 209–18.

51. Hutchins GD, Schwaiger M, Rosenspire KC, Krivokapich J, Schelbert H, Kuhl DE. Non-invasive quantification of regional blood flow in the human heart using N-13 ammonia and dynamic positron emission tomographic imaging. *J Am Coll Cardiol* 1990; 15(5): 1032–42.

52. Herrero P, Markham J, Shelton ME, Weinheimer CJ, Bergmann SR. Non-invasive quantification of regional myocardial perfusion with rubidium-82 and positron emission tomography. Exploration of a mathematical model. *Circulation* 1990; 82(4): 1377–86.

53. Nekolla SG, Reder S, Saraste A, Higuchi T, Dzewas G, Preissel A, et al. Evaluation of the novel myocardial perfusion positron-emission tomography tracer 18F-BMS-747158-02: comparison to 13N-ammonia and validation with microspheres in a pig model. *Circulation* 2009; 119(17): 2333–42. Epub 2009/04/ 22.

54. Maddahi J, Czernin J, Lazewatsky J, Huang SC, Dahlbom M, Schelbert H, et al. Phase I, first-in-human study of BMS747158, a novel 18F-labelled tracer for myocardial perfusion PET: dosimetry, biodistribution, safety, and imaging characteristics after a single injection at rest. *J Nucl Med* 2011; 52(9): 1490–8. Epub 2011/08/19.

55. Berman DS, Maddahi J, Tamarappoo BK, Czernin J, Taillefer R, Udelson JE, et al. Phase II safety and clinical comparison with single-photon emission computed tomography myocardial perfusion imaging for detection of coronary artery disease: flurpiridaz F 18 positron emission tomography. *J Am Coll Cardiol* 2013; 61(4): 469–77. Epub 2012/12/ 26.

56. Anagnostopoulos C, Almonacid A, El Fakhri G, Curillova Z, Sitek A, Roughton M, et al. Quantitative relationship between coronary vasodilator reserve assessed by 82Rb PET imaging and coronary artery stenosis severity. *Eur J Nucl Med Mol Imaging.* 2008; 35(9): 1593–601.

57. Lortie M, Beanlands RS, Yoshinaga K, Klein R, Dasilva JN, DeKemp RA. Quantification of myocardial blood flow with 82Rb dynamic PET imaging. *Eur J Nucl Med Mol Imaging.* 2007; 34(11): 1765–74.

58. Lautamaki R, George RT, Kitagawa K, Higuchi T, Merrill J, Voicu C, et al. Rubidium-82 PET-CT for quantitative assessment of myocardial blood flow: validation in a canine model of coronary artery stenosis. *Eur J Nucl Med Mol Imaging.* 2009; 36(4): 576–86. Epub 2008/11/06.

59. Huang SC, Williams BA, Krivokapich J, Araujo L, Phelps ME, Schelbert HR. Rabbit myocardial 82Rb kinetics and a compartmental model for blood flow estimation. *Am J Physiol.* 1989; 256(4 Pt 2): H1156–64.

60. Araujo L, Schelbert HR. Dynamic positron emission tomography in ischaemic heart disease. *Am J Cardiac Imag* 1984; 1: 117–24.

61. Dorbala S, Di Carli MF, Beanlands RS, Merhige ME, Williams BA, Veledar E, et al. Prognostic value of stress myocardial perfusion positron emission tomography: results from a multicenter observational registry. *J Am Coll Cardiol* 2013; 61(2): 176–84. Epub 2012/12/12.

62. Murthy VL, Naya M, Foster CR, Hainer J, Gaber M, Di Carli G, et al. Improved cardiac risk assessment with non-invasive measures of coronary flow reserve. *Circulation* 2011; 124(20): 2215–24. Epub 2011/10/19.

63. Shah A, Schelbert HR, Schwaiger M, Henze E, Hansen H, Selin C, et al. Measurement of regional myocardial blood flow with N-13 ammonia and positron-emission tomography in intact dogs. *J Am Coll Cardiol* 1985; 5(1): 92–100.

64. Schaefers K, Spinks TJ, Camici PG, Bloomfield PM, Rhodes CG, Law MP, Baker CS, Rimoldi O Absolute quantification of myocardial blood flow with $H_2^{15}O$ and 3-dimensional PET: an experimental validation. *J Nucl Med* 2002; 43(8):1031–40.

65. Kaufmann PA, Gnecchi-Ruscone T, Yap JT, Rimoldi O, Camici PG. Assessment of the reproducibility of baseline and hyperemic myocardial blood flow measurements with 15O-labelled water and PET. *J Nucl Med* 1999; 40(11): 1848–56.

66. Uren NG, Camici PG, Melin JA, Bol A, de Bruyne B, Radvan J, et al. Effect of aging on myocardial perfusion reserve. *J Nucl Med* 1995; 36(11): 2032–6.

67. Chareonthaitawee P, Kaufmann PA, Rimoldi O, Camici PG. Heterogeneity of resting and hyperemic myocardial blood flow in healthy humans. *Cardiovasc Res* 2001; 50(1): 151–61.

68. Lorenzoni R, Rosen SD, Camici PG. Effect of alpha 1-adrenoceptor blockade on resting and hyperemic myocardial blood flow in normal humans. *Am J Physiol* 1996; 271(4 Pt 2): H1302–6.

69. Kaufmann PA, Gnecchi-Ruscone T, di Terlizzi M, Schafers KP, Luscher TF, Camici PG. Coronary heart disease in smokers: vitamin C restores coronary microcirculatory function.[see comment]. *Circulation* 2000; 102(11): 1233–8.

70. Kaufmann PA, Gnecchi-Ruscone T, Schafers KP, Luscher TF, Camici PG. Low density lipoprotein cholesterol and coronary microvascular dysfunction in hypercholesterolemia. *J Am Coll Cardiol* 2000; 36(1): 103–9.

71. Sdringola S, Patel D, Gould KL. High prevalence of myocardial perfusion abnormalities on positron emission tomography in asymptomatic persons with a parent or sibling with coronary artery disease. *Circulation* 2001; 103(4): 496–501.

72. Momose M, Abletshauser C, Neverve J, Nekolla SG, Schnell O, Standl E, et al. Dysregulation of coronary microvascular reactivity in asymptomatic patients with type 2 diabetes mellitus. *Eur J Nucl Med Mol Imaging.* 2002; 29(12): 1675–9.

73. Uren NG, Melin JA, De Bruyne B, Wijns W, Baudhuin T, Camici PG. Relation between myocardial blood flow and the severity of coronary-artery stenosis. *N Engl J Med* 1994; 330(25): 1782–8.

74. Herzog BA, Husmann L, Valenta I, Gaemperli O, Siegrist PT, Tay FM, et al. Long-term prognostic value of 13N-ammonia myocardial perfusion positron emission tomography added value of coronary flow reserve. *J Am Coll Cardiol* 2009; 54(2): 150–6. Epub 2009/07/ 04.

75. Danad I, Raijmakers PG, Appelman YE, Harms HJ, de Haan S, van den Oever ML, et al. Hybrid imaging using quantitative H215O PET and CT-based coronary angiography for the detection of coronary artery disease. *J Nucl Med* 2013; 54(1): 55–63. Epub 2012/12/13.

76. Rimoldi O, Schafers KP, Boellaard R, Turkheimer F, Stegger L, Law MP, et al. Quantification of subendocardial and subepicardial blood flow using 15O-labelled water and PET: experimental validation. *J Nucl Med* 2006; 47(1): 163–72. Epub 2006/01/05.

77. Rajappan K, Rimoldi OE, Dutka DP, Ariff B, Pennell DJ, Sheridan DJ, et al. Mechanisms of coronary microcirculatory dysfunction in patients with aortic stenosis and angiographically normal coronary arteries. *Circulation* 2002; 105(4): 470–6. Epub 2002/01/ 30.

78. Camici PG, Ferrannini E, Opie LH. Myocardial metabolism in ischaemic heart disease: basic principles and applications to imaging by positron tomography. *Prog Cardiovasc Dis* 1989; 32: 217–38.

79. Camici PG, Marraccini P, Marzilli M. Coronary haemodynamics and myocardial metabolism during and after pacing stress in normal humans. *Am J Physiol* 1989; 257: E309–E17.

80. Schelbert HR, Henze E, Schon HR. C-11 palmitic acid for the non-invasive evaluation of regional myocardial fatty acid metabolism with positron computed tomography. IV. In vivo demonstration of impaired fatty acid oxidation in acute myocardial ischaemia. *Am Heart J* 1983; 106: 736–50.

81. Buxton DB, Schwaiger M, Nguyen A, Phelps M, Schelbert HR. Radiolabelled acetate as a tracer of myocardial tricarboxylic acid cycle flux. *Circ Res* 1988; 63: 628–34.

82. Armbrecht JJ, Buxton DB, Schelbert HR. Validation of [1-¹¹C]acetate as a tracer for non-invasive assessment of oxidative metabolism with positron emission tomography in normal, ischaemic, postischaemic and hyperaemic canine myocardium. *Circulation* 1990; 81: 1594–605.

83. Buxton DB, Nienaber CA, Luxen A. Non-invasive quantitation of regional myocardial oxygen consumption in vivo with [1-¹¹C]acetate and dynamic positron emission tomography. *Circulation* 1989; 79: 134–42.

84. Bing RJ. *The Metabolism of the Heart*. Harvey Lecture Series 50. Orlando, FL/New York: Academic Press; 1954, pp. 22–70.

85. Armbrecht JJ, Buxton DB, Brunken R, Phelps M, Schelbert HR. Regional myocardial oxygen consumption determined non-invasively in humans with [1-¹¹C] acetate and dynamic positron tomography. *Circulation* 1989; 80: 863–72.

86. Walsh MN, Geltman EM, Brown MA. Non-invasive estimation of regional myocardial oxygen consumption by positron emission tomography with carbon-11 acetate in patients with myocardial infarction. *J Nucl Med* 1989; 30: 1798–808.

87. Gallagher BM, Fowler JS, Gutterson NI, MacGregor RR, Wan C-N., Wolf AP. Metabolic trapping as a principle of radiopharmaceutical design: some factors responsible for the biodistribution of [¹⁸F]2-deoxy-2-fluoro-D-glucose. *J Nucl Med* 1978; 19: 1154–61.

88. Huang SC, Phelps ME. Principles of tracer kinetic modelling in positron emission tomography and autoradiography. In: Phelps ME, Mazziotta JC, Schelbert HR, editors. *Positron Emission Tomography and Autoradiography Principles and Applications for the Brain and Heart*. New York: Raven; 1986, pp. 287–346.

89. Botker HE, Bottcher M, Schmitz O, Gee A, Hansen SB, Cold GE, et al. Glucose uptake and lumped constant variability in normal human hearts determined with [18F]fluorodeoxyglucose. *J Nucl Cardiol*. 1997; 4: 125–32.

90. Ferrannini E, Santoro D, Bonadonna R, Natali A, Parodi O, Camici PG. Metabolic and hemodynamic effects of insulin on human hearts. *Am J Physiol* 1993; 264(2 Pt 1): E308–15.

91. Ghosh N, Rimoldi OE, Beanlands RS, Camici PG. Assessment of myocardial ischaemia and viability: role of positron emission tomography. *Eur Heart J* 2010; 31(24): 2984–95. Epub 2010/10/ 23.

92. Goldstein DS, Chang PC, Eisenhofer G, Miletich R, Finn R, Bacher J, et al. Positron emission tomographic imaging of cardiac sympathetic innervation and function. *Circulation* 1990; 81(5): 1606–21.

93. Wieland DM, Rosenspire KC, Hutchins GD, Van Dort M, Rothley JM, Mislankar SG, et al. Neuronal mapping of the heart with 6-[18F]fluorometaraminol. *J Med Chem* 1990; 33(3): 956–64.

94. Schwaiger M, Kalff V, Rosenspire K, Haka MS, Molina E, Hutchins GD, et al. Non-invasive evaluation of sympathetic nervous system in human heart by positron emission tomography [see comment]. *Circulation* 1990; 82(2): 457–64.

95. Munch G, Nguyen NTB, Nekolla SG, Ziegler S, Muzik O, Chakraborty P, et al. Evaluation of sympathetic nerve terminals with [¹¹C]epinephrine and [¹¹C]hydroxyephedrine and positron emission tomography. *Circulation* 2000; 101: 516–23.

96. Yu M, Bozek J, Lamoy M, Kagan M, Benites P, Onthank D, et al. LMI1195 PET imaging in evaluation of regional cardiac sympathetic denervation and its potential role in antiarrhythmic drug treatment. *Eur J Nucl Med Mol Imaging* 2012; 39(12): 1910–9. Epub 2012/08/ 07.

97. Syrota A. Positron emission tomography: evaluation of cardiac receptors. In: Marcus ML, Schelbert HR, Skorton DJ, Wolf GL, editors. *Cardiac Imaging a Companion to Braunwald's Heart Disease*. Philadelphia: W B Saunders; 1991, pp. 1256–70.

98. Staehelin M, Hertel C. [3H]CGP-12177, a beta-adrenergic ligand suitable for measuring cell surface receptors. *J Recept Res* 1983; 3(1–2): 35–43.

99. Lefroy DC, de Silva R, Choudhury L, Uren NG, Crake T, Rhodes CG, et al. Diffuse reduction of myocardial beta-adrenoceptors in hypertrophic cardiomyopathy: a study with positron emission tomography. *J Am Coll Cardiol* 1993; 22(6): 1653–60.

100. Schafers M, Dutka D, Rhodes CG, Lammertsma AA, Hermansen F, Schober O, et al. Myocardial presynaptic and postsynaptic autonomic dysfunction in hypertrophic cardiomyopathy. *Circ Res* 1998; 82(1): 57–62.

101. Bristow MR, Ginsburg R, Minobe W, Cubicciotti RS, Sageman WS, Lurie K, et al. Decreased catecholamine sensitivity and beta-adrenergic-receptor density in failing human hearts. *N Engl J Med* 1982; 307(4): 205–11.

102. Esler M, Kaye D, Lambert G, Esler D, Jennings G. Adrenergic nervous system in heart failure. *Am J Cardiol* 1997; 80(11A): 7L–14L.

103. Merlet P, Delforge J, Syrota A, Angevin E, Maziere B, Crouzel C, et al. Positron emission tomography with 11C CGP-12177 to assess beta-adrenergic receptor concentration in idiopathic dilated cardiomyopathy. *Circulation* 1993; 87(4): 1169–78.

104. Delforge J, Janier M, Syrota A, Crouzel C, Vallois JM, Cayla J, et al. Non-invasive quantification of muscarinic receptors in vivo with positron emission tomography in the dog heart. *Circulation* 1990; 82(4): 1494–504.

105. Le Guludec D, Cohen-Solal A, Delforge J, Delahaye N, Syrota A, Merlet P. Increased myocardial muscarinic receptor density in idiopathic dilated cardiomyopathy: an in vivo PET study. *Circulation* 1997; 96(10): 3416–22.

106. Le Guludec D, Delforge J, Syrota A, Desruennes M, Valette H, Gandjbakhch I, et al. In vivo quantification of myocardial muscarinic receptors in heart transplant patients. *Circulation* 1994; 90(1): 172–8.

107. Garcia EV, Faber TL. New trends in camera and software technology in nuclear cardiology. *Cardiol Clin* 2009; 27(2): 227–36.

108. Patton JA, Slomka PJ, Germano G, Berman DS. Recent technologic advances in nuclear cardiology. *J Nucl Cardiol*. 2007; 14(4): 501–13.

109. Sharir T, Slomka PJ, Hayes SW, DiCarli MF, Ziffer JA, Martin WH, et al. Multicenter trial of high-speed versus conventional single-photon emission computed tomography imaging: quantitative results of myocardial perfusion and left ventricular function. *J Am Coll Cardiol* 2010; 55(18): 1965–74. Epub 2010/05/01.

110. Einstein AJ, Moser KW, Thompson RC, Cerqueira MD, Henzlova MJ. Radiation dose to patients from cardiac diagnostic imaging. *Circulation* 2007; 116(11): 1290–305. Epub 2007/09/12.

111. Slomka PJ, Dey D, Duvall WL, Henzlova MJ, Berman DS, Germano G. Advances in nuclear cardiac instrumentation with a view towards reduced radiation exposure. *Current Cardiology Reports* 2012; 14(2): 208–16. Epub 2012/02/14.

112. Bengel FM, Higuchi T, Javadi MS, Lautamaki R. Cardiac positron emission tomography. *J Am Coll Cardiol* 2009; 54(1): 1–15. Epub 2009/06/27.

113. Hofmann M, Steinke F, Scheel V, Charpiat G, Farquhar J, Aschoff P, et al. MRI-based attenuation correction for PET/MRI: a novel approach combining pattern recognition and atlas registration. *J Nucl Med* 2008; 49(11): 1875–83. Epub 2008/10/18.

114. Hofmann M, Pichler B, Scholkopf B, Beyer T. Towards quantitative PET/MRI: a review of MR-based attenuation correction techniques. *Eur J Nucl Med Mol Imaging* 2009; 36 Suppl 1: S93–104. Epub 2008/12/24.

115. Schmidt M, Voth E, Schneider CA, Theissen P, Wagner R, Baer FM, et al. F-18-FDG uptake is a reliable predictory of functional recovery of akinetic but viable infarct regions as defined by magnetic resonance imaging before and after revascularization. *Magn Reson Imaging* 2004; 22(2): 229–36. Epub 2004/03/11.

116. Knuuti J, Bengel FM. Positron emission tomography and molecular imaging. *Heart* 2008; 94(3): 360–7.

117. Schwaiger M, Bengel FM. From thallium scan to molecular imaging. *Mol Imaging Biol* 2002; 4 (6): 387–98.

118. Wu JC, Bengel FM, Gambhir SS. Cardiovascular molecular imaging. *Radiology* 2007; 244(2): 337–55.

119. Thackeray JT, Bengel FM. Assessment of cardiac autonomic neuronal function using PET imaging. *J Nucl Cardiol* 2013; 20(1): 150–65. Epub 2012/11/28.

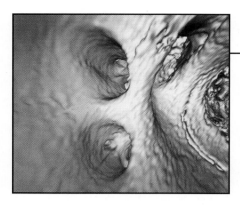

CHAPTER 3

Cardiac CT—basic principles

Filippo Cademartiri, Erica Maffei, Teresa Arcadi, Orlando Catalano, and Gabriel Krestin

Contents

Introduction

Since 2004 multi-detector computed tomography (MDCT) scanners have been available, which enable the simultaneous acquisition of 64 slices per rotation. The additional improvement in number of slices per rotation, spatial and temporal resolution that followed has already provided excellent results in the field of cardiac imaging. Nowadays we further optimize technical aspects that may provide new clinical insight and applications.

Basic cardiac CT technique

The most important components of a CT system are the X-ray tube and the system of detectors (⊃ Fig. 3.1). The combination of a fast rotation time and multi-slice acquisitions is particularly important for cardiac applications [1, 2]. The latest generation of 64-MDCT scanners meets these requirements. They are able to acquire 64 sub-millimetre slices per rotation and routinely achieve excellent image quality and the visualization of small-diameter vessels of the coronary circulation, combining isotropic spatial resolution (0.4 mm³) with gantry rotation speeds of 330 ms. They also redefine the MDCT methodology of analysing coronary plaque and evaluating stent lumens.

Until a few years ago, CT systems had only a single row of detectors, which meant that for each rotation they were able to acquire only one slice. These systems were followed by others known as multi-slice or multi-detector-row, featuring many detector rows positioned in a two-dimensional array. During a rotation, numerous contiguous slices are acquired. As a result, a broader region of the body can be acquired in the same timeframe, with an improvement in image quality. This also has the advantage of drastically reducing examination times, which is an important factor given that thoracic and abdominal examination requires the patient to maintain breath-hold to guarantee that image quality is not compromised by chest motion. The clinical impact of the new technology lies in the improvement in image quality in terms of both spatial and temporal resolution. The improvement in spatial resolution includes numerous features of non-invasive coronary imaging:

◆ it increases the ability to visualize small-diameter vessels (e.g. the distal coronary branches) [3];

◆ it increases the ability to quantify calcium, in that it reduces blooming artefacts;

◆ it enables the reduction of blooming artefacts in stents and therefore enables the visualization of the stent lumen;

◆ it improves the definition of the presence of coronary plaques and better quantifies their characteristics (volume, attenuation, etc.).

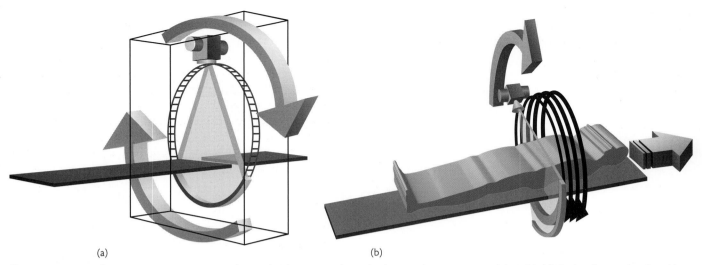

(a)   (b)

Fig 3.1 Geometry of a CT scanner. A CT scanner is designed with an X-ray tube and a detector that rotate around the table (a). During the rotation the table moves in order to generate the volume dataset (b).

The improvement in temporal resolution influences many other aspects of non-invasive coronary imaging:

- it increases the ability to freeze images in the cardiac cycle;
- it enables additional reconstruction windows to be found within the cardiac cycle;
- it increases the performance of the system when left ventricular function needs to be evaluated;
- it reduces scan time.

The technical characteristics of each scanner vary according to the model, and their technological development is ongoing and rapid. The precise temporal resolution of the images obtained by MDCT scanners depends on many factors: gantry rotation speed, size and position of the field of view in the scan volume, and the image reconstruction and post-processing algorithms. In reality, the data acquired at half a rotation of the gantry are enough to reconstruct a single tomographic image with retrospective or prospective ECG control (◑ Fig. 3.2). The temporal resolution of the latest MDCT scanners therefore approximate 165 ms [4–6]. This can be enough to obtain images of the heart during the diastolic phase (when cardiac motion is at a minimum) free of obvious motion artefacts, if the heart rate (HR) is <70 beats per minute.

Definition of CT parameters

A brief list of the main parameters used to create cardiac CT images includes:

- Spatial resolution—the capability to separate two neighbouring points.
- Coverage resolution—the minimum time required to complete a single volumetric acquisition.
- Temporal resolution—the minimum time required to generate one single axial image.
- Contrast resolution—the capability to separate two neighbouring attenuation values (Hounsfield Units) with a given background noise.

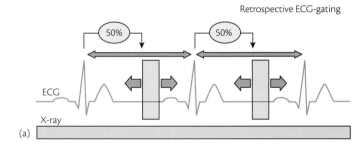

Retrospective ECG-gating

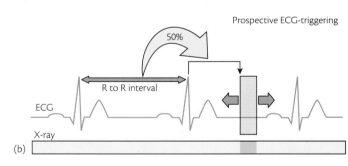

Prospective ECG-triggering

Fig 3.2 Retrospective ECG gating vs. prospective ECG triggering. The two main techniques for cardiac CT ECG synchronization are displayed. In (a) we can observe retrospective ECG gating. It is based on spiral continuous X-ray delivery at low pitch while recording the ECG track. Afterwards the operator is able to arbitrarily decide which phase of the cardiac cycle is worth reconstructing. In (b) we can observe the prospective ECG triggering. It is based on sequential scanning (also called 'step and shoot' mode). Radiation is delivered only within the phase of the cardiac cycle that has been decided prior to the initiation of the scan. It requires very low heart rate and/or very high temporal resolution to guarantee adequate image quality.

- Collimation (i.e. X-ray beam collimation)—the beam width along the longitudinal axis at the scanner iso-centre.
- Pitch (◑ Fig. 3.3)—reflects how wide is the helix created by the rotating gantry and table feed.
- Scan pitch—conventionally defined as beam/volume pitch (table feed/slice collimation) and it is not affected by the number of detectors that characterizes the scanner.

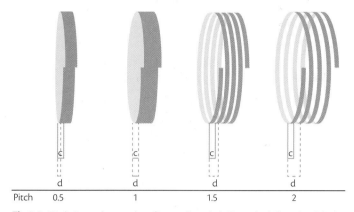

| Pitch | 0.5 | 1 | 1.5 | 2 |

Fig 3.3 Pitch. Several examples of increasing pitch. From the left to the right we can see the unravelling of the helical geometry of volumetric CT acquisition. Abbreviations: c = slice thickness; d = distance between 2 points at 360° rotation.

- Table feed—the speed of a patient's translation along the z-axis. A fast table feed determines a faster scan speed.

- MilliAmpere per second (mAs) of the X-ray beam represents the number of photons that are produced and that actually run through the patient. A higher mAs improves the contrast-to-noise ratio (e.g. image quality).

- KiloVolt (kV) represents the energy of the photons (usually 120–140 kV for cardiac CT). Recently, it has been suggested that MSCT could be performed with a lower patient dose using protocols with 80/100 kV and increasing the mAs. Another recent development in the field of kV concerns the so called 'dual energy' scan mode. In this setting, the energy of the photons is different (usually 80 kV and 120–140 kV) during the scans (by switching intermittently or with dual sources); the result is that it is possible to obtain multi-parametric imaging due to the different absorption properties of iodine, calcium, water, and so forth.

- Effective slice width refers to the thickness in the longitudinal axis from which the image is generated.

- Reconstruction increment—the distance between consecutive reconstructed axial slices. It affects mainly spatial resolution in the longitudinal axis. Reconstruction increment is usually set in order to obtain 50% overlapping slices.

- Field of view (FOV)—the size of the image that is going to be reconstructed.

- Image matrix—the number of pixels that are reconstructed in one image and is generally constant for CT (i.e. 512 × 512 pixels). A small FOV increases in-plane spatial resolution.

- Interpolation—an algorithm by which the software estimates a missing value from known surrounding points. This operation is used for image reconstruction in spiral CT and in three-dimensional reconstruction.

- Kernels—convolution filters that modify the value of a voxel according to the values of the surrounding voxels. Convolution kernels may smoothen or sharpen CT images. Sharp kernels and filters are used to enhance the edges of high-contrast structures (e.g. calcifications and stents).

Patient selection

Inclusion criteria

Normally inclusion criteria for the scan are HR <65 bpm (spontaneous or induced by drugs) and ability to maintain breath-hold for a period compatible with the scan time [2, 3, 7]. Both these criteria are aimed at avoiding motion artefacts. Even though MDCT coronary angiography can be diagnostic with a higher HR, motion artefacts progressively reduce the number of segments that can be correctly visualized [8]. The second criterion aims at avoiding artefacts associated with respiratory motion.

Exclusion criteria

Patients with a HR ≥70 bpm, known allergies to iodinated contrast agent, renal insufficiency (serum creatinine >120 mmol/l), pregnancy, respiratory failure, unstable clinical conditions, and severe heart failure are excluded from the MDCT coronary angiography study.

In case of mild renal failure, the administration of contrast agent may be better tolerated if a smaller amount and an iso-osmolar agent is used and/or if the patient is adequately hydrated prior to contrast agent injection [9].

Scan parameters

The ideal protocol enables high spatial resolution (thin collimation), high temporal resolution (fast gantry rotation), and low radiation dose (prospective modulation of the tube current synchronized to the ECG [10]) compatible with a good signal-to-noise ratio. The main scan parameters for 64-slice CT of the heart are presented in ⊃ Table 3.1.

Regardless of the number of slices used, spatial and temporal resolutions need to be as high as possible, all the while remaining compatible with the other scan parameters. The final objective is to obtain a scan during an easily performed breath-hold. The duration of the scan is essentially linked to the number of slices and the pitch: generally <0.5 and more often <0.3. This allows for the oversampling of data that characterize CT of the heart. Multi-segment reconstructions should be avoided, because there is no evidence to suggest that they are able to compensate for the lack of temporal resolution at higher heart rates.

Retrospective gating

The acquisition of image data in the MDCT coronary angiography scan is continuous during the cardiac cycle, such that the data corresponding to the phase when cardiac motion is at a minimum need to be retrospectively extracted to minimize blurring and motion artefacts (⊃ Figs 3.4 and 3.5) [5, 6]. This process is called *cardiac gating* (⊃ Fig. 3.2). Once the data have been acquired, they can be reconstructed with retrospective gating in any phase of the cardiac cycle by shifting the initial point of the image reconstruction window relative to the R-wave. Therefore, the combination of z-interpolation and cardiac gating enable a stack of parallel tomographic images to be generated that represent the heart in

Table 3.1 Scan and reconstruction parameters with 64-slice CT

Scan	Sensation 64
Detectors	64 (32 × 2)
Collimation	0.6 mm
KiloVolt	120
MilliAmpere/s (range)	900
Rotation time	330 ms
Tube current modulation	Systolic
Effective temporal resolution	165 ms
Maximum temporal resolution	83 ms*
Effective spatial resolution	0.3 × 0.3 × 0.4 mm
Feed/rotation	3.84 mm
Feed/second	11.63 mm
Pitch	0.2
Scan time	12 s
Reconstruction	
Effective slice width	0.6–0.75 mm
Reconstruction increment	0.3–0.4 mm
Temporal windows ('hot spots')	End-diastole/end-systole
FOV	140–180 mm
Convolution filter/Kernel	Medium
Contrast Material	
Synchronization	Test bolus/bolus tracking
Region of interest (ROI)	Ascending aorta
Threshold in the ROI	+ 100 HU
Pre-delay	10 s
Transition time (breath-hold instructions)	4–6 s
CM volume	80–100 ml
CM rate	4–6 ml/s
Administration time	15–20 s
Iodine concentration	350–400 mgI/ml
Bolus chaser	40 ml @ 4–6 ml/s
Venous access	Antecubital
Total administration time	23–28 s

*Multi-segment algorithm.

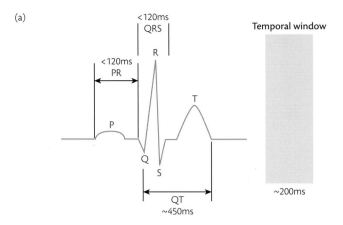

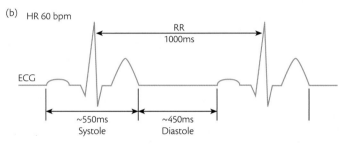

Fig 3.4 Baseline ECG in MDCT coronary angiography. The cardiac cycle is composed of a systole and a diastole. Systole involves contraction of the atria, followed by contraction of the ventricles. The synchronized contraction is guided by a conducting system, which arises from the sinoatrial node in the right atrium. The impulse then propagates to the atrio-ventricular node via the walls of the atria. From the atrio-ventricular node the impulse is transmitted via the conducting system across the septum and the ventricular walls. This phenomenon is depicted by the ECG trace, which shows the typical sequence of waves. (a) P-wave (atrial contraction), QRS complex (ventricular contraction), T-wave (ventricular repolarization). Normally the P–R interval is <120 ms, the QRS complex is <80 ms and the Q–T interval is ~320 ms. Therefore, the duration of a complete systolic contraction with repolarization wave is ~550 ms. The diastolic period is ~450 ms. This means that for a HR of 60 bpm systole and diastole account for 55% and 45% of the cardiac cycle, respectively (b). The ~200-ms windows for the ECG retrospectively gated reconstruction obtainable with MDCT coronary angiography is generally placed in the diastolic phase (a). The most generally favourable position extends from mid- to end-diastole just prior to the P-wave.

the same phase of the cardiac cycle [5, 6]. A real optimization of retrospective gating is yet to be achieved.

To obtain images in the diastolic phase, some operators reconstruct the images in relation to the phase (i.e. a percentage) of the cardiac cycle (typically between 50% and 60% of the R–R interval), whereas others use the time window of the absolute interval prior to the peak of the next R-wave (typically 300–400 ms; ⊃ Fig. 3.6) [11, 12]. Multiple reconstructions are usually performed in different time windows, and the physician/operator successively selects the dataset where motion artefacts are minimal, paying particular attention to the visualization of the right coronary artery [13]. In MDCT coronary angiography, different time windows can be optimized and used in the same patient for the visualization of the left and right coronary arteries [4, 12,

13]. Improving the temporal resolution of the MDCT coronary angiography scan by increasing gantry rotation speed is subject to obvious limitations. To overcome these difficulties new data post-processing strategies have been proposed to further increase temporal resolution. With the simultaneous acquisition of multiple slices using an MDCT coronary angiography scanner and the relative overlapping of the volume acquired, multi-segment reconstructions can be created.

In a multi-segment reconstruction data acquired in the same cardiac phase but from different cardiac cycles are combined in a single image. In this case the temporal resolution will depend on the number and size of the segments used for the creation of a single image, but it will be higher than that derived from a single segment [5]. This technique is sensitive to variations in beat-per-beat HR and the current implementation of these algorithms does not always improve image quality [14].

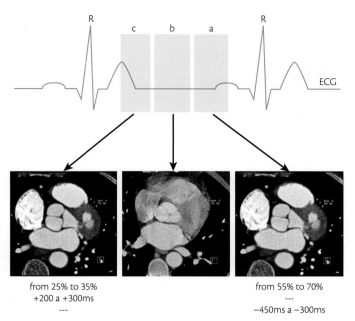

from 25% to 35%   from 55% to 70%
+200 a +300ms   ---

                         −450ms a −300ms

Fig 3.5 Positioning the reconstruction time window. Several principles need to be borne in mind regarding the positioning of the time window when performing image reconstruction in MDCT coronary angiography. The operator should concentrate on three main areas of the ECG trace. The first (a) is the end-diastolic phase. In this phase the ventricle has completed filling, just prior to atrial systole and motion is at a minimum. The second phase (b) is the early-mid diastolic phase. In this phase the heart is filling and there is generally residual motion which does not allow adequate coronary artery imaging. The third phase (c) is end-systole. In this phase the heart is in isovolumetric contraction and motion is at a minimum. The images obtained in this phase can be just as valid as those obtained at end-diastole and in a number of cases even better.

Prospective triggering and radiation dose

The first geometry for ECG synchronization applied to tomographic equipment was prospective ECG triggering. In particular, this technique was applied to an older technology (i.e. electron beam computed tomography) that could rely on a very high temporal resolution in the range of 50–100 ms. This technique suffered from low spatial resolution and the field of application was mainly calcium score. In the last 8 years CT technology has developed newer scanners with newer software and/or very high temporal resolution (i.e. 2nd-generation dual-source CT with 70 ms temporal resolution). New software applications allow prospective scanning using a 'pad' (a temporal window that can be modified according to the operator's experience and the patient's heart rate). Combining these newer technologies with aggressive heart rate control, it is possible to obtain diagnostic image quality with prospective ECG triggering (◒ Fig. 3.2). Due to the improvement of CT hardware and software it has been reported that CT of the coronary arteries can be performed with radiation doses below 1 mSv.

In fact radiation dose has been one, if not the main, issue of cardiac CT since the first reports. The increase in spatial resolution brought an increase in radiation dose. With 64-slice CT and no special means for reduction, the range of dose was between 10 mSv and 25 mSv. The first means to reduce radiation dose was applied to retrospective ECG gating and relied on ECG-controlled

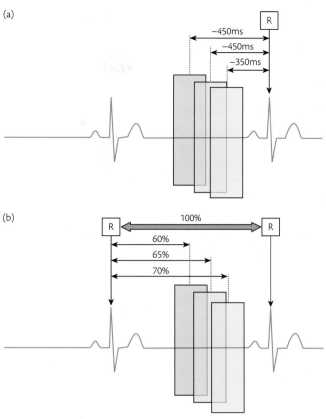

Fig 3.6 End-diastolic positioning of temporal windows. In (a) the temporal windows are positioned in the end-diastolic phase consecutively prior to the next R wave at 50 ms distance each. In (b) the temporal windows are positioned in the end-diastolic phase at 5% R–R interval distance.

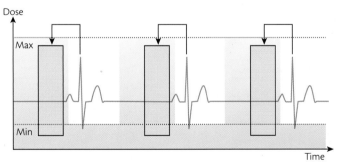

Fig 3.7 Prospective tube current modulation. While the reconstruction can be reliably performed in the end-diastolic phase (especially at low and regular heart rates), tube current can be modulated and reduced to 4–20% of the peak during the systolic phase.

prospective tube current modulation (◒ Fig. 3.7). Using this technique it is possible to reduce radiation dose by up to 50%, depending on the patient's heart rate (the lower the heart rate, the lower the dose).

The implementation of prospective ECG triggering, single-beat acquisition (320-slice CT equipments), or high-pitch prospective ECG triggering (dual-source CT equipment) techniques has led to a dramatic reduction of radiation dose due to the capability of exposing the patient to radiation of only the desired phase, without significant deterioration of image quality (range: 1–4 mSv; optimal conditions <1 mSv).

Currently, the preferred strategy for MDCT coronary angiography is to have an optimal patients' selection, create the best scan conditions, and then apply prospective ECG triggering.

Image reconstruction

According to the literature, the techniques able to provide diagnostic images are based on few reconstructions concentrated from the mid- to end-diastole (the time windows are positioned at about 400 ms prior to the next R-wave or at 60% of the R–R interval). A variety of approaches can be used for the reconstructions. At least four different strategies can be listed (⟳ Fig. 3.8):

1. Relative delay strategy, whereby the delay time is a percentage of the R–R interval [15].

2. Absolute delay strategy, whereby the delay time is constant after the previous R wave [15].

3. Absolute reverse delay strategy, whereby the delay time is constant prior to the next R-wave [15].

4. End of the time window positioned at the peak of the P-wave [16].

All four strategies can be used, but this will largely depend on the degree of experience of the operator and, to a lesser extent, on the capabilities of the software/hardware, the type of change in the HR, and the time available for the reconstructions.

Other reconstruction parameters are relevant for obtaining an image of diagnostic quality. The effective slice thickness is usually slightly wider than the minimum possible collimation, so as to improve the signal-to-noise ratio of the image. The reconstruction increment should be about 50% of the effective slice thickness, so as to improve spatial resolution and the overlap in the z-axis. The field of view should be as small as possible to include the entire heart, so as to fully exploit the image matrix, which is constant (512×512 pixels). The convolution kernel should be half-way between noise and image quality. In general, medium convolution kernels are used for coronary artery imaging. When the coronary arteries are highly calcified or stents are present, sharper convolution kernels may be used: although they tend to increase image noise, they usually improve the visualization of the vessel wall or the structure of the stent and its lumen.

A recent development in reconstruction technique is the introduction of iterative reconstructions. These algorithms are closer to what was defined as 'exact method' and they are very demanding in terms of computer power. Today they are available on all new high-end CT scanners. The main advantage is the gain in image smoothness, which allows further reduction of mAs during the scan and, ultimately, the total radiation dose down by 20–30%. As an alternative, with the same radiation, they improve significantly the capability of CT in the visualization of the inner lumen of coronary stents.

Image evaluation

The stack of axial images resulting from the reconstruction will be fused into a continuous volume of data (⟳ Fig. 3.9).

There is still no standardized technique for the evaluation of MDCT coronary angiography images. In terms of repeatability, the performance of MDCT coronary angiography is currently operator-dependent [17]. The evaluation is generally performed with the American Heart Association classification in 15 or 16 coronary segments [18]. With this classification in mind, the operator carefully observes the clinically more important segments (⟳ Fig. 3.10). The studies conducted to date have demonstrated the ability of MDCT coronary angiography to identify significant stenoses, which are defined as a reduction in lumen diameter ≥50% [2, 3, 7]. The evaluation is always done in a semiquantitative fashion. The first step is to observe the axial images by scrolling the dataset to evaluate whether

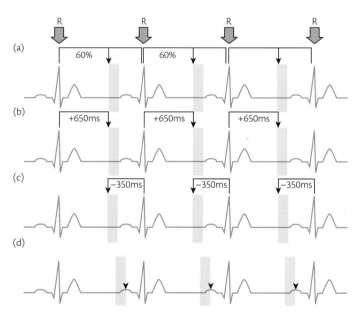

Fig 3.8 Retrospective cardiac gating techniques. The figure depicts different strategies for cardiac gating in MDCT coronary angiography. (a) Probably the most widely used strategy: percentage relative delay. The software calculates the distance from one R-wave to the next and positions the time window at a defined point based on the percentage of the entire R–R interval. (b) Absolute delay. With this strategy the time window is placed according to a fixed delay time after the previous R-wave. (c) Absolute reverse delay. With this strategy the time window is placed with a fixed time delay prior to the next R-wave. (d) With this strategy the final portion of the time window is positioned at the peak of the P-wave. The aim of this approach is to 'strike' the final moment of cardiac akinesia prior to systolic contraction.

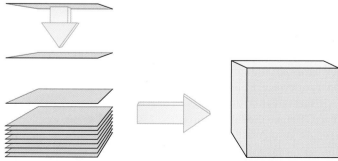

Fig 3.9 Volume dataset. The stack of axial images derived from the reconstruction platform are interpolated (or 'fused') into a continuous volume.

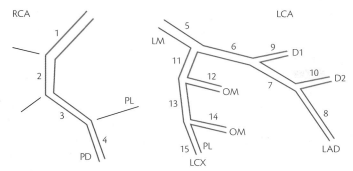

Fig 3.10 Classification of coronary artery segments. The figure shows a diagram of the coronary tree divided into 15 segments, according to the modified American Heart Association classification [18]. The classification includes most of the segments with diameter greater than 1.5 mm. Abbreviations: LCA, left coronary artery; LCX, left circumflex coronary artery; LAD, left anterior descending coronary artery; LM, left main coronary artery; OM, obtuse marginal branch; RCA, right coronary artery; D1, first diagonal branch; D2, second diagonal branch; PL, posterolateral branch; PD, posterior descending branch.

there are any pertinent findings that do not regard the coronary arteries. At the same time, the location of the cardiac structures can be checked (e.g. the great thoracic vessels, the cardiac valves, the atria, the ventricles, etc.), including the coronary arteries, to identify the presence of significant morphologic anomalies.

The next step involves the evaluation of the multi-planar reconstructions (MPR). For each vessel there is a dedicated plane that facilitates its correct and complete visualization. The main planes for the evaluation of the coronary arteries are: (1) the plane parallel to the atrio-ventricular groove, which enables the longitudinal visualization of the right coronary artery and the left circumflex artery; and (2) the plane parallel to the inter-ventricular groove, which enables the visualization of the left anterior descending coronary artery. Once the best evaluation plane has been obtained, in the event the vessel has a tortuous course, the reconstruction algorithm for maximum intensity projections (MIP) can be used. If vascular calcifications are absent or present in only minimal quantities, an MIP with a thickness between 5 and 8 mm is usually excellent, whereas if the calcifications are present in great quantity, the slice thickness needs to be reduced to 3 mm. Manually or automatically tracing the centreline of the vascular lumen to produce a curved MPR reconstruction may be useful when the vessel is only partially visualized, but also when it can be completely visualized in a plane. When dedicated software is used, the resulting image

may be rotated 360° on its own axis. At the same time, a cross-sectional plane of the vessel is visualized. This modality of visualization is particularly useful for the evaluation of stenoses with a semiquantitative system. Volume-rendering images are usually reconstructed to obtain a global view and for teaching purposes.

Limitations in MDCT coronary angiography

Patients with a HR higher than 70 bpm should not undergo MDCT coronary angiography unless very fast CT scanners are available. Patients with slightly irregular cardiac rhythms can be included (e.g. early beat, atrial fibrillation, left bundle-branch block, prolonged QRS complex, HR less than 40 bpm, etc.); in some cases and with some equipment, event patients with atrial fibrillation can undergo CT [10]. In the presence of an abnormal HR the location of the period with lowest dose will be variable and can be included within diastole. In addition, the presence of rhythm irregularities, with the exclusion of low HR (<40bpm), does not allow the application of multi-segment reconstruction algorithms [19, 20]. This is due to the variability in diastolic filling, which hampers the combination of data originating from contiguous cardiac cycles.

Future developments and outlook

The newer technical developments are all aiming in the following directions:

- Reduce radiation dose.
- Increase image quality.
- Extend the spectrum of applications.

The reduction of radiation exposure is already a reality since the latest solutions allow an average dose of <1 mSv. We expect further radiation dose reduction by the implementation of new detectors, further improvement in iterative reconstructions, and more temporal resolution. Image quality will increase due to the improvement of detector technology (more sensitivity and speed). The final objective would be flat panel technology with 0.2 mm³ resolution. The spectrum of applications is widening with the implementation of dual-energy. The possibility of obtaining multi-parametric imaging of the heart with CT will enhance plaque characterization, delayed enhancement, and perfusion capabilities without significant impact in radiation dose.

References

1. Flohr TG, Schoepf UJ, Kuettner A, et al. (2003) Advances in cardiac imaging with 16-section CT systems. *Acad Radiol* 10: 386–01.
2. Nieman K, Cademartiri F, Lemos PA, et al. Reliable non-invasive coronary angiography with fast submillimetre multi-slice spiral computed tomography. *Circulation* 2002; 106: 2051–54.
3. Ropers D, Baum U, Pohle K, et al. Detection of coronary artery stenoses with thin-slice multi-detector row spiral computed tomography and multiplanar reconstruction. *Circulation* 2003; 107: 664–66.
4. Achenbach S, Ulzheimer S, Baum U, et al. Non-invasive coronary angiography by retrospectively ECG-gated multi-slice spiral CT. *Circulation* 2000; 102: 2823–28.
5. Ohnesorge B, Flohr T, Becker C, et al. Cardiac imaging by means of electrocardiographically gated multisection spiral CT: initial experience. *Radiology* 2000; 217: 564–71.
6. Kachelriess M, Kalender WA. Electrocardiogram-correlated image reconstruction from subsecond spiral computed tomography scans of the heart. *Med Phy* S 1998; 25: 2417–31.

7. Mollet NR, Cademartiri F, Nieman K, et al. Multi-slice spiral computed tomography coronary angiography in patients with stable angina pectoris. *J Am Coll Cardiol* 2004; 43: 2265–70.

8. Nieman K, Rensing BJ, van Geuns RJ, et al. Non-invasive coronary angiography with Multi-slice spiral computed tomography: impact of heart rate. *Heart* 2002; 88: 470–74.

9. Aspelin P, Aubry P, Fransson SG, et al. Nephrotoxic effects in high-risk patients undergoing angiography. *N Engl J Med* 2003; 348: 491–99.

10. Jakobs TF, Becker CR, Ohnesorge B, et al. Multi-slice helical CT of the heart with retrospective ECG gating: reduction of radiation exposure by ECG-controlled tube current modulation. *Eur Radiol* 2002; 12: 1081–86.

11. Nieman K, Oudkerk M, Rensing BJ, et al. Coronary angiography with multi-slice computed tomography. *Lancet* 2001; 357: 599–03.

12. Georg C, Kopp A, Schroder S, et al. [Optimizing image reconstruction timing for the RR interval in imaging coronary arteries with multi-slice computerized tomography]. *Rofo Fortschr Geb Rontgenstr Neuen Bildgeb Verfahr* 2001; 173: 536–41.

13. Hong C, Becker CR, Huber A, et al. ECG-gated reconstructed multi-detector row CT coronary angiography: effect of varying trigger delay on image quality. *Radiology* 2001; 220: 712–17.

14. Flohr T, Ohnesorge B. Heart rate adaptive optimization of spatial and temporal resolution for electrocardiogram-gated multi-slice spiral CT of the heart. *J Comput Assist Tomogr* 2001; 25: 907–23.

15. Cademartiri F, Luccichenti G, Marano R, et al. Non-invasive angiography of the coronary arteries with multi-slice computed tomography: state of the art and future prospects. *Radiol Med (Torino)* 2003; 106: 284–96.

16. Sato Y, Matsumoto N, Kato M, et al. Non-invasive assessment of coronary artery disease by Multi-slice spiral computed tomography using a new retrospectively ECG-gated image reconstruction technique. *Circ J* 2003; 67: 401–05.

17. Cademartiri F, Mollet NR, Lemos PA, et al. Standard vs. user-interactive assessment of significant coronary stenoses with multi-slice computed tomography coronary angiography. *Am J Cardiol* 2004; 94: 1590–93.

18. Austen WG, Edwards JE, Frye RL, et al. A reporting system on patients evaluated for coronary artery disease. Report of the Ad Hoc Committee for Grading of Coronary Artery Disease, Council on Cardiovascular Surgery, American Heart Association. *Circulation* 1975; 51 (Suppl 4): 5–40.

19. Dewey M, Laule M, Krug L, et al. Multi-segment and halfscan reconstruction of 16-slice computed tomography for detection of coronary artery stenoses. *Invest Radiol* 2004; 39: 223–29.

20. Halliburton SS, Stillman AE, Flohr T, et al. Do segmented reconstruction algorithms for cardiac multi-slice computed tomography improve image quality? *Herz* 2003; 28: 20–31.

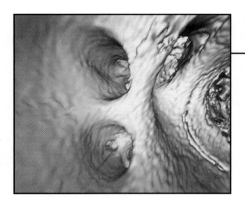

CHAPTER 4

CMR—basic principles

Jeremy Wright and Jan Bogaert

Contents

Introduction to MRI physics

Magnetic resonance imaging (MRI), formerly called nuclear magnetic resonance (NMR), relies on the physical properties of hydrogen nuclei (protons). These protons, abundantly present in the human body, have an intrinsic 'spin'. When a patient is brought into a high-strength magnetic field, the 'spins' of the human body align with the direction of the magnetic field [1]. Application of a radiofrequency (RF) pulse can excite the spins and perturb their alignment, with vector components in line with the magnetic field (longitudinal magnetization) and perpendicular to the field (transverse magnetization). These spins gradually return to their resting state (relax), and in the process create RF signals, which are used to create an image. The magnitude of signal arising from the tissue is mainly influenced by two relaxation times (T1 and T2), proton density, and movement of the protons (blood flow) [2].

T1 is the time constant describing the return of longitudinal magnetization to baseline, and T2 is the time constant describing return of transverse magnetization to baseline. Note that T1 and T2 of a proton are independent, and vary according to the local environment of the proton (i.e. the tissue). This phenomenon enables the excellent soft-tissue discrimination seen in MRI images. Fat and water are at the extremes of T1 and T2 relaxation times. Fat has short T1 and T2, whereas water has long T1 and T2 times. T1-weighted images exploit the differences in T1-relaxation behaviour between tissues. For instance, fat has a hyper-intense ('bright') appearance, fluid has a hypo-intense ('dark') appearance, while myocardial tissue is iso-intense ('grey'). In comparison, on T2-weighted images, fluid has a bright appearance, while fat has a less bright appearance.

Image formation also requires understanding of the origin of a particular signal in the patient. This is achieved by application of magnetic field gradients in a process called spatial encoding, a detailed discussion of this can be found in any basic MR textbook. For any image 'slice' the raw data acquired are called 'K-space' [3], and consist of multiple 'lines' of data (typically between 128 and 256). To generate an image, the K-space data undergo a complex mathematical process called Fourier transformation. The key concept of this transformation is that the centre of K-space contains image contrast information, while image resolution is governed by the periphery of K-space [4].

Contraindications to MRI

The main contraindications to MRI relate to the presence of metal implanted within the patient. Non-magnetic material has a risk of heating and electric current induction, and ferromagnetic material may move in the magnetic field. An implanted programmable device (neurostimulator, insulin pump, cochlear implant, etc.) can malfunction when exposed to magnetic fields and RF pulses. Sternal wires, most prosthetic cardiac valves, coronary stents, orthopaedic implants, and surgical clips are *not* contraindications to

MRI. The situation with implantable cardiac devices is complex. Permanent pacemakers and defibrillators are a contraindication to routine MRI, as deaths and device malfunction have been reported [5]. However, many studies report safe MRI scanning of patients with pacemakers and defibrillators. The new MRI conditional pacemaker generator and lead systems can safely have MRI [6]. Older pacemakers and all current defibrillators are classified as MRI unsafe, but under certain circumstances can still undergo MRI [7]. Implanted loop recorders (e.g. Reveal©) are MRI conditional, though data may be erased by the scan. All implants must be confirmed as MRI safe, conditional, or unsafe before the patient enters the scanner. Image artefacts are usually seen around implanted devices, so MRI is not useful for assessment of a device, but diagnostic data can usually be obtained about other aspects of cardiac structure/function.

Pregnancy is not a contraindication to MRI, and no harm to a developing foetus has been documented. However, it is prudent to only perform MRI on pregnant patients if the information is required prior to delivery and ultrasound is inadequate [5].

MRI contrast agents

Contrast agents are often used in assessing heart disease patients with CMR.

The most commonly used contrast agents contain chelates of the lanthide metal element gadolinium with multi-dentate ligands (e.g. Gd-DTPA or Gd-DOTA). These are non-specific contrast agents that distribute throughout the extracellular space, and are renally excreted in an unchanged form. They shorten the T1 relaxation times of tissues, and therefore result in an increase in signal intensity on T1-weighted images (lesser effect on T2). The typical dose is 0.1–0.2 mmol/kg (~15–30 ml). Side-effects are very rare, and these contrast agents have proven to be much safer than the iodinated contrast agents used for conventional X-ray. However, precautions are still necessary. Gadolinium-containing contrast agents do not cause renal dysfunction, but should be avoided in patients with GFR <30 ml/min because of the recently observed association with nephrogenic systemic fibrosis [8]. Gadolinium should be avoided in patients with haemolytic and sickle cell anaemia, and use during pregnancy is discouraged. In lactating women a small amount of gadolinium may be excreted into breast milk and absorbed by the infant, so it is prudent to express and discard breast milk for 24 hours after injection. It is important to note that assessment of cardiac structure, global and regional myocardial function, valve function, coronary angiography, and flow quantification can be performed without administration of contrast.

Pulse sequences

A pulse sequence is a carefully timed series of RF pulses and magnetic field gradients, and provides the raw information filling K-space—the 'echo'. The two broad families of pulse sequences are spin-echo and gradient-echo.

In spin-echo sequences, a 90° RF pulse is applied to the selected slice, so that the resting longitudinal magnetization (Z) is entirely flipped into the transverse (XY) plane. The transverse magnetization begins to diphase, then a 180° RF pulse is applied. This causes the transverse magnetization to partially rephase and produce a spin 'echo', filling one line of K-space. This rephasing 180° pulse can be repeated multiple times to acquire multiple lines of K-space, this is known as fast or turbo-spin echo. Excellent quality images can be obtained, with T1, T2, or proton-density weighting. The main drawback of these sequences is the long time required to fill K-space.

In contrast, gradient-echo pulse sequences utilize a smaller initial RF pulse (usually between 10° and 90°), and then apply magnetic field gradients to rephase the magnetic moments to produce a signal known as a 'gradient' echo. These sequences can produce images with T1, T2, or proton density weighting. The main advantage of gradient echo sequences is that gradient-echoes can be generated very quickly, so that scan times are reduced. The main disadvantage is an increased susceptibility to artefacts.

Imaging speed is a key concern in cardiac MRI, and parallel imaging is often used to reduce scan times or improve temporal resolution [9, 10]. The vendors have slightly different parallel imaging techniques—SENSE (Philips), ASSET (General Electric), GRAPPA (Siemens). They all rely upon multiple-element coils, which allow under-sampling of K-space, and allow for a 2–3-fold reduction in scan times. The main disadvantage of parallel imaging is a reduced signal-to-noise ratio (SNR).

Cardiac motion

As with other imaging modalities, CMR data acquisition is synchronized to cardiac motion using the electrical activity of the heart. The magnetic field exerts a significant magneto-hydrodynamic effect on the surface ECG, resulting in a voltage artefact in the ST segment of the ECG. Reliable R-wave detection is possible using a vector cardiogram [11] (VCG), but reliable ST/T wave monitoring is not possible. The VCG can be used for either prospective triggering or retrospective gating.

Prospective triggering is typically used for single-phase acquisitions, i.e. a static image of the heart at a single point in the cardiac cycle. Information is acquired at a specific interval after the R-wave, usually chosen to coincide with diastasis (when the heart is relatively still). Typically the data for a single slice are obtained in a ~10-s breath-hold.

Multi-phase acquisitions are used to acquire dynamic information such as cine MRI. Typically data are acquired throughout the cardiac cycle, and are reconstructed with retrospective reference to the VCG. Usually the cardiac cycle is divided into 20–30 phases. One image is reconstructed for each phase, and the resulting images are displayed as a cineloop. A single-slice cineloop is acquired during a ~10 s breath-hold.

Real-time cine MRI images can be acquired by increasing the parallel imaging factor and reducing the spatial resolution. With these sequences it is possible to obtain diagnostic images in patients who cannot breath-hold, and in those with very irregular cardiac rhythms (when normal cine images are often sub-optimal).

Respiratory motion

Most CMR images are obtained during breath-holds, typically of 10–15-s duration. In general, an end-inspiratory breath-hold is more comfortable and able to be held longer. However, a breath-hold at the end of gentle expiration tends to be more consistent (minimizing slice misregistration) and is less likely to provoke ectopy. We generally commence with inspiratory breath-holds, but have a low threshold for changing to expiration. Administration of oxygen is helpful for patients experiencing shortness of breath.

The use of a navigator-echo during free breathing is an alternative method of image acquisition, and is typically used for high-resolution imaging such as coronary angiography. The navigator-echo is typically positioned on the right hemidiaphragm to monitor respiratory motion. The patient is instructed to breathe regularly and consistently, and image information is only acquired when the diaphragm is in a pre-determined position (e.g. end expiration). Depending on the scan prescribed and navigator efficiency, these scans take 5–15 min to acquire.

We will now discuss the specific sequences used for assessment of cardiac function, cardiac morphology, perfusion, viability, and MR angiography.

Cardiac function

The balanced steady-state free precession (b-SSFP) sequence is the mainstay of functional assessment [12]. There are several monikers for such pulse sequences: balanced FFE (Philips), FIESTA (General Electric), TrueFISP (Siemens). The resultant images are not T1- or T2-weighted, rather the signal intensity depends upon the ratio of T2/T1 in addition to flow; therefore, blood, water, and fat all appear bright.

First, a set of single-phase localizer scout views are obtained in the axial, coronal, and sagittal planes. Next, a cine sequence is obtained in the vertical long axis (VLA)—a plane prescribed on the axial images through the apex of the LV and the middle of the mitral valve (⊃ Fig. 4.1a). On this image a second cine sequence is prescribed in the horizontal long axis (HLA)—transecting the LV apex and the middle of the mitral valve (⊃ Fig. 4.1b). Now the LV short axis can be prescribed, perpendicular to both the VLA and HLA. The ventricles are encompassed in a stack of 10–12 contiguous slices in short-axis direction (⊃ Fig. 4.1c–d). The end-diastolic and end-systolic frames are selected, and then the endocardial and epicardial contours are delineated. This

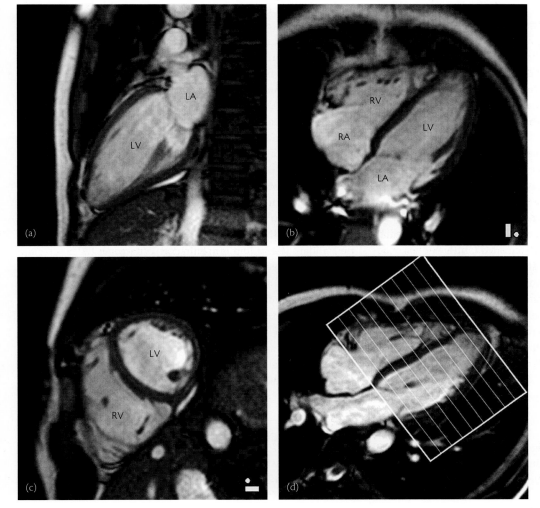

Fig. 4.1 Assessment of cardiac function. A b-SSFP cine sequence is used for functional assessment (only end diastolic frames are shown here). From the localizer scout images the VLA plane is prescribed (a). A plane perpendicular to the VLA produces the HLA (b). The LV short-axis plane can now be prescribed, perpendicular to both the VLA and HLA (c). The LV is encompassed by a stack of slices in the short-axis plane (d) to enable quantification of ventricular volumes and assessment of global and regional systolic function. LV, left ventricle; LA, left atrium; RV, right ventricle; RA, right atrium; VLA, vertical long axis; HLA, horizontal long axis.

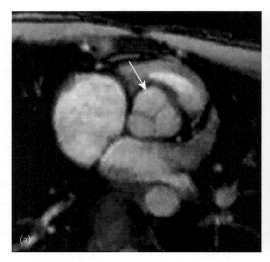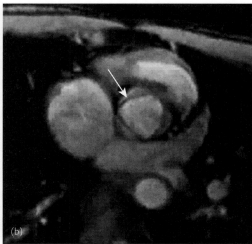

(a) (b)

Fig. 4.2 Assessment of valve morphology. Valve morphology and function can be qualitatively assessed with b-SSFP cine imaging. Short-axis images of the aortic valve at end-diastole (a) and mid-systole (b) demonstrate a trileaflet aortic valve with thin leaflets that open normally.

allows calculation of global functional parameters: end-diastolic volume (EDV), end-systolic volume (ESV), stroke volume (SV) and ejection fraction (EF), and myocardial mass. This is the reference standard for *in vivo* assessment of myocardial volume, global function, and mass [13–16]. Regional function is assessed qualitatively and quantitatively. In addition to short-axis slices, the standard echocardiographic views can be prescribed: 2-chamber, 4-chamber, and apical long-axis views. Qualitative evaluation of LV contractility is reported using the 17-segment model proposed by the American Society of Echocardiography.

It is also possible to perform volumetric quantification of the right ventricle (RV) on the stack of short-axis slices. However, it can be challenging to recognize the plane of the tricuspid valve. Therefore, we prefer to perform quantification of RV function on a stack of contiguous axial images that encompasses the heart.

Valvular function can also be assessed with cine imaging. The valve leaflets are easily seen (⊃ Fig. 4.2) and mechanisms of dysfunction identified. Although the b-SSFP sequence is designed to be relatively flow 'insensitive', turbulent flow through stenotic or regurgitant valves is visible. The regurgitant fraction of an isolated valve lesion can be calculated from the difference between LV and RV stroke volume. Further assessment of valve dysfunction will be discussed in the section on velocity encoded CMR.

Myocardial tagging is another CMR technique useful in functional analysis [17]. A grid or tag of lines on the myocardium is transiently created, and these lines track the underlying myocardial deformation. These images can be analysed qualitatively and quantitatively, e.g. strain analysis, but the elaborate post-processing required for quantitative analysis has largely limited their use to the research setting.

Cardiac morphology and tissue characterization

Important information regarding cardiac structure is obtained from pulse sequences that produce non-cine images. Optimal depiction of cardiac anatomy is achieved by making the flowing blood appear black by using two 180° inversion pre-pulses (double

inversion recovery) [18]. A third inversion pre-pulse can also be applied, to suppress the signal arising from fat. The images can be T1- or T2-weighted. T1-weighted images typically provide excellent delineation of cardiac anatomy (⊃ Fig. 4.3a). In contrast, T2-weighted images provide unique information about free-water content—MRI is the only imaging modality that can non-invasively detect and quantify myocardial oedema, for example, in patients with acute myocardial infarction [19] (⊃ Fig. 4.3b).

In addition to producing images, these sequences enable absolute quantification of T1 and T2* relaxation times (T2* is the time constant reflecting T2 relaxation and dephasing owing to local magnetic field inhomogeneities). The same principles apply to T1 and T2* mapping, though different sequences are required. A single-phase LV short-axis slice is acquired multiple times (usually 6–9), each at a different echo time. A region of interest is delineated, signal intensity vs. echo time is plotted, the resulting curve used to calculate the absolute relaxation time.

T1 mapping pre- and post-gadolinium contrast is useful for assessment of myocardial fibrosis because gadolinium-contrast distributes throughout extracellular space and reduces T1 of fibrotic tissue relative to normal myocardium. This technique is especially important for diffuse interstitial fibrosis, which may not be visible on standard late gadolinium enhancement images [20].

T2* mapping sequences enable estimation of tissue iron content [21]. This is possible because iron within tissue becomes 'magnetized', and causes a reduction in T2 and T2* relaxation time. T2* has been extensively validated for assessment of iron content in the liver and myocardium [22], and at present is the preferred method, as the available T2 sequences require long scan times and have poor signal-to-noise ratio (SNR). However, as use of 3T systems increases we are likely to see more interest in T2 mapping.

Delayed contrast enhancement

Delayed contrast enhancement, also known as contrast enhanced MRI, late gadolinium enhancement, or contrast-enhanced IR (CE-IR), is a key strength of CMR and is considered the reference

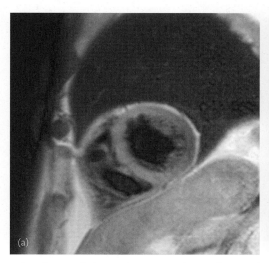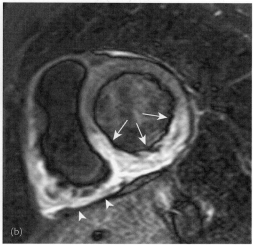

Fig. 4.3 Assessment of cardiac morphology with fast spin-echo. Cardiac morphology can be assessed with fast spin-echo sequences and 'black-blood' pre-pulses. A single-phase image in mid-diastole is usually acquired, to minimize motion artefact. These images can be T1- or T2-weighted, with or without fat suppression. (a) T1-weighted short-axis image (without fat suppression) of a normal heart. (b) T2-weighted short-axis image (with fat suppression) of a patient with a large inferior myocardial infarction. Note the marked increase in signal intensity (white) in the inferior, infero-lateral, and infero-septal segments of the left ventricle (arrows), as well as the extensive involvement of the inferior wall of the right ventricle (arrowheads).

standard for *in vivo* assessment of myocardial infarction in both the acute and chronic phases, as well as the assessment of scar resulting from non-ischaemic disease. It has been extensively evaluated in animal and human studies [23–25] and can accurately measure infarction within 1 g. The technique is called 'late' or 'delayed' because images are typically obtained 10–20 min after injection of contrast. This is the optimal time to discriminate between normal and abnormal myocardium, with the maximum difference in gadolinium-contrast concentration between normal and abnormal tissue. The usual dose of contrast is 0.15–0.2 mmol/kg.

The mechanism of accumulation of contrast within infarcted tissue is incompletely understood. Regarding acute infarction, it is thought that myocardial cell membrane rupture allows gadolinium to diffuse into the intracellular space (it must be noted that gadolinium is an extracellular contrast agent). The greater distribution area, concomitant myocardial oedema, and altered contrast kinetics result in hyper-enhancement relative to the normal myocardium [26]. The mechanism of contrast accumulation within chronic infarcts is thought due to increased interstitial space between collagen fibres, combined with slower wash-in and wash-out contrast kinetics of infarct tissue compared to normal myocardium [27].

The technique consists of first applying an inversion RF prepulse [28]. As the 'spins' of a tissue 'relax' towards their resting state, they pass through a point where they have zero longitudinal magnetization. If image information is acquired at this point no signal will arise from these spins, which are 'nulled' and appear dark on the resultant image. This delay between the inversion pre-pulse and image acquisition is called the inversion time (TI). Typically, we choose to null the signal of normal myocardium, while infarcted or scarred myocardium has a bright signal because of the gadolinium within it (⊃ Fig. 4.4a). The TI to null

normal myocardium is variable and depends upon patient weight, contrast dose, renal function, and time-point after injection of the contrast. It is usually between 200 and 250 ms for the first images and 250–300 ms for later images. Choosing the correct TI is crucial to maximize the contrast between normal and abnormal myocardium and to prevent image artefacts. Experienced users can usually satisfactorily estimate the TI, but in difficult cases (and for inexperienced users), pulse sequences are available to help choose the ideal TI (Look Locker, TI-scouting). A new type of pulse sequence, called phase-sensitive inversion-recovery (PS-IR) has been developed to overcome the difficulty of choosing TI [29]. These sequences enable the TI to be arbitrarily chosen with no adverse effect on the resultant image.

2D- and 3D-acquisition schemes are available. 3D acquisitions enable imaging of the entire heart in a single breath-hold with a high SNR, but are prone to image blurring [30]. In contrast, 2D sequences acquire one slice per breath-hold (more tiring for the patient) and has lower SNR. However, despite more image 'noise', the 2D images usually provide greater spatial resolution. We recommend commencing with a 3D sequence, and to examine abnormal areas with a 2D sequence.

It is important to emphasize that enhancement on contrast-enhanced CMR images is not specific for ischaemic injury (⊃ Fig. 4.4a); it can also be seen in myocarditis (⊃ Fig. 4.4b), infiltrative disorders (e.g. amyloid, sarcoid), and cardiomyopathies (e.g. hypertrophic, arrhythmogenic right ventricular dysplasia) [31]. It is the pattern of enhancement that is used to distinguish between the different aetiologies. The other main limitation of delayed enhancement imaging is the reduced ability to depict diffuse myocardial fibrosis, because signal intensity may be uniform with no 'normal' myocardium for comparison [20].

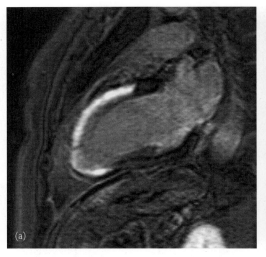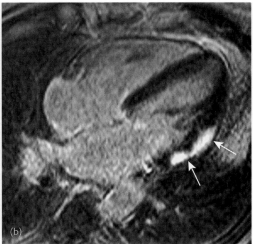

Fig. 4.4 Contrast enhanced CMR. A vertical long slice of the left ventricle showing nearly complete transmural hyper-enhancement of the anterior wall and LV apex due to acute myocardial infarction (a). Figure (b) shows extensive sub-epicardial enhancement of the lateral wall due to myocarditis (arrows).

Myocardial perfusion

'First-pass' imaging after intravenous injection of a small dose of contrast is the standard CMR method of assessing myocardial perfusion (perfusion-CMR) [32]. It is performed at rest and during pharmacologic vasodilator stress (adenosine or dipyridamole). Usually, 3–5 short-axis slices of the LV are obtained to encompass all myocardial segments. An ultra-fast acquisition scheme is required because each slice is imaged once per heartbeat immediately after gadolinium contrast (usually injected at 2 ml/s followed by a saline flush). The optimal dose of gadolinium is 0.03–0.1 mmol/kg, depending on the sequence used and whether visual analysis (higher dose) or semi-quantitative analysis is planned.

Visual analysis is the most frequently used approach. A perfusion defect is identified as a region of non-enhancing myocardium during the first pass of contrast (⊃ Fig. 4.5). A defect is most pronounced in the sub-endocardium and has variable trans-mural

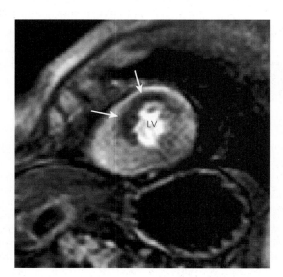

Fig. 4.5 Adenosine stress first-pass myocardial perfusion imaging. A short-axis slice of the left ventricle at mid-ventricular level is shown during the first pass of intravenous gadolinium during adenosine vasodilator stress. There is a large perfusion defect in the mid anterior and antero-septal segments (arrows).

spread. It is critical to differentiate true defects from frequently encountered dark rim artefacts [33]. Semi-quantitative assessment is usually performed by analysis of signal intensity–time curves. The myocardial perfusion reserve index (MPRI) is calculated by comparing the myocardial perfusion upslope between rest and stress [34–36]. Absolute quantitative assessment of perfusion can be performed, but is largely confined to the research setting.

Velocity encoded CMR

Velocity-encoded CMR, also known as phase-contrast flow quantification, is an established fast and simple method of measuring blood flow [37]. It is based upon the phenomenon that as 'spins' flow along a magnetic field gradient, they acquire a 'shift' in their transverse (XY) magnetization. This shift is proportional to the strength of the magnetic field gradient, as well as the flow velocity, which can thus be calculated. Comparisons with invasive measurements and phantom studies have demonstrated that the overall error in flow measurement is <10% [38–40].

To measure flow through a vessel, first an image slice is prescribed perpendicular to the flow direction. It is important this slice is within 15° of the true perpendicular plane, otherwise flow will be significantly underestimated (similar to the principle of Doppler line-up in echocardiography). Second, an appropriate encoding velocity (VENC) is selected, which must be greater than the highest velocity in the flow. Otherwise aliasing will make the data unreliable. The images are acquired during a 15–20-s breath-hold, and minor post-processing produces flow and velocity data (⊃ Fig. 4.6). Flow in any vessel can be assessed, though in clinical imaging vessels smaller than the pulmonary veins are rarely quantified.

There are many applications of flow quantification, including calculation of RV and LV stroke volumes, shunt quantification (Qp:Qs), calculation of valvular regurgitant fraction [41], and assessment of diastolic function (mitral inflow, pulmonary vein flow, mitral annular velocities, tricuspid inflow, caval flow). In addition, velocity data enable assessment of pressure gradients, which are crucial for the assessment of stenotic valvular lesions [42].

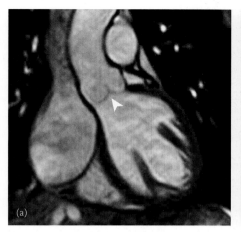
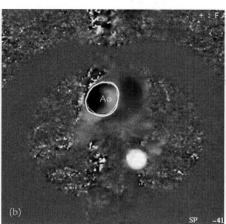
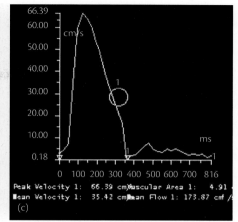

Fig. 4.6 Velocity encoded CMR flow quantification of aortic flow. A long-axis view of the aortic valve (a) is used to prescribe an imaging plane perpendicular to aortic flow. On the resultant image the vessel is delineated (b). Flow through the vessel is calculated (c). Ao, aorta.

MR angiography

Gadolinium contrast-enhanced MR angiography is widely used for evaluation of the great vessels of the thorax. The standard technique is a 3D gradient-echo acquisition during the first pass of contrast, resulting in a 3D volume of high spatial-resolution images [43]. A 'bolus-tracker' is used to ensure optimal timing of image acquisition relative to arrival of the contrast [44]. Usually 0.1–0.2 mmol/kg of gadolinium is injected at 2 ml/s followed by a saline flush. Post-processing techniques can be used to explore the 3D datasets—including maximum intensity projections (MIP), multi-planar reformatting (MPR), and volume rendering (Fig. 4.7a).

Coronary artery imaging with MRI is much more challenging, and has extensively been investigated. The principal challenges are the small size of the coronaries (2–5 mm), their long tortuous course, motion (respiratory, cardiac and individual artery), and flow. Many techniques have been used, but despite promising results in the literature [45], coronary artery imaging by CMR is clinically only performed to assess the anomalous

coronary origins and to follow the aneurysms of Kawasaki disease (Fig. 4.7b).

An important factor is the fast-growing availability of multi-detector computer tomography (CT) scanners, which offer fast and reliable imaging of the coronary arteries. This makes coronary CMR somewhat redundant, though it remains an appealing option when nephrotoxic contrast agents must be avoided (e.g. severe renal dysfunction). Technical developments in the near future may renew the interest for this exciting field of cardiac imaging (e.g. coronary wall or plaque imaging).

Conclusions

MRI is a powerful tool for assessment of the cardiovascular system; indeed, it is the reference standard for the assessment of many aspects of cardiac structure and function. A wide variety of pulse sequences are available, and the full potential of CMR is realized when data from all the relevant sequences is integrated in a comprehensive manner.

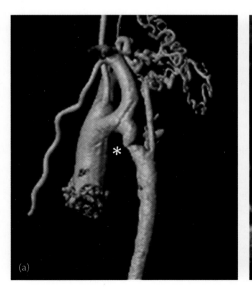
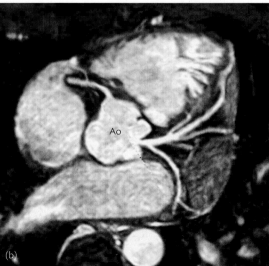

Fig. 4.7 Magnetic resonance angiography. 3D MRA was performed following injection of a gadolinium-containing contrast agent. Post-processing of the data with volume rendering (a) showing significant aortic coarctation (*) with extensive collateral formation. (b) Magnetic resonance coronary angiography. A tangential view showing normal origin and proximal courses of the left and right coronary arteries. Ao, aorta.

References

1. Hendrick RE. The AAPM/RSNA physics tutorial for residents. Basic physics of MR imaging: an introduction. *Radiographic* S 1994; 14: 829–46.
2. Van Guens RJ, Wielopolski PA, de Bruin HG, et al. Basic Principles of magnetic resonance imaging. *Prog Cardiovasc Dis* 1999; 42: 149–56.
3. Petersson JS, Christoffersson JO, Golman K. MRI simulation using the K-space formalism. *Magn Reson Imaging* 1993; 11: 557–68.
4. Henning J. K-space sampling strategies. *Eur Radiol* 1999; 9: 1020–31.
5. Kanal E, Barkovich AJ, Bell C, et al. ACR guidance document on MR safe practices: 2013. *J Magn Reson Imaging* 2013; 37: 501–30.
6. Shinbane JS, Colletti PM, Shellock FG. Magnetic resonance imaging in patients with cardiac pacemakers: era of 'MR conditional' designs. *J Cardiovasc Magn Reson* 2011; 13: 63.
7. Shinbane JS, Colletti PM, Shellock FG. MR in patients with pacemakers and ICDs: defining the issues. *J Cardiovasc Magn Reson* 2011; 9 (1): 5–13.
8. Morcos SK. Nephrogenic systemic fibrosis following the administration of extracellular gadolinium based contrast agents: is the stability of the contrast agent molecule an important factor in the pathogenesis of this condition? *Br J Radiol* 2007; 80: 73–6.
9. Sodickson DK, Manning WJ. Simultaneous acquisition of spatial harmonics (SMASH): fast imaging with radiofrequency coil arrays. *Magn Reson Med* 1997; 38: 591–603.
10. Pruessmann KP, Weiger M, Scheidegger MB, Boesiger P. SENSE: sensitivity encoding for fast MRI. *Magn Reson Med* 1999; 42: 952–62.
11. Fischer SE, Wickline SA, Lorenz CH. Novel real-time R-wave detection algorithm based on the vector cardiogram for accurate gated magnetic resonance acquisitions. *Magn Reson Med* 1999; 42: 361–70.
12. Thiele H, Nagel E, Paetsch I, et al. Functional cardiac MR imaging with steady-state free precession (SSFP) significantly improves endocardial border delineation without contrast agents. *J Magn Reson Imaging* 2001; 14: 362–367.
13. Bogaert J, Bosmans H, Rademakers FE, et al. Left ventricular quantification with breath-hold MR imaging: comparison with echocardiography. *Magma* 1995; 3: 5–12.
14. Sakuma H, Fujita N, Foo TK, et al. Evaluation of left ventricular volume and mass with breath-hold cine MR imaging. *Radiology* 1993; 188: 377–80.
15. Grothues F, Smith GC, Moon JC, et al. Comparison of interstudy reproducibility of cardiovascular magnetic resonance with two-dimensional echocardiography in normal subjects and in patients with heart failure or left ventricular hypertrophy. *Am J Cardiol* 2002; 90: 29–34.
16. Myerson SG, Bellenger NG, Pennell DJ. Assessment of left ventricular mass by cardiovascular magnetic resonance. *Hypertension* 2002; 39: 750–5.
17. Zerhouni EA, Parish DM, Rogers WJ, et al. Human Heart: Tagging with MR Imaging—a method for non-invasive assessment of myocardial motion. *Radiology* 1988; 169: 59–63.
18. Stehling MK, Holzknecht NG, Laub G, et al. Single shot T1-and T2-weighted magnetic resonance imaging of the heart with black blood: preliminary experience. *Magma* 1996; 4: 231–40.
19. Friedrich MG, Abdel-Aty H, Taylor A, Schulz-Menger J, Messroghli D, Dietz R. The salvaged area at risk in reperfused acute myocardial infarction as visualised by cardiovascular magnetic resonance. *J Am Coll Cardiol* 2008; 51: 1581–87.
20. Mewton N, Liu CY, Croisille P, Bluemke D, Lima J. Assessment of myocardial fibrosis with cardiovascular magnetic resonance. *J Am Coll Cardiol* 2011; 57: 891–903.
21. Anderson LJ, Holden S, Davis B, et al. Cardiovascular T2* magnetic resonance for the early diagnosis of myocardial iron overload. *Eur Heart J* 2001; 22: 2171–79.
22. Carpenter JP, He T, Kirk P, et al. On T2* magnetic resonance and cardiac iron. *Circulation* 2011; 123: 1519–28.
23. Kim RJ, Fieno DS, Parrish TB, et al. Relationship of MRI delayed contrast enhancement to irreversible injury, infarct age, and contractile function. *Circulation* 1999; 100: 1992–2002.
24. Wu E, Judd RM, Vargas JD, Klocke FJ, Bonow RO, Kim R. Visualization of presence, location, and transmural extent of healed Q-wave and non-Q wave myocardial infarction. *Lancet* 2001; 357: 21–28.
25. Wagner A, Mahrholdt H, Holly TA, et al. Contrast-enhanced MRI and routine single photon emission computed tomography (SPECT) perfusion imaging for detection of subendocardial myocardial defects: an imaging study. *Lancet* 2003; 361: 374–9.
26. Judd RM, Lugo-Oliveri CH, Arai M, et al. Physiological basis of myocardial contrast enhancement in fast magnetic resonance images of 2-day old reperfused canine infarcts. *Circulation* 1995; 92: 1902–10.
27. Lima JA, Judd RM, Bazille A, Schulman SP, Atalar E, Zerhouni EA. Regional hetereogeneity of human myocardial infarcts demonstrated by contrast-enhanced MRI. Potential mechanisms. *Circulation* 1993; 92: 1117–25.
28. Simonetti OP, Kim RJ, Fieno DS, et al. An improved method for the visualisation of myocardial infarction. *Radiology* 2001; 218: 215–23.
29. Kellman P, Arai AE, McVeigh ER, et al. Phase-sensitive inversion recovery for detecting myocardial infarction using gadolinium-delayed hyperenhancement. *Magn Reson Med* 2002; 47: 372–83.
30. Kuhl HP, Papavasiliu TS, Beek AM, et al. Myocardial viability: rapid assessment with delayed contrast-enhanced MR imaging with three dimensional inversion-recovery prepared pulse sequence. *Radiology* 2004; 230: 576–82.
31. Bogaert J, Taylor AM, Kerkhove Fvan, Dymarkowski S. Use of inversion recovery contrast-enhanced MRI for cardiac imaging: spectrum of applications. *Am J Roentgenol* 2004; 182: 609–15.
32. Ishida N, Sakuma H, Motoyasu M, et al. Non-infarcted myocardium: correlation between dynamic first-pass contrast-enhanced myocardial MR and quantitative coronary angiography. *Radiology* 2003; 229: 209–16.
33. Gerber BL, Raman SV, Nayak K, et al. Myocardial first-pass perfusion cardiovascular magnetic resonance: history, theory, and current state of the art. *J Cardiovasc Magn Reson* 2008; 10 (1): 18.
34. Wilke N, Jerosch-Herold M, Wang Y, et al. Myocardial perfusion reserve: assessment with multisection, quantitative, first-pass MR imaging. *Radiology* 1997; 204: 373–84.
35. Cullen JHS, Horsfield MA, Reek CR., et al. A myocardial perfusion reserve index in humans using contrast enhanced magnetic resonance imaging. *J Am Coll Cardiol* 1999; 33: 1386–94.
36. Al-Saadi N, Nagel E, Gross M, et al. Non-invasive detection of myocardial ischaemia from perfusion reserve based on cardiovascular magnetic resonance. *Circulation* 2000; 101: 1379–183.
37. Spritzer CE, Pelc NJ, Lee JN, et al. Rapid MR imaging of blood flow with a phase sensitive, limited flip angle, gradient recalled pulse sequence: preliminary experience. *Radiology* 1990; 176: 255–62.
38. Kondo C, Caputo GR, Semelka R, et al. Right and left ventricular stroke volume measurements with velocity encoded cine MR imaging: in vitro and in vivo validation. *Am J Roentgenol* 1991; 157: 9–16.
39. Hoeper MM, Tongers J, Leppert A, et al. Evaluation of right ventricular performance with a right ventricular ejection fraction thermodilution catheter and magnetic resonance imaging in patients with pulmonary hypertension. *Chest* 2001; 120: 502–507.

40. Lee VS, Spritzer CE, Caroll BA, et al. Flow quantification using fast cine phase-contrast MR imaging, conventional cine phase-contrast MR imaging,and Doppler sonography: in vitro and in vivo validation. *Am J Roentgenol* 1997; 12: 1952–53.

41. Kozerke S, Schwitter J, Pedersen EM, Boesiger P. Aortic and mitral regurgitation: quantification using moving slice velocity mapping. *J Magn Reson Imaging* 2001; 14: 106–12.

42. Eichenberger AC, Jenni R, Schulthess GK von. Aortic valve pressure gradients in patients with aortic valve stenosis: quantification with velocity-encoded cine MR imaging. *Am J Roentgenol* 1993; 160: 971–7.

43. Prince MR, Narasimham DL, Jacoby WT, et al. Three-dimensional gadolinium-enhanced MR angiography of the thoracic aorta. *Am J Roentgenol* 1996; 166: 1387–97.

44. Riederer SJ, Bernstein MA, Breen JF, et al. Three-dimensional contrast-enhanced MR angiography with real-time fluoroscopic triggering: design specifications and technical reliability in 350 patient studies. *Radiology* 2000; 215: 584–93.

45. Kim YW, Danias PG, Stuber M, et al. Coronary magnetic resonance angiography for the detection of coronary stenoses. *N Engl J Med* 2001; 345: 1863–9.

SECTION II

New technical developments in imaging techniques

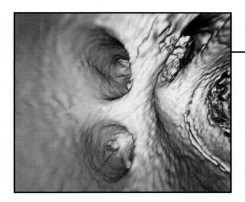

CHAPTER 5

New developments in echocardiography/ advanced echocardiography

Silvia Gianstefani, Jens-Uwe Voigt, and Mark J. Monaghan

Contents

Three-dimensional echocardiography

Development of the 3D technique

The concept of, and indeed the ability to, perform three-dimensional echocardiography (3DE), has been around for some time now. It was back in 1974 that investigators first reported the acquisition of 3D ultrasound images of the heart [1], but it has not been until the last decade that 3DE has started to enter clinical practice. The early attempts at this form of imaging were based around computerized reconstruction from multiple 2D slices, achieved by carefully tracking a transducer through a number of 2D acquisitions over many cardiac cycles. Over subsequent years, the technique was gradually refined and improved upon; ECG gating was introduced and free hand scanning gave way to motorized rotary transducers, whose location in space was continually tracked. This approach appeared to produce accurate volumes [2] and impressive images; however, the time involved for reconstruction and the labour-intensive analysis, not to mention the requisite computing capabilities, meant that it was the preserve of dedicated research departments.

The advent of a sparse matrix array transducer in the early 1990s [3] represented a marked improvement. The transducer was capable of obtaining direct volumetric data at volume rates high enough to demonstrate cardiac motion. Images were presented as 2D orthogonal planes, and both spatial and temporal resolutions were low.

Transducer technology continued to advance and fully sampled matrix array technology facilitated the integration of 3DE into clinical practice. These transducers allowed rapid ECG-gated or real-time 3D image acquisition with temporal and spatial resolution sufficient for clinical applications.

The last technical advancement consists of the introduction of broadband (1–5 MHz) monocrystal transducers. The electromechanical efficiency of these monocrystals is 80–100% better than that of the currently used piezoelectric crystals making them twice as sensitive. This results in a better penetration, resolution, and signal-to-noise ratio. These transducers allow high-resolution harmonic imaging with improved cavity delineation. The efficiency of the monocrystal matrix array transducers and miniaturization has also led to the introduction of transoesophageal (TEE) real time 3D echocardiography (RT3DE).

Acquisition techniques

Improvements in workflow have meant that 3D data acquisition now can be completely incorporated into a standard 2D examination. Integrated 2D/3D probes for transthoracic echocardiography (TTE) have recently been commercially available. During an examination it is only necessary to press a button on the screen to switch between 2D and 3D modes.

The current generation of matrix-phased array transducers facilitates five main types of image acquisition, which are available on both TTE and TEE 3D probes. Each of them differs in spatial and temporal resolution profiles, as well as the number of cardiac cycles required for image capture. A complete understanding of these different live modes and of their potential and their limitations is crucial in order to appropriately use them in every specific clinical setting [4–5] (see ⊃ Fig. 5.1):

- Simultaneous multi-plane mode.
- Real-time 3D mode—narrow sector.
- Focused wide sector—'zoom'.
- Full volume—gated acquisition.
- 3D colour Doppler.

Simultaneous multi-plane mode

Simultaneous multi-plane mode allows the simultaneous presentation of several 2D slices captured in a single cardiac cycle. It is based on the capability to acquire two/three perpendicular scan planes simultaneously. 3D matrix transducer technology facilitates multi-directional beam steering. The exact angle of these slices can be adjusted depending on the structures being imaged. Colour flow Doppler imaging can also be superimposed onto the 2D images.

Real-time 3D mode

Real-time 3D mode permits the acquisition of a real-time, beat-by-beat 3D image that can be manipulated live. The field sector is narrow at about 30° in the elevation plane and about 65° in lateral plane. Due to high line density and relatively narrow scan volume, this 3D mode has a high spatial and high temporal resolution. It is particularly useful for visualization of minute structures (valves, small masses) or to guide interventional procedures where real-time 3D imaging is required. However, due to the pyramidal shape of the volume, additional cropping may be required to obtain an 'en face' view of the structure of interest during scanning.

Focused wide sector '3D zoom' mode

Focused wide sector '3D zoom' mode provides a magnified dataset of a specific volume. The region of interest can be manually defined during scanning to obtain a direct view of the structures and eliminating the need of cropping the volume. This facility makes 3D zoom the most commonly used acquisition mode during 3D TEE. 3D zoom mode is obtained in one beat acquisition; therefore it is not limited by stitching artefacts. Nevertheless, it is characterized by a relatively low temporal resolution (wide scan volume) and a low spatial resolution (lower line density).

'Full-volume' mode

'Full-volume' mode allows the 3D dataset to be wide enough to include the entire heart. The acquisition can be performed over 4–7 cardiac cycles gated to the R-wave and with suspended respiration; or in true real-time with one beat full volume acquisition (which has become commercially available in the last couple of years). In the first scenario, the final volume consists of multiple 3D volumes stitched together (thereby not permitting live 3D viewing). The dataset needs cropping and and needs to be analysed off-line.

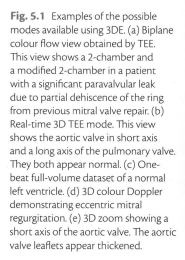

Fig. 5.1 Examples of the possible modes available using 3DE. (a) Biplane colour flow view obtained by TEE. This view shows a 2-chamber and a modified 2-chamber in a patient with a significant paravalvular leak due to partial dehiscence of the ring from previous mitral valve repair. (b) Real-time 3D TEE mode. This view shows the aortic valve in short axis and a long axis of the pulmonary valve. They both appear normal. (c) One-beat full-volume dataset of a normal left ventricle. (d) 3D colour Doppler demonstrating eccentric mitral regurgitation. (e) 3D zoom showing a short axis of the aortic valve. The aortic valve leaflets appear thickened.

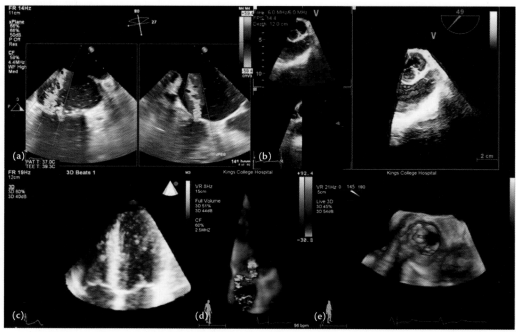

Images can then be displayed in a number of ways to facilitate viewing and analysis of cardiac structures. The stitched full-volume mode provides relatively high temporal resolution; however, it is prone to stitching artefacts mainly caused by translation of the heart during respiration or irregular R–R intervals during the volume acquisition time. These limitations have been overcome by one-beat full-volume modality. The disadvantage of this acquisition modality is a reduced volume rate and/or spatial resolution.

Full volume is the most appropriate mode for transthoracic acquisition and quantitative analysis of large volumes, such as cardiac cavities. In transoesophageal examinations it can be used to include multiple valves or large structures (such as intra-cardiac masses).

3D colour Doppler

3D colour Doppler combines volume imaging with colour Doppler and it is ideal for assessing valve regurgitation. It can be used in full volume, zoom modality, and real-time 3D. However, it currently suffers with low volume rates (temporal resolution).

Display of 3D datasets

Each 3D dataset can be displayed in different ways, accordingly to the operator's needs and preferences. This allows one to accurately visually analyse the structure of interest or to obtain exact measurements of dimensions and volumes.

Cropping

Once the 3D dataset has been acquired and manually rotated to provide the best view of the cardiac structures, the volume has to be cropped in order to expose the region of interest. The procedure consists of manually moving a free cutting tool, cropping the 3D dataset along virtually infinite planes, or in performing the cropping along three perpendicular axes during or after the acquisition (see ⊃ Fig. 5.2).

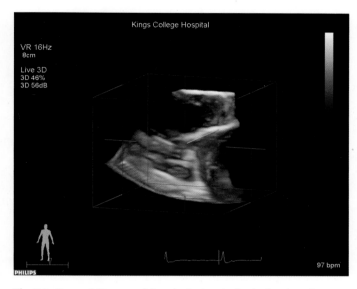

Fig. 5.2 Cropped 3D zoom of the mitral valve obtained using the yellow cropping box characterized by three perpendicular cropping planes (red, green and blue).

Post-acquisition display

After the acquisition, a 3DE dataset can be visualized interactively using a number of 3D visualization and rendering software packages. 3DE images can be viewed as volume rendered images, surface rendered or wire-frame display images, and 2D tomographic slices.

Volume rendered images

Volume rendering provides an 'en face' view of the structure of interest and of its anatomical spatial relationships, not obtainable by 2DE. It is particularly useful for evaluating valves and adjacent anatomic structures. Shading techniques, such as opacification, brightness, and smoothing, and various colour maps are used to generate a 3D display improving the perception of depth and enhancing the texture of cardiac structures (see ⊃ Fig. 5.3).

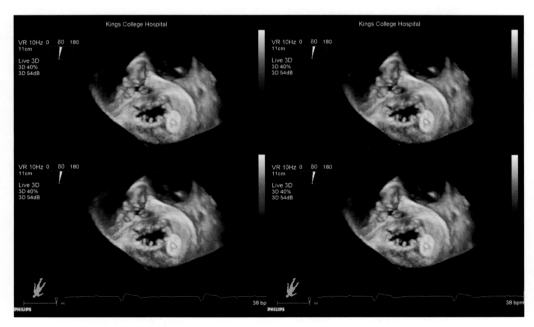

Fig. 5.3 An example of different volume rendering of the mitral valve obtained by changing the colour map and the shading techniques. The mitral valve is imaged in the surgical view. A posterior mitral valve ring can be appreciated. Furthermore an occluder plug used to close a paravalvular leak can also be seen at the level of the P3 segment.

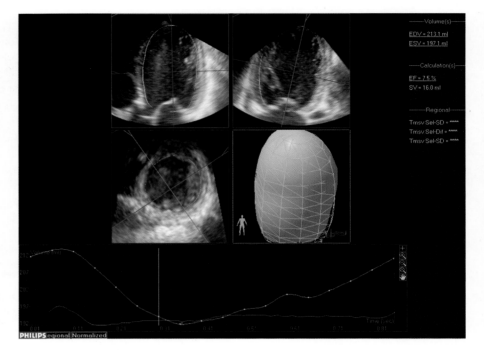

Fig. 5.4 3D analysis of the left ventricle. Semi-automatically detected LV contours are combined together in order to generate a 3D model of the left ventricle. The wireframe surface-rendering technique is used to visualize the endocardial border during diastole and improve the appreciation of left ventricular contraction. In this case the LV is severely dilated with severely impaired systolic function.

Surface rendered images

Surface rendering allows the visualization of structures in a solid appearance. It is mainly used to display models of the ventricles and of the left atrium (LA), improving the visual assessment of their volumes and function. Solid and wire-frame surface-rendering techniques can be combined to appreciate the extent of cardiac chambers' motion and their changes in volume during the cardiac cycle. In order to obtain the 3D render the endocardium can be traced manually in cross-sectional views generated from the 3D dataset or using a semiautomatic border detection algorithm. These contours are combined together to produce a 3D shape that can be visualized as a solid object or a wireframe (see ➲ Fig. 5.4). See 📹 Video 5.2.

2D tomographic slices

2D tomographic slices' mode consists of perpendicular 2D views (coronal, sagittal, and transverse) obtained from the same 3D dataset displayed simultaneously in a cineloop format; or of multiple 2D parallel tomographic slices. This technique is particularly useful in 3D stress echocardiography (see ➲ Fig. 5.5).

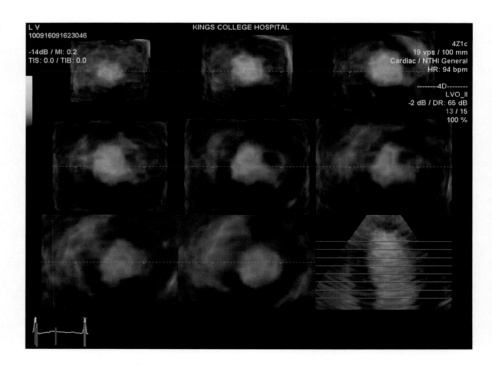

Fig. 5.5 Representation of tomographic slices obtained by cutting the left ventricle across multiple parallel short-axis planes. This is useful to analyse regional wall motion as during this case of dobutamine stress echocardiogram (DSE) with the use of contrast.

Pitfalls

Patient selection

In order to obtain a good-quality 3D dataset it is important to understand which acquisition modality is most appropriate for each specific clinical setting. This capability comes with experience and frequent use of 3D technology. We have described two common clinical scenarios as examples.

In patients not capable of breath-holding or in the presence of arrhythmia, such as atrial fibrillation, 3D zoom represents the modality of choice, as it provides a reasonable volume rate without stitching artefacts. These are related to translation of the heart during breathing or to irregular cardiac cycles. One beat (real-time) full-volume acquisition can also be used in this setting; however, there are some compromises required, as previously discussed. On the other hand, in patients in sinus rhythm and capable of breath-holding, the stitched 3D full-volume is the method of choice to image a large structure (e.g. left ventricle), as it provides in 3–5 beats excellent temporal resolution with a dataset volume wide enough to contain all the required information.

Dataset optimization

It is not possible to produce a high-quality diagnostic 3D dataset if the 2D dataset is not optimized. Optimal-gain setting is mandatory. Low gain could result in dropout, with the risk of eliminating information. On the other hand, a high-gain setting could lead to a decrease in resolution, loss of 3D perspective, and artefacts.

The 'ideal' quality 3D dataset is a compromise between the spatial and temporal maximum resolutions achievable. An increased scan line density will improve spatial resolution; however, this results in a longer acquisition phase (susceptible to stitching artefacts). To improve the temporal resolution (volume rate), the sector size should be minimized, focusing on the volume of interest.

Optimal views of acquisition

3D TTE examination should be performed from multiple transducer positions. However, there are specific 3D views that enable higher temporal and spatial resolutions due to the closer position of the structure of interest to the transducer. For example, to image the mitral valve, the best approach is from the parasternal long-axis window. For the aortic valve, the parasternal approach also allows higher spatial resolution, while the apical approach allows the '*en face*' visualization of the valve. Apical window is the most appropriate for the LV and LA volume acquisition.

Artefacts

Knowledge of the main artefacts in 3D echocardiography is important for correct interpretation of the acquired images. The principal types of artefacts consist of:

◆ Stitching artefacts.
◆ Dropout artefacts.
◆ Blurring and blooming artefacts.
◆ Artefacts related to gain settings.

Stitching artefacts

One of the main limitations of the full-volume and colour Doppler modes is the potential for thin 'fault lines' to appear between the sub-volumes after reconstruction. These lines, known as stitching artefacts, can be caused by irregular R–R intervals or by any movement of the heart relative to the transducer during image acquisition. Stitching artefacts not only impair image quality, but also hinder analysis and make it challenging to image patients with an arrhythmia. This is a problem that has been overcome by the latest generation of transducers and software, which have recently been released. Acquisition times have now been reduced to such an extent that they are capable of high frame rate and full volume 90° by 90° acquisitions, including 3D colour Doppler, all in one cardiac cycle. This abolishes the potential for stitching artefacts, making it easier to accurately image patients with arrhythmias. See 🎦 Video 5.1.

Dropout artefacts

Dropout artefacts are caused by loss of 3D surface information related to poor echo-signal intensity of delicate intra-cardiac structures (i.e. inter-atrial septum). This typically results in a false 'hole'. Discriminating between a true defect or a dropout can be very challenging and requires experience. To achieve a correct interpretation of dropout artefact, it is useful to compare 3D volume with 2D views of the same structure with and without colour Doppler. To minimize this kind of artefact, it is important to use an appropriate gain setting (avoiding overgain), high frequency, and to orientate the structure of interest perpendicular to the transducer.

Blurring and blooming artefacts

These are mainly caused by inaccurate voxel interpolation between distant image lines and are inversely proportional to line density [5]. Blurring refers to the thicker representation of thin structures (i.e. mitral valve leaflets, mitral subvalvular apparatus). Blooming refers more to unsharp representation of high echo-density structures, mainly artificial structures (i.e. mechanical prosthesis or pacemaker leads). However, blooming and blurring artefacts commonly coexist.

Gain artefacts

Gain artefacts are related to overgaining, which may cause an effect of smoke or noise that can completely obscure the structure of interest. In order to avoid this phenomena, and to achieve an optimal representation, it is advisable to turn up the gain setting until the smoke appears, then turn it down just to the point where the smoke has disappeared (see ➲ Fig. 5.6).

Advantages and limitations of 3D versus conventional 2D echocardiography

Clinical research in 3DE concentrated at first on chamber quantification. Following the development of 'interventional echocardiography', the focus has moved mainly on the assessment of valve disease and on other conditions, such as patent foramen ovale (PFO) and atrial septal defect (ASD). The principal advantage of a direct volumetric acquisition is overcoming image foreshortening and any geometric assumptions on cardiac structures. Moreover, 3DE supplies volumetric information of the structure of interest

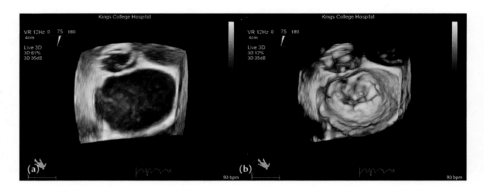

Fig. 5.6 (a) 3D zoom of the mitral valve obtained with high gain setting where structure detail has been obscured by noise (smoke) artefacts. (b) The gain setting has been turned down in the same dataset. The mitral valve anatomy can now be fully appreciated (stenotic, rheumatic valve).

in relation to contiguous cardiac structures. We have summarized the main current applications of 3D echocardiography, comparing it with conventional 2D echocardiography.

Left ventricle

One of the most important, widely researched, and current clinical applications of 3DE TTE is LV quantification. The main forms of analysis that can be performed are LV mass, global function (volumes and ejection fraction), and regional function, for which a number of off-line software packages are available. In addition, most vendors have some form of on-cart quantification package available. 3D LV mass analysis can be done from a full volume by using an anatomically corrected biplane technique and semi-automated border detection. Not only is this technique relatively quick and easy, but it has been proven to be more accurate than 2D or M–mode calculations when compared to cardiac magnetic resonance imaging (CMR) [6, 7], which the current gold standard for mass and volumes. In order to obtain global LV function, semi-automated border tracking software can be used to create a mathematical cast of the LV throughout the cardiac cycle and from this volumes and ejection fraction are extracted, completely dispelling the need for geometric assumptions (see ⊃ Fig. 5.4).

In this context, multiple research publications have proven the superiority of this technique over 2D and M-mode measurements when compared to CMR. Correlation has been very good with the gold standard technique, albeit with a tendency for echocardiography to slightly underestimate volumes, probably because of the difference in endocardial border visualization [8]. Furthermore, 3DE has better inter-observer, intra-observer, and test–retest variability [9] than 2D, and has been shown to have significant clinical impact when assessing patients for interventions [10]. The mathematical cast described can also be used to provide regional information. It can be divided into the American Society of Echocardiography 16 or 17 segment models, and for each segment a regional ejection fraction can be obtained, as well as a time to minimum volume. From this data a systolic dyssynchrony index can be calculated [11], which is based on the time to minimum volume of all the segments. This technique gives a measure of the intra-ventricular mechanical dyssynchrony and there is a mounting body of evidence supporting its use in the selection of patients for cardiac resynchronization therapy. Further subdivision of this model, into over 800 segments, can be performed with the time to peak contraction of each one colour-coded. This information

can be merged to give a dynamic parametric image known as a contraction front map. This technique offers an intuitive display of mechanical contraction, with an ability to rapidly demonstrate significant areas of myocardial delay (see ⊃ Fig. 5.7).

Another important aspect of LV assessment is stress imaging, which can now be performed with 3DE, with or without contrast enhancement. 3D stress echocardiography has the potential to overcome the major limitations of 2D stress echocardiography, such as LV foreshortening and difficulties in matching the same myocardial segment during the different stages of the acquisition protocol [12]. A 3D dataset allows a multi-plane view with the simultaneous display of all major orthogonal planes as well as a multi-slice view with multiple short-axis images extracted from LV apex to base. See 🎥 Video 5.3. The overall wall motion is simultaneously assessed in different planes, whereas in 2DE the various planes are imaged at different times. For these reasons the accuracy in diagnosis of regional wall motion abnormalities (RWMA) is potentially greater than in 2D stress echocardiography. 3D is also less operator-dependent and has reduced inter-observer variability compared to 2D [13–17]. However, 3D stress requires a longer analysis time, and temporal and spatial resolutions are lower than in 2D. Nevertheless, in the latest generation of single-beat acquisition and smaller footprint matrix transducers, the frame rate has improved (40 frames/s with good temporal resolution); single-beat acquisition also avoids stitching artefacts and reduces the acquisition time. Dedicated 3D stress echo viewers provide semi-automated, side-by-side analysis of multiple cross-sections during different stress stages; this will save data analysis time and may help 3D stress echo become more clinically attractive.

3D myocardial perfusion imaging has also been investigated in the setting of dobutamine and adenosine stress echocardiography, producing good preliminary results; however, this technique is still limited to dedicated research departments [18–20].

Right ventricle

The complicated geometrical structure and asymmetry of the RV, both in health and disease, has significantly limited 2D quantification of size and function. This chamber is often not explored enough with the standard RV projections and is subject to misinterpretation with the modified ones. 3D analysis has been shown to be more accurate, as it does not rely on geometrical assumptions that may be applied to the right ventricle improperly. There are two different ways to analyse an RV dataset: a 3D summation-of-disks method, based

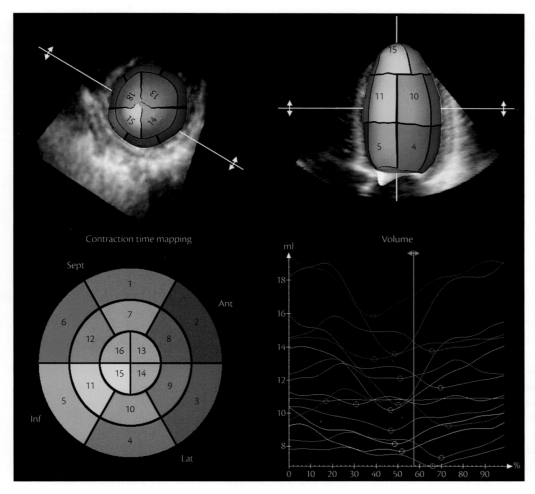

Fig. 5.7 A semi-automated border tracking software is used to create a mathematical cast of the left ventricle. This can then be segmented for regional analysis (16-segments model). Regional time–volume curves are seen in the bottom right of the LV providing a visual assessment of LV dyssynchrony.

on manual tracing of six to ten parallel cross-sectional RV planes [21, 22], or dedicated analysis software, which creates a mathematical cast and global time–volume curves similar to the one that can be created for the LV. Again global volumes can be obtained and ejection fraction calculated. This technique has been validated *in vitro* [23] and *in vivo* in children and adults in different clinical settings, and is accurate when compared to CMR [24]. The advantages of 3D imaging over 2D are improved inter-observer variability and a reduced underestimation of the RV end-diastolic and end-systolic volumes compared to CMR both in healthy subjects [2] and in RV pathology [25–28]. However, 3D analysis is still time-consuming and requires experienced operators and very good quality datasets in order to produce reliable measurements.

Left atrium

The LA has an important role in cardiac performance due to its capability to dilate and remodel in relation to the LV filling pressures. It represents a good marker of the magnitude and duration of LV systolic and diastolic dysfunction, and a validated prognostic marker [29–32]. In the most recent guidelines on chamber quantification [33], volume determinations have been advised over linear dimensions, as they allow accurate assessment of any asymmetric remodelling of the LA. 3D TTE has been demonstrated to be more accurate and reproducible than 2D TTE compared to CMR [34] and cardiac CT [35] (see ⊃ Fig. 5.8).

3D TEE has now an important role in the assessment of the LA before ablation procedures [36] and percutaneous closure of LA

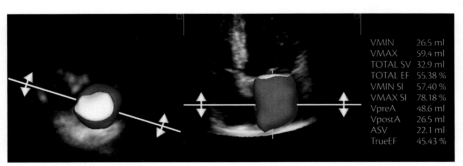

VMIN	26.5 ml
VMAX	59.4 ml
TOTAL SV	32.9 ml
TOTAL EF	55.38 %
VMIN SI	57.40 %
VMAX SI	78.18 %
VpreA	48.6 ml
VpostA	26.5 ml
ASV	22.1 ml
TrueEF	45.43 %

Fig. 5.8 Accurate LA systolic and diastolic volumes and ejection fraction obtained by 3D analysis and volumetric spatial representation of the LA.

appendage. 3D TEE provides an accurate anatomical visualization of the atrial structures, such as the LA ridge, LA isthmus, LA appendage, and pulmonary veins.

The LA appendage is complex in shape, elongated, often multilobar, and usually heavily trabeculated with pectinate muscles. A 3D TEE assessment can be very useful in this setting. The acquisition of a single 3D volume overcomes the need to obtain multiple views of the appendage from different angles, as the 3D dataset can be cropped in the post-processing phase through an infinite number of planes. This potentially reduces the study length. In the setting of percutaneous LA appendage closure, 3D TEE has an important role in identifying an accurate appendage orifice area, which is essential for the subsequent sizing of the closure device [37]. Moreover, 3D TEE is very useful in monitoring the percutaneous closure procedure and in the assessment of its results once completed.

Mitral valve

The mitral valve (MV) and the mitral subvalvular apparatus are optimally imaged by 3DE with an 'en face' view of the valve from both LV and LA perspectives. The view of the MV imaged with an LA perspective is called 'surgical view', as it represents what a surgeon sees standing on the right side of the patient and looking at the MV from an open LA (see ⊃ Fig. 5.9). In MV imaging, a 3D transoesophageal approach provides significantly better images compared to TTE; however, both of the methods can be used for a detailed assessment of the MV. 3D echo visualizes the spatial relationship of the valve with the surrounding structures. In the post-processing phase, it is possible to perform a segmental analysis of each scallop, achieving an anatomically correct orifice area and obtaining functional data with 3D colour Doppler (see ⊃ Fig. 5.10). It is also feasible to image the MV annulus, which it is not possible to assess in its shape and perimeter by 2D echo.

Data have suggested that a good 3D TTE can abolish the need for 2D TEE in conditions such as MV prolapse [38].

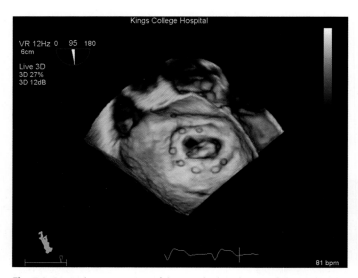

Fig. 5.9 Surgical 3D zoom view of the mitral valve. There is a full ring placed during previous mitral valve repair. The A2 segment of the mitral valve is flail and prolapsing into the LA.

3D is considered superior to 2D in evaluating the extent and location of MV disease, especially in the presence of commissural pathology and cleft, as well as in defining the exact mechanism of valve dysfunction. Moreover, the direct comparison between the 3D surgical view and the intra-operative findings, facilitates an effective communication with cardiothoracic surgeons, both in the pre-operative assessment of valve pathology and in evaluation of the surgical results.

In the context of prosthetic valves, 3D colour Doppler is very useful in identifying the exact origin and severity of a paravalvular leak, which can be very challenging with 2D TEE.

3DE is also superior to 2DE for the quantification of mitral valve stenosis (MVS). MV 3D planimetry is a direct, accurate, and relatively haemodynamically independent measurement of mitral valve area (MVA) and it is recommended as the method of choice for assessment of MVS by the recent European guidelines on the management of valve disease [39]. With the simultaneous display of the three orthogonal planes, it is often possible to optimally position a plane at the MV leaflets' tip, obtaining the smallest MV orifice area (see ⊃ Fig. 5.11a).

This measurement can be very challenging with 2DE due to calcification, distortion of the MV anatomy, and significant LA enlargement. Moreover, in the setting of MV regurgitation, 3D colour Doppler can add important information on the effective regurgitant orifice area, and on the shape and dimension of the vena contracta, eliminating any geometrical assumption on its shape, which is elliptical in many patients. The 3D vena contracta area correlates also more closely with Doppler-derived effective regurgitant orifice area, than 2D vena contracta diameter [40].

Finally, MV quantification software offers a multitude of measurements, not obtainable by 2DE, such as annular areas, leaflet tenting volumes, and mitral aortic offset angle. These measurements could potentially have a role in improving the planning of mitral valve replacement (MVR).

Aortic valve

Currently, the gold standard technique to assess the effective AV area (AVA) in AV stenosis (AVS) is the continuity equation, which implies measurement of the transvalvular velocity and of the LV outflow tract (LVOT) by 2DE. However, the continuity equation is based on the geometric assumption of LVOT circularity, which can make the AVA calculation not completely accurate, as it has been shown to be elliptical in many patients [41, 42]. Therefore, with an accurate 3D measurement of the LVOT area, it is possible to overcome geometrical assumptions and obtain a more reliable estimation of the AVA in the continuity equation.

A correct estimation of AVS can also be achieved by 3D planimetry of the valve [43, 44]. This post-processing method is based on an accurate positioning of one of the three orthogonal planes at the level of the tips of the aortic valve cusps in systole, where AVA is smallest. The true AVA will be displayed in the perpendicular plane. It is possible to measure it by manual tracing. This could also lead to correct measurement in valves of unusual geometries (degenerated or bicuspid valves) (see ⊃ Fig. 5.11b).

An accurate assessment of the aortic valve can be challenging due to its small size and to frequent thickening and calcification

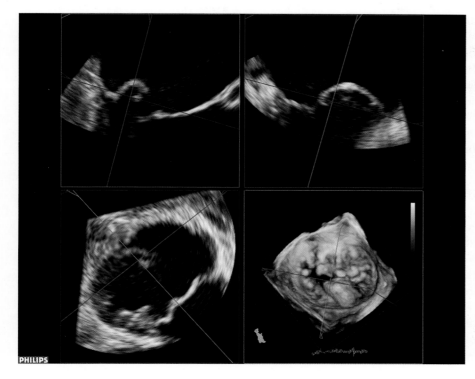

Fig. 5.10 Multi-planar reconstruction of a mitral valve imaged with zoomed, 3D TEE echocardiography. Orthogonal cut planes are used to accurately identify a flail P2 segment.

of the leaflets. With the development of TAVI, AV assessment by 3D TEE has acquired a fundamental role as guidance for choosing the optimal prosthesis size. 3D TEE enables the operator to accurately assess annulus dimensions and shape, location and amount of calcifications, aortic root dimensions and distance between the coronary arteries and the aortic annulus providing invaluable information [45].

Tricuspid and pulmonary valve

3D transthoracic assessment of tricuspid and pulmonary valves is considerably more challenging, primarily because of their locations and the thinness of the leaflets. Clinical roles have been researched, but they are less well-delineated.

Transoesophageal echocardiography for guidance of non-coronary trans-catheter interventions

3D TEE has gained a new important field of application after the recent development and diffusion of non-coronary trans-catheter interventions. 3D echo has become an invaluable diagnostic tool in procedures such as TAVI, mitral valve clip, ASD, PFO, LA appendage percutaneous closure, and percutaneous occluder implantation for paravalvular leaks.

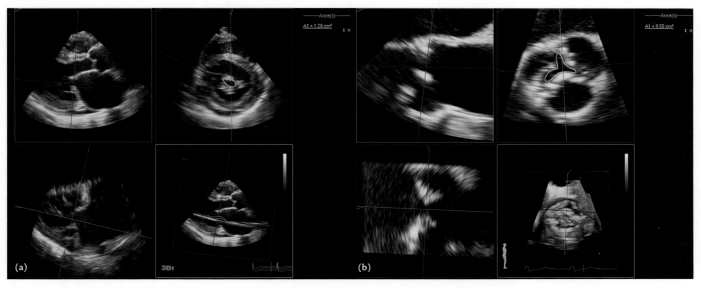

Fig. 5.11 Measurement of the MV area (a) and AV area (b) through an optimal plane position at the leaflet tips. On the red plane the minimum valve orifices are displayed and the valve orifice areas measured. There is moderate rheumatic mitral stenosis (a) and severe aortic stenosis in a restricted and calcified valve (b).

The rationale behind the use of 3D TEE in these settings is the need of an optimal pre-procedural structural assessment, and continuous soft-tissue imaging during the intervention (which cannot be provided by fluoroscopy alone). It also provides prompt monitoring of the final result and possible complications. 3D compared to 2D provides accurate visualization of devices, balloons, guide wires, and catheters assessing their position in relation to the surrounding cardiac anatomy [46]. It allows continuous real-time imaging of structures of interest, avoiding the necessity to constantly change the angle of acquisition in order to detect the position of catheters, wires, and balloons.

Trans-catheter closure of PFO and ASD

PFO and ASD closure are now widely performed procedures. In the majority of the cases a combination of fluoroscopy and TEE is used to guide and monitor the device deployment and to assess the final result. 3D TEE has great capability in this setting as it provides anatomical views and leads to an accurate estimation of the shape and dimensions of the defect without the necessity of mental reconstruction. Moreover 3DE supplies information about surrounding structures (such as the aortic rim and pulmonary veins, etc.) representing the most accurate peri-procedural imaging tool (see ⊃ Fig. 5.12).

Percutaneous aortic valve implantation

The recent guidelines on the Use of Echocardiography in New Transcatheter Interventions for Valvular Heart Disease [45] recommend TEE prior to TAVI if there are any concerns on the assessment of the aortic root anatomy, aortic annular size, or number of cusps. Accurate sizing of the prosthesis is also critical to TAVI

procedural success. The views obtained by 2D TEE are limited to a short-axis view and a long-axis view of the structures (annulus, aortic root). 3D TEE overcomes this limitation by providing an anatomical visualization leading to a more accurate sizing. It is also fundamental in determining the distance between the annulus and the ostium of the right and left coronary arteries obtained to avoid ostial occlusion during the valve deployment. 3D TEE measurements have been shown to correlate very well with CT and the two techniques can be considered interchangeable. During the procedure, 3D TEE supplies continuous monitoring of the prosthesis position. Once the valve is implanted, 3D colour flow provides invaluable information on presence, location, and severity of residual valvular and paravalvular leaks.

Mitral valve clip

Mitral valve clip is now a treatment option in the setting of severe degenerative (prolapse or flail of A2/P2) or functional MV regurgitation in patients unsuitable for open heart surgery [47, 48]. The device is delivered via percutaneous femoral venous transseptal access. The mitral clip grasps the scallops of the MV creating a double orifice, which increases the leaflets' coaptation and reduces the degree of regurgitation. This technique is an echocardiographically guided interventional procedure, as TEE guides the transseptal puncture and the optimal alignment of the device in the LA. 3D TEE compared with 2D furnishes an anatomical view of the inter-atrial septum for the inter-atrial puncture and provides an 'en face' view of the MV, which is particularly helpful in monitoring the perpendicular orientation of the clip to the MV coaptation line. Moreover, with 3D colour Doppler it is possible to more accurately assess the severity and the position of the regurgitant jets

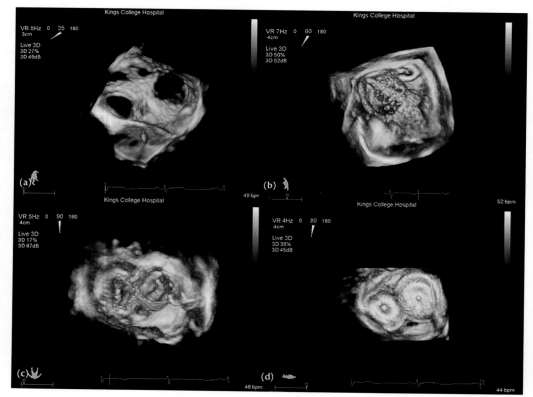

Fig. 5.12 A selection of 3D TEE pictures during a percutaneous closure of two ASDs. (a) The two defects (ostium secundum and sinus venosus) are visualized in their 3D shape. (b) A balloon used to measure the defect size is already inflated in the ostium secundum ASD. A guide wire is passed through the sinus venosus ASD from the right to the left atrium (c) Both balloons are inflated in the two ASDs. (d) The two closure devices are *in situ* with an excellent final result.

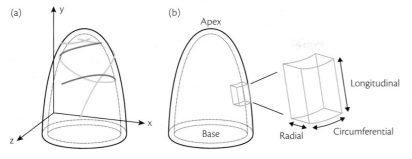

Fig. 5.13 (a) Myocardial fibres of the LV wall are arranged in layers of different helical fibre orientation which results in a complex LV deformation. (b) For clinical use, LV deformation is reported relative to the LV itself as longitudinal, radial (transverse) and circumferential. In addition, torsion occurs.

before and after clip positioning and to determine if a second clip is needed.

Paravalvular leak closure

In paravalvular leak closure, 3D colour Doppler is particularly useful for correctly identifying the location of the leak(s). Obtaining an optimal dataset without echo dropout is crucial to avoid misdiagnosis. The superiority of 3D TEE over 2D TEE in the procedure monitoring relies on obtaining anatomical views of the closure device in relation to the surrounding structures.

Technical issues and future perspective

Before the advent of one-beat acquisition capability, 3D echocardiography was mainly limited by translation of the heart during respiration or by irregular heart rate. This new technique has overcome these issues, with the disadvantage of reduced temporal and spatial resolutions. Research efforts in this setting are to achieve the highest spatial and volume rates in a single-beat acquisition. Intelligent software promises fully automated analyses, potentially further reducing subjectivity and improving workflow.

The advent of dedicated stress viewing packages will facilitate the application of clinical 3D stress echo, and 3D perfusion offers the hope of volumetric quantification of perfusion defects. 3D speckle tracking has now also been developed and promises to give us true 3D myocardial deformation. Direct volumetric acquisitions also allow the possibility of fusion imaging with CMR, computed tomography, and SPECT. In the crowded setting of the cardiac catheter lab, integrated small 3D imaging consoles will allow better use of space and better access to the patients by the team involved in the procedure. It should also reduce the radiation exposure of the echocardiographer.

Deformation imaging: 2D and 3D techniques

Key concepts of myocardial function quantification

The evaluation of myocardial function by echocardiography is based on observing and interpreting the motion of tissue within the scan-plane or volume by either Doppler-based velocity measurements or tracking-based displacement measurements. All other function parameters, such as deformation, rotation, or torsion are directly or indirectly derived from what has been discussed.

All echocardiographically derived functional parameters are load-dependent. Therefore, their appropriate clinical interpretation requires considering the load of the myocardial fibres, which may vary according to chamber geometry, wall curvature, wall thickness, or cavity pressures. In a clinical setting, combining parameters under an opposite influence of loading (e.g. E/e') is, in some cases, a practical solution.

LV myocardial architecture and deformation

Myocardial fibre architecture of the LV is characterized by helical layers of different fibre direction. The resulting deformation of the myocardium is three-dimensional and complex. For practical reasons, LV deformation is usually described relative to the LV long axis, by reporting the longitudinal, radial, and circumferential deformation component. The rotational deformation or torsion of the entire LV is reflected in regional shear (see ➲ Fig. 5.13).

Tissue Doppler

Principles and data acquisition

Tissue Doppler is available as spectral and colour Doppler. A so-called 'wall filter' distinguishes signals from tissue and blood motion, depending on signal strength and velocity. Handling, optional settings, and aliasing issues are comparable with blood pool Doppler (see ➲ Fig. 5.14). Colour Doppler is the imaging modality with the best temporal resolution (frame rate) in clinical cardiology. The frame rate can be optimized by reducing depth and sector width of both grey scale and Doppler sector, and by selecting a low line density at the cost of low lateral resolution. During acquisition, care should be taken to avoid reverberation artefacts, which will particularly disturb strain rate estimations over a wide area (see ➲ Fig. 5.15). The motion direction of the interrogated myocardium should be aligned with the ultrasound beams. Data should be acquired unsparingly over at least three beats (i.e. covering at least four QRS) and stored in a raw data format for post-processing. The additional acquisition of blood-flow Doppler spectra of the in- and outlet valves of the interrogated ventricle is recommended since that allows exact definition of cardiac time intervals (see ➲ Fig. 5.17).

Post-processing

Spectral Doppler data cannot be further processed. Peak values or slopes are measured directly on the spectral display. ➲ Figure 5.16

Fig. 5.14 Settings for spectral and colour Doppler acquisition and display. (a) high (green) and low (red) frame rate acquisition of the same velocity curve. Note the blunting of the sharp diastolic peaks. Isovolumic peaks are not valid any more. (b) Tissue priority high (left) and low (right) as well as (c) Transparency high (left) and low (right) influence the display of colour data compared to the underlying grey scale image. Data content of the acquisition is not affected. (d) Low velocity reject low (left) and high (right) removes clutter signals around baseline. (e) A threshold setting low (left) and high (right) suppresses weak signals in the background.

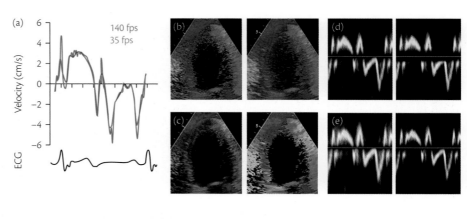

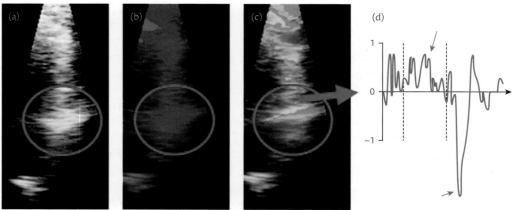

Fig. 5.15 Reverberation artefacts (red circles), visible as white stationary lines in the grey scale image (a) lead to wrong velocity estimates (b) and disturb strain/~rate calculation (c and d).

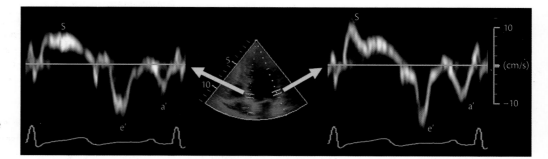

Fig. 5.16 Normal tissue Doppler spectra from the basal septum (left) and the basal lateral wall (right). Note the different amplitude and shape of the curves.

shows normal curve patterns from the basal septum and lateral wall.

Colour Doppler data can be post-processed in many ways. They are either visualized as reconstructed curves of regional function parameters or as colour-coded images (2D or as straight or curved M-mode) (see ➲ Figs 5.17 and 5.27). Particularly curved M-mode displays provide easy visual access to the regional and temporal distribution of a parameter within the interrogated wall. Curve reconstructions are possible from any point within a stored dataset (see ➲ Fig. 5.17) with the advantage that the sample volume position can track the motion of the myocardium throughout the entire cardiac cycle. The time course of a spectral Doppler velocity curve is similar to a colour-derived one. However, absolute values cannot be used interchangeably, since most labs measure on the outer edge of the spectrum, while colour Doppler data approximate the median velocity of a region.

Parameters of myocardial function

Colour Doppler datasets can be used to calculate derived parameters, such as motion (displacement), deformation and deformation rate (strain and strain rate), rotation, rotational deformation (twist, torsion), as well as to display the temporal course of events, such as the time of appearance of velocity peaks (tissue synchronicity imaging; see ➲ Fig. 5.19) or phase differences between myocardial regions (VVI phase map; see ➲ Fig. 5.20).

Velocity

By default, colour Doppler imaging delivers velocity values, comparable to spectral Doppler. Data are given in [cm/s] (see ➲ Fig. 5.17a).

Motion

Motion or displacement is the temporal integral of the tissue velocity. It describes the motion component of the tissue in the

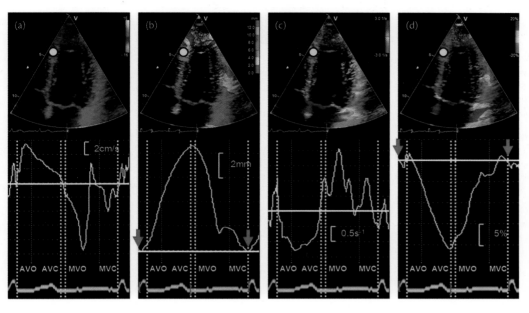

Fig. 5.17 Different function parameters, derived from one region of interest within the same colour Doppler dataset. Top panels: colour coded display, below curves, bottom: ECG. (a) velocity, (b) displacement, (c) strain rate, (d) strain. Note that in this case the baseline is—arbitrarily— set to the curve value (red arrows) at the automatically recognized beginning of QRS (red opening bracket).

sample volume towards and away from the transducer during the cardiac cycle (see ⊃ Fig. 5.17b).

Strain rate

Strain rate is the temporal derivative of myocardial deformation. It describes how fast the tissue changes its length. Strain rate is given in 1/s (see ⊃ Fig. 5.17c).

Strain

Strain or deformation describes the relative regional length or thickness change of myocardium. When interrogated with tissue Doppler echocardiography, it is calculated as temporal integral of strain rate. Strain is unitless and usually given as a percentage (see ⊃ Fig. 5.17d). In most cases, a potential baseline drift is automatically compensated by the analysis software (see ⊃ Fig. 5.18).

For the calculation of deformation and deformation rate one can refer to a baseline value (Lagrangian strain/~rate) or sum up the instantaneous changes (natural strain/~rate). Both approaches differ in values but can be converted into each other. The type of strain/~rate used needs to be reported.

Motion and deformation of the myocardium are cyclic processes with no natural beginning or end. Therefore, the position of the baseline (zero line) is arbitrary. Most analysis packages define zero automatically as the value at the beginning of the QRS complex (red arrows in ⊃ Fig. 5.17b; ⊃ Fig. 5.17d) and report in measurements the actual position or length change relative to that. This approach may be inappropriate under certain circumstances (e.g. bundle branch blocks). The definition used must always be considered and reported.

Tissue synchronicity

Tissue synchronicity imaging uses regular velocity data. Only the colour coding of the 2D display is changed to a colour scale, which codes the time of the first occurrence of a positive velocity

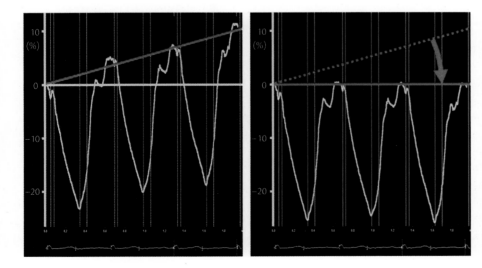

Fig. 5.18 Integration of velocity or strain rate data often results in considerable baseline shifts of the resulting motion or strain (left panel) curves. Most software allows a linear correction (right panel). Note that both systolic and diastolic values are influenced by this correction.

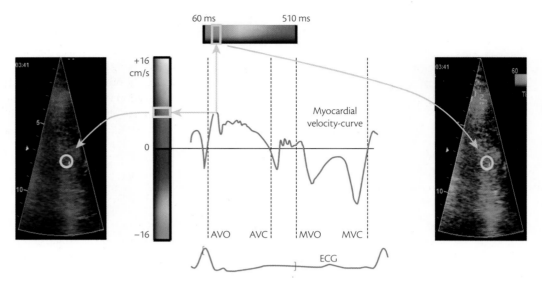

Fig. 5.19 Principle of tissue synchronicity imaging. While regular colour Doppler displays encode the velocity of the myocardium (left panel), tissue synchronicity imaging (TSI) detects the first positive velocity peak in a certain time window (given by the red brackets on the ECG) and uses a green-red colour scale to encode the time to appearance of this peak, resulting in a motion delay display (right panel). Motion delays do not necessarily display contraction delays.

peak after a certain point in time (begin QRS, aortic valve opening, etc.; see ➲ Fig. 5.19). Measurement results are therefore given in ms.

Speckle tracking

Principles and data acquisition

Speckle tracking is based on image analysis. A software algorithm recognizes patterns in the images (e.g. 'speckles') and measures their displacement frame by frame. Since the frame rate of the echo loop is known, the velocity of one speckle and—using several speckles—the regional deformation of the myocardium can be estimated (see ➲ Fig. 5.21). In contrast to Doppler measurements, tissue tracking works in all directions within the image plane, i.e. it also identifies the direction of motion. With this, additional parameters, such as rotation, become directly available.

Tissue tracking requires regular grey-scale data of excellent quality. Reverberation artefacts, noise, and shadowing have to be avoided by all means.

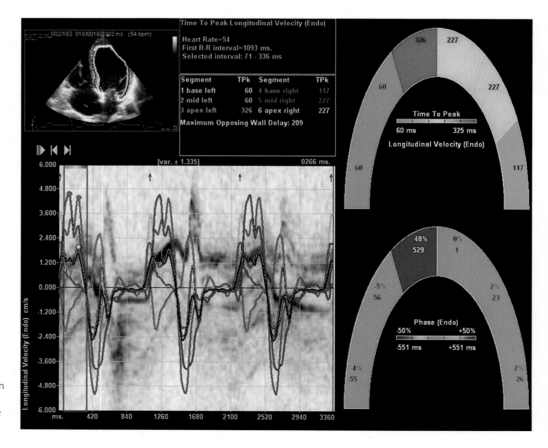

Fig. 5.20 Phase imaging (lower graph on the right) is another way of displaying inhomogeneous timing of ventricular motion. The off-set is given in percent of the cycle length and displayed in colour depending on the average value per segment.

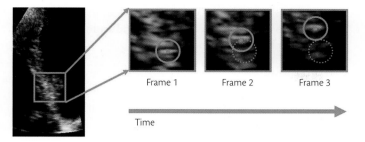

Fig. 5.21 Prominent speckles in the image are recognized and followed frame by frame. The measured displacement between frames allows calculation of velocity and direction of motion. Tracking several speckles allows the calculation of two-dimensional deformation.

Like in tissue Doppler imaging, sector width and depth have to be optimized to allow high frame rates. Unlike tissue Doppler, however, lateral resolution needs to be preserved to allow good tracking across the beams. Therefore, typical frame rates rarely exceed 80 frames/s, which limits the technique mainly to the analysis of systolic events (see ⮌ Fig. 5.14a). For the same reason, tracking-derived velocity and deformation rate data should be used with caution.

A three-beat acquisition is recommended, although most software uses single beats for analysis.

Post-processing

The different steps of post-processing are vendor-specific but usually comprise a semi-automated selection of the region to be interrogated, a short waiting time for processing by the tracking algorithm, and a subsequent display of the tracking result.

The tracking result must be carefully checked on a sub-segment scale by visually comparing the motion of the tracking points to the motion of the underlying grey-scale data. Software that does not allow this control step should not be used. Estimates on tracking quality provided by the software may be considered, but cannot replace a careful visual inspection (see ⮌ Fig. 5.22, 📹 Video 5.4, Video 5.5).

Complex regularization algorithms are usually applied to derive clinically meaningful velocity, motion, and deformation estimates from the initially very noisy tracking data. This post-processing is vendor-specific and usually cannot be controlled by the user. The underlying algorithms influence the measurements of a certain myocardial region and may lead to an under- or overestimation of the interrogated parameter.

On the other hand, automated post-processing, with limited user interaction is convenient and allows fast data analysis and a higher reproducibility of tracking results compared to tissue Doppler and other 'manual' echocardiographic measurements. See 📹 Video 5.6.

Tracking-derived parameters of myocardial function

Tissue tracking can provide all parameters known from tissue Doppler, such as velocity, motion, deformation rate, and deformation. Limitations due to frame rate and tracking quality have to be considered. Data are available in all directions within the image plane. In general, however, tracking results along the ultrasound beam are more reliable than those perpendicular to it. By default, most tracking software provide options to select a display of results along or perpendicular to the endocardial contour. Tracking measurements may differ from Doppler due to data quality and due to the differing segmentation of the ventricle, which usually includes the very apical region. Vendor-specific differences are still common and prevent a direct comparison of measurements. The following additional information can be derived by tracking (see ⮌ Fig. 5.23):

- Rotation, twist, and torsion. Rotation is usually understood as an in-plane turning of the entire ventricular slice [49] and is given in degrees (°). The term 'twist' (given in degrees) should be used to describe the difference in apical and basal rotation of a ventricle. When normalized to the distance between the rotating planes the term 'torsion' should be used (given in degrees/cm).

- Rotation rate, twist rate, and torsion rate. Temporal derivatives are possible from all mentioned parameters but critical due to the limited frame rate of tracking data.

The described parameters of rotational deformation refer to the entire ventricle. On a regional level, they are better represented by cirumferential strain/~rate and CL shear strain/~rate. The concept of describing rotational deformation of the LV by means of 2D speckle tracking is challenged by the fact that apical and basal image planes are never truly parallel and that their distance cannot be determined. Therefore, measurements vary a lot and are currently not recommended for clinical use [50].

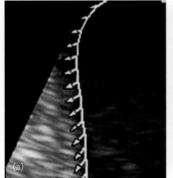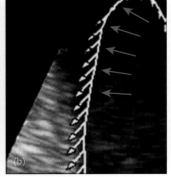

Fig. 5.22 Careful visual inspection of the tracking result is mandatory. Detail of endocardial tracking in the apex: (a) good tracking, (b) bad tracking, since the line does not follow the myocardium.

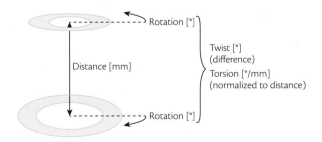

Fig. 5.23 Parameters describing rotational deformation. Grey rings indicate apical and basal short-axis planes in which rotation is measured. Twist and torsion can be calculated as described in the text.

Global function assessment by tracking

Tracking techniques can favourably be applied to global LV function assessment. Combining a semi-automated contouring and tracking of the LV with the method of discs (Simpson) results in a faster volume and ejection fraction assessment with improved reproducibility and inter-observer variability [51]. Global longitudinal strain is defined as deformation of the entire LV contour, either mid-wall or endocardial (vendor-specific). It has been shown to be sensitive to subtle LV function changes and to be more reproducible compared to classic ejection fraction assessments. Values may differ between vendors, depending on the definition of the parameter and on the algorithm used.

Three-dimensional regional function estimation

Principles

With the evolution of real-time 3D imaging, 'full-volume' datasets have become available. In 3D post-processing, LV endocardial contouring is usually fully automated and allows fast and accurate volume and global function estimates in patients with a good imaging window [52].

Tracking 3D datasets would potentially allow one to describe the complex regional ventricular motion and deformation completely. However, current 3D datasets have limited temporal and spatial resolution, which makes tracking challenging [53]. Further technological progress needs to be observed and the added value of 3D regional function assessment remains to be determined.

3D-derived parameters

In addition to all parameters mentioned, 3D tracking could provide principal strain, i.e. the regional direction and magnitude of the highest and lowest deformation of the myocardium. Further, true torsion estimates would become possible. On a regional level, myocardial shear in relation to normal strain components may be an interesting study subject.

Clinical applications

The feasibility, validity, and clinical value of quantitative function assessment has been demonstrated in numerous experimental,

animal and clinical studies [54, 55]. However, in many clinical situations, the role of these techniques in addressing the management of patients remains to be clarified [50].

Diastolic function

LV myocardial velocities measured by TVI may serve for non-invasive estimation of LV filling pressures [56]. Early studies have shown a correlation between LV filling pressure and the ratio between mitral inflow velocity (E) and the early diastolic mitral annular velocity (E') [57, 58]. Later experience has suggested that this relation does not hold in all clinical scenarios [59]. Current guidelines, therefore, suggest a comprehensive assessment combining E/E' and other parameters of diastolic function in a decision tree (see ⊃ Fig. 5.24a and b).

In addition, E' velocity can help to distinguish patients with constrictive pericarditis from those with a restrictive cardiomyopathy [60] or it may discriminate between physiologic and pathologic hypertrophy.

Global systolic function

2D global systolic strain is a new, sensitive marker of global LV function. It has been shown to be more sensitive to subtle changes in LV function and to be better and more reproducible than classic EF% measurements [61, 62] (see ⊃ Fig. 5.25). Although global strain often behaves concordantly with EF [63], it usually reflects mostly longitudinal LV function and may therefore reveal abnormal LV function in patients with normal EF, particular in hypertrophic cardiomyopathy [64, 65] or infiltrative cardiac disease, such as amyloidosis [66, 67].

In patients with good imaging windows, 3D-derived volume and EF estimates have reached an accuracy that is similar to MR [68]. To what extent this higher accuracy can contribute to a better patient stratification remains to be determined.

Regional systolic function

Strain imaging allows one to analyse the time course of regional myocardial deformation. Post-systolic shortening (PSS), a longitudinal shortening after aortic valve closure, is of particular interest since it indicates, with high sensitivity, regional inhomogeneities

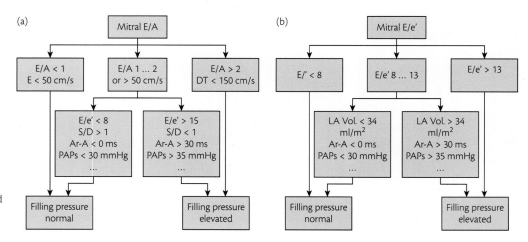

Fig. 5.24 Current guideline recommendations for the estimation of filling pressures (a) in an LV with reduced function (EF<50%) and (b) in an LV with good function (EF>50%).

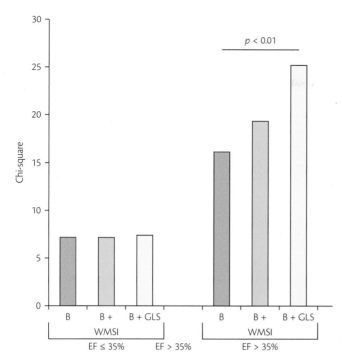

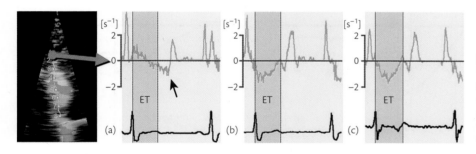

Fig. 5.25 Prediction of mortality by global strain. A subanalysis of patients with mildly or moderately reduced EF (right) reveals the significant added value of global longitudinal strain (GLS) compared to baseline EF assessment (B) and wall motion scoring (WMSI).

of myocardial contractility. It is regularly found in ischaemia and chronic scar (see ➲ Figs 5.26 and 5.27). A newly occurring PSS during a stress echo is always a marker of ischaemia [69] (see ➲ Fig. 5.28), while pre-existing PSS is only then likely to be pathologic if systolic shortening is reduced and PSS exceeds *c.* 20% of the total deformation amplitude [50, 70] (see ➲ Fig. 5.29). PSS contributes to the dispersion of myocardial function in ischaemic disease, which can be used as prognostic marker for arrhythmic events [71]. Whether PSS can be used to predict viability remains subject to debate.

Dyssynchrony

Multiple Doppler- and tracking-based indexes have been proposed for quantitation of intra-ventricular dyssynchrony for the selection of candidate-patients for resynchronization therapy. While it is rather easy to detect LV dyssynchrony, it has been shown to be challenging to define a single parameter that reflects the specific motion and deformation patterns (see ➲ Figs 5.30 and 5.31, 📹 Video 5.7), which predict therapy success. Therefore, a lot of previously suggested echocardiographic dyssynchrony parameters do not have added predictive value for CRT patient selection and approximately one-third of CRT patients remain non-responders [72].

Specific parameters need to retain both local and temporal information. Delay in anteroseptal vs. posterior radial strain, septal

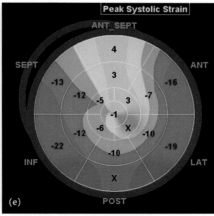

Fig. 5.26 Strain rate traces from the area at risk in (a) the acute myocardial infarction, (b) one day after revascularization and (c) two weeks after revascularization. Note the reduced systolic function and the typical post-systolic shortening (red arrow) in the acute phase, while strain rate patterns normalize with reperfusion.

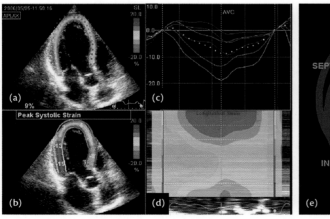

Fig. 5.27 Different displays of chronic scar by 2D speckle tracking. (a) Colour-coded longitudinal strain, (b) numeric display of segmental peak systolic strain, (c) segmental strain curves (note the reduced systolic function and post-systolic shortening in the infarct region), (d) curved M-mode, representing the regional and temporal distribution of longitudinal strain in this echocardiographic view, (e) bull's eye view colour-coded for peak systolic strain showing the anteroseptal dysfunction after myocardial infarction.

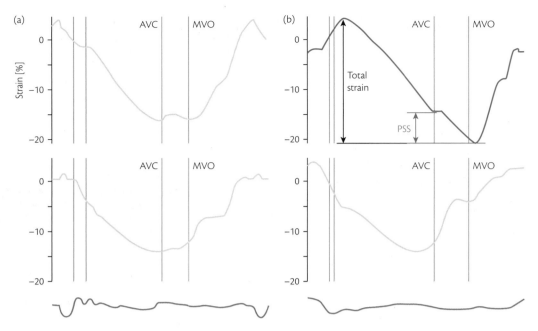

Fig. 5.28 Longitudinal strain during stress echocardiography. Top panels: segment with ischaemic response. Bottom panels: segment with normal response. (a) Baseline strain curves with normal patterns in both segments. (b) Under peak dobutamine stress the normal segment shows still a normal curve pattern. The ischaemic response of the upper segment can be clearly seen by the newly developed marked post systolic shortening (PSS).

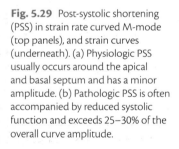

Fig. 5.29 Post-systolic shortening (PSS) in strain rate curved M-mode (top panels), and strain curves (underneath). (a) Physiologic PSS usually occurs around the apical and basal septum and has a minor amplitude. (b) Pathologic PSS is often accompanied by reduced systolic function and exceeds 25–30% of the overall curve amplitude.

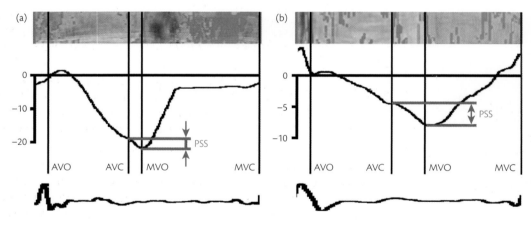

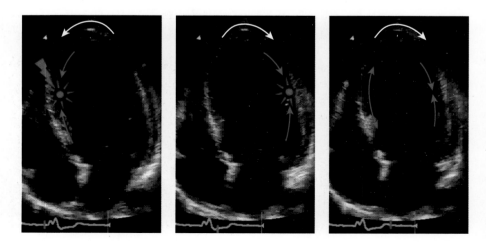

Fig. 5.30 Typical contraction sequence in LBBB: A short initial (apical) septal contraction causes the apex to move septally. The lateral wall is activated with delay, pulling the apex laterally and stretching the septum.

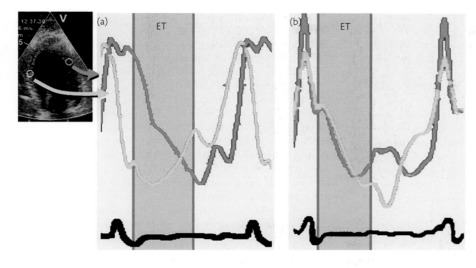

Fig. 5.31 Longitudinal strain curves clearly show the asynchronous shortening of the different walls of the LV. (a) CRT off: note the off-phase shortening in the septum and the lateral wall resembling a typical LBBB pattern. (b) CRT on: mostly synchronous shortening in both walls during ejection time (ET) indicating a more effective LV function under CRT.

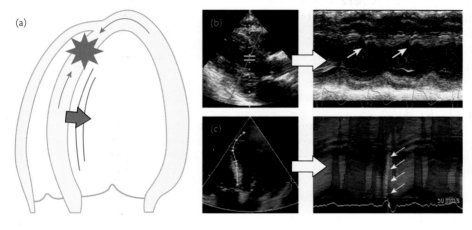

Fig. 5.32 Common mechanism underlying septal flash and apical rocking: the early septal activation leads to a contraction during the end of filling, i.e. against low load. This allows the apex to be pulled over towards the septum and the septum to bounce inward.

flash and apical rocking are examples of such specific parameters [73, 74] (see ⊃ Figs 5.30 and 5.32). This is not yet reflected in current practice guidelines [75].

Conclusion

Functional imaging supplements clinical echocardiography since it allows one to quantify the traditionally visual assessment of regional myocardial function. Tissue Doppler-based imaging currently offers the highest temporal resolution in cardiac imaging. New tracking methods offer new parameters and allow semi-automated post-processing. Current applications of functional imaging comprise diastolic function assessment, the detection of scar and acute ischaemia, as well as subtle function changes and dyssynchrony. Three-dimensional applications allow volume and EF estimates with high accuracy. In several other areas, further studies are needed before the routine implementation of the technique. Future developments may utilize tracking in high volume rate 3D echo datasets.

Acknowledgements

Antonis Ioannidis for his fundamental graphic support, Peter Pearson, Joseph Reiken and Nicola Walker for acquiring, selecting and providing excellent quality 3DE images.

References

1. Dekker DL, Piziali RL, Dong E. A system for ultrasonically imaging the human heart in three dimensions. *Comput Biomed Re* S 1974; 7: 544–53.

2. Siu SC, Rivera JM, Guerrero JL, et al. Three-dimensional echocardiography. In vivo validation for left ventricular volume and function. *Circulation* 1993; 88: 1715–23.

3. von Ramm OT, Smith SW. Real time volumetric ultrasound imaging system. *J Digit Imaging* 1990; 3: 261–6.

4. Lang RM, Badano LP, Tsang W, et al. EAE/ASE Recommendations for image acquisition and display using three-dimensional echocardiography. *Eur Heart J Cardiovasc Imaging* 2012; 13 (1): 1–46.

5. Buck T, Franke A, Monaghan MJ (eds) (2011) *Three-Dimensional Echocardiography*. Springer, Berlin Heidelberg New York.

6. Mor-Avi V, Sugeng L, Weinert L, et al. Fast measurement of left ventricular mass with real-time three-dimensional echocardiography: comparison with magnetic resonance imaging. *Circulation* 2004; 110: 1814–18.

7. Takeuchi M, Nishikage T, Mor-Avi V, et al. Measurement of left ventricular mass by real-time three-dimensional echocardiography: validation against magnetic resonance and comparison with two-dimensional and m-mode measurements. *J Am Soc Echocardiogr* 2008; 21: 1001–5.

8. Mor-Avi V, Jenkins C, Kuhl HP, et al. Real-time 3-dimensional echocardiographic quantification of left ventricular volumes: multicenter study for validation with magnetic resonance imaging and investigation of sources of error. *J Am Coll Cardiol Img* 2008; 1: 413–23.

9. Jenkins C, Bricknell K, Hanekom L, Marwick TH. Reproducibility and accuracy of echocardiographic measurements of left ventricular parameters using real-time three-dimensional echocardiography. *J Am Coll Cardiol* 2004; 44: 878–86.

10. Hare JL, Jenkins C, Nakatani S, Ogawa A, Yu CM, Marwick TH. Feasibility and clinical decision-making with 3D echocardiography in routine practice. *Heart* 2007; 94 (4): 440–5.

11. Kapetanakis S, Kearney MT, Siva A, Gall N, Cooklin M, Monaghan MJ. Real-time three-dimensional echocardiography: a novel technique to quantify global left ventricular mechanical dyssynchrony. *Circulation* 2005; 112: 992–1000.

12. Abusaid G, Ahmad M. Real time three-dimensional stress echocardiography advantages and limitations echocardiography 2012; 29: 200–6.

13. Ahmad M, Xie T, McCulloch M, et al. Real-time three-dimensional dobutamine stress echocardiography in assessment stress echocardiography in assessment of ischemia: Comparison with two-dimensional dobutamine stress echocardiography. *J Am Coll Cardiol* 2001; 37: 1303–9.

14. Pulerwitz T, Hirata K, Abe Y, et al. Feasibility of using a real-time 3-dimensional technique for contrast dobutamine stress echocardiography. *J Am Soc Echocardiogr* 2006; 19: 540–5.

15. Nemes A, Leung KY, van Burken G, et al. Side-by-side viewing of anatomically aligned left ventricular segments in three-dimensional stress echocardiography. *Echocardiography* 2009; 26: 189–95.

16. Badano LP, Muraru D, Rigo F, et al. High volume-rate three-dimensional stress echocardiography to assess inducible myocardial ischemia: A feasibility study. *J Am Soc Echocardiogr* 2010; 23: 628–35.

17. Aggeli C, Giannopoulos G, Misovoulos P, et al. Realtime three-dimensional dobutamine stress echocardiography for coronary artery disease diagnosis: validation with coronary angiography. *Heart* 2007; 93: 672–7.

18. Bhan A, Kapetanakis S, Rana BS, et al. Real-time three-dimensional myocardial contrast echocardiography: is it clinically feasible? *Eur J Echocardiogr* 2008; 9: 761–65.

19. Aggeli C, Felekos I, Roussakis G, et al. Value of real-time three-dimensional adenosine stress contrast echocardiography in patients with known or suspected coronary artery disease. *Eur J Echocardiogr* 2011; 12: 648–55.

20. Abdelmoneim SS, Bernier M, Dhoble A, et al. Assessment of myocardial perfusion during adenosine stress using real time three-dimensional and two-dimensional myocardial contrast echocardiography: Comparison with single-photon emission computed tomography. *Echocardiography* 2010; 27: 421–9.

21. Niemann PS, Pinho L, Balbach T, et al. Anatomically oriented right ventricular volume measurements with dynamic three-dimensional echocardiography validated by 3-Tesla magnetic resonance imaging. *J Am Coll Cardiol* 2007; 50: 1668–76.

22. Khoo NS, Young A, Occleshaw C, Cowan B, Zeng IS, Gentles TL. Assessments of right ventricular volume and function using three-dimensional echocardiography in older children and adults with congenital heart disease: comparison with cardiac magnetic resonance imaging. *J Am Soc Echocardiogr* 2009; 22: 1279–88.

23. Chen G, Sun K, Huang G. In vitro validation of right ventricular volume and mass measurement by real-time three-dimensional echocardiography. *Echocardiography* 2006; 23: 395–9.

24. Gopal AS, Chukwu EO, Iwuchukwu CJ, et al. Normal values of right ventricular size and function by real-time 3-dimensional echocardiography: comparison with cardiac magnetic resonance imaging. *J Am Soc Echocardiogr* 2007; 20: 445–55.

25. Grewal J, Majdalany D, Syed I, Pellikka P, Warnes CA. Three-dimensional echocardiographic assessment of right ventricular volume and function in adult patients with congenital heart disease: comparison with magnetic resonance imaging. *J Am Soc Echocardiogr* 2010 23: 127–33.

26. Tamborini G, Brusoni D, Torres Molina JE, et al. Feasibility of a new generation three-dimensional echocardiography for right ventricular volumetric and functional measurements. *Am J Cardiol* 2008; 102: 499–505.

27. Prakasa KR, Dalal D, Wang J, et al. Feasibility and variability of three dimensional echocardiography in arrhythmogenic right ventricular dysplasia/cardiomyopathy. *Am J Cardiol* 2006; 97: 703–9.

28. Leibundgut G, Rohner A, Grize L, Bernheim A, et al. Dynamic assessment of right ventricular volumes and function by realtime three-dimensional echocardiography: a comparison study with magnetic resonance imaging in 100 adult patients. *J Am Soc Echocardiogr* 2010; 23: 116–26.

29. Rossi A, Cicoira M, Bonapace S, et al. Left atrial volume provides independent and incremental information compared with exercise tolerance parameters in patients with heart failure and left ventricular systolic dysfunction. *Heart* 2007; 93 (11): 1420–5.

30. Beinart R, Boyko V, Schwammenthal E, et al. Long-term prognostic significance of left atrial volume in acute myocardial infarction. *J Am Coll Cardiol* 2004; 44 (2): 327–34.

31. Pritchett AM, Mahoney DW, Jacobsen SJ, Rodeheffer RJ, Karon BL, Redfield MM. Diastolic dysfunction and left atrial volume: a population-based study. *J Am Coll Cardiol* 2005; 45 (1): 87–92.

32. Benjamin EJ, D'Agostino RB, Belanger AJ, Wolf PA, Levy D. Left atrial size and the risk of stroke and death. The Framingham Heart Study. *Circulation* 1995; 92 (4): 835–41.

33. Lang RM, Bierig M, Devereux RB, Flachskampf FA, Foster E, Pellikka PA, et al. Recommendations for chamber quantification: a report from the American Society of Echocardiography's Guidelines and Standards Committee and the Chamber Quantification Writing Group, developed in conjunction with the European Association of Echocardiography, a branch of the European Society of Cardiology. *Eur J Echocardiogr* 2006; 7: 79–108.

34. Khankirawatana B, Khankirawatana S, Lof J, Porter TR. Left atrial volume determination by three-dimensional echocardiography reconstruction: validation and application of a simplified technique. *J Am Soc Echocardiogr* 2002; 15 (10 Pt 1): 1051–6.

35. Miyasaka Y, Tsujimoto S, Maeba H, Yuasa F, Takehana K, Dote K, et al. Left atrial volume by real-time three-dimensional echocardiography: validation by 64-slice multidetector computed tomography. *J Am Soc Echocardiogr* 2011; 24: 680–6.

36. Faletra FF, Ho SY, Regoli F., et al. Real-time three dimensional transoesophageal echocardiography in imaging key anatomical structures of the left atrium: potential role during atrial fibrillation ablation. *Heart* 2013; 99: 133–42.

37. Shah SJ, Bardo DM, Sugeng L, et al. Real-time three-dimensional transesophageal echocardiography of the left atrial appendage: initial experience in the clinical setting. *J Am Soc Echocardiogr* 2008; 21: 1362–8 (12).

38. Gutiérrez-Chico JL, Zamorano Gómez JL, Rodrigo-López JL, et al. Accuracy of real-time 3-dimensional echocardiography in the assessment of mitral prolapse. Is transesophageal echocardiography still mandatory? *Am Heart J* 2008; 155: 694–8.

39. Vahanian A, Alfieri O, Andreotti F, et al. Guidelines on the management of valvular heart disease (version 2012): The Joint Task Force on the Management of Valvular Heart Disease of the European Society of Cardiology (ESC) and the European Association for Cardio-Thoracic Surgery (EACTS). *Eur Heart J* 2012; 33: 2451–96.

40. Kahlert P, Plicht B, Schenk IM, Janosi RA, Erbel R, Buck T. Direct assessment of size and shape of noncircular vena contracta area in functional versus organic mitral regurgitation using real-time three-dimensional echocardiography. *J Am Soc Echocardiogr* 2008; 21: 912–21.

41. Doddamani S, Bello R, Friedman MA, et al. Demonstration of left ventricular outflow tract eccentricity by real time 3D echocardiography: implications for the determination of aortic valve area. *Echocardiography* 2007; 24: 860–6.

42. Khaw AV, von Bardeleben RS, Strasser C, et al. Direct measurement of left ventricular outflow tract by transthoracic real-time 3D-echocardiography increases accuracy in assessment of aortic valve stenosis. *Int J Cardiol* 2009; 136: 64–71.

43. Menzel T, Mohr-Kahaly S, Kolsch B, et al. Quantitative assessment of aortic stenosis by three-dimensional echocardiography. *J Am Soc Echocardiogr* 1997; 10: 215–23.

44. Handke M, Schafer DM, Heinrichs G, Magosaki E, Geibel A. Quantitative assessment of aortic stenosis by three-dimensional anyplane and three-dimensional volume-rendered echocardiography. *Echocardiography* 2002; 19: 45–53.

45. Zamorano JL, Badano LP, Bruce C, et al. EAE/ASE recommendations for the use of echocardiography in new transcatheter interventions for valvular heart disease. *J Am Soc Echocardiogr* 2011; 24 (9): 937–65.

46. Smith LA, Dworakowski R, Bhan A, et al. Real-time three-dimensional transesophageal echocardiography adds value to transcatheter aortic valve implantation. *J Am Soc Echocardiogr* 2013; 26 (4): 359–69.

47. Feldman T, Kar S, Rinaldi M, et al. Percutaneous mitral repair with the MitraClip system: safety and midterm durability in the initial EVEREST (Endovascular Valve Edge-to-Edge REpair Study) cohort. *J Am Coll Cardiol* 2009; 54: 686–94.

48. Feldman T, Foster E, Glower DD, et al. EVEREST II Investigators. Percutaneous repair or surgery for mitral regurgitation. *N Engl J Med* 2011; 364 (15): 1395–406. doi: 10.1056/NEJMoa1009355. Epub 2011 Apr 4. Erratum in: N Engl J Med 2011; 365 (2): 189.

49. Helle-Valle T, Crosby J, Edvardsen T, et al. New noninvasive method for assessment of left ventricular rotation: speckle tracking echocardiography. *Circulation*. 2005; 112: 3149–56.

50. Mor-Avi V, Lang RM, Badano LP, et al. Current and evolving echocardiographic techniques for the quantitative evaluation of cardiac mechanics: ASE/EAE consensus statement on methodology and indications endorsed by the Japanese Society of Echocardiography. *Eur J Echocardiogr*. 2011; 12 (3): 167–205. doi: 10.1093/ejechocard/jer021.

51. Szulik M, Pappas CJ, Jurcut R, et al. Clinical validation of a novel speckle-tracking-based ejection fraction assessment method.

J Am Soc Echocardiogr 2011; 24 (10): 1092–100. doi: 10.1016/j.echo.2011.05.004. Epub 2011 Jun 23.

52. Muraru D, Badano LP, Peluso D, et al. Comprehensive analysis of left ventricular geometry and function by three-dimensional echocardiography in healthy adults. *J Am Soc Echocardiogr* 2013; 26 (6): 618–28.

53. Badano LP, Cucchini U, Muraru D, Al Nono O, SaraisC, Iliceto S. Use of three-dimensional speckle tracking to assess left ventricular myocardial mechanics: inter-vendor consistency and reproducibility of strain measurements. *Eur Heart J Cardiovasc Imaging* 2013; 14 (3): 285–93.

54. Edvardsen T, Gerber BL, Garot J, Bluemke DA, Lima JA, Smiseth OA. Quantitative assessment of intrinsic regional myocardial deformation by Doppler strain rate echocardiography in humans: validation against three-dimensional tagged magnetic resonance imaging. *Circulation* 2002; 106: 50–6.

55. Sutherland GR, Hatle L (eds). Doppler Myocardial Imaging—A Textbook. BSWK bvba, Hasselt 2006 (ISBN978-90-810592-1-3) [Voi01] Heimdal A, Stoylen A, Torp H, Skjaerpe T. Real-time strain rate imaging of the left ventricle by ultrasound. *J Am Soc Echocardiogr* 1998; 11, 1013–9.

56. Nagueh SF, Appleton CP, Gillebert TC, et al. Recommendations for the evaluation of left ventricular diastolic function by echocardiography. *Eur J Echocardiogr* 2009; 10 (2): 165–93. doi: 10.1093/ejechocard/jep007.

57. Nagueh SF, Middleton KJ, Kopelen HA, Zoghbi WA, Quiñones MA. Doppler tissue imaging: a noninvasive technique for evaluation of left ventricular relaxation and estimation of filling pressures. *J Am Coll Cardiol* 1997; 30 (6): 1527–33.

58. Ommen SR, Nishimura RA, Appleton CP, et al. Clinical utility of Doppler echocardiography and tissue Doppler imaging in the estimation of left ventricular filling pressures: a comparative simultaneous Doppler-catheterization study. *Circulation* 2000; 102 (15): 1788–94.

59. Mullens W, Borowski AG, Curtin RJ, Thomas JD, Tang WH. Tissue Doppler imaging in the estimation of intracardiac filling pressure in decompensated patients with advanced systolic heart failure. *Circulation* 2009; 119 (1): 62–70.

60. Rajagopalan N, Garcia MJ, Rodriguez L, et al. Comparison of new Doppler echocardiographic methods to differentiate constrictive pericardial heart disease and restrictive cardiomyopathy. *Am J Cardiol* 2001; 87: 86–94.

61. Erven K, Florian A, Slagmolen P, et al. Subclinical cardiotoxicity detected by strain rate imaging up to 14 months after breast radiation therapy. *Int J Radiat Oncol Biol Phy* S 2013; 85 (5): 1172–8. doi: 10.1016/j.ijrobp.2012.09.022. Epub 2012 Nov 10.

62. Stanton T, Leano R, Marwick TH. Prediction of all-cause mortality from global longitudinal speckle strain: comparison with ejection fraction and wall motion scoring. *Circ Cardiovasc Imaging* 2009 Sep; 2 (5): 356–64.

63. Brown J, Jenkins C, Marwick TH. Use of myocardial strain to assess global left ventricular function: a comparison with cardiac magnetic resonance and 3-dimensional echocardiography. *Am Heart J* 2009; 157 (1): 102.

64. Serri K, Reant P, Lafitte M, et al. Global and regional myocardial function quantification by two-dimensional strain: application in hypertrophic cardiomyopathy. *J Am Coll Cardiol* 2006; 47: 1175–81.

65. Kato TS, Noda A, Izawa H, et al. Discrimination of nonobstructive hypertrophic cardiomyopathy from hypertensive left ventricular hypertrophy on the basis of strain rate imaging by tissue Doppler ultrasonography. *Circulation* 2004; 110: 3808–14.

66. Lindqvist P, Olofsson BO, Backman C, Suhr O, Waldenstrom A. Pulsed tissue Doppler and strain imaging discloses early signs of

infiltrative cardiac disease: a study on patients with familial amyloidotic polyneuropathy. *Eur J Echocardiogr* 2006; 7: 22–30.

67. Al Zahrani GB, Bellavia D, Pellikka PA, et al. Doppler myocardial imaging compared to standard 2-dimensional and doppler echocardiography for assessment of diastolic function in patients with systemic amyloidosis. *J Am Soc Echocardiogr* 2008; 22 (3): 290–8.

68. Van der Heide JA, Kleijn SA, Aly MF, Slikkerveer J, Kamp O. Three-dimensional echocardiography for left ventricular quantification: fundamental validation and clinical applications. *Neth Heart J* 2011; 19 (10): 423–31. doi: 10.1007/s12471-011-0160-y.

69. Voigt JU, Lindenmeier G, Exner B, et al. Incidence and characteristics of segmental postsystolic longitudinal shortening in normal, acutely ischemic, and scarred myocardium. *J Am Soc Echocardiogr* 2003; 16 (5): 415–23.

70. Voigt JU, Exner B, Schmiedehausen K, et al. Strain-rate imaging during dobutamine stress echocardiography provides objective evidence of inducible ischemia. *Circulation* 2003; 107 (16): 2120–6. Epub 2003 Apr 7.

71. Haugaa KH, Smedsrud MK, Steen T, et al. Mechanical dispersion assessed by myocardial strain in patients after myocardial infarction for risk prediction of ventricular arrhythmia. *JACC Cardiovasc Imaging* 2010; 3 (3): 247–56. doi: 10.1016/j.jcmg.2009.11.012.

72. Chung ES, Leon AR, Tavazzi L, et al. Results of the Predictors of Response to CRT (PROSPECT) trial. *Circulation* 2008; 117: 2608–16.

73. Szulik M, Tillekaerts M, Vangeel V, et al. Assessment of apical rocking: a new, integrative approach for selection of candidates for cardiac resynchronization therapy. *Eur J Echocardiogr* 2010; 11 (10): 863–9.

74. Parsai C, Bijnens B, Sutherland GR, et al. Toward understanding response to cardiac resynchronization therapy: left ventricular dyssynchrony is only one of multiple mechanisms. *Eur Heart J* 2009; 30 (8): 940–9.

75. McMurray JJ, Adamopoulos S, Anker SD, et al. ESC Committee for Practice Guidelines. ESC Guidelines for the diagnosis and treatment of acute and chronic heart failure 2012: The Task Force for the Diagnosis and Treatment of Acute and Chronic Heart Failure 2012 of the European Society of Cardiology. Developed in collaboration with the Heart Failure Association (HFA) of the ESC. *Eur Heart J* 2012; 33 (14): 1787–847. doi: 10.1093/eurheartj/ehs104. Epub 2012 May 19. No abstract available. Erratum in: Eur Heart J 2013 Jan; 34 (2): 158.

⮩ **For additional multimedia materials, please visit the online version of the book** (🖰 **http://www.esciacc.oxfordmedicine.com**)

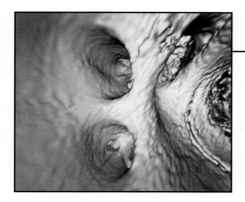

CHAPTER 6

Hybrid imaging: combination of PET, SPECT, CT, and MRI

Juhani Knuuti and Philipp A. Kaufmann

Contents

Introduction

Hybrid scanners combining PET or SPECT with high resolution multi-detector CT are becoming the standard for almost all commercially available nuclear imaging systems. In addition, the newest generation of scanners offers combination of PET with MRI. Hybrid scanners offer the ability to assess the anatomy of the heart and coronary arteries, and the functional evaluation either at stress (for assessment of induced ischaemia), or at rest (for viability) in association with the left ventricular systolic function. Therefore, combining functional information with anatomy by using hybrid systems is appealing [1].

Definition of cardiac hybrid imaging

The term cardiac hybrid imaging has been proposed if images are fused combining two datasets, whereby both modalities are equally important in contributing to image information. Mostly this refers to combining CT with a nuclear myocardial perfusion imaging technique. Some reports have referred to X-ray based attenuation correction of perfusion imaging as hybrid imaging, raising confusion about its exact meaning because in such settings the CT or MRI data do not provide added anatomical information, but are simply used to improve image quality of the PET or SPECT modality. Similarly, the parametric maps obtained from low-dose CT do not provide image information beyond that needed for attenuation correction, although it could be used to obtain calcium scoring [2, 3].

Others have used the term hybrid imaging for the mere side-by-side analysis of perfusion and CT or MRI images. To avoid confusion we suggest using the term hybrid imaging to describe any combination of structural and functional information beyond that offered by attenuation correction or side-by-side analysis, by fusion of the separate datasets, for example, from CT coronary angiography and from SPECT or PET into one image. Similarly, separate acquisition of structural information, as well as functional data such as, for example, perfusion on two separate scanners or on one hybrid device, would allow mental integration of side-by-side evaluation but only fusion of both pieces of information would result in what should be considered a hybrid image (⊃ Fig. 6.1).

Rationale for cardiac hybrid imaging

The field of cardiac imaging has witnessed an enormous development in the past years and is now offering an ever-increasing spectrum of tools and options to the clinicians. The potential disadvantage is that the patients may now be exposed to multiple, sequential, time-consuming, and costly diagnostic tests and procedures, which may deliver occasionally

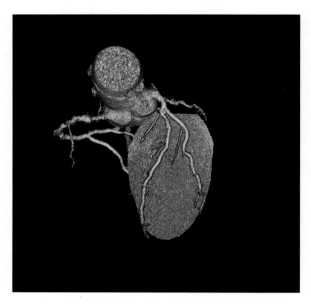

Fig. 6.1 Three-dimensional cardiac hybrid PET-CT image providing a panoramic view of stress perfusion MPI (red and yellow colours indicate normal perfusion) in relation to the coronary territories. Despite several calcifications in the proximal segments of the left and right coronary arteries there is no relevant ischaemia.

even contradicting results. This may have contributed to the fact that the majority of patients are referred to diagnostic invasive coronary angiography and, consequently, to percutaneous coronary interventions (PCI) in the absence of any sort of functional evaluation [4, 5], although professional guidelines call for objective documentation of ischaemia prior to elective PCI [6, 7]. It is this background that has paved the way for the conceptual search of a non-invasive technique to assess coronary artery disease in which the detected perfusion abnormalities can be immediately and accurately associated with the individual's coronary anatomy.

Although CT coronary angiography with multi-detector scanners has proven to be a valuable alternative to diagnostic invasive coronary angiography for the evaluation of many subgroups of patients with known or suspected coronary artery disease, it currently provides purely morphological information. The limitations of morphologic measures for delineating the physiologic implications of stenoses are well-described [8]. The vasomotor

tone and coronary collateral flow, both of which are known to affect myocardial perfusion, cannot be estimated by measures of stenosis severity. The percent diameter stenosis is only a weak descriptor of coronary resistance, as it does not take into account the length and shape of stenosis. Lastly, CTA is limited in its ability to accurately define the severity of stenosis.

Accordingly, the major drawback of the CT has been found to be the relatively low positive predictive value and that the estimation of the haemodynamic significance of the detected stenosis is difficult [9–11]. In contrast, myocardial perfusion imaging provides a simple and accurate integrated measure of the effect of all of these parameters on coronary resistance and tissue perfusion, thereby optimizing selection of patients who may ultimately benefit from revascularization. This has triggered the idea of obtaining combined anatomic and functional non-invasive imaging of the coronary circulation in a single session through hybrid instrumentation.

Early studies conducted with image fusion of invasive coronary angiography and myocardial perfusion imaging from SPECT showed limited success due to the disadvantages inherent in warping a planar 2D angiogram into a fusion with a 3D perfusion dataset. Furthermore, the fusion process was time-consuming and, therefore, not helpful for rapid decision-making during an ongoing intervention. Alternatively, combined information can be gained by mental integration of the information, e.g. from invasive or CT angiography and SPECT. However, the planar projections of coronary angiograms and axial slice-by-slice display of cardiac perfusion studies make a subjective integration difficult. This may lead to inaccurate allocation of the coronary lesion to its subtended myocardial territory, particularly in patients with multi-vessel disease and intermediate severity lesions. In addition, standard distribution of myocardial territories corresponds with the real anatomic coronary tree in only 50–60% of cases, which may cause misleading interpretation.

Therefore, the concept of hybrid imaging to deliver comprehensive integrated morphological and functional information is particularly appealing. In addition to being intuitively convincing, these images provide a panoramic view of the myocardium, the regional myocardial perfusion or viability, and the coronary artery tree, thus eliminating uncertainties in the relationship of perfusion defects, scar regions, and diseased coronary arteries in watershed regions (➲ Fig. 6.2). This may be particularly helpful

Fig. 6.2 Three-dimensional cardiac hybrid SPECT-CT image: a volume rendered CT coronary angiography image is fused with the stress perfusion SPECT. The left panel shows a basal inferior ischaemic area (blue area, black arrow heads). The middle panel reveals a lesion in the right coronary artery (white arrow), with otherwise unremarkable coronaries and normal perfusion. Invasive coronary angiography confirms a significant lesion in the RCA (white arrow).

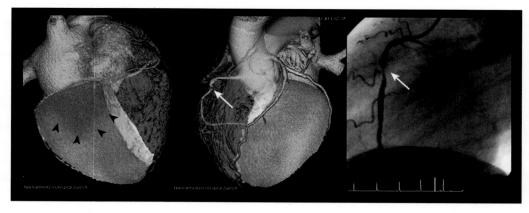

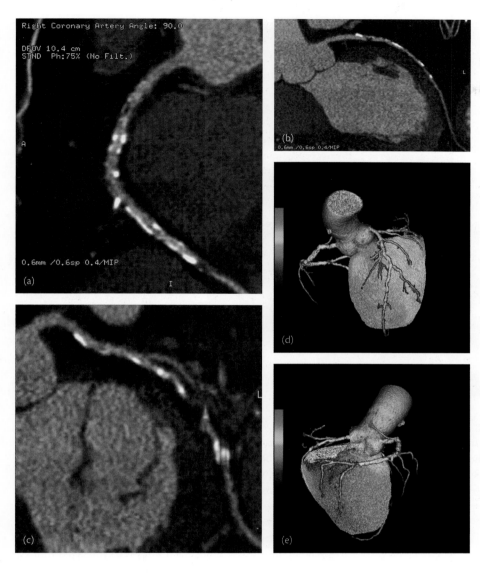

Fig. 6.3 CT coronary angiography images (curved multi-planar reconstructions) of a male patient with effort angina. The images of RCA (a), LAD (b), and LCX (c) show several calcified and non-calcified plaques, which suggest significant multi-vessel disease. Three-dimensional cardiac hybrid PET-CT images of anterior (d) and right lateral view (e) show very different stress perfusion patterns in each vessel region. Perfusion in the region supplied by LCX was normal (red and yellow colour), slightly reduced in the region supplied by LAD (green colour), and severely compromised in the region supplied by RCA (blue colour).

in patients with multiple perfusion abnormalities (⊃ Fig. 6.3) and complex CAD, including situations after bypass surgery (⊃ Fig. 6.4). Combining anatomical information with perfusion also helps to identify and correctly register the subtle irregularities in myocardial perfusion (⊃ Fig. 6.5).

Also, the combination of MR volumetric perfusion has been fused with three-dimensional volume rendered CTA into hybrid images [12]. However, the new PET/MR scanners enable combination of ventricular function, perfusion, viability, and infarct scar for evaluation of ischaemic heart disease. There are also other

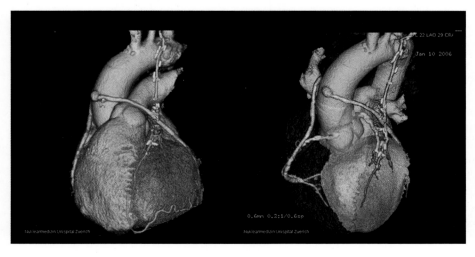

Fig. 6.4 In situations of complex coronary CAD, and after bypass surgery, hybrid cardiac imaging provides added value. CT coronary angiography may allow visualization of patent bypass grafts but the evaluation of the anastomoses remains difficult. A conclusion about haemodynamically relevant lesions can only be reached in conjunction with perfusion. The image documents residual ischaemia in the distal left anterior descending artery territory.

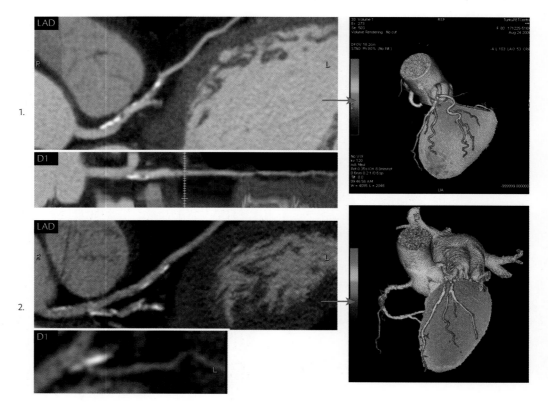

Fig. 6.5 Examples of two clinically similar symptomatic patients who had also similar findings in LAD and the first diagonal branch (D1) in CT angiography (left panels). The patient 1 (upper row) showed in hybrid PET/CT imaging (right panel) only subtle reduction in territory supplied by D1. The patient 2 (lower row) showed large poorly perfused region covering whole anterior wall supplied by both LAD and D1.

promising future applications that involve molecular imaging of cardiac targets, and these may further enhance the clinical utility of hybrid imaging using PET/CT or PET/MR [13].

Integrated scanners versus software fusion

The potential added value of hybrid imaging originates from the spatial correlation of structural and functional information on the fused images, which facilitates a comprehensive interpretation of coronary lesions and their pathophysiologic relevance. An important prerequisite of hybrid imaging is accurate image coregistration, as misalignment may result in erroneous allocation of perfusion defects to coronary artery territories. From a technical perspective, image coregistration can be achieved by a software-based or hardware-based approach.

Hardware-based image coregistration permits the acquisition of fused anatomical and functional images using hybrid scanners (such as PET/CT, SPECT/CT or PET/MRI devices) with the capability to perform imaging acquisition almost simultaneously with the patient's position fixed. Inherently, image fusion is performed fully or semi-automatically by superposition of image datasets. The real benefit of fusing different imaging modalities is also in the ability of using the anatomical information acquired *in situ* to improve the scan efficiency and to use the CT or MRI images for attenuation correction of the nuclear scan. Last but not least, the very important benefit for the patient is that comprehensive study can be performed in a short single session of scans. The drawback

is that the sequential procedure requires careful planning of logistics to enable efficient patient throughput.

Alternatively, with software-based coregistration, image datasets can be obtained on standalone scanners and fused manually through the use of landmark-based coregistration techniques. Intuitively, the hardware-based approach appears preferable since manual coregistration may be hampered by issues of accuracy and user interaction. While hybrid devices are the preferred tool for whole-body imaging predominantly used in oncology, the routine use of fully automated hardware-based image coregistration for cardiac hybrid applications is challenged by certain organ-specific characteristics. First, minor beat-to-beat variations in the heart's position may interfere with accurate image coregistation, despite fixation of the patient's position and orientation. Second, CT and MRI image acquisition and analysis requires electrocardiographical gating. With CT and often with MRI, the images are acquired during breath-hold. With SPECT and PET in some protocols also non-gated datasets are used resulting in a slight mismatch of ventricular size between the image sets. Furthermore, the position of the heart is susceptible to respiratory motion; SPECT and PET images are typically acquired during normal breathing. These facts can result in misalignment of the heart between PET/SPECT and superimposed CT/MRI and can also lead to diagnostic errors [14]. Therefore, nowadays software realignment of cardiac image sets is performed, even if the scans were acquired in a single session using a hybrid device.

Despite the integration of high-end devices with nuclear scanners to form dedicated cardiac hybrid scanners, software-based image coregistration may still remain a common form of hybrid

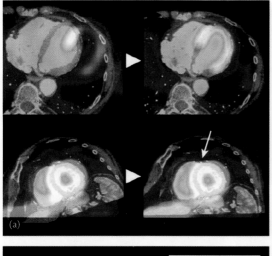
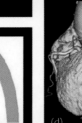
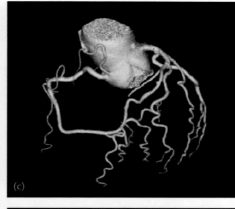
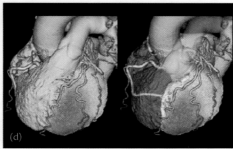

Fig. 6.6 Illustration of the main steps for creating a cardiac hybrid SPECT-CT image from standalone systems. The main steps include (a) image coregistration, (b) epicardial contour detection, (c) coronary artery segmentation, and (d) MPI and CT image superposition. The same steps are also performed even if hardware based hybrid imaging (PET/CT or SPECT/CT) device were used. *European Journal of Nuclear Medicine*, 34: 2007. Validation of a new cardiac image fusion software for three-dimensional integration of myocardial perfusion SPECT and stand-alone 64-slice CT angiography, Oliver Gaemperli, with kind permission from Springer Science and Business Media.

imaging. Dedicated cardiac fusion software packages are now commercially available allowing hybrid imaging with an excellent inter-observer reproducibility and short processing durations. Image transfer processes to workstations performing coregistration is currently simple and fast. A recent validation study has documented that 3D SPECT/CT image fusion (➲ Fig. 6.6) from image sets obtained on standalone scanners with such a software package is feasible and reliable, allowing correct superposition of PET/SPECT segments onto cardiac CT anatomy. Such software is used irrespective of whether the images are acquired on a hybrid device or on two different standalone scanners.

Indeed, with SPECT the standalone scanner setting may appear favourable in view of the fact that, with latest generation multi-detector CT scanners, coronary angiography is acquired within seconds, while emission scans for stress plus rest gated SPECT takes 20–45 min [15]. Thus, in a hybrid cardiac device, the high-end CT facilities will be blocked during long emission scan periods and therefore operate at low capacity. Advances in nuclear medicine, such as newly developed dedicated cardiac detectors systems and novel image reconstruction algorithms [16], may contribute to reduce emission scan times considerably and may eventually help to shift the balance in favour of hybrid scanners in the future.

With PET there are several advantages of hybrid imaging using hardware-based image fusion. The efficiency of imaging is enhanced. The PET imaging protocols are short, allowing both CT angiography and perfusion imaging to be performed in a single session of 15–30 min total scan duration. It is expected that PET/CT will be increasingly used, at least in traditionally difficult patient populations, such as obese and diabetic subjects. There are also other promising future applications that involve molecular imaging of cardiac targets and these may further enhance the clinical utility of hybrid imaging using PET/CT or PET/MRI.

As explained in earlier chapters, PET imaging offers a unique possibility to measure myocardial perfusion quantitatively in absolute terms. This is useful in patients with diffuse CAD or balanced disease, where relative assessment of myocardial perfusion cannot uncover global reduction in perfusion (➲ Fig. 6.7). Typically, in relative analysis of perfusion, only the regions supplied with the most severe stenosis are detected. Quantification of myocardial perfusion using dynamic PET provides a high performance level for the detection and localization of CAD [17]. The incremental value of quantitative analysis was also recently studied and it was found that the accuracy of PET was further improved by quantitative analysis [18–21].

Imaging protocols for hybrid imaging

The patient preparation for hybrid study is mostly the same as for the individual scans. It is important that the patient's heart rate is controlled for CT and that caffeine-containing drinks are avoided during at least the preceding 12 h, since pharmacological stressors are commonly used in hybrid imaging. There are several options for hybrid imaging, which each have certain advantages and disadvantages.

In the protocols where the need of perfusion study is individually decided upon the findings in CT angiography, the protocol naturally starts with CT. This procedure is powerful since it utilizes the high negative predictive value of CT and only that fraction of patients that had suspicious findings in CT will continue

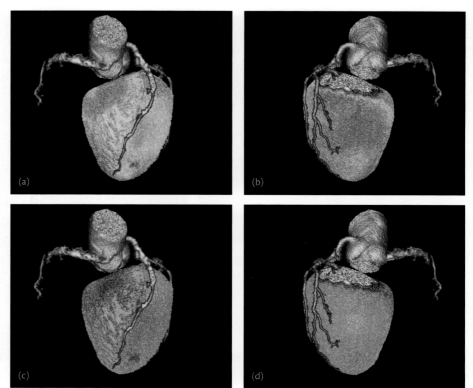

Fig. 6.7 Hybrid images from stress PET/CT with extensive coronary artery disease. The images (a, b) scaled to relative scale where the best perfused region is set to maximum and has the brightest colour (in rainbow scale lowest = blue and highest = red). The hybrid images of anterior (a) and posterior (b) views suggested only minor perfusion abnormalities in the anterior wall. The images scaled according to absolute scale (c and d) (0 ml/g/ min = blue and 3.5 ml/g/min = red) uncovered global reduction of perfusion. The hybrid images of anterior (c) and posterior (d) views showed severely reduced stress perfusion in the anterior wall but also abnormally low perfusion in other myocardial territories (green colour).

with perfusion imaging. Depending on the selected patient population, this fraction is about 25–50% and, thus, on the average one perfusion session is needed for each three patients. The potential limitation is that the premedication needed for CT angiography may also affect the perfusion results, although in a recent study [21] beta blockers had no influence on the results when adenosine was used.

If perfusion study is performed first, the mentioned potential problem is avoided but currently the analysis of perfusion images is not fast enough to be used for immediate decision-making (whether to leave out CT angiography in the case of completely normal perfusion result). Thus, in this protocol, both studies are usually performed in all patients.

The positioning of the patient to the scanner bed is critical to prevent any motion artefacts. It is strongly recommended that hands are supported upright and not within the field of view. The calcium score study can be performed first, followed by the CT angiography study. The detailed protocol of CT angiography depends on the system used. Thereafter, low-dose CT for attenuation correction scan is performed, if needed (in some systems a calcium score study can be used for this).

The perfusion imaging protocol depends on whether PET or SPECT or which tracer is used. In hybrid imaging, the stress study is performed using pharmacologic stressors, such as adenosine, dipyridamole, or dobutamine. With PET tracers, such as ^{82}Rb and ^{15}O-water studies (half-lives 76 s and 112 s), the stress study can be performed practically without delay after the rest study. With ^{13}N-ammonia, stress testing is delayed for about 30 min to allow

tracer decay. If no method for correcting patient motion between stress and rest studies is available, a second low-dose CT scan for attenuation correction is needed. In all studies, a quality control process is needed to ensure optimal alignment of the CT attenuation and PET emission scans and, if necessary, misalignment needs to be corrected (◑ Fig. 6.6).

If the system is capable of list mode acquisition, the data can be collected in ECG-gated mode, which allows the simultaneous assessment of regional and global left ventricular wall motion from the same scan data. This is particularly practical in ^{82}Rb and ^{13}N-ammonia studies. The total time required for the whole study session depends on the tracer used. With ^{15}O-water and ^{82}Rb, the whole session can be finished in 30 min and with ^{13}N-ammonia in 80 min. In patients without previous myocardial infarction, only single stress perfusion imaging seems to be enough when using quantification [21, 22] and the hybrid protocols are very short (15–25 min). If hybrid imaging is used to assess myocardial viability, the standard patient preparations and procedures are used as in standalone imaging.

Image analysis and interpretation of hybrid imaging

The analysis of CT angiography includes the standard processes and techniques, such as visual assessment of original transaxial slices, multi-planar reconstructions, and utilization of quantitative tools available. The analysis of PET/SPECT studies also follows the standard procedures that have been explained in detail in the guidelines [23–25]. However, to utilize the true power of hybrid imaging, an analysis system that is able to handle fused images and data should be also used. In this way the individual coronary anatomy can be visualized together with functional information enabling accurate association between coronary anatomy and, for example, perfusion. The most advanced analysis also includes visualization of perfusion in diagnostic quality multi-planar reconstructions of CT. If quantitative measurement of flow has been performed, the absolute stress flow values should be also included in the analysis (➲ Fig. 6.7).

Radiation safety aspects

Utilizing hybrid imaging, the patient radiation dose will further increase, since the 'additional' imaging techniques utilize also ionizing radiation. The dose for a patient from CT angiography has been reported to be in the range of 1 to 20 mSv, depending on the system and protocol used. Recently, techniques that reduce patient dose have been developed and the doses have been reduced as low as 1–7 mSv [26]. The radiation doses from single SPECT perfusion imaging range from 5 to 8 mSv (^{99m}Tc-based tracers). The radiation dose from PET perfusion studies is small, e.g. radiation dose from single PET perfusion study is 0.8 mSv ^{15}O-water and 1 mSv for ^{13}N-ammonia. Therefore, although the use of hybrid imaging obviously causes increased radiation dose for the patient, the recent technical development has improved the radiation safety tremendously and a complete hybrid imaging can now be performed with radiation dose clearly below 10 mSv [27–29].

Clinical impact of cardiac hybrid imaging

As mentioned, it is well established that a comprehensive assessment of CAD requires not only morphologic information about coronary artery stenosis location and degree, but also functional information on pathophysiologic lesion severity. Eventually, many factors that cannot fully be assessed with coronary luminology determine whether a given lesion really induces a myocardial perfusion defect (➲ Fig. 6.8) (see also ➲ Figs 6.3, 6.5, and 6.7). It has been repeatedly shown that only about half of the lesions classified as significant in CT are linked with abnormal perfusion [9–11, 22].

In a study by Namdar et al. [30], the concept was evaluated in patients with suspected CAD yielding a sensitivity and specificity of 90% and 98%, respectively, to detect haemodynamically important coronary lesions (as compared to the combination of stress-rest PET perfusion imaging and invasive coronary angiography). In a recent study using PET/CT systems with a 64-slice CT scanner, it was found that the positive predictive value of stenosis in CT was low (around 50%) in predicting stress-inducible perfusion abnormalities in PET, but the negative predictive value was over

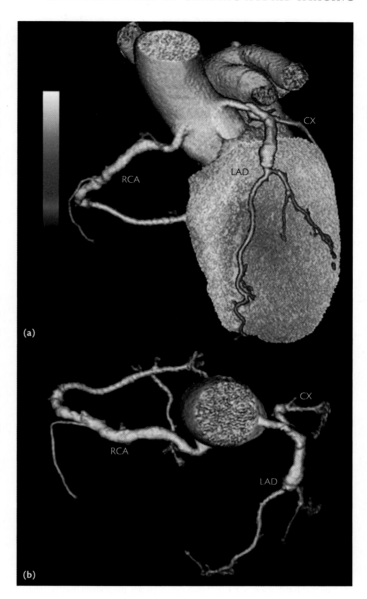

Fig. 6.8 (a) Hybrid images from stress SPECT MPI fused with the CT coronary angiography indicating that the territory subtended by the ectatic left anterior descending (LAD) is ischaemic (blue area). (b) CT coronary angiography shows the extent of the ectatic coronary disease involving also the right (RCA) and the circumflex (CX) coronary arteries.

European Journal of Nuclear Medicine, 35: 2008, Coronary artery ectasia causing ischemia, Husmann et al., with kind permission from Springer Science and Business Media.

90% [31]. This indicates that the assessment of functional consequences of coronary stenosis is difficult with CT, and that perfusion imaging provides useful complementary information.

Although these studies provide important clinical information about the performance of different imaging modalities, they do not directly show the incremental value of the hybrid imaging. Hybrid images may offer superior diagnostic information with regard to identification of the culprit vessel and, therefore, increase diagnostic confidence [22, 32–34]. The combined SPECT perfusion imaging and CT coronary angiography studies indicate that in almost one-third of patients the fused SPECT/CT analysis provided added diagnostic information on pathophysiologic lesion severity not obtained on side-by-side analysis [31]. The incremental value was most pronounced for functionally relevant lesions in distal segments and diagonal branches, and in vessels with extensive CAD or substantial calcification on CT. Similar results have been also obtained using hybrid PET/CT imaging [22, 35, 36]. Due to the variant coronary anatomy in each individual and the complex disease pattern in these patients, correct allocation of perfusion defect and subtending coronary artery was only achieved by the hybrid images. As hybrid images offered superior information with regard to identification of the culprit vessel, the diagnostic confidence for categorizing intermediate lesions and equivocal perfusion defects was significantly improved. Interestingly, most of the lesions that were originally found to be equivocal with regard to pathophysiologic severity on side-by-side analysis (due to the fact they could not be firmly assigned to a perfusion defect) were classified with high confidence by hybrid image evaluation. From these results one can conclude that the greatest added value appears to be the firm exclusion of haemodynamic significance of coronary abnormalities seen on CT coronary angiography, which might be useful to avoid unnecessary interventional procedures.

Another group of patients in whom hybrid imaging is possibly clinically useful are those with multi-vessel CAD. Typically, myocardial perfusion analysis is based on relative assessment of perfusion distribution. This technique, however, often uncovers only the coronary territory supplied by the most severe stenosis. In multi-vessel disease, coronary flow reserve may be abnormal in all territories, thereby reducing the heterogeneity of flow between 'normal' and 'abnormal' zones (➲ Fig. 6.7). This is obviously limiting the ability of relative perfusion analysis to delineate the presence of multi-vessel CAD.

There are several alternatives to solve this problem. The response of left ventricular ejection fraction to stress can be measured from perfusion data, and a decrease in peak stress indicates multi-vessel disease [37]. PET has here some benefit since the acquisition is done during stress, unlike with SPECT where post-stress imaging is performed. Another solution would be using quantification of myocardial perfusion in absolute terms (in ml/g/min), which is readily possible with PET [18–21] and provides independent information about all myocardial territories. In addition, integrated PET/CT offers an opportunity to assess the presence and magnitude of the subclinical atherosclerotic disease burden and to measure absolute myocardial blood flow as a marker of endothelial health and atherosclerotic disease activity. Last but not least, anatomical information from CT is able to identify the patients with severe balanced multi-vessel disease, despite globally reduced but relatively homogenous myocardial perfusion.

The prognostic value of CTA combined with perfusion imaging was studied in a study including 541 patients at intermediate risk of CAD [38]. After adjusting for clinical risk factors, CTA and myocardial perfusion information were independent predictors of events. The prediction of risk was improved by the combination of the two modalities compared with either modality alone. These findings were confirmed in another, recent study using SPECT-CT hybrid imaging [39].

One of the strengths of hybrid imaging is that it can guide selection of the most appropriate treatment strategy (medical conservative vs. percutaneous vs. surgical revascularization) [40, 41]. Therefore, it can be anticipated that in the patients with multi-vessel disease, hybrid imaging can be helpful for the evaluation of the extent of disease and for localizing the culprit flow-limiting lesions. ➲ Figure 6.9 shows the potential new algorithm for how hybrid imaging could help in detection and guiding the therapy of CAD.

Although assessment of myocardial viability using standalone systems is well established, the hybrid imaging provides clear benefits. The detected dysfunctional but viable or scar regions can be directly linked with the individual's coronary anatomy and linked with coronary stenoses. The limitation of the hybrid approach in this patient group is that a substantial fraction of the patients have other diseases that prevent the use of iodinated contrast agents. In this application, PET/MRI systems can be expected to be promising [13].

Future perspectives

Although the role of hybrid imaging in daily clinical routine remains to be determined, it appears that this approach may have the potential to become the central decision-making element in future diagnostic and therapeutic strategies for patients with coronary artery disease. Studies assessing the cost-effectiveness of hybrid imaging are warranted.

Currently, the position of nuclear imaging in cardiovascular research and patient care is primarily based on its capacity for image perfusion and glucose metabolism. However, the methods allow for imaging and quantification of molecular interactions and pathways with picomolar sensitivity. Thus, a number of cellular processes can be studied, e.g. receptor density, enzyme activity, inflammatory processes, and gene expression.

Rupture of vulnerable coronary atherosclerotic lesions accounts for one-third of all deaths worldwide and constitutes a major source of disability and healthcare costs. Non-invasive techniques, such as multi-slice CT, can characterize morphologic criteria associated with high risk of atherosclerotic plaque rupture. In contrast, PET and SPECT utilize radiolabelled molecules designed to specifically target individual inflammatory activities in atherosclerotic plaques. This approach is possible only with high-resolution morphological imaging of the coronary arteries using hybrid imaging.

Hybrid imaging, combining MR with PET or SPECT, is potentially desirable for many reasons, including lack of additional ionizing radiation, tissue characterization properties of MR, and the possibility to do simultaneous acquisition with MRI and PET. Hybrid scanners containing MR and PET scanners have been available for a short period of time and there are still technical issues to be resolved before their potential in cardiac applications can be fully explored [13].

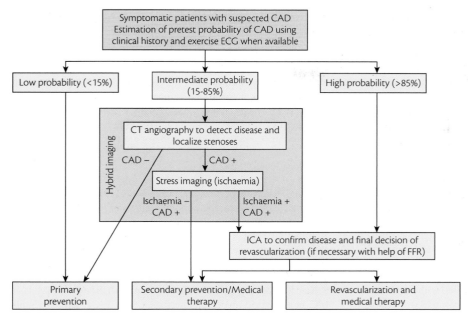

Fig. 6.9 The new proposed diagnostic path including hybrid imaging starts with the similar selection process based on the pre-test probability of CAD. The first imaging test in patients with intermediate probability would be CT angiography (CTA). The patient without CAD in CTA can be recommended for primary prevention, whereas the patients with suspicion of obstructive CAD continue with non-invasive test to detect ischaemia in a region supplied by the corresponding vessel. Those with CAD, but no ischaemia can be recommended aggressive secondary prevention. Those patients with both anatomical evidence of epicardial CAD and ischaemia have highest likelihood to benefit from revascularization and can be referred to ICA to make final decision on treatment. (with permission from [40])

Conclusion

The newest generation of hybrid imaging devices have matured to the level where they can be successfully used for clinical cardiovascular imaging. In addition, software-based image fusion has become readily available, allowing robust and fast image merging.

It is likely that in the near future the primary clinical use of hybrid imaging will be in the detection of coronary artery disease using CT coronary angiography and nuclear perfusion imaging, but in long term also, other molecular imaging applications are entering into clinical cardiology.

References

1. Bax JJ, Beanlands RS, Klocke FJ, Knuuti J, Lammertsma AA, Schaefers MA, et al. Diagnostic and clinical perspectives of fusion imaging in cardiology: is the total greater than the sum of its parts? *Heart* 2007; 93 (1): 16–22.

2. Schepis T, Gaemperli O, Koepfli P, Ruegg C, Burger C, Leschka S, et al. Use of coronary calcium score scans from stand-alone multislice computed tomography for attenuation correction of myocardial perfusion SPECT. *Eur J Nucl Med Mol Imaging* 2007; 34 (1): 11–9.

3. Koepfli P, Hany TF, Wyss CA, Namdar M, Burger C, Konstantinidis AV, et al. CT attenuation correction for myocardial perfusion quantification using a PET/CT hybrid scanner. *J Nucl Med* 2004; 45 (4): 537–42.

4. Lin GA, Dudley RA, Lucas FL, Malenka DJ, Vittinghoff E, Redberg RF. Frequency of stress testing to document ischaemia prior to elective percutaneous coronary intervention. *JAMA* 2008; 300 (15): 1765–73.

5. Topol EJ, Ellis SG, Cosgrove DM, Bates ER, Muller DW, Schork NJ, et al. Analysis of coronary angioplasty practice in the United States with an insurance-claims data base. *Circulation* 1993; 87(5): 1489–97.

6. Hendel RC, Berman DS, Di Carli MF, Heidenreich PA, Henkin RE, Pellikka PA, et al. ACCF/ASNC/ACR/AHA/ASE/SCCT/SCMR/SNM 2009 appropriate use criteria for cardiac radionuclide imaging: a report of the American College of Cardiology Foundation Appropriate Use Criteria Task Force, the American Society of Nuclear Cardiology, the American College of Radiology, the American Heart Association, the American Society of Echocardiography, the Society of Cardiovascular Computed Tomography, the Society for Cardiovascular Magnetic Resonance, and the Society of Nuclear Medicine. *Circulation* 2009; 119 (22): e561–87.

7. Montalescot G, Sechtem U, Achenbach S, Andreotti F, Arden C, Budaj A, et al. 2013 ESC guidelines on the management of stable coronary artery disease: the Task Force on the management of stable coronary artery disease of the European Society of Cardiology. *Eur Heart J* 2013; 34 (38): 2949–3003.

8. Boden WE, O'Rourke RA, Teo KK, Maron DJ, Hartigan PM, Sedlis SP, et al. Impact of optimal medical therapy with or without percutaneous coronary intervention on long-term cardiovascular end points in patients with stable coronary artery disease (from the COURAGE Trial). *Am J Cardiol* 2009; 104 (1): 1–4.

9. Rispler S, Keidar Z, Ghersin E, Roguin A, Soil A, Dragu R, et al. Integrated single-photon emission computed tomography and computed tomography coronary angiography for the assessment of hemodynamically significant coronary artery lesions. *J Am Coll Cardiol* 2007; 49 (10): 1059–67.

10. Di Carli MF, Hachamovitch R. New technology for non-invasive evaluation of coronary artery disease. *Circulation* 2007; 115 (11): 1464–80.

11. Meijboom WB, Meijs MF, Schuijf JD, Cramer MJ, Mollet NR, van Mieghem CA, et al. Diagnostic accuracy of 64-slice computed tomography coronary angiography: a prospective, multicenter, multivendor study. *J Am Coll Cardiol* 2008; 52 (25): 2135–44.

12. Manka R, Kuhn FP, Kuest SM, Gaemperli O, Kozerke S, Kaufmann PA. Hybrid cardiac magnetic resonance/computed tomographic imaging: first fusion of three-dimensional magnetic resonance perfusion and low-dose coronary computed tomographic angiography. *Eur Heart J* 2011; 32 (21): 2625.

13. Rischpler C, Nekolla SG, Dregely I, Schwaiger M. Hybrid PET/MR imaging of the heart: potential, initial experiences, and future prospects. *J Nucl Med* 2013; 54 (3): 402–15.

14. Gould KL, Pan T, Loghin C, Johnson NP, Guha A, Sdringola S. Frequent diagnostic errors in cardiac PET/CT due to misregistration of CT attenuation and emission PET images: a definitive analysis of causes, consequences, and corrections. *J Nucl Med* 2007; 48 (7): 1112–21.

15. Hansen CL, Goldstein RA, Berman DS, Churchwell KB, Cooke CD, Corbett JR, et al. Myocardial perfusion and function single photon emission computed tomography. *J Nucl Cardiol* 2006; 13: e97–120.

16. Borges-Neto S, Pagnanelli RA, Shaw LK, Honeycutt E, Shwartz SC, Adams GL, et al. Clinical results of a novel wide beam reconstruction method for shortening scan time of Tc-99m cardiac SPECT perfusion studies. *J Nucl Cardiol* 2007; 14 (4): 555–65.

17. Muzik O, Duvernoy C, Beanlands RS, Sawada S, Dayanikli F, Wolfe ER,Jr, et al. Assessment of diagnostic performance of quantitative flow measurements in normal subjects and patients with angiographically documented coronary artery disease by means of nitrogen-13 ammonia and positron emission tomography. *J Am Coll Cardiol* 1998; 31 (3): 534–40.

18. Yoshinaga K, Katoh C, Noriyasu K, Iwado Y, Furuyama H, Ito Y, et al. Reduction of coronary flow reserve in areas with and without ischaemia on stress perfusion imaging in patients with coronary artery disease: a study using oxygen 15-labeled water PET. *J Nucl Cardiol* 2003; 10 (3): 275–83.

19. Parkash R, deKemp RA, Ruddy TD, Kitsikis A, Hart R, Beauchesne L, et al. Potential utility of rubidium 82 PET quantification in patients with 3-vessel coronary artery disease. *J Nucl Cardiol* 2004; 11 (4): 440–9.

20. Kajander S, Ukkonen H, Joutsiniemi E, Maki M, Saraste A, Ala-Kruuttila E, et al. The clinical value of absolute quantification of myocardial perfusion in the detection of coronary artery disease. A study using positron emission tomography to detect multi-vessel disease. *Circulation* 2008; 118 (18): S1010–S1.

21. Joutsiniemi E, Saraste A, Pietila M, Maki M, Kajander S, Ukkonen H, et al. Absolute flow or myocardial flow reserve for the detection of significant coronary artery disease? *Eur Heart J Cardiovasc Imaging* 2014; 15(6): 659–65.

22. Kajander S, Joutsiniemi E, Saraste M, Pietila M, Ukkonen H, Saraste A, et al. Cardiac positron emission tomography/computed tomography imaging accurately detects anatomically and functionally significant coronary artery disease. *Circulation* 2010; 122 (6): 603–13.

23. Hesse B, Tagil K, Cuocolo A, Anagnostopoulos C, Bardies M, Bax J, et al. EANM/ESC procedural guidelines for myocardial perfusion imaging in nuclear cardiology. *Eur J Nucl Med Mol Imaging* 2005; 32 (7): 855–97.

24. Bacharach SL, Bax JJ, Case J, Delbeke D, Kurdziel KA, Martin WH, et al. PET myocardial glucose metabolism and perfusion imaging: Part 2—Guidelines for data acquisition and patient preparation. *J Nucl Cardiol* 2003; 10 (5): 543–56.

25. Schelbert HR, Beanlands R, Bengel F, Knuuti J, DiCarli M, Machac J, et al. PET myocardial perfusion and glucose metabolism imaging: Part 2—Guidelines for interpretation and reporting. *J Nucl Cardiol* 2003; 10 (5): 557–71.

26. Kazakauskaite E, Husmann L, Stehli J, Fuchs T, Fiechter M, Klaeser B, et al. Image quality in low-dose coronary computed tomography angiography with a new high-definition CT scanner. *Int J Cardiovasc Imaging* 2013; 29 (2): 471–7.

27. Husmann L, Herzog BA, Gaemperli O, Tatsugami F, Burkhard N, Valenta I, et al. Diagnostic accuracy of computed tomography coronary angiography and evaluation of stress-only single-photon emission computed tomography/computed tomography hybrid imaging: comparison of prospective electrocardiogram-triggering vs. retrospective gating. *Eur Heart J* 2009; 30 (5): 600–7.

28. Herzog BA, Husmann L, Landmesser U, Kaufmann PA. Low-dose computed tomography coronary angiography and myocardial perfusion imaging: cardiac hybrid imaging below 3mSv. *Eur Heart J* 2009; 30 (6): 644.

29. Kajander S, Ukkonen H, Sipila H, Teras M, Knuuti J. Low radiation dose imaging of myocardial perfusion and coronary angiography with a hybrid PET/CT scanner. *Clin Physiol Functional Imaging* 2009; 29 (1): 81–8.

30. Namdar M, Hany TF, Koepfli P, Siegrist PT, Burger C, Wyss CA, et al. Integrated PET/CT for the assessment of coronary artery disease: a feasibility study. *J Nucl Med* 2005; 46 (6): 930–5.

31. Gaemperli O, Schepis T, Valenta I, Koepfli P, Husmann L, Scheffel H, et al. Functionally relevant coronary artery disease: comparison of 64-section CT angiography with myocardial perfusion SPECT. *Radiology* 2008; 248 (2): 414–23.

32. Santana CA, Garcia EV, Faber TL, Sirineni GK, Esteves FP, Sanyal R, et al. Diagnostic performance of fusion of myocardial perfusion imaging (MPI) and computed tomography coronary angiography. *J Nucl Cardiol* 2009; 16 (2): 201–11.

33. Slomka PJ, Cheng VY, Dey D, Woo J, Ramesh A, Van Kriekinge S, et al. Quantitative analysis of myocardial perfusion SPECT anatomically guided by coregistered 64-slice coronary CT angiography. *J Nucl Med* 2009; 50 (10): 1621–30.

34. Schaap J, de Groot JA, Nieman K, Meijboom WB, Boekholdt SM, Post MC, et al. Hybrid myocardial perfusion SPECT/CT coronary angiography and invasive coronary angiography in patients with stable angina pectoris lead to similar treatment decisions. *Heart* 2013; 99 (3): 188–94.

35. Sampson UK, Dorbala S, Limaye A, Kwong R, Di Carli MF. Diagnostic accuracy of rubidium-82 myocardial perfusion imaging with hybrid positron emission tomography/computed tomography in the detection of coronary artery disease. *J Am Coll Cardiol* 2007; 49 (10): 1052–8.

36. Danad I, Raijmakers PG, Appelman YE, Harms HJ, de Haan S, van den Oever ML, et al. Hybrid imaging using quantitative H215O PET and CT-based coronary angiography for the detection of coronary artery disease. *J Nucl Med* 2013; 54 (1): 55–63.

37. Dorbala S, Vangala D, Sampson U, Limaye A, Kwong R, Di Carli MF. Value of vasodilator left ventricular ejection fraction reserve in evaluating the magnitude of myocardium at risk and the extent of angiographic coronary artery disease: a 82Rb PET/CT study. *J Nucl Med* 2007; 48 (3): 349–58.

38. van Werkhoven JM, Schuijf JD, Gaemperli O, Jukema JW, Boersma E, Wijns W, et al. Prognostic value of multislice computed tomography and gated single-photon emission computed tomography in patients with suspected coronary artery disease. *J Am Coll Cardiol* 2009; 53 (7): 623–32.

39. Pazhenkottil AP, Nkoulou RN, Ghadri JR, Herzog BA, Buechel RR, Kuest SM, et al. Prognostic value of cardiac hybrid imaging integrating single-photon emission computed tomography with coronary computed tomography angiography. *Eur Heart J* 2011; 32 (12): 1465–71.

40. Knuuti J, Saraste A. Combined functional and anatomical imaging for the detection and guiding the therapy of coronary artery disease. *Eur Heart J* 2013; 34: 1954–7.

41. Pazhenkottil AP, Nkoulou RN, Ghadri JR, Herzog BA, Kuest SM, Husmann L, et al. Impact of cardiac hybrid single-photon emission computed tomography/computed tomography imaging on choice of treatment strategy in coronary artery disease. *Eur Heart J* 2011; 32 (22): 2824–9.

42. Gaemperli O, Schepis T, Koepfli P, Valenta I, Soyka J, Leschka S, et al. Accuracy of 64-slice CT angiography for the detection of functionally relevant coronary stenoses as assessed with myocardial perfusion SPECT. *Eur J Nucl Med Mol Imaging* 2007; 34 (8): 1162–71.

43. Husmann L, Herzog BA, Burkhard N, Valenta I, Weber K, Kaufmann PA. Coronary artery ectasia causing ischaemia. *Eur J Nucl Med Mol Imaging* 2008; 35 (11): 2142.

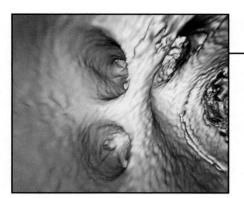

CHAPTER 7

New technical developments in cardiac CT

Stephan Achenbach

Contents

Introduction

Computed tomography (CT), in the context of cardiac imaging, faces numerous challenges. The heart is a complex, three-dimensional organ, which moves very rapidly and has small dimensions. Especially the coronary arteries, the main target of cardiac CT imaging, are difficult to visualize by any non-invasive technique. All the same, technology progress has made the use of CT for cardiac and coronary diagnosis possible. For selected applications, including ruling out coronary artery stenoses in low-risk individuals, CT has become a clinical tool [1, 2].

Historical development

In order to be useful for cardiac imaging, several prerequisites must be fulfilled (see ➲ Table 7.1). The first commercially available CT scanner that permitted visualization of the heart with high temporal and spatial resolution was the 'electron beam tomography' system introduced in the late 1980s. Instead of an X-ray tube, which needs to rotate mechanically around the patient, it used an electron beam that was deflected by electromagnetic coils to sweep across semi-circular targets arranged around the patient where the X-rays were created. The radiation passed through the patient and attenuation was recorded by stationary detectors arranged on the opposite side. Temporal resolution was 100 ms, but slice thickness was limited to 1.5 or 3.0 mm, images were relatively noisy, and cost was high. The electron beam system is no longer available, but it demonstrated the utility of CT imaging for coronary artery calcium assessment and even early CT coronary angiography [3]. This prompted the development of cardiac applications for mechanical CT systems.

Around the year 2000, the first multi-detector row spiral (or 'helical') CT systems were introduced, permitting acquisition of up to four cross-sections with sub-mm thickness simultaneously along with ECG-synchronized image reconstruction. A relatively low pitch (table feed) was used, so that every level of the heart was covered during the entire cardiac cycle by at least one of the four detectors (this acquisition mode is called 'retrospectively ECG-gated spiral acquisition' and is still in use today). It allows all data acquired in systole to be discarded and images to be reconstructed based solely on X-ray attenuation data acquired during phases of slow cardiac motion in diastole. Multi-row acquisition was necessary to cover the complete volume of the heart within one breath-hold, and with four-slice systems, acquisition typically required 35 to 40 s. Imaging the coronary arteries was cumbersome, but possible [4, 5]. It was soon reported that low heart rates substantially improve image quality (since the diastolic phase of slow motion is

Table 7.1 Prerequisites for cardiac imaging using CT

Prerequisite	Achieved through
High spatial resolution	High resolution detector technology Thin slice thickness Relatively high radiation exposure (to reduce noise)
High temporal resolution	High rotation speed Half-scan reconstruction algorithms Dual-source CT Multi-cycle reconstruction algorithms
Synchronization to heart beat	Retrospectively ECG-gated image reconstruction Prospectively ECG-triggered image acquisition
Short overall image acquisition time (one breath-hold)	Multi-detector row technology

Table 7.2 Hardware improvements in cardiac CT and their effect on image quality

Hardware improvement	Effect
Smaller detector elements	Higher spatial resolution
Thinner detector rows	Higher spatial resolution
More detector rows	Faster coverage of the volume of the heart (fewer heart beats), no influence on temporal resolution or spatial resolution
Faster gantry rotation	Higher temporal resolution
Dual-source CT	Higher temporal resolution
Stronger X-ray tube	Lower image noise. Necessary to offset higher noise which would be introduced through thinner slices and faster rotation

prolonged) and short-acting medication to control the heart rate has been recommended for cardiac CT ever since [6].

During subsequent years, the technology of CT evolved substantially. The main achievements were: faster rotation, which immediately translates to better temporal resolution; thinner slices, which improve spatial resolution; and stronger tubes, which are necessary to limit image noise, and are a prerequisite to achieve constant image quality while increasing temporal and spatial resolution. Furthermore, wider detectors were constructed, initially from 4 to 16 and 64 detector rows. A further increase of the number of simultaneously acquired slices was achieved through tubes that have two focal points, so that by rapidly alternating X-ray emission between the two focal points, the number of cross-sectional slices that are acquired is twice as high as the number of detector rows.

Currently, the widest detectors have 320 rows. At a slice thickness of 0.5 mm, a scan volume of 16 cm can be covered, which is sufficient to cover the heart in 'one sweep', so that, unless a combination of data acquired during several cardiac cycles is used to improve temporal resolution, the entire heart can be imaged in one single diastolic phase [7]. This limits the potential for artefacts, permits short breath-holds, and through the shorter

data acquisition time, reduces the amount of contrast agent that is required to achieve intravascular enhancement during the acquisition.

Another major hardware achievement is dual-source CT. It combines two X-ray tubes and two detectors arranged at an angle of approximately 90° [8]. Since X-ray attenuation data acquired over an angle of approximately 180° are necessary to reconstruct one cross-sectional image, dual-source CT permits collection of the required data during a quarter rotation of the X-ray gantry, while single-source CT requires one-half rotation. Dual-source CT, therefore, improves temporal resolution by a factor of two. With a gantry rotation time of 0.28 s, the temporal resolution of each acquired slice is 75 ms (it does not exactly correspond to one-quarter rotation time because the two tubes and detectors are not exactly aligned at a 90° angle). ⊃ Table 7.2 lists hardware advancements and their influence on image quality.

Currently, four manufacturers provide high-end CT systems capable of cardiac imaging. Gantry rotation time is 0.27 to 0.35 s, the number of detector rows ranges from 64 to 320, minimum slice thickness ranges from 0.5 to 0.625 mm, and X-ray tube output from 72 to 100 kW (see ⊃ Table 7.3).

Table 7.3 Comparison of technical properties of currently available high-end cardiac CT systems

	GE Healthcare Revolution	Philips Healthcare iCT	Siemens Healthcare Somatom FORCE	Toshiba Medical Systems Aquilion One
Gantry rotation time	0.28 s	0.27 s	0.25 s	0.35 s
Minimum reconstructed slice width	0.625 mm	0.625	0.5 s	0.5 mm
Number of rows	256	128 (256 slices)	2x196	320
Detector width	160 mm	80 mm	2x58 mm	160 mm
X-ray tube output	120 kW	120 kW	2x120 kW	72 kW
Gantry aperture	80 cm	70 cm	78 cm	72 cm

Areas for improvement

At present, the main application of cardiac CT is coronary artery imaging. Without contrast agent, coronary artery calcification can be detected and quantified, an application that does not require technology to be stretched to its limits. After intravenous injection of contrast, CT permits visualization of the coronary artery lumen. In this context, the spatial and temporal resolution of current CT scanners is just about sufficient to achieve adequate image quality. However, in order to achieve stable image quality, the patient's heart rate should be lowered to 60 beats/min or less, motion artefacts can still be present, and the limited spatial resolution causes problems, e.g. with severely calcified coronary arteries, in the presence of coronary artery stents and in small vessels. Image noise can furthermore be a problem and in the interplay of temporal resolution, spatial resolution, and image noise, false-positive findings can occur, which limit the specificity of coronary CT angiography, especially in difficult-to-image patients (patients with high heart rate, severe calcification, and high body weight) [9, 10]. A further issue is radiation exposure. Especially with spiral acquisition and retrospectively ECG-gated image reconstruction, radiation exposure can be high and unless specific measures are taken to limit exposure, the effective dose can reach 25 mSv or more [11]. Numerous measures have been introduced to reduce dose, but they can increase image noise (such as the use of lower tube current and lower tube voltage), or limit the options to obtain motion-free images (such as the use of prospectively ECG-triggered axial acquisition). The use of low- and very-low dose image acquisition protocols therefore need to be carefully balanced against the need to maintain appropriate image quality.

A completely different aspect is the fact that the limitations of purely anatomic imaging of the coronary artery system are increasingly realized. The extent of ischaemia that a lesion produces is substantially more relevant than the mere anatomic degree of luminal stenosis. Pure anatomic imaging—as provided, for example, by coronary CT angiography—is therefore quite useful to *rule out* haemodynamically relevant coronary artery disease, but in order to identify lesions that require revascularization, information on inducible ischaemia is often desired.

New technical developments—both regarding hardware and especially software—in cardiac CT address the problems outlined and it can be expected that they will increase the applicability of coronary CT angiography and cardiac CT in general.

Prospectively ECG-triggered axial acquisition

The traditional image acquisition mode in coronary CT angiograph has been retrospectively ECG-gated spiral (or 'helical') acquisition. X-ray data are acquired continuously throughout the cardiac cycle, and using the simultaneously recorded ECG, only X-ray data during a specified time interval—usually diastole—are utilized for image reconstruction. Any desired time interval of the cardiac cycle can be used for image reconstruction, so that the 'best time instant' can systematically be searched to minimize motion artefact. Also, dynamic datasets can be reconstructed, which allow analysis of ventricular function. However, much of the acquired X-ray data are not used for image reconstruction and hence, radiation exposure is relatively high.

For this reason, all CT manufacturers have implemented prospectively ECG-triggered axial acquisition modes. In this scan mode, no 'spiral' or 'helical' acquisition is performed. Instead, X-ray data are acquired without table movement, at a pre-specified short time-interval within the cardiac cycle, and then the X-ray tube is switched off and the table moved to the next position [6]. The possibility to perform this data acquisition mode hinges on some hardware requirements: the detector must be of sufficient width so that the complete volume of the heart can be covered within a few steps. Typically, at least 64 slices must be acquired simultaneously (approximately 3 cm), so that the 12–15-cm scan range can be covered in 4 to 5 steps. Depending on heart rate, this amounts to 4 to 10 heart beats (in higher heart rates, images can only be acquired in every other cardiac cycle). Also, scanners must have a sufficiently fast rotation time to guarantee motion-free images in the pre-specified cardiac phase. Especially when heart rate is well-controlled (less than 60 to 65 beats/min), very high image quality can robustly be achieved with prospectively ECG-triggered axial acquisition and the associated radiation exposure is low (typically 1.5 to 3.5 mSv; see ➲ Fig. 7.1). Prospectively ECG-triggered axial acquisition, often termed 'step-and-shoot'

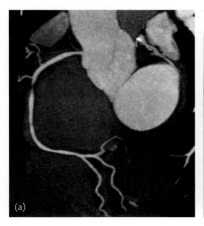
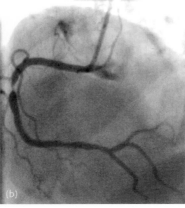

Fig. 7.1 Coronary CT angiography using prospectively ECG-triggered axial acquisition. In patients with low heart rates, high image quality can robustly be achieved. This example was acquired using 100 kV tube voltage, at an effective dose of 1.4 mSv, and shows a high-grade stenosis of the right coronary artery, both in coronary CT angiography (a) and invasive coronary angiography (b).

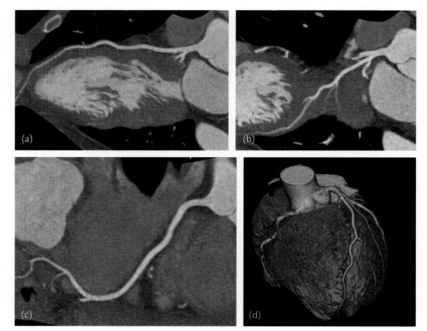

Fig. 7.2 Single-beat coronary CT angiography using prospectively ECG-triggered high-pitch acquisition. Visualization of the left anterior descending coronary artery (a), left circumflex coronary artery (b), right coronary artery (c), and a 3-dimensional reconstruction of the heart and coronary arteries (d). With 100 kV tube voltage, the estimated effective dose was 0.84 mSv.

acquisition, has become the standard scan mode for coronary CT angiography in many institutions.

Single-beat acquisition

Acquisition of the entire cardiac dataset in one single cardiac cycle is attractive because it eliminates 'misalignment' artefacts that can occur when the dataset is pieced together from several cardiac cycles—as typically done in retrospectively ECG-gated spiral acquisition or prospectively ECG-triggered axial acquisition. There are two options to acquire a dataset of the entire heart within one cardiac cycle: If the detector is wide enough, a single prospectively ECG-triggered axial acquisition may provide enough coverage to visualize the entire volume of the heart. This is typically possible with 320-slice scanners [7]. Another option is high-pitch spiral (or 'helical') acquisition, where the table is moved with such a high speed that the entire volume of the heart is covered during spiral acquisition in a period of about 200 ms [12]. This scan mode is well established and validated for dual-source CT and, providing that heart rate is low and very stable, achieves good image quality at very low radiation exposure (see ➲ Fig. 7.2).

Single-beat acquisitions are also attractive for myocardial perfusion studies since they provide a uniform dataset of the complete left ventricle, with all data acquired at the same time interval after contrast injection.

Iterative reconstruction

The conventional method of reconstructing images based on the acquired X-ray attenuation data is called 'filtered back projection'. This method does not make full use of the information in the X-ray data, but is computationally efficient and therefore

widely used in order to keep image reconstruction time acceptable in clinical practice. 'Iterative reconstruction' is a more elaborate image reconstruction method, which makes better use of the information in the X-ray attenuation data, but requires substantially longer times for reconstruction when compared to filtered back projection. However, with modern computers, processing power has increased so that iterative reconstruction methods can now be used clinically. While they alter the visual impression of the reconstructed image data, their substantial advantage is lower image noise (see ➲ Fig. 7.3). Hence, they can be used in combination

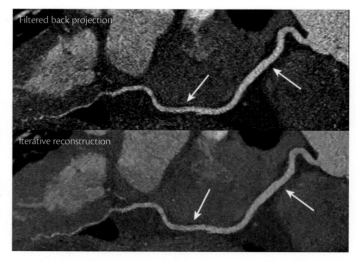

Fig. 7.3 Visualization of the right coronary artery in a low-dose coronary CT angiography dataset acquired at 80 kV (effective dose: 0.3 mSv). Comparison of image noise in conventional filtered back projection and iterative reconstruction. Based on the same raw dataset, iterative reconstruction—although at the cost of longer reconstruction times and visually altered image impression—achieves lower image noise. It may therefore be suited to preserve image quality in low-dose acquisitions.

with low-dose tube settings in order to maintain an acceptable contrast-to-noise ratio while substantially reducing radiation exposure [13, 14]. The potential of iterative reconstruction has not been fully explored yet, but it can be expected to be disseminated widely very soon and to help keep radiation exposure of cardiac CT in an acceptable range.

Dual-energy CT

The tissue-specific absorption of X-ray photons depends on their energy. Therefore, tissue type (even when its concentration is unknown) can be identified based on its relative absorption at different X-ray energies. This effect is utilized in dual-energy CT. X-ray photons with different peak energy levels are sent through the tissue, and based on the differential absorption, specific materials—such as iodine—can be recognized. Specifically, dual-energy CT can be performed by rapidly switching between tube voltages using a single X-ray tube, or by using two tubes (dual-source CT) that simultaneously emit X-rays, the attenuation of which are recorded by two different detectors.

In cardiac imaging, dual-energy CT is infrequently applied. Its use has been suggested to improve the assessment of iodine concentration in the myocardium (see ➲ Fig. 7.4), for example for perfusion imaging or late enhancement [15]. In peripheral vascular CT, dual-energy CT has been used to improve the identification of iodine-filled vessel lumen next to severely calcified plaque [16]. In cardiac and coronary artery imaging, this has not been fully explored, mainly since it would not remove all negative effects that are created by calcium, such as aggravated motion artefacts.

Functional assessment of coronary artery lesions

Relevant coronary stenoses can be ruled out very reliably if a coronary CT angiography dataset shows a completely normal coronary artery lumen or very slight deposition of plaque. However, if luminal narrowing is present, CT does not provide for an accurate assessment of lesion severity. It is even less accurate for identifying lesions that cause ischaemia, since the degree of luminal narrowing and the effects on blood flow at rest and exercise do not correlate closely. All the same, ischaemia is the main reason to treat a coronary artery lesion and the inability to separate 'functionally relevant' (= ischaemia-causing) lesions from stenoses that do not cause ischaemia has been an area of critique.

In order to improve the ability of CT to identify ischaemia-causing lesions, and also to possibly make lesion assessment more independent from image quality, several new developments are undertaken.

CT myocardial perfusion imaging

In a fashion very similar to SPECT myocardial perfusion, CT imaging can be performed before and after adenosine medication, and intravenous iodine-based contrast is injected to enhance the left ventricular myocardium [17] (see ➲ Fig. 7.5). Acquisition can either be 'static' or 'dynamic'. In static acquisitions, a CT dataset of the heart is acquired 3 to 5 min into a continuous adenosine infusion, at a single time instant (typically, at peak enhancement) after injection of i.v. contrast [18]. In 'dynamic' CT myocardial perfusion, image acquisition is repeated, for example, at every heart beat or every other heart beat during a certain time interval [19]. At the price of increased radiation exposure, information on the upslope

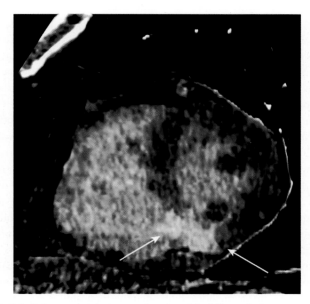

Fig. 7.4 Colour-coded dual-energy imaging of the left ventricular myocardium in a dataset obtained 12 min after contrast injection. 'Late enhancement' (arrows) in the inferior region can clearly be delineated in the iodine concentration map based on dual-energy CT acquired simultaneously at 100kV and 140kV peak tube voltage.

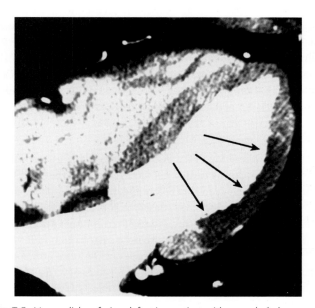

Fig. 7.5 Myocardial perfusion defect in a patient with an occluded intermediate branch of the left main coronary artery. The hypo-perfused myocardium can clearly be delineated (arrows).

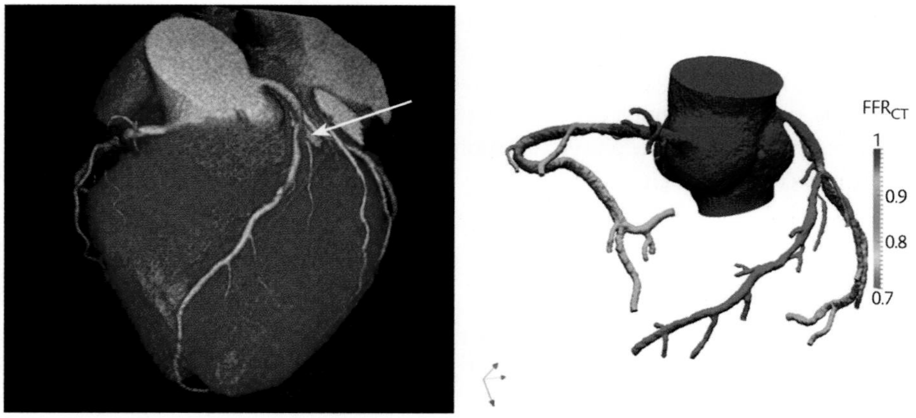

Fig. 7.6 Determination of FFR$_{CT}$. Left: 3-dimensional reconstruction of a coronary CT angiography dataset that shows a high grade stenosis of the left anterior descending coronary artery (arrow). Right: Determination of FFR$_{CT}$ shows that the FFR distal to the lesion is below 0.75, indicating a haemodynamically significant stenosis.

of myocardial attenuation after contrast injection can be obtained. CT myocardial perfusion imaging is still undergoing clinical validation. Superiority of one acquisition method over another, and many methodological details, such as the best form of contrast injection or pharmacological stress, the best algorithms for evaluation, the use of iterative reconstruction or dual-energy protocols, have not yet been clarified. Comparisons to other methods that assess the functional relevance of coronary artery lesions have been performed and indicate relatively good agreement [18, 19, 20]. The best clinical algorithms to combine coronary CT angiography and CT myocardial perfusion imaging remain to be defined.

Transluminal attenuation gradient

The 'transluminal attenuation gradient' has been suggested to extract information on the haemodynamic relevance of a coronary artery lesion from the coronary CT angiography dataset acquired at rest [21, 22]. CT attenuation is measured in short, fixed intervals along the course of a coronary artery from its proximal part to the distal segment. Smoothing functions correct for variations due to spotty calcified lesions, image noise, and measurement variability. It is assumed that 'haemodynamically relevant' stenoses are associated with a steeper decline of intraluminal contrast attenuation than non-relevant stenoses or lesions which, because of artefacts, appear more severely narrowed than they actually are. The 'transluminal attenuation gradient' has been evaluated in a small number of studies [21–23] and its role has not yet been firmly established.

FFR$_{CT}$

Fractional flow reserve (FFR) can be measured with intra-coronary pressure probes during cardiac catheterization. It is the gradient of mean intra-coronary pressure before and distal to a coronary artery lesion during adenosine stress. Based on the 'FAME' study results [24, 25], FFR values >0.80 are considered to represent a non-significant lesion, which does not require revascularization. FFR values ≤0.75 indicate a 'haemodynamically relevant' lesion, a grey zone of indeterminate relevance lies between FFR values of 0.75 and 0.80.

Using computational fluid dynamics, the effect of coronary artery geometry obtained by coronary CT angiography at rest on FFR during adenosine stress can be modelled. The resulting values are referred to as FFR$_{CT}$ and are displayed in a colour-coded, continuous

fashion alongside the coronary artery tree (see ⤷ Fig. 7.6). FFR$_{CT}$ has been validated against invasively measured FFR in two multi-centre trials. The initial 'Discover-Flow' trial comprised 104 patients and demonstrated a high accuracy of FFR$_{CT}$ to identify coronary arteries with an invasively measured FFR <0.80 (sensitivity 88%, specificity 82%) [26]. The advantage as compared to purely anatomic, visual analysis of the CT angiography dataset was most pronounced in lesions of intermediate severity. In a second, larger trial of 252 patients with known or suspected stable coronary artery disease, in which less rigorous constraints were applied concerning image quality, per-patient sensitivity was 90% and specificity was 54% [27]. The possibility of obtaining functional information out of purely static coronary CT angiography datasets has raised considerable attention. Clinical application depends on further, intensive validation.

Automated plaque analysis

One of the very interesting properties of coronary CT angiography is its ability to visualize—and, with certain limitations, to characterize—non-stenotic coronary atherosclerotic plaque. Currently, the most frequently used parameter to quantify the extent of coronary atherosclerosis in CT angiography is the 'segment involvement score' (SIS) first proposed in 2007 [28]. Optimally, however, evaluation of plaque burden and plaque characteristics would be fully quantitative and include the entire coronary artery tree. Manual identification and tracing of plaque along the entire coronary artery system is not feasible and is subject to high variability. Hence, global quantification of coronary atherosclerotic plaque would only be possible with an automated approach. Algorithms for this purpose are challenging because of the low difference in tissue densities between non-calcified atherosclerotic plaque and adjacent peri-vascular tissue. However, they are under development and in validation and can be expected to become clinically available soon [29] (see ⤷ Fig. 7.7).

In summary, the technical progress of cardiac CT, and especially coronary CT angiography, is continuous and rapid. One major aim is to improve image quality and broaden the applicability of coronary CT angiography, while at the same time achieving lower radiation doses. The other major aim is to extract more than purely anatomic information out of the dataset and to complement the information in luminal narrowing with information on downstream ischaemia.

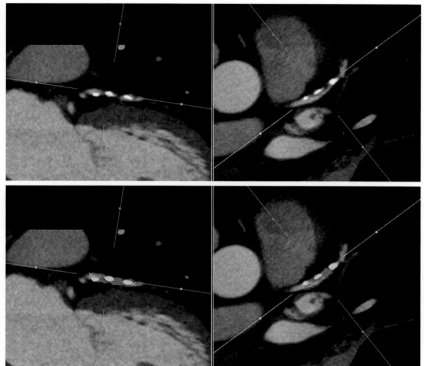

Fig. 7.7 Automated plaque analysis: automated determination of calcified plaque (yellow) and non-calcified plaque (red) in a lesion of the left anterior descending coronary artery. Total plaque volume is 187 mm³, calcified plaque volume is 43 mm³ and non-calcified volume is 144 mm³. The volume of non-calcified plaque with a density below 30 HU (often assumed to indicate plaque vulnerability) is 37mm³.

References

1. Taylor AJ, Cerqueira M, Hodgson JM, et al. American College of Cardiology Foundation Appropriate Use Criteria Task Force; Society of Cardiovascular Computed Tomography; American College of Radiology; American Heart Association; American Society of Echocardiography; American Society of Nuclear Cardiology; North American Society for Cardiovascular Imaging; Society for Cardiovascular Angiography and Interventions; Society for Cardiovascular Magnetic Resonance. ACCF/SCCT/ACR/AHA/ASE/ASNC/NASCI/SCAI/SCMR 2010 Appropriate Use Criteria for Cardiac Computed Tomography. A Report of the American College of Cardiology Foundation Appropriate Use Criteria Task Force, the Society of Cardiovascular Computed Tomography, the American College of Radiology, the American Heart Association, the American Society of Echocardiography, the American Society of Nuclear Cardiology, the North American Society for Cardiovascular Imaging, the Society for Cardiovascular Angiography and Interventions, and the Society for Cardiovascular Magnetic Resonance. *J Am Coll Cardiol* 2010; 56 (22): 1864–94.

2. Hamm CW, Bassand JP, Agewall S, et al. ESC Committee for Practice Guidelines. ESC guidelines for the management of acute coronary syndromes in patients presenting without persistent ST-segment elevation: The Task Force for the management of acute coronary syndromes (ACS) in patients presenting without persistent ST-segment elevation of the European Society of Cardiology (ESC). *Eur Heart J* 2011; 32 (23): 2999–3054.

3. Achenbach S, Moshage W, Ropers D, Nossen J, Daniel WG. Value of electron-beam computed tomography for the noninvasive detection of high-grade coronary-artery stenoses and occlusions. *N Engl J Med* 1998; 339: 1964–71.

4. Achenbach S, Ulzheimer S, Baum U, et al. Non-invasive coronary angiography by retrospectively ECG-gated multi-slice spiral CT. *Circulation* 2000; 102: 2823–28.

5. Achenbach S, Giesler T, Ropers D, et al. Detection of coronary artery stenoses by contrast-enhanced, retrospectively ECG-gated, multi-slice spiral CT. *Circulation* 2001; 103: 2535–38.

6. Abbara S, Arbab-Zadeh A, Callister TQ, et al. SCCT guidelines for performance of coronary computed tomographic angiography: a report of the Society of Cardiovascular Computed Tomography Guidelines Committee. *J Cardiovasc Comput Tomogr* 2009; 3: 190–204.

7. Dewey M, Zimmermann E, Deissenrieder F, et al. Noninvasive coronary angiography by 320-row computed tomography with lower radiation exposure and maintained diagnostic accuracy: comparison of results with cardiac catheterization in a head-to-head pilot investigation. *Circulation* 2009; 120: 867–75.

8. Flohr TG, McCollough CH, Bruder H, et al. First performance evaluation of a dual-source CT (DSCT) system. *Eur Radiol* 2006; 16: 256–68.

9. Paech DC, Weston AR. A systematic review of the clinical effectiveness of 64-slice or higher computed tomography angiography as an alternative to invasive coronary angiography in the investigation of suspected coronary artery disease. *BMC Cardiovasc Disord* 2011; 11: 32.

10. Westwood ME, Raatz HD, Misso K, et al. Systematic review of the accuracy of dual-source cardiac CT for detection of arterial stenosis in difficult to image patient groups. *Radiology* 2013; 267 (2): 387–95.

11. Hausleiter J, Meyer T, Hermann F, et al. Estimated radiation dose associated with cardiac CT angiography. *JAMA* 2009; 301: 500–7.

12. Achenbach S, Marwan M, Ropers D, et al. Coronary computed tomography angiography with a consistent dose below 1 mSv using prospectively ECG-triggered high-pitch spiral acquisition. *Eur Heart J* 2010; 31: 340–46.

13. Leipsic J, Labounty TM, Heilbron B, et al. Estimated radiation dose reduction using adaptive statistical iterative reconstruction in

coronary CT angiography: the ERASIR study. *AJR Am J Roentgenol* 2010; 195: 655–60.

14. Bittencourt MS, Schmidt B, Seltmann M, et al. Iterative reconstruction in image space (IRIS) in cardiac computed tomography: initial experience. *Int J Cardiovasc Imaging* 2011; 27: 1081–87.

15. Schwarz F, Ruzsics B, Schoepf UJ, et al. Dual-energy CT of the heart—principles and protocols. *Eur J Radiol* 2008; 68: 423–33.

16. Huang SY, Nelson RC, Miller MJ, et al. Assessment of vascular contrast and depiction of stenoses in abdominopelvic and lower extremity vasculature: comparison of dual-energy MDCT with digital subtraction angiography. *Acad Radiol* 2012; 19: 1149–57.

17. Blankstein R, Shturman LD, Rogers IS, et al. Adenosine-induced stress myocardial perfusion imaging using dual-source cardiac computed tomography. *J Am Coll Cardiol* 2009; 54: 1072–84.

18. Rocha-Filho JA, Blankstein R, Shturman LD, et al. Incremental value of adenosine-induced stress myocardial perfusion imaging with dual-source CT at cardiac CT angiography. *Radiology* 2010; 254: 410–19.

19. Ho KT, Chua KC, Klotz E, Panknin C. Stress and rest dynamic myocardial perfusion imaging by evaluation of complete time-attenuation curves with dual-source CT. *JACC Cardiovasc Imaging* 2010 Aug; 3 (8): 811–20.

20. Wang Y, Qin L, Shi X, Zeng Y, Jing H, Schoepf UJ, Jin Z. Adenosine-stress dynamic myocardial perfusion imaging with second-generation dual-source CT: comparison with conventional catheter coronary angiography and SPECT nuclear myocardial perfusion imaging. *AJR Am J Roentgenol* 2012 Mar; 198 (3): 521–9.

21. Steigner ML, Mitsouras D, Whitmore AG, et al. Iodinated contrast opacification gradients in normal coronary arteries imaged with prospectively ECG-gated single heart beat 320-detector row computed tomography. *Circ Cardiovasc Imaging* 2010; 3: 179–86.

22. Choi JH, Koo BK, Yoon YE, et al. Diagnostic performance of intra-coronary gradient-based methods by coronary computed tomography angiography for the evaluation of physiologically significant coronary artery stenoses: a validation study with fractional flow reserve. *Eur Heart J Cardiovasc Imaging* 2012; 13 (12): 1001–7.

23. Yoon YE, Choi JH, Kim JH, et al. Noninvasive diagnosis of ischaemia-causing coronary stenosis using CT angiography: diagnostic value of transluminal attenuation gradient and fractional flow reserve computed from coronary CT angiography compared to invasively measured fractional flow reserve. *JACC Cardiovasc Imaging* 2012; 5: 1088–96.

24. Tonino PA, De Bruyne B, Pijls NH, et al. FAME Study Investigators. Fractional flow reserve versus angiography for guiding percutaneous coronary intervention. *N Engl J Med.* 2009; 360: 213–24.

25. De Bruyne B, Pijls NH, Kalesan B, et al. FAME 2 Trial Investigators. Fractional flow reserve-guided PCI versus medical therapy in stable coronary disease. *N Engl J Med.* 2012; 367: 991–1001.

26. Koo BK, Erglis A, Doh JH, et al. Diagnosis of ischaemia-causing coronary stenoses by noninvasive fractional flow reserve computed from coronary computed tomographic angiograms results from the prospective multicenter DISCOVER-FLOW (diagnosis of ischaemia-causing stenoses obtained via noninvasive fractional flow reserve) Study. *J Am Coll Cardiol* 2011; 58: 1989–897.

27. Min JK, Leipsic J, Pencina MJ, et al. Diagnostic accuracy of fractional flow reserve from anatomic CT angiography. *JAMA* 2012; 308: 1237–45.

28. Min JK, Shaw LJ, Devereux RB, et al. Prognostic value of multidetector coronary computed tomographic angiography for prediction of all-cause mortality. *J Am Coll Cardiol* 2007; 50: 1161–70.

29. Dey D, Schepis T, Marwan M, Slomka PJ, Berman DS, Achenbach S. Automated three-dimensional quantification of noncalcified coronary plaque from coronary CT angiography: comparison with intravascular US. *Radiology* 2010; 257: 516–22.

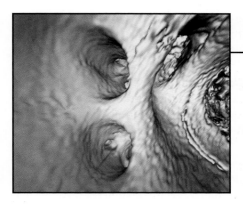

CHAPTER 8

New technical developments in CMR

Reza Razavi, Manav Sohal, Zhong Chen, and James Harrison

Contents

T1 mapping

Structure, function, regional myocardial scar assessment, and, recently, perfusion assessment have become the cornerstones of routine clinical cardiac magnetic resonance (CMR) imaging applications. In the last two years there has been a tremendous growth in clinical research in the area of T1 mapping to address the need for better myocardial tissue characterization. There is great potential in T1 mapping and its related forms being used as biomarkers for detection and monitoring of disease pathology, response to treatment, and as prognostic indicators to clinical outcomes.

The first medical application of magnetic resonance imaging measured longitudinal proton relaxation time, T1, was to detect and characterize tumour [1]. A myocardial T1 map is a parametric reconstructed image where the signal intensity of each pixel represents the T1 longitudinal relaxation time of the corresponding myocardial voxel. The voxel-by-voxel T1 estimation is derived from multiple samplings along the recovery curve following a specific preparation sequence (see ⊃ Fig. 8.1). It allows true quantitative signal quantification on a standardized scale of image voxel to characterize tissue heterogeneity. This eliminates the influence of imprecise inversion time selection, which is needed to null the apparently normal remote myocardium with standard delayed enhanced CMR.

T1 mapping methods

There are many ways of assessing T1. Two methods, based on the standard Look-Locker method, have largely been adopted and validated for T1 mapping in the literature [2, 3]. The Modified Look-Locker Inversion recovery sequence (MOLLI), proposed by Messroghli et al., merges images sampled from eleven different inversion times (TI) from three consecutive inversion–recovery (IR) experiments into one dataset in a 17-heartbeat breath-hold; whereas Shortened Modified Look-Locker Inversion recovery (ShMOLLI), proposed by Piechnik et al., samples from seven different TIs in a 9-heartbeat breath-hold. Both methods have been readily applied in T1 mapping data acquisition in patients with a variety of cardiac pathologies. However, both methods are susceptible to underestimation of the true T1 values. Especially at high T1 values, MOLLI demonstrated a greater dependence on heart rate requiring adjustment whereas ShMOLLI required only an empirical adjustment [3–5].

Myocardial fibrosis detection by delayed contrast enhancement CMR sequence is dependent on a greater distribution volume and slower wash-out of contrast agents within tissues of greater extracellular space. The delayed contrast-enhanced CMR pulse sequence has been the gold standard in detecting regional fibrosis. An important drawback of the method is the need for manual selection of IR time to generate an image with signal contrasts between the fibrotic region and apparently non-fibrotic region. Delayed-enhancement imaging thus is good at differentiating between 'normal' and diseased

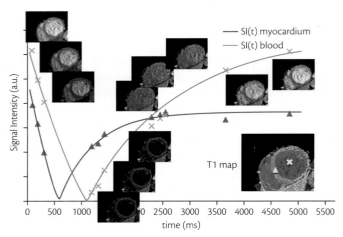

Fig. 8.1 Illustration of T1 mapping using Modified Look-Locker Inversion recovery imaging (MOLLI) sequence. The final T1 map merges images sampled from eleven different inversion times (TI). T1 value is determined by fitting a 3-parameter exponential model to the measured data on a voxel-by-voxel basis.

myocardium but less good at looking at diffuse processes that affect the myocardium in a more homogeneous way. T1 mapping by assessing the voxel signal intensity on a standardized scale, rather than an arbitrary scale, does not depend on a 'normal' reference and therefore has the advantage of detecting diffuse fibrosis.

In addition to the type of acquisition sequence, heart rate and scanner field strength, the post-contrast T1 value in T1 mapping measurements is also largely dependent on the properties of the gadolinium contrast agents, the dose of contrast, the time delay of the T1 mapping after contrast injection, the haemocrit level, which affects the partition coefficient of the gadolinium contrast agent, the contrast kinetics between regions of fibrosis and normal myocardium, and the contrast wash-out rate, which is also influenced by the renal clearance rate. Myocardial contrast volume of distribution ($VD_{(m)}$) or extracellular volume (ECV) quantification has been therefore proposed as a measure of myocardial fibrosis in order to circumvent some of these confounding factors related to standalone post-contrast T1 measurement.

ECV is estimated from the concentration of extracellular contrast agent such as gadolinium in the myocardium relative to the blood in a dynamic steady state:

$$ECV = (1 - \text{haematocrit}) \times ((1/\text{Post-contrast T1myocardium} - 1/\text{Pre-contrast T1myocardium})/(1/\text{Post-contrast T1blood} - 1/\text{Pre-contrast T1blood}))$$

The formula holds true when the extracellular contrast concentration in the blood and the myocardium reaches equilibrium.

Kehr et al. demonstrated a correlation between ECV and collagen volume fraction (CVF) in human myocardium *in vitro* [6]. Using a bolus injection followed by a slow infusion of contrast protocol to ensure a steady contrast equilibrium when post-contrast T1 is measured, Flett et al. have demonstrated a close correlation between ECV and CVF measured on histological samples indicating diffuse fibrosis from a group of patients with either aortic stenosis or hypertrophic cardiomyopathy (HCM) [7].

There is an ongoing debate whether, instead of infusion, a bolus injection of contrast can achieve a steady state between the intravascular compartment and the myocardial interstitial compartment. A single bolus injection would make the CMR protocol simpler and easier to integrate into daily clinical practice. Schelbert et al. demonstrated that there is no significant difference between the measured ECV 12–50 min after a bolus injection of contrast compared with an infusion protocol in 10 volunteers with an age range between 20 and 81 [8]. However, Kawal et al. demonstrated that serial measurements between 5 and 45 min after bolus injection of contrast revealed a small but significant increase in measured ECV in a group of younger healthy volunteers, implying that post-contrast T1 values for the estimation of ECV should be made at the same intervals post-bolus injection in order to improve the accuracy of ECV as a biomarker for diffuse fibrosis [9]. Messroghli et al. demonstrated a moderate correlation of ECV, estimated with post-contrast T1 measured 20 min after bolus injection of contrast, with CVF found on cardiac histology in a rat model of cardiac diffuse interstitial fibrosis [10].

T1 mapping requires a fundamental post-imaging processing, which is a voxel-by-voxel registration between the different T1 images taken at different IR times; in addition, in order to generate ECV maps and analysis, further registration is required to match the pre- and post-contrast T1 maps. In its clinical application, we are likely to encounter image motions due to body movement given the significant time-lapse between the pre- and post-contrast T1 maps acquisition (typically 15-30 min apart), respiratory motion artefact due to inadequate breath-hold, as well as cardiac motion due to arrhythmia and heart rate variability. Xue et al. has described and validated a method that is non-rigid, fully automated, and integrated to the image acquisition and processing of T1 mapping [11]. Incorporating this method, Kellman et al. has devised a workflow that integrates the motion correction and coregistration of breath-holds to improve the accuracy of ECV mapping/calculation, which make its translation to clinical application feasible [12]. They correlated the ECV on a continuous scale with the severity of fibrosis in a variety of disease pathologies that included myocarditis, non-ischaemic dilated cardiomyopathy (NIDCM), HCM, amyloidosis, and chronic myocardial infarction [13].

Clinical applications of T1 mapping

The initial research into the clinical applications of T1 mapping has focused on post-contrast T1 values. Iles et al. first demonstrated a correlation between post-contrast T1 values with a quantitative histological measure of fibrosis, CVF, in patients with heart failure of various aetiologies [14]. Lower post-contrast T1 values were correlated with a higher histological percentage of collagen and associated with worsening diastolic function markers detected by transthoracic echocardiograph. Recently, in a larger cohort of 45 patients with cardiomyopathies of mixed aetiologies, most of whom had evidence of diffuse fibrosis on histology, Sibley et al. also found that post-contrast T1 values had a significant correlation with histological measure of fibrosis [15]. Ng et al. also found lower global post-contrast T1 correlated with diastolic dysfunction in diabetic patients free of coronary artery disease and regional fibrosis [16]. Sparrow et al. showed that segmental post-contrast T1 values were increased in regions with impaired wall motion in a small number of patients with chronic aortic regurgitation [17].

T1 measurements can also be performed in regional fibrosis caused by scar post-myocardial infarction. Messroghli et al. found lower post-contrast T1 values in the infarct region compared with non-infarct region in acute and chronic myocardial infarction [5]. Increases in the interstitial space can also be caused by processes such as the protein deposition in amyloidosis, and Maceira et al. found an association of lower sub-endocardial post-contrast T1 in patients with amyloidosis compared with controls [18]. However, the application of T1 measurements in these areas with regional changes is potentially problematic because the derived ECV measurement relies on the prerequisite of a two-compartment model with contrast equilibrium between the blood and the myocardium. An assumption is made that there is a constant myocardial plasma volume fraction, reflecting homogeneous capillary density in the myocardium, which is not necessarily the case in conditions such as amyloidosis and replacement fibrosis post-myocardial infarction.

It was recognized early on that converse to post-contrast T1, non-contrast T1 is higher in infarct regions compared with non-infarct regions in ischaemic cardiomyopathy [3, 5]. Though still susceptible to the influence of acquisition sequence and magnetic field strength, native non-contrast T1 can remove the dependence on contrast kinetics and avoid the potential of contrast-associated nephrogenic systemic fibrosis. In two separate studies, Puntmann et al. and Dass et al. have both recently demonstrated significantly higher non-contrast T1 values in hypertrophic cardiomyopathy (HCM) and non-ischaemic dilated cardiomyopathy (NIDCM) compared with normal controlled group with T1 mapping acquired on 3Tesla scanners [19, 20]. Dass et al. not only noticed a difference between regions with late gadolinium enhancement (LGE), but also regions without LGE, in the cardiomyopathy group and the normal control group. Both studies suggest the potential implication of non-contrast native T1 being a useful biomarker in detecting diffuse disease in cardiac pathologies. Puntmann et al. further demonstrated a higher non-contrast native T1 in systemic lupus erythematosus patients with normal myocardial function, implying that native T1 mapping can be a sensitive detector of subclinical myocardial disease [21]. Indeed, Karamitsos et al. found a higher non-contrast T1 value in patients with amyloid light-chain (AL) amyloidosis in the absence of definitive cardiac manifestations [22]. The scale of T1 value correlated with markers of cardiac systolic and diastolic function. Others have found non-contrast native T1 value to be useful for assessing areas of myocardial oedema in Takotsubo cardiomyopathy and quantifying areas-at-risk in acute myocardial infarction, comparable with the conventional T2-weighted images [23–25]. In a systematic analysis and an attempt to establish a normal reference range of non-contrast T1 values acquired with ShMOLLI on 1.5T scanner (a cohort of 342 healthy volunteers, 50% females, age 11–69), Piechnik et al. found the non-contrast T1 to be a highly reproducible and stable biomarker for characterizing the myocardium [26].

Potential promise and limitations of T1 mapping

Given the reported correlation of non-contrast native T1 with disease pathology, we must, however, be cautious in interpreting the value of native T1. We know that T1 increases with increased water content. We therefore speculate that the increase in native non-contrast T1 is due to an expansion of extracellular volume and change in extracellular matrix composition. This assumption seems to be in accordance with the trend observed with post-contrast T1 and ECV, for example, Scholz et al., demonstrated a correlation between T1 with the amount of free-water content and collagen in canine hearts [27]. Bull et al. also found a correlation between native T1 with CVF on histology samples from patients with moderate and severe aortic stenosis [28]. This, however, may not be the complete picture. Puntmann et al. did not find a significant difference in non-contrast T1 value between the regions with and without LGE in the septum in patients with HCM or NIDCM [19] and Dass et al. found a stronger correlation of non-contrast T1 with impaired myocardial energetics measured by magnetic resonance spectroscope than with LGE, suggesting that non-contrast T1 may additionally reflect intracellular metabolic state associated with myocardial disease [20].

As with any emerging technique, we can only explore the potentials of T1 mapping through a better understanding of its limitations. Though differences in T1 mapping acquisition sequences and protocols make the absolute T1 values difficult to compare across studies, the evidence presented so far demonstrated that T1 mapping can be used as a sensitive tool for characterizing myocardial tissue. It shows great promise in becoming another cornerstone in the clinical application of CMR, but needs to be performed in rigorous conditions with accurate post-processing registration in order to improve its efficacy. We are waiting to demonstrate the correlation of T1 mapping and ECV with clinical outcomes and new acquisition sequences that will allow us to characterize the myocardium in high resolution in a three-dimensional scale in patients.

Atrial CMR

In recent years, radiofrequency (RF) catheter ablation has emerged as an effective and potentially curative approach for patients with symptomatic paroxysmal and persistent atrial fibrillation (AF), who have failed drug therapy [29]. The demonstration that paroxysmal AF is frequently triggered by ectopy arising from within the pulmonary veins (PV) has led to the emergence of PV isolation as a widely practised therapy for this arrhythmia and even as a first-line therapy in selected patients [30, 31]. These procedures require trans-septal access to the left atrium (LA) and identification of the PV ostia, following which ablation lesions are deployed in a continuous and circumferential manner to isolate the left and right PVs, either individually or in pairs, with the endpoint of electrical disconnection from the LA. Incomplete or non-transmural circumferential ablation lesions may lead to immediate or delayed reconnection of the PVs, which can be documented in the majority of cases of AF recurrence [32]. These gaps in ablation lines are thought to be one of the reasons for the relatively modest success rates of AF ablation.

Accordingly, there has been an increasing interest in the use of cardiac magnetic resonance (CMR) to provide pre- and post-procedural non-invasive atrial tissue characterization to assess patient suitability and response to catheter ablation [33–42] and to guide both repeat catheter ablation [39, 43] and real-time CMR-guided electrophysiology procedures [44–47]

CMR of ablation injury

Several animal studies have shown that atrial and ventricular ablation lesions can be acutely visualized with CMR following thermal injury. Lardo et al. described the spatial and temporal extent of ablation lesions created at the right ventricular apex of six mongrel dogs using T2-weighted and contrast enhanced T1-weighted CMR and found a strong correlation between lesion size, according to CMR, and macroscopic examination [48]. Dickfeld et al. described the gadolinium enhanced T1-weighted CMR appearances of acute RF ablation lesions created on the right ventricular epicardium of eight mongrel dogs using a power-controlled, cooled-tip ablation system [49]. Four distinct phases of signal enhancement were observed over a follow-up period of 10 h, which correlated well with pathological findings. In a further study, they were also able to visualize lesions with non-enhanced T2-weighted CMR from 30 min to 12 h after ablation [50].

However, visualizing lesions in the thinner walled atria is inherently more challenging. Even at the current limits of CMR spatial resolution, the atrial wall is covered by only a few voxels and the contrast between acute injury or chronic scar/fibrosis and healthy atrium is less easily visualized than in the ventricle. Published studies investigating acute atrial CMR lesion measurements in comparison with pathological examination are limited and have been in the context of real-time CMR-guided electrophysiology [44–46]. Vergara et al. showed a correlation between the size of four focal atrial ablation lesions, measured by T2-weighted CMR and macroscopic examination, but only 30% of lesions could be visualized [45]. Nordbeck et al. demonstrated a correlation between the size of eight focal atrial and ventricular ablation lesions measured by T2-weighted and late gadolinium enhancement (LGE) CMR and

macroscopic examination, with a trend towards larger lesion size measured by T2-weighted CMR [46]. Most recently, Ranjan et al. demonstrated the ability of CMR to visualize deliberate gaps in acute ablation lesions up to 1.4 mm in size with a strong correlation between gap length identified using CMR and gross pathology [44].

Left atrial CMR

Over the past few years, technological developments and novel imaging sequences [38–41] have made LA LGE CMR possible. A recent series of studies has suggested that LA LGE, both before and after catheter ablation, can help predict the chance of recurrence of AF by identifying the extent of pre-existing fibrosis and post-ablation scar [33, 34, 38–41, 51]. It is proposed that this may allow a more individualized approach to AF ablation.

Imaging sequences for LA LGE imaging vary between institutions. In summary, they involve planning scans, an anatomical scan for LA and PV segmentation, and a 3D inversion–recovery (IR) LGE sequence following the injection of a gadolinium-based contrast agent.

In our institution [36, 37], scans are performed in a 1.5T Philips Achieva MR scanner (Philips Medical Systems, Best, The Netherlands) using a 32-channel surface coil. First, survey and sensitivity encoding (SENSE) reference scans are obtained, followed by a 2D multi-cardiac phase cine scan acquired in a 4-chamber orientation. From this scan, the trigger delay is determined for all subsequent scans in order to minimize artefacts from atrial wall motion. The anatomical sequence is a respiratory navigated, ECG-triggered 3D balanced steady-state free precession (b-SSFP) scan acquired in a sagittal orientation with whole heart coverage (typical echo time, TE, is 30 ms; isotropic resolution 2 mm). Twenty minutes after the administration of 0.2 ml/kg Gadovist (Bayer HealthCare Pharmaceuticals, Berlin, Germany), 3D LGE imaging is performed with a respiratory navigated, ECG-triggered IR turbo field echo (TFE) acquisition with a spatial resolution of $1.3 \times 1.3 \times 4$ mm^3, reconstructed to $0.6 \times 0.6 \times 2$ mm^3, using TE/TR of 3.0/6.2 ms and a flip angle of 25°. The inversion time (TI) is determined using a preceding Look-Locker sequence, to achieve optimal suppression of ventricular myocardium. The scan is acquired in an axial orientation, typically with 30–40 slices to achieve complete coverage of the LA (◑ Fig. 8.2). The length of

Fig. 8.2 An axial slice from a 3D LGE CMR (left) and a 3D left atrial reconstruction (right) from a patient with previous pulmonary vein isolation for paroxysmal atrial fibrillation. The 3D reconstruction is created by segmenting a whole heart b-SSFP acquisition and displaying the LGE scan on the segmented left atrial shell using a maximum intensity projection (signal intensities are expressed as the number of standard deviations (SD) from the mean signal intensity of the atrial blood pool).

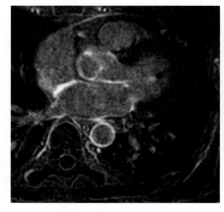
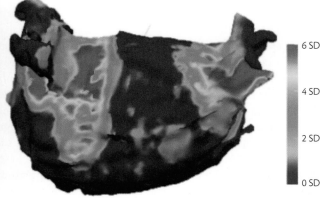

the acquisition window is set to a maximum of 150 ms to mini-mize motion artefacts.

The entire scan takes approximately 45 min. The two most important predictors of poor LA LGE image quality are the presence of AF (particularly with a rapid ventricular response rate) and an inconsistent respiratory navigator signal.

Pre-ablation imaging

Irreversible remodelling of the LA is thought to limit the effectiveness of PV isolation for AF and to be an important factor impacting the success of the procedure [52]. Endomyocardial atrial biopsies in patients with lone AF show fibrosis in the left atrial wall [53]. A non-invasive method of detecting the location and extent of these fibrotic areas before AF ablation might be able to predict the long-term success of the procedure in an individual patient.

Oakes et al. first studied the role of LA LGE CMR in detecting the extent of atrial remodelling in 118 patients before AF ablation for either paroxysmal or persistent AF [33]. Image quality was insufficient in 37 patients, leaving 81 patients in the study. They identified varying degrees of LGE in the LA wall, with 43 patients having mild enhancement (<15% of the LA wall area), 30 with moderate enhancement (15–35% of the LA wall area) and 8 with severe enhancement (>35% of the LA wall area). At 6 months follow-up, AF recurrence increased with pre-ablation enhancement, with 14% recurrence in the mild enhancement group, 43% in the moderate enhancement group, and 75% in the severe enhancement group. They concluded that LA LGE CMR is able to offer a non-invasive means of predicting disease severity and response to AF ablation.

The same group later revised the extent of LA enhancement into a four-stage classification system: Utah I (<5% enhancement), Utah II (5–20% enhancement), Utah III (21–35% enhancement), and Utah IV (>35% enhancement) [34, 40]. These studies once again suggested that the extent of pre-existing LGE is proportional to the incidence of AF recurrence, despite there being comparable LGE across the four Utah stages on follow-up scans 3 months after ablation. There was no difference in this finding between patients with lone and those with non-lone AF. They further stated that a more extensive ablation strategy was appropriate in those with more enhancement, although in Utah IV ablation was unlikely to be successful.

This non-invasive pre-ablation imaging has recently been extended to predicting the risk of stroke in AF. It is known that LA structural remodelling in AF increases the risk of thrombo-embolism [54] and, therefore, the extent of LGE in the LA wall may be a predictor of stroke risk. Daccarett et al. [55] used the Utah staging system to show that patients with more LA enhancement were more likely to have had a previous stroke and have a higher $CHADS_2$ score [56] than those with less LA enhancement. However, this has not yet been assessed prospectively.

Post-ablation imaging

Peters et al. first described the technique of LA LGE CMR after catheter ablation for AF in 2007 in 23 patients [35] and attempted to quantify the extent of circumferential enhancement of the PVs on 2D reconstructions of the PV ostia. They did not show pre-ablation LGE in any patients, which is inconsistent with the published findings of the University of Utah group mentioned in the previous section.

A similar technique was then used by the Utah group to assess the relationship between AF recurrence and the extent of post-ablation LGE at 3 months [41, 51]. These studies, in cohorts of 46 and 86 patients, reported significantly less total LA wall enhancement in patients with AF recurrence. They also showed complete encirclement of only 39% of PVs at 3 months post-ablation, with the number of PVs encircled being proportional to procedural success.

The authors suggested that certain patients may be more 'resistant' to scar formation, although the mechanisms responsible are not understood. It may be that those with more pre-existing LA remodelling are less likely to form scar, although this would not be consistent with the finding of comparable LGE at 3 months across the four Utah stages [34]. Insights into the temporal formation of left atrial scar have also been revealed by LGE imaging [38]. CMR scans at 24 h post-ablation were repeated at 3 months in 10 patients (and at 6 and 9 months in 16 patients). This showed that LGE imaging within 24 h of ablation overestimates the extent of enhancement at 3 months, suggesting a transient inflammatory response, which then resolves. This is probably due in part to LA wall oedema, shown on T2-weighted imaging, which has resolved by 3 months [37].

Potential promise and limitations of atrial imaging

Recent technical advances and novel sequence development have brought LA LGE CMR to the clinical arena, with a potential role in predicting the outcome of AF ablation by assessing pre-existing LA remodelling and in assessing post-ablation scar formation and the variable response to RF injury. However, the thin atrial wall is at the limits of current CMR resolution and artefacts and poor image quality are not uncommon, particularly in those with uncontrolled AF or erratic breathing. We therefore have to be cautious about interpreting findings particularly in patients where image quality is not of a high standard. However, the rapid developments over the past few years are certain to continue, with increasing resolution and decreasing scan duration. This is sure to produce better insights into the mechanisms of atrial remodelling in AF and the variable success of AF ablation.

MRI of cardiac implantable electric devices

Magnetic resonance imaging (MRI) is rapidly becoming the preferred imaging modality for a variety of clinical indications, providing unparalleled soft-tissue resolution and the ability to image in virtually any plane without the need for ionizing radiation. The number of clinically indicated MRI scans is increasing, as is the number of cardiac implantable electric device (CIED) implants.

This presents an important clinical problem as it is estimated that between 50% and 75% of patients with CIEDs will have a clinical indication for an MRI scan in their lifetime [57]. The presence of a CIED has historically been seen as an absolute contraindication to MRI scanning given the potential for MRI–CIED interaction within the scanner. This notion is no longer felt to be the case and several studies have reported the safety of MRI with selected CIEDs when performed with appropriate safeguards. Conversely, some older devices have been associated with major complications when exposed to an MR environment and as such it is important to understand: (a) the nature of potential MRI–CIED interactions and the status of research into the safety of CIEDs within an MR environment; (b) the fact that there is a marked heterogeneity in the response of CIEDs to the MR environment; and (c) advances in scanning protocols to optimize scan quality.

Potential interactions of MRI–CIEDs

Force

Contemporary pacing systems consist of a generator and leads comprising connectors, circuitry, and a power source. Each of these components will have some ferromagnetic material and, thus, will be potentially liable to magnetic field interactions and transfer of electromagnetic energy. The strong static and gradient magnetic fields of MR scanners can lead to the application of force and torque, thereby leading to possible device movement. The amount of force to which any device is exposed is dependent on the inherent ferromagnetic properties of the device, distance of the CIED from the magnet bore, and the magnetic field strength. In an *in vitro* and *in vivo* canine study of multiple ICD and pacemaker models scanned at 1.5T, damage to the generator was only seen in ICDs manufactured before 2000. Amongst the (as of 2004) newer devices, the maximal force acting on the device was <100g [58]. This level of force is unlikely to be clinically significant in chronically implanted devices. This has been borne out by prospective studies in humans that have not demonstrated problems with device or lead migration [59, 60]. The fact that some force is applied has led to many institutions adopting a 6-week delay rule prior to allowing MRI scanning after CIED implant.

Heating

MRI-induced heating of metallic implants is a well-described phenomenon [61]. The radiofrequency current of MR scanners induces high currents that coalesce and form hot spots at the tip of CIED leads. This results from a drop in impedance from the adjacent myocardium to the lead tip. There have been conflicting reports on the degree of heating encountered, with one study of pigs with chronically implanted leads demonstrating temperature rises of up to 20°C, as well as significant alterations in capture threshold and impedance [62]. Interestingly, there was no histological evidence of necrosis at the lead–myocardium interface in this study and also no concomitant rise in troponin. The lack of troponin rise has been borne out by several prospective studies and significant heating would be expected to cause a degree of myocardial necrosis, such that troponin release might be expected [63–65].

Electrical current induction

Electrical currents may be induced by the RF current and pulsed gradient magnetic fields within the MR environment. Canine experiments with implanted leads have found that the induced current is usually of insufficient magnitude to effect capture (≤0.5 mA) but, with the addition of extra loops, a current of 30 mA is possible and this can result in capture [66]. This has not been observed in humans but could be the cause of death in those cases of fatality in patients with CIEDs undergoing MRI scanning under unmonitored conditions.

The effect of electromagnetic interference

CIEDs may receive electromagnetic interference (EMI) and this may lead to inappropriate tracking of RF noise, asynchronous pacing, inhibition of demand pacing, inappropriate delivery of ICD therapies, programming changes, or loss of function [67].

Reed-switch behaviour

The reed switch is a feature of most CIEDs designed to program a device by means of a magnet placed over the generator. The response of the switch to the magnet is to commit to an asynchronous pacing mode so as to avoid problems with EMI during procedures, such as surgery involving the use of electro-cautery. The static magnetic field of MR scanners is capable of activating the reed switch and the subsequent response can be unpredictable.

MRI scanning of non-MR conditional CIEDs

Several centres have developed protocols for performing MRI in patients with conventional CIEDs (both pacemakers and ICDs). The literature amounts to scans in over 1000 patients in whom the complication rate is low [63, 68, 69]. Such protocols are performed at centres with clinical expertise in MRI–CIED interaction, where there are established links with specialists in CIED programming and trouble-shooting. It is imperative that scans are performed in an environment with suitable monitoring during the scan. Pacing dependent patients are generally programmed to an asynchronous pacing mode and non-dependent patients are programmed to inhibited modes to prevent problems with electromagnetic interference. Other pacing modes, such as rate response and tachyarrhythmia detection, are deactivated. Given the vast permutations in terms of device and lead model and manufacturer there is no single scanning protocol that is applicable to every patient and so there has been much emphasis on designing devices that are MR conditional.

MRI conditional CIEDs

The potential for MRI–CIED interaction and the expanding need for clinical MRI scans in a significant number of patients with CIEDs has led device manufacturers to invest heavily in the development of devices that are specifically designed to operate in an MRI environment. Adaptations have focused on reducing the ferromagnetic content and on modifications to the leads to minimize heating. There has also been a move towards replacing reed switches with a Hall sensor. The Hall sensor behaves much more predictably within the MR environment. The ability of MR conditional devices to perform their primary function, i.e. pacing, was verified in a prospective, controlled study of 107 patients implanted with either an MRI conditional system (EnRhythm MRI SureScan and CapSureFix MRI leads, Medtronic, Inc.) or a conventional dual-chamber pacing system. Both systems fared equally well with a 100% implant success rate and excellent pacing parameters at up to 1-year follow-up [70]. The same system then underwent further testing with 464 patients implanted with the EnRhythm device randomized to either undergo MRI scans of the brain/lumbar spine at 1.5T or not [71]. No MRI-related complications occurred and pacemaker sensing and capture thresholds were similar between both study groups. Given that the scans were limited such that the isocentre of the RF coil had to be above C1 vertebra or below T12, the next aim was to test MR conditional systems such that they safely permit scanning of thoracic structures. The Advisa MRI pacemaker and CapSureFix lead system (Medtronic) were developed to enable safe scanning at 1.5T without anatomical restriction. Patients randomized to undergo MRI scanning were scanned with 16 commonly run head and chest sequences up to a specific absorption rate (SAR) of 2 W/kg. Total static field exposure averaged 60 min with a total scan time of 30 min [72]. No MRI-related complications occurred during or after MR scanning and the minimal differences in sensing and capture threshold after MRI were comparable with the group that did not undergo scanning. The data from well-designed studies, therefore, reflects favourably on the safety profile of MR conditional pacemakers regardless of scan location but only to a field strength of 1.5T.

Effect of CIEDS on scan quality

The impact of conditional MR CIEDs on image quality during thoracic scans remains an issue. The ferromagnetic components cause variation in the surrounding magnetic field, which can lead to image distortion, areas of signal void, and poor fat suppression. Artefacts appear to be most problematic with SSFP cine images and inversion–recovery sequences. Using imaging planes perpendicular to the plane of the device, shortening echo time, and using fast-spin echo sequences may all help to reduce the extent of artefact [73]. The Advisa MRI randomized clinical multicentre study results looked specifically at image quality of cardiac MRI scans in patients with implanted Advisa MRI systems (Medtronic)

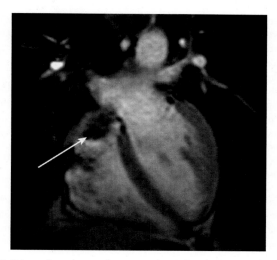

Fig. 8.3 Balanced steady-state free-precession 4-chamber image taken from a patient with a dual chamber MRI-conditional pacemaker (Medtronic Ensura DR; Medtronic, USA). The patient had no underlying rhythm and was paced in a committed dual-chamber pacing mode. Device parameters were unchanged after the scan. The white arrow points to artefact produced by the right atrial lead.

[74]. The SSFP long-axis cine images of the LV were of diagnostic quality in 95% of cases and those of the RV in 98% of cases. The presence of the device did not affect the tracking of tagged images from systole into early diastole in all segments. ➲ Figure 8.3 demonstrates a 4-chamber balanced steady-state free precession image in a patient with a dual-chamber Medtronic Ensura MR conditional pacemaker scanned at 1.5T at our institution.

Potential promise and limitations of MRI of patients with CIEDs

MR imaging is at the forefront of diagnostic medicine given its excellent temporal and spatial resolution and lack of ionizing radiation. The presence of a CIED need not be seen as an absolute contraindication to MR scanning, provided stringent safety and scanning protocols are followed. The development of MR conditional devices is a major step forward and is likely to lead to more patients with CIEDs being scanned. Image artefacts are encountered but are usually not sufficient to affect diagnostic value.

References

1. Damadian R. Tumour detection by nuclear magnetic resonance. *Science* 1971; 171: 1151–3.
2. Messroghli DR, Greiser A, Fröhlich M, Dietz R, Schulz-Menger J.Optimization and validation of a fully-integrated pulse sequence for Modified Look_Locker Inversion-Recovery (MOLLI) T1 mapping of the heart. *J Magn Reson Imaging* 2007; 26: 1081–86.
3. Piechnik SK, Ferreira VM, Dall'Armellina E, et al. Shortened Modified Look-Locker Inversion recovery (ShMOLLI) for clinical myocardial T1-mapping at 1.5 and 3 T within a 9 heartbeat breath-hold. *J Cardiovasc Magn Reson* 2010; 12: 69.
4. Messroghli DR, Plein S, Higgins DM, et al. Human myocardium single breath-hold MR T1 Mapping with high spatial resolution—reproducibility study. *Radiology* 2006; 235: 1004–12.
5. Messroghli DR, Walters K, Plein S, et al. Myocardial T1 Mapping: Application to patients with acute and chronic myocardial infarction. *Magn Reson Med* 2007; 58: 34–40.
6. Kehr E, Sono M, Chugh S, Jerosch-Herold M. Gadolinium-enhanced magnetic resonance imaging for detection and quantification of fibrosis in human myocardium in vitro. *Int J Cardiovasc Imaging* 2008; 24: 61–68.

7. Flett AS, Hayward MP, Ashworth MT, et al. Equilibrium contrast car-diovascular magnetic resonance for the measurement of diffuse myo-cardial fibrosis: preliminary validation in humans. *Circulation* 2010; 122: 138–44.

8. Schelbert E, Testa SM, Meier CG, et al. Myocardial Extracellular Volume Fraction Measurement by Gadolinium Cardiovascular Magnetic Resonance in Humans: Slow Infusion versus Bolus. *J Cardiovasc Magn Reson* 2011; 13: 16.

9. Kawel N, Nacif M, Zavodni A, et al. T1 mapping of the myocardium: intra-individual assessment of post-contrast T1 time evolution and extracellular volume fraction at 3T for Gd-DTPA and Gd-BOPTA. *J Cardiovasc Magn Reson* 2012; 14: 27.

10. Messroghli DR, Nordmeyer S, Dietrich T, et al. Assessment of diffuse myocardial fibrosis in rats using small-animal Look-Locker inversion recovery T1 mapping. *Circ Cardiovasc Imaging* 2011; 4 (6): 636–40.

11. Xue H, Shah S, Greiser A, et al. Motion correction for myocardial T1 mapping using image registration with synthetic image estimation. *Magn Reson Med* 2012; 67(6): 1644–55.

12. Kellman P, Wilson JR, Xue H, Ugander M, Arai AE. Extracellular vol-ume fraction mapping in the myocardium, part 1: evaluation of an automated method. *J Cardiovasc Magn Reson* 2012; 14: 63.

13. Kellman P, Wilson JR, Xue H, et al. Extracellular volume fraction mapping in the myocardium, part 2: initial clinical experience. *J Cardiovasc Magn Reson* 2012: 14: 64.

14. Iles L, Pfluger H, Phrommintikul A, et al. Evaluation of diffuse myo-cardial fibrosis in heart failure with cardiac magnetic resonance con-trast-enhanced T1 mapping. *J Am Coll Cardiol* 2008; 52: 1574–80.

15. Sibley CT, Noureldin RA, Gai N, et al. T1 Mapping in cardiomyopathy at cardiac MR: comparison with endomyocardial biopsy. *Radiology* 2012; 265(3): 724–32.

16. Ng AC, Auger D, Delgado V, et al. Association between diffuse myo-cardial fibrosis by cardiac magnetic resonance contrast-enhanced T_1 mapping and subclinical myocardial dysfunction in diabetic patients: a pilot study. *Circ Cardiovasc Imaging* 2012; 5(1): 51–9.

17. Sparrow P, Messroghli DR, Reid S, Ridgway JP, Bainbridge G, Sivananthan MU. Myocardial T1 mapping for detection of left ven-tricular myocardial fibrosis in chronic aortic regurgitation: pilot study. *AJR Am J Roentgenol* 2006; 187: W630–L 5.

18. Maceira AM, Joshi J, Prasad SK, et al. Cardiovascular magnetic reso-nance in cardiac amyloidosis. *Circulation* 2005; 111: 186–93.

19. Puntmann VO, Voigt T, Chen Z, et al. Native T1 mapping in differen-tiation of normal myocardium from diffuse disease in hypertrophic and dilated cardiomyopathy. *JACC Cardiovasc Imaging* 2013: 6(4): 475–84.

20. Dass S, Suttie JJ, Piechnik SK, et al. Myocardial tissue characterization using magnetic resonance noncontrast T1 mapping in hypertrophic and dilated cardiomyopathy. *Circ Cardiovasc Imaging* 2012; 5(6): 726–33.

21. Puntmann VO, D'Cruz D, Smith Z, Pastor A, Choong P, Voigt T, Carr-White G, Sangle S, Schaeffter T, Nagel E. Native myocardial T1 mapping by cardiovascular magnetic resonance imaging in subclini-cal cardiomyopathy in patients with systemic lupus erythematosus. *Circ Cardiovasc Imaging* 2013; 6(2): 295–301.

22. Karamitsos TD, Piechnik SK, Banypersad SM, et al. Noncontrast T1 mapping for the diagnosis of cardiac amyloidosis. *JACC Cardiovasc Imaging* 2013; 6(4): 488–97.

23. Dall'Armellina E, Piechnik SK, Ferreira VM, et al. Cardiovascular magnetic resonance by non contrast T1-mapping allows assessment of severity of injury in acute myocardial infarction. *J Cardiovasc Magn Reson* 2012; 14: 15.

24. Ugander M, Bagi PS, Oki AJ, et al. Myocardial edema as detected by pre-contrast T1 and T2 CMR delineates area at risk associated with acute myocardial infarction. *JACC Cardiovasc Imaging* 2012; 5(6): 596–603.

25. Ferreira VM, Piechnik SK, Dall'Armellina E, et al. Non-contrast T1-mapping detects acute myocardial edema with high diagnostic accuracy: a comparison to T2-weighted cardiovascular magnetic resonance. *J Cardiovasc Magn Reson* 2012; 14: 42.

26. Piechnik SK, Ferreira VM, Lewandowski AJ, et al. Normal variation of magnetic resonance T1 relaxation times in the human population at 1.5 T using ShMOLLI. *J Cardiovasc Magn Reson* 2013; 15: 13.

27. Scholz TD, Fleagle SR, Burns TL, Skorton DJ. Nuclear magnetic reso-nance relaxometry of the normal heart: relationship between colla-gen content and relaxation times of the four chambers. *Magn Reson Imaging* 1989; 7(6): 643–8.

28. Bull S, White SK, Piechnik SK, Flett AS, Ferreira VM, Loudon M, Francis JM, Karamitsos TD, Prendergast BD, Robson MD, Neubauer S, Moon JC, Myerson SG. Human non-contrast T1 values and cor-relation with histology in diffuse fibrosis. *Heart* 2013; 99(13): 932–7.

29. Calkins H, Kuck KH, Cappato R, et al. 2012 HRS/EHRA/ECAS expert consensus statement on catheter and surgical ablation of atrial fibrillation: recommendations for patient selection, proce-dural techniques, patient management and follow-up, definitions, endpoints, and research trial design: a report of the Heart Rhythm Society (HRS) Task Force on Catheter and Surgical Ablation of Atrial Fibrillation. Developed in partnership with the European Heart Rhythm Association (EHRA), a registered branch of the European Society of Cardiology (ESC) and the European Cardiac Arrhythmia Society (ECAS); and in collaboration with the American College of Cardiology (ACC), American Heart Association (AHA), the Asia Pacific Heart Rhythm Society (APHRS), and the Society of Thoracic Surgeons (STS). Endorsed by the governing bodies of the American College of Cardiology Foundation, the American Heart Association, the European Cardiac Arrhythmia Society, the European Heart Rhythm Association, the Society of Thoracic Surgeons, the Asia Pacific Heart Rhythm Society, and the Heart Rhythm Society. *Heart Rhythm* 2012; 9(4): 632–96 e 21.

30. Haissaguerre M, Jais P, Shah DC, et al. Spontaneous initiation of atrial fibrillation by ectopic beats originating in the pulmonary veins. *N Engl J Med* 1998; 339(10): 659–66.

31. Verma A, Natale A. Should atrial fibrillation ablation be considered first-line therapy for some patients? Why atrial fibrillation ablation should be considered first-line therapy for some patients. *Circulation* 2005; 112(8): 1214–22; discussion 1231.

32. Nanthakumar K, Plumb VJ, Epstein AE, Veenhuyzen GD, Link D, Kay GN. Resumption of electrical conduction in previously isolated pulmonary veins: rationale for a different strategy? *Circulation* 2004; 109(10): 1226–9.

33. Oakes RS, Badger TJ, Kholmovski EG, et al. Detection and quanti-fication of left atrial structural remodeling with delayed-enhance-ment magnetic resonance imaging in patients with atrial fibrillation. *Circulation* 2009; 119(13): 1758–67.

34. Akoum N, Daccarett M, McGann C, et al. Atrial fibrosis helps se-lect the appropriate patient and strategy in catheter ablation of atrial fibrillation: a DE-MRI guided approach. *J Cardiovasc Electrophysiol* 2011. 22(1): 16–22.

35. Peters DC, Wylie JV, Hauser TH, et al. Detection of pulmonary vein and left atrial scar after catheter ablation with three-dimensional nav-igator-gated delayed enhancement MR imaging: initial experience. *Radiology* 2007; 243(3): 690–5.

36. Knowles BR, Caulfield D, Cooklin M, et al. 3-D visualization of acute RF ablation lesions using MRI for the simultaneous determination of the patterns of necrosis and edema. *IEEE Trans Biomed Eng* 2010; 57(6): 1467–75.

37. Arujuna A, Karim R, Caulfield D, et al. Acute pulmonary vein isola-tion is achieved by a combination of reversible and irreversible atrial injury after catheter ablation: evidence from magnetic resonance im-aging. *Circ Arrhythm Electrophysiol* 2012; 5(4): 691–700.

38. Badger TJ, Oakes RS, Daccarett M, et al. Temporal left atrial lesion formation after ablation of atrial fibrillation. *Heart Rhythm* 2009; 6(2): 161–8.

39. Badger TJ, Daccarett M, Akoum NW, et al. Evaluation of left atrial lesions after initial and repeat atrial fibrillation ablation: lessons learned from delayed-enhancement MRI in repeat ablation procedures. *Circ Arrhythm Electrophysiol* 2010; 3(3): 249–59.

40. Mahnkopf C, Badger TJ, Burgon NS, et al. Evaluation of the left atrial substrate in patients with lone atrial fibrillation using delayed-enhanced MRI: implications for disease progression and response to catheter ablation. *Heart Rhythm* 2010; 7(10): 1475–81.

41. McGann CJ, Kholmovski EG, Oakes RS, et al. New magnetic resonance imaging-based method for defining the extent of left atrial wall injury after the ablation of atrial fibrillation. *J Am Coll Cardiol* ,2008; 52(15): 1263–71.

42. Peters DC, Wylie JV, Hauser TH, et al. Recurrence of atrial fibrillation correlates with the extent of post-procedural late gadolinium enhancement: a pilot study. *JACC Cardiovasc Imaging* 2009; 2(3): 308–16.

43. Reddy VY, Schmidt EJ, Holmvang G, Fung M. Arrhythmia recurrence after atrial fibrillation ablation: can magnetic resonance imaging identify gaps in atrial ablation lines? *J Cardiovasc Electrophysiol* 2008; 19(4): 434–7.

44. Ranjan R, Kholmovski EG, Blauer J, et al. Identification and acute targeting of gaps in atrial ablation lesion sets using a real time MRI system. *Circ Arrhythm Electrophysiol* 2012.

45. Vergara GR, Vijayakumar S, Kholmovski EG, et al. Real-time magnetic resonance imaging-guided radiofrequency atrial ablation and visualization of lesion formation at 3 Tesla. *Heart Rhythm* 2011; 8(2): 295–303.

46. Nordbeck P, Hiller KH, Fidler F, et al. Feasibility of contrast-enhanced and nonenhanced MRI for intraprocedural and postprocedural lesion visualization in interventional electrophysiology: animal studies and early delineation of isthmus ablation lesions in patients with typical atrial flutter. *Circ Cardiovasc Imaging* 2011; 4(3): 282–94.

47. Sommer P, Grothoff M, Eitel C, et al. Feasibility of real-time magnetic resonance imaging-guided electrophysiology studies in humans. *Europace* 2013; 15(1): 101–8.

48. Lardo AC, McVeigh ER, Jumrussirikul P, et al. Visualization and temporal/spatial characterization of cardiac radiofrequency ablation lesions using magnetic resonance imaging. *Circulation* 2000; 102(6): 698–705.

49. Dickfeld T, Kato R, Zviman M, et al. Characterization of radiofrequency ablation lesions with gadolinium-enhanced cardiovascular magnetic resonance imaging. *J Am Coll Cardiol* 2006; 47(2): 370–8.

50. Dickfeld T, Kato R, Zviman M, et al. Characterization of acute and subacute radiofrequency ablation lesions with nonenhanced magnetic resonance imaging. *Heart Rhythm* 2007; 4(2): 208–14.

51. Segerson NM, Daccarett M, Badger TJ, et al. Magnetic resonance imaging-confirmed ablative debulking of the left atrial posterior wall and septum for treatment of persistent atrial fibrillation: rationale and initial experience. *J Cardiovasc Electrophysiol* 2010; 21(2): 126–32.

52. Verma A, Wazni OM, Marrouche NF, et al. Pre-existent left atrial scarring in patients undergoing pulmonary vein antrum isolation: an independent predictor of procedural failure. *J Am Coll Cardiol* 2005; 45(2): 285–92.

53. Frustaci A, Chimenti C, Bellocci F, Morgante E, Russo MA, Maseri A. Histological substrate of atrial biopsies in patients with lone atrial fibrillation. *Circulation* 1997; 96(4): 1180–4.

54. Abhayaratna WP, Seward JB, Appleton CP, et al. Left atrial size: physiologic determinants and clinical applications. *J Am Coll Cardiol* 2006; 47(12): 2357–63.

55. Daccarett M, Badger TJ, Akoum N, et al. Association of left atrial fibrosis detected by delayed-enhancement magnetic resonance imaging and the risk of stroke in patients with atrial fibrillation. *J Am Coll Cardiol* 2011; 57(7): 831–8.

56. Gage BF, Waterman AD, Shannon W, Boechler M, Rich MW, Radford MJ. Validation of clinical classification schemes for predicting stroke: results from the National Registry of Atrial Fibrillation. *JAMA* 2001; 285(22): 2864–70.

57. Kalin R, Stanton MS. Current clinical issues for MRI scanning of pacemaker and defibrillator patients. *Pacing Clin Electrophysiol* 2005; 28(4): 326–8.

58. Roguin A, Zviman MM, Meininger GR, et al. Modern pacemaker and implantable cardioverter/defibrillator systems can be magnetic resonance imaging safe: in vitro and in vivo assessment of safety and function at 1.5 T. *Circulation* 2004; 110(5): 475–82.

59. Del Ojo JL, Moya F, Villalba J, et al. Is magnetic resonance imaging safe in cardiac pacemaker recipients? *Pacing Clin Electrophysiol* 2005; 28(4): 274–8.

60. Naehle CP, Meyer C, Thomas D, et al. Safety of brain 3-T MR imaging with transmit-receive head coil in patients with cardiac pacemakers: pilot prospective study with 51 examinations. *Radiology* 2008; 249(3): 991–1001.

61. Buchli R, Boesiger P, Meier D. Heating effects of metallic implants by MRI examinations. *Magn Reson Med* 1988; 7(3): 255–61.

62. Luechinger R, Zeijlemaker VA, Pedersen EM, et al. In vivo heating of pacemaker leads during magnetic resonance imaging. *Eur Heart J* 2005; 26(4): 376–83; discussion 325–7.

63. Sommer T, Naehle CP, Yang A, et al. Strategy for safe performance of extrathoracic magnetic resonance imaging at 1.5 tesla in the presence of cardiac pacemakers in non-pacemaker-dependent patients: a prospective study with 115 examinations. *Circulation* 2006; 114(12): 1285–92.

64. Mollerus M, Albin G, Lipinski M, Lucca J. Cardiac biomarkers in patients with permanent pacemakers and implantable cardioverter-defibrillators undergoing an MRI scan. *Pacing Clin Electrophysiol* 2008; 31(10): 1241–5.

65. Boilson BA, Wokhlu A, Acker NG, et al. Safety of magnetic resonance imaging in patients with permanent pacemakers: a collaborative clinical approach. *J Interv Card Electrophysiol* 2012; 33(1): 59–67.

66. Tandri H, Zviman MM, Wedan SR, Lloyd T, Berger RD, Halperin H. Determinants of gradient field-induced current in a pacemaker lead system in a magnetic resonance imaging environment. *Heart Rhythm* 2008; 5(3): 462–8.

67. Gimbel JR. Unexpected asystole during 3T magnetic resonance imaging of a pacemaker-dependent patient with a 'modern' pacemaker. *Europace* 2009; 11(9): 1241–2.

68. Nazarian S, Hansford R, Roguin A, et al. A prospective evaluation of a protocol for magnetic resonance imaging of patients with implanted cardiac devices. *Ann Intern Med* 2011; 155(7): 415–24.

69. Martin ET, Coman JA, Shellock FG, Pulling CC, Fair R, Jenkins K. Magnetic resonance imaging and cardiac pacemaker safety at 1.5-Tesla. *J Am Coll Cardiol* 2004; 43(7): 1315–24.

70. Forleo GB, Santini L, Della Rocca DG, et al. Safety and efficacy of a new magnetic resonance imaging-compatible pacing system: early results of a prospective comparison with conventional dual-chamber implant outcomes. *Heart Rhythm* 2010; 7(6): 750–4.

71. Wilkoff BL, Bello D, Taborsky M, et al. Magnetic resonance imaging in patients with a pacemaker system designed for the magnetic resonance environment. *Heart Rhythm* 2011; 8(1): 65–73.

72. Rod Gimbel J, Bello D, Schmitt M, et al. Randomized trial of pacemaker and lead system for safe scanning at 1.5 Tesla. *Heart Rhythm* 2013.

73. Nazarian S, Halperin HR. How to perform magnetic resonance imaging on patients with implantable cardiac arrhythmia devices. *Heart Rhythm* 2009; 6(1): 138–43.

74. Schwitter J, Kanal E, Schmitt M, et al. Impact of the Advisa MRI Pacing System on the diagnostic quality of cardiac MR images and contraction patterns of cardiac muscle during scans: Advisa MRI randomized clinical multicenter study results. *Heart Rhythm* 2013; 10(6): 864–72.

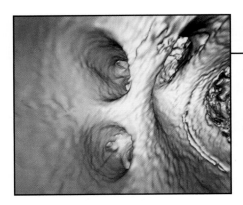

CHAPTER 9

Imaging during cardiac interventions

Luis M. Rincón and José L. Zamorano

Contents

Introduction

Interventional cardiology has evolved during the last decades and the number of procedures and indications has increased. This offers a new therapeutic option for conditions that previously required surgery or that were not amenable to any intervention. In parallel, cardiac imaging has experienced a similar technological development and it is commonly required in the catheterization laboratory to evaluate, guide and improve results of several percutaneous procedures [1] (⮕ Table 9.1).

Percutaneous treatment can offer an alternative to surgery in many cases of non-valvular structural heart diseases, such as atrial septal defects (ASDs) and patent foramen ovale (PFO), with cardiac imaging routinely used in this context.

Atrial fibrillation with pulmonary veins ablation and left atrial appendage percutaneous occlusion are commonly guided by cardiac imaging. Other supraventricular and ventricular tachyarrhythmias ablation procedures performed in the electrophysiology laboratory (EP) have become clinical settings in which imaging can be useful.

Echocardiography is routinely used for evaluation, guidance, and follow-up of patients undergoing alcohol septal ablation for hypertrophic cardiomyopathy (HCM).

Trans-catheter interventions for valvular heart disease, such as aortic stenosis or mitral regurgitation, are in constant evolution due to their clinical importance and high prevalence. The use of echocardiography in this context is discussed in a separate chapter.

Catheterization laboratory procedures

Patent foramen ovale

Diagnosis and indications of PFO closure

The foramen ovale plays a role by letting the blood flow across the atrial septum before birth. Afterwards, right heart pressures and pulmonary resistances decrease due to breathing and left atrial pressure rises with the beginning of pulmonary venous return. Septum primum is then shoved against the septum secundum, and a permanent fusion can be seen by the age of two in most children. Patent foramen ovale (PFO) can occur as a result of an absence in the fusion of the septum primum with the septum secundum, and can be seen in 24–27% of adult population. This persistence can cause a blood flow from the right to the left atrium whenever the pressure is higher in the first. Approximately 30% of survivors of stroke are said to be cryptogenic, and PFO by TEE has been reported to be present in around 50% in comparison with 24% for the general population. This has led clinicians to think that the underlying cause of the stroke was frequently a PFO. In the last two years several clinical trials such as RESPECT, PC Trial, and CLOSURE I have tried

Table 9.1 Imaging techniques used for guidance in percutaneous procedures

Procedure	TTE	ICE	2D-TEE	3D-TEE
Trans-septal catheterization	+	++	++	+++
PFO and ASDs closure	+	+++*	++	+++
VSDs closure	+	+	+++	+++
Alcohol septal ablation in HCM	++		+	+
LAA occlusion		++	++	+++
Myocardial biopsy	++	+	+	+
Pericardiocentesis	+++			

+small benefit; ++moderate benefit, use if possible; +++recommended use.
*Depending on centre experience and availability.

to shed light into this matter, although none of them has shown a significantly lower rate of their primary end points with closure than with medical therapy, despite evidence of a favourable trend. Indications for PFO closure are now uncertain and the question is still open [2–7]. Current ESO guidelines recommend PFO closure after recurrent stroke or for high-risk patients in whom paradoxical embolism is suspected, leaving an open definition for 'high risk' [8].

Diagnosis of PFO can be reached using TTE, TEE, or transcranial Doppler (TCD). Apical 4-chamber view TTE is considered positive when atrial septum is bowed towards the left atrium (LA) with Valsalva manoeuvre. Contrast is often needed in order to make the diagnosis, which is positive if three or more microbubbles are seen in the left chambers within the first three cardiac cycles after the opacification of the right chambers. A classification of severity can be performed by counting the number of bubbles in a single frame, being considered as mild from 3 to 9 bubbles, moderate from 10 to 30, and severe if more than 30 bubbles. Contrast TCD can be used as a screening test, and in case of a positive result (3 or more bubbles seen in the first 20 s), TTE is then indicated [9]. TEE remains as the gold-standard and can be used to confirm the diagnosis when better image definition is needed or prior to a PFO closure procedure [10].

Echocardiographic guidance of PFO

Unless there is a formal contraindication, trans-catheter devices are the first choice for PFO closure. The initial approach consists of a single femoral venous puncture. A catheter with the device is placed up to its position through it. This is usually done using both X-rays and TEE guidance, although some operators use X-rays alone for the deployment of an Amplatzer device. TEE, especially 3D-TEE, gives a very precise definition of PFO anatomy and its relationship with structures in the vicinity. It can be very useful in complex PFOs. Intra-cardiac echocardiography (ICE) can be used as an alternative to TEE; among its advantages, it makes general anaesthesia unnecessary and its use in this context in the United States is widespread [11]. Both techniques are able to assess the following items:

* PFO morphology: size, location, length of the tunnel and rim dimensions.

* Spatial relation of the defect to the aortic root and the cava vein.
* Comprehensive evaluation of the atrial septum to discard atrial septum aneurysm and other atrial septal defects. Thickness of the residual septum.
* Guide the placement of the device.

Factors related to PFO complexity are: presence of multiple orifices, other congenital heart defects (such as prominent Eustachian valve and Chiari network that can impair the adequate expansion of the device), tunnel length ≥8 mm, septal thickness >10 mm, and atrial septum aneurysm.

Trans-catheter closure of PFO is performed by approaching the right atrium from the inferior vena cava and sliding a catheter along the septum primum. In order to select the device size, the double of the maximum PFO diameter is taken as reference. TEE can be used to guide the advance of the delivery system into the left atrium and monitor the adequate expansion after the left-sided disc or umbrella of the device is deployed and retracted, evaluating its stability prior to the release.

Follow-up after PFO percutaneous closure

Major intra-procedural complications are rare (1.5%). They include device embolization, symptomatic air embolism, and chamber perforation. Among late complications, special mention to thrombus formation on the device, and also embolization, infection, atrial arrhythmias, allergic reactions, or erosion of adjacent structures, usually related to bigger devices whose rims can perforate the aorta or pericardium.

Prior to discharge and at 6-months follow-up, a TTE using saline contrast is recommended to exclude any residual shunt or possible complication.

Atrial septal defects (ASDs)
Evaluation and indications of ASD closure

Atrial septal defects (ASDs) represent the most frequent congenital cardiac abnormality in the adult population after bicuspid aortic valve, accounting for 10% of the total of congenital cardiac abnormalities. They are usually classified into five types: ostium secundum (OS), ostium primum (OP), superior sinus venous, inferior sinus venous, and unroofed coronary sinus. Currently only OS is amenable to percutaneous closure. The protocol for ASD assessment is the same as for PFO. Despite the fact that TTE can usually evaluate the rims, it is compulsory to perform a TEE in order to improve the anatomic resolution. Possible haemodynamic consequences should be excluded, with special focus on right ventricular overload causing Eisenmenger's physiology and calculation of the ratio of pulmonary flow (Qp) to systemic flow (Qs), which gives information of the shunt. The echocardiographic study should also exclude other possible congenital heart defects and any other abnormality that might interfere with the procedure, like inadequate septal rims, small distance to inferior vena cava or coronary sinus, and maximal ASD diameter >40 mm; the presence of any of them contraindicates percutaneous closure in favour of surgery.

Clinical indications for ASD closure include cryptogenic stroke in which a paradoxical embolic event is suspected, and haemodynamic significance, usually defined as right chamber enlargement or Qp/Qs ≥1.5. Some of the clinical contraindications for ASD percutaneous closure include impossibility or contraindication to receive an anticoagulant or antiplatelet treatment and severe pulmonary hypertension with Eisenmenger's physiology, in which ASD closure would eliminate the only 'pump-off' valve available [12].

Echocardiography is necessary in order to evaluate and assess the haemodynamic significance of ASD and to perform patient selection in order to improve the results. Diameter assessments have been reported to be systematically smaller if 2D-TEE is used in comparison with 3D-TEE, probably due to difficulties in obtaining the maximal diameter with 2D-TEE. One study comparing 2D-TEE with 3D-TEE has shown association between the usage of smaller devices as indicated by 2D-TEE with the presence of residual shunts that could have been avoided by 3D-TEE. This was especially important in the presence of complex ASDs or non-circular defects. Therefore, 3D-TEE usage has improved the evaluation of atrial septum and it is the elective technique for the selection of candidates. 3D-TEE can avoid the need of balloon sizing of the defect during the procedure. Several morphological features have to be assessed in order to establish if a percutaneous device closure is feasible, which is in approximately 80% of patients (⊃ Table 9.2). It must be noted that ASD size varies during the cardiac cycle and the measurements should be done during atrial diastole. 3D-TEE allows the visualization of all the parts of the inter-atrial septum in the same image, and performance of 3D zoom or full volume is recommended. Gain and acquisition parameters must be optimized in order to avoid loss of visualization of the inferior rim and the fossa ovalis, and in some cases colour 3D-TEE can be used to confirm ASD measurements. Current guidelines for grown-up congenital heart diseases place special care in the measurement of cardiac rims, as an aortic rim of less than 3 mm or other rim <5 mm can increase the erosion risk and cause interference with other structures. This risk is also increased if the maximal disc diameter is >90% of the inter-atrial septum or if the device is shoved against the aorta [13].

Echocardiographic guidance of ASDs

The addition of intra-procedural echocardiography offers significant advantages to monitor procedural efficacy and possible complications as compared to fluoroscopy alone. TTE, 2D-TEE, 3D-TEE, and ICE are amenable to be used during the procedure, and each of them can offer advantages. TEE remains as the most extended method used in Europe. Maximal diameter and rims should be reassessed, and 3D-TEE can be used in order to choose the device size [14]. Therefore, 3D-TEE can avoid the intra-procedural use of invasive balloon sizing that can lead to distortion of the anatomy of the defect because of the deformation caused by the balloon (⊃ Figs 9.1 and 9.2).

Although there are several devices currently used for ASD closure, and each one implies small variations in the implantation method, they all involve crossing the ASD from the right atrium and stenting the defect. 3D-TEE can monitor the wire position

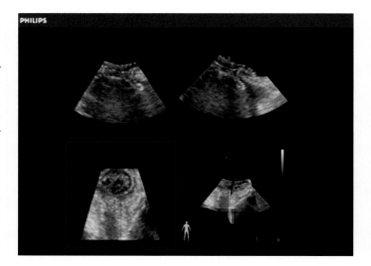

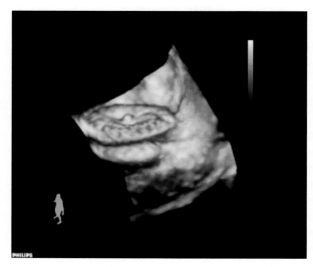

Figs 9.1 and 9.2 Trans-catheter ASD closure. 3D-transoesophageal echocardiographic evaluation of the atrial discs of an Amplatzer device released from the delivery catheter.

Table 9.2 Morphological items to be assessed prior to ASD percutaneous closure

ASD type	Only OS ASDs percutaneous closure are indicated
Diameter of the defect	Maximal diameter <38 mm
Rims	Required at least 5 mm except towards the aorta (≥3 mm)
Total length and width of inter-atrial septum	Erosion risk increases if device size is >90% of the inter-atrial septum length
Shape and number	Percutaneous closure must be avoided if other congenital heart defects are present
Location	Contraindicated if ASD is in close proximity to coronary sinus or inferior vena cava
Haemodynamic consequences	Eisenmenger physiology contraindicates ASD closure

in the atrium and may be especially helpful in dilated atriums or if multiple orifices are present [15, 16]. Once the device is deployed, echocardiographic monitoring must be used to confirm the position of both discs between the inter-atrial septum, exclude residual shunt or interferences with other structures, and confirm the stability of the device prior to the liberation [17].

TEE is the more common imaging technique used in this context but it requires additional sedation or general anaesthesia. Recent studies have described the successful usage of ICE for the guidance of percutaneous closure of ASDs and PFOs, overcoming these particular limitations (Table 9.3). ICE has proved to be reliable to assess the inter-atrial crossing and to optimize the device positioning and deployment. Potential complications of the procedure can also be observed with ICE, such as perforation, interference with other structures or presence of residual shunts.

Follow-up recommendations

Current clinical guidelines recommend the usage of echocardiography prior to hospital discharge in order to exclude residual shunt and to assess RV size and function, TR and PAP. TTE is usually enough for this purpose, and regular follow-up during the first 2 years is recommended. Afterwards it can be used every 2–4 years, depending on the results, focusing on possible residual problems and their severity.

Ventricular septal defects (VSDs)

Ventricular septal defects (VSDs) are the most common congenital malformation at birth after bicuspid aortic valve. It can appear as an isolated finding or associated with other malformations, and it is usually diagnosed before adulthood. They are subdivided in different groups depending on their location; the most frequent VSDs are peri-membranous, accounting for 80%, and muscular/trabecular for up to 20%. When there is a significant haemodynamic repercussion, surgery is usually indicated, although percutaneous trans-catheter closure can be considered in a subgroup of high-risk patients or those with multiple previous surgeries. In centrally located muscular VSDs, trans-catheter closure is considered an alternative to surgery and it has also been described to be a feasible alternative for peri-membranous VSDs [18]. Transthoracic and transoesophageal echocardiography are essential for the diagnosis of VSD and the assessment of severity and morphological features; they can also detect ventricular overload. There are several reports regarding the use of ICE during the percutaneous closure of peri-membranous VSDs, but experience is limited. Therefore, ICE is currently investigational in this context.

Post-infarction ventricular septal rupture occurs in approximately 0.2% of cases of myocardial infarction, and it is associated with high mortality risk. Surgery remains as the standard treatment for large defects and in the setting of acute ruptures. After the improvement of procedural success rates with trans-catheter closure of congenital VSDs, percutaneous repair was suggested as an alternative in the setting of myocardial infarction. Although there are no adequate clinical trials in this context, percutaneous closure has shown a similar rate of mortality as surgery. It can be the preferred option for simple defects with diameter <15 mm in the sub-acute (>3.5 weeks) or chronic stage [12]. MRI, CT, or TEE must be performed prior to the procedure in order to establish the number of defects, size, margins, and, if possible, viability of the surrounding tissues. Almost all published studies describe TEE as the imaging technique used for guidance. Intra-procedure TEE can be used to assess the device size. The device size is usually chosen to have a diameter 50% greater than the defect, as the septum can suffer laceration, especially in the acute setting of myocardial infarction. Once it is deployed, residual shunts or entrapment of the apparatus of the atrioventricular valves must be excluded. Procedural success rate varies from 74% to 91%, and complications, such as device embolization or myocardial rupture, can reach up to 20% in the sub-acute setting.

Table 9.3 Advantages and limitations of techniques used to guide ASD percutaneous interventions

	Advantages	Limitations
TTE	– Sedation or general anaesthesia not required – Real-time imaging	– Limited ability to visualize the lower rim of atrial septum after device deployment – Suboptimal colour doppler imaging – Limited acoustic window in most cases – Interference with interventional cardiologist
2D-TEE	– Real-time, highly precise imaging of the inter-atrial septum and other structures – Small interference with the procedure – Low risk in expert hands	– Conscious sedation or general anaesthesia required – Catheter tips not well defined
3D-TEE	– Stable and precise real-time imaging – Better guidance of complex cardiac ASDs than 2D-TEE – Good visualization of the catheter tips and surrounding structures – Reduction of fluoroscopy usage	– Lower spatial resolution as compared with 2D-TEE
ICE	– Stable and precise imaging of intra-cardiac anatomy with imaging quality comparable to 2D-TEE – Additional sedation or general anaesthesia not required – Reduction of radiation exposure – Real-time imaging of catheters and intra-cardiac devices	– Monoplane image – High cost – Small increase of vascular-related complications rate

Echocardiography in trans-septal catheterization

Trans-septal catheterization is the initial approach used in all procedures that involve left-sided heart structures. This includes percutaneous mitral valvuloplasty, PFO closure, placement of LAA occlusion devices, EP procedures such as radiofrequency ablation of AF or other arrhythmias, percutaneous mitral valve repair, or anterograde aortic balloon valvuloplasty. In expert hands, the risk of severe complications, such as perforation and mortality, remain low but still significant (1% and 0.15%, respectively). Fluoroscopy has been traditionally the only technique used, but there are several conditions, such as lipomatous hypertrophy of the septum, dilated atria, previous trans-septal catheterizations, inter-atrial septum aneurysm, double layer septum, and/or cardiac rotation, that can make echocardiography useful in this context.

TTE, TEE, and ICE can be helpful to identify the fossa ovalis, the trans-septal catheter, and the surrounding structures, although TTE quality is often cumbersome. Once the tip of the catheter is pressing the inter-atrial septum, the bulging or tenting of the fossa ovalis can be used to define the optimal place for puncture. Although TTE is usually unable to precisely assess the best location, saline contrast can be used to confirm the needle position in the right atrium. ICE offers the advantage that it does not require additional sedation and it has become the standard technique whenever it is required to guide this procedure and no complex monitoring is required afterwards. ICE catheter is oriented in order to visualize the long axis of the atrial septum perpendicular to the ultrasound beam and the right side of the fossa shows a clear ridge. Bicaval view at 70–90° with 2D-TEE and 3D-TEE can perfectly support this task and both can be the elective technique when this procedure is done for percutaneous mitral valvuloplasty, LAA closure, or paravalvular leaks closure [19]. Adequate placement of the trans-septal dilator is confirmed by the tenting of the septum at the fossa ovalis. It is important to exactly locate the tip of the catheter and its direction prior to the puncture;

3D-TEE is superior to 2D-TEE and ICE for this task. Systems that integrate 3D-TEE and X-ray imaging into a coherent view can enhance navigation and reduce the use of fluoroscopy (⊃ Fig. 9.3).

Usage of echocardiography to guide trans-septal catheterization increases the safety of the procedure, and although not required, it is recommended, especially in difficult clinical settings. Both 3D-TEE and ICE can be reliable for this purpose, and ICE has the advantage that it does not require additional sedation or different personnel involved [20].

Alcohol septal ablation for hypertrophic obstructive cardiomyopathy

Patients with hypertrophic cardiomyopathy and symptoms of advanced limiting heart failure due to an outflow obstruction with a gradient of at least 50 mmHg at rest or with provocation manoeuvres who do not respond to medical therapy must be evaluated in order to be referred to septal reduction intervention. Surgical septal myectomy is the elective technique and has a good safety profile. It obtains good long-term clinical results and a permanent reduction of the left-ventricular outflow obstruction, mitral regurgitation, and intra-ventricular pressures, with the same rate of survival as the general population. Nevertheless, percutaneous septal ablation can be an alternative to surgery in a subgroup of patients with high surgical risk due to comorbidities, elder age, or reluctance towards surgery; it has been increasingly used in Europe since it was first described in 1995 [21].

Septal myectomy is the preferred treatment option, although data comparing alcohol septal ablation and septal myectomy are not adequate to fully inform about the best option in certain cases. Patient selection is influenced by clinical parameters such as age, significant comorbidity, or concerns about airway management; echocardiography can provide information useful to establish the best treatment option, and patients with a septal thickness of 30 mm or more may experience little or no benefit from alcohol septal ablation.

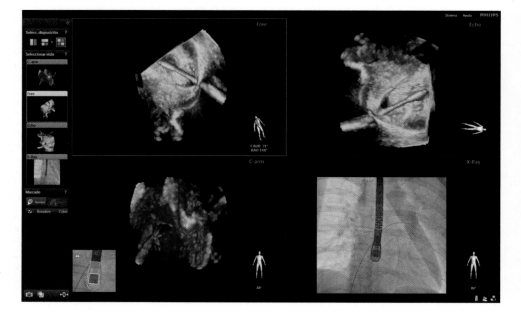

Fig. 9.3 Trans-septal puncture using integrated X-ray and 3D-transoesophageal echocardiography with the EchoNavigator system.

Percutaneous alcohol septal ablation creates a localized transmural infarction of the basal septum by the infusion of absolute alcohol into the first major septal perforator branch of the left anterior descending coronary artery. It simulates the results of the surgical myectomy and has been successfully performed in a large number of patients. Myocardial scar at the point of contact of the anterior mitral leaflet reduces the LV-outflow tract obstruction and the associated mitral regurgitation [21, 22].

The conventional approach for intra-procedural monitoring of percutaneous alcohol septal ablation involves TTE using contrast enhancement to delineate the myocardial distribution of the septal perforator artery. TEE has been described to be useful as well for this purpose, obtaining higher definition of the structures involved. ICE has not been extensively used, although it could be used as an alternative.

The target territory includes the basal septum at the point of contact with the anterior mitral leaflet where the colour Doppler shows the maximal flow acceleration. In order to determine the adequate selection, contrast injection through the inflated balloon central lumen can help delimitate the affected area under continuous TTE or TEE. Both agitated angiographic contrast or 1–2 ml of diluted echocardiographic contrast agent followed by 1–2 ml of saline flush can be used in order to obtain a good myocardial opacification with low attenuation. It must be ensured that the papillary muscles, free wall, and right ventricle are not opacified (➲ Fig. 9.4) Standard views for TTE include apical 4-chamber and 3-chamber views; additionally, parasternal long-axis and short-axis views may be useful. Once alcohol is infused, the intra-cavitary gradient must be measured. If 2D-TEE is used, 0° apical 4-chamber and 120–130° longitudinal views can help to determine the right ventricular opacification; transgastric views can complement the previous with a short-axis view. A mid-oesophageal long-axis view or a deep transgastric view can be also used to measure the intra-cavitary gradient.

Approximately 1–3 ml of alcohol are infused into the selected perforator branch, and echocardiography should be used to monitor the alcohol injection and to evaluate the results of the procedure before it is finished. The infarcted region is typically echo dense and a decrease in resting and forced gradients can be observed immediately after alcohol is injected, due to stunning, with reduced thickening and contractility. There must be a reduction of the systolic anterior motion of the anterior mitral leaflet and mitral regurgitation shortly after the alcohol delivery (➲ Figs 9.5 and 9.6). In case of incomplete results, echocardiography can be used to assess the occlusion of other septal branches, avoiding potential secondary effects or unnecessary additional scar. Long-term echocardiographic results should be evaluated at least over the first 3 months after the procedure, as myocardial scar retraction, widening of the outflow tract, and ventricular remodelling can improve the results and decrease the intra-cavitary gradient.

Percutaneous closure of left atrial appendage (LAA)

Approximately 90% of thromboembolic events in patients with AF arise in the left atrial appendage (LAA). In some cases this

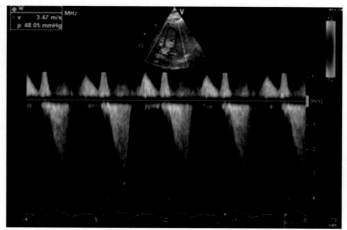

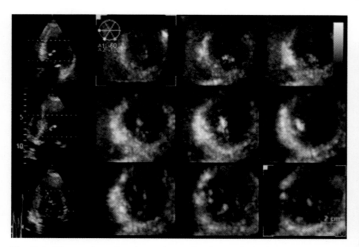

Fig. 9.4 3D transthoracic echocardiography during alcohol septal ablation for hypertrophic obstructive cardiomyopathy. Cross-sectional images obtained from an apical view after the injection of angiographic contrast. Opacified regions demonstrate the perfused territory supplied by the selected septal artery.

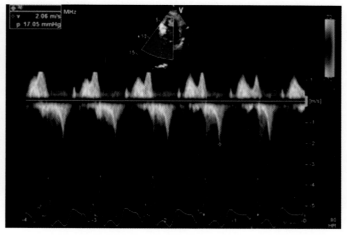

Figs 9.5 and 9.6 Transthoracic echocardiography. Continuous Doppler demonstrating a significant reduction of the intra-cavitary gradient during the procedure before alcohol injection (Fig. 9.5) and immediately after (Fig. 9.6).

observation was used to justify prophylactic intra-operative liga-tion of the LAA during cardiac surgery, regardless of the indica-tion. Percutaneous placement of LAA occluders is an effective alternative for the prophylaxis of embolic events for patients in AF who cannot receive anticoagulant therapy. It has a good safety profile when it is performed in experienced centres.

There are currently two devices available in Europe for the clo-sure of LAA: WATCHMAN (Boston Scientific Natick, MA, USA) and Amplatzer Cardiac Plug (ACP) (St Jude Medical Inc., MN, USA). Both of them are able to seal the communication between the LAA and the left atrium.

Patient selection

TEE is the screening method used for percutaneous closure of LAA and should be performed prior to the procedure, as the presence of a thrombus inside the LAA contraindicates it. LAA ostium tends to be elliptic, therefore increasing the importance of using TEE for its evaluation. LAA diameter should be drawn under the circumflex artery when using an ACP device, in order to avoid disc compres-sion after deployment (◒ Fig. 9.7). Measurement of LAA ostium with 2D-TEE and delineation of the full extent of LAA (with possi-ble multiple lobes) raises more difficulties and it has to be assessed in multiples planes in order to obtain reliable results [19]. Never-theless, 2D-TEE is only recommended for expert sonographers, as it has proven inferior to 3D-TEE and cardiac CT [23, 24].

Echocardiographic guidance in the placement of LAA occluders

TEE has been used in all clinical trials published up to date with these devices, as fluoroscopy alone is not enough for LAA loca-tion and guidance [25]. In percutaneous closure, LAA is accessed through a trans-septal approach using fluoroscopy and TEE

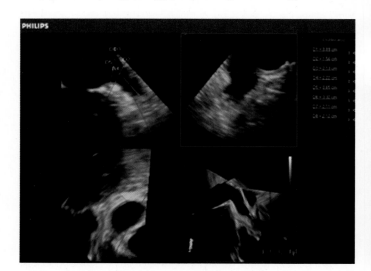

Fig. 9.7 3D-transoesophageal echocardiography for the assessment of LAA prior to percutaneous closure. Three orthogonal planes can be seen. Orifice diameters and depth must be measured and thrombus excluded in order to establish feasibility of the procedure and calculation of the device size. Diameters are taken from the origin of the left circumflex coronary artery to the roof of the left atrial appendage 1 cm below the ligament of Marshall. For an Amplatzer device, size must be at least 2 mm larger than the diameter of the anchoring zone.

guidance (◒ Figs 9.8 and 9.9). 3D-TEE is preferred over fluor-oscopy for calculation of the device size, and once it is chosen, 3D-TEE can guide the introduction, expansion, and liberation of the device [26]. Meticulous cropping can also be used to ensure that no portion of the device is spread out of the LAA. Prior to the liberation, echocardiography must be used to ensure that there are no interferences with the left inferior pulmonary vein and the mitral valve. The device disc should occupy all the ostium without residual defect. It is important to note that there is no interference with the circumflex artery. Once adjacent structures have been evaluated and the device is considered to be stable it is liberated from the catheter. After the liberation, TEE must be used to deter-mine any residual shunt and reassess the device stability. Pericar-dial effusion must be excluded after this process.

Follow-up

An echocardiogram must be performed prior to hospital dis-charge in order to confirm stability of the device. Possible complications, such as residual defects, thrombus, migration,

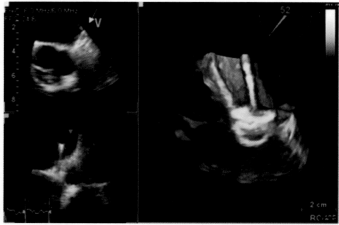

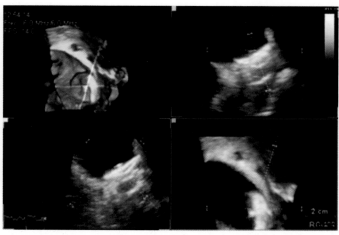

Figs 9.8 and 9.9 3D-transoesophageal echocardiography during percutaneous closure of LAA. Fig. 9.8: LAA occluder expanded prior to its liberation. Fig. 9.9: post-deployment image. The device fully covers the orifice of LAA with no compromise of surrounding structures; correct apposition and stability is confirmed.

mitral regurgitation, pulmonary vein interference, or pericardial effusion, have to be excluded. Procedure success rates have been reported to be high (96%) with a relatively low rate of serious complications (7%). Despite TEE as the ideal technique for initial follow-up, TTE can be enough for certain patients. Echocardiographic follow-up is recommended on at least the first month, sixth month, and annually [25].

Use of echocardiography to guide myocardial biopsy

Myocardial biopsies are usually performed for the diagnosis and follow-up of several cardiac conditions, such as heart transplant, infiltrative cardiomyopathies, and, less frequently, myocarditis. This procedure is usually guided by fluoroscopy alone, but it is not uncommon to use echocardiography to complement or substitute fluoroscopic images. TTE is the elective echocardiographic technique, although some reports indicate that both TEE and ICE have been successfully used to guide cardiac biopsies, especially for biopsy of intra-cardiac masses [27].

When using TTE, the optimal views in order to guide right ventricular biopsies are apical 4-chamber and subxiphoid 4-chamber view. One of the main limitations of TTE for guiding cardiac biopsies is the poor acoustic window that is frequently obtained caused by supine position in the catheterization laboratory. In optimal conditions, TTE can assess the best site to perform the biopsy, directing it to the target region (i.e. ventricular septum, right ventricular apex, or free wall), reducing the procedure and fluoroscopy times and the risk of complications, such as perforation or displacement of the tip of the catheter towards the right atrium or tricuspid valve. ICE has also been used for the evaluation of cardiac masses, guidance of the biopsy needle, and monitoring of complications.

TEE using a mid-oesophageal 4-chamber view or transgastric short- and long-axis views, and ICE from any of the right chambers, are feasible techniques that overcome the limitation of a poor acoustic window. However, both of them entail an additional risk because of the need of additional sedation and vascular access, respectively, and must be reduced for selected patients that require a highly precise cardiac biopsy [28].

Use of echocardiography to guide pericardiocentesis

Pericardial effusion can develop as a result of several conditions that affect the pericardium. There is a wide variety of aetiological causes that can lead to pericardial effusion, such as pericarditis, malignancies, autoimmune disorders, tuberculosis, thyroid disease, or chronic renal insufficiency, and their prevalence can vary depending on the area. Pericardiocentesis is an invasive procedure that can be performed to evacuate and resolve symptoms when there is a severe or symptomatic effusion, or with diagnostic purposes to obtain aetiological confirmation. Transthoracic echocardiography is the main technique and gold-standard for diagnosis of pericardial effusion and evaluation of its consequences.

Initial evaluation of a pericardial effusion should be made to establish its size, location, and haemodynamic consequences, grade its severity, and discard possible causes of effusion that may contraindicate pericardiocentesis, such as myocardial rupture secondary to myocardial infarction or aortic dissection. Echocardiographic signs of tamponade, such as respiratory alterations of AV flows, right chamber collapse, and inferior vena cava plethora, should be correlated with clinical signs and symptoms of cardiac tamponade.

Transthoracic echocardiography is essential for confirmation of severe pericardial effusion or cardiac tamponade and selecting the optimal site for needle entry, with enough margins as to prevent myocardial laceration. It can also be used for confirming the location of the needle in the pericardial cavity, and has overcome fluoroscopy avoiding radiation exposure and improving the logistics related to the procedure. The use of echocardiography during pericardiocentesis has been shown to increase the success rate and especially the safety of this procedure. Reports from the Mayo Clinic state a 97% successful rate of procedures with 1.2% of major complications, such as severe pneumothorax, chamber laceration, or death, and 3.2% of minor complications like minor pneumothorax, transient perforation, or non-sustained arrhythmia.

Once the indication of pericardiocentesis is made, location of the ideal site for puncture should be performed on the basis of identifying the point where the fluid collection is largest and the distance to the surface is shortest, avoiding vital structures. 2D transthoracic echocardiographic imaging at the apical, subxiphoid, and left parasternal views should be performed, assessing the site with the biggest echo-free space.

There are three possible sites for needle entry: the subxiphoid approach has been the classical site prior to echocardiography era, but higher procedure-related complications, such as damage to the liver, pleura, or diaphragm lesions, have made other approaches generally more adequate. Echocardiography has been directly involved in the development of the left parasternal approach, in which the needle is inserted in the 5th or 6th intercostal space close to the sternum; this site frequently offers a direct route, closer to the pericardial cavity and with wide echo-free margins. Although there is risk of pneumothorax it has been reported to have a better safety profile. Finally, the left apical approach must be always performed with echocardiographic guidance and it is not usually indicated in emergency situations due to the risk of complications. If the location of the tip of the catheter is not surely defined or there are reasonable questions, injection of agitated saline can confirm the position of the catheter in the pericardial cavity by opacification of the pericardial sac.

Use of echocardiography in electrophysiological procedures

Introduction

Recent advances performed during the last decade have revolutionized the electrophysiology (EP) laboratories, as ablation of supraventricular and ventricular arrhythmias have proven to be safe and reliable procedures. This has led to an increase in the number and complexity of cases performed in EP laboratories, and a new set of imaging tools have been developed to improve the efficacy and safety of these procedures. Miniaturization of ultrasound transducers mounted on flexible and thin catheters allowed the inclusion of intra-cardiac ultrasound among these imaging techniques. More recently, the advent of 3D-TEE has raised the interest of echocardiographic monitoring and guidance for EP procedures [24, 29].

Echocardiographic monitoring can not only be useful for guiding the trans-septal catheterization, but also for visualizing the tip of the catheters and their relation with anatomic structures such as the triangle of Koch, the terminal crest, the cavo-tricuspid isthmus, or the coronary sinus. TTE utility during EP procedures is limited due to the low imaging resolution in supine position and difficulty to maintain sterility of the procedural field. ICE and TEE can support and guide procedures such as ablation of atrial fibrillation, complex ablation procedures in patients with congenital heart diseases, and ablation of atrial flutter or ventricular tachycardia. ICE imaging has shown superiority to the use of impedance monitoring to identify safe sites for ablation and can reduce or completely avoid radiation exposure. Reduction of fluoroscopic time is particularly important in some groups of patients, such as pregnant women or children. Therefore, ICE has spread in the EP laboratories as it overcomes some of the limitations of TEE, such as the need of an additional operator and increased risk due to requirement of sedation and oesophageal intubation [30]. While ICE can also provide images with excellent intra-cardiac resolution comparable to those obtained with TEE, it is exposed too to a series of limitations like vascular events secondary to the additional catheter insertion (bleeding from the puncture site, thrombus formation, pulmonary embolism, cardiac perforation have been described, although they are infrequent); other limitations inherent to ICE include difficulty to visualize the tip of the catheter in real time, as it provides 2D images and can force the usage of 3D-TEE in selected cases; finally, there are no current guidelines that standardize the usage and views for ICE [11].

There are several ICE catheters available that have been used for EP procedures. There are two different ICE technologies. One uses a mechanical non-steerable catheter that incorporates a 360° rotating single-element ultrasound transducer at the tip (e.g. Boston Scientific Corp, San José, CA, USA); it provides real-time imaging of all surrounding structures, although its depth is reduced (approximately 5 cm) as compared with other catheters. This forces the operator to displace it to the coronary sinus or to the left atrium, depending on the target, in order to be able to see left-sided structures. Doppler capabilities are not available with these catheters. Other options are the steerable catheters with a phased-array multi-element transducer and variable frequency (e.g. AcuNav, Siemens, Mountain View, CA, USA). They improve the resolution obtained for left-sided structures, including pulmonary veins or LAA. They provide a 90° longitudinal monoplane sector image that reaches up to 16 cm of depth and support colour and pulse or continuous-wave Doppler. Manoeuvrability is higher in comparison with mechanical catheters and due to their increased tissue penetration they are able to visualize left-sided structures

with the catheter placed in the right heart. Some of these catheters have included a special sensor of electromagnetic field designed to merge the information obtained by ICE with electro-anatomical mapping navigation systems, which improves their performance.

Use of echocardiography for cardiac catheter ablation of atrial fibrillation

Ablation of atrial fibrillation was one of the first clinical settings in which the paradigm shift in electrophysiology was confirmed: some anatomical structures proved necessary for arrhythmia initiation or maintenance. Subsequently, ablation targets were not only defined by electrophysiological recordings, but also by their relation with anatomical structures. There are conventional interventional procedures that can be performed using only electrophysiological recordings and fluoroscopy guidance, such as the ablation of atrioventricular nodal re-entry or accessory pathways. On the other hand, ablation of complex arrhythmias raises the need to establish an anatomical relationship in order to increase the success rate. ICE has become the main echocardiographic method used for this purpose.

TEE and ICE can be used to ensure adequate contact between the tip of the catheter and the tissue, prematurely detecting tissue injury, thrombus formation, or potential complications such as pulmonary veins stenosis, perforation, thromboembolic events, or atrio-oesophageal fistula. Identification of pulmonary venous ostia is a key feature in catheter ablation of atrial fibrillation. There is high inter-subject variability in the anatomy of pulmonary veins and their junction with the left atrium; previous studies have shown that the prevailing pattern for the left side pulmonary veins is to have a common antrum, and this can be seen in approximately 80% of cases. There are other anatomical variants both for the left and right side pulmonary veins, and ICE is able to identify and delineate them with a high degree of precision.

There are different strategies available for 3D reconstruction when ICE is used. Integration of electro-anatomical mapping and echocardiography can be feasible with a phased-array ICE catheter. The information that comes from both techniques will be used to perform a semi-automatic delineation of the region of interest in different planes. A phased-array ICE catheter located in the right atrium or right ventricle can be highly accurate to provide contour points for the 3D electro-anatomical map of the left atrium or left ventricle, respectively.

Images of rotational scanning using conventional phased-array ICE catheters can also be used to perform a 3D reconstruction. Semi-automatic 3D-ICE images of the left atrium are obtained by means of a motor that rotates from 90 to 360° the transducer array around the longitudinal axis of the catheter placed in the right atrium, using a respiration and ECG trigger. 2D images are then postprocessed in order to obtain the 3D reconstruction (e.g. Tomtec software, Germany). This method has been mainly used for the left atrium and allows a very precise definition of pulmonary vein anatomy and width. Nevertheless its use has also been described for guidance of complex ablation procedures in the left ventricle [31].

3D reconstructed images for the guidance of atrial fibrillation ablation procedures can also be obtained using a mechanical single-element ultrasound with a pull-back device with external control that moves the ICE catheter linearly. The main limitation for the usage of this technique for ablation of atrial fibrillation is the limited imaging depth, but it has been successfully employed in other EP procedures for visualization of structures such as triangle of Koch, fossa ovalis, or coronary sinus [32].

Use of echocardiography for other EP ablation procedures

ICE has been used to support and guide complex atrial flutter ablation, especially in patients with congenital heart disease or known abnormal cardiac anatomy. ICE guidance can complement fluoroscopy by identifying the cavo-tricuspid isthmus, the Eustachian ridge, and the terminal crest.

ICE has been extensively described during ventricular tachycardia ablation procedures, establishing three goals for its use: identification of the arrhythmogenic substrate, monitoring of the position of the catheter and cardiac structures, and exclusion of complications. Myocardial scars secondary to ischaemic heart disease are the main aetiology of the cases referred for ablation due to ventricular tachycardia. ICE can easily identify the akinetic regions and guide the position of the catheter. ICE has been described as the best imaging method to guide ablation of idiopathic VTs originating in the left ventricular outflow tract or in the right ventricle secondary to arrhythmogenic right ventricular cardiomyopathy.

In addition, 3D transthoracic echocardiography usage has been also described in complex ventricular tachycardia ablation procedures by identifying the origin of ventricular ectopic activity, especially when a ventricular outflow tract origin is suspected.

Identification of the region with earliest contraction during ventricular premature beats using tissue-tracking imaging can help to fix the target of the ablation and reduce the procedure time.

As for patients undergoing epicardial complex ablation procedures, percutaneous intra-pericardial cardiac echo (PICE) has been described as a feasible and safe imaging technique, capable of providing real-time high-resolution images thanks to a phased-array ultrasound transducer. It has been reported to provide additional valuable information for epicardial ablation procedures. Despite this, its use is currently limited to investigation.

Echocardiography in cardiac resynchronization therapy procedures

Cardiac resynchronization therapy (CRT) has become a key element in the treatment of advanced chronic heart failure with reduced systolic function. However, approximately 25% of patients undergoing CRT are considered to be non-responders, which has led to the search of patterns that can help the identification of appropriate candidates.

Echocardiography has the capability to identify dyssynchronic areas. This could potentially be used to select the optimum pacing site and to guide the placement of the left ventricle lead. Regional display of time to maximum contraction can be useful for the identification of the site of maximum regional mechanical delay and subsequently the best place for LV pacing. In this sense 3D-echocardiography has a higher potential to identify dyssynchrony and several studies have described the use of 3D-TTE and 3D-TEE for resynchronization guidance and the effect on remodelling of the left ventricle [29]. Although 3D-ICE has been suggested for this purpose, there is not enough evidence to evaluate its current usefulness.

References

1. Zamorano JL, Badano LP, Bruce C, et al. EAE/ASE recommendations for the use of echocardiography in new trans-catheter interventions for valvular heart disease. *Eur Heart J* [Internet] 2011 [cited 2013 Apr 18]; 32: 2189–214. Available from: http://www.ncbi.nlm.nih.gov/pubmed/21885465

2. Carroll JD, Saver JL, Thaler DE, et al. Closure CNY of patent foramen ovale versus medical therapy after cryptogenic stroke. *N Engl J Med* [Internet] 2013 [cited 2013 Mar 20]; 368: 1092–100. Available from: http://www.ncbi.nlm.nih.gov/pubmed/23514286

3. Tullio MR, Sacco RL, Sciacca RR, et al. Patent foramen ovale and the risk of ischemic stroke in a multiethnic population. *JACC* 2007; 49: 797–802.

4. Furlan AJ, Reisman M, Massaro J, et al. Closure or medical therapy for cryptogenic stroke with patent foramen ovale. *N Engl J Med* [Internet] 2012 [cited 2013 Apr 9]; 366: 991–9. Available from: http://www.ncbi.nlm.nih.gov/pubmed/22417252

5. Meier B, Kalesan B, Mattle HP, et al. Percutaneous closure of patent foramen ovale in cryptogenic embolism. *N Engl J Med* [Internet] 2013 [cited 2013 Mar 20]; 368: 1083–1091. Available from: http://www.ncbi.nlm.nih.gov/pubmed/23514285

6. Meissner I, Khandheria BK, Heit J, et al. Patent foramen ovale: innocent or guilty? Evidence from a prospective population-based study. *JACC* 2006; 47: 440–445.

7. Messé SR, Kent DM. Still no closure on the question of PFO closure. *N Engl J Med* [Internet] 2013 [cited 2013 Mar 20]; 368: 1152–3. Available from: http://www.ncbi.nlm.nih.gov/pubmed/23514293

8. European Stroke Organisation (ESO) Executive Committee EWC. Guidelines for management of ischaemic stroke and transient ischaemic attack 2008. *Cerebrovasc Di* S2008; 25: 457–507.

9. Pepi M, Evangelista A, Nihoyannopoulos P, et al. Recommendations for echocardiography use in the diagnosis and management of cardiac sources of embolism: European Association of Echocardiography (EAE) (a registered branch of the ESC). *Eur J Echocardiogr* [Internet] 2010 [cited 2013 Mar 3]; 11: 461–76. Available from: http://www.ncbi.nlm.nih.gov/pubmed/20702884

10. Davison P, Clift PF SR. The role of echocardiography in diagnosis, monitoring closure and post-procedural assessment of patent foramen ovale. *Eur J Echocardiogr* 2010; 11: i27–i34.

11. Ali S, George LK, Das P, Koshy SKG. Intra-cardiac echocardiography: clinical utility and application. *Echocardiography* [Internet] 2011

[cited 2013 Apr 20]; 28: 582–90. Available from: http://www.ncbi.nlm.nih.gov/pubmed/21564275

12. Kenny D, Hijazi ZM. Trans-catheter approaches to non-valvar structural heart disease. *Int J Cardiovasc Imaging* [Internet] 2011 [cited 2013 Apr 28]; 27: 1133–41. Available from: http://www.ncbi.nlm.nih.gov/pubmed/21331612

13. Baumgartner H, Bonhoeffer P, Groot NMS De, et al. ESC guidelines for the management of grown-up congenital heart disease (new version 2010). *Eur Heart J* [Internet] 2010 [cited 2013 Mar 7]; 31: 2915–57. Available from: http://www.ncbi.nlm.nih.gov/pubmed/20801927

14. Roberson DA, Cui W, Patel D, et al. Three-dimensional transoesophageal echocardiography of atrial septal defect: a qualitative and quantitative anatomic study. *J Am Soc Echocardiogr* [Internet] 2011 [cited 2013 Apr 28]; 24: 600–10. Available from: http://www.ncbi.nlm.nih.gov/pubmed/21477991

15. Balzer J, Kelm M, Kühl HP. Real-time three-dimensional transoesophageal echocardiography for guidance of non-coronary interventions in the catheter laboratory. *Eur J Echocardiogr* [Internet] 2009 [cited 2013 Apr 28]; 10: 341–9. Available from: http://www.ncbi.nlm.nih.gov/pubmed/19211569

16. Saric M, Perk G, Purgess JR, Kronzon I. Imaging atrial septal defects by real-time three-dimensional transesophageal echocardiography: step-by-step approach. *J Am Soc Echocardiogr* [Internet] 2010 [cited 2013 Apr 28]; 23: 1128–35. Available from: http://www.ncbi.nlm.nih.gov/pubmed/20833505

17. Vaidyanathan B, Simpson JM KR. Transesophageal echocardiography for device closure of atrial septal defects. *JACC.* 2009; 2: 1238–1242.

18. Kim MS, Klein AJ, Carroll JD. Trans-catheter closure of intra-cardiac defects in adults. *J Interv Cardiol* [Internet] 2007 [cited 2013 Apr 28]; 20: 524–45. Available from: http://www.ncbi.nlm.nih.gov/pubmed/18042058

19. Lang RM, Badano LP, Tsang W, et al. EAE/ASE recommendations for image acquisition and display using three-dimensional echocardiography. *Eur Heart J Cardiovasc Imaging* [Internet] 2012 [cited 2013 Mar 29]; 13: 1–46. Available from: http://www.ncbi.nlm.nih.gov/pubmed/22275509

20. Silvestry FE, Kerber RE BM. Echocardiography-guided interventions. *JASE* 2009; 22: 213–26.

21. Gersh BJ, Maron BJ, Bonow RO, et al. 2011 ACCF/AHA guideline for the diagnosis and treatment of hypertrophic cardiomyopathy: a report of the American College of Cardiology Foundation/American Heart Association Task Force on Practice Guidelines. *Circulation* [Internet] 2011 [cited 2013 Mar 9]; 124: e783–831. Available from: http://www.ncbi.nlm.nih.gov/pubmed/22068434

22. Mor-Avi V, Lang RM, Badano LP, et al. Current and evolving echocardiographic techniques for the quantitative evaluation of cardiac mechanics: ASE/EAE consensus statement on methodology and indications endorsed by the Japanese Society of Echocardiography. *Eur J Echocardiogr* [Internet] 2011 [cited 2013 Apr 9]; 12: 167–205. Available from: http://www.ncbi.nlm.nih.gov/pubmed/21385887

23. Flachskampf FA, Badano L, Daniel WG, et al. Recommendations for transoesophageal echocardiography: update 2010. *Eur J Echocardiogr* [Internet] 2010 [cited 2013 Mar 3]; 11: 557–76. Available from: http://www.ncbi.nlm.nih.gov/pubmed/20688767

24. Gonçalves A, Zamorano JL. Valve anatomy and function with transthoracic three-dimensional echocardiography: advantages and limitations of instantaneous full-volume color Doppler imaging. *Ther Adv Cardiovasc Dis* [Internet] 2010 [cited 2013 May 8]; 4: 385–94. Available from: http://www.ncbi.nlm.nih.gov/pubmed/20965949

25. Lockwood SM, Alison JF, Obeyesekere MN, Mottram PM. Imaging the left atrial appendage prior to, during, and after occlusion. *JACC Cardiovasc Imaging* [Internet] 2011 [cited 2013 Apr 3]; 4: 303–6. Available from: http://www.ncbi.nlm.nih.gov/pubmed/21414580

26. Joshi D, Mazimba S, Neal Kay G, et al. Role of live/real time three-dimensional transesophageal echocardiography in the percutaneous epicardial closure of the left atrial appendage. *Echocardiography* [Internet] 2012 [cited 2013 Mar 21]; Available from: http://www.ncbi.nlm.nih.gov/pubmed/23016575

27. Miglioranza MH, Leiria TLL, Haertel JC, Winkler M, Fernández-Golfin C, Zamorano JL. The role of three-dimensional echocardiography in interventricular mass evaluation. *Echocardiography* [Internet] 2013 [cited 2013 May 8]; 30: E125–7. Available from: http://www.ncbi.nlm.nih.gov/pubmed/23489108

28. Pérez de Isla L, Castro R de, Zamorano JL, et al. Diagnosis and treatment of cardiac myxomas by transesophageal echocardiography. *Am J Cardiol* [Internet] 2002 [cited 2013 May 8]; 90: 1419–21. Available from: http://www.ncbi.nlm.nih.gov/pubmed/12480063

29. Kautzner J, Peichl P. 3D and 4D echo—applications in EP laboratory procedures. *J Interv Card Electrophysiol* [Internet] 2008 [cited 2013 Apr 28]; 22: 139–144. Available from: http://www.ncbi.nlm.nih.gov/pubmed/18421574

30. Banchs JE, Patel P, Naccarelli G.V, Gonzalez MD. Intra-cardiac echocardiography in complex cardiac catheter ablation procedures. *J Interv Card Electrophysiol* [Internet] 2010 [cited 2013 Apr 28]; 28: 167–84. Available from: http://www.ncbi.nlm.nih.gov/pubmed/20480388

31. Govil A, Calkins H, Spragg DD. Fusion of imaging technologies: how, when, and for whom? *J Interv Card Electrophysiol* [Internet] 2011 [cited 2013 Apr 26]; 32: 195–203. Available from: http://www.ncbi.nlm.nih.gov/pubmed/21964620

32. Ho JK, Nakahara S, Shivkumar K, Mahajan A. Live three-dimensional transesophageal echocardiographic imaging of novel multielectrode ablation catheters. *Heart Rhythm* [Internet] 2010 [cited 2013 Apr 28]; 7: 570–1. Available from: http://www.ncbi.nlm.nih.gov/pubmed/19875342

SECTION III

Valvular heart disease

CHAPTER 10

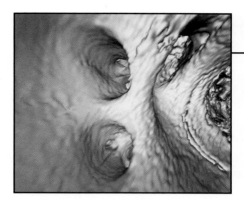

Aortic valve stenosis

Helmut Baumgartner, Erwan Donal, Stefan Orwat, Axel Schmermund, Raphael Rosenhek, and David Maintz

Contents

Echocardiographic assessment of morphology and severity with its pitfalls and limitations

Assessment of morphology

Site of left ventricular outflow obstruction—differential diagnosis

Aortic stenosis (AS) is most commonly valvular. However, left ventricular outflow tract obstruction also occurs subvalvular and can then be either fixed in case of congenital malformation (discrete membrane or muscular band; or dynamic in the case of hypertrophic obstructive cardiomyopathy (see section on Cardiomyopathies) or supravalvular as rare congenital condition . Because of the fundamental differences in treatment strategies it is essential to correctly identify the level of left ventricular outflow tract obstruction. Echocardiography allows distinction of these entities by morphologic assessment, Doppler determination of the site of velocity increase, and analysis of its time course (early, mid, late systolic peak; see ➲ Fig. 10.4). Typical examples are shown in ➲ Fig. 10.1.

Assessment of AS aetiology

Calcific AS is the most common form and is characterized by thickened and calcified cusps (bicuspid or tricuspid valve) with reduced mobility [1]. Congenital AS presents most commonly with bicuspid and less frequently with unicuspid, tricuspid, or quadricuspid valves. The two cusps of bicuspid valves are typically of different size and the larger cusp often contains a raphe (fusion line of two cusps). Typically the cusps are oriented either in an anterior/posterior (fusion of right and left coronary cusp; 80%) or right/left manner (fusion of right and non-coronary cusp). Rheumatic aortic stenosis is characterized by commissural fusion, thickening of the cusp edges, and sometimes cusp retraction. It is commonly associated with aortic regurgitation and mitral valve involvement. Typical examples are shown in ➲ Fig. 10.2. In advanced disease stages, congenitally malformed and rheumatic valves develop calcification. Once the valve is extensively calcified, the exact determination of underlying morphology and aetiology becomes difficult.

Assessment of aortic valve calcification

Aortic valve calcification is best assessed in a short-axis view, although the presence of extensive calcification may also be noted in the 5-chamber view. The degree of calcification (see ➲ Fig. 10.3) can be classified into mild (isolated, small spots), moderate (multiple bigger spots), and severe (extensive thickening/calcification of all cusps). It has prognostic implications (see Calcification of the aortic valve) [2].

Assessment of the aorta

Assessment of the ascending aorta is crucial as aneurysms are not uncommon. In particular, congenital AS is frequently associated with dilatation of the ascending aorta. Its extent

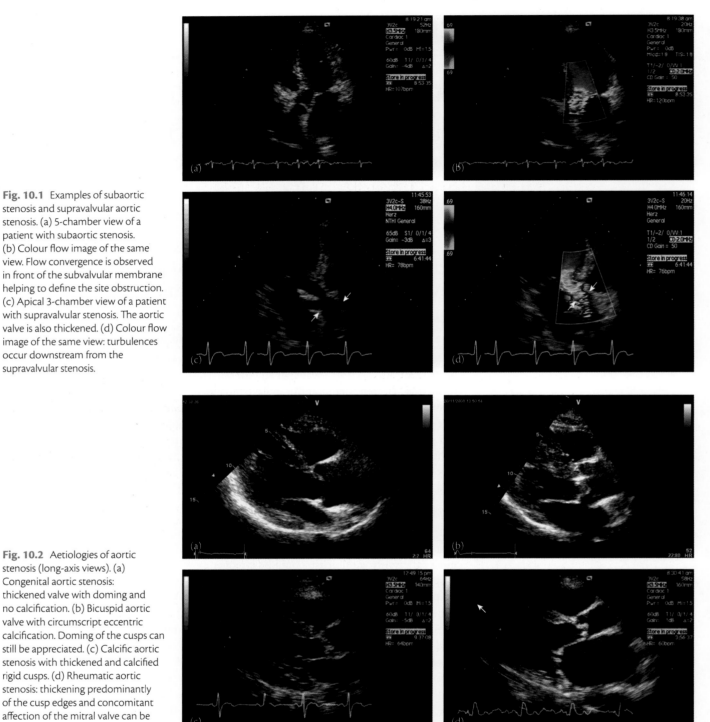

Fig. 10.1 Examples of subaortic stenosis and supravalvular aortic stenosis. (a) 5-chamber view of a patient with subaortic stenosis. (b) Colour flow image of the same view. Flow convergence is observed in front of the subvalvular membrane helping to define the site obstruction. (c) Apical 3-chamber view of a patient with supravalvular stenosis. The aortic valve is also thickened. (d) Colour flow image of the same view: turbulences occur downstream from the supravalvular stenosis.

Fig. 10.2 Aetiologies of aortic stenosis (long-axis views). (a) Congenital aortic stenosis: thickened valve with doming and no calcification. (b) Bicuspid aortic valve with circumscript eccentric calcification. Doming of the cusps can still be appreciated. (c) Calcific aortic stenosis with thickened and calcified rigid cusps. (d) Rheumatic aortic stenosis: thickening predominantly of the cusp edges and concomitant affection of the mitral valve can be appreciated.

is not related to the haemodynamic severity of AS. Dilation at the level of sinuses is in general easily recognized. However, aneurysms distal to the sinotubular junction are more difficult to image and require special care generating atypical long-axis views with angulation towards the ascending aorta.

Additional findings

The echocardiographic assessment must also include the determination of concomitant left ventricular hypertrophy and

dysfunction, coexisting mitral valve disease, and pulmonary hypertension.

Quantification of stenosis severity

A normal aortic valve has an orifice area of 3–4 cm² and a laminar normal transvalvular flow with a peak velocity of less than 2 m/s. While several other parameters have been proposed for the AS quantification, peak transvalvular velocity, mean Doppler gradient, and effective orifice area, as derived from the continuity

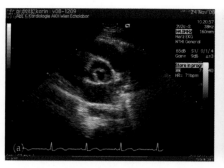
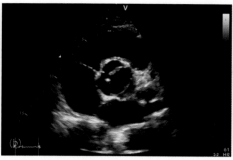
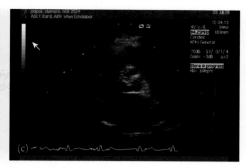

Fig. 10.3 Degree of aortic valve calcification. (a) Parasternal short-axis view of a unicuspid stenotic aortic valve without calcification. (b) Parasternal short-axis view of a bicuspid aortic stenosis with minimal calcification. (c) Parasternal short-axis view of a moderately calcified stenotic aortic valve (right-noncoronary fusion pattern). (d) Parasternal short-axis view of a severely calcified stenotic aortic valve with extensive thickening and calcification of all cusps.

equation, have been best validated and are currently recommended for clinical assessment of AS [3–5].

Transvalvular velocity and gradients

Transvalvular velocity continuously increases with AS severity as long as cardiac output is maintained.

Transvalvular gradients (ΔP) are calculated from continuous-wave Doppler derived transvalvular velocities (v) using the Bernoulli equation, which is based on the conservation of energy principle. In clinical practice, the simplified Bernoulli equation:

$$\Delta P = 4v^2, \tag{10.1}$$

which ignores viscous losses and the effects of flow acceleration, is used [6]. It also ignores the flow velocity proximal to the stenosis, which is an acceptable assumption as long as the transvalvular velocity is significantly greater than the proximal flow velocity and in particular when ≤1 m/s. However, if proximal velocity is increased (narrow outflow tract or increased flow rate caused by high cardiac output or aortic regurgitation) the less simplified version:

$$\Delta P = 4\left(v_2^2 - v_1^2\right) \tag{10.2}$$

should be used, where v_2 and v_1 represent the transvalvular and the proximal flow velocities, respectively.

The peak transaortic pressure gradient corresponds to the maximum instantaneous difference between the pressure in the aorta and the ventricle. With increasing stenosis severity, the peak of the gradient occurs later during systole (see ⊃ Fig. 10.4). Note that the peak gradient is different from the 'peak-to-peak' gradient that is determined by catheter and corresponds to the difference between peak aortic pressure and peak left ventricular pressure. The latter is not a physiologic measure, since these two peaks do not occur simultaneously and it cannot be determined by Doppler echocardiography.

The mean gradient is calculated by averaging the instantaneous gradients throughout the ejection period.

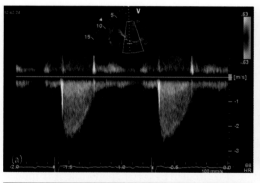
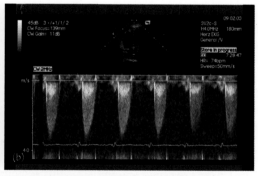
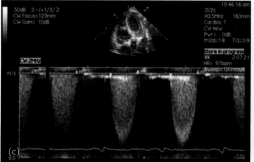
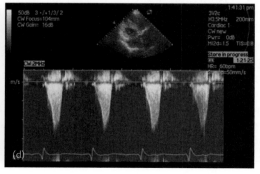

Fig. 10.4 Continuous-wave Doppler velocity spectrum. (a) Mild aortic stenosis with immediate peak. (b) Moderate aortic stenosis with early peak. (c) Severe aortic stenosis with midsystolic peak. (d) Dynamic obstruction in the setting of a hypertrophic obstructive cardiomyopathy with late peak.

Fig. 10.5 Continuous-wave Doppler recordings of a patient with severe aortic stenosis (AS): the recording from the apical window provides a peak velocity of 3.4 m/s consistent with moderate AS (a), whereas the right parasternal window provides 4.3 m/s consistent with severe AS (b) emphasizing the importance of the use of multiple transducer positions.

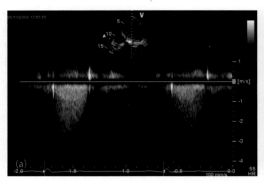 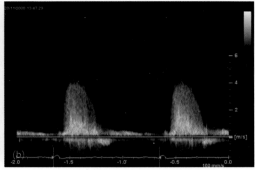

Technical considerations and pitfalls

Besides the neglect of an increased subvalvular velocity (see gradient calculation) a number of other sources of error may occur. A correct alignment of the Doppler beam with the direction of the stenotic jet is essential. Malalignment leads to an underestimation of the Doppler gradient and hence of the severity of AS. Multiple transducer positions (i.e. right parasternal, suprasternal, apical, and sometimes even subcostal) have to be used, to obtain the accurate velocity. For that purpose, the use of a small, dedicated continuous-wave Doppler transducer (pencil probe) is mandatory (see ➲ Fig. 10.5). When the rate of haemodynamic progression is determined, one has to make sure that measurements are recorded from the same window.

Another potential source of error that needs to be avoided is the confusion of the AS signal with a signal originating from another obstruction or from mitral or tricuspid regurgitation. In the presence of arrhythmias, such as atrial fibrillation, several consecutive beats have to be averaged and beats after long R–R intervals or post-extrasystolic beats must be avoided.

The phenomenon of pressure recovery may also cause pitfalls and may explain discrepancies between catheter and Doppler derived pressure gradients [7]. Obstruction of flow in any kind of stenosis causes flow velocity increase and pressure drop corresponding to a conversion of potential energy to kinetic energy. Pressure is lowest and velocity is greatest at the level of the vena contracta, the site of minimum cross-sectional flow area. The jet expands and decelerates downstream from the stenosis. Although some of the kinetic energy dissipates into heat due to turbulences and viscous losses, some of it will be reconverted into potential energy and pressure will increase again to some degree (= pressure recovery). The Doppler gradient corresponds to the maximum pressure drop from proximal to the vena contracta and overestimates the net pressure drop as usually given by catheter measurement in the case of significant pressure recovery. In AS, the magnitude of pressure recovery is frequently small since the abrupt widening from the small valve orifice to a generally normally sized or enlarged aorta causes a lot of turbulence. However, the effects of pressure recovery may be significant in the presence of a small ascending aorta (<30mm) [7].

Doppler velocites and pressure gradients are highly flow-dependent. In the presence of high cardiac output or significant aortic regurgitation consideration of these measurements alone may cause significant overestimation of AS severity. On the other hand, in the presence of low flow rates, most commonly caused by an impaired left ventricular function but also e.g. in the presence of mitral stenosis or small hypertrophied ventricles, AS severity may be underestimated. Thus, valve area, as a less flow-dependent parameter, is required for appropriate AS quantification.

Valve area calculation by the continuity equation

The continuity equation has gained most acceptance for valve area calculation [8, 9]. It is based on the fact that the stroke volume passing through the left ventricular outflow tract (LVOT) must equal the stroke volume crossing the stenotic aortic valve:

$$AVA \times VTI_{AS} = CSA_{LVOT} \times VTI_{LVOT}, \qquad (10.3)$$

where AVA is the aortic valve area, VTI_{AS} and VTI_{LVOT} are the velocity time integrals in the LVOT and effective valve orifice, respectively and CSA_{LVOT} is the cross-sectional area of the LVOT (see ➲ Fig. 10.6).

A simplified version of the continuity equation that uses peak aortic jet and outflow tract velocities instead of the velocity time integral has also been proposed.

The cross-sectional area (CSA) of the LVOT is calculated using the formula:

$$CSA_{LVOT} = \pi(D/2)^2, \qquad (10.4)$$

where D is the diameter of the LVOT measured in the parasternal long-axis view at mid-systole.

This assumption of a circular LVOT shape (while it is indeed frequently oval) and the requirement of measuring LVOT size and velocity exactly at the same site are important limitations of the method that may cause error.

The LVOT flow velocity is measured from an apical approach using pulsed Doppler ultrasound with the assumption of laminar flow and a flat velocity profile. The fact that these assumptions may not be fulfilled also limits the accuracy of the method.

Despite these limitations, the continuity equation has been shown to be currently the best technique of valve area estimation and yields valuable measurements for AS quantification as a basis

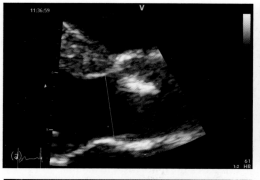
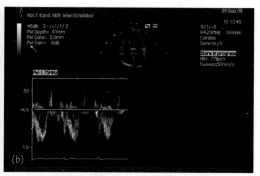
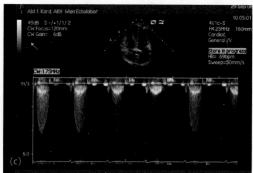
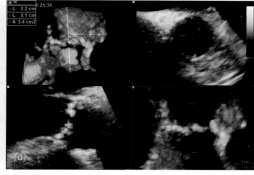

Fig. 10.6 Continuity equation: required recordings. (a) Zoomed parasternal long-axis view with the left ventricular outflow tract diameter measurement. (b) Pulsed-wave Doppler recording of LVOT velocity obtained from an apical 5-chamber view. (c) Continuous-wave Doppler recording of the aortic jet velocity (apical transducer position). (d) Measurement of LVOT area using 3D TEE in systole.

for patient decision-making when sources of error are carefully considered.

Velocity ratio

In order to reduce the error related to LVOT measurements it has been proposed to remove it from the continuity equation. The so determined dimensionless velocity ratio expresses the size of the effective valve area as a proportion of the cross-sectional area of the LVOT:

$$\text{Velocity ratio} = V\text{LVOT} / V\text{AS}. \qquad (10.5)$$

Both velocity time integrals and peak velocities have been used. Severe stenosis is present when the velocity ratio is 0.25 or less, corresponding to a valve area 25% of normal. To some extent, velocity ratio normalizes for body size because it reflects the ratio of the actual valve area to the expected valve area in each patient, regardless of body size. However, this measurement ignores variability in LVOT size beyond variation in body size and has gained less acceptance for routine use than the combination gradients and continuity equation valve area.

Valve area planimetry

Planimetry of the valve area, primarily by 2D TEE has also been proposed. However, the orifice of a stenotic aortic valve frequently represents a complex 3-dimensional structure that cannot be reliably assessed with a planar 2D-image. The presence of valvular calcification further limits an accurate delineation of the aortic valve orifice. Thus, this method has not been accepted as a routine measurement. Nevertheless, it might be useful in selected patients when additional information is needed [5].

Three-dimensional echocardiography has been reported to allow valve area planimetry but has not sufficiently been validated yet.

Dobutamine echocardiography

Dobutamine echocardiography is indicated in the setting of low flow–low gradient AS, which is defined by a small calculated valve area (<1.0 cm^2), in the presence of a reduced transaortic gradient (<30 to 40 mmHg) and a reduced left ventricular function determined by a low-stroke volume index (<35 mL/m^2) [10]. It is performed at a low dobutamine dose that is gradually increased up to a maximum dose of 10–20 μg/kg/min by steps of 5 μg/kg/min per 3–5 min, trying not to exceed a heart rate of 100 beats/min.

It allows the determination of the presence of a contractile reserve or a 20% relative increase in ejection fraction (defined as an increase of stroke volume ≥20%), which has been shown to be of prognostic value. In the presence of a contractile reserve it allows a further differentiation between pseudosevere stenosis (compared to baseline, the gradients remain small, whereas the valve area increases significantly with increasing flow, indicating that AS is non-severe and severely reduced opening passively caused by diminished driving forces) and true severe stenosis (gradients increase, whereas the valve area remains small indicating a fixed small valve orifice with a low gradient caused by secondary LV dysfunction and flow reduction).

Experimental methods of AS quantification

Several additional parameters such as valve resistance, stroke work loss, or the energy loss coefficient have been proposed to quantify aortic stenosis severity. Since their complexity adds sources

Table 10.1 Recommendations for classification of AS severity (3-5) [3-5]

	Aortic sclerosis	Mild	Moderate	Severe
Aortic jet velocity (m/s)	≤ 2.5 m/s	2.6–2.9	3–4	>4
Mean gradient (mmHg)	—	<20	20–40	>40
AVA (cm²)	—	>1.5	1.0–1.5	<1.0
Indexed AVA (cm²/m²)		>0.85	0.60–0.85	<0.6
Velocity ratio		>0.50	0.25–0.50	<0.25

of error and since they lack solid prognostic validation, they are still considered experimental and not recommended for routine clinical use [5].

Definition of AS severity

By current recommendations, severity of AS is assessed by combining aortic jet velocity, mean gradient and valve area (see ⊃ Table 10.1) [3–5]. Because of prognostic implications, the differentiation between severe and non-severe stenosis is of particular importance. In the presence of normal transvalvular flow, severe AS is considered with a peak aortic jet velocity greater than 4 m/s and a mean gradient greater than 40 mmHg. Outcome worsens with increasing velocity and event rates have been shown to be particularly high when peak velocities exceed 5.5 m/s. Current recommendations define severe AS by using a cut-off of <1 cm² for the valve area. It has also been suggested to index aortic valve area to body surface area (cut-off 0.6 cm²/m²). However, there is no linear relation between body surface area and valve area, and there is particular distortion at the extremes of the spectrum.

Diagnosis of severe AS is easy when peak velocity, mean gradient, and valve area are consistent but becomes a challenge if they are inconsistent, in particular when valve area is less than 1 cm² but peak velocity less than 4 m/s and mean gradient less than 40 mmHg. One reason for this constellation is a reduced flow in the presence of LV dysfunction. In this situation, 'classical' low flow–low gradient AS with reduced ejection fraction (EF) must be assumed and dobutamine echocardiography can help to distinguish between pseudosevere and true severe AS (see section Dobutamine echocardiography). The most challenging finding in clinical practice is a valve area smaller than 1 cm² with a peak velocity less than 4 m/s and mean gradient less than 40 mmHg, despite normal LV EF. The new entity of severe 'paradoxical' low flow–low gradient AS with preserved EF has recently been introduced and refers to patients with hypertrophied, small ventricles resulting in reduced transvalvular flow (stroke volume index <35 ml/m²) despite normal EF [11, 12]. However, this entity has to be diagnosed with particular care since other more frequent reasons for the finding of a small valve area and low gradients in

the presence of normal EF have to be excluded. The continuity equation may underestimate the valve area because of flow underestimation caused by the underestimation of the LVOT area when assuming a circular shape while it is indeed oval and other measurement errors [13]. Transoesophageal 3D echocardiography may prove to be useful in measuring the definite LVOT cross-sectional area to obtain more accurate values [14] (⊃ Fig. 10.6d). Furthermore, it has to be emphasized that current cut-offs for valve area and velocity/gradient are not really consistent to begin with. To generate a mean gradient of 40 mmHg with a normal stroke volume, the valve area must be closer to 0.8 than to 1.0 cm² [15–17]. Finally, small stature of the patient may be another reason for a small valve area and low gradient in the presence of normal EF. Severe 'paradoxical' low flow–low gradient AS with preserved EF has in general been described in elderly patients with hypertrophied ventricles of small volume. Reduced longitudinal LV function and fibrosis were found. However, the vast majority of these patients had a history of hypertension that may have caused the LV pathology [11, 12]. In addition, it remains so far unclear how to distinguish between pseudosevere and true severe AS in this setting. Dobutamine echocardiography may be less helpful in these ventricles with small volumes and normal EF. The degree of valve calcification may then be a final important hint to identify true severe AS [18].

Thus, definition of severe AS remains challenging and current guidelines emphasize that diagnosis in clinical practice must be based on an integrated approach including transvalvular velocity/gradient, valve area, valve morphology, transvalvular velocity, LV morphology and function, blood pressure and symptoms [19].

Role of MRI and CT

Although echocardiography remains the standard modality for the diagnosis and quantification of AS, MRI and CT are gaining importance, both for valve assessment and adjunct cardiovascular evaluation.

The role of MRI in patients with AS may be 4-fold: (1) assessment of valve morphology, (2) assessment of valve function, (3) assessment of LV function, and (4) assessment of aortic disease.

For the assessment of valve morphology, cine imaging is applied in at least two orthogonal planes through the aortic valve, usually in the orientation of the aortic ring and in the LVOT orientation. Usually cine imaging is performed using steady-state-free-precession sequences with an effective temporal resolution of c. 35 ms. Cine images in LVOT orientation show a flow jet during systole extending from the valve into the ascending aorta. This jet is due to phase dispersion in increased flow velocities. To quantify the aortic valve area by planimetry, systolic images through the aortic ring are needed (see ⊃ Fig. 10.7). Computer programs are available to perform planimetry semi-automatically on most workstations. Measurements of the aortic valve area based on steady-state free-precession images have been shown to correlate better with TEE than conventional spoiled gradient echo images [20].

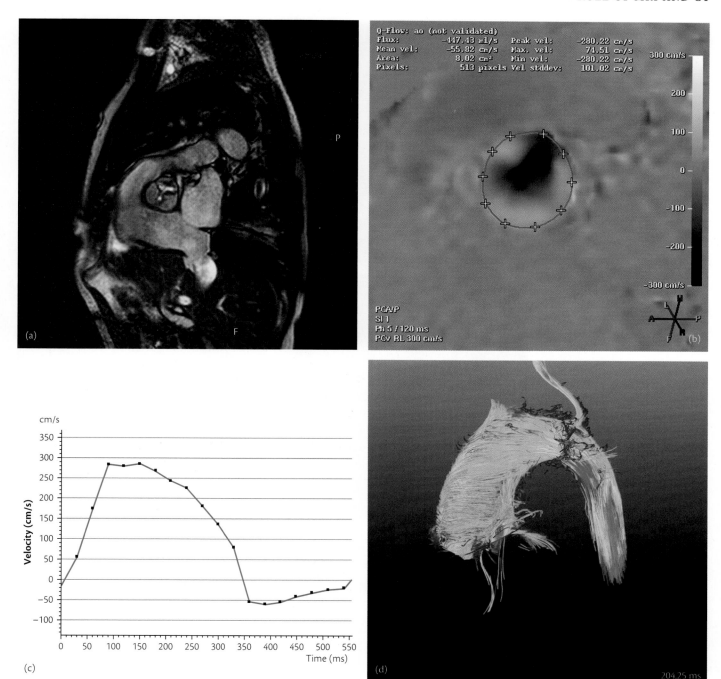

Fig. 10.7 MRI of aortic stenosis: steady-state free-precession MR images in systole. (a) Impaired opening of the valve and reduced valve area. (b) A phase contrast image at a level 2 cm above the valve. (c) A time curve of peak flow velocity measurements. (d) Time-resolved 3D phase contrast (4D flow) CMR provides aortic flow characterization in a patient with bicuspid aortic valve (right-left fusion pattern). Velocity streamlines show a right-handed helix flow jet pattern in the ascending aorta.

One advantage of MRI (vs. CT) is that in addition to the assessment of valve morphology in cine images, flow can be measured in phase-contrast sequences. The background of these techniques is the fact that the phase shift in moving spins is proportional to their velocity. By measuring the peak velocity one can derive the pressure gradient by the use of the Bernoulli equation (see ⊃ Fig. 10.7). Prerequisite for exact measurements in phase contrast sequences is that the expected maximum velocity is provided, otherwise aliasing artefacts may occur. Valve area can also be calculated from MRI data using the continuity equation.

MRI is the method of highest accuracy for the assessment of LV function and LV mass. At the same time, the LV can be evaluated for the presence of fibrotic changes by the use of late-enhancement imaging. The detection of diffuse fibrosis has recently been demonstrated using T1 mapping [21]. Pathology of the aorta

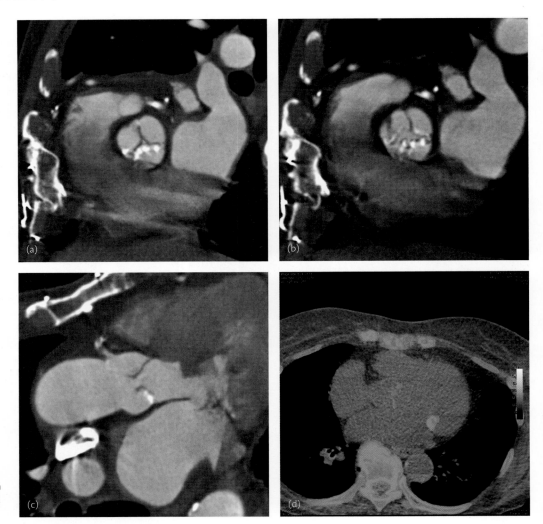

Fig. 10.8 Computed tomography (CT) of aortic stenosis: diastolic and systolic reformations through the aortic valve show impaired opening of the heavily calcified posterior and left cusp of the valve. (a, b) short-axis views. (c) 3-chamber view. (d) Non-contrast CT acquisition with calculation of the aortic valve calcium score (Agatston equivalent; threshold 130 HU).

(aneurysm, coarctation) may be investigated using contrast-enhanced magnetic resonance angiography or 3D cine velocity acquisitions (see ⊃ Fig. 10.7).

With the advent of 64-slice CT scanners, the assessment of valve morphology and function using CT has become feasible. CT has the advantage of a high spatial resolution and a very high sensitivity for the detection of calcific changes of the valves (see ⊃ Fig. 10.8). Despite its inferior temporal resolution compared to echo and MRI, CT is able to acquire systolic and diastolic images of the aortic valve that allow for the assessment of valve morphology, as well as planimetry of the aortic valve area (AVA). In recent comparisons of CT and echocardiography, a good correlation of both methods was found with a tendency of CT to measure larger values for AVA [22, 23].

The quantification of valve calcification has been proposed to identify severe AS (>1651 Agatston units: 82% sensitivity, 80% specificity, 88% negative-predictive value and 70% positive-predictive value for the diagnosis of severe AS) in the setting of low flow–low gradient AS [18] (see ⊃ Fig. 10.8). While it cannot provide haemodynamic data, CT has the important advantage over MRI and echo that it may also assess the coronary

arteries in the same scan. The method has been shown to detect significant coronary artery disease in patients prior to valve surgery [24].

Prognostic information provided by imaging

Severity of AS

Imaging techniques allow the detection and quantification of AS. Even the presence of aortic sclerosis without haemodynamic obstruction is associated with an increased morbidity and mortality. With an increasing severity of AS, outcome is further impaired. In fact, peak aortic jet velocity is an important predictor of outcome in asymptomatic patients with AS. With increasing velocity, subsequent necessity of an aortic valve replacement becomes more likely [15] (see ⊃ Fig. 10.9). A peak velocity >5.5 m/s has been reported to be associated with a particularly high event rate, mostly valve replacement required because of symptom development [25].

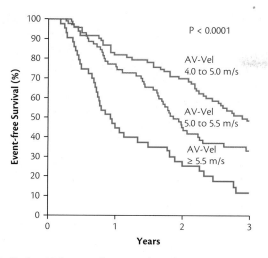

Fig. 10.9 Kaplan–Meier event-free survival rate for patients with a peak aortic jet velocity (AV-Vel) between 4.0 and 5.0 m/s (red line) vs between 5.0 and 5.5 m/s (blue line) vs >5.5 m/s (green line). Modified from: Raphael Rosenhek et al, Natural History of Very Severe Aortic Stenosis, *Circulation*, 121:1, with permission from Wolters Kluwer Health.

Haemodynamic progression

Faster rates of haemodynamic progression are associated with an increased event rate, both in patients with severe, but also in patients with mild-to-moderate, aortic stenosis [2, 26]. Haemodynamic progression is actually indirectly related to AS severity. While there is great inter-individual variability in the rates of haemodynamic progression, the presence of a calcified aortic valve was shown to predict faster haemodynamic progression.

Calcification of the aortic valve

The presence of a moderate-to-severe calcified aortic valve on echocardiography is a significant predictor of outcome in patients with mild-to-moderate AS [26] (see ➲ Fig. 10.10). More importantly, in patients with severe AS, the presence of a moderate-to-severe calcified aortic valve is associated with an event-rate of 80% within 4 years with events defined as symptom onset warranting aortic valve replacement or death [2] (see ➲ Fig. 10.10). The presence of a calcified aortic valve in combination with a rapid haemodynamic progression (defined as an increase in peak aortic jet velocity of more than 0.3 m/s within one year) identifies a high-risk population with an event-rate of 79% within 2 years (see ➲ Fig. 10.10).

Left ventricular function

Although LV function has a high tendency to improve after valve replacement, poor LV function is known to be associated with a worse outcome. However, reduced LVEF is extremely rare in asymptomatic patients (<1% of severe AS). A recent study reported a poor outcome of such patients, even after valve replacement, leading to the suspicion that impaired LV function may have been due to other associated yet not identified disease [27]. Global longitudinal LV strain, as measured with echo speckle tracking,

may be more sensitive for detecting early LV dysfunction and has been reported to predict events in asymptomatic patients, as well as mortality in aortic stenosis [28]. Furthermore, impaired strain prior to valve replacement has recently been reported to predict worse post-operative outcome with regard to rehospitalization for heart failure and mortality [29]. These new data still require multicentric validation studies.

Left ventricular hypertrophy

The impact of left ventricular hypertrophy (LVH) on outcome has been studied for a long time with inconclusive results. A recent study reported excessive LVH to be associated with a significantly higher event rate in asymptomatic patients [30] (see ➲ Fig. 10.13).

Myocardial fibrosis

Focal myocardial fibrosis in AS, as demonstrated by CMR late gadolinium enhancement, has been reported to be associated with worse post-operative outcome in particular residual symptoms but also mortality in patients undergoing valve replacement [31]. Whether the search for fibrosis in asymptomatic patients can help to optimize the time of surgery remains unknown. CMR T1 mapping has recently been reported to identify diffuse fibrosis in AS and can be found even in asymptomatic patients [32]. However, the clinical relevance of such findings remains to be shown.

Pulmonary hypertension

Pulmonary hypertension (PH) is known to be associated with an increased operative mortality and has therefore been included in current surgical risk scores. PH at rest and with exercise has recently been shown to predict events, mostly symptom development in asymptomatic patients [33, 34].

Exercise haemodynamics

An exercise-induced increase of the mean transaortic gradient of more than 18mmHg was proposed as a predictor of poor outcome [35] and this has been confirmed in a second study using a cut-off for the increase in mean gradient of 20 mmHg [36] (see ➲ Fig. 10.11).

Dobutamine echocardiography in low flow–low gradient aortic AS

The absence of contractile reserve in low flow–low gradient aortic stenosis is a predictor of poor outcome [10] (see ➲ Fig. 10.12). When patients with contractile reserve have true severe AS, they generally benefit from aortic valve surgery. However, although they have a markedly higher operative mortality, even patients without contractile reserve may frequently improve in left ventricular function after surgery. A recent study has confirmed that patients with pseudosevere AS followed conservatively have a markedly better outcome than those with true severe AS or without contractile reserve [37]. Management decisions remain

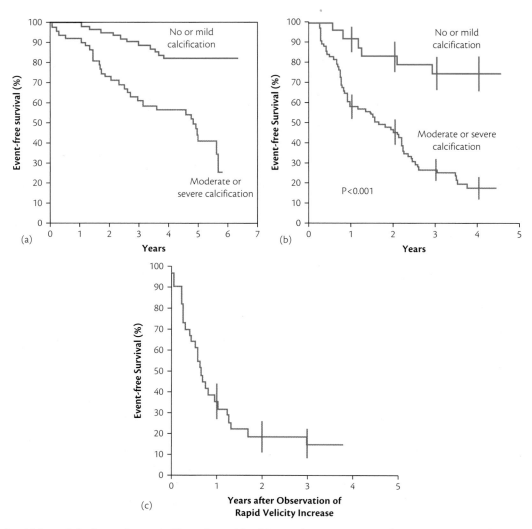

Fig. 10.10 (a) Kaplan−Meier analysis of event-free survival for patients with mild or moderate aortic stenosis having no or mild calcification compared with patients having moderate or severe aortic valve calcification ($P = 0.0001$). Modified from: Raphael Rosenhek et al, European Heart Journal, Mild and moderate aortic stenosis: Natural history and risk stratification by echocardiography, Vol. 25: 199−205, Copyright 2004 by permission of Oxford University Press. (b) Kaplan−Meier analysis of event-free survival for patients with severe aortic stenosis (aortic jet velocity of at least 4 m/s at study entry) having no or mild aortic valve calcification compared with patients having moderate or severe calcification ($P<0.001$). The vertical bars indicate standard errors. (c) Kaplan−Meier analysis of event-free survival patients with moderate or severe calcification of their aortic valve and a rapid increase in aortic jet velocity (at least 0.3 m/s within one year). In this analysis, follow-up started with the visit at which the rapid increase was identified. The vertical bars indicate standard errors. Modified from: Raphael Rosenhek, Thomas Binder, Gerold Porenta, et al, The New England Journal of Medicine, Predictors of Outcome in Severe, Asymptomatic Aortic Stenosis, 343: 611−617, Copyright 2000. Massachusetts Medical Society. Reprinted with permission from Massachusetts Medical Society.

difficult in this patient population and need to be taken on an individual basis.

Imaging in clinical decision-making

Indications for surgery

Echocardiography is the gold standard for diagnosis and quantification of AS as the basis for the decision-making process in this disease. The strongest indication for valve replacement is given by the occurrence of symptoms in the presence of severe AS. In asymptomatic patients, otherwise unexplained left

ventricular systolic dysfunction, as detected by echo, is considered an indication for surgery [3, 4]. Exercise testing has been shown to be helpful for selecting patients who might benefit from surgery while still reporting to be asymptomatic. The incremental value of exercise echo as compared with regular stress testing still requires validation, although an increase in mean gradient >20 mmHg on exercise has been added as a IIb indication in the recent ESC guidelines and surgery may be considered in asymptomatic patients with low operative risk. The echocardiographically provided criterion of moderate to severe aortic valve calcification and a rapid haemodynamic progression (increase of peak aortic jet velocity >0.3 m/s

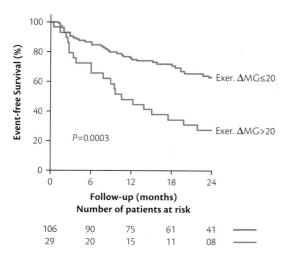

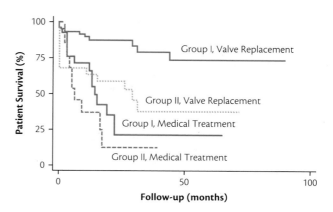

Fig. 10.12 Kaplan–Meier survival estimates of 136 consecutive patients with low-flow low-gradient aortic stenosis. Group I ($n = 92$) represents patients with contractile reserve determined by low-dose dobutamine echocardiography, Group II represents the group of patients with absent contractile reserve ($n = 44$). Survival estimates are represented according to contractile reserve and treatment strategy (aortic valve replacement versus medical therapy). Modified from: Jean-Luc Monin et al, Low-Gradient Aortic Stenosis: Operative Risk stratification and predictors for long-term outcome: A multicenter study using dobutamine stress hemodynamics, *Circulation*, 108: 319–24, copyright 2003 with permission from Wolters Kluwer Health.

Fig. 10.11 Event-free survival curves according to exercise-induced changes in mean transaortic pressure gradient (MPG) in 69 consecutive patients with severe aortic stenosis ($P = 0.0001$). Event-free. Modified from: Sylvestre Maréchaux et al, Usefulness of exercise-stress echocardiography for risk stratification of true asymptomatic patients with aortic valve stenosis, *European Heart Journal*, 31: 1390–97, copyright 2010, by permission of Oxford University Press.

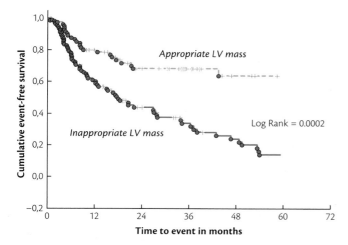

Fig. 10.13 Event-free survival curves in patients with appropriate (dotted line) or inappropriately high (continuous line) left ventricular (LV) mass. Modified from: Giovanni Cioffi et al, Prognostic effect of inappropriately high left ventricular mass in asymptomatic severe aortic stenosis, 97: 301–7, copyright 2011, with permission from BMJ Publishing Group Ltd.

within 12 months) is a class IIa indication for elective surgery in asymptomatic patients as is a peak velocity >5.5 m/s and surgery should be considered because of a high likelihood of symptom development within a short time. Excessive LVH has also been added as a IIb indication in the recent ESC guidelines and surgery may be considered in asymptomatic patients with low operative risk.

Scheduling follow-up intervals

Intervals for follow-up visits of asymptomatic patients with AS can be scheduled based on the severity of AS. Generally patients with a severe stenosis should be seen every 6 months and patients with moderate AS on a yearly basis. In addition, factors such as the previous rate of haemodynamic progression and the degree valve calcification (important calcification is associated with more rapid disease progression) help to optimize the timing of follow-up visits.

References

1. Roberts WC, Ko JM. Frequency by decades of unicuspid, bicuspid, and tricuspid aortic valves in adults having isolated aortic valve replacement for aortic stenosis, with or without associated aortic regurgitation. *Circulation* 2005; 111(7): 920–5.

2. Rosenhek R, Binder T, Porenta G, et al. Predictors of outcome in severe, asymptomatic aortic stenosis. *NEJM* 2000; 343(9): 611–7.

3. American College of Cardiology, American Heart Association Task Force on Practice Guidelines (Writing Committee to revise the 1998 guidelines for the management of patients with valvular heart disease), Society of Cardiovascular Anesthesiologists, Bonow RO, Carabello BA, Chatterjee K, et al. ACC/AHA 2006 guidelines for the management of patients with valvular heart disease: a report of the American College of Cardiology/American Heart Association Task Force on Practice Guidelines (writing Committee to Revise the 1998 guidelines for the management of patients with valvular heart disease) developed in collaboration with the Society of Cardiovascular Anesthesiologists endorsed by the Society for Cardiovascular Angiography and Interventions and the Society of Thoracic Surgeons. *J Am Coll Cardiol* 2006;114, e1–148.

4. Joint Task Force on the Management of Valvular Heart Disease of the European Society of Cardiology (ESC), European Association for Cardio-Thoracic Surgery (EACTS), Vahanian A, Alfieri O, Andreotti F, Antunes MJ, et al. Guidelines on the management of valvular heart disease (version 2012). *Eur Heart J* 2012: 2451–96.

5. Baumgartner H, Hung J, Bermejo J, et al. Echocardiographic assessment of valve stenosis: EAE/ASE recommendations for clinical practice. *J Am Soc Echocardiogr* 2009: 1–23; quiz 101–2.

6. Currie PJ, Seward JB, Reeder GS, et al. Continuous-wave Doppler echocardiographic assessment of severity of calcific aortic stenosis: a simultaneous Doppler-catheter correlative study in 100 adult patients. *Circulation* 1985; 71(6): 1162–9.

7. Baumgartner H, Stefenelli T, Niederberger J, Schima H, Maurer G. 'Overestimation' of catheter gradients by Doppler ultrasound in patients with aortic stenosis: a predictable manifestation of pressure recovery. *J Am Coll Cardiol* 1999; 33(6): 1655–61.

8. Otto CM, Pearlman AS, Comess KA, Reamer RP, Janko CL, Huntsman LL. Determination of the stenotic aortic valve area in adults using Doppler echocardiography. *JAC* 1986; 7(3): 509–17.

9. Oh JK, Taliercio CP, Holmes DR, et al. Prediction of the severity of aortic stenosis by Doppler aortic valve area determination: prospective Doppler-catheterization correlation in 100 patients. *JAC* 1988; 11(6): 1227–34.

10. Monin J-L, Quéré J-P, Monchi M, et al. Low-gradient aortic stenosis: operative risk stratification and predictors for long-term outcome: a multicenter study using dobutamine stress hemodynamics. *Circulation* 2003; 108(3): 319–24.

11. Hachicha Z, Dumesnil JG, Bogaty P, Pibarot P. Paradoxical low-flow, low-gradient severe aortic stenosis despite preserved ejection fraction is associated with higher afterload and reduced survival. *Circulation* 2007 115(22): 2856–64.

12. Pibarot P, Dumesnil JG. Low-flow, low-gradient aortic stenosis with normal and depressed left ventricular ejection fraction. *J Am Coll Cardiol* 2012; 60(19): 1845–53.

13. Baumgartner H, Kratzer H, Helmreich G, Kuehn P. Determination of aortic valve area by Doppler echocardiography using the continuity equation: a critical evaluation. *Cardiology* 1990; 77(2): 101–11.

14. Gaspar T, Adawi S, Sachner R, et al. Three-dimensional imaging of the left ventricular outflow tract: impact on aortic valve area estimation by the continuity equation. *J Am Soc Echocardiogr* 2012; 25(7): 749–57.

15. Carabello BA. Clinical practice. Aortic stenosis. *N Engl J Med* 2002; 346(9): 677–82.

16. Minners J, Allgeier M, Gohlke-Baerwolf C, Kienzle R-P, Neumann F-J, Jander N. Inconsistent grading of aortic valve stenosis by current guidelines: haemodynamic studies in patients with apparently normal left ventricular function. *Heart* 2010; 96(18): 1463–8.

17. Minners J, Allgeier M, Gohlke-Baerwolf C, Kienzle R-P, Neumann F-J, Jander N. Inconsistencies of echocardiographic criteria for the grading of aortic valve stenosis. *Eur Heart J* 2008; 29(8): 1043–8.

18. Cueff C, Serfaty J-M., Cimadevilla C, et al. Measurement of aortic valve calcification using multislice computed tomography: correlation with haemodynamic severity of aortic stenosis and clinical implication for patients with low ejection fraction. *Heart* 2011; 97(9): 721–6.

19. Authors Task Force Members, Vahanian A, Alfieri O, Andreotti F, et al. Guidelines on the management of valvular heart disease (version 2012): The Joint Task Force on the Management of Valvular Heart Disease of the European Society of Cardiology (ESC) and the European Association for Cardio-Thoracic Surgery (EACTS). *Eur Heart J* 2012, 33, 2451–96.

20. Schlosser T, Malyar N, Jochims M, et al. Quantification of aortic valve stenosis in MRI-comparison of steady-state free precession and fast low-angle shot sequences. *Eur Radiol* 2007; 17(5): 1284–90.

21. Bull S, White SK, Piechnik SK, et al. Human non-contrast T1 values and correlation with histology in diffuse fibrosis. *Heart* 2013, 99, 932–7.

22. Lembcke A, Thiele H, Lachnitt A, et al. Precision of forty slice spiral computed tomography for quantifying aortic valve stenosis: comparison with echocardiography and validation against cardiac catheterization. *Invest Radiol* 2008; 43(10): 719–28.

23. Pouleur A-C, le Polain de Waroux J-B, Pasquet A, Vanoverschelde J-LJ, Gerber BL. Aortic valve area assessment: multidetector CT compared with cine MR imaging and transthoracic and transesophageal echocardiography. *Radiology* 2007; 244(3): 745–54.

24. Pouleur A-C, le Polain de Waroux J-B, Kefer J, Pasquet A, et al. Usefulness of 40-slice multidetector row computed tomography to detect coronary disease in patients prior to cardiac valve surgery. *Eur Radiol* 2007; 17(12): 3199–207.

25. Rosenhek R, Zilberszac R, Schemper M, et al. Natural history of very severe aortic stenosis. *Circulation* 2010; 121(1): 151–6.

26. Rosenhek R, Klaar U, Schemper M, et al. Mild and moderate aortic stenosis. Natural history and risk stratification by echocardiography. *Eur Heart J* 2004; 25(3): 199–205.

27. Henkel DM, Malouf JF, Connolly HM, et al. Asymptomatic left ventricular systolic dysfunction in patients with severe aortic stenosis: characteristics and outcomes. *J Am Coll Cardiol* 2012; 60(22): 2325–9.

28. Kearney LG, Lu K, Ord M, et al. Global longitudinal strain is a strong independent predictor of all-cause mortality in patients with aortic stenosis. *Eur Heart J Cardiovasc Imaging* 2012; 13(10): 827–33.

29. Dahl JS, Videbæk L, Poulsen MK, Rudbæk TR, Pellikka PA, Møller JE. Global strain in severe aortic valve stenosis: relation to clinical outcome after aortic valve replacement. *Circ Cardiovasc Imaging* 2012; 5(5): 613–20.

30. Cioffi G, Faggiano P, Vizzardi E, et al. Prognostic effect of inappropriately high left ventricular mass in asymptomatic severe aortic stenosis. *Heart* 2011; 97(4): 301–7.

31. Weidemann F, Herrmann S, Störk S, et al. Impact of myocardial fibrosis in patients with symptomatic severe aortic stenosis. *Circulation* 2009; 120(7): 577–84.

32. Bull S, Suttie JJ, Willis H et al. Circumferential strain predicts major adverse cardiac events independent of myocardial perfusion in asymptomatic aortic stenosis. *J Cardiovasc Magn Reson*; 2012 Feb (14), 90.

33. Mutlak D, Aronson D, Carasso S, Lessick J, Reisner SA, Agmon Y. Frequency, determinants and outcome of pulmonary hypertension in patients with aortic valve stenosis. *Am J Med. Sci* 2012; 343(5): 397–401.

34. Lancellotti P, Magne J, Donal E, et al. Determinants and prognostic significance of exercise pulmonary hypertension in asymptomatic severe aortic stenosis. *Circulation* 2012; 126(7): 851–9.

35. Lancellotti P, Lebois F, Simon M, Tombeux C, Chauvel C, Piérard LA. Prognostic importance of quantitative exercise Doppler echocardiography in asymptomatic valvular aortic stenosis. *Circulation* 2005; 112(9 Suppl): I377–82.

36. Maréchaux S, Hachicha Z, Bellouin A et al. Usefulness of exercise-stress echocardiography for risk stratification of true asymptomatic patients with aortic valve stenosis. *Eur Heart J* 2010; 31(11): 1390–7.

37. Fougères E, Tribouilloy C, Monchi M, et al. Outcomes of pseudo-severe aortic stenosis under conservative treatment. *Eur Heart J* 2012; 33(19): 2426–33.

38. Otto CM, Burwash IG, Legget ME, et al. Prospective study of asymptomatic valvular aortic stenosis. Clinical, echocardiographic, and exercise predictors of outcome. *Circulation* 1997; 95(9): 2262–70.

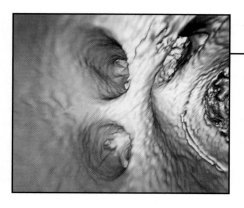

CHAPTER 11

Aortic regurgitation

Raphael Rosenhek

Introduction

The presentation of aortic regurgitation encompasses the spectrum from asymptomatic patients in different disease stages to symptomatic patients who may present with preserved or already depressed ventricular function. While echocardiography is the method of choice permitting a comprehensive non-invasive diagnostic workup of these patients, more advanced imaging techniques are helpful to ascertain the diagnosis and assess the ascending aorta.

Imaging of the aortic valve

The most detailed morphological assessment of the aortic valve is performed in a parasternal short-axis view. Additional information on aortic valve morphology and mobility can be obtained from the parasternal long-axis, the 3- and 5-chamber views. CT and CMR may allow a detailed assessment of valve morphology.

Aortic regurgitation may be the result of a valvular lesion or may be of functional origin in pathologies involving the aortic root. In the assessment of patients with aortic regurgitation, the fact that aortic valve surgery may be indicated, either due to reasons related directly to the valve or to reasons related to aortic root pathology, should be considered [1].

Assessing the ascending aorta

The ascending aorta should be routinely assessed in patients with aortic regurgitation, since a dilation of the ascending aorta is frequently present. In particular, patients with bicuspid aortic valves tend to have associated aortic aneurysms. The assessment is performed in a parasternal long-axis view and includes measurements at the levels of the aortic annulus, the sinuses of valsalva, the sinotubular junction, and the ascending aorta. While the aortic annulus is measured as an inner diameter, the other measures of the ascending aorta are measured from leading edge to leading edge. The aortic arch can be visualized from a suprasternal view. Transoesophageal echocardiography (TOE) is of additional diagnostic value in selected cases. A limitation of echocardiography is that it is not possible to visualize the entire ascending aorta.

When an ascending aneurysm is detected by echocardiography, or when the echocardiographic visualization is insufficient, the systematic use of additional imaging methods such as CMR or CT are indicated.

Aortic regurgitation aetiology

Valvular aortic regurgitation

The most frequent aetiology of aortic regurgitation is bicuspid aortic valve disease. Other aetiologies include rheumatic aortic regurgitation, endocarditis, and also degenerative forms. Patients with Marfan syndrome have a high likelihood of developing aortic regurgitation.

Congenital aortic regurgitation

Congenital aortic regurgitation is typically encountered in patients with a bicuspid aortic valve, although unicuspid, tricuspid, and quadricuspid forms are encountered [2]. The most common type of bicuspidity is a fusion between the right and left coronary cusps (~80%), followed in incidence by a fusion of the right and the non-coronary cusps (~19%), while a fusion between the left and the non-coronary cusps is rare (~1%) [3]. A raphe, which corresponds to an area of thickening at the site of the fused leaflets, may be present. The distinction between a tricuspid and a bicuspid aortic valve with a raphe is not always unequivocal. Suggestive signs of a bicuspid aortic valve are a sigmoid shape of the aortic valve in the parasternal long-axis view or an eccentric closure line in the M-mode.

Rheumatic aortic regurgitation

Rheumatic aortic regurgitation is nowadays rarely encountered in developed countries but still a major health issue on a global scale. The valve is characterized by thickening at the leaflet borders and commissural fusion. Frequently, concomitant aortic stenosis and affection of the mitral valve are present.

Degenerative aortic regurgitation

Degenerative aortic regurgitation is increasingly observed in adult patients. The valve is characterized by thickening and calcification of the leaflets and is frequently associated with some degree of stenosis. Also bicuspid aortic valves tend to calcify and the distinction between a bi- and tricuspid valve may be difficult when extensive calcification is present.

Aortic root pathology with functional aortic regurgitation

A direct anatomical relationship exists between the aortic valve and the aortic root. Pathologies of the latter in the form of an aneurysm or of an aortic dissection may cause secondary or functional aortic regurgitation. The following forms of functional aortic regurgitation can be differentiated:

Sinotubular junction dilation

This results from a dilation of the sinotubular junction relative to the annulus and involves leaflet tethering. Aortic root dilatation may be of congenital origin (such as in patients with bicuspid aortic valve disease, Marfan syndrome, or other connective tissue disorders), as well as related to inflammatory or infectious aortitis. Degenerative causes of aortic root dilatation that are associated with atherosclerosis and hypertension are increasingly observed.

Aortic leaflet prolapse

An aortic dissection extending into the aortic root may cause a disruption of the normal leaflet attachment and thereby cause an aortic leaflet prolapse resulting in aortic regurgitation.

Dissection flap prolapse

In the presence of an aortic dissection, a dissection flap may prolapse through intrinsically normal leaflets thereby leading to aortic regurgitation despite an anatomically normal aortic valve.

Functional classification of aortic regurgitation

A systematic description of the mechanism of aortic regurgitation is important, particularly when aortic repair procedures are considered. In analogy to the Carpentier classification proposed for mitral regurgitation, a functional classification has been proposed for aortic regurgitation [4]:

Type 1:   Enlargement of the aortic root with normal cusps

Type 2:   Cusp prolapse or fenestration

Type 3:   Poor cusp tissue quality or quantity

The extent of aortic valve calcification can be quantified as in patients with aortic stenosis.

Left ventricular response to aortic regurgitation

In aortic regurgitation, the left ventricle is subject to volume overload that is a direct result of regurgitant flow. In addition, the ejection of a larger stroke volume into the aorta results in left ventricle pressure overload. In chronic aortic regurgitation, the left ventricle dilates and develops eccentric hypertrophy, as an adaptive response. This compensatory mechanism permits the maintenance of a normal wall stress and systolic function. In acute regurgitation, compensatory mechanisms are absent.

The assessment of left ventricular function and size is an integrative component of the echocardiographic exam. Ejection fraction using the biplane Simpson method should be routinely determined in patients with severe aortic regurgitation. It is recognized that ejection fraction is an imperfect measure of left ventricular systolic function, in particular in regurgitant lesions. Nevertheless it has been shown to be of important prognostic value and is thus an integral part of the echocardiographic assessment of patients with aortic regurgitation. Strain and strain rate may also be assessed, although they do not have a validated clinical prognostic value in this indication.

Left ventricular diameters should be measured in 2D- and M-mode echocardiography and values of diameters indexed to body surface area should be reported. In the M-mode measurement, both the end-systolic and the end-diastolic diameters should be recorded, because of direct implications on management decisions.

Quantification of aortic regurgitation severity

Quantification of aortic regurgitation severity should be based on an integrative approach of qualitative and quantitative parameters using colour-flow, pulsed-wave, and continuous-wave Doppler imaging [5, 6] (⊃ Table 11.1).

Table 11.1 Quantification of aortic regurgitation severity

	Mild	Moderate	Severe
Qualitative Structural and Doppler Parameters			
Valve morphology (2D/3D)	Normal or abnormal	Normal or abnormal	Abnormal/flail or coaptation defect
Jet width (Colour flow)	Small	Intermediate	Large (central jets) Variable (eccentric jets)
Jet density (CW)	Faint	Dense	Dense
Diastolic flow reversal in descending aorta (PW)	Early diastolic	Intermediate	Holodiastolic
Indirect Quantitative Parameters			
Pressure half-time, ms (CW)	>500	200 to 500	<200
Vena contracta width, mm (Colour flow)	<3	3 to 6	>6
Quantitative Parameters			
EROA, cm²	<10	10 to 30	≥30
Regurgitant volume, ml	<30	30 to 60	≥60
Regurgitant fraction, %	<30	30 to 50	≥50

CW = continuous wave Doppler, PW = pulsed wave Doppler, EROA = effective regurgitant orifice area.
Modified from [5 and 6].

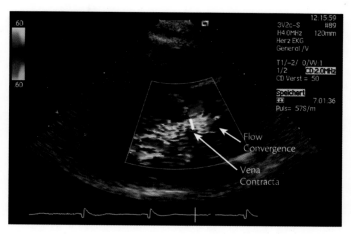

Fig. 11.1 Colour flow imaging in a parasternal long-axis view in a patient with severe aortic regurgitation. The flow convergence zone and the vena contracta width are indicated.

Colour flow Doppler

Jet size

Regurgitant flow can be directly visualized by colour-flow Doppler imaging. Regurgitant jet length and area depend on the pressure difference between the aorta and the left ventricle, as well as on left ventricular compliance, and are only poorly related with aortic regurgitation severity—hence their use for quantification of regurgitation severity is discouraged. The proximal jet width or the cross-sectional jet area is measured just below the aortic valve. It is recommended to calculate the ratio between the proximal jet width and the left ventricular outflow tract, or the ratios between the cross-sectional area and the outflow tract area: ratios of 65% and 60% are suggestive of severe aortic regurgitation. A limitation of this measure is the potential underestimation of eccentric jets and the overestimation of central jets, which expand fully.

Vena contracta

The vena contracta width represents the narrowest regurgitant jet width and is measured at the level of the aortic valve in the parasternal long-axis view (⊃ Fig. 11.1). For an accurate assessment of the vena contracta, the three jet components: flow convergence, vena contracta, and regurgitant jet, should all be visualized. A vena contracta of less than 3 mm is compatible with mild, a vena contracta of 3 to 6 mm is suggestive of moderate, and a vena contracta of more than 6 mm has the highest specificity and sensitivity

for the diagnosis of severe aortic regurgitation. The vena contracta is not reliable in the presence of multiple regurgitant jets.

Flow convergence

The flow convergence zone can be visualized from apical imaging windows, the parasternal long axis, or an upper right-parasternal view (⊃ Fig. 11.1). It is important to zoom on the area of interest and to adjust the Nyquist limit so as to obtain a round and defined PISA radius. After measuring the peak regurgitant velocity and the velocity time integral from a CW-Doppler recording, the effective regurgitant orifice area (EROA) can be calculated. The regurgitant volume (RVol) can be derived by multiplying the RVol by the aortic regurgitant jet time velocity integral (AR_{TVI}):

$$\text{Flow rate} = 2\pi r^2 \times \text{Aliasing Velocity}$$
$$\text{EROA (mm}^2) = \text{Flow rate} / \text{Peak AR velocity}$$
$$\text{RVol (ml)} = \text{EROA} \times AR_{TVI}$$

Severe aortic regurgitation is defined by an EROA ≥0.30 cm² and an RVol ≥60 ml. In aortic regurgitation, the PISA method is only reliably performable in a limited number of patients due to technical and anatomical limitations resulting in suboptimal visualization of the flow convergence zone. Aortic regurgitation severity may be underestimated in the presence of an aortic aneurysm. A planar convergence zone is mandatory since the method is based on the assumption of a hemispheric flow convergence.

Pulsed wave Doppler

Diastolic aortic flow reversal

The flow in the descending aorta is measured from a suprasternal approach using a PW-Doppler probe. A prominent holodiastolic flow reversal is suggestive of severe aortic regurgitation (⊃ Fig. 11.2). An end-diastolic reverse flow velocity ≥18 cm/s is suggestive of severe AR. Measurement of holodiastolic flow reversal in the abdominal aorta is an even more specific indicator of severe aortic regurgitation. A mild flow reversal early in diastole is not a pathological finding.

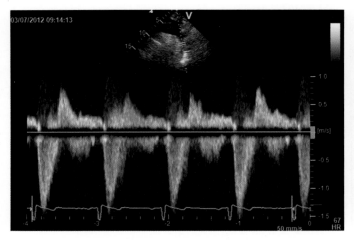

Fig. 11.2 Pulsed wave Doppler imaging in the descending aorta: the holodiastolic flow reversal is indicative of severe aortic regurgitation.

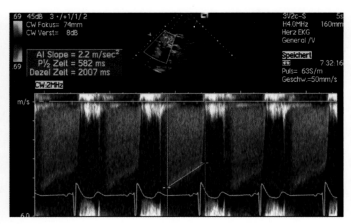

Fig. 11.4 Continuous wave Doppler recording showing the deceleration slope in a patient with mild-to-moderate aortic regurgitation, recorded from an atypical suprasternal view.

Flow reversal may be extended when aortic compliance is reduced in the presence of a stiff aorta. In the case of severe acute AR, there is a fast equalization of the aortic and the left ventricular diastolic pressure, and hence no end-diastolic flow reversal may be observed. A colour M-mode imaging in the descending aorta can also be used to illustrate the duration of retrograde flow (➲ Fig. 11.3).

Calculation of volume flow

Stroke volume can be determined across the aortic valve and across the mitral valve (in the absence of relevant mitral regurgitation) or the pulmonary valve as measures of systemic stroke volume. A regurgitant fraction of more than 50% is compatible with severe aortic regurgitation. Aortic regurgitant volume may also be calculated as the difference of transaortic and transmitral flow.

Continuous wave Doppler

Diastolic jet deceleration: pressure half-time

The pressure half-time is determined by measuring the diastolic flow deceleration across the aortic valve on a CW-Doppler

recording (➲ Fig. 11.4). For an accurate recording, the CW-beam needs to be aligned with the regurgitant jet. With increasing aortic regurgitation severity, the pressure drop in the aorta and the rise of left ventricular diastolic pressure will occur more rapidly. A pressure half-time of less than 200 ms corresponds to severe aortic regurgitation and a pressure half-time of more than 500 ms, to mild regurgitation. However, the pressure half-time is not independent of left ventricular compliance and aortic pressure. An elevated left ventricular filling pressure may lead to a shortening, whereas chronic changes of left ventricular compliance due to aortic regurgitation may lead to a lengthening of the pressure half-time.

Signal density of the CW-Doppler signal

The CW-Doppler signal of aortic regurgitation can be measured from an apical 5-chamber view, although in eccentric jets, the signal may be more reliably recorded from a parasternal window. The density of the CW-Doppler signal is usually weak in the presence of mild aortic regurgitation. At the same time, it does not have a

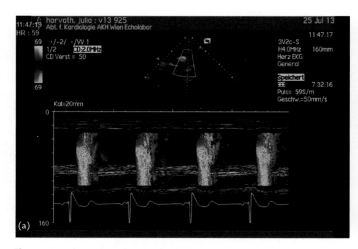

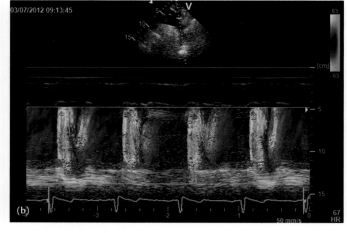

Fig. 11.3 Colour Doppler M-mode imaging of the descending aorta showing early diastolic retrograde flow in a patient with mild-to moderate aortic regurgitation (a) and holodiastolic retrograde flow in a patient with severe aortic regurgitation (b).

significant discriminatory power to distinguish between moderate and severe regurgitation and is thus of limited use in clinical practice.

Quantification of combined regurgitant and stenotic aortic valve disease

Patients with congenital, rheumatic, and increasingly also degenerative aortic disease may present with mixed disease, where aortic regurgitation and stenosis coexist in the same valve. The quantification of disease severity in this condition poses specific challenges because of the interdependency of measures of disease severity. The coexistence of aortic stenosis may lead to left ventricular hypertrophy and to an impaired relaxation, which has been shown to result in longer pressure half-time measures for a given aortic regurgitation severity [7]. On the other hand, aortic regurgitation leads to an increased transaortic flow rate, which is reflected in higher transvalvular gradients. While the vena contracta is a measure that is not significantly affected by aortic stenosis, aortic valve area, calculated by the continuity equation, is a flow-independent measure and thus a marker of aortic stenosis severity. An integrative approach using multiple parameters, ideally allows the quantification of the severity of the regurgitant and of the stenotic components. Aortic jet velocity, which reflects both stenotic and regurgitant severity, has been identified as an important predictor of the need for aortic surgery in previously asymptomatic patients [8].

The role of 3D-echocardiography

3D-TTE and, in particular, 3D-TEE permit a detailed assessment of the aortic valve morphology but also of the sub-and supra-aortic structures. Using 3D colour Doppler echocardiography, the vena contracta can be directly visualized in mid-diastole in an ideal cross-sectional view right under the aortic plane [9]. The 3D EROA can thus be determined by direct planimetry. The regurgitant volume is derived by multiplying the 3D-EROA by the velocity time integral of the aortic regurgitant jet. The quantification of aortic regurgitation by 3D echocardiography has been shown to be accurate and to compare well with velocity encoded magnetic resonance [10]. An advantage of quantitation by 3D-TTE as compared to 2D-TTE can be observed in particular in the presence of eccentric jets [10].

Quantification of AR severity by cardiac magnetic resonance

CMR permits assessment of aortic valve morphology, the aorta, left ventricular size and function, as well as the quantification of aortic regurgitation severity [11]. Although an appropriate quantification can be achieved in most cases by echocardiography, CMR is very useful when echocardiography is not unequivocal. In selected cases, and particularly when values close to thresholds indicating surgery are mentioned, it may also be useful to assess left ventricular function and size by a second method.

Quantification of AR is performed with flow mapping using through-plane phase-contrast velocity mapping. The imaging slice is placed just above the aortic valve in a long-axis left ventricular outflow tract view perpendicularly to the flow direction, which allows the measurement of forward and regurgitant flow across the aortic valve and thus also permits the calculation of the regurgitant fraction (RF) using the following formula:

$$RF(\%) = \text{Regurgitant flow (ml) / Forward flow (ml)} \times 100.$$

Quantitative assessment of AR severity by CMR and, in particular, a regurgitant fraction >33% has been shown to be predictive of the development of a surgical indication [12]. AR may also be quantified by subtraction of left and right ventricular stroke volumes using cine-imaging and under the condition of the absence of shunt-lesions or other valve incompetencies [13]. While a direct visual assessment of the regurgitant jet signal void allows a gross estimation of AR severity based on the jet width at the origin, it is not a very precise method and should thus be interpreted with caution.

Imaging of the aorta by computed tomography and cardiac magnetic resonance

Both computed tomography and magnetic resonance imaging allow the visualization of the thoracic aorta in detail. A detailed imaging of the thoracic aorta is indicated when echocardiography provides the suspicion of a dilated aorta or when the echocardiographic imaging quality is not satisfactory. In particular, in patients with bicuspid aortic valves who have a high likelihood of an associated aortopathy, a comprehensive visualization of the ascending aorta is mandatory. Computed tomography, which is frequently used in the pre-operative workup of patients scheduled to undergo aortic valve surgery, may provide additional relevant information on previous bypass grafts and atheromatous aortic plaques. However, in younger patients, and particularly when serial exams are expected to be required, magnetic resonance is favoured since it has the advantage of avoiding radiation. Both techniques may also assess the morphology of the aortic valve.

Risk stratification and clinical implications: timing of surgery in aortic regurgitation

Many of the criteria that define the timing of aortic valve surgery were identified in studies assessing the prognostic value of pre-operative variables on post-operative survival. Long-term outcome after aortic valve surgery is significantly better in patients who are operated in an asymptomatic or mildly symptomatic

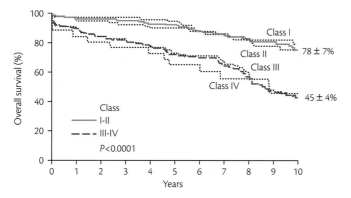

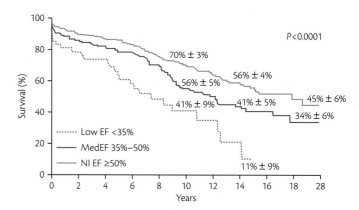

Fig. 11.5 Long-term post-operative survival after aortic valve replacement in patients with severe aortic regurgitation stratified according to pre-operative symptoms. Patients in NYHA functional classes III or IV ($n = 128$) had a significantly worse outcome than patients in classes I or II ($n = 161$).
Myerson SG. Heart valve disease: investigation by cardiovascular magnetic resonance. J Cardiovasc Magn Reson. 2012; 14: 7.

Fig. 11.6 Survival after aortic valve replacement in patients with severe aortic regurgitation stratified according to ejection fraction ($n = 450$). Patients with markedly low ejection fraction had significantly lower survival rates than those with normal ejection fraction and moderately reduced ejection fraction before aortic valve replacement.
Reproduced from SR Underwood et al. Magnetic resonance assessment of aortic and mitral regurgitation. Heart 56: 455-462. Copyright 1986, with permission from BMJ Publishing Group Ltd.

stage (NYHA classes I or II), as compared to severely symptomatic patients (NYHA classes III or IV) (⊅ Fig. 11.5) [14]. A pre-operative end-systolic left ventricular diameter of more than 55mm is associated with a poor long-term outcome [15]. Furthermore, a pre-operative impairment of left ventricular function of less than 50% is associated with a reduced outcome (⊅ Fig. 11.6) [16]. The necessity of surgery indicated by the development of symptoms or left ventricular dysfunction is predicted by the presence of left ventricular dilatation with an end-systolic left ventricular diameter >50mm and an end-diastolic diameter >70mm (⊅ Fig. 11.7) [17]. These criteria are incorporated into current ESC/EACTS practice guidelines [18], which recommend surgery in patients with severe aortic regurgitation who are symptomatic (class I) or present with an impaired left ventricular fraction (≤50%) or with end-systolic and

end-diastolic diameters of more than 50 (or >25 mm/m² indexed to body surface area) and 70mm, respectively (class IIa). A severely regurgitant aortic valve should be operated when surgery of the aorta or other heart surgery is performed (class I)—in this setting replacement of a moderately regurgitant valve may be considered but constitutes only a class IIb indication according to ESC guidelines.

Once the criteria indicating aortic valve surgery, defined in current guidelines, are reached, surgery should no longer be postponed, since more advanced symptoms, left ventricular enlargement, or dysfunction are associated with worse long-term post-operative outcome, as compared to patients being operated 'early' according to the guidelines (⊅ Fig. 11.8) [19].

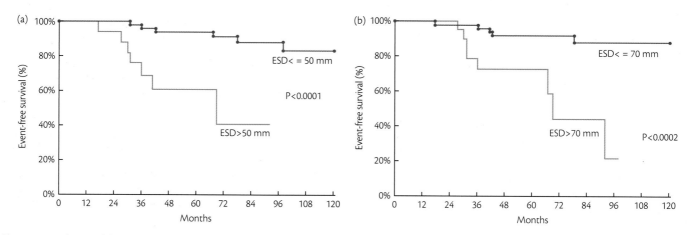

Fig. 11.7 Predictors of the need of aortic valve replacement surgery indicated by left ventricular dysfunction or the development of symptoms in patients with severe aortic regurgitation ($n = 101$). The need of subsequent surgery was predicted by a left ventricular end-systolic diameter >50 mm (a) and an end-diastolic diameter >70 mm (b).
Reprinted from Klodas E, Enriquez-Sarano M, Tajik AJ, Mullany CJ, Bailey KR, Seward JB. Optimizing timing of surgical correction in patients with severe aortic regurgitation: role of symptoms. J Am Coll Cardiol 30: 746-752. Copyright 1997 with permission from Elsevier.

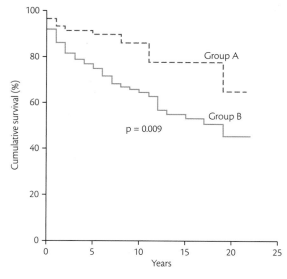

Fig. 11.8 Survival after aortic valve replacement in patients with severe aortic regurgitation operated according to a guidelines-based strategy. Patients operated 'early' according to the guidelines (*n* = 60, NYHA I–II, EF 45–50%, LVESD 50–55mm) had a significantly better survival than those operated 'late' according to the guidelines (*n* = 110, NYHA III–IV, EF <45%, LVESD >55mm).

Reproduced from Hari PC, Mohty D, Avierinos J-F, et al. Outcomes after aortic valve replacement in patients with severe aortic regurgitation and markedly reduced left ventricular function. *Circulation*, 106:21, 2687-2693, Copyright 2002 with permission from Wolters Kluwer Health.

References

1. Roberts WC, Ko JM, Moore TR, Jones WH, III. Causes of pure aortic regurgitation in patients having isolated aortic valve replacement at a single US tertiary hospital (1993 to 2005). *Circulation* 2006; 114: 422–29.

2. Roberts WC, Ko JM. Frequency by decades of unicuspid, bicuspid, and tricuspid aortic valves in adults having isolated aortic valve replacement for aortic stenosis, with or without associated aortic regurgitation. *Circulation* 2005; 111: 920–25.

3. Schaefer BM, Lewin MB, Stout KK, et al. The bicuspid aortic valve: an integrated phenotypic classification of leaflet morphology and aortic root shape. *Heart* 2008; 94: 1634–38.

4. le Polain de Waroux JB, Pouleur AC, Goffinet C, et al. Functional anatomy of aortic regurgitation: accuracy, prediction of surgical repairability, and outcome implications of transesophageal echocardiography. *Circulation* 2007; 116: I264–69.

5. Zoghbi WA, Enriquez-Sarano M, Foster E, et al. Recommendations for evaluation of the severity of native valvular regurgitation with two-dimensional and Doppler echocardiography. *J Am Soc Echocardiogr* 2003; 16: 777–802.

6. Lancellotti P, Tribouilloy C, Hagendorff A, et al. European Association of Echocardiography recommendations for the assessment of valvular regurgitation. Part 1: aortic and pulmonary regurgitation (native valve disease). *Eur J Echocardiogr* 2010; 11: 223–44.

7. de Marchi SF, Windecker S, Aeschbacher BC, Seiler C. Influence of left ventricular relaxation on the pressure half time of aortic regurgitation. *Heart* 1999; 82: 607–13.

8. Zilberszac R, Gabriel H, Schemper M, et al. Outcome of combined stenotic and regurgitant aortic valve disease. *J Am Coll Cardiol* 2013; 61: 1489–95.

9. Perez de Isla L, Zamorano J, Fernandez-Golfin C, et al. 3D colour-Doppler echocardiography and chronic aortic regurgitation: a novel approach for severity assessment. *Int J Cardiology* 2013; 166: 640–45.

10. Ewe SH, Delgado V, van der Geest R, et al. Accuracy of three-dimensional versus two-dimensional echocardiography for quantification of aortic regurgitation and validation by three-dimensional three-directional velocity-encoded magnetic resonance imaging. *Am J Cardiology* 2013; 112: 560–66.

11. Myerson SG. Heart valve disease: investigation by cardiovascular magnetic resonance. *J Cardiovasc Magn Reson* 2012; 14: 7.

12. Myerson SG, d'Arcy J, Mohiaddin R, et al. Aortic regurgitation quantification using cardiovascular magnetic resonance: association with clinical outcome. *Circulation* 2012; 126: 1452–60.

13. Underwood SR, Klipstein RH, Firmin DN, et al. Magnetic resonance assessment of aortic and mitral regurgitation. *British Heart Journal* 1986; 56: 455–62.

14. Klodas E, Enriquez-Sarano M, Tajik AJ, Mullany CJ, Bailey KR, Seward JB. Optimizing timing of surgical correction in patients with severe aortic regurgitation: role of symptoms. *J Am Coll Cardiol* 1997; 30: 746–52.

15. Bonow RO, Rosing DR, Kent KM, Epstein SE. Timing of operation for chronic aortic regurgitation. *Am J Cardiol* 1982; 50: 325–36.

16. Chaliki HP, Mohty D, Avierinos JF, et al. Outcomes after aortic valve replacement in patients with severe aortic regurgitation and markedly reduced left ventricular function. *Circulation* 2002; 106: 2687–93.

17. Tornos MP, Olona M, Permanyer-Miralda G, et al. Clinical outcome of severe asymptomatic chronic aortic regurgitation: a long-term prospective follow-up study. *Am Heart J* 1995; 130: 333–39.

18. Vahanian A, Alfieri O, Andreotti F, et al. Guidelines on the management of valvular heart disease (version 2012): The Joint Task Force on the Management of Valvular Heart Disease of the European Society of Cardiology (ESC) and the European Association for Cardio-Thoracic Surgery (EACTS). *Eur Heart J* 2012.

19. Tornos P, Sambola A, Permanyer-Miralda G, Evangelista A, Gomez Z, Soler-Soler J. Long-term outcome of surgically treated aortic regurgitation: influence of guideline adherence toward early surgery. *J Am Coll Cardiol* 2006; 47: 1012–17.

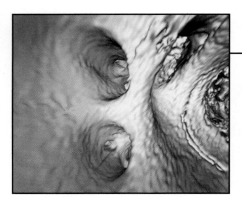

CHAPTER 12

Valvular heart disease: mitral valve stenosis

Eric Brochet and Alexandra Gonçalves

Introduction

Rheumatic fever is still the predominant aetiology of mitral stenosis (MS) [1] particularly in underdeveloped countries. Less often it can be degenerative, congenital, or the result of inflammatory or drug-induced valve diseases [2].

Echocardiography, using M- mode, 2-dimensional echocardiography (2DE) and 3DE is the main method to diagnose and assess severity and consequences of MS [3]. In degenerative MS, the main lesion is calcification of the annulus and base of the leaflets, which usually has few haemodynamic consequences. Conversely, in rheumatic MS, the main mechanism is commissural fusion. Additionally, leaflet thickening and superimposed calcification, chordal shortening, and fusion contribute to the restriction of leaflet motion. Classically, the posterior leaflet is restricted and immobile, and the anterior leaflet has a hockey-stick appearance. The recognition and comprehensive assessment of rheumatic morphology is fundamental for the treatment strategy. 2DE evaluation provides the best assessment of leaflets' mobility and calcification. 3DE, particularly transoesophageal echocardiography (TEE) improves the visualization of the leaflet motion, commissures and submitral apparatus involvement, which is of particular interest in candidates to percutaneous mitral commissurotomy (PMC). Lately, cardiac magnetic resonance imaging (MRI) and multi-slice computed tomography (MSCT) are increasing adjuncts to echocardiography, but the experience in MS is still limited.

Role of echo and MRI in quantifying mitral stenosis. How to do it?

The evaluation of MS severity depends on an integrative approach, combining all echocardiographic and Doppler parameters [2]. Mitral valve area (MVA) is the main parameter, assessed through direct valve planimetry or estimated by pressure time (PT) or eventually by calculation using the continuity equation or proximal isovelocity surface area (PISA) method. Doppler mitral transvalvular gradient is also a reflection of severity of MS but should be interpreted according to loading conditions and heart rate MVA by planimetry performed using 2DE, by direct tracing of the mitral orifice, including opened commissures, in parasternal short-axis mid-diastole view. It has the advantage of being a direct anatomic measurement of MVA independently of flow conditions; consequently it is considered the reference measurement [4]. Nonetheless, it requires left ventricle scanning from the apex to the base to ensure the measurement at the leaflet tips, perpendicular to the mitral orifice. Given the absence of anatomical landmarks to ensure that the short-axis view used to trace the orifice is the smallest one, 2DE planimetry of the mitral valve has the inherent error of misplacement, leading to frequent overestimation of valve area. Using 3DE, any orientation of the cardiac structures can be obtained, independently of the stenotic valve opening angle, assessing the optimal plane of the smallest mitral valve orifice (+ Fig. 12.1). This methodology shows the best agreement with the mitral orifice area

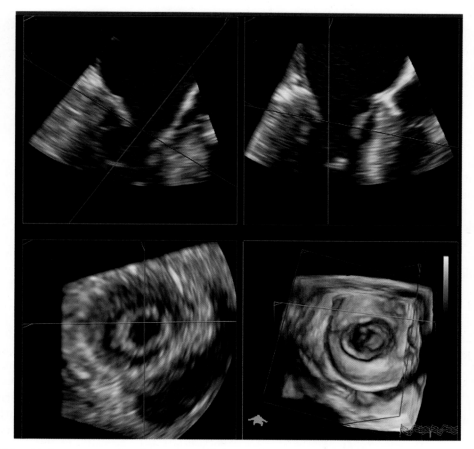

Fig. 12. 1 Real-time 3D TEE multi-plane reconstruction allowing correct alignment of the plane to perform planimetry of the mitral valve orifice.

calculations, derived from the Gorlin formula, and it is currently suggested as the new standard for mitral valve area quantification [5].

Accurate planimetry measurements require optimal gain settings for the visualization of the whole contour of the mitral orifice, as too much gain may cause underestimation of valve area, principally if the leaflet tips are calcified, which is usually encountered in degenerative MS. Moreover, either 2DE or 3DE MVA planimetry require technical expertise.

The determination of the MVA by PHT method, uses the equation:

$$MVA = 220/PHT. \qquad 12.1$$

PHT is defined as the time interval in milliseconds between the maximum mitral gradient in early diastole and the time point where the gradient is half the maximum initial value. It is measured by tracing the deceleration slope of the E-wave on Doppler spectral display of transmitral flow using the same Doppler signal used for the measurement of mitral gradient. The deceleration slope can be bimodal; in these cases it is recommended to measure in mid-diastole, instead of the early deceleration slope. This equation should not be used immediately after balloon valvuloplasty or for patients who have severe aortic regurgitation or high filling pressures by decreased left ventricle compliance, as in these cases MS severity might be underestimated.

MVA can also be estimated using the continuity equation. However, this method is less often used, hampered by the risk of error from the multiple measurements needed. Moreover, this equation cannot be used in cases of atrial fibrillation or if there is marked aortic or mitral valve regurgitation, as aortic regurgitation can cause underestimation of mitral stenosis severity while mitral regurgitation can cause its overestimation.

$$MVA = LVOT D^2 \times 0.785 \times (VTI_{LVOT}/VTI_{MV}), \qquad 12.2$$

where D is the diameter of the LVOT (in cm) and VTI is in cm.

The PISA method uses colour Doppler hemispherical shape of the convergence of diastolic mitral flow on the atrial side of the mitral valve to estimate MVA, according to the following formula:

$$MVA = \pi(r2)(Valiasing)/Peak\ Vmitral \bullet \alpha/1800 \qquad 12.3$$

r, the radius of the convergence hemisphere (in cm), Valiasing, aliasing velocity (in cm/s), peak Vmitral, peak CWD velocity of mitral inflow (in cm/s), and α, the opening angle of mitral leaflets relative to flow direction.

This method is rarely used in daily practice, as it is technically demanding, particularly at the measurement of the radius of the convergence hemisphere. However, if the aliasing velocity is high, PISA can become small enough not to be confined by the mitral leaflets. In this case, angle correction may not be needed at the

equation. Additionally, it can be used in the presence of significant mitral regurgitation [6].

The estimation of the diastolic pressure gradient is derived from the transmitral velocity flow curve, using the simplified Bernoulli equation:

$$P = 4v^2. \qquad\qquad 12.4$$

The Doppler gradient is assessed by the apical window using colour Doppler to identify the best orientation of diastolic mitral jets, followed by continuous wave Doppler (CWD), to ensure maximal velocities and parallel alignment of the ultrasound beam on the mitral inflow. Mean gradient is dependent on MVA, but also on heart rate, cardiac output, and associated mitral regurgitation. It is important to notice that patients with low cardiac output or bradycardia may have a low mean gradient, even in the presence of severe MS and vice versa. However, diastolic pressure gradient is useful to check reliability in the assessment of severity, particularly in patients in sinus rhythm. In patients with atrial fibrillation, the mean gradient should be calculated as the average of five cycles with the least R–R variation. Maximal gradient is not used as it derives from peak mitral velocity, which is influenced by left atrial (LA) compliance and left ventricle (LV) diastolic function.

In summary, MVA should be measured using planimetry as the method of choice, complemented with PHT and transvalvular mean gradient. Finally, echocardiography comprehensive evaluation of concomitant valve disease and pulmonary artery pressures disease is mandatory.

Cardiac magnetic resonance imaging (MRI) may be helpful for patients with MS, if echocardiography data are insufficient or are inconsistent, particularly in cases of complex congenital heart disease. Its large spatial resolution with no acoustic window constrains provides accurate evaluation of MS aetiology, LA size, and the eventual presence of thrombus, right ventricle size, left and right ventricle systolic function, and the coexisting mitral regurgitation or aortic valve disease. The thickening of the subvalvular apparatus and leaflet calcification is frequently suboptimal when compared to echocardiography, but using MRI steady-state free-precession (SSFP) cine pulse sequence, valvular apparatus anatomy, and motion can be assessed throughout the entire cardiac cycle. The pulse sequence has excellent blood-to-myocardium contrast and a high intrinsic signal-to-noise ratio. It produces 2D ECG-gated imaging with a usual temporal resolution of 25 to 50 ms, obtained in a single breath-hold (6 to 12 s) [7].

Similarly to echocardiography, direct planimetry of the MS orifice area can be performed by placing an imaging plane at the mitral valve tips during diastole. This method has good agreement with echocardiography but care must be taken to put the plane positioned at the real tips of the mitral valve in order to obtain an accurate valve area (⊃ Fig. 12.2; 🎞 Video 12.1). CMR was found to have a sensitivity of 89% and a specificity of 75% for diagnosing mitral stenosis in adults, when a cut-off of 1.65 cm² or less was used for MVA [8, 9].

SSFP and gradient echo cine pulse sequences can visualize flow turbulence, locate the jets, and optimize the place for velocity sampling. SSFP provides improved visualization of valve anatomy, but it is less sensitive for showing flow disturbances.

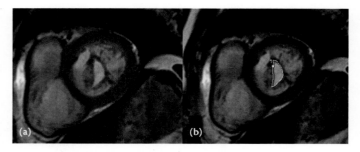

Fig. 12. 2 Cardiac magnetic resonance imaging view of mitral orifice (a) and measurement by direct planimetry of the MS orifice area (b). Courtesy of Dr P Ou, Bichat Hospital.

Phase-contrast pulse sequences (velocity-encoded cine, Q flow, or velocity mapping) are used for velocity measurements. Approximately 1.5 cm above the mitral leaflets, ECG-triggered series are obtained in the short-axis orientation. Similar to echocardiography, peak mitral early diastolic velocity (E) and late diastolic velocity (A) waves are determined from the flow velocity curve and using the formula (MVA = 220/PHT) and MVA is calculated [1]. Peak and mean transvalvular gradients are obtained from the same series. Velocity mapping produces magnitude image that is used for anatomic orientation of the imaging slice and phase velocity maps. The turbulent flow is depicted with signal loss within the magnitude image and the phase map encodes the velocities within each pixel. Using both images, the region of interest can be traced on each time frame of the dataset and the peak instantaneous velocity (V_{max}) and the peak instantaneous gradient ($4V^2_{max}$) can be obtained. Mean MS pressure gradients are obtained by averaging all of the instantaneous velocities over diastole [7]. However, MRI flow measurement is time-consuming and MRI limited temporal resolution reduces the accuracy of velocity measurements. Lower frame rates may not be able to capture high velocities of short duration, resulting in underestimation of peak velocities. In addition, it is crucial that the imaging slice is oriented perpendicular to the flow of blood, because if the angle of intercept is not 90°, it is prone to inaccurate velocity measurements. Moreover, the presence of dysrhythmia as atrial fibrillation reduces the accuracy of MRI flow measurements [10].

The assessment of the MVA in patients with MS can also be performed by multi-slice computed tomography (MSCT). This

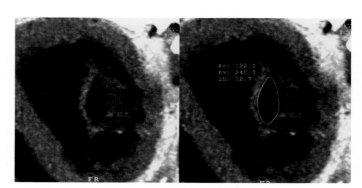

Fig. 12. 3 Assessment of mitral valve area by multi-slice computed tomography.
Courtesy of Dr D Messika-Zeitoun, Bichat Hospital.

technique is widely used for coronary artery assessment, but there a limited experience in the study of patients with MS (➲ Fig. 12.3). However, MSCT allows 3D acquisition of the entire heart throughout the cardiac cycle and using multiple plane reconstructions and it can provide an accurate MVA evaluation [11]. The main constraint can be the presence of atrial fibrillation, which may significantly limit image quality. Even so, MSCT can be considered an alternative technique available for MS severity assessment.

Prognostic information provided by echo

The prediction of long-term outcome and event-free survival following percutaneous mitral commissurotomy (PMC) is based not only on morphological characteristics of the valve, but also on a number of clinical and procedural variables, including age, NYHA functional class, effective balloon dilating area, and the final valve area [12–14]. Morphologic detailed data with significance on procedure success is described in the section Echocardiography during percutaneous mitral commissurotomy (PMC).

Exercise echocardiography is useful in patients whose symptoms are equivocal with the severity of MS. It is recommended in patients with MVA<1.5 cm² who claim to be asymptomatic or with doubtful symptoms. Semi-supine exercise echocardiography allows the monitoring of gradient and pulmonary pressure at each step of increasing workload (➲ Fig. 12.4). However, up to now there are no results showing this data impact on MS mid- or long-term prognosis. Dobutamine stress echocardiography has shown prognostic value but is a less physiological approach than exercise echocardiography [15]. The cutpoint of 18 mmHg mean diastolic gradient in dobutamine stress best detected those patients who would have

a clinical event on follow-up [5]. The measurement of pulmonary pressure during exercise or dobutamine echocardiography can help to distinguish those patients that would benefit from invasive intervention from those who should continue in medical treatment. (This issue is fully discussed in the next section.)

Thus far there are no data available on the prognostic value of MSCT or MRI in MS.

Imaging in the decision-making: echo, MRI, and CT

Echocardiography

In addition to clinical evaluation, echocardiography plays a central role for the choice of the most appropriate intervention. The management of MS has been described comprehensively in the recently updated ESC/EASCTS guidelines and in the AHA/ACC guidelines [16, 17].

The first role of echocardiography is to confirm the severity of MS, as intervention is considered only in patients with significant MS (moderate to severe MS with an MVA<1.5 cm²) [17]. The second role is to assess valve anatomy, which is essential for the selection of candidates for PMC [3, 17, 18].

TTE examination should provide a comprehensive description of the different anatomic features of the mitral valve apparatus. The assessment of commissural fusion is the most important parameter to report, and it is best evaluated in short-axis TTE view [18, 19] (➲ Fig. 12.5a). Real-time 3D TTE, when available, provides a more comprehensive assessment of the completeness and extent of commissural fusion [5, 20] (➲ Fig. 12.5b) Commissural assessment is also critical in patients presenting with restenosis after

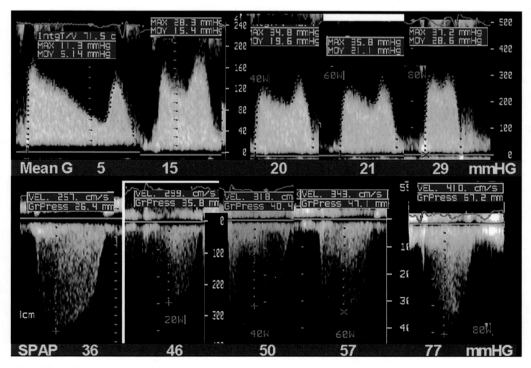

Fig. 12. 4 Exercise echocardiography in a patient with severe asymptomatic mitral stenosis. Showing rapid elevation of mean mitral gradient (mean G) and systolic pulmonary pressure (SPAP) with exercise.

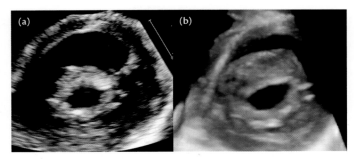

Fig. 12. 5 An example of rheumatismal mitral stenosis with bicommissural fusion viewed in short-axis view using 2D TTE (a) and real-time 3D TTE (b).

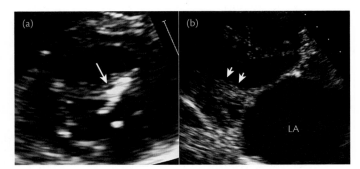

Fig. 12. 6 Calcifications of the anterolateral commissure (arrow) viewed in short-axis view using 2D TTE (a) Severe thickening and fusion of the subvalvular apparatus (arrows) viewed in the parasternal long-axis view using TTE (b).

previous surgical commissurotomy or PMC, allowing restenosis to be differentiated due to commissural fusion from restenosis due to valve rigidity in which there is no commissural fusion [19].

The main anatomic features of MS to be assessed are leaflet thickening, mobility and pliability, presence and location of calcifications, and impairment of the subvalvular apparatus. (⊃ Fig. 12.6a and b).

Different scoring systems have been developed in order to predict immediate and long-term results of PMC. The most widely used is the Wilkins' score (⊃ Table 12.1) [21] in which anatomic components are graded from 1 to 4. Summation of these grades provides a score between 4 and 16, a score of ≤8 being considered favourable for PMC. A simpler score is the Cormier score [22], which relies on a global assessment of mitral valve anatomy (⊃ Table 12.2). Other scores have been described but are more

rarely used. Recently, a new scoring system has been proposed, using real-time 3D TTE in patients with MS candidate for PMC [23]. Nevertheless, all scoring systems have limitations, in particular concerning their predictive value of the final result and risk of procedural complications (PCR) [22]. In clinical practice, it is recommended to use one scoring system that the clinician is familiar with and to provide in the echo report an accurate description of the extent and location of valve abnormalities, in particular with regard to commissural areas [16].

TEE may be useful to assess valve anatomy, but its main indication is to exclude LA thrombus before performing PMC [3], which is a main contraindication for the procedure. LA thrombi are usually, but not exclusively, located in the LA appendage, which must be excluded by the systematic performance of TEE immediately before PMC [19, 24]. Dense LA spontaneous contrast is an important thromboembolic risk-factor but is not a contraindication to PMC.

Additional contra-indications (⊃ Table 12.3) are the presence of more than mild mitral regurgitation, severe or bicommissural valve calcifications, absence of commissural fusion, or restenosis after previous balloon or surgical commissurotomy, which is an indication for valve replacement [16].

MS is frequently associated with other valve diseases (i.e. severe aortic or severe organic tricuspid disease, as well as severe functional tricuspid regurgitation). The presence of severe valvular disease requiring intervention is a contraindication to PMC. Tricuspid valve should be carefully assessed, as moderate functional tricuspid regurgitation is frequent and is not a contraindication for PMC [16].

Decision-making

The presence of symptoms is a class I indication for intervention in patients with severe MS [16]. The choice of the therapeutic technique depends on the suitability for PMC and contraindications or risks inherent to PMC or surgery. PMC is definitely the preferred treatment in patients with favourable valve anatomy, i.e. with a Wilkins' score of ≤8 or a Cormier class 1. In patients with less favourable valve anatomy (Wilkins' score >8 or Cormier class 2 or 3), the decision should be individualized and take into account for the prediction of the short- and long-term results for patient selection [12, 18].

PMC should be considered as an initial treatment for selected patients with mild-to-moderate calcification or unfavourable

Table 12.1 Wilkins' score

Grade	Mobility	Subvalvular thickening	Thickening	Calcification
1	Highly mobile valve with only leaflet tips restricted	Minimal thickening just below the mitral leaflets	Leaflets near normal in thickness (4–5 mm)	A single area of increased echo brightness
2	Leaflet mid and base portions have normal mobility	Thickening of chordal structures extending up to one-third of the chordal length	Mid-leaflets normal, considerable thickening of margins (5–8 mm)	Scattered areas of brightness confined to leaflet margins
3	Valve continues to move forward in diastole mainly from the base	Thickening extending to the distal third of the chords	Thickening extending through the entire leaflet (5–8 mm)	Brightness extending into the mid-portions of the leaflets
4	No or minimal forward movements of the leaflets in diastole	Extensive thickening and shortening of all chordal structures extending down to the papillary muscles	Considerable thickening of all leaflet tissue (>8–10 mm)	Extensive brightness throughout much of the leaflet tissue

Table 12.2 Cormier score

Echocardiographic group	Mitral valve anatomy
Group 1	Pliable non-calcified anterior mitral leaflet and mid subvalvular disease (i.e., thin chordae ≥10 mm long)
Group 2	Pliable non-calcified anterior mitral leaflet and severe subvalvular disease (i.e., thin chordae <10 mm long)
Group 3	Calcification of mitral valve of any extent, as assessed by fluoroscopy, whatever the state of subvalvular apparatus

Adapted with permission from [22].

Table 12.3 Contraindications to PMC

Contraindications for percutaneous mitral commissurotomy
Left atrial thrombus
More than mild mitral regurgitation
Absence of commissural fusion
Severe or bicommissural calcification
Combined severe aortic valve disease and severe tricuspid stenosis and regurgitation
Coronary disease requiring bypass surgery

subvalvular apparatus, who have otherwise favourable clinical characteristics, especially young patients in whom it allows the deference of valve replacement [16]. PMC may be also performed in selected patients with unfavourable anatomy but with high risk for surgery, or as a bridge to surgery in critically ill patients, or to avoid re-intervention in patients with previous surgery (i.e. previous surgical commissurotomy or aortic valve replacement) [25]. Surgery is indicated in patients who are unsuitable for PMC. Considering the small but definite risk inherent to the procedure, PMC is generally not indicated in asymptomatic patients with severe mitral stenosis (including exercise evaluation) [16].

Exercise echocardiography in decision-making

In patients with severe MS with no symptoms at rest, exercise echocardiography identifies patients who develop dyspnoea during exercise or have exaggerated haemodynamic changes early during exercise. Although an elevation of pulmonary artery systolic pressure (sPAP) >60 mmHg is generally retained as pathologic, this sPAP threshold, as stated in guidelines to consider intervention in asymptomatic patients, relies on low levels of evidence [3, 16, 26]. Exercise echocardiography is also useful in the subgroup of patients with only mild MS but who describe limiting symptoms such as dyspnoea. PMC can be proposed in patients with a valve area >1.5 cm² who, during exercise, exhibit a transmitral mean gradient >15 mmHg or sPAP >60 mm Hg (class IIb, level of evidence C, according to the ACC/AHA guidelines) [17]. Dobutamine stress echocardiography is a less physiological approach than exercise echocardiography and is rarely used [27, 28]. It may be useful in patients presenting discrepancy between symptoms and severity of MS who cannot exercise. An absolute increase in the mean transmitral gradient >18 mmHg,

during the test has been shown in one study to be the best cut-off value to predict clinical deterioration or the need to operate [28].

Role of CT

Although not recommended as a first-intention method for MS severity assessment, MSCT may provide accurate and reproducible planimetry of the mitral valve orifice and reliably detects MV calcification in patients with MS [11, 29]. Therefore, CT may be useful in the decision-making process in selected cases, especially in patients with poor echocardiographic windows.

Role of MRI

To date, few investigations have been made on the role of magnetic resonance imaging (MRI) in decision-making in MS. Preliminary data suggest a potential role of MRI in assessing the severity of MS, especially by measuring planimetry of the mitral orifice, although it tends to overestimate MVA when compared with TTE and cardiac catheterization [1, 8]. This can be of interest as an alternative to echo measurements in patients with poor echocardiographic windows.

Echocardiography during percutaneous mitral commissurotomy (PMC)

PMC, using the stepwise single balloon Inoue technique, has become the first-line treatment for symptomatic patients with severe MS and favourable anatomy [16]. Echocardiography plays a key role during PMC to monitor commissural opening and to detect the presence of complications. Different echo techniques can be used. In many centres PMC is performed under local anaesthesia and TTE guidance [30]. Advantages of TTE are wide availability and the fact that it can be performed in conscious patients. According to this strategy, TEE may be restricted to the cases of difficult trans-septal puncture, or during pregnancy to avoid radiation exposure [31]. TEE guidance under general anaesthesia is preferred in some centres [31]. Advantages of TEE use are the potential to enhance safety during trans-septal puncture, good visualization of the balloon position as it is advanced into the mitral orifice, and a rapid assessment of the severity and mechanism of mitral regurgitation [32]. Real-time 3D TEE further improves the quality of guidance, allowing better visualization of the positioning of the balloon relative to the mitral valve orifice (Video 12.2) and facilitating the assessment of commissural splitting immediately after balloon inflation [33, 34]. The main limitation of TEE is that it generally requires general anaesthesia during long procedures.

Intra-cardiac echocardiography (ICE) is another imaging alternative during PMC, avoiding the need for general anaesthesia [35]. ICE has a well-established role for trans-septal puncture guidance and may also help to monitor balloon positioning and inflation. Limitations of ICE are a less optimal visualization of the mitral valve orifice than with TEE, and the high cost of the catheter.

During PMC, echocardiography is performed after each balloon inflation to assess commissural splitting, appearance or increment of mitral regurgitation [14] and presence of complications, such as pericardial effusion or severe mitral regurgitation. Commissural opening is the main parameter, assessed in the parasternal short-axis view during TTE. Echo examination should precise the symmetry and completeness of commissural opening (⊃ Fig. 12.7).

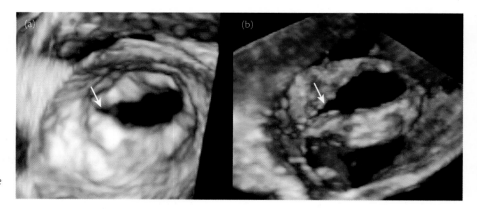

Fig. 12. 7 Monitoring of commissural opening during PMC in short-axis 2D TTE view. Before PMC (a), opening of the postero-medial commissure (arrow) (b) opening of both commissures (arrows) (c).

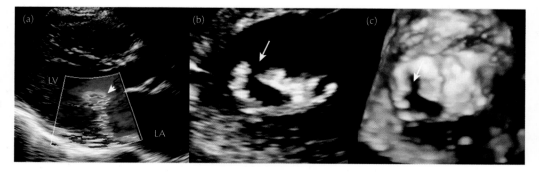

Fig. 12. 8 Real-time 3D TEE *'en face'* view of the mitral valve showing opening of the commissure (arrow) from the left atrial perspective (a) and from the left ventricular perspective (b).

RT 3D TTE using parasternal short-axis views and RT 3D TEE *en face* views of the mitral valve further improve assessment of the extent of commissural splitting from the left atrial or the left ventricular perspective (Fig. 12.8) [33, 34]. Changes in the degree of mitral regurgitation should be assessed carefully with colour Doppler, paying attention to the mechanism and location of the mitral regurgitation jet. If mitral valve opening is insufficient and MR has not increased, inflation should be repeated with the balloon diameter increased by 1–2 mm, according to the symmetry or not of commissural splitting [3]. Planimetry of mitral valve area performed in short-axis view using 2D TTE is the method of choice to assess the result. Opened commissural areas should be included in the planimetry area in order to avoid underestimation of the result. Planimetry can also be performed using 3D TEE using multi-plane reconstruction [36] (Fig. 12.1). Mitral gradient is less reliable to assess the result, by its dependency to changes in the heart rate or cardiac output.

Desired end point of the procedure is (a) mitral valve area >1 cm²/m² of body surface area; (b) complete opening of at least one commissure; or (c) appearance or increase of mitral regurgitation >¼ [36, 37].

Detection of complications

Procedural complications are rare with the Inoue technique [37–39] but echocardiography should be immediately performed when complication is suspected. This stresses the importance of the immediate availability of echocardiography in the catheterization laboratory when performing PMC [37].

Haemopericardium may be related to trans-septal catheterization or, more rarely, to left ventricular perforation by the guide wire or the balloon. Immediate pericardiocentesis is ideally performed under echocardiographic guidance.

Severe mitral regurgitation is relatively rare, with a frequency ranging from 2–19% mostly related to non-commissural leaflet tearing, sometimes associated with chordal or more rarely papillary muscle rupture [38, 39]. Although anatomic factors are important, this complication remains largely unpredictable in any given patient [40, 41]. Immediate TTE and/or TEE should assess the mechanism and severity of mitral regurgitation and short-axis views using 2D/3D TTE or 3D TEE *en face* are the best views for identifying anterior leaflet tear (Fig. 12.9) [32].

Fig. 12. 9 Severe mitral regurgitation (MR) due to anterior leaflet tear during PMC. Note the eccentric posteriorly directed MR jet in long-axis 2D TTE view (a) and the identification of the anterior tear in short-axis 2D TTE view (b) even better assessed with 3D TTE (c).

Echocardiography after the procedure

Comprehensive TTE examination should be performed early after PMC, generally the day after the procedure, to assess the final result. The most accurate evaluation of the result is valve area, measured by planimetry, using 2D or RT 3D TTE [42]. In difficult cases, RT 3D TTE has been shown to increase the ability to perform an accurate MVA planimetry immediately after PMC [20, 42]. In addition to the valve area, the completeness and symmetry of the commissural opening should be systematically reported after PMC [20]. As previously explained, the PHT method is not reliable in this acute setting, due to changes in atrio-ventricular compliance [43].

Final echo report should also address mean mitral gradient, severity of residual mitral regurgitation, with a particular attention to eccentric commissural jets, and level of pulmonary pressure.

If mitral regurgitation is more than moderate, TEE should be needed to precise the exact mechanisms of MR. Left to right inter-atrial shunt is often small and will disappear in the majority of cases at follow-up. Pericardial effusion is rare.

In addition to pre-procedural clinical and anatomical parameters, some of these early post-PMC features have been shown to have an impact on late functional outcome, such as the degree of valve opening, post-procedural MVA, and a small mean mitral gradient. Both the degree of commissural opening and mitral valve area have been shown to be independent predictors of good late functional results [20, 44, 45].

Acknowledgements

Alexandra Gonçalves receives funds from Portuguese Foundation for Science and Technology Grant HMSP-ICS/007/2012.

References

1. Lin SJ, Brown PA, Watkins MP, et al. Quantification of stenotic mitral valve area with magnetic resonance imaging and comparison with Doppler ultrasound. *J Am Coll Cardiol* 2004; 44(1): 133–7. PubMed PMID: 15234421. Epub 2004/07/06. eng.

2. Iung B, Baron G, Butchart EG, et al. A prospective survey of patients with valvular heart disease in Europe: The Euro Heart Survey on Valvular Heart Disease. *Eur Heart J* 2003; 24(13): 1231–43. PubMed PMID: 12831818. Epub 2003/07/02. eng.

3. Baumgartner H, Hung J, Bermejo J, et al. Echocardiographic assessment of valve stenosis: EAE/ASE recommendations for clinical practice. *Eur J Echocardiogr* 2009; 10(1): 1–25. PubMed PMID: 19065003. Epub 2008/12/10. eng.

4. Faletra F, Pezzano A, Jr, Fusco R, et al. Measurement of mitral valve area in mitral stenosis: four echocardiographic methods compared with direct measurement of anatomic orifices. *J Am Coll Cardiol* 1996; 28(5): 1190–7. PubMed PMID: 8890815. Epub 1996/11/01. eng.

5. Zamorano J, Cordeiro P, Sugeng L, et al. Real-time three-dimensional echocardiography for rheumatic mitral valve stenosis evaluation: an accurate and novel approach. *J Am Coll Cardiol* 2004; 43(11): 2091–6. PubMed PMID: 15172418. Epub 2004/06/03. eng.

6. Messika-Zeitoun D, Fung Yiu S, Cormier B, et al. Sequential assessment of mitral valve area during diastole using colour M-mode flow convergence analysis: new insights into mitral stenosis physiology. *Eur Heart J* 2003; 24(13): 1244–53. PubMed PMID: 12831819. Epub 2003/07/02. eng.

7. Cawley PJ, Maki JH, Otto CM. Cardiovascular magnetic resonance imaging for valvular heart disease: technique and validation. *Circulation* 2009; 119(3): 468–78. PubMed PMID: 19171869. Epub 2009/01/28. eng.

8. Djavidani B, Debl K, Buchner S, et al. MRI planimetry for diagnosis and follow-up of valve area in mitral stenosis treated with valvuloplasty. *RöFo* 2006; 178(8): 781–6. PubMed PMID: 16862504. Epub 2006/07/25. eng.

9. Djavidani B, Debl K, Lenhart M, et al. Planimetry of mitral valve stenosis by magnetic resonance imaging. *J Am Coll Cardiol* 2005; 45(12): 2048–53. PubMed PMID: 15963408. Epub 2005/06/21. eng.

10. Christiansen JP, Karamitsos TD, Myerson SG. Assessment of valvular heart disease by cardiovascular magnetic resonance imaging: a review. *Heart Lung Circ* 2011; 20(2): 73–82. PubMed PMID: 20956088. Epub 2010/10/20. eng.

11. Messika-Zeitoun D, Serfaty JM, Laissy JP, et al. Assessment of the mitral valve area in patients with mitral stenosis by multi-slice computed tomography. *J Am Coll Cardiol* 2006; 48(2): 411–3. PubMed PMID: 16843196.

12. Palacios IF, Sanchez PL, Harrell LC, Weyman AE, Block PC. Which patients benefit from percutaneous mitral balloon valvuloplasty? Prevalvuloplasty and postvalvuloplasty variables that predict long-term outcome. *Circulation* 2002; 105(12): 1465–71. PubMed PMID: 11914256. Epub 2002/03/27. eng.

13. Fawzy ME, Shoukri M, Al Buraiki J, et al. Seventeen years' clinical and echocardiographic follow up of mitral balloon valvuloplasty in 520 patients, and predictors of long-term outcome. *J Heart Valve Dis* 2007; 16(5): 454–60. PubMed PMID: 17944115. Epub 2007/10/20. eng.

14. Ben-Farhat M, Betbout F, Gamra H, et al. Predictors of long-term event-free survival and of freedom from restenosis after percutaneous balloon mitral commissurotomy. *Am Heart J* 2001; 142(6): 1072–9. PubMed PMID: 11717614. Epub 2001/11/22. eng.

15. Reis G, Motta MS, Barbosa MM, Esteves WA, Souza SF, Bocchi EA. Dobutamine stress echocardiography for noninvasive assessment and risk stratification of patients with rheumatic mitral stenosis. *J Am Coll Cardiol* 2004; 43(3): 393–401. PubMed PMID: 15013120. Epub 2004/03/12. eng.

16. Vahanian A, Alfieri O, Andreotti F, et al. Guidelines on the management of valvular heart disease (version 2012). *Eur Heart J* 2012; 33(19): 2451–96. PubMed PMID: 22922415. Epub 2012/08/28. eng.

17. Bonow RO, Carabello BA, Chatterjee K, et al. 2008 focused update incorporated into the ACC/AHA 2006 guidelines for the management of patients with valvular heart disease: a report of the American College of Cardiology/American Heart Association Task Force on Practice Guidelines (Writing Committee to revise the 1998 guidelines for the management of patients with valvular heart disease). Endorsed by the Society of Cardiovascular Anesthesiologists, Society for Cardiovascular Angiography and Interventions, and Society of Thoracic Surgeons. *J Am Coll Cardiol* 2008; 52(13): e 1–142. PubMed PMID: 18848134.

18. Prendergast BD, Shaw TR, Iung B, Vahanian A, Northridge DB. Contemporary criteria for the selection of patients for percutaneous balloon mitral valvuloplasty. *Heart* 2002; 87(5): 401–4. PubMed PMID: 11997400. Pubmed Central PMCID: 1767103.

19. Garbarz E, Iung B, Cormier B, Vahanian A. Echocardiographic criteria in selection of patients for percutaneous mitral commissurotomy.

Echocardiography 1999; 16(7, Pt 1): 711–21. PubMed PMID: 11175213.

20. Messika-Zeitoun D, Brochet E, Holmin C, et al. Three-dimensional evaluation of the mitral valve area and commissural opening before and after percutaneous mitral commissurotomy in patients with mitral stenosis. *Eur Heart J* 2007; 28(1): 72–9. PubMed PMID: 16935871.

21. Wilkins GT, Weyman AE, Abascal VM, Block PC, Palacios IF. Percutaneous balloon dilatation of the mitral valve: an analysis of echocardiographic variables related to outcome and the mechanism of dilatation. *Br Heart J* 1988; 60(4): 299–308. PubMed PMID: 3190958. Pubmed Central PMCID: 1216577.

22. Iung B, Cormier B, Ducimetiere P, et al. Immediate results of percutaneous mitral commissurotomy. A predictive model on a series of 1514 patients. *Circulation* 1996; 94(9): 2124–30. PubMed PMID: 8901662.

23. Anwar AM, Attia WM, Nosir YF, et al. Validation of a new score for the assessment of mitral stenosis using real-time three-dimensional echocardiography. *J Am Soc Echocardiogr* 2010; 23(1): 13–22. PubMed PMID: 19926444. Epub 2009/11/21. eng.

24. Vahanian A. Balloon valvuloplasty. *Heart* 2001; 85(2): 223–8. PubMed PMID: 11156680. Pubmed Central PMCID: 1729609.

25. Iung B, Garbarz E, Doutrelant L, et al. Late results of percutaneous mitral commissurotomy for calcific mitral stenosis. *Am J Cardiology* 2000; 85(11): 1308–14. PubMed PMID: 10831945.

26. Brochet E, Detaint D, Fondard O, et al. Early haemodynamic changes versus peak values: what is more useful to predict occurrence of dyspnea during stress echocardiography in patients with asymptomatic mitral stenosis? *J Am Soc Echocardiogr* 2011; 24(4): 392–8. PubMed PMID: 21324641.

27. Hecker SL, Zabalgoitia M, Ashline P, Oneschuk L, O'Rourke RA, Herrera CJ. Comparison of exercise and dobutamine stress echocardiography in assessing mitral stenosis. *Am J Cardiology* 1997; 80(10): 1374–7. PubMed PMID: 9388122.

28. Reis G, Motta MS, Barbosa MM, Esteves WA, Souza SF, Bocchi EA. Dobutamine stress echocardiography for noninvasive assessment and risk stratification of patients with rheumatic mitral stenosis. *J Am Coll Cardiol* 2004; 43(3): 393–401. PubMed PMID: 15013120.

29. Mahnken AH, Muhlenbruch G, Das M, et al. MDCT detection of mitral valve calcification: prevalence and clinical relevance compared with echocardiography. *American J Roentgenology* 2007; 188(5): 1264–9. PubMed PMID: 17449769.

30. Chen CR, Cheng TO. Percutaneous balloon mitral valvuloplasty by the Inoue technique: a multicenter study of 4832 patients in China. *Am Heart J* 1995; 129(6): 1197–203. PubMed PMID: 7754954.

31. Himbert D, Brochet E, Messika-Zeitoun D, Vahanian A. Current status of percutaneous valvular procedures. *Curr Treat Option CV Med* 2006; 8(6): 435–42. PubMed PMID: 20848347.

32. Park SH, Kim MA, Hyon MS. The advantages of On-line transesophageal echocardiography guide during percutaneous balloon mitral valvuloplasty. *J Am Soc Echocardiogr* 2000; 13(1): 26–34. PubMed PMID: 10625828.

33. Eng MH, Salcedo EE, Quaife RA, Carroll JD. Implementation of real time three-dimensional transesophageal echocardiography in percutaneous mitral balloon valvuloplasty and structural heart disease interventions. *Echocardiography* 2009; 26(8): 958–66. PubMed PMID: 19968682.

34. Perk G, Lang RM, Garcia-Fernandez MA, et al. Use of real time three-dimensional transesophageal echocardiography in intracardiac catheter based interventions. *J Am Soc Echocardiogr* 2009; 22(8): 865–82. PubMed PMID: 19647156.

35. Green NE, Hansgen AR, Carroll JD. Initial clinical experience with intracardiac echocardiography in guiding balloon mitral valvuloplasty: technique, safety, utility, and limitations. Catheterization and cardiovascular interventions: *Catheterization and Cardiovascular Interventions;* 2004 Nov; 63(3): 385–94. PubMed PMID: 15505848.

36. Dreyfus J, Brochet E, Lepage L, et al. Real-time 3D transoesophageal measurement of the mitral valve area in patients with mitral stenosis. *Eur J Echocardiogr* 2011; 12(10): 750–5. PubMed PMID: 21824874.

37. Vahanian A, Palacios IF. Percutaneous approaches to valvular disease. *Circulation* 2004; 109(13): 1572–9. PubMed PMID: 15066960.

38. Nobuyoshi M, Arita T, Shirai S, et al. Percutaneous balloon mitral valvuloplasty: a review. *Circulation* 2009; 119(8): e 211–9. PubMed PMID: 19106383.

39. Hernandez R, Macaya C, Banuelos C, et al. Predictors, mechanisms and outcome of severe mitral regurgitation complicating percutaneous mitral valvotomy with the Inoue balloon. *Am J Cardiology* 1992; 70(13): 1169–74. PubMed PMID: 1414941.

40. Nair M, Agarwala R, Kalra GS, Arora R, Khalilullah M. Can mitral regurgitation after balloon dilatation of the mitral valve be predicted? *Br Heart J* 1992; 67(6): 442–4. PubMed PMID: 1622691. Pubmed Central PMCID: 1024883.

41. Iung B, Nicoud-Houel A, Fondard O, et al. Temporal trends in percutaneous mitral commissurotomy over a 15-year period. *Eur Heart J* 2004; 25(8): 701–7. PubMed PMID: 15084376.

42. Zamorano J, Perez de Isla L, Sugeng L, et al. Non-invasive assessment of mitral valve area during percutaneous balloon mitral valvuloplasty: role of real-time 3D echocardiography. *Eur Heart J* 2004; 25(23): 2086–91. PubMed PMID: 15571823.

43. Thomas JD, Wilkins GT, Choong CY, et al. Inaccuracy of mitral pressure half-time immediately after percutaneous mitral valvotomy. Dependence on transmitral gradient and left atrial and ventricular compliance. *Circulation* 1988; 78(4): 980–93. PubMed PMID: 3168200.

44. Ben-Farhat M, Betbout F, Gamra H, et al. Predictors of long-term event-free survival and of freedom from restenosis after percutaneous balloon mitral commissurotomy. *Am Heart J* 2001; 142(6): 1072–9. PubMed PMID: 11717614.

45. Bouleti C, Iung B, Laouenan C, et al. Late results of percutaneous mitral commissurotomy up to 20 years: development and validation of a risk score predicting late functional results from a series of 912 patients. *Circulation* 2012; 125(17): 2119–27. PubMed PMID: 22456478.

⊃ **For additional multimedia materials please visit the online version of the book (⏎ http://www.esciacc.oxfordmedicine.com)**

CHAPTER 13

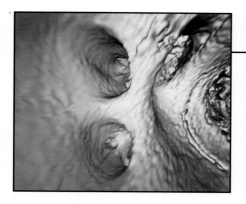

Mitral valve regurgitation

Patrizio Lancellotti and Julien Magne

Contents

Introduction

The prevalence of mitral regurgitation (MR) is increasing in Western countries despite the reduced incidence of rheumatic disease [1]. MR is the second most frequent valvular heart disease requiring surgery [2]. According to the aetiology, MR can be classified as organic (i.e. due to an organic lesion of the mitral valve or subvalvular apparatus) or functional (i.e. due to a disease of the left ventricle). The updated European Society of Cardiology (ESC) guidelines have classified MR as primary (organic) or secondary (functional, ischaemic, or non-ischaemic). Causes of primary MR include, most commonly, degenerative disease (Barlow's, fibroelastic degeneration, Marfan, Ehlers–Danlos, annular calcification), rheumatic disease, toxic valvulopathy, and infective endocarditis. Mitral regurgitation due to ruptured (complete/partial) or scarred/retracted papillary muscle secondary to myocardial infarction has been included among primary ischaemic MR. Causes of secondary MR include ischaemic heart disease and cardiomyopathies. Because these two typologies of MR are easy to identify and fundamentally opposed in their pathophysiology, prognosis, and management, the present chapter will refer to this classification. In the uncommon cases of mixed mechanisms (i.e. concomitant primary and secondary MR), the predominant one will guide management and treatment.

In high volume and experienced centres, the excellent results obtained by mitral valve repair, since its introduction in the early 1970s, have radically changed the prognosis and management of patients presenting with severe MR. The possibility of repairing the mitral valve imposes new responsibilities on the assessment of MR by imaging, which should provide precise information on type and extent of anatomical lesions, mechanisms of regurgitation, aetiology, amount of regurgitation, and reparability of the valve.

Anatomy and function of the mitral valve

The structure of the entire mitral valve apparatus, which include the mitral leaflets, annulus, chordae tendinae attachment, papillary muscles, and the supporting ventricular walls, affect overall mitral valve function. ○ Figure 13.1 illustrates the anatomy and the morphology of the mitral valve using a 3-dimensional transthoracic echocardiographic model.

Valvular leaflets

The normal mitral valve has two leaflets that are attached at their bases to the fibromuscular annulus, and by their free edges to the subvalvular apparatus. The posterior leaflet has a quadrangular shape and is attached to approximately two-thirds of the annular circumference; the anterior leaflet attaches to the remaining one-third. The posterior leaflet typically has two well-defined indentations, which divide the leaflet into three individual scallops identified as P1, P2, and P3. The anterior leaflet has a semicircular shape and is in continuity with the non-coronary cusp of the aortic valve, referred to as the intervalvular

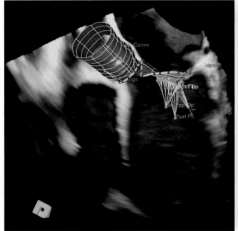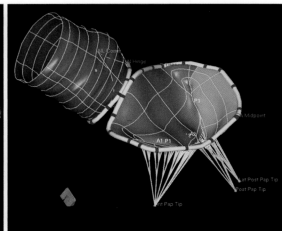

Fig. 13.1 Anatomy and morphology of the mitral valve anatomy using a 3-dimensional transthoracic echocardiographic model.

fibrosa. The free edge of the anterior leaflet is usually continuous, without indentations. It is artificially divided into three portions A1, A2, and A3, mirroring the posterior scallops P1, P2, and P3. The commissures define a distinct area where the anterior and posterior leaflets come together at their insertion into the annulus.

Mitral annulus

Mitral annulus is D- and saddle-shaped. Its anterior portion is flat and rigid. The posterior two-thirds may contribute to annular dilatation. The anterior posterior diameter can be measured using either 3D or conventional 2D echo in the parasternal long-axis view. The diameter is compared to the length of the anterior leaflet in diastole. Annular dilatation is present when the ratio antero-posterior annulus diameter/anterior leaflet length in diastole is >1.3 or when the antero-posterior annulus diameter is >35 mm [3]. The presence and extent of annular calcification is an important parameter to describe.

Chordae tendinae and papillary muscles

The analysis of the subvalvular apparatus includes the measurement of the chordal length, the description of calcification, fusion, elongation, and rupture. The possible displacement of the papillary muscles needs to be quantified. Two measures are usually performed: (1) apical displacement of the posterior papillary muscle (distance between the papillary muscle head and the intervalvular fibrosa, and (2) inter-papillary distance measured in the short-axis view.

Pathophysiology of MR

MR is the systolic retrograde flow, which results from the incomplete mitral valve closure and from the pressure gradient between the left ventricle (LV) and the left auricle (LA). It may occur in the presence of the dysfunction of one or, more often, several of the components of mitral apparatus. The Carpentier's classification has subcategorized the mechanisms of MR according to leaflet motion and it is useful to assess valve function, specifically

when mitral valve repair is contemplated. Three types of MR are described:

Type I: The leaflet motion is normal. MR is determined by leaflet perforation (infective endocarditis) or, more frequently, by annular dilatation.

Type II: Increased and excessive leaflet mobility accompanied by displacement of the free edge of one or both leaflets beyond the mitral annular plane (mitral valve prolapse).

Type III: Reduced mobility of one or both leaflets. The type III is subdivided into type IIIa, implying restricted leaflet motion during both diastole and systole due to shortening of the chordae and/or leaflet thickening, such as in rheumatic disease, and type IIIb when leaflet motion is restricted only during systole.

Mixed mechanisms may be involved in the pathophysiology of MR.

The MR severity may be quantified by the assessment of both regurgitant volume (R Vol) and the effective regurgitant orifice area (EROA). Nevertheless, despite well-correlated, R Vol and EROA are not similar. The former is a parameter of the volume overload burden, whereas the latter represents the extent of the valvular lesion. In addition, R Vol is determined by the EROA, the systolic pressure gradient across the mitral valve and duration of cardiac systole. In the presence of small EROA, MR is often not holosystolic and predominates in early systole. In mitral valve prolapse, the EROA may increase throughout the systole and is generally markedly higher at end-systole. Conversely, in secondary ischaemic MR, there is a frequent reinforcement of the MR severity at early and late systole, with a decrease in EROA in mid-systole, when the closing forces are the highest.

The physiologic and haemodynamic impact of significant MR differ in acute and chronic regurgitation. Acute MR mainly results from chordae rupture, leaflet tear or perforation, and leads to an instantaneous marked decrease in LV afterload, increase in LV emptying, and in LA pressure and, in turn, in pulmonary arterial pressure. The LV ejection fraction remains normal but the LV forward stroke volume is decreased, requiring tachycardia in

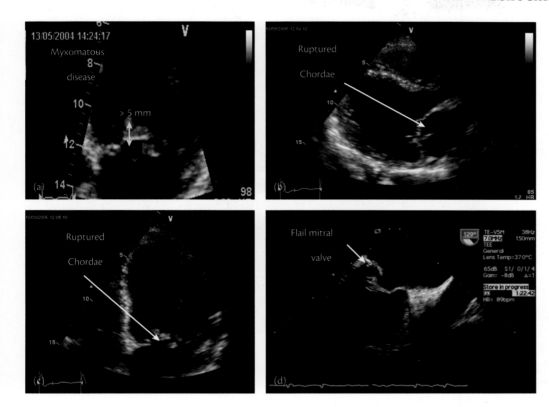

Fig. 13.2 Aetiology and mechanisms of primary mitral regurgitation.

order to maintain normal cardiac output. In its chronic phase, MR generates an LV volume overload leading to increased total LV stroke volume and thus, maintained LV forward stroke volume. The LV volume overload progressively produces LV eccentric hypertrophy and, in parallel, the LA enlarges and becomes more compliant, allowing LA pressure and pulmonary pressures to remain in the normal range. When this compensated phase is overcome, symptoms, LA fibrillation, pulmonary hypertension, and impairment in LV systolic and diastolic function may occur.

By definition, primary MR results from the organic alteration of one or more of the components of mitral valve and mitral subvalvular apparatus (⊃ Fig. 13.2). By contrast, secondary MR is functional and results from the alteration of the geometry and function of LV following remodelling occurring after myocardial infarction or during the clinical course of cardiomyopathies (⊃ Fig. 13.3). Indeed, LV remodelling and myocardial contractility impairment may create a repositioning and displacement of the papillary muscles, which may, in turn, generate a tethering of the mitral valve leaflet and the displacement of the coaptation within the LV by the intercessor of chordae tendinae. This geometrical remodelling of the valve limits its leaflet coaptation and leads to MR. Hence, secondary MR results from an imbalance between closing forces (generated by the LV during systole) and tethering forces. Nevertheless, recent studies tend to show that secondary MR is not solely functional and may be accompanied by a morphological mitral valve tissue increase, as a compensatory process aiming at limiting the mitral valve tethering impact [45].

Echocardiographic evaluation

Transthoracic echocardiography (TTE) is the modality of choice to assess and monitor MR and global cardiac function and remodelling. However, transoesophageal echocardiography (TOE) plays a major role when TTE is non-diagnostic, when further diagnostic refinement is required, or when mitral valve surgery is contemplated. The short-axis view can be obtained by TTE or TOE, using the classical parasternal short-axis view and the transgastric view at 0°. These views permit in diastole the assessment of the six scallops and the two commissures (⊃ Fig. 13.4). In systole, the localization of prolapse may be identified by the localization of the origin of the regurgitant jet. With TTE, a classical apical 4-chamber view is obtained and explores the anterior leaflet: the segments A3 and A2 and the posterior leaflet in its external scallop P1. With TOE, different valvular segments are observed, which depend on the position of the probe in the oesophagus when progresses from up to down. This permits observation of, successively A1 and P1 close to the anterolateral commissure, A2 and P2, and finally A3 and P3 close to the posteromedial commissure (at 40–60°). Parasternal long-axis view with TTE and sagittal view at 120° with TOE show the medium portions of the leaflets (A2 and P2) (⊃ Fig. 13.5a). A bi-commissural view can be obtained in the apical 2-chamber view with TTE (⊃ Fig. 13.5d) and a view at 40° to 60° with TOE showing the two commissural regions and from left to right P3, A2 and P1 (⊃ Fig. 13.4, lower, right panel). A 2-chamber view from the transgastric position, perpendicular to the subvalvular apparatus permits to measure the length

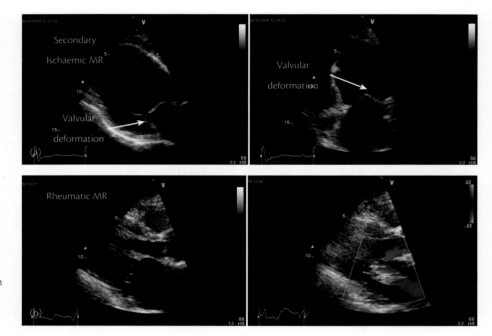

Fig. 13.3 Mitral valve geometry and deformation in a patient with secondary mitral regurgitation (a) and in a patient with rheumatic mitral regurgitation (b).

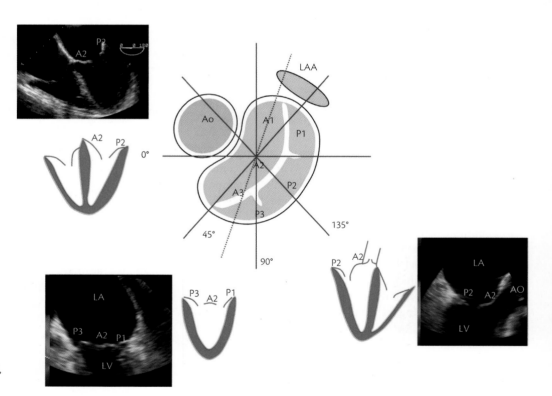

Fig. 13.4 Transoesophageal echocardiographic segmental analysis of the mitral valve. Anterior leaflet (A1, A2, A3), posterior leaflet (P1, P2, P3).

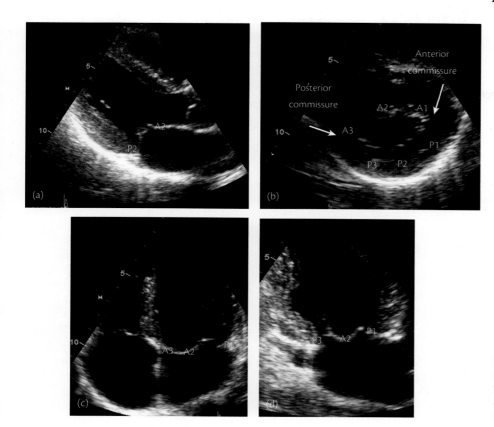

Fig. 13.5 Mitral valvular segmentation: (a) parasternal long-axis view, (b) short-axis view, (c) apical 4-chamber view, and (d) apical 2-chamber view. Anterior leaflet (A1, A2, A3), posterior leaflet (P1, P2, P3).

of the chordae and the distances between the head of the papillary muscle and the mitral annulus.

Three-dimensional (3D) echocardiography

It is reasonable to perform a 3D TTE/TOE in complex mitral valve pathology. 3D echocardiography has demonstrated its superiority over 2D for the accurate localization of valvular abnormalities (⊃ Fig. 13.6). Simultaneous multi-plane imaging permits precise determine of the localization and extent of leaflet lesions. Colour flow Doppler imaging can be superimposed onto these 2D images, which may make easier the identification of commissural jets. With the use of real-time 3D imaging, the mitral valve is best imaged when obtained in zoom mode to avoid stitch artefacts that may occur during gated multi-beat acquisition. With both TEE and TOE, the unique 'en face' view from the atrium, which is similar to the surgical view after left atriotomy, can be displayed. To simulate the surgeon's view of the valve, the 3D images are reoriented to exhibit the aortic valve at the 11-o'clock position (⊃ Fig. 13.6). The subvalvular apparatus is, on the opposite, best imaged from the LV perspective. To note, the gated full-volume modality (wide-angled acquisition of 4 to 7 ECG-gated pyramidal volumes) is the ideal way for imaging the entire mitral valve apparatus (chordae, papillary muscles, LV). Recently, new, dedicated software for advanced 3D analysis of the mitral valve has been developed to be incorporated into clinical practice. It provides a 3D realistic model of the mitral valve and allows the calculation of a wide range of potentially useful parameters (annulus, anterior and posterior leaflet, leaflet segmentation, coaptation line and potential coaptation defects, mitral valve spatial relationship with the papillary muscles and aortic valve). The possibility of measuring the surface of the anterior leaflet to estimate, in a beating heart, the size of the annular ring, ranks among the most interesting features. The added value of these parameters still needs to be defined.

The use of 3D colour flow volumetric imaging allows direct assessment of the size and shape of the regurgitant orifice, preventing the geometric assumptions applied by 2D imaging. With manual cropping of the image plane perpendicularly orientated to the jet direction, the narrowest cross-sectional area of the MR jet can be obtained in an 'en face' view and measured by planimetry in systole. In primary MR, the shape of the regurgitant orifice has been shown to be relatively rounder. Several studies using 3D TOE for planimetry of the anatomical regurgitant orifice (the vena contracta area) have found a high correlation with the 2D vena contracta and the PISA method [23]. A recent study showed its superiority over the PISA method in eccentric jets [24]. Of note, new 3D/4D ultrasound probe generations will allow automatic visualization of 3D PISA surface and anatomic orifice area, with expected higher accuracy of the subsequent regurgitant volume calculation (⊃ Fig. 13.7).

The assessment of LV volumes by 3D echocardiography is discussed in another chapter. In MR, 3D echocardiographic

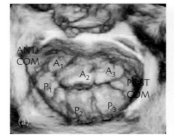 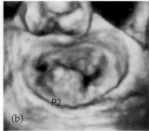 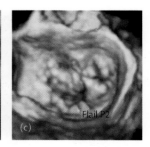

Fig. 13.6 Real-time 3D transoesophageal echocardiography volume rendering of the mitral valve. (a) Surgical 'en-face' view. (b) Mitral valve prolapse of P2. (c) Flail (ruptured chordae) of P3. A1, A2, A3, anterior mitral valve scallops; P1, P2, P3, posterior mitral valve scallops; ANT COM, anterolateral commissure; POST COM, posteromedial commissure.

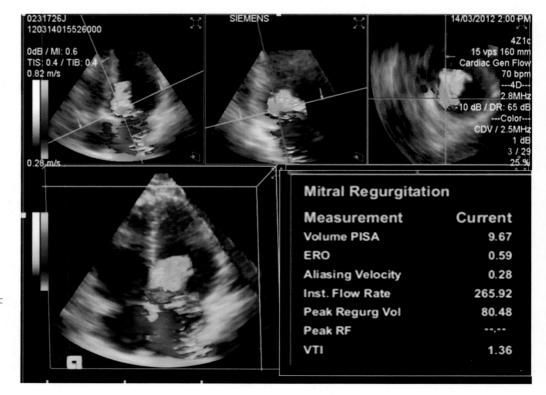

Fig. 13.7 Real-time 3D transthoracic echocardiography for the 3-dimensional assessment of the flow convergence zone of the mitral regurgitation and the calculation of the effective regurgitant orifice area (EROA) using the 3D PISA method.

assessment of LV function provides more accurate and reproducible data than 2D.

Predictors of successful mitral valve repair

Several echocardiographic parameters that characterize the extent or the severity of the disease can help to identify patients at risk of treatment failure (⮞ Table 13.1) [89]. In primary MR, a series of questions should be highlighted: which scallop is affected?; are the commissures involved?; is there any calcification?; what is the extent of calcification?; is there a lack of mitral valve tissue?; is there any abnormality of the subvalvular apparatus? In primary MR, some predictors of recurrent MR after surgery have been reported: the presence of a large central regurgitant jet, severe annular dilatation (>50 mm), involvement of ≥3 scallops, especially if the anterior leaflet is involved, and extensive valve calcification. In secondary

MR, the severity of mitral valve deformation and the extent of LV remodelling largely affect MR persistence or recurrence after repair. A coaptation distance >1 cm, a systolic tenting area >2.5 cm² (alternatively, tenting volume may be measured using 3D echocardiography), a posterior leaflet angle ≥45° (indicating a high posterior leaflet restriction), a central regurgitant jet (indicating a severe restriction of both leaflets in patients with severe functional ischaemic MR), the presence of complex jets originating centrally and posteromedially, and a severe LV enlargement >65 mm (low likelihood of reverse LV remodelling after repair and poor late outcome) increase the risk of mitral valve repair failure.

Assessment of MR severity

There are many echocardiographic approaches to assess the severity of MR. Emphasis should be put on an integrative approach and the evaluation of ventricular performance (⮞ Tables 13.2 and 13.3).

Table 13.1 Probability of successful mitral valve repair in MR based on echo findings

Aetiology	Dysfunction	Calcification	Mitral annulus dilatation	Probability of repair
Degenerative	II: Localized prolapse (P2 and/or A2)	No/Localized	Mild/Moderate	**Feasible**
Secondary	I or IIIb	No	Moderate	**Feasible**
Barlow	II: Extensive prolapse (≥3 scallops, posterior commissure) IIIa but pliable anterior leaflet	Localized (annulus)	Moderate	**Difficult**
Rheumatic	II: Extensive prolapse	Localized	Moderate	**Difficult**
Severe Barlow	(≥3 scallops, anterior commissure)	Extensive (annulus + leaflets)	Severe	**Unlikely**
Endocarditis	II: Prolapse but destructive lesions	No	No/Mild	**Unlikely**
Rheumatic	IIIa but stiff anterior leaflet	Extensive (annulus + leaflets)	Moderate/Severe	**Unlikely**
Secondary	IIIb but severe valvular deformation	No	No or Severe	**Unlikely**

Adapted from Lancellotti et al. [3] (*Eur Heart J Cardiovasc Imaging* 2013).

Colour flow imaging

Colour Doppler is the basic tool to start the MR evaluation. It allows fast screening for MR and identifies lesions that require further quantitation. Although, the size of the jet has a good correlation with the degree of MR, measurements of the jet size (jet area, jet area/LA area ratio) are not recommended to quantitate MR severity. Indeed, jet size is affected by several physical and technical factors that lead to over- or underestimation of MR severity.

Vena contracta width

For MR, imaging of the vena contracta—the regurgitant jet as it traverses the mitral orifice or the effective regurgitant area—is obtained from the parasternal long-axis or the apical 4-chamber view [16–18]. To properly identify the vena contracta, the

three components of the regurgitant jet should be visualized (◗ Fig. 13.8). A narrow colour sector scan coupled with the zoom mode is recommended to improve measurement accuracy. Using a Nyquist limit of 40–70 cm/s, a vena contracta width <3 mm correlates with mild MR, whereas a width ≥7 mm indicates severe MR. Intermediate values are not accurate at distinguishing moderate from mild or severe MR (large overlap); they require the use of another method for confirmation.

The flow convergence method (the proximal isovelocity surface area or PISA method)

The flow convergence method is the most recommended quantitative approach to evaluate the degree of MR (◗ Fig. 13.8) [24]. Imaging of the flow convergence zone is obtained from the apical 4-chamber or the parasternal long- or short-axis view. The

Table 13.2 Grading the severity of primary MR

Parameters	Mild	Moderate	Severe
Qualitative			
MV morphology	Normal/Abnormal	Normal/Abnormal	Flail leaflet/Ruptured PMs
Colour flow MR jet	Small, central	Intermediate	Very large central jet or eccentric jet adhering, swirling and reaching the posterior wall of the LA
Flow convergence zone	No or small	Intermediate	Large
CW signal of MR jet	Faint/Parabolic	Dense/Parabolic	Dense/Triangular
Semi-quantitative			
VC width (mm)	<3	Intermediate	≥7 (>8 for biplane)*
Pulmonary vein flow	Systolic dominance	Systolic blunting	Systolic flow reversal
Mitral inflow	A wave dominant	Variable	E wave dominant (>1.5 m/s)
TVI mit/TVI Ao	<1	Intermediate	>1.4
Quantitative			
EROA (mm²)	<20	20–29; 30–39**	≥40
R Vol (ml)	<30	30–44; 45–59**	≥60
+ LV and LA size and the systolic pulmonary pressure			

* For average between apical 4-and 2- chamber views.

** Grading of severity of organic MR classifies regurgitation as mild, moderate or severe, and sub-classifies the moderate regurgitation group into 'mild-to-moderate' (EROA of 20–29 mm or an R Vol of 30–44 ml) and 'moderate-to-severe' (EROA of 30–39 mm² or an R Vol of 45–59 ml). In secondary MR, the thresholds of severity, which are of prognostic value, are 20 mm² and 30 ml, respectively.

Adapted from Lancellotti et al.[3] (*Eur Heart J Cardiovasc Imaging* 2013).

Table 13.3 Echocardiographic parameters used to quantify MR severity: recordings

Parameters	Recordings
Mitral valve morphology	1. Visual assessment 2. Multiple views
Colour flow MR jet	1. Optimize colour gain/scale 2. Evaluate in two views 3. Measure blood pressure
VC width	1. PT-LAX and/or apical 4-chamber view 2. Optimize colour gain/scale 3. Identify the 3 components of the regurgitant jet (VC, PISA, Jet into LA) 4. Reduce the colour sector size and imaging depth to maximize frame rate 5. Expand the selected zone (Zoom) 6. Use the cine-loop to find the best frame for measurement 7. Measure the smallest VC (immediately distal to the regurgitant orifice, perpendicular to the direction of the jet)
PISA method	1. Apical 4-chamber 2. Optimize colour flow imaging of MR 3. Zoom the image of the regurgitant mitral valve 4. Decrease the Nyquist limit (colour flow zero baseline) 5. With the cine mode select the best PISA 6. Display the colour off and on to visualize the MR orifice 7. Measure the PISA radius at mid-systole using the first aliasing and along the direction of the ultrasound beam 8. Measure MR peak velocity and TVI (CW) 9. Calculate flow rate, EROA, R Vol
Doppler volumetric method (PW)	Flow across the mitral valve 1. Measure the mitral inflow by placing the PW sample volume at the mitral annulus (apical 4-chamber view) 2. Measure the mitral annulus diameter (apical 4-chamber view) at the maximal opening of the mitral valve (2-3 frames after the end-systole) Flow across the aortic valve 3. Measure the LV outflow tract flow by placing the PW sample volume 5 mm below the aortic cusps (apical 5-chamber view) 4. Measure the LV outflow tract diameter (parasternal long-axis view)
CW MR jet profile	1. Apical 4-chamber
Pulmonary vein flow	1. Apical 4-chamber 2. Sample volume of PW places into the pulmonary vein 3. Interrogate the different pulmonary veins when possible
Mitral peak E velocity	1. Apical 4-chamber 2. Sample volume of PW places at mitral leaflet tips
Atrial and LV size	1. Use preferably the Simpson method

CW: continuous-wave; LA: left atrium, EROA: effective regurgitant orifice area; LV: left ventricle; MR: mitral regurgitation; PT-LAX: parasternal long-axis; PW: pulse wave; R Vol: regurgitant volume; VC: vena contracta.
Adapted from Lancellotti et al. [3] (*Eur Heart J Cardiovasc Imaging* 2013)

area of interest is reduced by using the zoom mode, the sector size is reduced as narrow as possible to maximize frame rate, and the Nyquist limit is reduced to obtain a clearly visible, round, and measurable PISA radius (15–40 cm/s) (⊃ Fig. 13.8). Qualitatively, the presence of flow convergence at a Nyquist limit of 50–60 cm/s should alert to the presence of severe MR. Quantitative assessment classifies MR as mild (EROA is <20 mm² and R Vol <30 ml), moderate or severe (EROA is ≥40 mm² and R Vol ≥60 ml), and sub-classifies the moderate regurgitation group into 'mild-to-moderate' (EROA of 20–29 mm or R Vol of 30–44 ml) and 'moderate-to-severe' (EROA of 30–39 mm² or R Vol of 45–59 ml). In secondary MR, the thresholds of severity, which

are of prognostic value, are 20 mm² and 30 ml, respectively [25]. EROA is the most robust parameter as it represents a marker of lesion severity. A large EROA can lead to large regurgitant kinetic energy (large R Vol) but also to potential energy, with low R Vol but high LA pressure.

The flow convergence method has several advantages. Instrumental and haemodynamic factors do not seem to substantially influence flow quantification by this approach. The aetiology of regurgitation or the presence of concomitant valvular disease does not affect the regurgitant orifice area calculation. Although less accurate, this method can still be used in eccentric jet without significant distortion in the isovelocity contours.

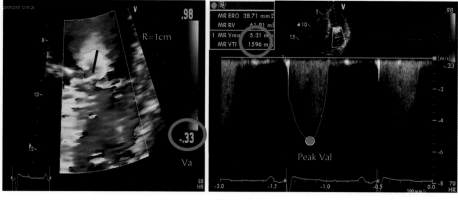

EROA = Flow/Peak velocity
EROA = (2πr² x Va)/Peak velocity

EROA = (2x3.14x1x33)/531
EROA = 207/531 = 0.39 cm²

R Vol = EROA x TVI
R Vol = 0.39 cm² x 159 cm = 61mL

Fig. 13.8 Method of calculation of the effective regurgitant orifice area (EROA) and of the regurgitant volume (R vol) using the PISA method.

Nevertheless, the flow convergence method also has some limitations. The shape of the PISA changes as the aliasing velocity changes. The convergence zone is flatter with higher aliasing velocities and becomes more elliptical with lower aliasing velocities. Practically, the aliasing velocity is set between 20 and 40 cm/s. Another limitation regards variation in the regurgitant orifice during the cardiac cycle. This is particularly important in mitral valve prolapse, where the regurgitation is often confined to the last half of systole. The precise location of the regurgitant orifice can be difficult to evaluate, which may cause an error in the measurement of the PISA radius (a 10% error in radius measurement will cause more than 20% error in flow rate and regurgitant orifice area calculations). A more important limitation is the distortion of the isovelocity contours by encroachment of proximal structures on the flow field. In this situation, an angle correction for wall constraint has been proposed but it is difficult in practice and thus not recommended. 3D echocardiography has been shown to overcome some of these limitations. Although promising, further 3D experience remains still required.

Doppler volumetric method

Quantitative pulsed wave Doppler method can be used as an additive or alternative method, especially when the PISA and the vena contracta are not accurate or not applicable (Fig. 13.9). This approach is time-consuming and is associated with several drawbacks [29]. Briefly, the regurgitant volume may be derived from the following formula: RVol = LV stroke volume (obtained from the Simpson method or 3D echocardiography)–LV forward stroke volume (from the pulsed-wave Doppler in the outflow tract). Similarly, regurgitant volume may be obtained by subtracting the mitral valve inflow (using the pulsed-wave Doppler in the mitral annulus) by the LV forward stroke volume.

Anterograde velocity of mitral inflow—mitral to aortic VTI ratio

In the absence of mitral stenosis, a peak mitral E velocity >1.5 m/s suggests severe MR. Conversely, a dominant A wave (atrial contraction) basically excludes severe MR. The pulsed Doppler mitral to aortic velocity time integral (VTI) ratio is also used as an easily measured index for the quantification of isolated pure organic MR. Mitral inflow Doppler tracings are obtained at the

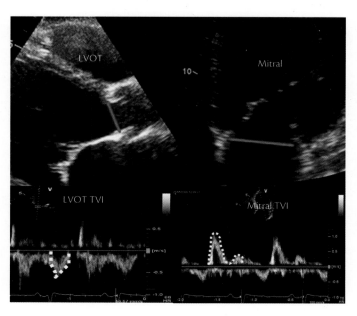

Fig. 13.9 Quantitative assessment of mitral regurgitation severity using the Doppler volumetric method requiring the measurements of left ventricular outflow tract diameter, the mitral annulus diameter, and of two pulse-wave velocity profiles (outflow tract and mitral inflow velocities).

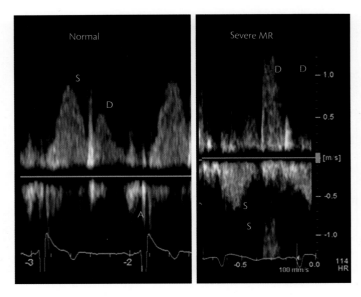

Fig. 13.10 Normal pulmonary vein flow pattern (a). Reversed systolic pulmonary flow in a patient with severe mitral regurgitation (b).

mitral leaflet tips and aortic flow at the annulus level in the apical 4-chamber view. A VTI ratio >1.4 strongly suggests severe MR, whereas a VTI ratio <1 is in favour of mild MR [30].

Pulmonary venous flow

Pulsed Doppler evaluation of pulmonary venous flow pattern is another aid for grading the severity of MR [31]. In normal individuals, pulmonary venous flow tracing is characterized by a positive systolic wave (S) followed by a smaller diastolic wave (D) and a reverse negative wave following atrial contraction (Ar) (⊃ Fig. 13.10). In severe MR, the S wave becomes frankly reversed if the jet is directed into the sampled vein. Atrial fibrillation and elevated LA pressure from any cause can blunt forward systolic pulmonary vein flow. Therefore, blunting of pulmonary venous flow lacks specificity for the diagnosis of severe MR.

Continuous wave (CW) Doppler of MR jet

Peak MR jet velocities by CW Doppler typically range between 4 and 6 m/s. This reflects the high systolic pressure gradient between the LV and LA. The velocity itself does not provide useful information about the severity of MR. Conversely, the signal intensity (jet density) of the CW envelope of the MR jet can be a qualitative guide to MR severity. A dense MR signal with a full envelope indicates more severe MR than a faint signal. The CW Doppler envelope may be truncated (notch) with a triangular contour and an early peak velocity (blunt). This indicates elevated LA pressure or a prominent regurgitant pressure wave in the LA due to severe MR. In eccentric MR, it may be difficult to record the full CW

envelope of the jet because of its eccentricity, while the signal intensity shows dense features.

Consequences of MR

The presence of severe MR has significant haemodynamic effects, primarily on the LV and LA and pulmonary pressures (⊃ Fig. 13.11).

LV size and function

MR imposes additional volume load on the LV. In acute MR, the LV is classically not enlarged, while in the chronic situation, the LV progressively dilates and irreversible LV dysfunction may occur. In the current guidelines, surgery is recommended in asymptomatic patients with severe MR when the LV ejection fraction is ≤60% and/or when the end-systolic diameter (less preload dependent) is ≥45 mm. New parameters are currently available for a better assessment of LV systolic function. A systolic tissue Doppler velocity measured at the lateral annulus <10.5 cm/s has been shown to identify subclinical LV dysfunction and to predict post-operative LV dysfunction in patients with asymptomatic primary MR [10]. Similarly, a global longitudinal strain <18% (2D-speckle tracking) has been associated with post-operative LV dysfunction [12]. More recently, LV global longitudinal strain <20% was associated with reduced cardiac event-free survival in asymptomatic patients with primary MR and no LV dysfunction/dilatation.

Left atrial size and function

The LA dilates in response to chronic volume and pressure overload. LA remodelling (diameter >40–50 mm or LA volume index >60 ml/m²) may predict onset of atrial fibrillation and poor prognosis in patients with organic MR [16, 17]. Conversely, MV repair leads to LA reverse remodelling, the extent of which is related to pre-operative LA size and to procedural success [18]. ESC guidelines recommend surgery in asymptomatic patients with severe MR due to flail mitral leaflet and no LV dysfunction/dilatation when the likelihood of durable repair is high, the surgical risk is low and LA volume is >40 ml/m² (class IIa, evidence C).

Systolic pulmonary arterial pressure

The excess regurgitant blood entering in the LA may induce acutely or chronically a progressive rise in pulmonary pressure. Pulmonary hypertension (PH: systolic pulmonary arterial pressure >50mmHg) is associated with a worse outcome both in conservative and surgically treated group of patients with primary MR [20, 21]. However, PH is uncommon in asymptomatic patients with preserved LV function [22], leading to relatively weak usefulness for the management and clinical decision-making. Nevertheless, PH is a class IIa indication (evidence C) for surgery in asymptomatic severe MR in the ESC guidelines.

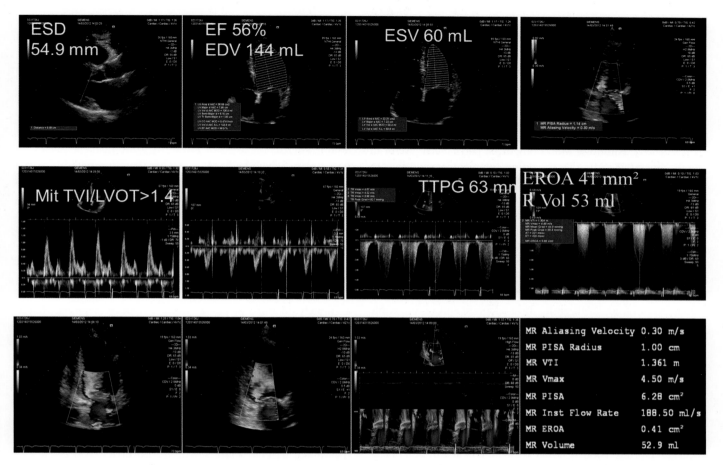

Fig. 13.11 Echocardiographic evaluation of a patient with 'moderate to severe' mitral regurgitation. Upper panels show the consequences of mitral regurgitation on left ventricular dilatation and dysfunction. Middle panels report the haemodynamic consequences of mitral regurgitation, mainly with elevated mitral E-wave velocity and markedly increased transtricuspid pressure gradient (TTPG). Lower panels show an eccentric jet, the classical pattern of convergence zone of primary mitral regurgitation using colour M-mode, and the effective regurgitant orifice area (EROA) and regurgitant volume (R vol) calculation.

Role of advanced multi-modality imaging

Role of exercise echocardiography

In asymptomatic patients with primary MR, exercise stress echocardiography may help to identify patients with unrecognized symptoms or subclinical latent LV dysfunction. Moreover, exercise echocardiography may also be helpful in patients with equivocal symptoms out of proportion to MR severity at rest. Worsening of MR severity (EROA >+ 10mm² or R Vol >+ 15ml), a marked increase in pulmonary arterial pressure (systolic pulmonary arterial pressure >60mmHg) and impaired contractile reserve (<4% increase in LV ejection fraction or exercise-induced <2% changes in longitudinal strain) can be useful findings to identify a subset of patients at higher risk who may benefit from early surgery [25]. Both the ACC/AHA and the ESC guidelines [28] recommend surgery in asymptomatic patients with preserved LV function, high likelihood of durable repair, low surgical risk, and exercise pulmonary hypertension. In secondary MR, large exercise-induced increases in MR (EROA ≥13 mm²) are associated with dyspnoea, recurrent acute pulmonary oedema, mortality, and hospitalization for heart failure. In the ESC guidelines, mitral valve repair is a class IIa indication in patients with LV systolic dysfunction, dynamic increase in secondary MR at exercise, pulmonary hypertension, and dyspnoea.

Multi-slice cardiac computed tomography (MSCT)

MSCT, from thin-section reconstructions, allows direct visualization of the thickening and calcification of the leaflets, mitral annulus, chordae, and papillary muscles. A recent study showed good correlation with 3D TOE concerning measurements of mitral valve geometry and leaflet lengths and angles. The extent of calcification of the mitral annulus might even be better demonstrated than by echo or cardiac magnetic resonance (CMR) [36]. The inner contour of the regurgitant orifice can manually be outlined on reconstructed cross-sectional images of the mitral valve in oblique short-axis. Two studies have demonstrated that MSCT-derived anatomical regurgitant orifice area correlates well with EROA measured by echocardiography. Chamber dimensions can be obtained after post-processing of the images with a contour-detection algorithm and manual correction if not satisfactory. The R Vol can be generated as the difference between the calculated stroke volume of the left and the right ventricle and has recently been shown to have a good correlation with the R Vol obtained by CMR [37]. Although MSCT might be particularly useful in the pre-operative setting by providing complementary information on the coronary arteries (high negative predictive value in patients who are at low risk of atherosclerosis), a routine clinical implementation is not yet recommended.

Cardiac magnetic resonance (CMR)

Practically, in patients with primary MR, CMR should be considered as the first choice alternative, when echocardiography is not conclusive. Indeed, CMR is the most accurate and reproducible non-invasive method for the assessment of LV volumes, LV ejection fraction, and torsional parameters. Basically, the LV dimensions are derived from a series of multi-sections perpendicular to the long axis of the LV (10–12 contiguous slices in short-axis direction). CMR can also be used for valve analysis using 'steady-state free-precession (SSFP)' sequences, which precisely discriminate blood from tissue (⊃ Fig. 13.12). First, mitral valve function can be assessed with cine imaging. Turbulent flow through mitral regurgitant orifice is easily visible with SSFP (visualization of signal voids due to spin dephasing in moving protons). Mitral valve anatomy can be imaged by acquisition of standard short-axis, 2-, 3- and 4-chamber long-axis views in combination with oblique long-axis cines orthogonal to the line of coaptation (⊃ Fig. 13.12). CMR has comparable diagnostic value to echocardiography for

identification of prolapsing scallops, but is inferior for imaging the subvalvular apparatus (torn chordae) due to lower spatial and temporal resolution. Only a few studies have used SSFP CMR for assessing the EROA by planimetry of the regurgitant orifice in a slice parallel to the valvular plane and perpendicular to the regurgitant jet at mid-systole (⊃ Fig. 13.13). Quantification of EROA was correlated well with angiographic and echocardiographic data. To note, CMR planimetry defines the anatomic regurgitant lesion, whereas the areas of EROA by PISA yield the narrowest flow stream, which tends to be smaller than the anatomic orifice area. It should also be underlined that the regurgitant orifice is frequently inconstant throughout systole in primary MR. This can potentially affect the estimation of the regurgitant severity. Lastly, planimetry of the MR regurgitant orifice is time consuming and remains challenging because appropriate plane alignment and angulation may be more difficult due to the longitudinal movement of the mitral annulus and in case of irregular shapes of regurgitant orifice. Furthermore, with CMR, blood flow and velocity can be accurately obtained by phase-contrast velocity mapping. Hence, R Vol can be measured indirectly as the difference between the total stroke volume and the aortic flow (forward stroke volume) (⊃ Fig. 13.13), as well as directly as the regurgitant flow across the mitral valve [38]. The latter, however, requires a specialized imaging sequence, which tracks the motion of the mitral valve annulus during the cardiac cycle. Lastly, it should be noted that all measurements with velocity imaging might be inaccurate in patients with high heart-rate variability. In the absence of other regurgitant lesions, a rare situation in primary MR, R Vol can also be calculated by subtracting the right ventricle stroke volume from the LV stroke volume. However, the calculation of the right ventricle stroke volume is less reproducible due to the extensive trabeculation of the right ventricle. Late gadolinium enhancement CMR (images obtained 10–20 min after injection of contrast) is

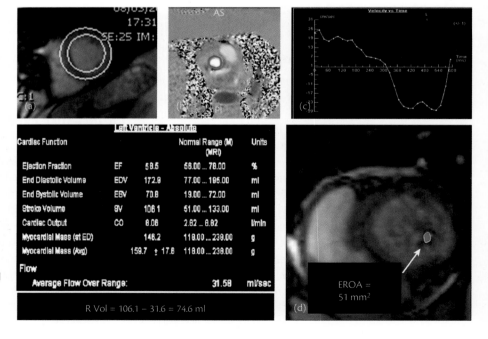

Fig. 13.12 Quantification of mitral regurgitation using cardiac magnetic resonance. (a) Total stroke volume derived from left ventricular volumes assessment. (b) Forward stroke volume derived from velocity-encoded cardiac magnetic resonance flow quantification of aortic flow. (c) Left ventricular outflow tract velocity measured throughout the cardiac cycle. (d) Planimetry of the anatomical regurgitant orifice area on a slice parallel to the valvular plane obtained by cardiac magnetic resonance. EROA indicates effective regurgitant orifice area and R Vol, regurgitant volume.

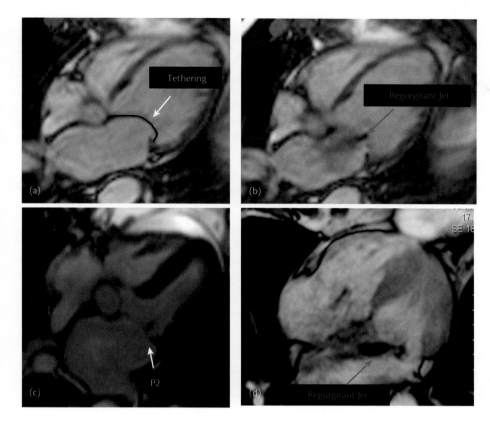

Fig. 13.13 Cardiac magnetic resonance imaging showing tethering of the mitral valve (a) and the regurgitant jet (red arrow, b). Mitral valve P2 prolapse (c). Eccentric regurgitant jet (d).

widely used to assess cardiac fibrosis in various cardiomyopathies. In contrast, there are practically no studies having investigated the prognostic role of cardiac fibrosis by CMR in primary MR. Perivalvular ventricular fibrosis and papillary muscle fibrosis have been well described in pathological studies, but not *in vivo*. Recently, Han and colleagues, using 3D high-resolution late gadolinium enhancement CMR imaging, have shown for the first time the presence of focal myocardial fibrosis in the papillary muscles in several patients with mitral valve prolapse [39]. Such a hyperenhancement of papillary muscles was more often associated with the presence of complex ventricular arrhythmias. In addition, the blood-to-leaflet contrast ratio was also increased in these patients, which may reflect the significantly expanded spongy layer with proteoglycans in the myxomatous valve. In secondary MR, CMR can play a major role for the evaluation of the extent of myocardial necrosis, which may limit the extent of functional recovery after revascularization or of functional recruitment in resynchronized patients.

In practice, the routine use of CMR is limited because of more difficult access to CMR than to echocardiography, and the need for specific expertise of radiologists and/or cardiologists in imaging. Other disadvantages of CMR are related to its potential incompatibility with pacemakers and the ECG-gated acquisition, which provokes problems in patients with arrhythmia.

References

1. Vahanian A, Alfieri O, Andreotti F, et al. Guidelines on the management of valvular heart disease (version 2012): The Joint Task Force on the Management of Valvular Heart Disease of the European Society of Cardiology (ESC) and the European Association for Cardio-Thoracic Surgery (EACTS). *Eur Heart J* 2012; 33: 2451–96.

2. Iung B, Baron G, Butchart EG, et al. A prospective survey of patients with valvular heart disease in Europe: The Euro Heart Survey on Valvular Heart Disease. *Eur Heart J* 2003; 24: 1231–43.

3. Lancellotti P, Tribouilloy C, Hagendorff A, et al. Recommendations for the Echocardiographic Assessment of Native Valvular Regurgitation: An Executive Summary from the European Association of Cardiovascular Imaging. *Eur Heart J Cardiovasc Imaging* 2013; 14: 611–44.

4. Chaput M, Handschumacher MD, Tournoux F, et al. Mitral leaflet adaptation to ventricular remodeling: occurrence and adequacy in patients with functional mitral regurgitation. *Circulation* 2008; 118: 845–52.

5. Beaudoin J, Handschumacher MD, Zeng X, et al. Mitral valve enlargement in chronic aortic regurgitation as a compensatory mechanism to prevent functional mitral regurgitation in the dilated left ventricle. *J Am Coll Cardiol* 2013; 61: 1809–16.

6. Monin JL, Dehant P, Roiron C, et al. Functional assessment of mitral regurgitation by transthoracic echocardiography using standardized imaging planes: diagnostic accuracy and outcome implications. *J Am Coll Cardiol* 2005; 46: 302–9.

7. Feneck R, Kneeshaw J, Fox K, et al. Recommendations for reporting perioperative transoesophageal echo studies. *Eur J Echocardiogr* 2010; 11: 387–93.

8. Kongsaerepong V, Shiota M, Gillinov AM, et al. Echocardiographic predictors of successful versus unsuccessful mitral valve repair in ischemic mitral regurgitation. *Am J Cardiol* 2006; 98: 504–8.

9. Omran AS, Woo A, David TE, Feindel CM, Rakowski H, Siu SC. Intraoperative transesophageal echocardiography accurately predicts mitral valve anatomy and suitability for repair. *J Am Soc Echocardiogr* 2002; 15: 950–7.

10. Agricola E, Galderisi M, Oppizzi M, et al. Pulsed tissue Doppler imaging detects early myocardial dysfunction in asymptomatic patients with severe mitral regurgitation. *Heart* 2004; 90: 406–10.

11. Marciniak A, Claus P, Sutherland GR, et al. Changes in systolic left ventricular function in isolated mitral regurgitation. A strain rate imaging study. *Eur Heart J* 2007; 28: 2627–36.

12. Lancellotti P, Cosyns B, Zacharakis D, et al. Importance of left ventricular longitudinal function and functional reserve in patients with degenerative mitral regurgitation: assessment by two-dimensional speckle tracking. *J Am Soc Echocardiogr* 2008; 21: 1331–6.

13. Magne J, O'Connor K, Mahjoub H, et al. Evaluation and impact on outcome of left ventricular contractile reserve in asymptomatic degenerative mitral regurgitation. *Eur Heart J* 2011; 32 [abstract supplement]: 170.

14. Mascle S, Schnell F, Thebault C, et al. Predictive value of global longitudinal strain in a surgical population of organic mitral regurgitation. *J Am Soc Echocardiogr* 2012; 25: 766–72.

15. Donal E, Mascle S, Brunet A, et al. Prediction of left ventricular ejection fraction 6 months after surgical correction of organic mitral regurgitation: the value of exercise echocardiography and deformation imaging. *Eur Heart J Cardiovasc Imaging* 2012; 13: 922–30.

16. Messika-Zeitoun D, Bellamy M, Avierinos JF, et al. Left atrial remodelling in mitral regurgitation—methodologic approach, physiological determinants, and outcome implications: a prospective quantitative Doppler-echocardiographic and electron beam-computed tomographic study. *Eur Heart J* 2007; 28: 1773–81.

17. Le Tourneau T, Messika-Zeitoun D, Russo A, et al. Impact of left atrial volume on clinical outcome in organic mitral regurgitation. *J Am Coll Cardiol* 2010; 56: 570–8.

18. Antonini-Canterin F, Beladan CC, Popescu BA, et al. Left atrial remodeling early after mitral valve repair for degenerative mitral regurgitation. *Heart* 2007; 28: 1773–81.

19. Cameli M, Lisi M, Righini FM, et al. Usefulness of atrial deformation analysis to predict left atrial fibrosis and endocardial thickness in patients undergoing mitral valve operations for severe mitral regurgitation secondary to mitral valve prolapse. *Am J Cardiol* 2013; 111: 595–601.

20. Barbieri A, Bursi F, Grigioni F, et al. Prognostic and therapeutic implications of pulmonary hypertension complicating degenerative mitral regurgitation due to flail leaflet: a multicenter long-term international study. *Eur Heart J* 2011; 32: 751–9.

21. Le Tourneau T, Richardson M, Juthier F, et al. Echocardiography predictors and prognostic value of pulmonary artery systolic pressure in chronic organic mitral regurgitation. *Heart* 2010; 96: 1311–7.

22. Magne J, Lancellotti P, Pierard LA. Exercise pulmonary hypertension in asymptomatic degenerative mitral regurgitation. *Circulation* 2010; 122: 33–41.

23. Breburda C, Griffin B, Pu M, Rodriguez L, Cosgrove D, Thomas J. Three-dimensional echocardiographic planimetry of maximal regurgitant orifice area in myxomatous mitral regurgitation: intraoperative comparison with proximal flow convergence. *J Am Coll Cardiol* 1998; 32: 432–7.

24. Lang RM, Mor-Avi V, Sugeng L, Nieman PS, Sahn DJ. Three-dimensional echocardiography: the benefits of the additional dimension. *J Am Coll Cardiol* 2006; 48: 2053–69.

25. Lancellotti P, Magne J. Stress testing for the evaluation of patients with mitral regurgitation. *Curr Opin Cardiol* 2012; 27: 492–8.

26. Magne J, Lancellotti P, Pierard LA. Exercise-induced changes in degenerative mitral regurgitation. *J Am Coll Cardiol* 2010; 56: 300–9.

27. Magne J, Lancellotti P, O'Connor K, Van de Heyning CM, Szymanski C, Pierard LA. Prediction of exercise pulmonary hypertension in asymptomatic degenerative mitral regurgitation. *J Am Soc Echocardiogr* 2011; 24: 1004–12.

28. Bonow RO, Carabello BA, Chatterjee K, et al. ACC/AHA 2006 guidelines for the management of patients with valvular heart disease: a report of the American College of Cardiology/American Heart Association Task Force on Practice Guidelines (Writing Committee to Revise the 1998 guidelines for the management of patients with valvular heart disease) developed in collaboration with the Society of Cardiovascular Anesthesiologists endorsed by the Society for Cardiovascular Angiography and Interventions and the Society of Thoracic Surgeons. *J Am Coll Cardiol* 2006; 48: e1–148.

29. Lee R, Haluska B, Leung DY, Case C, Mundy J, Marwick TH. Functional and prognostic implications of left ventricular contractile reserve in patients with asymptomatic severe mitral regurgitation. *Heart* 2005; 91: 1407–12.

30. Magne J, O'Connor K, Mahjoub H, et al. Evaluation and impact on outcome of left ventricular contractile reserve in asymptomatic degenerative mitral regurgitation. *Eur H J* 2014; 35: 1608–16.

31. Lebrun F, Lancellotti P, Pierard LA. Quantitation of functional mitral regurgitation during bicycle exercise in patients with heart failure. *J Am Coll Cardiol* 2001; 38: 1685–92.

32. Lancellotti P, Lebrun F, Pierard LA. Determinants of exercise-induced changes in mitral regurgitation in patients with coronary artery disease and left ventricular dysfunction. *J Am Coll Cardiol* 2003; 42: 1921–8.

33. Lancellotti P, Gerard PL, Pierard LA. Long-term outcome of patients with heart failure and dynamic functional mitral regurgitation. *Eur Heart J* 2005; 26: 1528–32.

34. Pierard LA, Lancellotti P. The role of ischemic mitral regurgitation in the pathogenesis of acute pulmonary edema. *N Engl J Med* 2004; 351: 1627–34.

35. Magne J, Sénéchal M, Mathieu P, Dumesnil JG, Dagenais F, Pibarot P. Restrictive annuloplasty for ischemic mitral regurgitation may induce functional mitral stenosis. *J Am Coll Cardiol* 2008; 51: 1692–701.

36. Van de Heyning CM, Magne J, Vrints CJ, Pierard L, Lancellotti P. The role of multi-imaging modality in primary mitral regurgitation. *Eur Heart J Cardiovasc Imaging* 2012; 13: 139–51.

37. Guo YK, Yang ZG, Ning G, et al. Isolated mitral regurgitation: quantitative assessment with 64-section multidetector CT—comparison with MR imaging and echocardiography. *Radiology* 2009; 252, 369–76.

38. Christiansen JP, Karamitsos TD, Myerson SG. Assessment of valvular heart disease by cardiovascular magnetic resonance imaging: a review. *Heart Lung Circ* 2011; 20: 73–82.

39. Han Y, Peters DC, Salton CJ, et al. Cardiovascular magnetic resonance characterization of mitral valve prolapse. *JACC Cardiovasc Imaging* 2008; 1: 294–303.

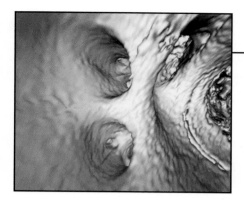

CHAPTER 14

Tricuspid and pulmonary valve disease

Bogdan A. Popescu, Maria Magdalena Gurzun, and Carmen Ginghina

Contents

Introduction

Although primary dysfunction of the tricuspid and pulmonary valves is rather infrequent, their secondary involvement is relatively common. The clinical and prognostic implications of right heart valve dysfunction are increasingly recognized. Therefore, the proper imaging assessment of tricuspid and pulmonary valves structure and function is of great interest for the best patient care.

Anatomy of the tricuspid and pulmonary valves

The tricuspid valve (TV) complex

This is formed by three leaflets (anterior, septal, and posterior), the tricuspid annulus (TA) and the subvalvular apparatus [1]. The anterior leaflet is the largest leaflet, while the posterior is the smallest one and commonly scalloped (see ⊃ Fig. 14.1a, 📷 Videos 14.1-14.2) [2]. The TV septal leaflet is inserted in a more apical position compared to the anterior mitral leaflet. This is an important discriminator between the tricuspid and the mitral valve and a reliable means to identify the anatomic right ventricle (RV) in

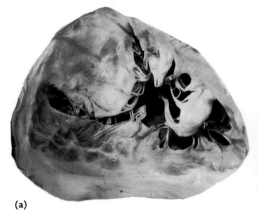

(a)

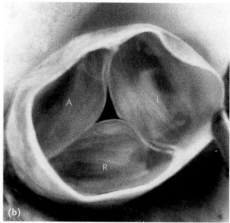

(b)

Fig. 14.1 (a) Anatomy of the normal TV. The three leaflets (septal-S, anterior-A, and posterior-P) are viewed from the right atrium. The anterior and the posterior leaflets correspond to the RV free wall, while the septal leaflet is attached to the ventricular septum (see 📷 Videos 14.1 and 14.2). (b) Anatomy of the normal PV. The three cusps (right-R, left-L, and anterior-A) are viewed from the pulmonary artery.
Reprinted with permission from Filipoiu FM [2].

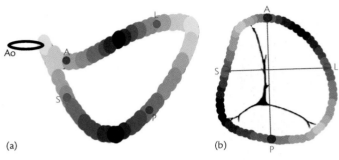

Fig. 14.2 (a) 3D drawing of the saddle-shaped TA. The high points (light grey) have antero-septal (adjacent to the aortic valve) and postero-lateral (180° from the aortic valve) locations. The low points (dark grey) have antero-lateral (90° from the aortic valve), and postero-septal location (aortic annulus, Ao; septal–lateral diameter, SL; antero-posterior diameter, AP). Modified after Fukuda et al. [4]. (b) 2D image of the oval-shaped TA. The antero-posterior diameter is larger than the septal-lateral one.

complex congenital heart disease [3]. The TA is normally an elliptic non-planar structure ('saddle-shaped'), having two high points (towards the atrium) and two low points (towards the RV) (see ➲ Fig. 14.2a) [4, 5]. The TA antero-posterior diameter is larger than the septal–lateral one (see ➲ Fig. 14.2b) [6, 7]. The TA changes its shape and size during the cardiac cycle [8], the annular dimensions and area decreasing significantly in systole compared to diastole [4]. The shortest TA diameter elongates significantly in diastole, while the longest diameter remains virtually unchanged. Therefore, the annulus becomes more circular in diastole [6]. The subvalvular apparatus is formed by three papillary muscles [7] and chordae supporting the leaflets during systole. A significant anatomical feature is that some third-degree chordae are attached directly to the ventricular septum, unlike the mitral valve [1].

The pulmonary valve (PV)

This consists of three cusps (right, left, and anterior/non-septal) (see ➲ Fig. 14.1b) [2]. It is inserted into the pulmonary artery annulus [3], which is supported entirely by freestanding musculature,

having no direct relation with the ventricular septum. The aortic and pulmonary valves normally lie at 90° planes to each other [9].

Imaging assessment: relative role, merits, and limitations of each technique

The goals of imaging the right heart valves are: detecting valvular disease, assessing severity, determining aetiology, evaluating consequences (e.g. RV size and function, pulmonary artery dimension, and pressure) (see ➲ Table 14.1).

Echocardiography

The main modality for imaging the right heart valves in clinical practice is transthoracic echocardiography (TTE). It allows the analysis of valvular morphology by 2- or 3-dimensional echo, detection and quantification of valvular dysfunction by Doppler techniques (colour, PW, CW), and evaluation of RV size and function [10–12] (see ➲ Table 14.1). The method is accurate, safe, available, and cost-effective. The main TTE views used to assess the tricuspid and pulmonic valve are presented in ➲ Figs 14.3 and 14.4 (see 📹 Videos 14.3-14.7). Routinely, only two leaflets of the tricuspid and pulmonary valves can be visualized simultaneously on a standard 2D view [13]. The 2D 'en face' views of the TV can sometimes be achieved from a modified subcostal short-axis view (see ➲ Fig. 14.5a, 📹 Video 14.8) [14]. In patients with a dilated right heart, recording the short-axis view of the TV or PV is feasible (see ➲ Fig. 14.5b and 14.5c, 📹 Videos 14.9-14.10). Due to the geometric assumptions about the RV, the accuracy of 2D echocardiography in evaluating RV function is limited [11]. TTE can appreciate RV inflow and outflow diameters, RV free wall thickness (see ➲ Fig. 14.6a, 📹 Video 14.11), and RV longitudinal systolic function (e.g. TAPSE, free wall S-wave velocity) (see ➲ Fig. 14.6b), or global systolic function (e.g. fractional area change) [11]. Although the right heart valves are located anteriorly, far from the transoesophageal echocardiography (TOE) probe, TOE can still provide additional information in selected cases [3, 9, 10, 12, 15] (see ➲ Figs 14.7 and 14.8, 📹 Videos 14.12-14.14).

Table 14.1 Comparison of echocardiography, multi-slice computed tomography, and cardiac magnetic resonance for characterization of right heart valves morphology and function

Parameter	Echocardiography	Multi-slice Computed Tomography	Cardiac Magnetic Resonance
Leaflet mobility	++++	++	+++
Valvular calcification	++	++++	+
Annular geometry	++	++++	+++
Stenotic orifice area	+++	+++	++
Transvalvular pressure gradients	++++	–	+++
Regurgitant jet morphology	++++	–	+++
Regurgitant volume	+++	+	++++
RV dimensions	++	+++	++++
RV function	++	+++	++++

Modified after [21].

(++++ excellent; +++ adequate; ++ marginal; + very limited; —unable)

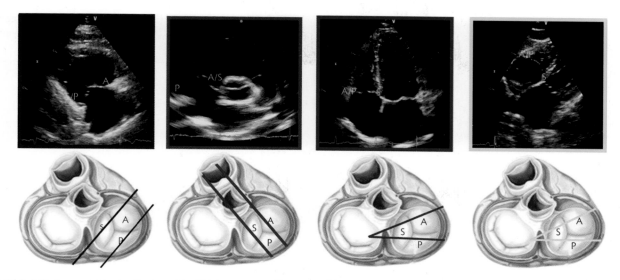

Fig. 14.3 TTE views used for visualization of the TV: the parasternal long-axis of the RV inflow view—blue box (obtained from the standard parasternal long-axis view by tilting the probe infero-medially and rotating it slightly clockwise) (see [icon], Video 14.3); the parasternal short-axis view—red box; (see [icon], Video 14.4); the apical 4-chamber view—green box; (see [icon], Video 14.5); and the subcostal 4-chamber view—yellow box. The TV leaflets visualized most often in each of these views are labelled (septal, S; anterior, A; and posterior, P).

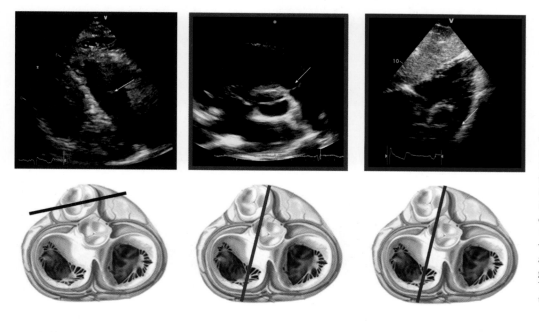

Fig. 14.4 TTE views used for visualization of the PV: the parasternal long-axis view of the RV outflow—blue box (obtained from the standard parasternal long-axis view by tilting the probe infero-laterally and rotating it slightly counter-clockwise); (see [icon], Video 14.6); the parasternal short-axis view—red box; (see [icon], Video 14.7); and the subcostal short-axis view—green box (more feasible in children). The white arrows are pointing to the PV.

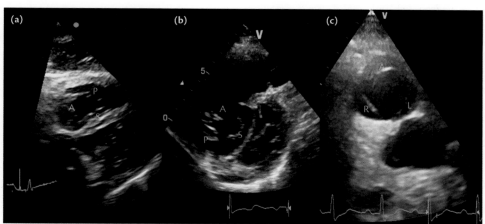

Fig. 14.5 (a) 2D 'en face' view of the TV from a modified subcostal short-axis view (from a standard subcostal view the probe is slightly rotated clockwise and tilted superiorly). All three leaflets (septal, S; anterior, A; and posterior, P) are visualized (see [icon], Video 14.8). (b) 2D 'en face' view of the TV from the parasternal short-axis view (at mitral valve level) in a patient with severe pulmonary hypertension, secondary TR, and dilated RV. All three leaflets (septal, S; anterior, A; and posterior, P) are visualized. (c) 2D 'en face' view of the PV from the parasternal basal short-axis view in a patient with severe pulmonary hypertension. All three cusps (right, R; left, L; and anterior, A) are visualized (see [icon], Video 14.10).

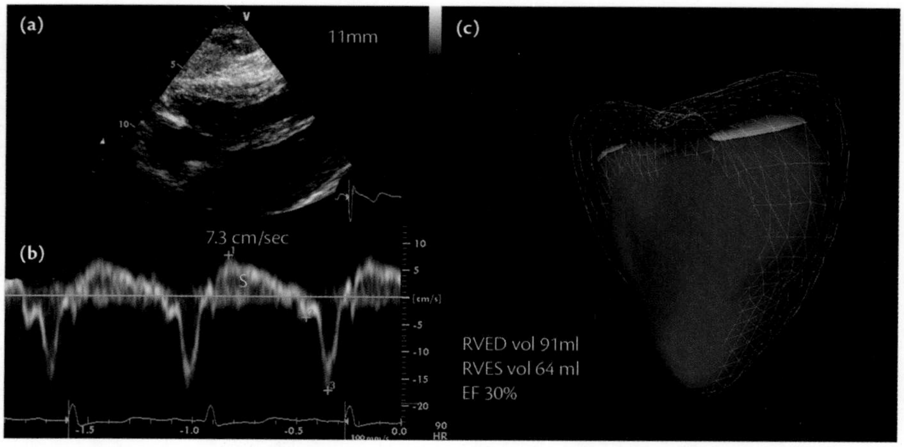

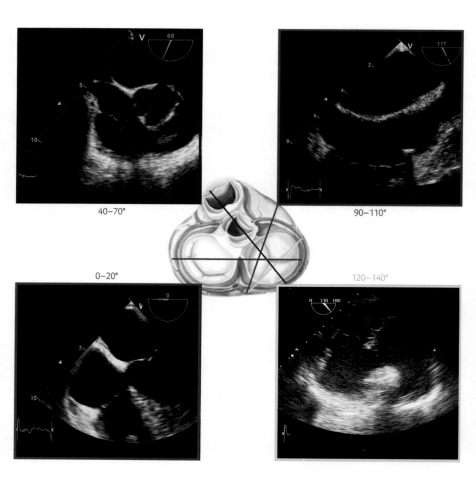

Fig. 14.6 (a) TTE, subcostal 4-chamber view in a patient with severe PS. There is increased diastolic thickness of the RV free wall (11 mm) indicating RV hypertrophy (see 📹 Video 14.11). (b) TTE, PW tissue Doppler examination of the RV free wall motion in a patient with PS. Peak S-wave velocity is reduced, indicating RV longitudinal systolic dysfunction. (c) 3-dimensional echocardiography measurement of the RV volumes and ejection fraction in a patient with pulmonary hypertension (see 📹 Video 14.15).

Fig. 14.7 TOE views used for visualization of the TV: mid-oesophageal 4-chamber view—green box (see 📹 Video 14.12); mid-oesophageal short-axis ('inflow-outflow') view—blue box; (see 📹 Video 14.13); the modified bicaval view—red box; (see 📹 Video 14.14); and the transgastric RV inflow view—yellow box.

Evaluation of the tricuspid and pulmonary valves using 3D is a useful and feasible tool [13, 16], allowing the visualization of all three leaflets and commissures simultaneously (📹 Videos 14.1-14.2). Moreover, 3D echocardiography provides accurate RV outflow tract measurements (supravalvular, subvalvular, and valvular) [9] and allows RV volumes and EF measurements without geometric assumption (see ⊃ Fig. 14.6c, 📹 Video 14.15).

Cardiac magnetic resonance (CMR) imaging

Cardiac magnetic resonance (CMR) imaging can provide complementary information to echocardiography and should be considered when echocardiography is technically limited or provides inconsistent results [17]. CMR visualizes all parts of the valve or valvular masses (e.g. vegetation, thrombus). However, echocardiography is superior to CMR for imaging structures that are thin and highly mobile (e.g. vegetations), due to its higher temporal resolution [18]. CMR allows the calculation of regurgitant volume and regurgitant fraction, mean and peak velocity or transvalvular gradient, and direct measurement of stenotic valve orifice or regurgitant orifice (see ⊃ Table 14.1) [19]. CMR does not involve geometric assumptions about the RV and allows accurate measurements of RV size and function being sensitive in

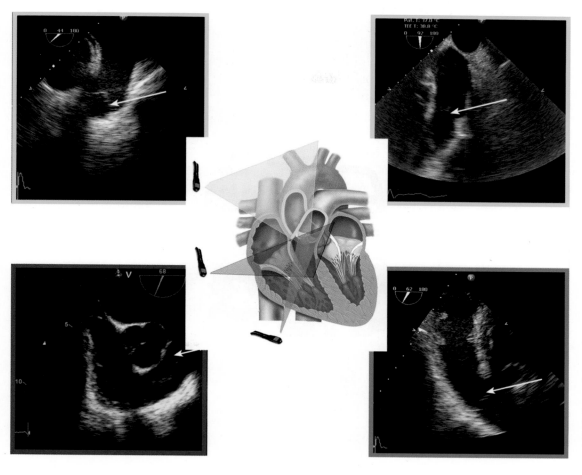

Fig. 14.8 TOE views used for visualization of the PV: mid-oesophageal short-axis ('inflow-outflow') view—blue box; transgastric RV outflow view—green box; mid-oesophageal ascending aorta short-axis view—left yellow box; and upper oesophageal aortic arch short-axis view—right yellow box. The white arrows are pointing to the PV.

detecting serial changes in these parameters. This feature is essential for the proper follow-up of patients with TR or PR.

Multi-slice computed tomography (MSCT)

Multi-slice computed tomography (MSCT) offers anatomic details of the valves due to its excellent spatial resolution and is useful especially in patients with complex congenital heart disease [20, 21]. This technique involves the use of ionizing radiation, which represents a limitation. It should only be used when the same amount of information cannot be obtained by non-radiating techniques (echocardiography, CMR).

Stenotic lesions of right heart valves: assessment and decision-making

Tricuspid stenosis (TS)

Tricuspid stenosis (TS), of rheumatic origin in 90% of cases, is rarely seen in developed countries [22]. Other possible causes of TS are: congenital tricuspid atresia, carcinoid syndrome, endomyocardial fibrosis, metabolic or enzymatic diseases, or right atrial tumours [22, 23] (see ⊃ Fig. 14.9).

Echocardiography enables a definitive diagnosis of the cause and severity of TS [22]. The rheumatic aetiology is suggested by commissural fusion and diastolic doming with thickened leaflets

and shortened chordate (see ⊃ Fig. 14.10a and 14.10b, ▣ Videos 14.16-14.17). Evaluation of TS severity by echocardiography is generally performed by CW Doppler (see ⊃ Fig. 14.10c). The clue of a stenotic TV is an increased transvalvular peak velocity (normally below 0.7 m/s but frequently exceeding 1 m/s in TS and approaching 2 m/s during inspiration) [24]. The echocardiographic findings suggestive of significant TS are presented in ⊃ Table 14.2.

The main advantage of 3DE in TS evaluation is its ability to image the valve '*en face*', allowing the analysis of leaflet morphology (thickness, calcifications, and mobility), relationship between leaflets, and the direct measurement of valve orifice (see ⊃ Fig. 14.10d and ▣ Video 14.18) [9, 25].

Although MSCT and CMR may be feasible in evaluating TS, they are not used routinely in this setting. Valve area can be assessed by placing of an image slice through the valve tips in diastole and measuring forward velocity through the valve [26].

Pulmonic stenosis (PS)

Pulmonic stenosis (PS), a congenital disorder in 95% of cases, may be isolated (abnormalities of the PV, subvalvular or supravalvular membrane), or a feature of complex congenital lesions (e.g. tetralogy of Fallot, complete atrio-ventricular canal, double outlet RV) [22, 24]. Rare acquired aetiologies of PS include rheumatic disease, carcinoid syndrome, and extrinsic compression. Subvalvular PS may be produced by infundibular muscular obstruction in RV hypertrophy [7, 24].

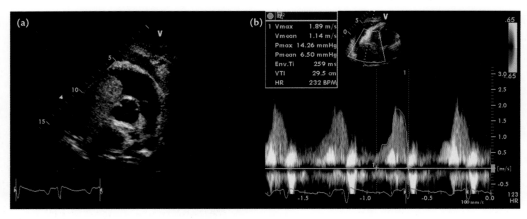

Fig. 14.9 (a) TTE, 2D parasternal short-axis view in a patient with a large RA tumour producing TV obstruction as a rare cause of TS. (a) TTE, CW Doppler exam in the same patient shows increased diastolic velocities through the TV (mean gradient of 6.5 mmHg), produced by the RA tumour. Reprinted with permission from Ginghina C [23].

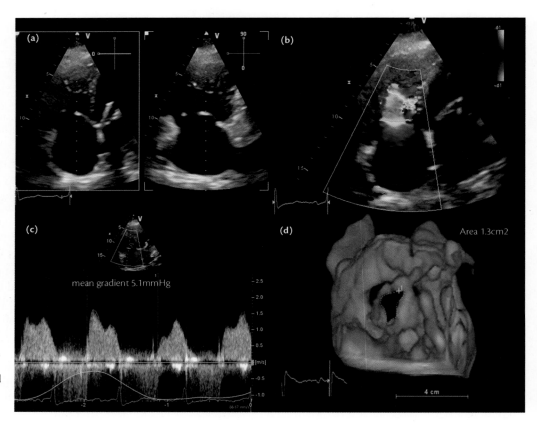

Fig. 14.10 TTE in a patient with rheumatic tricuspid valve stenosis. (a) Bi-plane view of the TV from the apical position. The leaflets are thickened, with diastolic doming, suggesting a rheumatic aetiology of TS in this patient (see ▣ Video 14.16). (b) Colour Doppler examination of the TV in the apical 4-chamber view. The diastolic flow through the valve is turbulent suggesting TS (see ▣ Video 14.17). (c) CW Doppler examination of the TV. The mean gradient through the valve is increased suggesting significant TS. There are typical respiratory variations of the diastolic inflow velocities. (d) 3D *'en face'* view of the TV seen from the RV. The opening of the leaflets is restricted, and the measured area (1.3 cm²) suggests moderate TS (see ▣ Video 14.18).

Table 14.2 Echocardiographic grading of tricuspid stenosis severity [24]

Findings indicative of haemodynamically significant tricuspid stenosis	
Mean pressure gradient	≥5 mmHg
Inflow velocity time integral	>60 cm
Pressure half time	≥190 ms
Valve area (by continuity equation)	≤1 cm²
Supportive findings	enlarged right atrium (≥moderate), dilated inferior vena cava

Echocardiography has an important role in the initial assessment and follow-up of patients with PS. 2D echocardiography allows the visualization of the obstruction site (subvalvular, valvular, supravalvular), the morphological features of the cusps (thickness, doming, reduced mobility), and RV evaluation (see ▣ Videos 14.19-14.22). Grading the severity of PS is primarily based on the peak velocity and gradient assessed by CW Doppler (see ➲ Table 14.3) (see ➲ Fig. 14.11) [24, 27]. Another useful index of severity is the estimated RV systolic pressure (based on the tricuspid regurgitant jet velocity and right atrial pressure) [24]. Moreover, the Doppler peak gradient measured by echocardiography is the main parameter for decision-making in PS (for a peak gradient greater than 64 mmHg intervention is indicated) [28].

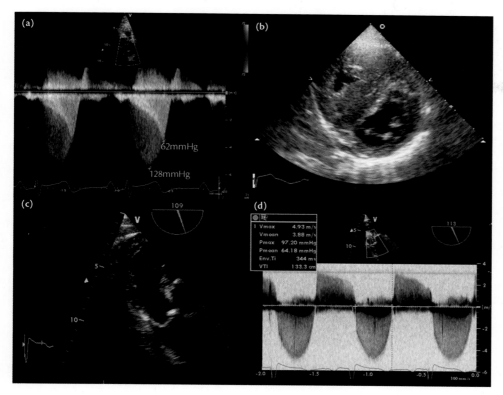

Fig. 14.11 (a) TTE, CW Doppler examination of the RV outflow. The envelope has a double contour, suggesting the presence of both valvular (peak gradient at 128 mmHg) and subvalvular dynamic (late peak at 62 mmHg) obstruction. (b) TTE, 2D short-axis view at mid-papillary level (end-diastolic frame) showing severe RV hypertrophy in the same patient (see 📹 Video 14.21). (c) TOE, 2D visualization of the PV from the transgastric view (systolic frame) in a patient with severe PS. The PV is thickened and calcified, with doming, while the RV outflow tract wall thickness is increased (see 📹 Video 14.22). (d) TOE, CW Doppler examination of the RV outflow tract in the patient shown in image (c). The peak gradient is increased at 97 mmHg, indicating severe valvular PS.

Reprinted with permission from Popescu BA, Ginghina C [27].

Table 14.3 Echocardiographic grading of pulmonary stenosis severity [24]

Parameter	Mild	Moderate	Severe
Peak velocity (m/s)	<3	3–4	>4
Peak gradient (mmHg)	<36	36–64	>64

3D echocardiography may offer more information regarding PV morphology, allowing the visualization of all three cusps in the same view. However, the assessment of PS by 3D echocardiography has not been reported [9].

The role of CMR and MSCT lies in the detailed anatomical evaluation.

CMR allows the identification of the location and severity of PS (see ⤷ Fig. 14.12, 📹 Videos 14.23–14.25). The recommended view is a cine RV outflow tract. A qualitative analysis of severity can be made by direct planimetry of the valve orifice (by cine image through the valve tips), or by peak velocity measurement. In-plane velocity mapping can be helpful in identifying the site of maximal velocity [26]. Another important role of CMR in PS is RV mass and function evaluation [2]. Concomitant pulmonary trunk or branch artery stenoses can be identified with either a thin-slice steady-state free-precession (SSFP) anatomical stack or MR angiography of the pulmonary arteries [26].

MSCT allows excellent visualization of the number, thickness, opening and closing of the valve leaflets, and valve calcification, while cine images may show the decreased valve mobility. Angio-CT findings suggestive of valvular PS are: post-stenotic enlargement of the main and left pulmonary arteries, and RV hypertrophy [30]. MSCT has an important role for pulmonary artery morphological characterization and supravalvular stenosis identification (see ⤷ Fig. 14.13).

Regurgitant lesions of right heart valves: assessment and decision-making

Tricuspid regurgitation (TR) is the most common right heart valve disease and is often secondary to TA enlargement due to RV dilatation (see 📹 Video 14.26) [7, 8]. Primary TR (anatomically abnormal valves) can be congenital (e.g. TV prolapse—see 📹 Video 14.27, Ebstein's anomaly, see ⤷ Fig. 14.14a and 4.14b, 📹 Videos 14.28-14.29, TV dysplasia), acquired (e.g. rheumatic valve disease; endocarditis, see ⤷ Fig. 14.14c, 📹 Video 14.30, carcinoid disease, see ⤷ Fig. 14.14d), or iatrogenic (e.g. pacemaker/defibrillator lead —see 📹 Videos 14.31-14.32, drugs; radiation) [7, 22].

Echocardiography is the main modality for detection and quantification of TR (see ⤷ Table 14.4 and ⤷ Fig. 14.15a–14.15d). Mild TR is frequently encountered in normal people (physiological TR). Physiological TR is characterized by normal leaflet morphology, thin, central TR colour jet, adjacent to valve closure [8, 10].

The 3D 'en face' view of the TV allows a better characterization of leaflet morphology and commissures. 3D echo is useful to indicate the aetiology and to quantify TR severity. Since the shape of vena contracta is ellipsoidal in secondary TR (similarly to secondary mitral regurgitation), the 3D measurements of its area and diameters may represent more reliable parameters for TR quantification [10, 31] (see ⤷ Fig. 14.15b).

Echocardiographic assessment of secondary TR—implications for surgical decision

Secondary (functional) TR is produced by TA dilatation and leaflet tethering [32]. These two parameters are useful to predict TR severity or residual TR after annuloplasty.

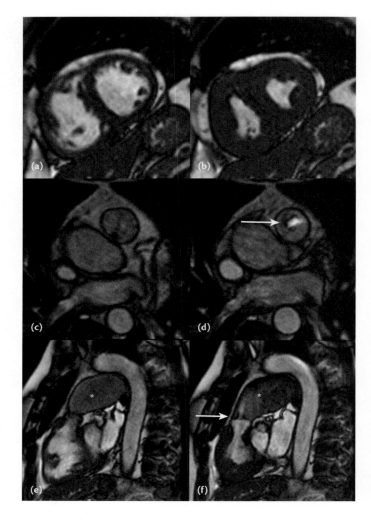

Fig. 14.12 Still frame cine CMR images at end-diastole (a, c, e) and end-systole (b, d, f) in a patient with severe pulmonary valve stenosis showing RV hypertrophy (RV mass of 82 g = 51 g/m²; normal values: 69 ± 14 g; 35 ± 7 g/m²) and normal RV systolic function (RV EF of 68%). The PV has limited opening (arrows)(d, f) and a measured area by planimetry of 0.6 cm²; there is post-stenotic dilatation (30 mm) of pulmonary artery trunk (asterixes) (e, f) (see 🖳 Videos 14.23-14.25).
Courtesy of Dr Anca Florian, Robert-Bosch KH Stuttgart.

The 2D echocardiographic evaluation of TA underestimates its actual size due to its elliptical shape. Therefore, the TA diameter measured in 4-chamber view (septal–lateral diameter) or short-axis view (oblique diameter) is smaller than the real antero-posterior diameter [13] (see ⊃ Fig. 14.2). The 3D 'en face' view of the TV allows a more accurate assessment of the TA than 2D echocardiography, being comparable to CMR [33]. The TA dilates, especially in the septal–lateral direction, resulting in a flat, more circular shape [5]) (see 🖳 Videos 14.33-14.34).

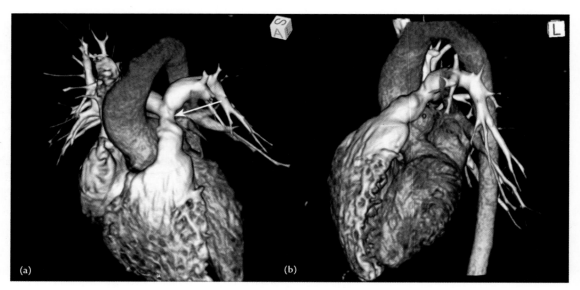

Fig. 14.13 3-Dimensional volume rendered CT images in left anterior oblique and left lateral projections in a patient with Ross intervention and pulmonary valved conduit implantation (Contegra® graft) showing high grade distal graft stenosis (peak to peak gradient of 55 mmHg) (white arrow).
Courtesy of Dr Stefan Orwat, Universitätsklinikum Münster.

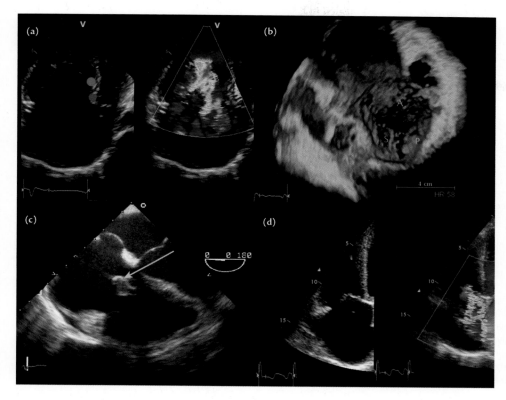

Fig. 14.14 (a) TTE, 2D and colour Doppler examination of the TV in a patient with Ebstein disease. The insertion of the septal tricuspid leaflet (red dot) is significantly displaced towards the apex compared with the insertion of the anterior mitral leaflet (blue dot) (see 👥 Video 14.28). (b) 3D '*en face*' view of the TV as seen from the RA, in the same patient (see 👥 Video 14.29). (c) TOE, 2D mid-oesophageal 4-chamber view showing a mass attached to TV septal leaflet (arrow). The mass is suggestive of vegetation, which was confirmed at surgery. There is also significant right heart cavities dilatation as the patient had severe TR (see 👥 Video 14.30). (d) TTE, 2D and colour Doppler examination of the TV (apical 4-chamber view, systolic frame) in a patient with carcinoid syndrome. The leaflets are thickened and fixed in an open position, determining severe primary TR.

Table 14.4 Echocardiographic grading of tricuspid regurgitation severity [10]

Parameters	Mild	Moderate	Severe
Qualitative			
TV morphology	Normal/abnormal	Normal/abnormal	Abnormal/flail/large coaptation defect
Colour flow TR jet	Small, central	Intermediate	Very large central jet or eccentric wall impinging jet
CW signal of TR jet	Faint/parabolic	Dense/parabolic	Dense/triangular with early peaking (peak <2 m/s in massive TR)
Semi-quantitative			
Vena contracta width (mm)	Not defined	<7	>7
PISA radius (mm)	≤5	6–9	>9
Hepatic vein flow	Systolic dominance	Systolic blunting	Systolic flow reversal
Tricuspid inflow	Normal	Normal	E wave dominant (≥1 m/s)
Quantitative			
EROA (mm²)	Not defined	Not defined	≥40
Regurgitant volume (ml)	Not defined	Not defined	≥45

The normal TA diameter in adults measured in the 4-chamber view in diastole is 28±5 mm. TA size correlates with TR severity: a diameter >32 mm in systole or >34 mm in diastole is a marker of significant TR [10].

The main clinical impact of TA measurement is related to the management of patients undergoing cardiac surgery for mitral valve disease. Late moderate-to-severe TR is frequent after mitral valve surgery [34]. TR is most commonly secondary to TA dilatation, which is progressive and may not be accompanied by TR initially. Outcome of isolated TV surgery late after mitral valve surgery is poor because most often RV dysfunction has already occurred. Therefore, TV repair with an annuloplasty ring should be performed at the time of initial mitral valve surgery, regardless of TR severity, if the TA is dilated. The cut-off value for recommending annuloplasty is 70 mm for the intra-operative measurement of TA (antero-septal to antero-posterior commisure, see ⮑ Fig. 14.16b) [35] and 40 mm for the apical 4-chamber view echo measurement (see ⮑ Fig. 14.16a) [36, 37]. Although there are no randomized clinical trials, some authors suggest the cut-off value of 35 mm (or 21 mm/m²) for the 4-chamber view TA measurement [34].

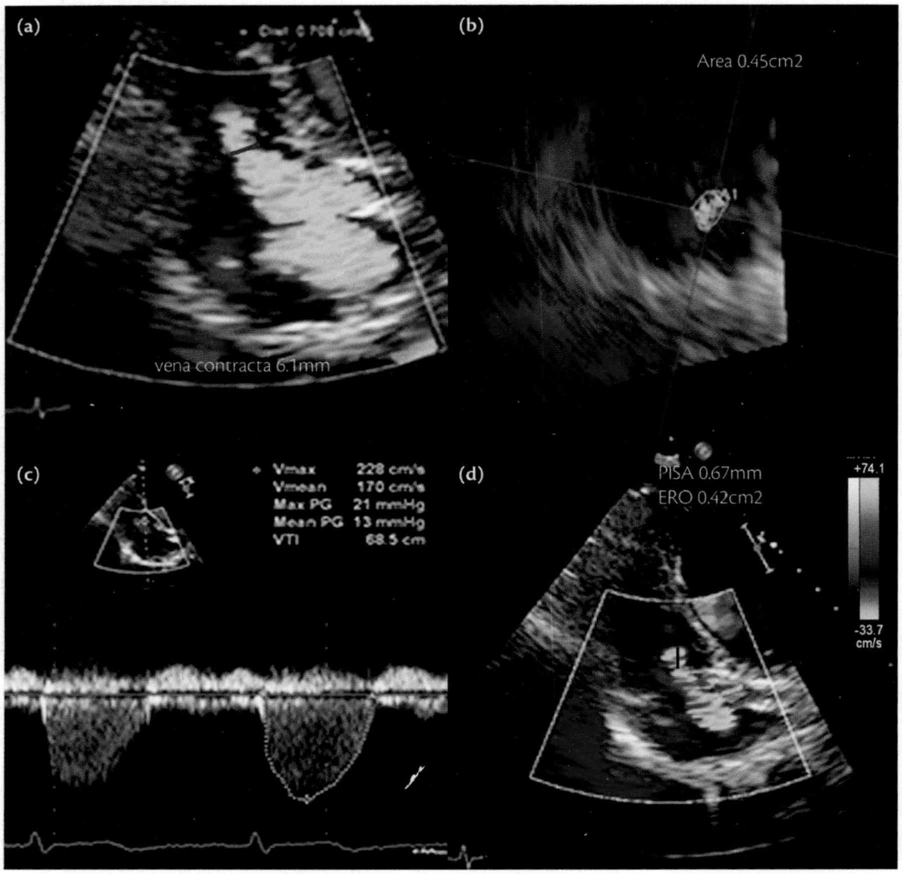

Fig. 14.15 TTE evaluation of TR severity. (a) Semi-quantitative TR assessment, TTE apical 4-chamber view modified for right heart cavities. The vena contracta width of the TR jet measures 6.1 mm, indicating moderate TR. (b) TR evaluation by Colour 3D. The regurgitant orifice has an elliptical shape and the smallest diameter corresponds to vena contracta measured by 2D echocardiography (green line). Therefore, TR severity can be underestimated by 2D vena contracta. The 3D vena contracta area is 0.45 cm^2, indicating severe TR. (c) CW Doppler across the TV. The signal has triangular shape, with early peaking and low peak velocity (2.2 m/s), suggesting significant TR. (d) Quantitative TR assessment by PISA method. To obtain a hemispherical PISA, the zero baseline is shifted in the blood flow direction. The PISA radius measured using the first aliasing is 0.67 mm, suggesting moderate to severe TR. The EROA calculated using peak TR velocity is 0.42 cm^2, consistent with severe TR.

The increased apical displacement of tricuspid leaflets (TV tethering) is evaluated by measuring the tenting area (tracing between the atrial surface of the leaflets and the TA plane at maximal systolic closure) and coaptation distance (distance between the TA plane and the point of coaptation) in the 4-chamber view [10] (see ⊃ Fig. 14.16d). The tenting volume can also be measured using 3D echocardiography [38].

Apical displacement of tricuspid leaflets is a determinant of TR severity: a tenting area >1 cm^2 is associated with severe TR [32]. TV tethering is also a predictor for residual TR after TV annuloplasty. A tethering distance >0.76 cm or a tethering area >1.63 cm^2 suggest the use of adjunctive surgical techniques to tricuspid annuloplasty or the use of TV replacement [39]. New data obtained by 3D echocardiography suggest that pre-annuloplasty tenting volume and the antero-posterior TA diameter are independent predictors of residual TR severity, but geometrical cut-off values have to be validated [38].

CMR can be used to assess TR, especially in patients with poor echocardiographic images or equivocal echo findings [8, 17]. CMR allows the visualization of leaflets' structure and function (SSFP cine sequences horizontal long-axis view) and evaluation of jet characteristics [26]. The quantification of TR can be done by calculation of regurgitant area or regurgitant volume. The regurgitant orifice is estimated by cine image through the leaflet tips in systole or by visualization of flow jet in cross-section

through-plane phase contrast velocity mapping in this plane. The regurgitant volume is estimated by calculating RV stroke volume and pulmonary forward flow. If TR is the only valvular leak, the difference between right and left ventricular stroke volumes may be used to estimate regurgitant volume [26]. CMR is the reference standard imaging modality in evaluating RV morphology and function [40], which are essential for TR mechanism detection and appropriate management of these patients (see ⊃ Fig. 14.17, 🎥 Videos 14.35-14.37). Echocardiography is superior to CMR for the estimation of pulmonary artery pressure using TR jet peak velocity (achievable even with trace/mild TR). Another utilization of CMR is in patients with Ebstein anomaly in whom valvular displacement and abnormality are well depicted, and RV function can be properly assessed [29].

Pulmonary regurgitation

Mild pulmonary regurgitation (PR) is particularly common in normal subjects (physiological PR), mild to moderate secondary PR is often seen in pulmonary hypertension, but more significant degrees are usually related to congenital heart disease (abnormal pulmonic valve leaflets, residual PR after surgical treatment of congenital disease: PS, Fallot tetralogy) [22, 23]. Primary PR is uncommon and can be produced by infective endocarditis, carcinoid syndrome, trauma, or rheumatic involvement [23].

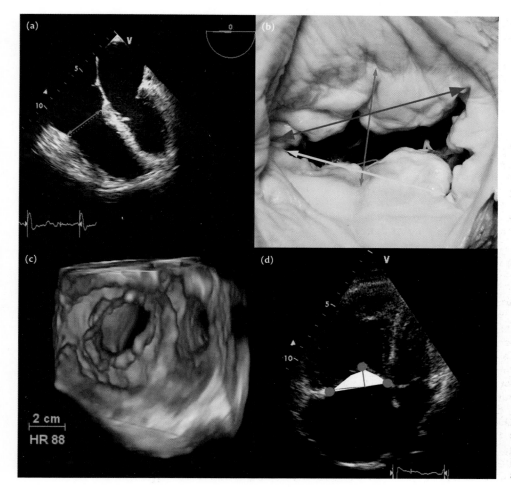

Fig. 14.16 (a) TOE, 2D mid-oesophageal 4-chamber view (diastolic frame). The TA measures 43 mm, indicating annulus dilatation. (b) Intra-operative measurement of the TA. The diameter between the antero-septal and the antero-posterior commissures (green line) is useful for intra-operative evaluation of TA dilatation and is larger than the one measured by echocardiography (red line). The distance between antero-septal and postero-septal commissures (yellow line) is essential for appreciation of prosthetic ring size. Because the TA dilates mainly in the septal-lateral direction, this distance remains essentially unchanged and can predict the appropriate ring size. Reprinted with permission from Filipoiu FM [2]. (c) TTE, 3D *'en face'* view of the TA in a patient with severe pulmonary hypertension. The TA is dilated and has changed from its normal elliptical shape (see 🎥 Video 14.33) into a round shape (see 🎥 Video 14.34). (d) TTE, 2D apical four chamber view in a patient with severe secondary TR. The leaflets coaptation point is displaced apically. The tenting area is measured in mid-systole between leaflets and TA.

Echocardiography can provide useful information regarding PV morphology, but grading of PR severity has been less validated (see ➲ Table 14.5). The echo assessment of PR severity is usually based on measuring jet diameter at its origin (see ➲ Fig. 14.18, 🎥 Video 14.38). A ratio between the width of PR colour jet immediately below the valve and the RV outflow tract dimension > 65% suggests significant PR [12]. 3D echocardiography may be a useful tool for PV morphology analysis and PR quantification. However, validation of this method is needed before recommending its routine use in this setting [41].

CMR allows an accurate assessment of PR and RV size and function. The anatomy of the valve is visualized in cine images of the RV outflow tract. Since the pressures in the right heart are low, the PR jet is poorly visualized on cine images, and in-plane phase contrast velocity mapping sequences are more adequate. CMR can accurately quantify the amount of regurgitation and regurgitant fraction using through-plane phase contrast velocity mapping. Placing the imaging slice for flow mapping just above the pulmonic valve allows quantification of both forward and regurgitant flow per cardiac cycle [26]. This method has been validated against right and left ventricular stroke volumes. The accurate measurement of RV volumes can guide the timing of valve surgery [26]. CMR is the method of choice, especially in patients with repaired tetralogy of Fallot and residual PR [42]. RV volumes (RV end-diastolic volume <160 ml/m² or RV end-systolic volume <82 ml/m²) are in this situation an indicator of the optimal timing for PV intervention [43, 44].

Conclusion

The imaging assessment of right heart valves has an important role for diagnosing valve dysfunction, grading of severity, and decision-making. Echocardiography is the main method used in clinical practice, usually able to provide all the information needed for patient care. CMR provides a more accurate evaluation of RV size and function, being able to detect serial changes in these parameters. MSCT has a very good spatial resolution being useful in selected, complex cases, but it is limited by the radiation involved.

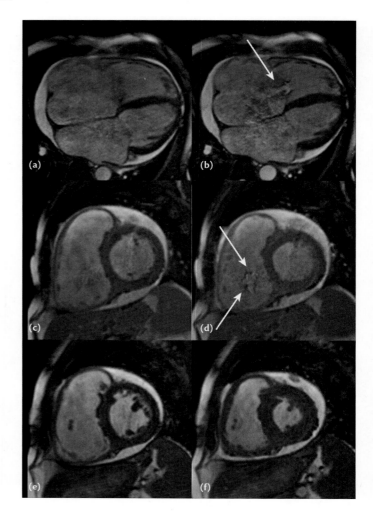

Fig. 14.17 Still frame cine CMR images in diastole (a, c, e) and systole (b, d, f) in a patient with severe TR showing a broad central regurgitant jet visualized as signal void (b, d) (arrows). There is severe RV dilatation (RV EDV 416 ml, RV ESV 250 ml) with impaired RV systolic function (RV EF 40%), and enlarged atria (right atrium 86 cm², left atrium 60 cm²). A mild to moderate pericardial effusion can also be seen (see 📹 Videos 14.35-14.37).
Courtesy of Dr Anca Florian, Robert-Bosch KH Stuttgart.

Table 14.5 Echocardiographic grading of pulmonary regurgitation severity [12]

Parameters	Mild	Moderate	Severe
Quantitative			
PV morphology	Normal	Normal/abnormal	Abnormal
Colour flow PR jet	Small (<10 mm)	Intermediate	Large, with a wide origin, may be brief in duration (rapid equalization of pressure between PA and RV)
CW signal of PR jet	Faint/slow deceleration	Dense/variable	Dense/steep deceleration, early termination of diastolic flow
Pulmonary vs aortic flow by PW	Normal or slightly increased	Intermediate	Greatly increased
Semi-quantitative			
Vena contracta width (mm)	Not defined	Not defined	Not defined
Quantitative			
EROA by 3D (mm²) Proposed cut-off values (41)	Not defined <20	Not defined 21–115	Not defined >115
Regurgitant volume by 3D (ml) Proposed cut-off values (41)	Not defined <15	Not defined 15–115	Not defined >115

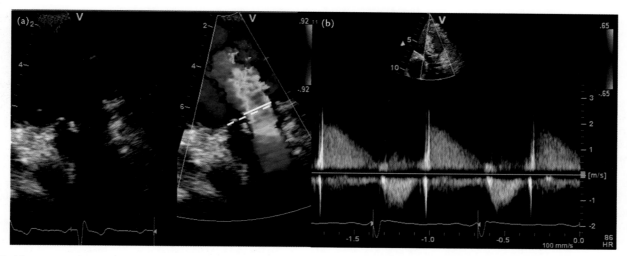

Fig. 14.18 (a) TTE, 2D and colour Doppler examination of the PV (diastolic frame). There is lack of leaflet coaptation in 2D and a broad jet of PR at colour Doppler (see 🎬 Video 14.38). (b) CW Doppler through the RV outflow tract in the same patient. Signal density of the regurgitant jet (similar to the forward flow) and the shape of the diastolic PR signal (with steep deceleration) suggest severe PR.
Reprinted with permission from Popescu BA, Ginghina C [27].

References

1. Taramasso M, Vanermen H, Maisano F, et al. The growing clinical importance of secondary tricuspid regurgitation. *J Am Coll Cardiol* 2012; 59: 703–10.

2. Filipoiu FM. Cordul. *Atlas Explicitat si Comentat.* Editura Prior & Books, Bucharest, 2012: 148–57.

3. Feigenbaum H, Armstrong W, Ryan T. *Tricuspid and Pulmonary Valves in Feigenbaum's Echocardiography.* Lippincott, Williams and Wilkins, Philadelphia, 2005: 353–74.

4. Fukuda S, Saracino G, Matsumura Y, et al. Three-dimensional geometry of the tricuspid annulus in healthy subjects and in patients with functional tricuspid regurgitation: a real-time, 3-dimensional echocardiographic study. *Circulation* 2006; 114: 1492–8.

5. Ton-Nu TT, Levine R, Handschumacher MD, et al. Geometric determinants of functional tricuspid regurgitation: insights from 3-dimensional echocardiography. *Circulation* 2006; 114: 143–9.

6. Maffessanti F, Gripari P, Pontone G, et al. Three-dimensional dynamic assessment of tricuspid and mitral annuli using cardiovascular magnetic resonance. *Eur Heart J Cardiovasc Imaging* 2013; 14: 986–95.

7. Pierard L, Moonen M, Lancellotti P. *Valvular Regurgitation in The ESC Textbook of Cardiovascular Imaging.* Springer, London, 2010: 149–77.

8. Badano LP, Muraru D, Enriquez-Sarano M. Assessment of functional tricuspid regurgitation. *Eur Heart J* 2013; 34: 1875–85.

9. Vegas V, Meineri M. Three-dimensional transesophageal echocardiography is a major advance for intraoperative clinical management of patients undergoing cardiac surgery: a core review. *Anesthesia & Analgesia* 2010; 6: 1548–73.

10. Lancellotti P, Moura L, Pierard LA, et al. European Association of Echocardiography recommendations for the assessmentof valvular regurgitation. Part 2: mitral and tricuspid regurgitation (native valve disease). *Eur J Echocardiogr* 2010; 11: 307–32.

11. Rudski LG, Lai WW, Afilalo J, et al. Guideliness for the echocardiographic assessment of the right hearts in adults: a report from the American Society of Echocardiography. *J Am Soc Echocardiogr* 2010; 23: 685–713.

12. Lancelotti P, Tribouilloy C, Hagendorff A, et al. European Association of Echocardiography recommendations for the assessment of valvular regurgitation. Part 1: aortic and pulmonary regurgitation (native valve disease). *Eur J Echocardiogr* 2010; 11: 223–44.

13. Anwar AM, Geleijnse ML, Soliman OI, et al. Assessment of normal tricuspid valve anatomy in adults by real-time three-dimensional echocardiography. *Int J Cardiovasc Imaging* 2007; 23: 717–24.

14. Stankovic I, Claus P, Jasaityte R, et al. Imaging the tricuspid valve—do we really need 3D echo? *Eur Heart J Cardiovasc Imaging* 2012; Abstracts Supplement: i 144.

15. Flachskampf FA, Badano L, Daniel WG, et al. European Association of Echocardiography; Echo Committee of the European Association of Cardiothoracic Anaesthesiologists. Recommendations for transoesophageal echocardiography: update 2010. *Eur J Echocardiogr* 2010; 11: 557–76.

16. Lang RM, Badano LP, Tsang W et al. EAE/ASE Recommendations for image acquisition and display using three-dimensional echocardiography. *Eur Heart J Cardiovasc Imaging* 2012; 13: 1–46.

17. Vahanian A, Alfieri O, Andreotti F, et al. Guidelines on the management of valvular heart disease (version 2012): the Joint Task Force on the Management of Valvular Heart Disease of the European Society of Cardiology (ESC) and the European Association for Cardio-Thoracic Surgery (EACTS). *Eur Heart J* 2012; 33: 2451–96.

18. Cawley P, Maki JH, Otto CM. Cardiovascular magnetic resonance imaging for valvular heart disease: technique and validation. *Circulation* 2009; 119: 468–78.

19. Masci PG, Dymarkowski S, Bogaert J. Valvular heart disease: what does cardiovascular MRI add? *Eur Radiol* 2008; 18: 197–208.

20. Vogel-Claussen J, Pannu H, Spevak P, et al. Cardiac valve assessment with MR imaging and 64-section multi-detector row CT. *RadioGraphics* 2006; 26: 1769–84.

21. Garcia M. Evaluation of valvular heart disease by cardiac magnetic resonance and computer tomography. In: Bonow R, Otto C (eds). *Valvular Heart Disease.* Saunders, Elsevier; Philadelphia, 2009: 101–12.

22. Bruce CJ, Connolly HM. Right-sided valve disease deserves a little more respect. *Circulation* 2009; 119: 2726–34.

23. Popescu BA, Calin A. Stenoza tricuspidiana in Ginghina C. *Mic tratat de cardiologie*. Editura Academiei, Bucharest, 2010: 469–74.

24. Baumgartner H, Hung J, Bermejo J, et al. Echocardiographic assessment of valve stenosis: EAE/ASE recommendations for clinical practice. *Eur J Echocardiogr* 2009; 22: 1–23.

25. Anwar AM, Geleijnse ML, Soliman OI, et al. Evaluation of rheumatic tricuspid valve stenosis by real-time three-dimensional echocardiography. *Heart* 2007; 93: 363–64.

26. Myerson SG. Heart valve disease: investigation by cardiovascular magnetic resonance. *J Cardiovasc Magn Reson* 2012; 14: 7.

27. Popescu BA, Ginghina C. *Ecocardiografia Doppler*. Editura Medicala, Bucharest, 2011.

28. Baumgartner H, Bonhoeffer P, De Groot NM, et al. ESC Guidelines for the management of grown-up congenital heart disease (new version 2010). *Eur Heart J* 2010; 31: 2915–57.

29. Pennel D. Cardiovascular magnetic resonance. *Circulation* 2010; 121: 692–705.

30. Chen JJ, Manning MA, Frazier AA, et al. CT angiography of the cardiac valves: normal, diseased, and postoperative appearances. *RadioGraphics* 2009; 29: 1393–1412.

31. Song JM, Jang MK, Choi YS, et al. The vena contracta in functional tricuspid regurgitation: a real-time three-dimensional color doppler echocardiography study. *J Am Soc Echocardiogr* 2011; 24: 663–70.

32. Kim HK, Kim YJ, Park JS, et al. Determinants of the severity of functional tricuspid regurgitation. *Am J Cardiol* 2006; 98: 236–42.

33. Anwar AM, Soliman OI, Nemes A, et al. Value of assessment of tricuspid annulus: real time three-dimensional echocardiography and magnetic resonance imaging. *Int J Cardiovasc Imaging* 2007; 23: 701–5.

34. Shiran A, Sagie A. Tricuspid regurgitation in mitral valve disease incidence, prognostic implications, mechanism, and management. *J Am Coll Cardiol* 2009; 53: 401–8.

35. Dreyfus GD, Corbi PJ, Chan KM, Bahrami T. Secondary tricuspid regurgitation or dilatation: which should be the criteria for surgical repair? *Ann Thorac Surg* 2005; 79: 127–32.

36. Benedetto U, Melina G, Angeloni E, et al. Prophylactic tricuspid annuloplasty in patients with dilated tricuspid annulus undergoing mitral valve surgery. *J Thorac Cardiovasc Surg* 2012; 143: 632–8.

37. Van de Veire NR, Braun J, Delgado V, et al. Tricuspid annuloplasty prevents right ventricular dilatation and progression of tricuspid regurgitation in patients with tricuspid annular dilatation undergoing mitral valve repair. *J Thorac Cardiovasc Surg* 2011; 141: 431–9.

38. Min SY, Song JM, Kim JH, et al. Geometric changes after tricuspid annuloplasty and predictors of residual tricuspid regurgitation: a real time three-dimensional echocardiography study. *Eur Heart J* 2010; 31: 2871–80.

39. Fukuda S, Song JM, Gillinov AM, et al. Tricuspid valve tethering predicts residual tricuspid regurgitation after tricuspid annuloplasty. *Circulation* 2005; 111: 975–79.

40. Kim HK, Kim YJ, Park EA, et al. Assessment of haemodynamic effects of surgical correction for severe functional tricuspid regurgitation: cardiac magnetic resonance imaging study. *Eur Heart J* 2010; 31: 1520–28.

41. Pothineni KR, Wells BJ, Hsiung MC, et al. Live/real time three-dimensional transthoracic echocardiographic assessment of pulmonary regurgitation. *Echocardiography* 2008; 25: 911–7.

42. Vliegen HW, van Straten A, de Roos A, et al. Magnetic resonance imaging to assess the hemodynamic effects of pulmonary valve replacement in adults late after repair of tetralogy of Fallot. *Circulation* 2002; 106: 1703–7.

43. Therrien J, Provost Y, Merchant N, et al. Optimal timing for pulmonary valve replacement in adults after tetralogy of Fallot repair. *Am J Cardiol* 2005; 95: 779–82.

44. Oosterhof T, van Straten A, Vliegen HW, et al. Preoperative thresholds for pulmonary valve replacement in patients with corrected tetralogy of Fallot using cardiovascular magnetic resonance. *Circulation* 2007; 116: 545–51.

⮑ **For additional multimedia materials, please visit the online version of the book (⮑ http://www.esciacc.oxfordmedicine.com).**

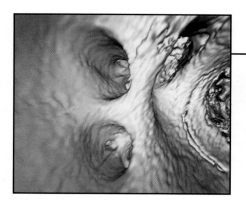

CHAPTER 15

Heart valve prostheses

Luigi P. Badano and Denisa Muraru

Contents

Prosthetic heart valves may be mechanical or bioprosthetic. Mechanical valves, which are composed primarily of metal or carbon alloys, are classified according to their design as ball-caged, single-tilting-disc, or bileaflet-tilting-disc valves (➲ Fig. 15.1). In ball-cage valves, the occluder is a sphere that is contained by a metal 'cage' when the valve is in its open position, and fills the orifice when the valve is in its closed position. In single-tilting-valves, the occluder is a single, circular disc that is constrained in its motion by a cage, a central strut, or a slanted slot in the valve ring, therefore it opens at an angle less than 90° to the sewing ring plane. In bileaflet-tilting-disc valves there are two occluders, two semicircular discs that open forming three orifices, a central one and two lateral ones.

Biological tissue valves prostheses may be heterografts, which are composed of porcine, bovine, or equine tissue (valvular or pericardial), or homografts, which are preserved human aortic valves. Heterografts include stented and stentless bioprostheses (➲ Fig. 15.2). In stented valves, the biological tissue of the valve is mounted on a rigid stent (plastic or metallic) covered with fabric. Conversely, stentless bioprostheses use the patient's native aortic root as the valve stent. The absence of a stent and sewing ring cuff make it possible to implant a larger valve for a given native annulus size, resulting in a larger effective orifice area (EOA).

Heart valve prostheses' specifications and functional parameters

The size of mechanical and stented biological valve prostheses can be described using geometrical and functional parameters. Geometrical parameters are measurements obtained by manufacturers and usually reported in product brochures. The sewing ring diameter (measured in mm) is the largest diameter of the sewing cuff (➲ Fig. 15.3). The internal orifice diameter (IOD, in mm) is the internal diameter of the stent. From the IOD, the geometric orifice area of the prosthesis (the internal valve area theoretically available for the bloodstream to pass through) can be calculated using the geometric formula:

$$\pi \cdot (IOD/2)^2. \qquad 15.1$$

The external diameter (ED, in mm) is the diameter of the stent plus fabric. From the ED, the mounting area of the prosthesis (the area that the prosthesis will occupy within the patient's native annulus) may be calculated using the geometric formula:

$$\pi \cdot (ED/2)^2. \qquad 15.2$$

The latter is rarely reported in product brochures, but it is needed in order to calculate the ratio between geometric orifice area and mounting area. This ratio depends on the prosthesis design and gives an indication of the space subtracted from the native annulus 'flow area' by the fixed structures (stent and cuff) of the prosthesis. This ratio also depends on the implant technique used. Generally, for a totally intra-annular prosthesis, this ratio

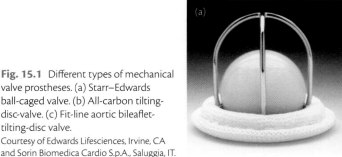

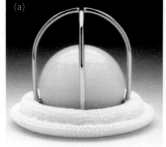

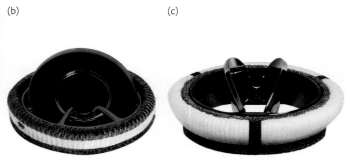

Fig. 15.1 Different types of mechanical valve prostheses. (a) Starr–Edwards ball-caged valve. (b) All-carbon tilting-disc-valve. (c) Fit-line aortic bileaflet-tilting-disc valve.
Courtesy of Edwards Lifesciences, Irvine, CA and Sorin Biomedica Cardio S.p.A., Saluggia, IT.

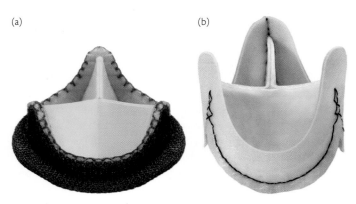

Fig. 15.2 Biological tissue valves. (a) Stented Soprano pericardial valve. (b) Stentless Solo pericardial valve.
Courtesy of Sorin Biomedica Cardio S.p.A., Saluggia, IT.

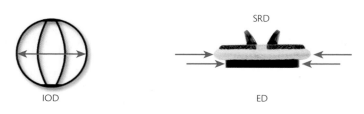

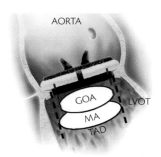

Fig. 15.3 Geometrical valve size specifications. The sewing ring diameter (SRD) is the maximum diameter of the sewing cuff. The external diameter (ED) is the diameter of the housing or housing plus fabric. From ED the area that the prosthesis will occupy within the patient annulus (mounting area, MA) is calculated (see text for details). The internal orifice diameter (IOD) is the internal diameter of the housing. From IOD, the internal valve area theoretically available for bloodstream to pass through (geometric orifice area, GOA) is calculated (see text for details). LVOT, left ventricular outflow tract; TAD, native tissue annulus diameter.

is 40–70% [1], it increases to 80–85% for partially supra-annular prostheses, and reaches 100% (resulting in a maximization of blood flow) for totally supra-annular prostheses.

Functional parameters of prosthesis size include both *in vitro* and *in vivo* EOA. *In vitro* EOA can be measured under static hydrodynamic conditions at a variety of flow rates, or under dynamic conditions with variable pulsatile waveforms and flow rates. Estimates of static EOA for bioprostheses vary by as much as 100%, as the steady flow rate increases. Dynamic pulsatile *in vitro* EOA data are non-standardized, unreproducible, and unavailable. Therefore, *in vitro* EOA is generally unsuitable for assessment of the clinical effect of prosthesis size [2]. *In vivo* EOA is always smaller than the geometric orifice area and corresponds to the smallest area of the jet passing through the prosthesis as it exits the valve (vena contracta). Both the shape of the inlet and the size of the orifice affect the ratio between the geometric and EOA (coefficient of orifice contraction) [3].

For clinical purposes, the size of a prosthesis is reported as labelled prosthesis size (i.e. 19 mm, 21 mm, etc.). However, labelled size is often the approximation of an integer number (i.e. labelled size = bicarbon 21 mm; actual size = 21.2 mm). The International Organization for Standardization (ISO) specification concerning the valve size labelling of heart valve prostheses (ISO/CD 5840) recommended that labelled prosthesis size should represent the tissue annulus diameter (TAD) of the patient into whom the valve is intended to be implanted.

Assessment of prosthetic valve function

Several imaging techniques can be used to assess valve prosthesis function.

Echocardiography

Echocardiography remains the imaging technique of choice for the assessment of prostheses' function. Two-dimensional transthoracic echocardiography can be used to assess sewing ring stability and occluder motion (➲ Fig. 15.4). The mechanical valves have a specific pattern of echoes that can help identify the type of prosthesis. A ball-caged valve will display a cage and the moving echo of the ball on the ventricular side. A single echo moving

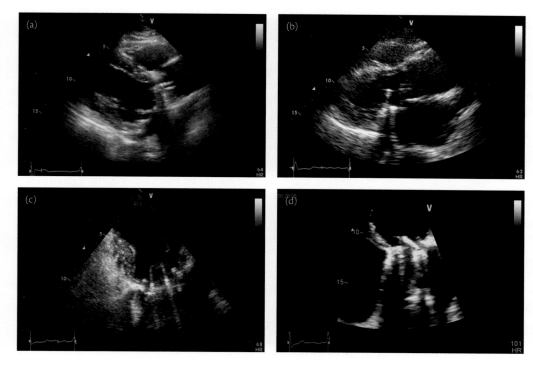

Fig. 15.4 Two-dimensional echocardiographic characteristic features of mechanical heart valve: (a) bileaflet tilting-disc valve in aortic position visualized from parasternal approach; (b) single tilting-disc valve in mitral position visualized from parasternal approach; (c) bileaflet tilting-disc valve in mitral position visualized from apical approach; (d) single tilting-disc valve in mitral position visualized from apical approach.

up and down on the ventricular side can be seen with tilting-disc valve (⊃ Fig. 15.4), and the two leaflets of the bileaflet valve can be visualized separately (⊃ Fig. 15.4). The transthoracic echocardiography has a higher sensitivity for demonstrating the motion of the two leaflets of a bileaflet-tilting disc valve in mitral position than for the aortic position. The heterograft bioprostheses (porcine or pericardial) are trileaflet structures. The two-dimensional and M-mode appearance of the leaflets of these valves is similar to those of the native aortic valve, which is a box-like opening in systole, if implanted in aortic position (⊃ Fig. 15.5), or diastole, if implanted in mitral position. However, similar to what happens with mechanical prosthesis, the sewing ring and the struts may limit the visualization of the leaflets. The stentless bioprosthetic aortic valves have an appearance similar to that of native aortic valves except for increased echogenicity in the aortic root (⊃ Fig. 15.5). An aortic homograft appears similar to a native aortic valve except for an increased thickness in the left ventricular outflow tract (LVOT) and the ascending aorta.

However, mechanical valve prostheses and stented bioprostheses are often difficult to visualize (prosthesis in aortic position more difficult than in mitral position) due to the presence of artificial components with far different acoustic properties than the surrounding cardiac tissue, which creates reverberations, artefacts and acoustic shadowing. The latter can be overcome with the use of the transoesophageal (TOE) approach and casting the shadowing in the opposite direction [4] (⊃ Fig. 15.6). In addition, since all echo systems are calibrated to measure distance on the velocity of ultrasound in the human body tissue, the presence of prosthetic material may alter the displayed size and location of the prosthesis, and can distort the appearance of its components.

Transthoracic Doppler echocardiography, by providing a complete haemodynamic assessment, is pivotal in assessing a valve prosthesis' function. The Bernoulli equation is used to calculate the peak and mean pressure gradients from the Doppler velocities. Although many assumptions are made in the derivation of the Bernoulli equation, an excellent correlation has been obtained

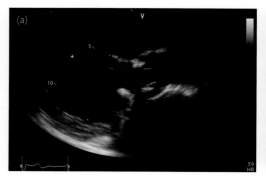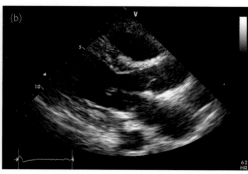

Fig. 15.5 Two-dimensional echocardiographic characteristics of bioprostheses: stented bioprosthesis (Mosaic 23 mm) in the aortic position visualized from parasternal approach (a) and stentless bioprosthesis (Freedom 21-mm) in the aortic position visualized from parasternal approach (b).

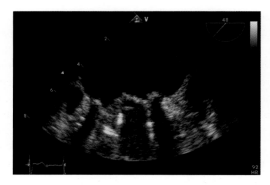

Fig. 15.6 Transoesophageal echocardiographic visualization of a normofunctioning bileaflet tilting-disc prosthesis in the mitral position. The metallic leaflet is visualized in systole in the closing position. An intense acoustic shadowing due to the highly reflective metallic leaflets can be appreciated on the left ventricular side.

between gradients obtained simultaneously with cardiac catheterization and Doppler echocardiography. The continuity equation is used to calculate the aortic EOA.

In general, the same principles used in native aortic valves are applicable to assess valve prosthesis function using echocardiography. However, the fluidodynamic characteristics of prosthetic valves are not exactly the same as those of native valves and proper formulae should be used to calculate reliable transprosthetic gradients and EOA. Although good agreement between Doppler-derived and catheter-derived pressure gradients for a variety of different valve prostheses has been reported (◯ Table 15.1), some investigators have found significant overestimation of pressure gradients by Doppler in the prosthetic valves [5, 6]. There are several reasons that may explain these apparent discrepancies between Doppler and catheter gradients. The presence of pressure recovery downstream from the prosthesis has been suggested as one potential cause [5]. Localized pressure gradients that may be recorded by selectively sampling velocity in the narrow 'slitlike' central orifice of some bileaflet-tilting-disc prostheses [5], but not

in all [7]. However, the most important cause of transprosthetic gradient overestimation using Doppler echocardiography is a methodological one.

Routine echocardiographic assessment of gradients through stenotic native or prosthetic valves in the aortic position is usually performed using the 'simplified' ($4V_2^2$), instead of the 'modified' Bernoulli equation:

$$[4 (V_2^2 - V_1^2)] \qquad 15.3$$

(the former does not take into account the velocity (V_1) in the LVOT). However, the simplified Bernoulli equation ignores the viscous friction and the energy required to overcome the initial forces caused by flow acceleration found in a pulsatile system and is only reliable for flow that is [8]:

(1) through a restrictive orifice (negligible inertial component); and

(2) with V_2 much greater than V_1.

Since new normofunctioning prosthetic valves (especially stentless and stented supra-annular bioprostheses) do not have a restrictive orifice and they show very low V_2 values (usually less than 2 m/s), the use of the simplified Bernoulli equation causes a significant overestimation of transprosthetic gradients also in patients with $V_1 < 1$ m/s. This overestimation may be negligible in stenotic native valves with a restrictive orifice and high V_2 values (from +3 to +5%), but it is clinically significant in normofunctioning bioprosthetic stentless valves (from +13 to +19%) [9].

In vivo EOA for prostheses in the aortic position is calculated from the continuity equation. The continuity equation assumes that flow coming into the narrowed orifice has a flat profile. The actual flow profile varies between prostheses, with mechanical tilting-disc prostheses having the greatest variance from a flat profile, and bioprosthetic valves showing a nearly flat profile of transprosthetic flow [1].

Similarly to stenotic native valves, the main source of error in calculating prosthesis EOA with the continuity equation is the measurement of the LVOT diameter. Due to the potential

Table 15.1 Studies that have validated transprosthetic gradients measured by Doppler echocardiography with cardiac catheterization data

Author, reference	Valve type/Position	Type of study (patients)	r	SEE (mmHg)
Sagar, *J Am Coll Cardiol* 1986; 7: 681	Hancock, Bjork–Shiley/Mitral	*in vivo* (19)	0.93	2.5
	Hancock, Bjork–Shiley/Aortic	*in vivo* (11)	0.94	7.4
Wilkins, *Circulation* 1986; 74: 786	Starr–Edwards, Bjork–Shiley, porcine/Mitral	*in vivo* (11)	0.96	
Burstow, *Circulation* 1989; 80: 504	Not specified/Aortic	*in vivo* (20)	0.94	3
	Not specified/Mitral	*in vivo* (20)	0.97	1.2
Baumgartner, *Circulation* 1990; 82: 1467	St Jude	*in vitro*	0.98	1.9
	Hancock	*in vitro*	0.98	1.4
Stewart, *J Am Coll Cardiol* 1991; 18: 769	Bioprostheses	*in vitro*	0.78–0.98	
Baumgartner, *J Am Coll Cardiol* 1992; 19: 324	St Jude	*in vitro*	0.98	2.0
	Medtronic–Hall	*in vitro*	0.99	0.5
	Starr–Edwards	*in vitro*	0.97	2.0
	Hancock	*in vitro*	0.99	1.5

errors (inner-edge-to-inner-edge measurement, foreshortening of left ventricular outflow tract) and limitations (interference of prosthesis shadowing) it was suggested that the nominal size of the replacement heart valve should be substituted for the direct measurement of the LVOT when applying the continuity equation [10, 11]. The assumption is that, regardless of manufacturer or model, all valves of a certain nominal size are interchangeable for a given patient tissue annulus diameter. However, this is not true. Studies attempting to assess the size of a valve by echocardiography show good agreement between LVOT diameter and valve size for stentless valves [12]. Conversely, as much as 2 mm difference was shown in one study on mechanical and stented biological valves [13]. Another study found a 95% confidence interval from –8.5 to +5.1 mm between LVOT measured by transthoracic echocardiography and nominal valve size [14]. Therefore, the external diameter of the prosthesis (if known), but not the labelled size, can be used as a surrogate for LVOT diameter. However, the external diameter of the prosthesis is rarely available, so the most convenient way is still to measure LVOT diameter during the baseline echocardiographic assessment of a given valve and then to use this constant value during follow-up echocardiographic controls.

Although the Hatle's method has been proposed to calculate the EOA for prosthetic valves in mitral position, and it should be theoretically applicable to such valves since pressure half-time is a physiologic measure of obstruction and does not require assumptions about inlet geometry and flow rate [15], there is now good evidence that the Hatle's method is not valid in normofunctioning prosthetic valves in mitral position [7, 16]. In such valves, with relatively large orifice areas, the pressure half-time is more dependent on other factors such as heart rate, transmitral pressure gradient at onset of diastole, stroke volume, and left atrial and ventricular compliance, than on prosthetic orifice area.

A complete echocardiographic study should include estimation of pressure peak and mean gradients, valve area, and mean transprosthetic flow rate. However, there are some peculiarities that should be taken into account to correctly interpret echocardiographic results.

First, prostheses are not all equal. Different types (i.e. mechanical bileaflet, mechanical tilting-disc, stented bioprosthesis, stentless bioprosthesis) show markedly different haemodynamics. For example, an EOA of 1.1 cm² may be normal in a 21-mm single-tilting-disc prosthesis [16], but it will be a pathologic finding in a 21-mm stentless bioprosthesis ($\circlearrowright$ Table 15.2). Different models of the same type show markedly different haemodynamics despite having the same labelled size and being made of the same tissue (i.e. bovine pericardium) [17]. The 21-mm Hancock II stented bioprosthesis shows a mean EOA (1.2±0.7 cm²) [18], which is significantly lower than the Pericarbon (1.5±0.4 cm²) [19]. Different sizes of the same valve model and type show different haemodynamics ($\circlearrowright$ Table 15.2) [17]. Therefore, the important message to the echocardiographer is the need to know the model, type, and size of the implanted valve in order to interpret echocardiographic haemodynamic data correctly.

Second, reference values reported in the literature about the haemodynamic performance of different valve prostheses represent a poor reference for the individual patient. This is particularly true for biological prostheses. Estimates of bioprosthesis *in vivo* EOA are particularly sensitive to cardiac output and blood pressure [20]. In addition, *in vivo* EOA of stentless bioprostheses has been observed to increase during the first year after implantation as haemodynamic data change and perivalvular hematoma and oedema resolve. Transprosthetic gradients are particularly sensitive to transprosthetic flow rate and change significantly with the haemodynamic state of the patient. Therefore, the second important message to the echocardiographer is to obtain a baseline full haemodynamic assessment of that prosthesis in a given patient together with his/her haemodynamic status (i.e. body surface area, cardiac rhythm, heart rate, blood pressure, haemoglobin level, and LV function) to use as a reference for interpreting follow-up studies.

The timing of baseline assessment of valve prosthesis haemodynamics is crucial. Ideally, it should be performed as soon as possible after the operation to make sure that the valve is actually normofunctioning (i.e. no tissue degeneration for biological valves or pannus formation for mechanical valves), but not too soon, in order to avoid misleading data. In patients undergoing aortic valve replacement, there is a relatively high output state immediately after the operation due to relative anaemia and sudden reduction of LV afterload, which affects transprosthetic gradients. Moreover, perivalvular oedema and haematoma may reduce prosthetic EOA. Finally, LV function will change significantly soon after aortic valve replacement due to regression of hypertrophy, and adaptation to the changed pre- and afterload conditions. Therefore, the optimal timing of the baseline assessment of valve prosthesis haemodynamics should be placed between the third and the sixth month (not later than 1 year) after surgery. The pre-discharge study should be used to assess post-operative LV function, exclude complications or early malfunction of the prosthesis, but not to assess normal function parameters of a certain valve in a given patient.

Follow-up examinations in asymptomatic patients without complications and with a 'normal' initial echocardiogram can be performed at yearly intervals and should consist of a detailed history and physical examination. Echocardiography should be performed whenever there is evidence of a new heart murmur, when there are doubts of prosthetic valve integrity or function, or there are concerns about ventricular or other valve function. There is no support in the literature for the strategy of performing an annual 'routine' Doppler echocardiogram in patients without complications [21].

Cinefluoroscopy

Cinefluoroscopy is a simple, rapid, inexpensive, and accurate technique to assess valve prosthesis function. The main indications for cinefluoroscopy are in patients with abnormally high aortic or mitral gradients or unusual regurgitant flow patterns observed with colour Doppler echocardiography.

Table 15.2 Published data about Doppler haemodynamic parameters of normofunctioning prosthetic valves in the aortic position

Type	Doppler parameter	Size (mm)									
		19	20	21	22	23	24	25	26	27	29
Single tilting-disc valves											
Starr–Edwards	GOA			1.41		1.67	1.79		1.94	2.16	2.57
(n = 79)	EOA			1.3		1.45	1.44		1.53	1.53	1.53
	Mean gr.			34±6		29±11	27±9		23±8	23±1	
Bjork–Shiley*	GOA	1.5		2		2.5		3.1		3.8	4.6
(n = 106)	EOA	0.7±0.2		1.1±0.1		1.6±0.3		2.0±0.4		2.6±0.4	
	Mean gr.	16±4		13±5		13±3		11±4		8±4	
Medtronic	GOA										
Hall (n = 108)	EOA			1.2±0.5		1.1±0.2		1.4±0.4		1.9±0.4	1.9±0.5
	Mean gr.			14±6		14±5		10±4		9±6	
Omnicarbon	GOA	1.63		2.11		2.55		3.14		3.80	3.80
(n = 49)	EOA			1.4±0.1		1.5±0.2		1.8±0.4		1.9±0.4	2.2±0.2
	Mean gr.			21±7		13±3		11±4		13±3	9±2
Allcarbon	GOA	1.5		2.0		2.5		3.1		3.8	4.5
(n = 83)	EOA	0.9±0.1		1.1±0.2		1.4±0.2		2.1±0.8		2.8±0.6	4.1±0.7
	Mean gr.	29±8		22±7		20±6		15±4		11±4	8±2
Bileaflet tilting-disc valves											
St Jude Medical	GOA	1.63		2.06		2.55		3.09		3.67	4.52
(n = 67)	EOA	1.0±0.2		1.3±0.2		1.3±0.3		1.8±0.4		2.4±0.6	2.7±0.3
	Mean gr.	17±7		14±5		16±6		13±6		11±5	7±1
St Jude Medical	EOA	1.7±0.2		2.2±0.3							
HP (n = 49)	Mean gr.	16±4		10±3							
Carbomedics	GOA	1.06		1.41		1.75		2.19		2.63	3.07
(n = 96)	EOA	1.0±0.4		1.5±0.3		1.6±0.3		2.0±0.4		2.4±0.5	2.6±0.4
	Mean gr.	19±6		12±4		10±4		8±4		9±3	6±3
Carbomedics Top-Hat	GOA										
(n = 65)	EOA	1±0.2		1.2±0.3		1.4±0.4					
	Mean gr.	20±2		17±6		13±4		11			
Duromedics Tekna	GOA	1.53		2.02		2.36		2.94		3.58	
(n = 90)	Mean gr.			8±5		7±2		5±2		6±3	
Bicarbon	GOA	1.76		2.27		2.83		3.45		4.14	5
(n = 166)	EOA	1.0±0.3		1.6±0.3		2.1±0.4		2.5±0.6		3.6±0.8	3.5±0.3
	Mean gr.	13±1		14±5		11±4		11±3		7±2	5±1
ATS Open Pivot	EOA	1±0.2		1.6±0.4		1.8±0.2		2.2±0.4		2.5±0.3	3.1±0.3
(n = 59)	Mean gr.	26±8		14±4		12±4		11±4		9±2	8±2

Type	Doppler parameter	Size (mm)									
		19	20	21	22	23	24	25	26	27	29
On X	EOA	1.5±0.2		1.7±0.4		2±0.6		2.4±0.8		3.2±0.6	
(n = 60)	Mean gr.	12±3		10±4		9±3		9±5		6±3	
Jyros (n = 23)	EOA				1.5		1.5		1.7		
	Mean gr.				11		11		8		
Stented bioprostheses											
Hancock I	EOA										
(n = 64)	Mean gr.					12±4		11±2		10±3	
Hancock II	EOA	1.2±0.3				1.4±0.2		1.5±0.2		1.6±0.2	1.6±0.2
(n = 376)	Mean gr.	15±4				17±7		3 17±7		–	–
Bio Medical°	EOA			1.3±0.4		1.6±0.6		2.1±0.7		3.2	
	Mean gr.			9±4		8±2		7±5		6	
Carpentier–Edwards	EOA	0.9±0.2		1.5±0.3		1.7±0.5		1.9±0.5		2.3±0.5	2.8±0.5
Porcine (n = 419)	Mean gr.	26±8		17±6		16±6		13±4		12±6	10±3
Carpentier–Edwards	EOA	1.2±0.1		1.5±0.4		1.8±0.3		–		–	
Pericardial (n = 75)	Mean gr.	24±9		20±9		2.3±0.5		9±2		6	
Carpentier–Edwards	EOA	1.1±0.1		1.1±0.2							
Supra-annular (n = 23)	Mean gr.			14±5							
Medtronic Intact	EOA			1.6±0.4		1.7±0.4		1.9±0.3		2.2±0.2	2.4±0.5
(n = 243)	Mean gr	24±9		19±8		19±6		16±6		15±4	16±2
Medtronic Mosaic	EOA			1.6±0.7		2.1±0.8		2.1±1.6			
(n = 279)	Mean gr.			12±7		12±7		10±5		9	
Mitroflow	EOA	1.1±o0.2									
(n = 21)	Mean gr.	10±3		15		8±3		11±7		7±2	
Pericarbon More	EOA	1.2±0.3		1.5±0.4		1.8±0.5					
(n = 22)	Mean gr.	23±9		18±8		16±5					
Soprano	EOA				1.9±0.5		2.1±0.5				
(n = 77)	Mean gr.				7±4		7±4				
Ionescu–Shiley	EOA	1.2±0.2									
(n = 95)	Mean gr.	20±9		15±2		10±3				9±6	

(Continued)

Type	Doppler parameter	Size (mm)									
		19	20	21	22	23	24	25	26	27	29
Stentless bioprostheses											
Toronto SPV	EOA	1.3±0.38		1.2±0.7	1.2	1.6±0.8		1.6±0.4		2.0±0.4	
(n = 554)	Mean gr.	8±4	5	8±4		7±4		6±4		5±2	
Medtronic Freestyle	EOA			1.6±0.3		1.9±0.5		2.0±0.4		2.5±0.5	
(n = 369)	Mean gr.	13		8±3		7±3		5±2		5±2	
O'Brien Angell	EOA			1.2±0.1		1.1±0.3		1.6±0.2		2.1±1.2	
(n = 50)	Mean gr.			15±8		19±13		18±13		12±7	
O'Brien Angell				1.6±0.6		2.4±0.2		2.9±0.9			
Supra-annular (n= 50)				9±1		8±1		9±1		7±1.4	
Cryolife O'Brien	EOA	1.3±0.1		1.6±0.6		2.2		2.3		2.7	
(n = 329)	Mean gr.	12±5		10±2		9		8		7	
Edwards Prima	EOA	1±0.3		1.3±0.3		1.5±0.5		1.7±0.6		2±0.6	2.5±0.5
(n = 253)	Mean gr.	15±7		16±11		12±5		11±9		7±4	5±5
Biocor	EOA			1.4±0.5		1.6±0.4		1.9±0.5			
(n = 331)	Mean gr.			18±4		19±7		18±7		18±2	
Biocor Extended	EOA	1.3±0.4		1.6±0.3		1.8±0.3					
(n = 50)	Mean gr.	10±4		8±3		8±2					
Homograft	EOA			2.1±1.3		3.6		2.4±0.7		2.6±1	
(n = 27)	Mean gr.			13±1		10		8±2		12±1	

*monostrut; GOA = geometric orifice area provided by the manufacturer in cm²; EOA = effective orifice area (continuity equation) in cm² ; Mean gr. = mean transprosthetic gradient in mmHg; *n* = examined patients.

The cinefluoroscopic exam usually begins by determining the valve's rotational orientation with a view perpendicular to the valve plane. By positioning the image intensifier in the right anterior oblique cranial position, the view is roughly perpendicular to either the aortic or mitral valve plane. Occasionally, a left anterior oblique caudal view is required to image the mitral valve. As an example, in a normally functioning bileaflet-tilting disc valve, two parallel lines appear and disappear intermittently (➲ Fig. 15.7b). If only one or if neither of the lines fails to appear or disappear, valve leaflet motion may be restricted or one leaflet has escaped. Then we should obtain a side view to assess leaflet opening and closing angles. To obtain this view, the image intensifier is moved longitudinally 90°, usually caudally and transversely to a position in line with the valve leaflet axis of rotation. Opening and closing angles are defined as the distance between the valve housing and the disc at its full opening and closing in single-disc valves (➲ Fig. 15.7a), and as the distance between leaflets in the fully open and closed positions for bileaflet valves (➲ Fig. 15.7b). ➲ Table 15.3 lists the approximate normal opening and closing angles of several heart valve prostheses. Deviation from the listed angles or differences between the open or closed angle of one leaflet relative to the other in bileaflet valves may indicate restricted leaflet motion. A slight asynchrony of leaflet motion is normal, especially in valves in mitral position.

Although it cannot visualize the leaflet of bioprostheses, it is very useful to assess the excursion of occluders in mechanical valves, a diminished motion of the disc or poppet suggest obstruction of the prosthesis from thrombus or ingrowth of tissue (➲ Fig. 15.8) [22]. Conversely, excessive tilt or rocking of the sewing ring is consistent with partial dehiscence of the valve (➲ Fig. 15.9).

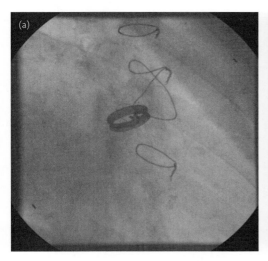

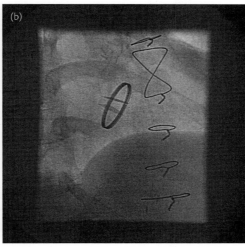

Fig. 15.7 Cinefluoroscopic side view of an Allcarbon single tilting-disc (a) and a St Jude Medical bileaflet tilting-disc (b) valve in open position. The disc of the Allcarbon valve forms an angle of 60° with the housing plane. The two hemidiscs of the St Jude Medical form a 10° angle. (See text for details.)

Table 15.3 Cinefluoroscopic opening and closing angles of commonly used normofunctioning mechanical heart valves (see text for details on how to measure angles)

Heart valve prosthesis	Specification	Opening angle (°)	Closing Angle (°)
Bileaflet-tilting disc valves			
St Jude Medical	19–25 mm	10	120
	27–33 mm	10	130
Carbomedics		12	118
Bicarbon		22	138
Edwards–Duromedics	Aortic	27	148
	Mitral	35	148
Jyros Valve		22	111
Single-tilting disc valves			
Bjork–Shiley		60	0
Medtronic–Hall	Aortic	75	0
	Mitral	70	0
Allcarbon		60	NA
Omniscience		80	12

NA, not available.

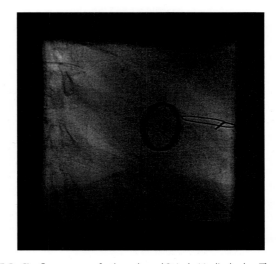

Fig. 15.8 Cinefluoroscopy of a thrombosed St Jude Medical valve. The left-sided leaflet is stuck in closed position during the entire cardiac cycle indicative of valve obstruction by a thrombus.

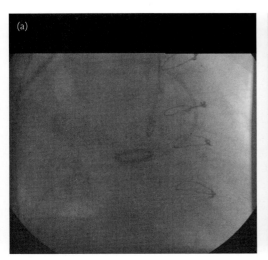

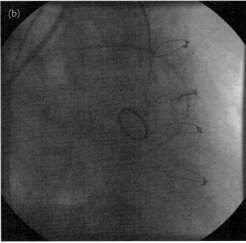

Fig. 15.9 Cine-angiography in a patient with partial dehiscence of a mechanical prosthesis in the aortic position. An excessive motion of the prosthetic housing from diastole (a) to systole (b) can be readily noticed.

Cardiac catheterization

Since cardiac catheterization is an invasive technique, it is indicated only when the information obtained by non-invasive techniques is inconclusive. With cardiac catheterization, the transprosthetic pressure gradients and flow can be measured and EOA calculated. A catheter can be passed safely through the orifice of a bioprosthesis without adverse effects. However, the catheter may become entrapped in the orifice of a single-tilting disc, sometimes requiring immediate surgical removal, or cause substantial valvular regurgitation if placed through the orifice of ball-caged valve.

Cardiac magnetic resonance

The low cost and wide availability of echocardiography makes it the primary clinical tool for the assessment of valvular heart disease and prostheses. However, cardiac magnetic resonance (CMR) may play a complementary role when transthoracic acoustic windows are poor and a TEE approach is undesirable. Therefore, its role is marginal when compared to ultrasounds. In the assessment of valve prostheses, CMR is limited due to the focal artefacts and signal loss relative to distortion of the magnetic field by the metal contained in the prostheses [23]. The artefacts are least pronounced on spin-echo images and more pronounced with gradient-echo cines. On the contrary, when the metal components are absent (as in biological valves), the CMR exam is similar to that performed on a native valve. However, incompatible prostheses to CMR are very rare. The major limitations of CMR for valve assessment are spatial and temporal resolution still sub-optimal and the need for a regular cardiac rhythm (⊃ Fig. 15.10).

Cardiac multi-detector computerized tomography

Cardiac multi-detector computerized tomography (MDCT) is an emerging technique in non-invasive cardiac imaging. Using data recorded during the cardiac cycle, it is possible to reconstruct multiple incremental datasets throughout the R–R interval. These datasets can be sequentially combined to provide functional imaging in a cine loop that allows evaluation of valvular leaflet morphology

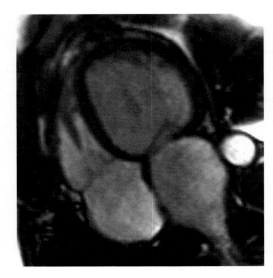

Fig. 15.10 Allcarbon single-disc prosthesis in mitral position. Horizontal long-axis steady-state free-precession cine magnetic resonance imaging.

and function (⊃ Fig. 15.11a and b). Even though its role is expanding in the evaluation of cardiac diseases, there is no clear indication for the use of MDCT for the assessment of valve diseases and prostheses. Moreover, concerns have been raised on the radiation burden of MDCT scanning. In fact, it has been estimated that about 0.4% of all cancers in the United States may be attributable to the radiation from MDCT studies. Therefore, the lack of a clear clinical benefit of CT for the assessment of prosthetic valve diseases should be weighed on the potential detrimental long-term risks.

Valve prostheses' normal function and dysfunction

Normal anterograde flow

From what has been written in the previous sections on heart valve prostheses' specifications and functional parameters (see also ⊃ Fig. 15.3), it is easy to understand why, compared to native valves, all normally functioning heart valve prostheses are inherently stenotic.

Fig. 15.11 St Jude Medical bileaflet valve in the mitral position. Sixty-four section multi-detector row CT scans show the mechanical bileaflet valve during diastole (left panel). A reconstructed 3-dimensional CT image using volumetric rendering method showing the same valve (right panel). Courtesy of Andrew Wood, Consultant Radiologist, University Hospital of Wales.

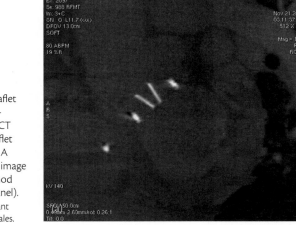

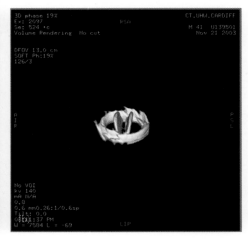

Table 15.4 Published data about Doppler haemodynamic parameters of normofunctioning prosthetic valves in the mitral position

Type	Doppler parameters	Size (mm) 23	25	27	29	31	33
Single tilting-disc prostheses							
Bjork– Shiley*	GOA	2.5	3.1	3.8	4.6	4.6	
(n = 237)	PHT	115	99±27	89±27	79±17	70±14	
	Mean gr.		6±2	5±2	3±1	2±2	
Medtronic-Hall	GOA	2.54	3.14	3.80	4.52		4.52
(n = 47)	PHT		78	69±15	77±17		
	Mean gr.		5±3	4±2	3±1		3±1
Omnicarbon	GOA	2.55	3.14	3.8	3.8	4.52	4.52
(n = 140)	PHT		102±16	105±33	120±40	134±31	
	Mean gr.	6±2	5±2	5±2	4±1	4±2	4
Allcarbon	GOA		3.1	3.8	4.5	4.5	
(n = 73)	PHT		105±29	89±14	85±23	88±27	
	Mean gr.		5±1	4±1	4±1	4±1	
Bileaflet tilting-disc prostheses							
St Jude Medical	GOA	2.55	3.09	3.67	4.52	5.18	
(n = 40)	PHT	160	76±4	72±11	74±15	71±14	
	EOA*	1.03	1.4±0.2	1.7±0.2	1.8±0.2	2.0±0.3	
	Mean gr.	4	3±1	5±2	3±1	4±2	
Duromedics	GOA			3.58			
(n = 69)	PHT			87±15	89±25	86±12	85
	Mean gr.			5±3	3±1	3±1	2
Carbomedics	GOA	1.75	2.19	2.63	3.07	3.07	3.07
(n = 75)	PHT	104	81±10	78±19	67±10	83±26	79±18
	EOA*	1.3	2.2±0.5	2.1±0.6	2.1±0.5	1.9±0.9	2.3±0.7
	Mean gr.	7	4±2	4±2	3±1	3±1	3±2
Bicarbon	GOA		3.45	4.14	5	5	5
(n = 68)	PHT		67±1	84±27	81±18	81±15	55
	Mean gr.		5±3	4±1	5±2	4±1	7
On X	PHT						
(n = 33)	Mean gr.		5±2	5±2	5±2	5±2	
Stented bioprostheses							
Medtronic–Intact	GOA		1.34	1.51	1.65	1.86	
(n = 26)	EOA*		1.4±0.1	1.5±0.1	1.6±0.1	1.8±0.2	
	Mean gr.		8±2	5±2	4±1	4±1	

(Continued)

Type	Doppler parameters	Size (mm) 23	25	27	29	31	33
Hancock I	PHT				115±20	95±17	90±12
(n = 46)	Mean gr.			5±2	2±1	5±2	4±2
Hancock II	PHT				105±63	81±23	
(n = 54)	Mean gr.			5±2	3±1	4±1	
Hancock pericardial	PHT				105±36	81±23	
(n = 22)	Mean gr.				3±1	4±1	
Ionescu–Shiley	PHT				80±30	79±15	75±19
(n = 45)	Mean gr.				3±1	3±1	4±1
Carpentier–Edwards	PHT			100	110±15	90±11	80
(n = 12)	Mean gr.			3.6	5±2	4±1	1
Mitroflow	PHT		90	90±20	102±21	91±22	
(n = 24)	Mean gr.		7	3±1	4±2	4±1	

*monostrut; GOA = geometric orifice area provided by the manufacturer in cm²; EOA = effective orifice area (continuity equation) in cm²; Mean gr. = mean transprosthetic gradient in mm Hg; n = examined patients.

Therefore, the anterograde velocities and pressure gradients across a normally functioning heart valve prosthesis will be higher, and prosthetic EOA will be smaller than the corresponding parameters measured in a normal native heart valve in the same position.

The expected velocities, pressure gradients, and EOAs depend on the specific type, size, and position of the heart valve prosthesis, and on transprosthetic flow rate across that valve (⮑ Tables 15.2 and 15.4). The strong dependency of pressure gradients on transprosthetic flow rate explains the wide standard deviation of reported values.

Different valve types show also different patterns of anterograde flow at colour Doppler examination (⮑ Fig. 15.12), which should be known because alterations of these patterns are early and sensitive markers of prosthetic valve obstruction, especially in single-disc tilting valves (⮑ Fig. 15.13).

Normal regurgitant flow

Normally functioning mechanical valves have physiologic regurgitant jets with a low velocity and limited penetration into the proximal chamber, generally less than 3 cm (⮑ Fig. 15.14). The normal regurgitant volume can be up to 10% of the stroke volume and very prominent, especially at TOE examination (⮑ Figs 15.15 and 15.16). The main reason for manufacturing these valves with a small amount of leakage is to prevent a sudden and irreversible occlusion. This physiologic regurgitation of mechanical valves is less likely to be detected in the mitral position than in the aortic position, which is due to the shielding of the regurgitant jets by the prosthetic valve in the mitral position. For the same reason, colour flow Doppler mapping is generally less sensitive than the continuous wave Doppler in detecting mechanical valve regurgitation in prostheses in the mitral position. Conversely, mitral valve 'physiologic' regurgitation patterns are visualized particularly well with transoesophageal colour Doppler because of its excellent image quality and spatial resolution.

The regurgitant flow (backflow) through a normally functioning valve prosthesis can be divided into 'closure backflow', occurring with the closure of the valve, and 'leakage backflow', occurring after the closure of the valve. The wide opening excursion of current mechanical valves may result in significant closure backflow as back pressure swings the leaflets through the long closing arc. Accordingly, a small jet occurring during the first 40–50 ms of systole can invariably be seen at TOE examination in a patient with tilting-disc mechanical valves. Bileaflet-tilting disc valves show two converging regurgitant jets from the pivot points (designed to reduce the likelihood of prosthesis thrombosis), one central jet and a variable number of peripheral jets [7]. Bjork–Shiley valves have a large central regurgitant jet originating from the central disc hole and a variable number of peripheral jets. The central regurgitant jet makes most of the colour Doppler signal but actually accounts for 30% of the regurgitant volume, the remaining 70% is from the less prominent peripheral jets. The Starr–Edwards ball-cage valves have very low regurgitant volumes because the ball completely occludes the primary flow orifice.

The stented bioprosthetic valves usually show only one centrally directed regurgitant jet originating from the central part of the valve. The prevalence of physiologic regurgitation across stented bioprosthetic valves is 19–25% and 26–30% for mitral and aortic positions, respectively. The newer generation stentless valves are being used frequently due to their excellent haemodynamic profile. The prevalence of mild aortic regurgitation with these valves may be up to 17% but the presence of significant amount of regurgitation is very low.

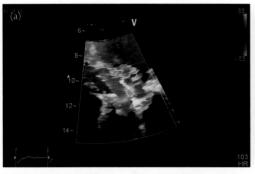

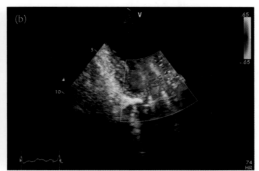

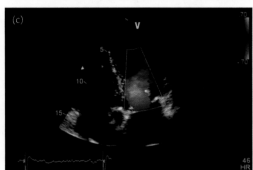

Fig. 15.12 Normal colour Doppler echocardiography appearance of anterograde flow across different valve types in the mitral position: a single tilting-disc valve with a major jet towards the lateral wall and a minor jet directed towards the canter of the cavity (a); a bileaflet-tilting disc valve in which flow passes through three well-separated orifices creating a near physiological flow pattern (b); and a bioprosthetic valve in which there is a single, central flow very similar to that of native valves (c).

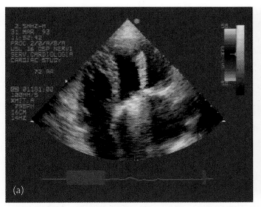

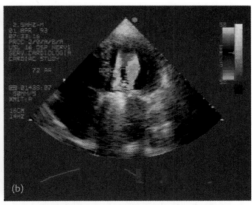

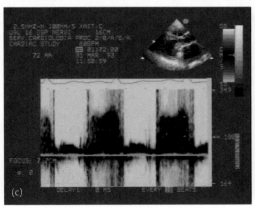

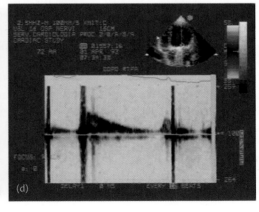

Fig. 15.13 Single tilting-disc valve thrombosis. Colour Doppler echocardiography at presentation (a) shows the absence of the central minor jet and increase of the velocity at CW spectral Doppler of the lateral major jet (c). After i.v. thrombolysis, the reappearance of the normal colour Doppler pattern of the anterograde flow (b) and a significance decrease of the anterograde flow velocity at CW spectral Doppler (d) was noted.

Prosthetic valve obstruction

Prosthetic heart valve obstruction may be caused by thrombus formation, fibrous tissue ingrowth (or pannus formation), or a combination of both, or by endocarditis. The aetiology may be difficult to determine and requires knowledge of the clinical presentation and findings on transthoracic and TOE echocardiography. The possibility of prosthetic valve thrombosis or endocarditis should be ruled out in patients with embolization.

Prosthetic heart valve thrombosis has a reported incidence of 13% in the first year in any valve position and even 20% for

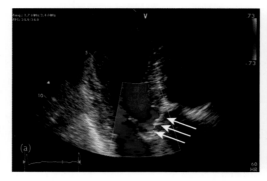 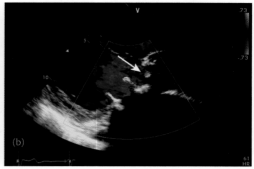

Fig. 15.14 Colour Doppler imaging during diastole showing the normal appearance of three 'physiologic' regurgitant jets (leakage backflow, white arrows) from a bileaflet valve (a) and a bioprosthesis (white arrow) (b) in aortic position.

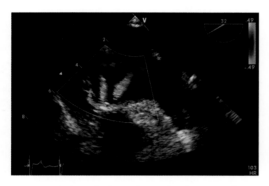

Fig. 15.15 Transoesophageal echocardiographic depiction of leakage backflow from a bileaflet valve in mitral position. These three jets represent the physiologic leakage from pivotal points (peripheral jets) and central closure line (central jets) and should not be interpreted as pathologic prosthetic regurgitation.

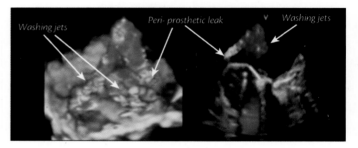

Fig. 15.16 Two- and three-dimensional colour Doppler imaging during diastole showing the normal appearance of 'physiologic' leakage jets as compared to a periprosthetic pathologic jet from a bileaflet valve in mitral position. Single tilting-disc valve obstruction. Colour Doppler echocardiography shows only one anterograde jet.

mechanical prostheses in the tricuspid position [24]. At any time, for prostheses in the mitral and/or aortic position, the overall incidence is 0.5–6% per patient-year, highest in the mitral position. The risk of thrombus in spite of adequate oral anticoagulation has been estimated at between 1% and 4% per year.

Echocardiography is the initial diagnostic approach in patients with suspected prosthetic heart valve obstruction. The increase of transprosthetic pressure gradients and a reduction of the effective area of the valve orifice, particularly in comparison with previous data in that patient, may be diagnostic (➲ Fig. 15.14). In experienced hands, transthoracic echocardiography can also detect an altered anterograde flow pattern at colour Doppler suggestive of intrinsic prosthesis obstruction (➲ Fig. 15.6). Increased anterograde transprosthetic flow velocities due to prosthesis obstruction should be differentiated from those due to high cardiac output state or coexisting prosthesis regurgitation, which may increase the anterograde volume flow rate across the prosthesis resulting in a high velocity and high transprosthetic gradients. However, in case of increased anterograde volume flow rate, the valve area remains relatively normal.

TOE is the most accurate diagnostic technique to assess alterations in the occlusive mechanism or the existence of thrombus on heart valve prostheses, especially for valves in the mitral position. Partial blockade of the prosthetic disc by thrombus can easily be detected by TOE as it usually holds it in a semi-open position, leaving an eccentric communication open in systole and diastole. The colour Doppler further facilitates more precise localization of prosthetic obstruction showing acceleration proximal to a stenosis and any associated degree

of regurgitation caused by lack of mobility of the occluder. In most cases, an echogenic mass is observed on the prosthetic valve surface at the site of the stenosis (➲ Fig. 15.17). Three-dimensional TOE allows a better spatial localization of the thrombus and its extension, as well as a more accurate assessment of the thrombotic burden (➲ Fig. 15.18). TOE may also be useful to differentiate thrombus from pannus as the mechanism of prosthetic obstruction. In prosthetic thrombosis, the movement of the disc is always abnormal, whereas in 40% of patients with obstruction due to pannus the mobility of the disc is normal. The visualization of an echogenic mass is almost diagnostic for thrombosis, but it can be detected in only 70% of obstructions caused by pannus. The echogenic characteristics of the mass are very important in differentiating thombus from pannus. The thrombus tends to be mobile, has soft ultrasound density, and is attached to the valve occluder (➲ Fig. 15.19). The pannus is firmly fixed, has bright ultrasound density, and is attached to the valve apparatus. In addition, finding of echo density around the sewing ring with bright reflective echoes and adequate anticoagulation heightens the suspicion of a pannus. A thrombotic mass is usually larger than pannus. In mitral prosthetic thrombosis the mass frequently extends into the atrial endocardial surface, a feature rarely seen in obstruction caused by pannus.

Prosthetic valve regurgitation

Echocardiography is highly useful in detecting prosthetic valvular regurgitation but with certain technical limitations, the most important of which are the problem of acoustic shadowing,

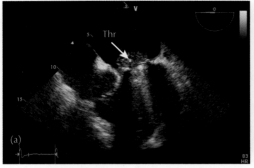

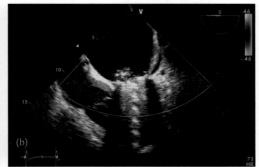

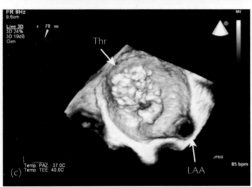

Fig. 15.17 Massive thrombosis on the atrial side of a bileaflet tilting-disc valve in the mitral position (white arrow) (a) at transoesophageal echocardiography. The presence of thrombus usually holds it in a semi-open position that creates an eccentric intra-prosthetic regurgitation (b). Real-time 3-dimensional transoesophageal echocardiography offers a better assessment of the extension and dimensions of the thrombus (c).

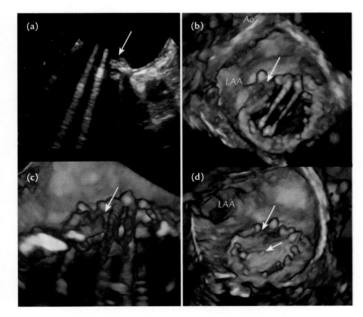

Fig. 15.18 Limited thrombosis partially obstructing one of the side holes of a bileaflet mechanical prosthetic valve in the mitral position. Transoesophageal 2-dimensional visualization of the thrombotic mass on the atrial side of the prosthesis (a) (arrow). A 3-dimensional *en face* view of the valve in the opening position from the atrial perspective allows a precise localization of the mass and its extension (b). Degree of obstruction and mobility of the thrombotic mass can be assessed more accurately with a longitudinal cut of the 3-dimensional dataset (c). An *en face* view of the prosthesis in the closing position from the atrial side allows the visualization of additional small thrombotic masses (d) (small arrow), which were not visualized using the 2-dimensional modality.

reverberation, and beam-width artefacts that occur when the ultrasound beam should traverse a reflective prosthesis before entering the cardiac chamber receiving the regurgitant jet. This occurrence may lead to non-visualization or underestimation of the severity of the regurgitation, especially with mechanical valves. In addition, colour artefacts are common in patients with heart valve prostheses and may alter detection of abnormal jets.

For prostheses in the aortic position, both parasternal and apical approaches may be useful since the ultrasound beam reaches the LVOT without crossing the prosthesis (⊃ Fig. 15.20). For prostheses in the mitral position, the parasternal approach may be helpful if a view in which the atrial side of the prosthesis can be obtained without acoustic shadowing. Apical views are rarely useful due to acoustic shadowing of the prostheses, even if in some cases a paraprosthetic regurgitant jet can be visualized from this approach (⊃ Fig. 15.21). Therefore, a transthoracic approach has a low sensitivity for detection and quantitation of prosthetic regurgitation of mitral valve prostheses and, usually, a transoesophageal approach is needed to visualize the left atrial size of the prosthesis. Sometimes colour Doppler may visualize proximal flow acceleration on the ventricular side of prostheses in the mitral position as a clue for raising the suspicion of a significant paravalvular regurgitation.

When a heart valve prosthesis regurgitation is detected, the first important question to the echocardiographer is whether 'physiologic' or pathologic prosthetic regurgitation is present. Differential characteristics of 'physiologic' from pathologic prosthetic valve regurgitation are uniform colour pattern rather than the mosaic flow disturbance, short extension into the receiving chamber (usually less than 2 cm), and the absence of supporting features like increased anterograde velocity, enlargement of cardiac chambers, and/or pulmonary hypertension.

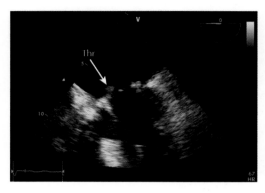

Fig. 15.19 Transoesophageal echocardiogram showing a thrombus (white arrow) visualized as a soft, small, and highly mobile mass on the atrial side of a mitral bioprosthetic valve entering the valve orifice during diastole.

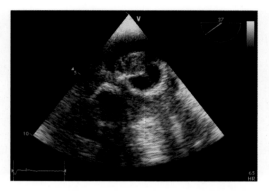

Fig. 15.20 Parasternal short-axis view by transthoracic approach showing a pathologic intra-prosthetic leakage of a bioprosthesis in the aortic position.

The most likely cause of intra-prosthetic pathologic regurgitation in mechanical valves is the incomplete closure of occluders due to pannus, ingrowth, thrombus formation, or vegetation (➲ Fig. 15.22). Pathologic intra-prosthetic regurgitation of bioprostheses is usually due to structural valve deterioration (➲ Fig. 15.22).

Paraprosthetic regurgitation is always pathological. Small paraprosthetic regurgitation around the circumference of a prosthetic valve between the sewing ring and the annulus of the native valve is common. The regurgitant jet is usually eccentric and it extends into the receiving chamber. More than one regurgitant jet may be simultaneously present. During the first year after valve replacement, these regurgitations are mostly related to surgical factors, are not associated with increased subclinical haemolysis, and are generally benign. Sometimes it may be difficult to distinguish intra- from paraprosthetic regurgitation using the transthoracic approach. In these cases, the transoesophageal approach is needed. Also in patients with paraprosthetic regurgitation, the three-dimensional modality allows a more precise localization and assessment of circumferential extent of the leak (➲ Fig. 15.23).

Structural valve deterioration

Structural deterioration is generally a problem for biological valves only and usually non-existent for the current generation of mechanical valves. However, in 1986 the Bjork–Shiley convexoconcave

single tilting disc valve was withdrawn from the market after reports of fracture of the valve ring strut, resulting in dislodgment and embolization of disc. Similarly, the TRI technologies' mechanical valve has been withdrawn from clinical use because of the high risk of structural failure after several cases of occluder escape [25]. Strut fracture usually results in the abrupt onset of dyspnoea, loss of consciousness, or cardiovascular collapse due to embolization of the disc and acute severe valvular regurgitation that can be demonstrated at echocardiography. Cinefluoroscopy may visualize the absence of the strut and the radiopaque disc marker within the housing of the valve. Cinefluoroscopy has also been used to identify patients implanted with the Bjork–Shiley convexoconcave single tilting disc valve who have outlet–strut separation without complete strut fracture. The valve prosthesis should be prophylactically replaced in these patients.

Structural deterioration of a bioprosthetic valve usually is the result of progressive tissue degeneration with fibrosis and calcification of valve leaflets resulting in increased resistance to open (stenosis) or failure to close properly (regurgitation). Regurgitation may also occur because of leaflet tear (➲ Fig. 15.24), or rupture of one or more of the valve cusps (➲ Fig. 15.25), and in these patients the clinical presentation is that of an acute regurgitation [26]. The risk of structural valve deterioration increases over time. Typically, failure of bioprostheses occurs after 10 years from implant.

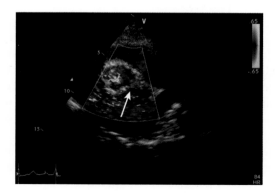

Fig. 15.21 Prosthetic mitral regurgitation jet (white arrow) detected by transthoracic echocardiography despite shadowing artefacts in the left atrium caused by the mechanical prosthesis.

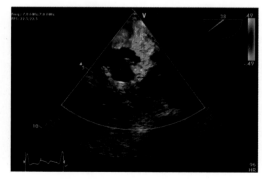

Fig. 15.22 Transoesophageal colour Doppler echocardiography showing an extensive intra-prosthetic leakage of a single tilting-disc prosthesis caused by pannus ingrowth.

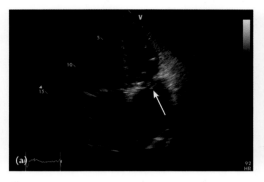
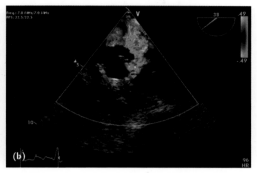

Fig. 15.23 Structural deterioration of a bioprosthetic valve in the mitral position causing fracture of one leaflet, which prolapses in the left atrium (white arrow) (a). An eccentric and turbulent jet into the left atrium is visualized in (b).

Prosthetic valve endocarditis and related complications

A prosthetic valve represents a foreign body within the circulatory system that is a potential site of infection. The characteristic lesion of valve prosthesis endocarditis is, similar to native valves, vegetation. When vegetations are small, they appear as irregular, immobile echogenic structures attached to the valve components

(Fig. 15.26). As they grow and become larger, they usually become sessile and move following the blood flow through the valve (Fig. 15.27). Due to the presence of the prosthetic material, the sensitivity of echocardiography (both transthoracic and transoesophageal) to detect vegetations on prosthetic valves is lower than in native valves. Large vegetations can occasionally cause prosthesis obstruction (Fig. 15.28). Taking into account the low

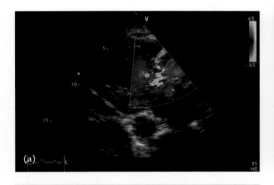
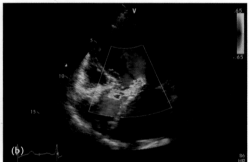
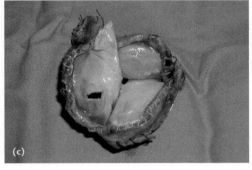

Fig. 15.24 Transthoracic colour Doppler echocardiography demonstrating severe regurgitation of a Cryolife O'Brien bioprosthesis from parasternal (a) and apical approach (b). The explanted valve (c) showed a tear within the body of the cusp in the non-coronary sinus of Valsalva.

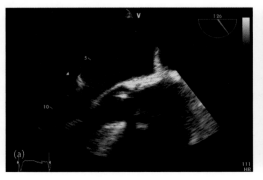
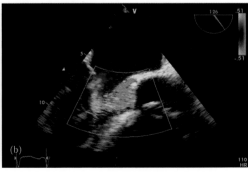

Fig. 15.25 Transoesophageal echocardiography showing degenerative calcification and rupture of a cusp (a) determining severe regurgitation (b) of a bioprosthesis in the aortic position.

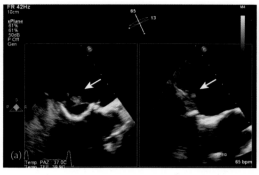
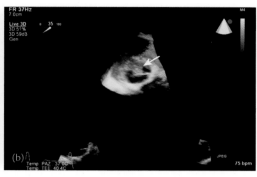

Fig. 15.26 Real-time three-dimensional transoesophageal echocardiography showing a small vegetation attached to the leaflet of a bioprosthetic valve in the mitral position. Multi-plane visualization of the vegetation (white arrows) (a). Rendering display of the vegetation allows better assessment of the size and shape of the vegetation (white arrow) (b).

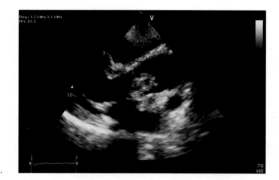

Fig. 15.27 Transthoracic echocardiography showing a large and highly mobile vegetation on the leaflet of a bioprosthesis in the aortic position.

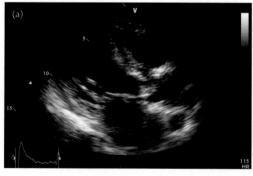
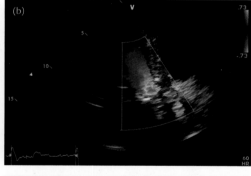
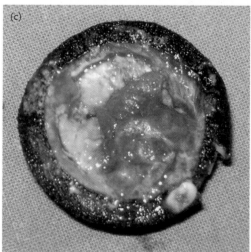
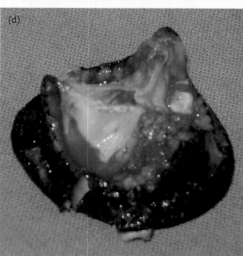

Fig. 15.28 Transthoracic echocardiography showing a large vegetation on the left ventricular side of a bioprosthesis in the aortic position. The vegetation enters the valve orifice during systole obstructing it (a) and (b). At surgery, the extensive obstruction of the bioprosthesis was confirmed (c, d).

sensitivity of the technique, a negative transthoracic study in a patient with moderate or high clinical suspicion of endocarditis does not exclude the diagnosis and transoesophageal examination should be warranted. It has also been reported that vegetations longer than 10 mm are associated with an increased risk of embolization, and vegetation size is a useful indicator to plan the urgency of surgical intervention. Three-dimensional echocardiography improves the assessment of vegetation size, localization of attachment point, and mobility (➲ Fig. 15.29)

Prosthetic valve endocarditis may evolve with paravalvular abscess formation. In the mitral position, a paravalvular abscess appears as an echo-free space adjacent to the sewing ring. However, often the only signs of abscess are indirect, as an increased prosthesis mobility resulting from suture dehiscence and lack of annular support. Frequently, ring or myocardial abscesses are only detected at surgery, suggesting the low sensitivity of the technique for valves in this position. For prostheses in the aortic position, increased thickening of the aortic root, with or without echo-free space inside confirmed in two views, suggests the presence of a ring abscess (➲ Fig. 15.30). Sometimes the diagnosis is difficult and the echo study should be repeated after a few days to look for an evolution of the finding (➲ Fig. 15.31). Fistolous communications with the right atrium, left atrium or right ventricle can be detected with colour Doppler.

Haemolysis

Although subclinical intravascular haemolysis (as evidenced by decreased serum haptoglobin, reticulocytosis, and increased lactate dehydrogenase concentrations) can be documented in most patients with normofunctioning mechanical heart valve

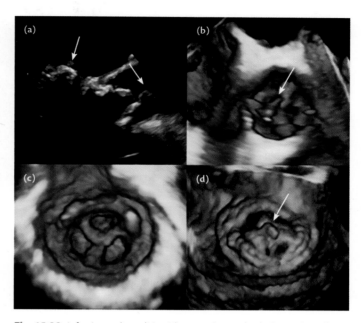

Fig. 15.29 Infective endocarditis with vegetation on both the aortic and mitral bioprostheses. Two-dimensional transoesophageal long-axis view showing vegetation (arrows) on both valve prostheses (a). Three-dimensional *en face* view of the aortic prosthesis from the aortic perspective showing the vegetation (b). Three-dimensional *en face* view of the mitral prosthesis from the ventricular perspective showing the prolapsing vegetation (c). Three-dimensional *en face* view of the mitral prosthesis from the atrial perspective showing the size, attachment and mobility of the vegetation (d).

prostheses, severe haemolytic anaemia is uncommon and suggests paravalvular leakage due to partial dehiscence of the valve, or infection or interaction of the jet with foreign bodies like annular rings (➲ Fig. 15.32).

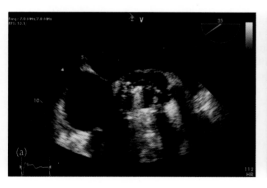
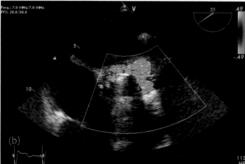

Fig. 15.30 Transoesophageal imaging of a short-axis view of the aortic root showing a prosthetic aortic valve endocarditis complicated by abscess and pseudoaneurysm formation. In the posterior part of the aortic root an echolucent space can be visualized suggesting the degeneration of the abscess in pseudoaneurysm of the mitral-aortic intervalvular fibrosa (a). By colour Doppler imaging, the blood flow is visualized exiting the pseudoaneurysm into the left ventricular outflow tract during diastole (b).

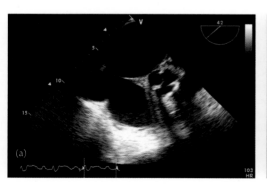
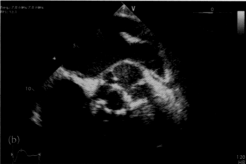

Fig. 15.31 At early stages, abscess appears as a thickening of the aortic wall, which is difficult to differentiate from hematoma (a). However, a transoesophageal echocardiogram repeated 5 days later showed evolution of the echocardiographic images with vacuolization confirming the original suspicion of an abscess (b).

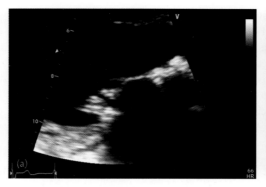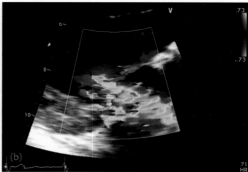

Fig. 15.32 Severe haemolysis in a female patient after mitral annuloplasty. Transthoracic echocardiography (a, b) showed a moderate regurgitant jet directed towards the annular ring, causing fragmentation of red cells and haemolysis.

References

1. Yoganathan AP, He Z, Casey J. Fluid mechanics of heart valves. *Annu Rev Biomed Eng* 2004; 6: 331–62.
2. Gillinov AM, Blackstone EH, Rodriguez LL. Prosthesis-patient size: measurement and clinical implications. *J Thorac Cardiovasc Surg* 2003; 126: 313–6.
3. Flaschkampf FA, Weyman AE, Guerrero JL. Influence of orifice geometry and flow rate on effective valve area: an in vitro study. *J Am Coll Cardiol* 1991; 15: 1173–80.
4. Van den Brink RBA. Evaluation of prosthetic heart valves by transoesophageal echocardiography: problems, pitfalls, and timing of echocardiography. *Semin Cardiothorac Vasc Anesth* 2006; 10: 89–100.
5. Baumgartner H, Khan S, DeRobertis M, et al. Discrepancies between Doppler and catheter gradients in aortic prosthetic valves in vitro: a manifestation of localized pressure gradients and pressure recovery. *Circulation* 1990; 82: 1467–75.
6. Rothbart RM, Smucker ML, Gibson RS. Overestimation by Doppler echocardiography of pressure gradients across Starr-Edwards prosthetic valves in the aortic position. *Am J Cardiol* 1988; 61: 475–6.
7. Badano LP, Mocchegiani R, Bertoli D, et al. Normal echocardiographic characteristics of the Sorin-Bicarbon bileaflet prosthetic heart valve in mitral and aortic position. *J Am Soc Echocardiogr* 1997; 10: 632–43.
8. Currie PJ, Seward JB, Reeder GS, et al. Continuous-wave Doppler echocardiographic assessment of severity of calcific aortic stenosis: a simultaneous Doppler-catheter correlative study in 100 adult patients. *Circulation* 1985; 71: 1162–9.
9. Badano LP, Zamorano JL, Pavoni D, et al. Clinical and haemodynamic implications of supra-annular implant of biological aortic valves. *J Cardiovasc Med* 2006; 7: 524–32.
10. 1McDonald ML, Daly RC, Schaff HV, et al. Haemodynamic performance of small aortic valve bioprostheses: is there a difference? *Ann Thorac Surg* 1997; 63: 362–6.
11. Chafizadeh ER, Zoghbi WA. Doppler echocardiographic assessment of the St Jude Medical prosthetic valve in the aortic position using the continuity equation. *Circulation* 1991; 83: 213–23.
12. Walther T, Falk V, Autschbach R, et al. Haemodynamic assessment of the stentless Toronto SPV bioprosthesis by echocardiography. *J Heart Valve Dis* 1994; 3: 657–65.
13. Caldwell RL, Girod DA, Hurwitz RA, Mahoney L, King H, Brown J. Pre-operative two-dimensional echocardiographic prediction of prosthetic aortic and mitral valve size in children. *Am Heart J* 1987; 113: 873–8.
14. Harpaz D, Shah P, Bezante G, Heo M, Stewart S, Hicks GL. Transthoracic and transoesophageal echocardiographic sizing of the aortic annulus to determine prosthesis size. *Am J Cardiol* 1993; 72: 1411–7.
15. Yoganathan AP, Cape EG, Sung H, Williams FP, Timoh A. Review of hydrodynamic principles for the cardiologist: application to the study of blood flow and jets by imaging techniques. *J Am Coll Cardiol* 1988; 12: 1344–53.
16. Badano LP, Bertoli D, Astengo D, et al. Doppler haemodynamic assessment of clinically and echocardiographically normal mitral and aortic Allcarbon valve prostheses: Valve Prosthesis Ligurian Cooperative Doppler study. *Eur Heart J* 1993; 14: 1602–9.
17. Rosenheck R, Binder T, Maurer G. Normal values for Doppler echocardiographic assessment of heart valve prostheses. *J Am Soc Echocardiogr* 2003; 16: 1116–27.
18. David TE, Armstrong S, Sun Z. Clinical and haemodynamic assessment of the Hancock II bioprosthesis. *Ann Thorac Surg* 1992; 54: 661–7.
19. Badano LP, Pavoni D, Musumeci S, et al. Stented bioprosthetic valve haemodynamics. How much is the supra-annular implant better than the intra-annular one? *J Heart Valve Dis* 2006; 15: 238–46.
20. Pibarot P, Dumesnil JG, Jobin J, Cartier P, Honos G, Durand LG. Haemodynamic and physical performance during maximal exercise in patients with an aortic bioprosthetic valve: comparison of stentless versus stented bioprostheses. *J Am Coll Cardiol* 1999; 34: 1609–17.
21. Seiler C. Management and follow-up of prosthetic heart valves. *Heart* 2004; 90: 818–2.
22. Muratori M, Montorsi P, Teruzzi G, et al. Feasibility and diagnostic accuracy of quantitative assessment of mechanical prostheses leaflet motion by transthoracic and transoesophageal echocardiography in suspected prosthetic valve dysfunction. *Am J Cardiol* 2006; 97: 94–100.
23. Pennel DJ, Sechtem UP, Higgins CB, et al. Society for Cardiovascular Magnetic Resonance; Working Group on Cardiovascular Magnetic Resonance of the European Society of Cardiology. Clinical indications for cardiovascular magnetic resonance (CMR): Consensus Panel report. *Eur Heart J* 2004; 25: 1940–65.
24. Caceres-Loriga FM, Perez-Lopez H, Santos-Garcia J, Morlans-Hernandez K. Prosthetic heart valve thrombosis: pathogenesis, diagnosis and management. *Int J Cardiol* 2006; 110: 1–6.
25. Bottio T, Casarotto D, Thiene G, Caprili L, Angelini A, Gerosa G. Leaflet escape in a new bileaflet mechanical valve: TRI technologies. *Circulation* 2003; 107: 2303–6.
26. Pavoni D, Badano LP, Ius F, et al. Limited long-term durability of the Cryolife O'Brien stentless porcine xenograft valve. *Circulation* 2007; 16: I-307–I-313.

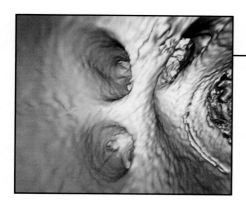

CHAPTER 16

Cardiovascular imaging in percutaneous valve therapy

Giovanni La Canna and Daniel Rodriguez Munoz

Contents

Introduction

Based on a large population study with systematic echocardiography, the overall age-adjusted prevalence of valvular heart disease (VHD) is estimated at 2.5%. However, prevalence increases significantly with age, from <2% below 65 years, to 8.5% between 65 and 75 years, and 13.2% over 75 years [1]. The degenerative form of mitral regurgitation (MR) and aortic stenosis (AS) is the most prevalent aetiology for primary VHD [1–3]. In addition, MR may be secondary to left ventricular dysfunction, and may be underestimated since the clinical picture is often dominated by heart failure symptoms. Secondary MR is a consequence of left ventricle (LV) remodelling, which causes the incomplete coaptation of normal valve apparatus. Due to the absence of a relevant murmur in a significant percentage of patients, Doppler echocardiography is essential for the detection and quantification of MR. Due to the increase of age-related epidemiologic burden, VHD is commonly associated with a greater frequency of comorbidity [4–6]. Consequently, a significant percentage of the elderly might be denied surgery due to high risk, although operated patients might show a favourable outcome. Following the surgical implantation of prosthetic valves, some patients may develop complications, such as recurrent paravalvular regurgitation, requiring high-risk redo surgery [7].

Over recent decades, the development of percutaneous valve therapy has opened a new pathway for the treatment of VHD, which can be considered a valid alternative to high-risk surgery [8, 9]. Owing to the changing face of the epidemiologic VHD burden, the impact of percutaneous treatment may be considered paramount.

Percutaneous techniques require multi-modality imaging for patient selection, procedure monitoring in the cardiac catheterization laboratory, and subsequent follow-up surveillance. Accurate visualization of the native valve, valve prosthesis or device, and their anatomic relationship is crucial before, during, and after percutaneous valve procedures. Several imaging modalities are available, including echocardiography using transthoracic (TTE), transoesophageal (TEE) and intra-cardiac (ICE) approaches, multi-slice computed tomography (MSCT), magnetic resonance imaging (MRI), and fluoroscopy. Echocardiography permits the imaging of soft radio-transparent structures, anatomic and physiologic real-time imaging with 2-dimensional (2D), 3-dimensional (3D) and Doppler techniques, and feasibility in the procedure room.

Patient selection and procedural risk assessment are crucial issues before percutaneous valve interventions. Imaging is essential for the assessment of valve functional anatomy, quantification of valve lesion severity, and the assessment of surrounding structures and vascular access. A routine TTE is the first imaging modality used for VHD assessment. However, in the case of TTE suboptimal image quality, TEE is required. TEE may be supplemented with real-time three-dimensional (RT3D) imaging to enhance VHD diagnostic balance by anatomic reconstruction. In addition, MSCT and MRI can also give detailed information on valve morphology and function. In particular, MSCT plays an important role in planning certain procedures, providing detailed information on feasibility and interventional access planes, and minimizing procedural-related complications.

Percutaneous valve therapies are usually performed in the catheterization laboratory, or in a hybrid operating room, and require the expertise of a multidisciplinary team. Several approaches can be used including anterograde trans-septal or retrograde trans-femoral artery and transapical left ventricle (LV) access.

To guide and monitor VHD percutaneous interventions, fluoroscopy and TEE are needed. Fluoroscopy can visualize a large area of the heart with excellent temporal and spatial resolutions. However, it projects 3D information onto a 2D screen, requiring multiple projections to determine the precise location of devices and structures in 3D space. Although information deriving from fluoroscopy remains essential, it does not permit visualization of cardiac soft-tissue structures and is inadequate to precisely delineate catheter course and location. Combined pre-procedural MSCT with fluoroscopy is a promising approach to enhance intra-procedural imaging during percutaneous valve therapy. TEE supplemented by RT3D, providing real-time anatomic imaging without radiation and contrast use, is the ideal technique for the guidance of certain procedures. TEE supplemented by RT3D imaging enables the visualization of soft cardiac structures and all intra-cardiac catheters throughout their entire course in the heart, thus improving procedural accuracy and safety. Its major disadvantage is that it sometimes requires general anaesthesia. The use of intra-procedural TEE has already been shown to reduce fluoroscopy time, thus decreasing radiation exposure for both patient and operator. ICE might play a role in trans-septal catheterization, but this role is limited during the subsequent steps of percutaneous valve therapy.

Percutaneous aortic valve replacement

Trans-catheter aortic valve implantation (TAVI) is a rapidly developing new technique for the treatment of severe AS. The implication of cardiovascular imaging in patient selection and during intervention guidance has led to numerous studies showing the usefulness of various techniques, and scientific societies producing detailed recommendations [10, 11], for imaging assessment before, during and after the intervention.

Before TAVI

Following AS diagnosis, patient eligibility for TAVI involves a series of considerations, including detailed evaluation of the dimensions and characteristics of the aortic valve, annulus, aortic root and ascending aorta, as well as the ilio-femoral vessels (⊃ Fig. 16.1). Accurate annulus measurement is particularly important to select prosthetic valve size to avoid potentially severe complications that can derive from the implantation of a valve that is either too small (paravalvular regurgitation, mismatch, valve migration, and embolism) or too large (incomplete deployment leading to valvular and paravalvular regurgitation, annular rupture) (⊃ Fig. 16.2). Measurement of the surrounding structures is also essential to determine its optimal positioning and therefore avoid the risks of implantation that is too high (aortic injury, valve antegrade embolization, coronary ostium occlusion, paravalvular regurgitation) or too low (mitral valve compromise, atrio-ventricular block, retrograde migration, paravalvular regurgitation), as well as ruling out exclusion criteria, such as severe hypertrophic basal septum, and insufficient distance between the annulus and coronary ostia. Echocardiography (2D-TTE, 2D-TEE, 3D-TEE), MSCT, and cardiac MRI can perform these measurements accurately. Two-dimensional TTE and TEE can accurately perform most of the mentioned measurements. Limitations to their accuracy may appear in heavily calcified cases, to differentiate tricuspid vs. bicuspid valves, and in markedly oval annulus, where single-plane measurements assuming circular shape may estimate erroneous dimensions. However, a 2D-TEE measurement-based strategy has shown to yield good clinical outcome when compared with MSCT [12]. Another limitation of 2D echocardiographic studies lies in the difficulty of measuring the distance between the annulus and left coronary ostium on a standard plane, which can be performed

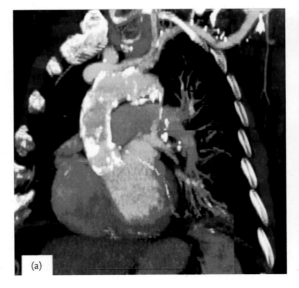

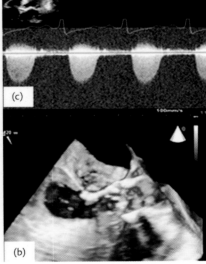

Fig. 16.1 3D-MSCT (a) and TEE (b) reconstruction in a patient with severe aortic stenosis (c, mean gradient 60 mmHg) showing extensive calcification of ascending aorta ('porcelain aorta').

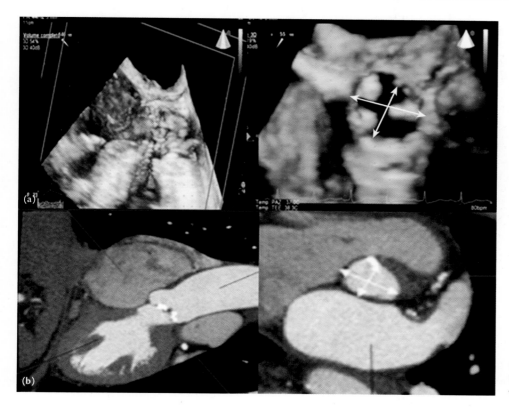

Fig. 16.2 Measurement of aortic annulus by short-axis view obtained with cropped full volume: (a) 3D-echocardiography; (b) MSCT.

with 3D reconstruction. The assessment of LV dynamic obstruction risk (extreme wall hypertrophy, papillary muscle malposition, mitral annular calcification) is an important issue when planning TAVI [13]. MSCT provides a clear added value in valve and annulus characterization in extensively calcified valves, especially through 3D systolic reconstruction [14]. Additionally, it can accurately measure the relationship of coronary ostia to the aortic annulus and leaflets [15], which is essential to avoid their occlusion when implanting the valve, and to provide useful information on aortic root angle, which optimizes alignment of the prosthetic valve, increasing precision and reducing duration and contrast usage compared to its aortographic evaluation [16]. MSCT also provides assessment of the aorta and iliofemoral vessels to define the transfemoral vs. transapical approach. In spite of its limitations, such as the use of radiation and iodinated contrast, MSCT has been widely incorporated into routine pre-TAVI evaluation at many centres.

Although MRI is able to accurately perform most of the necessary measurements in a pre-TAVI study [17, 18] without ionizing radiation, several limitations hinder its expansion as a widely used tool in this setting. Prolonged examination times, and common limitations in patients with pacemakers, etc., are particularly problematic in older patients. Its definition of vascular structures requires the use of gadolinium and can generate areas of missing information in densely calcified regions.

In summary: before TAVI a thorough evaluation and accurate measurement of the aortic valve and surrounding structures is essential for the success of the procedure. Two-dimensional

echocardiography, both transthoracic and transoesophageal, can adequately carry out the required measurements, but 3D-echocardiography, as well as MSCT and CMR, provide a significant added value in this process. Fusion imaging, allowing the use of these techniques in the catheterization laboratory, might optimize these studies in the future.

During TAVI

During the procedure, TEE is typically the preferred imaging guidance method due to the limitations of TTE, although the latter can be used to select the optimal location of thoracotomy in transapical approaches. In spite of the discomfort for patients in cases where general anaesthesia is considered unnecessary, and the possible interference with fluoroscopic images, TEE can contribute significantly to guidance during various steps of the procedure (⊃ Fig. 16.3):

– During initial balloon valvuloplasty, especially when the valve is not very calcified making fluoroscopic visualization more difficult, TEE can guide balloon positioning and stability, as well as cusp displacement and relationship with the coronary ostia.

– Immediately before its deployment, TEE can also complement fluoroscopy to confirm the correct positioning of the prosthetic valve, becoming the main guiding technique in placement selection in mildly calcified valves, or those implanted on a previous bioprosthetic valve.

– Immediately after deployment, TEE is used to confirm adequate positioning and function, mainly confirming correct stent

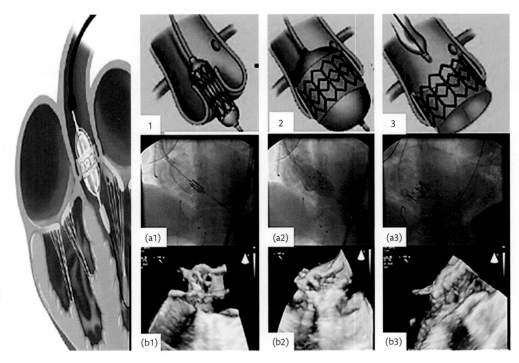

Fig. 16.3 Trans-catheter aortic valve implantation using the retrograde transfemoral approach. After aortic valve crossing and balloon dilatation, prosthetic valve is advanced and correctly positioned and deployed under rapid pacing with fluoroscopy (a1–3) and real-time 3D transoesophageal echocardiography (b1–3).

expansion, cusp motion, and the absence of significant paravalvular regurgitation. It is important to note that some regurgitation is normal during the first few minutes until the delivery device is removed and the prosthetic leaflets are fully expanded, and even subsequently. To ensure adequate detection of possible regurgitant jets, a complete evaluation of the valve from a transgastric view must be performed. Conventional quantification methods, such as jet dimension, vena contracta width, quantitative Doppler, or pressure half-time can be used in this context [19], while 3D-TEE can also contribute to a more precise evaluation [20].

– Following valve implantation, TEE also acquires an essential role in the detection of possible complications. As previously mentioned, prosthesis misplacement can result in severe complications, such as severe aortic regurgitation, antegrade or retrograde prosthetic embolism, acute mitral stenosis or regurgitation, cardiac tamponade or coronary ostial occlusion, dynamic LV obstruction [13, 21–24]. Early detection of these complications through TEE enables prompt treatment and can significantly influence outcome.

A large number of centres currently opt for the routine use of TEE during TAVI, based on its significant potential benefits and the manageable inconveniences.

After TAVI

Echocardiographic evaluation is recommended before discharge, 30 days after the procedure, at one-year follow-up, and thereafter annually [11]. Evaluation of trans-catheter-implanted valves is similar to that of those implanted surgically, although the presence of a stent, both proximal and distal to the implanted valve, can affect valve area calculations based on velocity measurements due to flow acceleration. It is therefore important to register velocity, both proximal and distal, to the stent [25]. An additional difficulty during follow-up lies in the evaluation of aortic regurgitation. Since paravalvular regurgitation is often eccentric and irregularly shaped, the percentage of the sewing ring occupied by the jet has been suggested as a method to estimate its severity, defining mild (<10% of the sewing ring), moderate (10–20%), or severe (>20%) regurgitation [26]. However, this method still has numerous limitations, such as assuming the continuity of the jet or overestimating the severity in cases of multiple small jets. Quantitative methods and, especially, 3D-echocardiography, have arisen as potential alternatives [27] during recent years, and may be more accurate in the assessment of trans-catheter prosthetic regurgitation.

Percutaneous mitral valve commissurotomy

Percutaneous mitral balloon valvuloplasty (PMBV) has proved to be a safe and effective alternative to surgical commissurotomy and mitral valve replacement in mitral stenosis (MS), especially since the introduction of the Inoue technique [28–30]. Imaging plays an essential role in adequate patient selection, wise decision-making during the procedure, and early detection of complications.

Before PMBV

Initial TTE evaluation aims to establish the degree of stenosis, followed by valve anatomy assessment. The Wilkins' score (see ⊃ Table 16.1) is the method most widely used to assess the anatomical features of MS, and the likelihood of successful PMBV [31]. RT3D-TEE increases accuracy in the characterization of

Table 16.1 Assessment of mitral valve anatomy according to the Wilkins' score

Grade	Mobility	Thickening	Calcification	Subvalvular Thickening
1	Highly mobile valve with only leaflet tips restricted	Leaflets near normal in thickness (4–5 mm)	A single area of increased echo brightness	Minimal thickening just below the mitral leaflets
2	Leaflet mid-portions and base portions have normal mobility	Midleaflets normal, considerable thickening of margins (5–8 mm)	Scattered areas of brightness confined to leaflet margins	Thickening of chordal structures extending to one-third of the chordal length
3	Valve continues to move forward in diastole, mainly from the base	Thickening extending through the entire leaflet (5–8 mm)	Brightness extending into the mid portions of the leaflets	Thickening extended to distal third of the chords
4	No or minimal forward movement of the leaflets in diastole	Considerable thickening of all leaflet tissue (>8–10 mm)	Extensive brightness throughout much of the leaflet tissue	Extensive thickening and shortening of all chordal structures extending down to the papillary muscles

Total score is the sum of the four items and ranges between 4 and 16.

commissures and subvalvular apparatus [32, 33], which have been described as the main determinants for the success of PBMV [34–36]. MSCT-based rather than TTE-based Wilkins' score has been reported to better predict area changes after PMBV [37].

During PMBV

TEE is typically the imaging method of choice during the procedure, especially if performed under general sedation or anaesthesia, since TTE interferes with the process and can compromise sterility. Initially, it is useful to rule out the presence of left atrial thrombus, that can develop quickly in MS patients. Also, although trans-septal puncture can be performed with fluoroscopic guidance, intra-cardiac or transoesophageal echocardiography can improve puncture-site selection and help avoid complications such as aortic puncture, especially in patients with anatomic variations. During the procedure, echocardiography provides useful information to optimize balloon placement, and lead progressive stepwise inflations through repeated measurement of valve area, gradient, regurgitation and commissural opening to achieve the best possible outcome (➲ Fig. 16.4). Additionally, RT3D seems to provide the most accurate information in estimating post-procedural valve area and the presence of complications, mainly those related to the subvalvular apparatus [38, 39]. TTE and TEE also enable the immediate detection of signs of complications, such as severe regurgitation and pericardial effusion (➲ Fig. 16.5).

After PMBV

Conventional TTE valve assessment is usually carried out during follow-up, mainly aimed at detecting the occurrence of restenosis. The time course of concomitant or (re-) development of tricuspid regurgitation is a relevant clinical problem after PMBV [40].

Percutaneous MitraClip treatment of mitral regurgitation

Conventional surgery is the consolidated approach to eliminate symptoms, and improve the life expectancy of patients with MR. However, many high-risk patients, especially the elderly or those

with comorbidities, are frequently denied surgery. Recently, the introduction of percutaneous MitraClip therapy has opened new frontiers in MR treatment, eliminating the need for thoracotomy and extracorporeal circulation [9, 41, 42] (➲ Fig. 16.6). MitraClip therapy can correct MR by intervening on the primary (degenerative) or secondary (functional) abnormalities of the mitral leaflets. The technique consists of approximating the free edge of the mitral leaflets on the site of the target lesion that is responsible for MR, and creating a double mitral orifice. It mimics Alfieri's surgical edge-to-edge approach, although the omission of prosthetic ring implantation is considered a potential weak point affecting

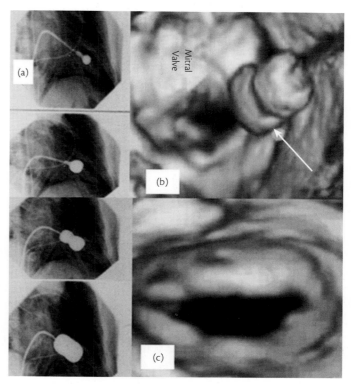

Fig. 16.4 Percutaneous mitral commissurotomy with stepwise Inoue technique: (a) fluoroscopy monitoring; (b) 3D transoesophageal echocardiography showing balloon position into mitral valve; and post-procedural valve area increase due to commissure splitting (c).

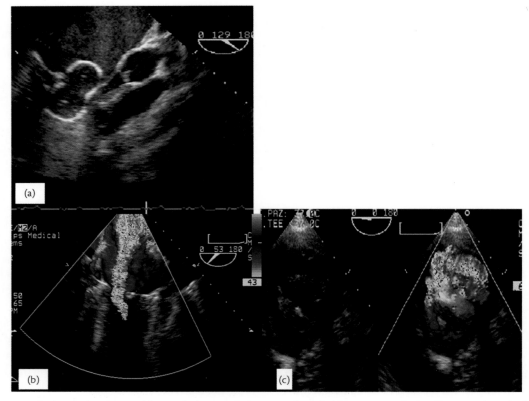

Fig. 16.5 Percutaneous mitral commissurotomy with stepwise Inoue technique complicated with severe regurgitation. Transoesophageal echocardiography showing balloon insufflation (a), severe mitral regurgitant jet (b, mid-oesophageal view) arising from postero-commissure drop-out due to laceration (c, transgastric view).

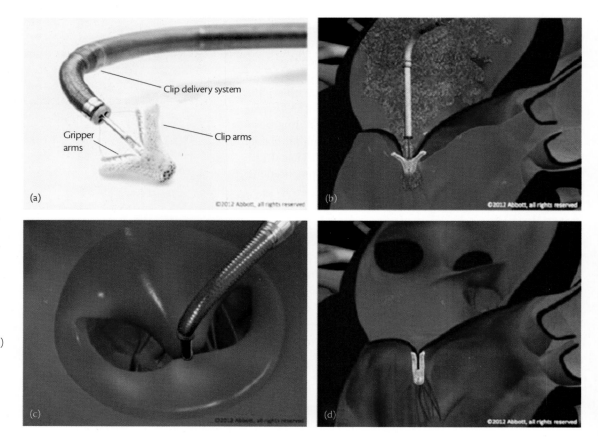

Fig. 16.6 MitraClip system for mitral repair (a) MitraClip components; (b), (c) and (d) clip implantation sequence creating double orifice with correction of mitral regurgitation.

EDGE-TO-EDGE THERAPY FOR MITRAL REGURGITATION

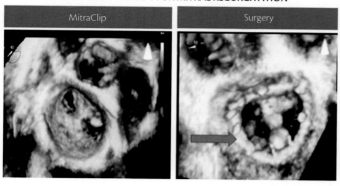

Fig. 16.7 MitraClip vs. surgical edge-to-edge therapy for MR. MitraClip is able to reproduce double orifice shape, although prosthetic ring is absent.

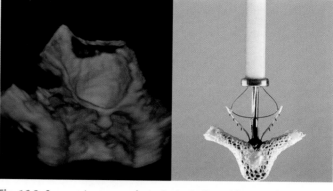

Fig. 16.8 Symmetric capture of mitral valve leaflets with optimal match between valve tissue and MitraClip device.

the durability of results (➲ Fig. 16.7). MitraClip therapy is based on fixed-length clip arms capable of antero-posterior leaflet capture up to 7 mm and latero-medial (intercommissural extension) width up to 4 mm. The success of the procedure depends on target valve lesion capture, involving both leaflets in a complete and symmetrical way, to eliminate MR without residual stenosis. To achieve this goal it is crucial to obtain an appropriate match between the varying valve functional anatomy and limited device capability (➲ Fig. 16.8).

Before MitraClip procedure

As with the surgical approach, the efficacy and feasibility of Mitra-Clip therapy depend on patient clinical selection, and on an accurate evaluation of the mechanism and severity of MR through the integrated use of Doppler echocardiography [43]. Characterization of the anatomo-functional mechanism of MR and feasibility analysis are based on the classification for surgical repair proposed by Carpentier (➲ Fig. 16.9):

– **Type I**. Loss of or incomplete leaflet systolic coaptation with preserved systo-diastolic mobility. The leaflets, despite normal apposition at annular surface level, do not coapt during systole due to annular dilatation.

– **Type II**. Loss of leaflet coaptation, due to excessive mobility (prolapse, chordal rupture).

– **Type III**. Leaflet apposition abnormality due to reduced systo-diastolic mobility (primary leaflet alterations) (Type IIIa), or to reduced systolic mobility only (Type IIIb) (functional malapposition, secondary to left-ventricular remodelling). Systolic coaptation of the leaflets may be incomplete or absent.

The rationale of echocardiographic selection is to identify the target valve lesion for capture, and the subsequent release of the MitraClip device without provoking mechanical lesions of the mitral apparatus. TTE is the first-line diagnostic approach, especially for patient exclusion from the procedure in the presence of evident valve calcification or extensive multiple mechanisms of MR. TEE evaluation is necessary to establish not only the ultimate suitability, but also the complexity of the MitraClip procedure. Different clinical-instrumental approaches are required for patients with functional/ischaemic MR and those with degenerative MR.

Appropriate selection of patients with degenerative MR (Carpentier's Type II) is based on a detailed evaluation of the target valve lesion. According to EVEREST criteria, the

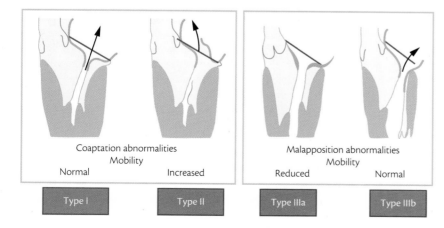

Fig. 16.9 Carpentier's nomenclature for MR mechanism.

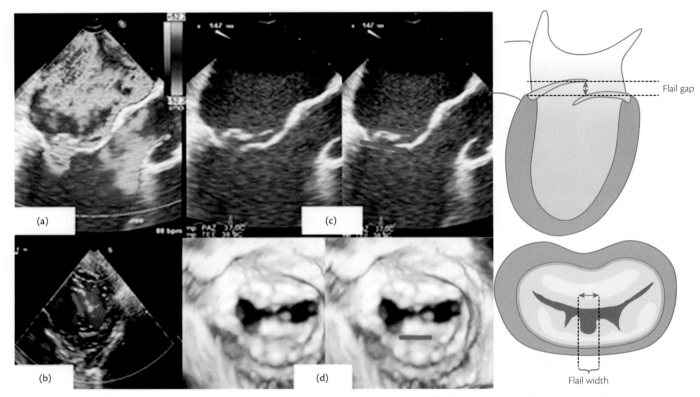

Fig. 16.10 Transoesophageal echocardiography in a patient with degenerative mitral regurgitation (MR) due to prolapse/flail of central scallop of posterior leaflet, suitable for MitraClip therapy. Colour Doppler shows severe MR (a, mid-oesophageal view) with central jet (b, transgastric view), flail gap 8 mm (c) and flail width 10 mm (d, 3D-TEE anatomic view).

following characteristics may be considered favourable for MitraClip therapy:

– Displacement of free-margin prolapsing segment (with or without chordal rupture) less than 10 mm from the annular plane, or the surrounding non-prolapsing mitral valve tissue (prolapse/flail gap).

– Central localization of the prolapsing segment with width less than 12 mm.

– Absence of calcification involving target lesion.

– Planimetric mitral valve area greater than 4 cm².

RT3D-TEE provides more detailed information on the site of maximum flail gap and target lesion width. ⊃ Figures 16.10 and 16.11 show Type II valve lesions, which may be considered optimal or adverse for MitraClip treatment, respectively. Team experience might facilitate, in selected cases, the correction of lesions defined suboptimal according to EVEREST criteria. However, excessive redundancy (Barlow syndrome), with multi-localized prolapse or with concomitant extreme leaflet retraction, represents an adverse anatomical condition, owing to clip fixed dimension, for potential leaflet capture mismatch, with the risk of early or late detachment or mechanical leaflet damage.

At present, MitraClip therapy cannot be considered equivalent to surgical repair in patients with degenerative MR, as regards applicability and durability. Patient selection for

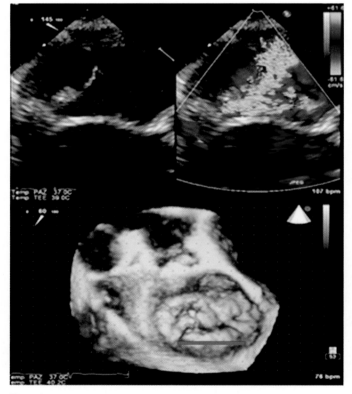

Fig. 16.11 Transoesophageal echocardiography in a patient with degenerative MR unsuitable for MitraClip therapy due to excessive flail gap (18 mm) and flail width (22 mm) of posterior leaflet.

percutaneous therapy has therefore to take this into account so as not to extend its application to those patients eligible for surgical repair with a low operative risk and the probability of optimal long-term results. Together with echocardiographic imaging, the selection of candidates for this percutaneous procedure requires careful clinical evaluation, including the surgical risk (⊃ Table 16.2).

The selection of patients with functional/ischaemic MR (Type IIIb) that can benefit from MitraClip treatment is complex and clinically challenging. Leaflet malapposition, measured as leaflet tenting area (TA), and coaptation-point displacement, measured as coaptation depth (CD) from the annulus, are the determinants of functional MR, which is strictly correlated, in terms of site and entity, to the interaction between remodelling type/grade and entity/asynchrony of LV coaptation forces. Leaflet malapposition can be asymmetric or symmetric as a consequence of LV regional or global remodelling, respectively. Owing to dynamic determinants, functional MR is affected by loading manipulations conditioning the degree of remodelling and LV contraction forces. MitraClip therapy feasibility consequently requires an integrated approach that considers all the variables underlying a certain MR severity and its correlated potential variability. Optimization of medical therapy and the identification of the so-called 'recoverable left ventricle', through the correction of asynchrony of contraction [44] and of ischaemic or tachycardia-dependent myocardial dysfunction, are essential before considering the feasibility and efficacy of MitraClip therapy in each patient. Doppler-echocardiography accurately defines the degree of MR. However, it requires an integrated and critical approach, which should take into account potentially misleading evidence regarding MR fluctuation. The site and direction of regurgitant jet geometry may differ, and can be central or eccentric according to the distribution of the functional tenting and coaptation abnormalities of the mitral valve tissue. In the presence of asymmetric lesions, the regurgitant jet moves away from the leaflet with the highest coaptation point compared to the contralateral leaflet, thus simulating a pseudo-prolapse.

The feasibility of MitraClip therapy in patients with functional/ischaemic MR depends on the following echocardiographic parameters:

- symmetric systolic leaflet tenting;
- systolic leaflet coaptation shape (CD <10 mm, longitudinal extension >2 mm).

According to the EVEREST study [9, 45], preserved systolic coaptation in the presence of symmetric tenting, facilitating complete leaflet capture, is the key point defining the feasibility and efficacy of MitraClip therapy. Vice versa, the loss of systolic leaflet coaptation, an expression of advanced LV remodelling or predominant annular dilation, may represent a suboptimal condition for MitraClip implantation, with the risk of intra-procedural mechanical complication or potential late displacement of the clip. Echo-Doppler mapping and intercommissural extension of the regurgitant lesion are essential to predict the site of clip implantation and the need for additional clips, avoiding the risk of post-procedural residual stenosis. The following criteria may be associated with an unsuccessful outcome or the non-feasibility of MitraClip therapy:

- Extended loss of coaptation and corresponding regurgitant jet (> 60% of intercommissural coaptation surface).
- Asymmetric malapposition involving commissure with dominant eccentric regurgitant jet.
- Extreme asymmetric malapposition with structural remodelling of mitral leaflet (leaflet hypoplasia, calcification involving target lesion, large cleft diastasis of posterior leaflet).
- Planimetric valve area <4 cm².

In selected conditions, an expert MitraClip team might attempt to perform a technically demanding procedure despite unfavourable mitral valve anatomy. However, this can be considered only in patients without absolute contraindication to eventual 'rescue' surgery (contractile reserve with dobutamine test, low comorbidity). 2D-TEE is sufficient to evaluate the functional anatomy

Table 16.2 Selection criteria for MitraClip therapy in patients with degenerative MR

Severe MR	ERO >0.4 cm², VC >7 mm
Type of valvular lesion	• Flail/prolapse gap <10 mm • Central origin and intercommissural width <12 mm • Absence of calcification at the target zone • Valve area >4 cm²

Clinical parameters	• Surgical indications with high operative risk
	  – left ventricle dysfunction (ESD >40 mm EF<60%)
	  – severe pulmonary artery hypertension
	  – comorbidities
	  – elderly patients
	• Mitral surgery contraindications
	  – porcelain aorta
	  – severe left ventricular dysfunction (EF<30%) without contractile reserve (dobutamine test)
	• Risk reduction for non-cardiac surgery, chemotherapy, high risk pregnancy

subtenting MR for MitraClip therapy, but 3D-TEE may add useful information regarding the feasibility and planning of the procedure, providing a more detailed depiction of functional anatomy. This information might be useful to predict unsuitability, or a technically demanding procedure, including the need for and sequence of additional clips and the risk of post-procedural mitral valve stenosis.

➲ Figure 16.12a–c shows MR functional mechanism, which can be considered optimal, suboptimal and unsuitable for MitraClip therapy. ➲ Table 16.3 summarizes the main points of the clinical-instrumental approach for the selection of patients with functional/ischaemic MR that might benefit from percutaneous MitraClip therapy.

During MitraClip procedure

MitraClip is delivered with trans-septal catheterization. The procedure is performed in a cardiac catheterization laboratory, or in a hybrid operating room, using general anaesthesia, fluoroscopy, and TEE guidance. 2D-TEE is an established method to monitor the MitraClip procedure, including:

– Trans-septal puncture site with a tailored distance from the mitral annular plane—guidance of the delivery system towards the mitral valve—adjustment of opened clip perpendicular to commissures in the left atrium and left ventricle.

– Match of MitraClip system with target mitral valve lesion for grasping and leaflet insertion.

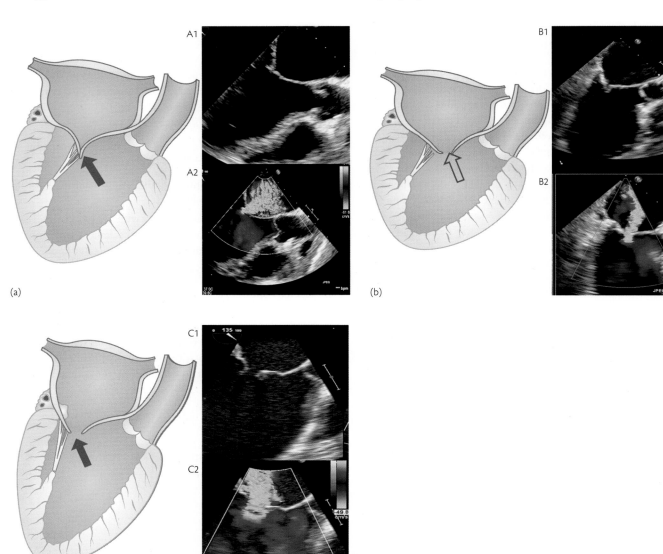

Fig. 16.12 Varying functional anatomy in patients with FMR. (a) Optimal valve lesion for MitraClip therapy: (A1) 2D-TEE showing symmetrical tethering of anatomically normal leaflets with preserved systolic coaptation (arrow); (A2) 2D-TEE colour Doppler showing severe MR with central regurgitant jet. (b) Suboptimal valve lesion for MitraClip therapy. 2D-TEE showing symmetric tethering of anatomically normal leaflet with coaptation loss (arrow) due to advanced LV remodelling (B1) and severe MR at colour Doppler (B2). (c) Adverse mitral valve anatomy for MitraClip therapy. 2D-TEE shows extreme tethering of partially calcified posterior leaflet (C1) and severe MR (C2).

Table 16.3 Clinical and echocardiographic selection criteria for MitraClip therapy in patients with functional/ischaemic MR

Clinical Evaluation
* **Signs and symptoms of heart failure**
  – dyspnoea, 'flash' pulmonary oedema, angina, systemic venous congestion
* **Medical optimal therapy**
  – ACE inhibitors, diuretics, beta-blockers (on–off)
* Identification of modifiable factors
  – Atrial fibrillation
  – Arterial hypertension
  – Anaemia
  – Water and sodium intake (diet, drug-mediated)
  – Ischaemic myocardial dysfunction
  – Asynchrony

Echocardiographic evaluation of MR
* **Significant regurgitation entity**
  – ERO >0.2 cm² (mid-systole), >0.4 cm² (proto-systole)
  – VC diameter >7 mm, area >0.4 cm² (multiple jet)
* **Anatomo-functional mechanisms**
  – Symmetric malapposition (tenting area)
  – Systolic coaptation depth (<1 cm)
  – Presence and longitudinal extension of coaptation (baseline and post-loading manipulation)
  – Central origin and intercommissural width of regurgitant jet <30%
  – Mitral valve area >4 cm²

MR: mitral regurgitation; ACE inhibitors: angiotensin-converting-enzyme inhibitors; ERO effective orifice area; VC vena contracta.

– Evaluation of effectiveness of leaflet capture on MR before clip deployment.

– Establishment of the need for additional clip(s) avoiding valve stenosis-effectiveness on MR and residual mitral valve area after clip implantation. Two-dimensional colour Doppler TEE can accurately guide step-by-step MitraClip implantation, although its relatively lower frame rate RT3D-TEE may add useful information optimizing the use of fluoroscopy exposure time and procedural results. The most important contribution of 3D-TEE includes the appropriate orientation of opened MitraClip to commissure plane, the evaluation of residual MR and accurate mitral valve area when additional clip implantation is considered (⊃ Figs 16.13 and 16.14).

The evaluation of residual MR after MitraClip implantation using conventional parameters is demanding, especially in the presence of multiple jets arising from a double-orifice mitral valve. Three-dimensional colour Doppler can accurately evaluate MR severity using the sum of single-jet vena contracta area [46] (⊃ Fig. 16.15). To avoid potential underestimation due to anaesthesia, evaluation of MR should be performed after the optimization of load conditions. Pulmonary vein flow pattern might be useful to assess the load conditions, even though this approach is limited in patients with atrial fibrillation. Accurate identification of the site of residual regurgitation is essential to guide additional clip implantation. Subsequent mitral valve area assessment, in addition to transvalvular gradient, can help predict stenosis following additional clip implantation. Using RT3D-TEE, the

smallest valve area can be accurately assessed before clip delivery. The prediction and recognition of MitraClip-related mitral valve stenosis is crucial in patients with severe pulmonary hypertension in the setting of end-stage cardiomyopathy to avoid left atrial pressure increase, despite the successful treatment of valve regurgitation.

⊃ Figure 16.16 shows MitraClip procedure in a patient with functional mitral regurgitation due to complex mechanism complicated by posterior leaflet laceration requiring emergency surgical mitral valve replacement.

After MitraClip procedure

After MitraClip implantation, echocardiographic examination, together with clinical evaluation, is indicated pre-discharge and at 6-monthly follow-up in patients with functional MR. In patients with degenerative MR an annual examination might be sufficient. TTE is recommended to evaluate the time-course of MitraClip efficacy. TEE is necessary to establish the mechanism of MitraClip failure, and the feasibility of a second MitraClip procedure or the need for surgical intervention (valve repair or replacement). In selected cases with recurrent symptoms without significant MR at rest, exercise TTE may be indicated to elicit fluctuant MR or to determine haemodynamically significant mitral stenosis. Finally, a relevant shunt arising from post-catheterization inter-atrial defect should also be excluded as a potential cause of symptoms.

Percutaneous mitral annuloplasty

There are several percutaneous techniques that have been tested in animal models mimicking surgical annuloplasty [47, 48]. Devices aiming to percutaneously reshape the mitral annulus can be separated into indirect types, which are positioned in the coronary sinus, and direct types, which directly address the mitral annulus. Indirect annuloplasty is when a device is placed into the coronary sinus to attempt favourable annulus remodelling. The Carillon™ Mitral Contour System (Cardiac Dimensions, Kirkland, WA, USA), which consists of two helical anchors interconnected by a nitinol bridge, is the most clinically tested device. Using right internal jugular access, the distal anchor is pledged in the great cardiac vein, and subsequent manual traction is applied to approximate the lateral and septal portion of the mitral annulus optimizing leaflet coaptation.

Direct annuloplasty consists of device implantation in the annulus, similar to surgical annuloplasty, using the retrograde, via the aorta into the left ventricle, or trans-septal approach. Apart from experimental models, the implantation in humans of some devices has been attempted to obtain MR reduction by direct annulus remodelling.

Before annuloplasty

Echocardiographic analysis of MR is crucial to select patients who might benefit from an annuloplasty procedure. As with surgical

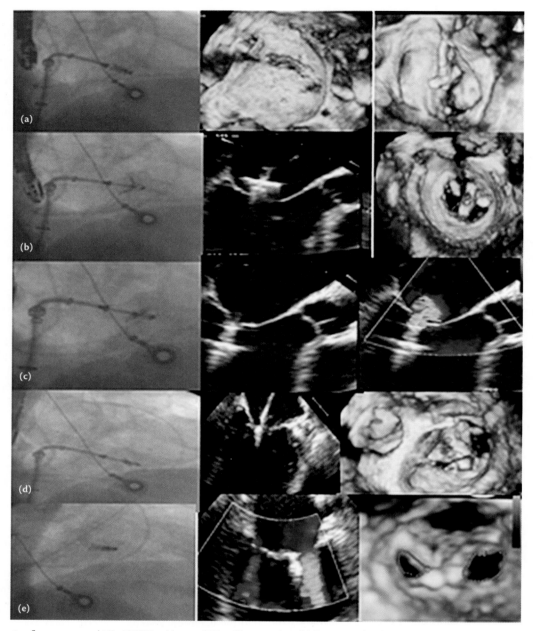

Fig. 16.13 Step-by-step fluoroscopy and 2D-, 3D-TEE guidance of MitraClip procedure. (a) Trans-septal catheterization and delivery system towards mitral valve. (b, c) Adjustment of opened MitraClip perpendicular to commissures in left atrium and left ventricle, MitraClip system/target mitral valve lesion matching. (d) Grasping and leaflet insertion, creating double valve orifice. (e) Effectiveness on MR without stenosis.

annuloplasty criteria, the ideal lesion includes Type I (incomplete copatation due to annular dilation/deformation) or Type IIIb (functional leaflet tethering) with symmetric leaflet malapposition and coaptation depth less than 1 cm. Mitral valve structural abnormalities (Type II, Type IIIa), or recognized tethering shapes that are predictive of unsuccessful surgical annuloplasty (asymmetric or extreme tethering), should be also excluded from the percutaneous approach. In addition, MSCT is essential for coronary sinus anatomy, surrounding coronary artery relationship [49]. Integrated analysis of annulus shape using MSCT and RT3D-TEE provides important information on the feasibility and planning of annuloplasty therapy.

During annuloplasty

Fluoroscopy and TEE are used to determine the final position of the device during indirect annuloplasty through the coronary sinus [50, 51]. Because of the close proximity of the circumflex artery, arteriograms are performed throughout the deployment sequence. Before the implant is decoupled, coronary arteriography is performed to confirm that coronary flow is not significantly compromised, and echocardiography is performed to confirm that a quantitative reduction in mitral regurgitation is achieved. In the event of coronary artery compromise or insufficient MR reduction, the implant should be recaptured by advancing the

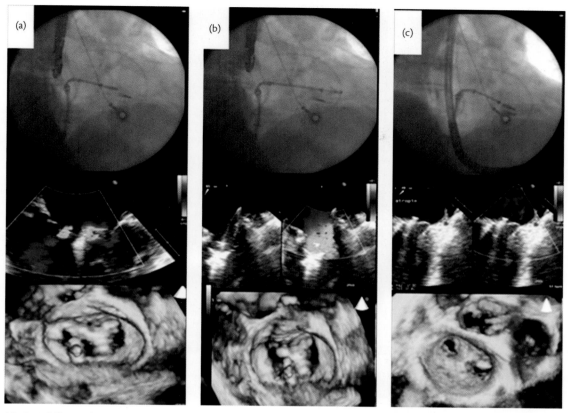

Fig. 16.14 Residual MR following first MitraClip implantation, which has been corrected by additional MitraClip. (a–c) Fluoroscopy, TEE colour flow mapping and 3D-TEE guidance for second MitraClip implantation abolishing the residual MR confined to lateral orifice.

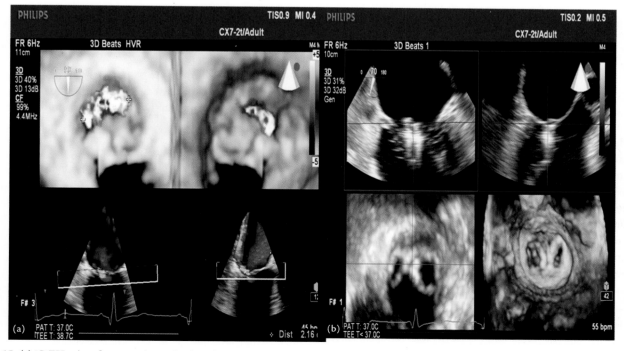

Fig. 16.15 (a) 3D-TEE colour flow mapping evaluation of vena contracta area of residual MR after MitraClip procedure; (b) 3D-TEE evaluation of planimetric smallest area after double-orifice creation.

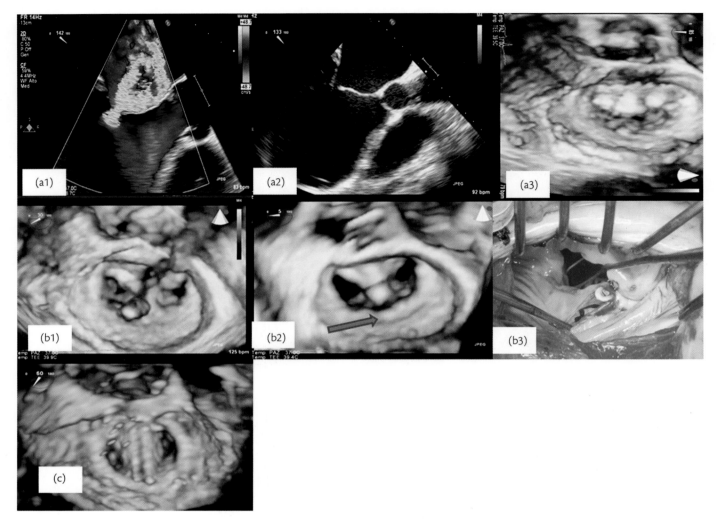

Fig. 16.16 MitraClip procedure in a patient with functional mitral regurgitation due to complex mechanism (extreme tethering of fibrotic posterior leaflet with complete loss of leaflet coaptation). (a1) 2D-TEE colour flow mapping; (a2) 2D-TEE; (a3) 3D-TEE. (b1) 3D-TEE during MitraClip implantation; (b2) 3D-TEE showing leaflet laceration (blue arrow) after MitraClip deployment, confirmed at surgical anatomic inspection. (c) 3D-TEE after mechanical prosthesis replacement.

delivery catheter to collapse the proximal anchor, followed by the distal anchor (➲ Fig. 16.17).

During direct annuloplasty, fluoroscopy and TEE are used to guide pledget positioning on the atrial side of the mitral annulus and assess annular downsizing efficacy on MR reduction. ➲ Figures 16.18 and 16.19 show a combined RT3D-TEE and fluoroscopy image of a direct percutaneous mitral annuloplasty device (Cardioband Valtech), the first in-man implantation (F Maisano, G La Canna, personal communication).

Percutaneous valve-in-ring implantation

In patients with failure of surgical mitral annuloplasty, transcatheter valve-in-ring implantation (TVIR) may be an alternative to high-risk re-operation. TVRI is feasible because the ring may be used as an anchor zone. Only the Edwards Sapien XT expandable

balloon prosthesis can be used for TVIR through the trans-septal catheterization or surgical LV transapical approach [52] (see ➲ Figs 16.20 and 16.21).

The selection of patients requires careful evaluation of MR site, which should be confined inside the ring, and exclusion of para-ring regurgitation. Fluoroscopy and 2D-, 3D-TEE are crucial to optimize prosthesis position to cover the mitral ring without paraprosthetic regurgitation or LV obstruction. In patients with non-radiopaque rings, a pigtail catheter may be positioned around the ring using 3D-TEE guidance in order to obtain fluoroscopy visibility.

Percutaneous treatment of para-prosthetic valve regurgitation

Paravalvular regurgitation (PVR) is a potential complication affecting 5–17% of surgically implanted prosthetic heart valves,

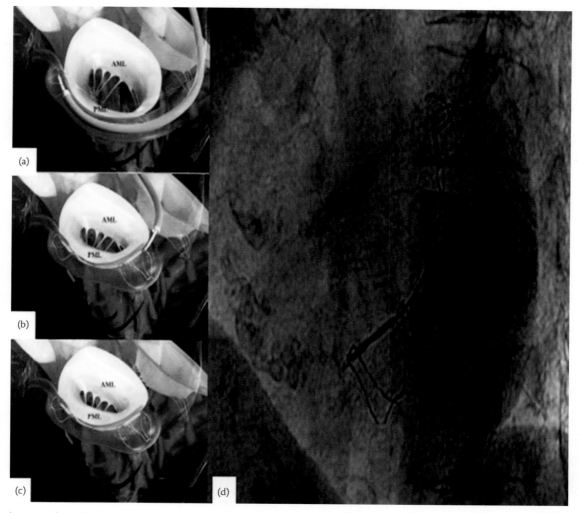

Fig. 16.17 Indirect mitral annuloplasty positioning Carillon device into coronary sinus. (a) Delivery catheter into coronary sinus. (b) Delivery of proximal and distal anchors of Carillon with significant reduction of septal-lateral dimension of mitral annulus. (c) Implantation of device. (d) Fluoroscopy imaging of final release of Carillon system into coronary sinus.

usually related to tissue friability, annular calcification, suture rupture, or endocarditis. The clinical course of patients with PVR may be asymptomatic, but can lead to heart failure or haemolytic anaemia, or even both. Recently, a percutaneous approach has been introduced for PVR treatment, therefore avoiding the high risk of surgical reoperation [7, 53]. Mitral PVR closure, with the positioning of one or more Amplatzer devices, is usually performed with an anterograde trans-septal approach. However, transapical left ventricular access has recently been introduced [54]. Aortic PVR treatment uses retrograde femoral artery access.

Before the procedure

Comprehensive colour Doppler echocardiographic imaging with TT and TEE provides diagnostic evidence of clinically suspected PVR and correlated haemodynamic burden. RT3D-TEE is crucial for depiction and anatomic PVR characterization regarding the defect's location, size, shape, and eventual number (see ➲ Figs 16.22–16.24). For mitral PVR defects, RT3D-TEE clearly identifies varying morphologic characteristics of leakage, which may show crescent, oblong, serpiginous, oval, or cylindrical morphology. This information is useful to establish the feasibility of percutaneous closure, based on optimal anatomic match between the occluder device (usually Amplatzer) and leak shape. Accurate identification of the leakage site is paramount. An *en face* 3D-TEE view can map the leak using the appendage, the aorta and the inter-atrial septum as anatomic references for lateral, anterior, and medial localization landmarks, respectively. ➲ Figure 16.22 shows a 3D-TEE patient with mitral paravalvular multiple leaks overlapping the anatomic specimen. TTE provides accurate diagnosis of para-aortic leakage that is located anteriorly, but is inaccurate when posteriorly confined, therefore requiring the TEE approach. MSCT is an emerging technique in adjunct to TEE for PVR, although artefacts from dense structures may affect image quality. When MR is severe due to large leaks, the patient commonly suffers from congestive heart failure. Therefore, even partial MR reduction might be advantageous. Complete closure should be targeted in cases of haemolysis, which is usually associated with a

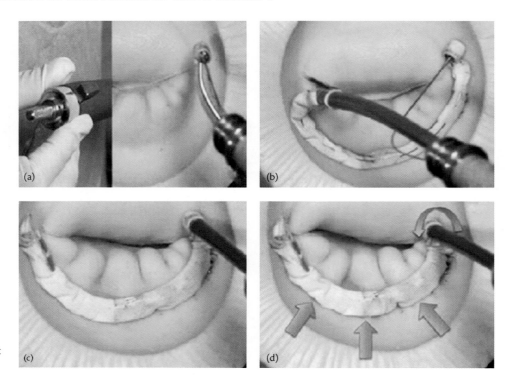

Fig. 16.18 (a) Direct annuloplasty with implantation of Cardioband device using a trans-septal approach and subsequent adjustment of annular constriction to attempt MR correction (b–d).

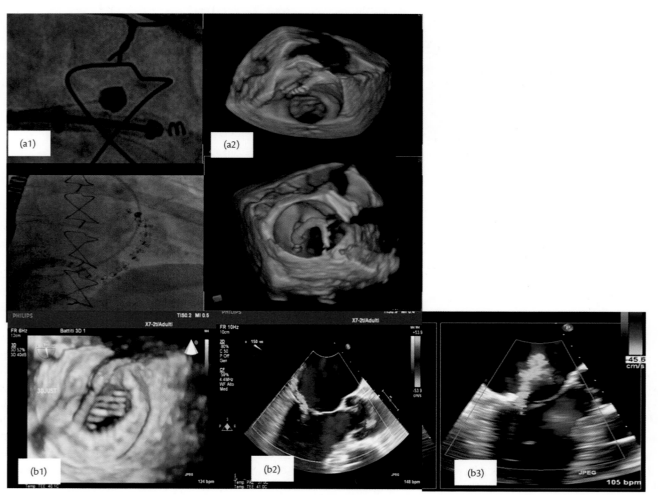

Fig. 16.19 First in-man implantation of Cardioband device using trans-septal approach with simultaneous fluoroscopy/3D-TEE guidance. (a1) Fluoroscopy imaging of delivery catheter implantation into the antero-lateral commissure and subsequent anchor release up to postero-medial commissure with 3D-TEE guidance (a2). (b1) 3D-TEE monitoring of ring adjustment to attempt reduction of MR (b2, baseline; b3 after ring adjustment).

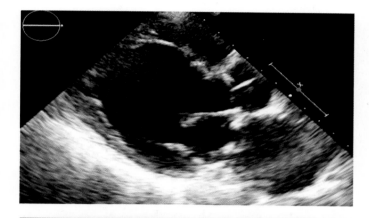

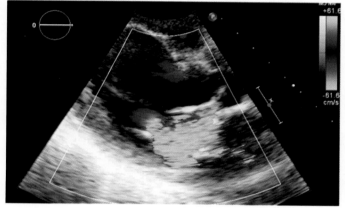

Fig. 16.20 Failure of surgical mitral annuloplasty with subannular malapposition and loss of systolic coaptation of mitral valve leaflets (TTE, top image) and related severe MR (TTE colour Doppler, bottom image).

smaller leak. Active endocarditis subtending PVR is considered a contraindication for percutaneous leak repair.

During the procedure

Percutaneous PVR closure is carried out under general anaesthesia, even though conscious sedation may be used for patients undergoing closure of para-aortic leak. Fluoroscopy and TEE, supplemented by RT3D-TEE, are requested to monitor the procedure [7]. Using an anterograde trans-septal approach for paramitral regurgitation, right anterior oblique and left anterior oblique fluoroscopy projections are used to image mitral prosthesis tangentially and *en face*, respectively. RT3D-TEE using an *en face* anatomic view gives a mapping nomenclature of the leak site (aorta at 12 o'clock, left atrial appendage at 9 o'clock, inter-atrial septum at 3 o'clock). To overcome the mirror imaging of fluoroscopy, 3D-TEE images may be displayed from a left ventricular view.

RT3D-TEE can guide the catheter system towards the quadrant in which the defect is located for subsequent crossing and advancement into the left ventricle (Fig. 16.25). Depending on the lateral or medial site of leakage, a different method for transseptal catheterization using the transfemoral or superior vena cava approach may be selected. Based on the shape and size of the defect, RT3D-TEE provides information for the selection of single or multiple device occluders. For smaller and cylindrical

shapes, usually determining haemolysis, a single device with an optimal match may be successful (Fig. 16.22). With crescent or oblong defects, multiple-device implantation is required. After the assessment of effective MR reduction without prosthetic leaflet malfunction, single or multiple occluder devices may be deployed. Recently, a retrograde approach has been introduced, which crosses the PVR through a transapical LV puncture. This approach, despite its more invasive nature, facilitates closure and limits fluoroscopy exposure, especially when the leak is located medially or in the presence of multiple defects (catheter manipulation and cannulation of defect from a trans-septal approach can be challenging). Figure 16.26 shows an effective 'rescue' paravalvular leak closure using a transapical approach subsequent to unsuccessful trans-septal occluder positioning. RT3D-TEE is useful to assess prosthesis malfunction before occluder deployment (Fig. 16.27), or to identify occluder migration in the left atrium (Fig. 16.28).

The retrograde femoral artery approach is used for para-aortic defect closure with one occluder, owing to its smaller dimension compared with para-mitral defects.

After the procedure

Pre-discharge and follow-up TTE, supplemented by TEE when necessary, is useful to establish long-term procedure effectiveness. Pulmonary artery pressure, prosthetic inflow, and transvalvular gradient, estimated by Doppler echocardiography, together with haemolysis assessment, provide clinically relevant information on the ultimate efficacy of percutaneous PVR closure. In selected cases, which reveal ineffective MR reduction, a second procedure may be considered.

Percutaneous pulmonary valve replacement

Intervention on the right ventricular outflow tract (RVOT) usually becomes necessary in patients with either pulmonary stenosis or regurgitation following repair of congenital heart disease. In the past, the treatment of regurgitation was often delayed as long as possible leading to chronic right ventricular overload, shown to be associated with adverse clinical outcome [55]. This, together with the development of new techniques allowing less invasive intervention with good mid- and long-term outcome, has led to a growing use of imaging techniques to contribute to the assessment of the optimal timing for intervention, and to its guidance [56, 57]. Although no specific guidelines for considering percutaneous pulmonary valve replacement (PPVR) have been established, the technique has been proposed in patients with right-ventricular-to-pulmonary-artery (RV–PA) conduit with moderate to severe associated stenosis or regurgitation, as well as in severe pulmonary regurgitation in symptomatic patients, or in those with RV dysfunction or dilatation associated with decreased exercise tolerance [58, 59]. PPVR in severe RVOT obstruction, whether in symptomatic or asymptomatic patients, has also been proposed [59].

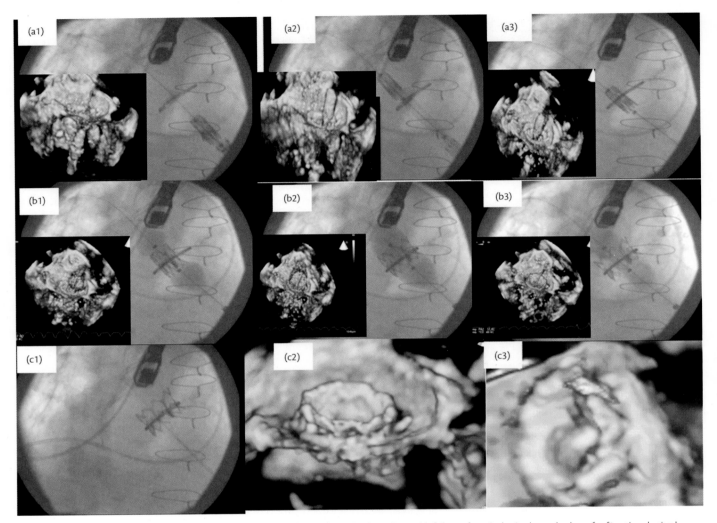

Fig. 16.21 Fluoroscopy and 3D-TEE monitoring of prosthetic valve implantation in patient with failure of surgical mitral annuloplasty for functional mitral regurgitation. (a1–3) Guidance to correctly position prosthesis in mitral ring. (b1–3) Expansion of prosthetic valve delivery catheter. (c1–3) Deployment of prosthesis with residual mild paravalvular regurgitation.

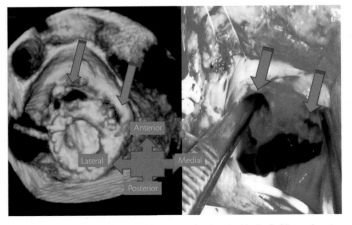

Fig. 16.22 3D-TEE localization of paraprosthetic mitral leaks (left), overlapping surgical anatomic findings (right).

Before PPVR

Optimal timing for the procedure and adequate patient selection are the means through which cardiovascular imaging can contribute to the success of PPVR. Accurate quantification of pulmonary stenosis and regurgitation, RV dimension and function are commonly assessed through TTE, TEE, and MRI and are, together with haemodynamic study, the key to selecting the appropriate timing for valve replacement (⊃ Fig. 16.29). MRI and echocardiography, as well as MSCT, can contribute to assessing patient eligibility through determination of RVOT shape, size, and relation to coronary arteries. An RV–PA conduit of a minimum diameter >16 mm and maximum diameter <22 mm is considered the ideal landing zone for the prosthetic valve [60], although successful implantation in non-conduit outflow tracts after pre-stenting to generate an appropriate implantation site have been reported [61, 62].

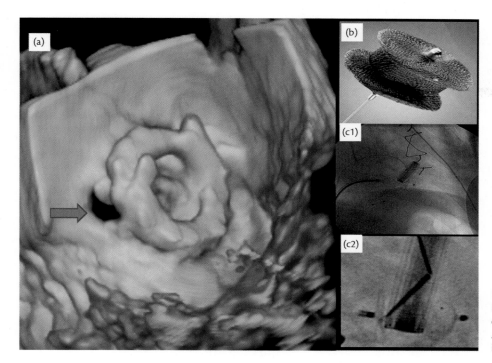

Fig. 16.23 (a) Pre-procedural mitral prosthetic leak (arrow) assessment by 3D-TEE, predicting an optimal Amplatzer/target lesion matching. (b) Amplatzer device. (c1, 2) Fluoroscopy imaging of implanted device.

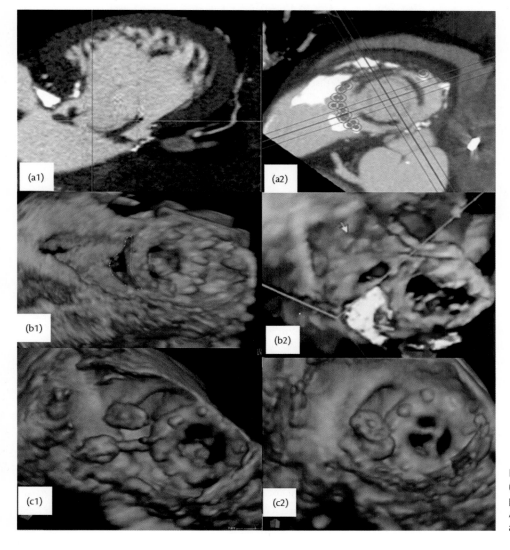

Fig. 16.24 MSCT (a1, 2) and 3D-TEE (b1, 2) showing a large (crescendo shape) paraprosthetic mitral leak, requiring double Amplatzer implantation with transapical approach (c).

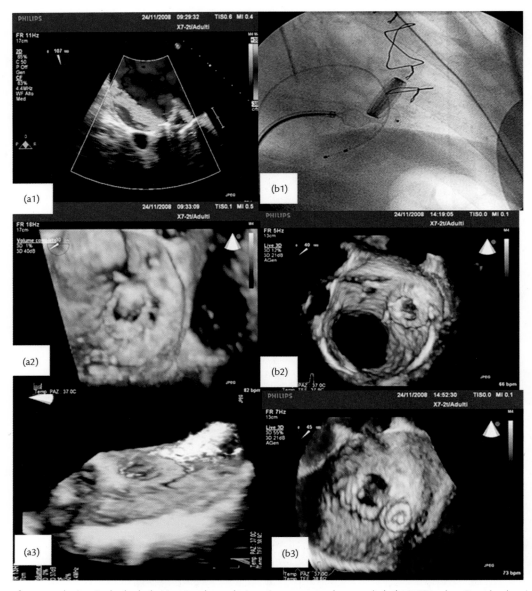

Fig. 16.25 Closure of paraprosthetic mitral valve leak using Amplatzer device using trans-septal approach. (a1) 2D-TEE colour Doppler showing severe MR arising from large medial paraprosthetic leak evident at 3D-TEE imaging (a2) and confirmed with 3D-TEE colour Doppler (a3). (b) Positioning of Amplatzer device guided by fluoroscopy (1) and 3D-TEE (2, 3).

It is, however, important to note that the determination of RVOT dimension based on averaged data can be misleading.

Pre-implantation imaging studies must focus on ruling out the risk of coronary artery compression, ideally done through MSCT or MRI, which is not uncommon and can lead to a fatal outcome, in the subset of patients more frequently requiring PPVR [63]. No specific data on minimum distance have been suggested, so additional intra-procedural assessment of potential coronary compression is recommended [59]. Echocardiographic assessment is indicated to rule out endocarditis before the procedure, and vascular ultrasound can be used to plan femoral or jugular access.

During PPVR

TEE can provide intra-procedural monitoring and guidance, in addition to angiographic images, in evaluating the potential displacement of the RVOT wall toward the coronary artery before valve implantation during previous balloon inflation. Subsequently, it can help optimize valve positioning before implantation, ensuring muscular RVOT is not covered by the stent, and that it lies away from the bifurcation. After implantation, TEE can be used to confirm adequate valve placement and the absence of complications, focusing especially on the detection of pericardial effusion, prosthesis migration, coronary occlusion, and pulmonary artery rupture.

After PPVR

Echocardiographic follow-up must focus on ruling out the presence of significant stenosis or regurgitation and endocarditis. Conventional X-ray or MSCT assessment can be used to detect stent fracture, a complication reported to occur in a considerable number of cases varying from 5% to 28% [64].

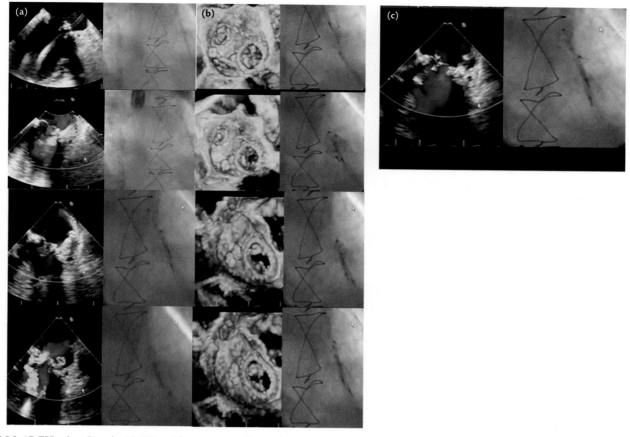

Fig. 16.26 2D-TEE colour Doppler, 3D-TEE and fluoroscopy guidance of transapical repair of MR due to a lateral paravalvular leak in patient with biological prosthesis who previously underwent multiple surgical procedures and ineffective trans-septal Amplatzer positioning. (a, b) Transapical implantation of double Amplatzer adjacent to previous trans-septal implanted device; (c) TEE colour Doppler showing complete closure of leak abolishing related MR.

Occluded Medial Prosthetic Orifice

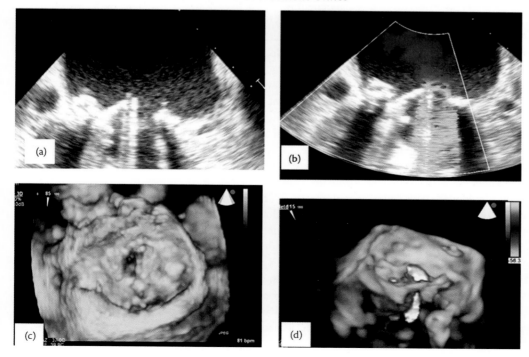

Fig. 16.27 2D- and 3D-TEE examination after repair of paravalvular mitral leak with Amplazter device, impeding opening of prosthetic disc (a, 2D-TEE; b, 3D-TEE) with occlusion of medial orifice and corresponding flow loss (c, 2D-TEE colour Doppler; d, 3D-TEE colour Doppler).

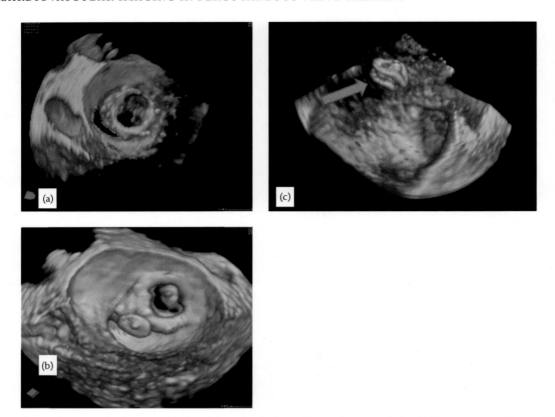

Fig. 16.28 3D-TEE showing large paraprosthetic mitral leak, with in crescendo shape (a), requiring transapical multiple Amplatzer positioning (b), with subsequent occluder migration in the left atrium (c).

Perspectives in the percutaneous treatment of tricuspid valve disease

Tricuspid regurgitation (TR) is commonly secondary to left-sided heart valve disease and may cause congestive heart syndrome with multi-organ failure [65]. TR may occur late despite successful correction of primary left-heart disease due to progressive right ventricular remodelling and dysfunction. As severe TR is often associated with late-stage myocardial damage, re-operation for recurrent TR is a particularly high-risk procedure. Percutaneous TR therapy, adapting some of the concepts that have been developed for MR treatment, might be promising, but at this time few or no data are available. For patients considered inoperable suffering from severe congestive right-venous syndrome, one possible approach is implantation of separate valves in the superior vena cava and in the inferior vena cava to block the distal transmission of right ventricular pressures to the body [66]. This might protect distal organs, such as the liver and the kidneys, but the effects of resultant high atrial distending pressure remain unclear.

The trans-catheter bioprosthesis Melody pulmonary valve has been implanted in patients with dysfunctional surgical bioprosthetic valves in the tricuspid position with clinical benefit [67].

Conclusion

Percutaneous VHD treatment requires multi-modality imaging for patient selection, procedure monitoring, and subsequent follow-up surveillance. A routine TTE is the first imaging modality used for VHD assessment. TEE supplemented with real-time 3-dimensional (RT3D) imaging may be required to enhance VHD diagnostic balance. MSCT plays an important role in planning certain procedures (e.g. TAVI, mitral annuloplasty, PVR repair) providing detailed information on feasibility and interventional access planes, and minimizing procedural-related complications. Fluoroscopy and TEE are needed to guide and monitor VHD percutaneous procedures, and combining pre-procedural MSCT information, its guidance capability may be optimized. Follow-up surveillance requires the use of echocardiography as a primary diagnostic approach, supplemented with additional multi-modality imaging when clinically necessary.

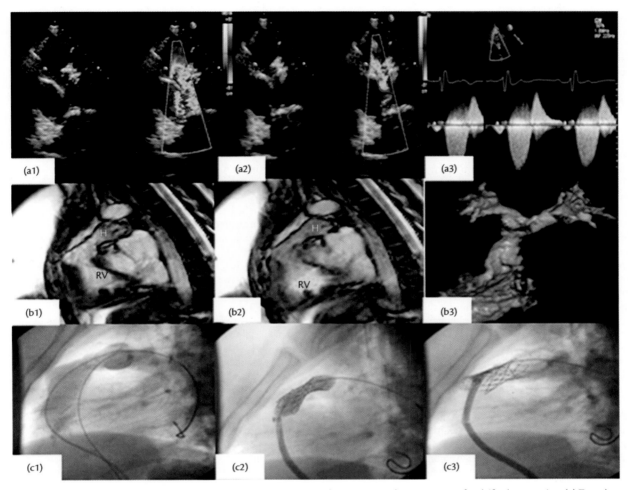

Fig. 16.29 Multi-modality imaging in a patient with severe pulmonary stenosis and regurgitation due to Homograft calcific degeneration. (a) Transthoracic echocardiogram showing pulmonary systolic turbulence (1), regurgitation (2), mean gradient 60 mmHg (3). (b) Magnetic resonance imaging with systolic (1), diastolic (2), and 3D reconstruction. (c1–3) Sequence of trans-catheter implantation of pulmonary Melody prosthesis.

References

1. Nkomo VT, Gardin JM, Skelton TN, et al. Burden of valvular heart diseases: a population-based study. *Lancet* 2006; 368: 1005–11.

2. Iung B, Baron G, Butchart EG, et al. A prospective survey of patients with valvular heart disease in Europe: the Euro heart survey on valvular heart disease. *Eur Heart J* 2003; 24: 1231–43.

3. Iung B, Baron G, Tornos P, et al. Valvular heart disease in the community: a European experience. *Curr Probl Cardiol* 2007; 32: 609–61.

4. Iung B, Cachier A, Baron G, et al. Decision making in elderly patients with severe aortic stenosis: why are so many denied surgery? *Eur Heart J* 2005; 26: 2714–20.

5. Mirabel M, Iung B, Baron G, et al. What are the characteristics of patients with severe, symptomatic, mitral regurgitation who are denied surgery? *Eur Heart J* 2007; 28: 1358–65.

6. Bach DS, Awais M, Gurm HS, Kohnstamm S. Failure of guideline adherence for intervention in patients with severe mitral regurgitation. *J Am Coll Cardiol* 2009; 54: 860–65.

7. Rihal CS, Sorajja P, Booker JD, et al. Principles of percutaneous paravalvular leak closure. *J Am Coll Cardiol* Intv 2012; 5: 121–30.

8. Leon MB, Smith CR, Mack M, et al. Trans-catheter aortic-valve implantation for aortic stenosis in patients who cannot undergo surgery. *N Engl J Med* 2010; 363: 1597–607.

9. Feldman T, Kar S, Rinaldi M, et al. Percutaneous mitral repair with the MitraClip system: safety and midterm durability in the initial EVEREST (Endovascular Valve Edge-to-Edge Repair Study) cohort. *J Am Coll Cardiol* 2009; 54: 686–94.

10. Zamorano JL, Badano LP, Bruce C, et al. EAE/ASE recommendations for the use of echocardiography in new trans-catheter interventions for valvular heart disease. *Eur Heart J.* 2011; 32 (17): 2189–214.

11. Holmes DR Jr, Mack MJ, Kaul S, et al. 2012 ACCF/AATS/SCAI/STS Expert consensus document on trans-catheter aortic valve replacement. *J Am Coll Cardiol* 2012; 59 (13): 1200–54.

12. Van de Veire N. Imaging to guide trans-catheter aortic valve implantation. *J Echocardiogr* 2010; 1–6.

13. Citro R, Mirra M, Baldi C, et al. Concomitant dynamic obstruction and endocarditis after 'valve-in-valve' TAVI implantation. *Int J Cardiol* 2013; 2.

14. Pontone G, Andreini D, Bartorelli AL, et al. Feasibility and accuracy of a comprehensive multidetector computed tomography acquisition for patients referred for balloon-expandable trans-catheter aortic valve implantation. *Am Heart J* 2011; 161 (6): 1106–13.

15. Akhtar M, Tuzcu EM, Kapadia SR, et al. Aortic root morphology in patients undergoing percutaneous aortic valve replacement: evidence of aortic root remodelling. *J ThoracCardiovasc Surg* 2009; 137 (4): 950–6.

16. Kurra V, Kapadia SR, Tuzcu EM, et al. Pre-procedural imaging of aortic root orientation and dimensions: comparison between x-ray angiographic planar imaging and 3-dimensional multidetector row computed tomography. *J Am Coll Cardiol Intv* 2010; 3 (1) 105–13.

17. Jabbour A, Ismail TF, Moat N, et al. Multi-modality imaging in trans-catheter aortic valve implantation and post-procedural aortic regurgitation: comparison among cardiovascular magnetic resonance, cardiac computed tomography and echocardiography. *J Am Coll Cardiol* 2011; 58 (21): 2165–73.

18. Yucel EK, Anderson CM, Edelman RR, et al. AHA scientific statement. Magnetic resonance angiography: update on applications for extracranial arteries. *Circulation* 1999; 100 (22): 2284–301.

19. Lancellotti P, Tribouilloy C, Hagendorff A, et al. European Association of Echocardiography recommendations for the assessment of valvular regurgitation. Part 1: aortic and pulmonary regurgitation (native valve disease). *Eur J Echocardiogr* 2010; 11 (3): 223–44.

20. Gonçalves A, Marcos-Alberca P, Zamorano JL. Echocardiography: guidance during valve implantation. *EuroIntervention* 2010 May; 6 Suppl G:G14-9. doi: 10.4244/. Review.

21. Tuzcu EM. Trans-catheter aortic valve replacement malposition and embolization: innovation brings solutions also new challenges. *Catheter Cardiovasc Interv* 2008; 72 (4): 570–80.

22. de Isla LP, Rodriguez E, Zamorano J. Transapical aortic prosthesis misplacement. *J Am Coll Cardiol* 2008; 52 (24): 2043.

23. Franco E, de Agustin JA, Hernandez-Antolin R, et al. Acute mitral stenosis after trans-catheter aortic valve implantation. *J Am Coll Cardiol* 2012; 60 (20): e 35.

24. Walther T, Falk V, Kempfert J, et al. Transapical minimally invasive aortic valve implantation: the initial 50 patients. *Eur J Cardiothorac Surg* 2008; 33 (6): 983–8.

25. Shames S, Kozco A, Hahn R, Jin Z, Picard MH, Gillam LD. Flow characteristics of the SAPIEN™ aortic valve: the importance of recognizing in-stent flow acceleration for the echocardiographic assessment of valve function. *J Am Soc Echocardiogr* 2011; 25 (6): 603–9.

26. Zoghbi WA, Chambers JB, Dumesnil JG, et al. Recommendations for evaluation of prosthetic valves with echocardiography and Doppler ultrasound: a report from the American Society of Echocardiography's Guidelines and Standards Committee and the Task Force on Prosthetic Valves, developed in conjunction with the American College of Cardiology Cardiovascular Imaging Committee, Cardiac Imaging Committee of the American Heart Association, the European Association of Echocardiography, a registered branch of the European Society of Cardiology, the Japanese Society of Echocardiography and the Canadian Society of Echocardiography, endorsed by the American College of Cardiology Foundation, American Heart Association, European Association of Echocardiography, a registered branch of the European Society of Cardiology, the Japanese Society of Echocardiography, and Canadian Society of Echocardiography. *J Am Soc Echocardiogr* 2009; 22 (9): 975–1014.

27. Pirat B, Little SH, Igo SR, et al. Direct measurement of proximal isovelocity surface area by real-time three-dimensional color Doppler for quantitation of aortic regurgitant volume: an in-vitro validation. *J Am Soc Echocardiogr* 2009; 22 (3): 306–13.

28. Reyes VP, Raju BS, Wynne J, et al. Percutaneous balloon valvuloplasty compared with open surgical commissurotomy for mitral stenosis. *N Engl J Med*. 1994; 331 (15): 961–7.

29. Ben Farhat M, Ayari M, Maatouk F, et al. Percutaneous balloon versus surgical closed and open mitral commissurotomy: seven-year follow-up results of a randomized trial. *Circulation* 1998; 97 (3): 245–50.

30. Inoue K, Owaki T, Nakamura T, Kitamura F, Miyamoto N. Clinical application of transvenous mitral commissurotomy by a new balloon catheter. *J ThoracCardiovasc Surg* 1984; 87 (3): 394–402.

31. Wilkins GT, Weyman AE, Abascal VM, Block PC, Palacios IF. Percutaneous balloon dilatation of the mitral valve: an analysis of echocardiographic variables related to outcome and the mechanism of dilatation. *Br Heart J* 1988; 60 (4): 299–308.

32. Valocik G, Kamp O, Mannaerts HF, Visser CA. New quantitative three-dimensional echocardiographic indices of mitral valve stenosis. *Int J Cardiovasc Imaging* 2007; 23 (6): 707–16.

33. Zamorano J, Cordeiro P, Sugeng L, et al. Real-time three-dimensional echocardiography for rheumatic mitral valve stenosis evaluation—an accurate and novel approach. *J Am Coll Cardiol* 2004; 43 (11): 2091–96.

34. Fatkin D, Roy P, Morgan JJ, Feneley MP. Percutaneous balloon mitral valvotomy with the Inoue single-balloon catheter: commissural morphology as a determinant of outcome. *J Am Coll Cardiol* 1993; 21 (2): 390–7.

35. Sutaria N, Northridge DB, Shaw TR. Significance of commissural calcification on outcome of mitral balloon valvotomy. *Heart* 2000; 84 (4): 398–402.

36. Turgeman Y, Atar S, Rosenfeld T. The subvalvular apparatus in rheumatic mitral stenosis: methods of assessment and therapeutic implications. *Chest* 2003; 124 (5): 1929–36.

37. White ML, Grover-McKay M, Weiss RM, et al. Prediction of change in mitral valve area after mitral balloon commissurotomy using cine computed tomography. *Invest Radiol* 1994; 29 (9): 827–33.

38. Zamorano J, Perez de Isla L, Sugeng L, et al. Non-invasive assessment of mitral valve area during percutaneous balloon mitral valvuloplasty: role of real-time 3D echocardiography. *Eur Heart J* 2004; 25 (23): 2086–91.

39. Applebaum RM, Kasliwal RR, Kanojia A, et al. Utility of three-dimensional echocardiography during balloon mitral valvuloplasty. *J Am Coll Cardiol* 1998; 32: 1405–9.

40. Lee S-P, Kim H-K, Kim K-H, et al. Prevalence of significant tricuspid regurgitation in patients with successful percutaneous mitral valvuloplasty for mitral stenosis: results from 12 years' follow-up of one centre prospective registry. *Heart* 2013; 99: 91–97.

41. Alfieri O, Maisano F, De Bonis M, et al. The double-orifice technique in mitral valve repair: a simple solution for complex problems. *J Thorac Cardiovasc Surg* 2001; 122: 674–81

42. Maisano F, La Canna G, Colombo A, Alfieri O. The evolution from surgery to percutaneous mitral valve interventions: the role of the edge to edge technique. *J Am Coll Cardiol* 2011; 58: 2174–82.

43. De Bonis M, Maisano F, La Canna G, Alfieri O. Treatment and management of mitral regurgitation. *Nat Rev Cardiol* 2011; 9: 133–46.

44. Auricchio A, Schillinger W, Meyer S, et al. Correction of mitral regurgitation in non-responders to cardiac resynchronization therapy by MitraClip improves symptoms and promotes reverse remodeling. *J Am Coll Cardiol* 2011; 58: 2183–89.

45. Feldman T, Foster E, Glower DG, et al. (2011) Percutaneous repair or surgery for mitral regurgitation. *N Engl J Med* 364: 1395–6.

46. Altiok E, Hamada S, Brehmer K, et al. Analysis of procedural effects of percutaneous edge-to-edge mitral valve repair by 2D and 3D echocardiography. *Circ Cardiovasc Imaging* 2012; 5: 748–55.

47. Fedak PW, McCarthy PM, Bonow RO. Evolving concepts and technologies in mitral valve repair. *Circulation* 2008; 117: 963–74.

48. Chiam PTL, Ruiz CE. Percutaneous transcatheter mitral valve repair. A classification of the technology. *J Am Coll Cardiol* Intv 2011; 4: 1–13.

49. Tops LF, Van de Veire NR, Schuijf JD, et al. Noninvasive evaluation of coronary sinus anatomy and its relation to the mitral valve annulus: implications for percutaneous mitral annuloplasty. *Circulation* 2007; 115: 1426–32.

50. Schofer J, Siminiak T, Haude M, et al. Percutaneous mitral annuloplasty for functional mitral regurgitation: results of the CARILLON Mitral Annuloplasty Device European Union Study. *Circulation* 2009; 120: 326–33.

51. Siminiak T, Wu JC, Haude M, et al. Treatment of functional mitral regurgitation by percutaneous annuloplasty: results of the TITAN Trial. *Eur J Heart Fail* 2012; 14: 931–38.

52. Descoutures F, Himbert D, Maisano F, et al. Trans-catheter valve-in-ring implantation after failure of surgical mitral repair. *Eur J Cardio-Thoracic Surgery* 2013: 1–8.

53. García-Fernandez MA, Cortes M, García-Robles JA, et al. Utility of real-time three-dimensional transoesophageal echocardiography in evaluating the success of percutaneous trans-catheter closure of mitral paravalvular leaks. *J Am Soc Echocardiogr* 2010; 23: 26–32.

54. Jelnin V, Dudiy Y, Einhorn BN, et al. Clinical experience with percutaneous left ventricular transapical access for interventions in structural heart defects. a safe access and secure exit. *J Am Coll Cardiol Intv* 2011; 4: 868–74.

55. Bouzas B, Kilner PJ, Gatzoulis MA. Pulmonary regurgitation: not a benign lesion. *Eur Heart J* 2005; 26 (5): 433–9.

56. Bonhoeffer P, Boudjemline Y, Saliba Z, et al. Percutaneous replacement of pulmonary valve in a right-ventricle to pulmonary-artery prosthetic conduit with valve dysfunction. *Lancet* 2000; 356 (9239): 1403–5.

57. Eicken A, Ewert P, Hager A, et al. Percutaneous pulmonary valve implantation: two-centre experience with more than 100 patients. *Eur Heart J* 2011; 32 (10): 1260–5.

58. Feltes TF, Bacha E, Beekman RH, et al. Indications for cardiac catheterisation and intervention in pediatric cardiac disease: a scientific statement from the American Heart Association. *Circulation* 2011; 123 (22): 2607–52.

59. Khambadkone S. Percutaneous pulmonary valve implantation. *Ann Pediatr Card* 2012; 5 (1): 53–60.

60. Khambadkone S, Coats L, Taylor A, et al. Percutaneous pulmonary valve implantation in humans: experience in 59 consecutive cases. *Circulation* 2005; 112 (8): 1189–97.

61. Momenah TS, El Oakley R, Al Najashi K, Khoshhal S, Al Qethamy H, Bonhoeffer P. Extended applications of percutaneous pulmonary valve implantation. *J Am Coll Cardiol* 2009; 53 (20): 1859–63.

62. Nordmeyer J, Lurz P, Khambadkone S, et al. Pre-stenting with a bare metal stent before percutaneous pulmonary valve implantation: acute and 1-year outcomes. *Heart* 2011; 97 (2): 118–23.

63. Lurz P, Coats L, Khambadkone S, et al. Percutaneous pulmonary valve implantation—Impact of evolving technology and learning curve on clinical outcome. *Circulation* 2008; 117 (15): 1964–72.

64. Lee YS, Lee HD. Percutaneous pulmonary valve implantation. *Korean Circ J* 2012; 42 (10): 652–6.

65. Taramasso M, Vanermen H, Maisano F, Guidotti A, La Canna G, Alfieri O. The growing clinical importance of secondary tricuspid regurgitation. *J Am Coll Cardiol* 2012; 59: 703–10.

66. Lauten A, Figulla HR, Willich C, et al. Percutaneous caval stent valve implantation: investigation of an interventional approach for treatment of tricuspid regurgitation. *Eu Heart J* (2010) 31, 1274–81.

67. Gurvitch R, Cheung A, Jian Ye J, et al. Transcatheter valve-in-valve implantation for failed surgical bioprosthetic valves. *J Am Coll Cardiol* 2011; 58: 2196–209.

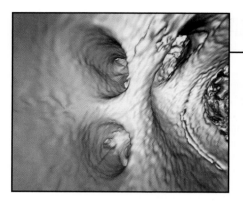

CHAPTER 17

Endocarditis

Gilbert Habib and Franck Thuny

Contents

Introduction

Infective endocarditis (IE) is a life-threatening disease associated with a high mortality rate [1, 2]. Despite major improvements in diagnostic and therapeutic procedures, both the diagnosis of IE and its management remain challenging. Several complications may occur during the course of IE, and are the cause of the persistent high morbidity and mortality of the disease [3]. Because of these very frequent and severe complications, about half of patients with IE are operated on during the active phase of the disease (early surgery) [4]. Imaging, particularly echocardiography, plays a key role in both the diagnosis and management of infective endocarditis. Echocardiography is also useful for the prognostic assessment of patients with IE, for their follow-up under therapy, and during and after surgery [5].

Echocardiography for diagnosis of infective endocarditis

When to perform echocardiography in IE?

Infective endocarditis is not a single disease but may present with several very different initial symptoms, including heart failure, cerebral embolism, pacemaker infection, or isolated fever. IE must be suspected in the presence of fever associated with regurgitant heart murmur, known cardiac disease, bacteraemia, new conduction disturbance, and embolic events of unknown origin [6]. In all these situations, echocardiography must be performed. ➲ Figure 17.1 is a proposed algorithm illustrating the respective indications of transthoracic (TTE) and transoesophageal (TOE) echocardiography. TTE must be performed first in all cases, because it is a non-invasive technique giving useful information both for the diagnosis and the assessment of severity of IE. TOE must also be performed in the majority of patients with suspected IE, because of its better image quality and better sensitivity, except in the case of good quality negative TTE associated with a low level of clinical suspicion.

Anatomic definitions—echocardiographic correlations

Anatomically, IE is characterized by a combination of vegetations and destructive lesions:

◆ Vegetations are typically attached on the low-pressure side of the valve structure, but may be located anywhere on the components of the valvular and subvalvular apparatus, as well as on the mural endocardium of the cardiac chambers or the ascending aorta. When large and mobile, vegetations are prone to embolism and less frequently to valve or prosthetic obstruction.

◆ Destructive lesions are very frequently associated with vegetations or may be observed alone. The consequences of this destructive process may include valve aneurysm, perforation, or prolapse, and chordae or, less frequently, papillary muscle rupture. The main consequences of these lesions are severe valve regurgitation and heart failure.

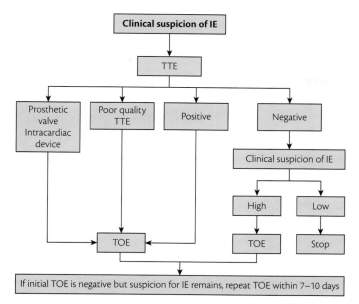

Fig. 17.1 Algorithm showing the role of echocardiography in the diagnosis and assessment of infective endocarditis. IE, infective endocarditis; TTE, transthoracic echocardiography; TOE, transoesophageal echocardiography. Reproduced by Habib G, Hoen B, Tornos P, Thuny F, Prendergast B, Vilacosta I, et al. Guidelines on the prevention, diagnosis, and treatment of infective endocarditis (new version 2009): The Task Force on the Prevention, Diagnosis, and Treatment of Infective Endocarditis of the European Society of Cardiology (ESC). *European Heart Journal* (2009) 30, 2369–2413 by permission of Oxford University Press.

◆ The third main anatomic feature of IE is abscess formation. Abscesses are more frequent in aortic and prosthetic valve IE and may be complicated by pseudoaneurysm or fistulization.

These three anatomic features are frequently present together and must be meticulously described by the echocardiographic

examination. Knowledge of these main anatomic and echocardiographic definitions is mandatory (⊃ Table 17.1).

Duke 'echocardiographic' criteria

In 1994, Durack proposed a new classification of criteria for IE called Duke criteria [7]. This new classification was a big step into the diagnosis of IE because it included echocardiography as a major criterion for IE. The major echographic criteria for IE are vegetation, abscess, and new dehiscence of a prosthetic valve.

Vegetation

Echocardiography is the reference method for the diagnosis of vegetation. Typically, vegetation presents as an oscillating mass attached on a valvular structure, with a motion independent to that of this valve (⊃ Figs 17.2, 17.3 ▤ Video 17.1). However, vegetation may also present as a non-oscillating mass and with an atypical location (▤ Video 17.2). Vegetations are usually localized on the atrial side of the atrioventricular valves, and on the ventricular side of the aortic and pulmonary valves. Less frequently, vegetations are localized on mural endocardium, papillary muscles, or ascending aorta. TTE has a sensitivity of about 75% for the diagnosis of vegetations. However, the sensitivity of TTE may be reduced in case of low echogenicity, very small vegetations, and in IE affecting intra-cardiac devices. TOE is mandatory in case of doubtful transthoracic examination, in prosthetic and pacemaker IE, and when an abscess is suspected. TOE enhances the sensitivity of TTE to about 85 to 90% for the diagnosis of vegetations. In addition, both TTE and TOE are useful to assess the size and mobility of the vegetation, as well as its evolution under antibiotic therapy [8].

Abscess formation

The second major echocardiographic criterion for endocarditis is the presence of peri-valvular abscesses. They are more frequently

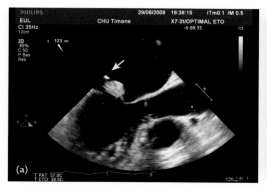
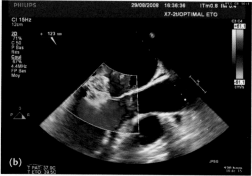

Fig. 17.2 TOE showing a large mitral vegetation on the anterior leaflet associated with a chordae rupture (a) and severe mitral regurgitation (b).

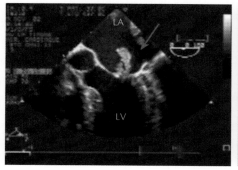
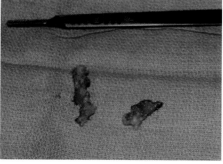

Fig. 17.3 Echo/anatomic correlations. TOE, large vegetations on the two mitral leaflets (arrow); LA, left atrium; LV, left ventricle.

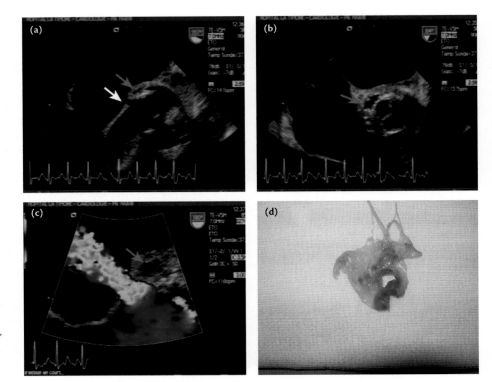

Fig. 17.4 TOE showing the peri-annular damage of an aortic bioprosthetic valve endocarditis. We can see the association of an annular abscess (a–c, red arrow) with a perforation of the basal area of the anterior mitral leaflet (a, white arrow; c, d) leading to a mitral regurgitation.

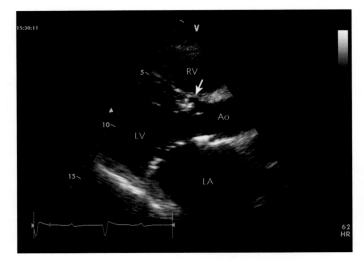

Fig. 17.5 TTE showing an anterior aortic annular abscess (arrow).

observed in aortic valve IE and in prosthetic valve IE. Abscess typically presents as a peri-valvular zone of reduced echo density, without colour flow detected inside. The diagnosis is easy in the presence of a clear free-space in the aortic root (◯ Figs 17.4 and 17.5), but may be much more difficult at the early stage of the disease when only a thickening of the aortic root is evidenced (◯ Figs 17.6 and 17.7). The sensitivity of TTE is about 50%, that of TOE 90%. The additional value of TOE is much higher for the diagnosis of abscess than for the diagnosis of vegetation. For this reason, TOE must be systematically performed in aortic valve IE, and as soon as an abscess is suspected.

Abscess formation is only one type of peri-valvular involvement in IE. Considering echographic and anomic definitions (◯ Table 17.1), three types of peri-valvular lesions may be described:

- Abscess is a non-communicating zone of necrosis with purulent material. Echographic appearance is a non-circulating peri-valvular zone of reduced echo density (◯ Fig. 17.8).
- Pseudoaneurysm is characterized anatomically by a perivalvular cavity communicating with the cardiovascular lumen. The echographic hallmark of pseudoaneurysm is the presence of a pulsatile peri-valvular echo free-space with colour Doppler flow inside (◯ Figs 17.9 and 17.10). The echographic appearance of partial systolic collapse proves that the abscess communicates with the cardiovascular lumen.
- Fistula may be a complication of both abscesses and pseudoaneurysm. They are defined anatomically by a communication between two neighbouring cavities and echographically by a colour Doppler communication between two adjacent cavities.

All these peri-valvular lesions are more frequently observed in aortic endocarditis and then involve the mitral-aortic inter-valvular fibrosa (◯ Fig. 17.11, ◙ Video 17.3) [9].

New dehiscence of a prosthetic valve

It represents the third main diagnostic criterion for IE [7]. IE must be suspected in the presence of a new peri-valvular regurgitation, even in the absence of vegetation or abscess. TOE has a better sensitivity than TTE for this diagnosis, especially in mitral prosthetic valve infective endocarditis (PVIE) (◯ Fig. 17.12). For this reason, systematic post-operative echocardiography must be performed after any valve replacement in order to serve as reference for better interpretation of future echocardiographic abnormalities.

Other echocardiographic findings in IE

Other echocardiographic features are not main criteria for IE but may be suggestive of the diagnosis. They include valve destruction

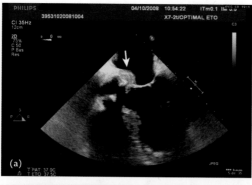
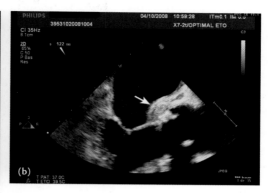
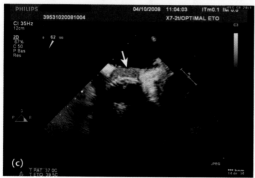

Fig. 17.6 TOE showing an echodense thickening around the annulus of a bioprosthetic valve corresponding to a peri-annular abscess (arrow) (a, b, c).

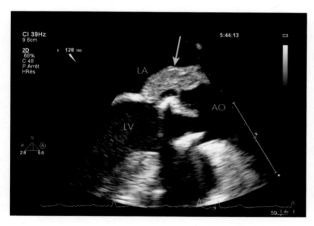

Fig. 17.7 Aortic bioprosthetic abscess, presenting as a thickening of the posterior aortic root (arrow). AO, aorta; LV, left ventricle; LA, left atrium.

and prolapse, aneurysm and/or perforation of a valve (➲ Fig. 17.13). The most frequent is anterior mitral valve perforation, which is usually a complication of aortic valve IE. It may be observed either isolated or as a complication of a mitral valve aneurysm (➲ Fig. 17.11). Perforation of the mitral valve may be the consequence of an infected aortic regurgitant jet and is best visualized by TOE [10].

In addition, both TTE and TOE are useful for the assessment of the underlying valve disease, and for the assessment of consequences of consequences of IE, including:

◆ Left ventricular size and function.

◆ Quantification of valve regurgitation/obstruction.

◆ Right ventricular function, estimation of pulmonary pressures.

Table 17.1 Echocardiographic definitions

	Surgery/Necropsy	Echocardiography
Vegetation	Infected mass attached to an endocardial structure or on implanted intracardial material	Oscillating or non-oscillating intra-cardial mass on valve or other endocardial structures or on implanted intra-cardial material
Pseudoaneurysm	Peri-valvular cavity communicating with the cardiovascular lumen	Pulsatile peri-valvular echo-free space with colour flow detected
Abscess	Peri-valvular cavity with necrosis and purulent material not communicating with the cardiovascular lumen	Peri-valvular zone of reduced echo density without colour flow
Perforation	Interruption of endocardial tissue continuity	Interruption of endocardial tissue continuity traversed by colour Doppler flow
Fistula	Communication between two neighbouring cavities through a perforation	Colour Doppler communication between two neighbouring cavities through a perforation
Valve aneurysm	Saccular outpouching of valvular tissue	Saccular bulging of valvular tissue (most usually affects the mitral valve)
New dehiscence of a prosthetic valve	Dehiscence of the prosthesis	New paravalvular regurgitation identified by TTE/TOE not present at a previous study

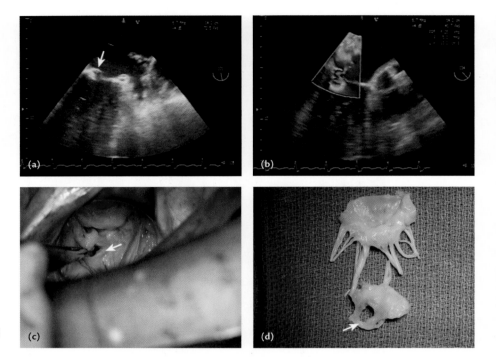

Fig. 17.8 TOE showing a mitral annular abscess (arrows, a) with perforation (b). (c and d) The valvular and peri-valvular damage observed during the operation.

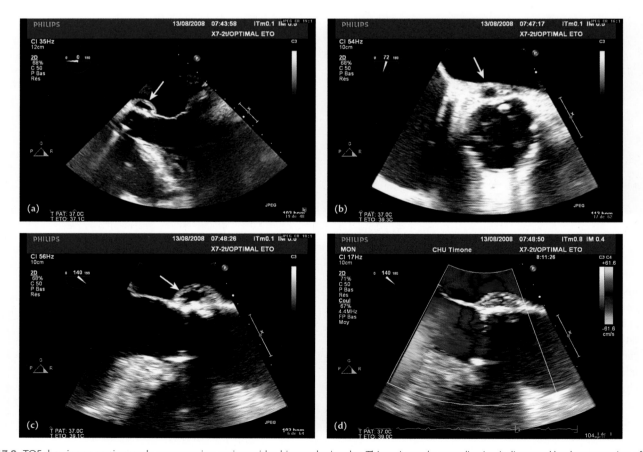

Fig. 17.9 TOE showing an aortic pseudo aneurysm in a patient with a bioprosthetic valve. This peri-annular complication is diagnosed by demonstration of an echolucent cavity within the posterior area of the valvular annulus (a–c, arrows) and a flow detected by colour Doppler into this cavity (d).

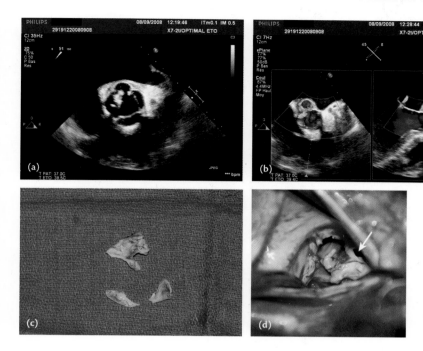

Fig. 17.10 TOE showing an aortic endocarditis with a destruction of the commissure between the non-coronary cusp and the left-anterior cusp (a). Large vegetation is seen on the non-coronary cusp (a). (b) Two orthogonal views of the aortic root during the same time by using the 3-dimensional TOE probe. There is a pseudo-aneurysm into the posterior wall of the aortic root. (c) The aortic cusp after surgical excision. (d) The gap of the pseudoaneurysm in the aortic wall (arrow).

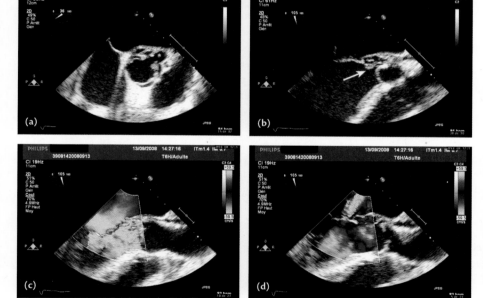

Fig. 17.11 TOE showing a mitral-aortic endocarditis with a pseudoaneurysm of the mitral-aortic fibrous inter-valvular area. Destruction of the posterior commissure of a bicuspid valve (a, white star). Large, mobile aortic vegetations prolapsing into the left ventricular outflow tract during diastole and contacting the ventricular aspect of the anterior mitral leaflet (b, arrow). These lesions lead to a severe aortic regurgitation (c) and a mitral perforation (d).

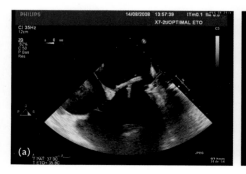
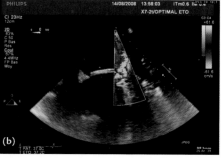

Fig. 17.12 TOE showing a large peri-valvular desinsertion on the lateral part of the annulus of mechanical prosthetic valve leading to a severe mitral regurgitation in a patient with an early prosthetic valve endocarditis (a, b).

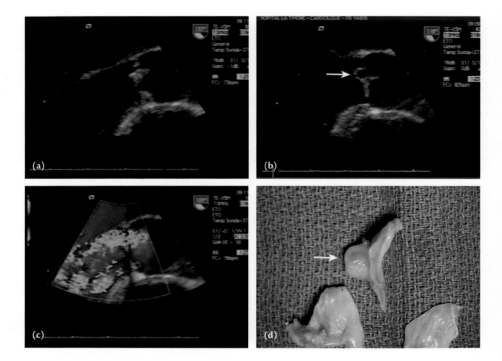

Fig. 17.13 TOE showing a native aortic valve endocarditis with a 'valvular aneurysm' (arrow) associated with a perforation leading to an acute aortic regurgitation (a, b, c, d).

Limitations and pitfalls of echocardiography

In clinical practice, the echocardiographic diagnosis of IE remains difficult in three main situations:

- In case of normal or doubtful echocardiography.
- In IE affecting intra-cardiac devices.
- In patients with PVIE.

In all these situations, echographic findings, positive or negative, must be interpreted with caution, taking into account the clinical presentation and the likelihood of IE.

Normal or doubtful echocardiography

A negative echocardiography may be observed in about 15% of IE. The most frequent explanations for negative echocardiography are very small or absent vegetations and difficulties in identifying vegetations in the presence of pre-existent severe lesions (mitral valve prolapse, degenerative lesions, and prosthetic valves). Similarly, diagnosis of IE may be more difficult in case of non-oscillating vegetation and in case of vegetations of atypical location (📷 Video 17.2). In addition, the diagnosis may be difficult at the early stage of the disease, when vegetations are not yet present or are too small to be identified. In one series [11], among 93 patients with anatomically confirmed IE, vegetation was observed by TOE in only 81%. In another series [12], among 105 patients with suspected IE, 65 had an initial negative TOE; in 3 cases, vegetation appeared on a repeat TOE. For this reason, repeat TTE/TOE examination must be performed 7/10 days after the first examination when the clinical level of suspicion is still high.

Conversely, false diagnosis of IE may occur in other situations; for example, it may be difficult to differentiate between vegetations and thrombi, cusp prolapse, cardiac tumours, myxomatous changes, Lambl's excrescences, strands, or non-infective vegetations (marantic endocarditis). Non-infective vegetations are impossible to differentiate from infective vegetations. They can be suspected in the presence of small and multiple vegetations, changing from one examination to another, and without associated abscess or valve destruction.

Similarly, diagnosis of a peri-valvular abscess may be difficult, even with the use of TOE, in case of small abscess (➲ Fig. 17.14), when echocardiography is performed very early in the course of the disease or in the immediate post-operative period after aortic root replacement or Bentall procedure. In these latter situations, a thickening of the aortic wall may be observed in the absence of

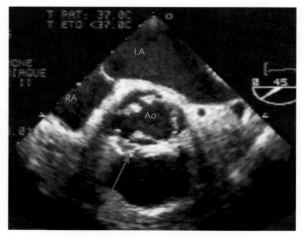

Fig. 17.14 Small abscess formation near the right coronary sinus (red arrow) in a patient with aortic endocarditis. LA, left atrium; Ao, aorta; RA, right atrium.

IE, mimicking abscess formation. Recent publications [13] underlined the discrepancies between the results of TOE and anatomical findings, particularly in patients with abscess localized around calcification in the posterior mitral annulus. Finally, a normal echocardiogram does not completely rule out IE, even if TOE is performed and even in expert hands, and a repeat examination has to be performed in case of high level of clinical suspicion.

Cardiac devices-related infective endocarditis (CDRIE)

CDRIE, including permanent pacemaker and implantable cardioverter defibrillators, is a severe disease associated with high mortality [14]. CDRIE is defined by an infection extending to the electrode leads, cardiac valve leaflets, or endocardial surface. CDRIE is probably one of the most difficult forms of IE to diagnose.

Similar to other forms of IE, echocardiography plays a key role in CDRIE and is helpful both for the diagnosis of lead vegetation, diagnosis of tricuspid involvement, diagnosis of tricuspid regurgitation, sizing of vegetations, as well as follow-up after lead extraction. Concerning diagnosis, although TOE has superior sensitivity and specificity than TTE, both must be systematically performed in suspected CDRIE. Vegetations may be observed both on the electrode leads, cardiac valve leaflets, or endocardial surface (Video 17.4). Careful examination of the entire leads is mandatory, from the superior vena cava to the apex of the right ventricle. However, both TTE and TOE may be falsely negative in CDRIE, and a normal echographic examination does not rule out CDRIE. Atypical findings are frequent, including thickening and 'sleeve-like' appearance of the pacemaker lead [14], and must be differentiated from normal findings.

The Duke criteria have been used for the diagnosis of infective endocarditis in cases of suspected CDRIE, but are difficult to apply in these patients, because of lower sensitivity, despite proposed modifications [14].

Prosthetic valve infective endocarditis (PVIE)

The anatomic involvement differs between PVIE affecting either mechanical or bioprosthetic valves [15]. In mechanical valves, the infection usually involves the junction between the sewing ring and the annulus, leading to peri-valvular abscess, dehiscence, pseudo-aneurysms, and fistula. Although similar mechanisms may also be observed in bioprosthetic PVIE, infection is more frequently located on the leaflets in those patients, leading to cusp rupture, perforation, and vegetations. Echocardiography, particularly TOE, plays a key role in the diagnosis and evaluation of PVIE (Fig. 17.15, Video 17.5). TOE is mandatory in PVE because of its better sensitivity and specificity for the detection of vegetations, abscesses, and peri-valvular lesions. However, the value of both TTE and TOE is lower in PVIE as compared with NVE because of both lower sensitivity and specificity, and because the presence of intra-cardiac material may hinder the identification of both vegetations and abscesses. Consequently, a negative echocardiography is frequently observed in PVIE [16], and does not rule out the diagnosis of PVIE. The Duke criteria cannot be applied in clinical practice in PVIE, because of their lower sensitivity in this setting [17].

Other imaging techniques

The evaluation of patients with infective endocarditis is no longer limited to conventional echocardiography, but must include several other imaging techniques.

Intra-cardiac echocardiography and three-dimensional (3D) echocardiography

Their use has been occasionally reported in case reports or short series.

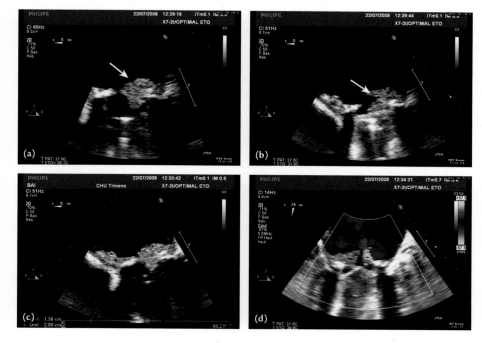

Fig. 17.15 TOE showing a large vegetation prolapsing into a mitral mechanical prosthetic valve (a–c, arrows). Disparition of two physiological regurgitations (d).

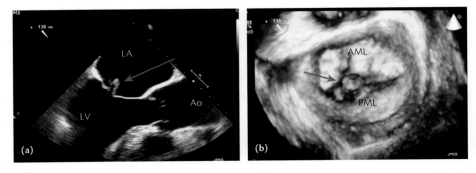

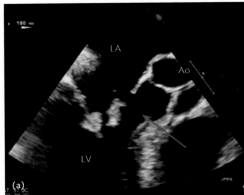

Fig. 17.16 Large vegetation on the posterior mitral leaflet (arrow) (TOE). (a) 2D-TOE. (b) 3D-TOE. LA, left atrium; LV, left ventricle; Ao, aorta; AML, anterior mitral leaflet; PML, posterior mitral leaflet.

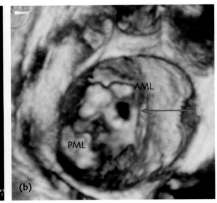

Fig. 17.17 Mitral valve infective endocarditis with a large vegetation and mitral perforation (arrows) by 2D-TOE (a) and 3D-TOE (b). LA, left atrium; LV, left ventricle; Ao, aorta; AML, anterior mitral leaflet; PML, posterior mitral leaflet.

Intra-cardiac echocardiography

This has recently been shown to be potentially useful for the diagnosis of cardiac device-related infective endocarditis [18], but its use cannot be recommended in clinical practice because of the paucity of published data and since this technique is not available in the majority of centres.

3D-echocardiography

This is not better than TTE or TOE for the diagnosis of vegetations, because of its lower spatial resolution, but is useful for the diagnosis and assessment of abscesses, false aneurysms, and anterior mitral valve perforation. In addition, 3D-TOE gives the opportunity to obtain 'surgical views' of the heart, particularly useful for discussion with the surgeon. ➲ Figures 17.16 to 17.19 illustrate the potential value of 3D-echocardiography in infective endocarditis.

Multi-slice computed tomography (CT) and magnetic resonance imaging (MRI)

CT scan of the heart can now be performed with high spatial and temporal resolution. Data in IE patients are scarce, but studies

have shown good results of multi-slice CT in detecting valvular abnormalities in both native and prosthetic valve endocarditis, as compared to operative findings, and with no significant difference with TOE (➲ Fig. 17.20) [19–20]. In addition, and probably more important, multi-slice CT allows diagnosis of extracardiac localisations of infection. Cerebral and abdominal CT scans are frequently used to diagnose embolic complications of IE. For example, splenic embolism is very frequent in IE. It may be silent and detected only by systematic abdominal CT scan (➲ Fig. 17.21). Finally, CT scan provides an anatomical assessment of the coronary bed, which is important in the preoperative evaluation. One limitation of multi-slice CT is that it cannot be used in patients with severe renal dysfunction and in severely allergic patients.

MRI, in addition to CT scan, is of utmost value for the diagnosis and management of cerebral complications of IE. MRI or conventional angiography may be used in case of suspected arterial mycotic aneurysm (➲ Fig. 17.22). MRI is particularly useful for the identification of silent cerebral complications of IE. Recent studies found that systematic MRI could detect subclinical

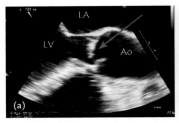

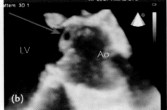

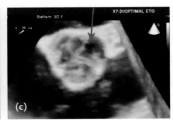

Fig. 17.18 Aortic valve infective endocarditis: case illustrating the additional role of 3D-TOE. (a) 2D-TOE showing a prolapse of the left coronary aortic leaflet. (b and c) 3D-TOE: long-axis and short-axis views revealing a perforation of the left coronary aortic leaflet (arrows). LA, left atrium; LV, left ventricle; Ao, aorta.

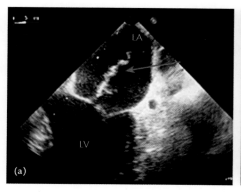

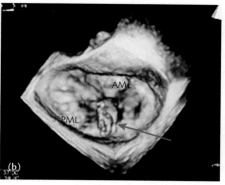

Fig. 17.19 Mitral valve infective endocarditis with a huge vegetation attached to the anterior mitral leaflet (arrows) by 2D-TOE (a) and 3D–TOE (b). LA, left atrium; LV, left ventricle; AML, anterior mitral leaflet; PML, posterior mitral leaflet.

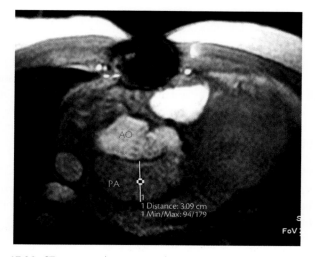

Fig. 17.20 CT scan: pseudoaneurysm of the ascending aorta. PA, pseudoaneurysm; AO, aorta.

cerebrovascular complications in about 50% of patients with IE [21–23], improves the diagnosis of IE, and may affect therapeutic strategies. MRI offers the advantages of being a non-ionizing imaging modality but is limited by its lower spatial resolution and availability in comparison with current CT scans [24].

18F-FDG PET/CT and other functional imaging modalities

These techniques aim to detect the inflammation and infection process and to evaluate the activity of IE. Positron emission tomography (PET)/CT using 18F-FDG allows detection of enhanced glucose metabolism within organs. It has been used in the diagnosis and follow-up of cancers and, more recently, for the detection of vascular prosthetic infection [24]. Recent studies showed that it could be of some value in the detection of infective endocarditis, particularly in cases of cardiac device-related IE (➲ Fig. 17.23) and in prosthetic valve endocarditis (➲ Fig. 17.24) [25]. In a recent prospective study on PVIE and 18F-FDG PET/CT, it was found that adding an abnormal FDG uptake around a prosthetic valve, as a new major criterion increases the sensitivity of the modified Duke criteria at admission from 70% to 97% [26]. An algorithm for evaluation of patients with suspected PVIE, including echocardiography and PET/CT, was suggested (➲ Fig. 17.25). 18F-FDG PET/CT is also useful in detection of peripheral embolic and metastatic infectious events in IE. However, 18F-FDG PET/CT seems of more limited value in native valve IE, in cases of small vegetations, and in patients who recently have undergone cardiac surgery [24].

Other functional imaging modalities, including gallium-67-, indium-111-, and technetium-99m-HMPAO-labelled leucocyte scintigraphy, have recently been proposed, but their value in IE need to be demonstrated [24].

Prognostic value of echocardiography

In addition to its role in diagnosing IE, echocardiography also has a major prognostic value in IE, for both prediction of death and embolic events.

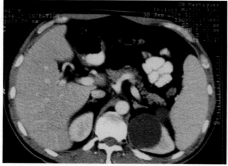

January 2006
Before antibiotic therapy

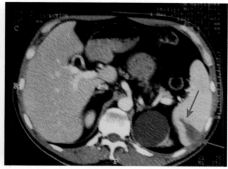

March 2006
After completion of antibiotic therapy

Fig. 17.21 Splenic embolism in a patient with infective endocarditis. January 2006: normal systematic CT scan on admission. March 2006: new asymptomatic splenic embolism detected by repeat examination.

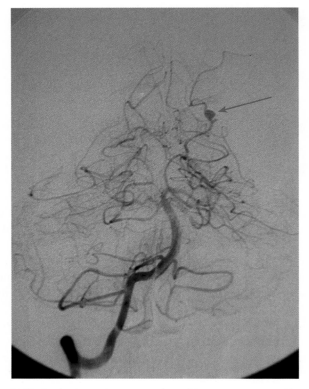

Fig. 17.22 Cerebral mycotic aneurysm (arrow) in a young woman with hypertrophic cardiomyopathy and staphylococcal endocarditis (same patient as ➲ Fig. 17.2).

Echocardiography predicts both in-hospital mortality and long-term prognosis in IE

Mortality is still high in IE, although it has declined in recent years. Several factors have been associated with an increased risk of death in IE including patients' characteristics (diabetes, comorbidity), presence or not of complications (heart failure, stroke, renal failure), and type of microorganism [27]. Echocardiography also plays a very important prognostic role in IE. Several echocardiographic features have been associated with worse prognosis, including peri-annular complications, severe valve regurgitation or obstruction, low LV ejection fraction, pulmonary hypertension, and premature mitral valve closure.

Premature mitral closure (➲ Fig. 17.26) is an old but still useful M-mode sign observed in severe aortic regurgitation, and indicates high left ventricular diastolic pressures and usually a need for early surgery. The presence of a vegetation, its size and its multivalvular location have been associated with a worse prognosis. In a recent series [28], large vegetations (>15 mm length) were associated with a worse prognosis. Echocardiography appears predictive of both the risk of embolism and death in IE.

Risk of embolism

Incidence of embolic events in IE

Embolic events (EE) are a frequent and life-threatening complication of IE, related to the migration of cardiac vegetations. Cerebral arteries and spleen are the most frequent sites of embolization in left-side IE, while pulmonary embolism is frequent in right-side and pacemaker lead IE. Stroke is a severe complication of cerebral embolism, which is the most frequent embolic complication, and is associated with an increased morbidity and mortality [1]. Conversely, embolic events may be totally silent in about 20% of patients with IE, especially in case of splenic or cerebral embolisms, and must be diagnosed by systematic non-invasive imaging. Total embolic risk is very high in IE, with EE occurring in 20–50% of IE. However, the risk of new EE (i.e. occurring after initiation of antibiotic therapy) is only 6–21% (1).

Predicting the risk of embolism

Echocardiography plays a key role in predicting embolic events, although this prediction remains difficult in the individual patient. Several factors have been associated with an increased risk of embolism, including the size and mobility of vegetations, the localization of the vegetation on the mitral valve, the increasing or decreasing size of the vegetation under antibiotic therapy, some microorganisms (staphylococci, *Streptococcus bovis*, *Candida* spp.), previous embolism, multi-valvular endocarditis, and biological markers [1]. Among them, the size and mobility of the vegetations are the most potent independent predictors of new embolic events in patients with IE. For example, in one study [29], a large number of patients (178) with strict criteria for IE were prospectively included. A significant relationship was found between presence of vegetation and occurrence of embolism, as well as between vegetation size and embolism, and between vegetation mobility and embolism. Embolic events were particularly frequent among patients with both severely mobile and very large vegetations (>15 mm). By multivariate analysis, mobility and size of the vegetation were the only independent predictors of embolism. Several studies subsequently confirmed that patients with

Fig. 17.23 Multi-modality imaging of a pacemaker lead endocarditis. (a) TOE: showing a severely thickened pacemaker lead with vegetations (arrow). (b) PET-CT showing increased 18F-Fluorodeoxyglucose uptake on the pacemaker lead (arrow). LA, left atrium; RA, right atrium; SVC, superior vena cava.

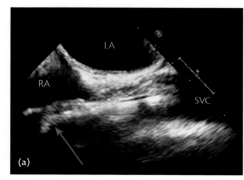
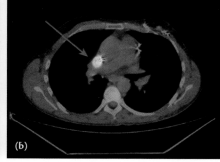

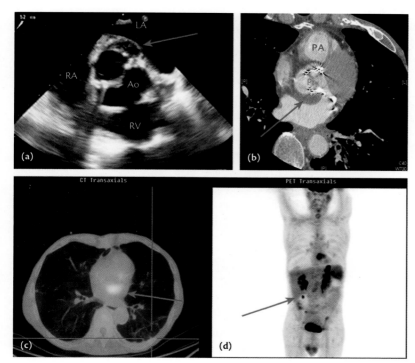

Fig. 17.24 Multi-modality imaging of a bioprosthetic aortic valve endocarditis. (a) TOE: showing a posterior aortic root abscess (arrow). (b) Posterior aortic root abscess visualized by CT-scan (arrow). (c and d) PET-CT showing increased 18F-Fluorodeoxyglucose uptake on both the aortic prosthesis (c) and on a colonic tumour (d). LA, left atrium; LV, left ventricle; Ao, aorta; PA, pulmonary artery; Pr, prosthesis.

large vegetations are at higher risk of embolism and this risk is particularly high in patients with very large (>15 mm) and mobile vegetations, especially in staphylococcal mitral valve endocarditis. It must be emphasized that the risk of new embolism is highest during the first days following the initiation of antibiotic therapy and decreases after 2 weeks [28, 30], although some degree of risk

persists indefinitely in the presence of a vegetation. However, even in studies focusing on new embolic events, the size and mobility of vegetations are still associated with an increased risk of embolism [28]. For this reason, the benefit of surgery to prevent embolization will be greatest during the first week of antibiotic therapy, when the embolic rate is highest.

Follow-up

Echocardiography must be used for follow-up of patients with IE under antibiotic therapy, along with clinical follow-up. The number, type, and timing of repeat examinations depend on the clinical presentation, the type of microorganism, and the initial echocardiographic findings. For example, only weekly TTE study may be sufficient to follow a non-complicated streptococcal native mitral valve IE. Conversely, early repeat TOE may be necessary in a patient with severe staphylococcal aortic IE, with suspected perivalvular involvement or large vegetation.

Few studies followed the outcome of vegetations under therapy. The results of such studies are difficult to interpret because the reduction in size of a vegetation may be due either to a healing of endocarditis or to the embolism of a part of the vegetation. Moreover, early surgical treatment may alter the course of the follow-up. In one study, failure to decrease vegetation size with antibiotic treatment was associated with an increased risk of embolism [8]. Conversely, Vilacosta [31] showed that most vegetation (83.8%) remains constant in size under therapy, and that this does not worsen prognosis. However in this study, both increase of vegetation size under antibiotic therapy (observed in 10.5% of patients with IE) and reduction of vegetation size under therapy were associated with an increased embolic risk. Thus, increasing

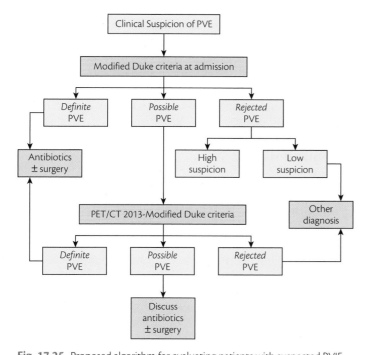

Fig. 17.25 Proposed algorithm for evaluating patients with suspected PVIE. Reprinted from *Journal of the American College of Cardiology*, 61:23, Ludivine Saby et al, Positron emission tomography/computed tomography for diagnosis of prosthetic valve endocarditis: increased valvular 18F-fluorodeoxyglucose uptake as a novel major criterion, 2374–2382. Copyright 2013, with permission from Elsevier.

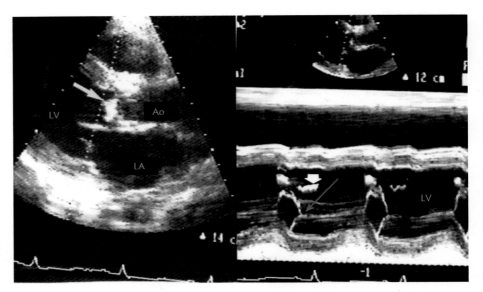

Fig. 17.26 Acute aortic endocarditis: M-mode recording showing a premature closure of the mitral valve (red arrow). LV, left ventricle; LA, left atrium; Ao, aorta.

vegetation size under therapy must be considered as a risk factor for new embolic event, while unchanged or reduced vegetation size under therapy may be more difficult to interpret [1].

Imaging and decision-making

Indications for surgery in IE may be subdivided in three categories—haemodynamic, infectious, and embolic indications [6]. Decision to operate is frequently difficult and must be discussed on an individual basis, using a multidisciplinary approach including cardiologist, infectious disease specialist, and cardiac surgeon. Imaging plays a central role in this decision, along with the clinical presentation. More specifically, echocardiography plays a central role in helping clinician to choose the optimal timing of surgery.

Haemodynamic indications

Presence of heart failure represents the main indication for surgery in IE. Recent European guidelines recommend early surgery to be performed in patients with acute regurgitation and congestive heart failure, as well as in patients with obstructive vegetations [6]. Echocardiography is useful in both situations. In acute regurgitation, it allows a detailed assessment of valve lesions, a quantification of valve regurgitation, and the evaluation of the haemodynamic tolerance of the regurgitation (cardiac output, pulmonary arterial pressures, left and right ventricular function). Some echocardiographic features suggest the need for urgent surgery including premature mitral valve closure (in aortic IE), massive regurgitation, and extensive destructive valvular lesions. The second haemodynamic indication is obstructive vegetation. In this situation, echocardiography is also useful for the assessment of mechanism and quantification of valve obstruction (➲ Fig. 17.15). Patients with initial heart failure not treated by urgent/emergency surgery must be closely followed by repeat clinical and echocardiographic examinations in order to detect worsening cardiac lesions.

Infectious indications

These represent the second most frequent indication for early surgery in Europe [4]. In the European guidelines, the infectious complications needing surgery include peri-valvular extension, persistent fever and some specific microorganisms with poor response to antibiotic therapy [6]. Echocardiography plays a key role in the assessment of peri-valvular lesions, including abscess, false aneurysm, fistula, and mitral valve aneurysm/perforation. Recent studies showed convincing evidence that aorto-cavitary fistulous tract formations are associated with bad prognosis [32], both in native and prosthetic valve aortic endocarditis. Early surgery must be performed in these high-risk subgroups when possible. In some situations, emergency surgery may be necessary because of extensive peri-valvular lesions associated with severe heart failure. Rarely, medical therapy alone may be attempted in patients with small non-staphylococcal abscesses (surface area less than 1 cm²) without severe valve regurgitation and without heart failure, in case of rapid and favourable response to antibiotic therapy. A careful clinical and echocardiographic follow-up is mandatory in this situation.

Embolic indications

The last reason for early surgery is because a high embolic risk is suspected. Again, echocardiography presents with a major value for the assessment of this risk. A careful measurement of the maximal vegetation size is crucial in IE, because this parameter is clearly related to the risk of new embolic event. However, prevention of emboli still represents the most controversial indication in IE. A recent randomized trial demonstrated that early surgery in patients with large vegetations significantly reduced the risk of death and embolic events, as compared with conventional therapy [33].

The ESC guidelines [6] recommend surgical therapy in case of large (>10 mm) vegetation following one or more embolic episodes, and when the large vegetation is associated with other predictors of complicated course (heart failure, persistent infection under therapy, abscess, and prosthetic endocarditis), indicating an earlier surgical decision. The decision to operate early in isolated very large vegetation (>15 mm) is more difficult. Surgery may be preferred when a valve repair seems possible, particularly in mitral valve IE. But the most important point is that the surgery, if needed, must be performed on an urgent basis. Finally, the benefit of surgery may be weighed against the operative risk and take into account the clinical status of the patient and the comorbidities.

Intra-operative echocardiography

Intra-operative echocardiography is mandatory in patients operated on for IE. It gives to the surgeon a final anatomic evaluation of the valvular and peri-valvular lesions, and is particularly useful to assess the immediate result of conservative surgery and in cases of complex peri-valvular repair [34]. Intra-operative TOE must be performed in homograft or autograft surgery, which is relatively frequently used in IE.

Conclusion

Imaging plays a key role in IE, both concerning its diagnosis, the diagnosis of its complications, its follow-up under therapy, and its prognostic assessment. Echocardiography is particularly useful for the initial assessment of embolic risk and in decision-making in IE. TOE plays a major role both before surgery and during surgery (intra-operative echocardiography). Other imaging techniques are complementary with echocardiography for the evaluation of patients with IE. Among them, FDG PET/CT imaging seems the most promising new imaging technique, particularly for the diagnosis of prosthetic valve endocarditis.

References

1. Habib G. Embolic risk in subacute bacterial endocarditis. Role of transesophageal echocardiography. *Curr Cardiol Rep* 2003; 5: 129–36.
2. Hoen B, Alla F, Selton-Suty C, et al. Changing profile of infective endocarditis: results of a 1-year survey in France. *JAMA* 2002; 288: 75–81.
3. Hasbun R, Vikram HR, Barakat LA, Buenconsejo J, Quagliarello VJ. Complicated left-sided native valve endocarditis in adults: risk classification for mortality. *JAMA* 2003; 289: 1933–40.
4. Tornos P, Iung B, Permanyer-Miralda G, et al. Infective endocarditis in Europe: lessons from the Euro heart survey. *Heart* 2005; 91: 571–75.
5. Habib G, Avierinos JF, Thuny F. Aortic valve endocarditis; is there an optimal surgical timing? *Curr Op Cardiol* 2007; 22: 77–83.
6. Habib G, Hoen B, Tornos P, et al. Guidelines on the prevention, diagnosis, and treatment of infective endocarditis (new version 2009): The Task Force on the Prevention, Diagnosis, and Treatment of Infective Endocarditis of the European Society of Cardiology (ESC). *Eur Heart J* 2009; 30, 2369–13.
7. Durack DT, Lukes AS, Bright DK. New criteria for diagnosis of infective endocarditis: utilization of specific echocardiographic findings. Duke Endocarditis Service. *Am J Med* 1994; 96: 200–9.
8. Rohmann S, Erbel R, Darius H, et al. Prediction of rapid versus prolonged healing of infective endocarditis by monitoring vegetation size. *J Am Soc Echocardiogr* 1991; 4: 465–74.
9. Karalis DG, Bansal RC, Hauck AJ, et al. Transesophageal echocardiographic recognition of subaortic complications in aortic valve endocarditis. Clinical and surgical implications. *Circulation* 1992; 86: 353–62.
10. Vilacosta I, San Roman JA, Sarria C, et al. Clinical, anatomic, and echocardiographic characteristics of aneurysms of the mitral valve. *Am J Cardiol* 1999; 84: 110–13, A119.
11. Habib G, Derumeaux G, Avierinos JF, et al. Value and limitations of the Duke criteria for the diagnosis of infective endocarditis. *J Am Coll Cardiol* 1999; 33: 2023–29.
12. Sochowski RA, Chan KL. Implication of negative results on a monoplane transesophageal echocardiographic study in patients with suspected infective endocarditis. *J Am Coll Cardiol* 199321: 216–21.
13. Hill EE, Herijgers P, Claus P, Vanderschueren S, Peetermans WE, Herregods MC. Abscess in infective endocarditis: the value of transesophageal echocardiography and outcome: a 5-year study. *Am Heart J* 2007; 154: 923–28.
14. Klug D, Lacroix D, Savoye C, et al. Systemic infection related to endocarditis on pacemaker leads: clinical presentation and management. *Circulation* 1997; 95: 2098–7.
15. Piper C, Korfer R, Horstkotte D. Prosthetic valve endocarditis. *Heart* 2001; 85: 590–593.
16. Habib G, Thuny F, Avierinos JF. Prosthetic valve endocarditis: current approach and therapeutic options. *Prog Cardiovasc Dis* 2008; 50: 274–81.
17. Lamas CC, Eykyn SJ. Suggested modifications to the Duke criteria for the clinical diagnosis of native valve and prosthetic valve endocarditis: analysis of 118 pathologically proven cases. *Clin Infect Dis* 1997; 25: 713–19.
18. Narducci ML, Pelargiono G, Russo E, et al. Usefulness of intra-cardiac echocardiography for the diagnosis of cardiovascular implantable electronic device-related endocarditis. *J Am Coll Cardiol* 2013; 61: 1398–405.
19. Feuchtner GM, Stolzmann P, Dichtl W, et al. Multi-slice computed tomography in infective endocarditis: comparison with transesophageal echocardiography and intraoperative findings. *J Am Coll Cardiol* 2009; 53: 436–44.
20. Fagman E, Perrotta S, Bech-Hanssen O, et al. ECG-gated computed tomography: a new role for patients with suspected aortic prosthetic valve endocarditis. *Eur Radiol* 2012; 22: 2407–14.
21. Cooper HA, Thompson EC, Laureno R, et al. Subclinical brain embolization in left-sided infective endocarditis: results from the evaluation by MRI of the brains of patients with left-sided intra-cardiac solid masses (EMBOLISM) pilot study. *Circulation* 2009; 120: 585–91.
22. Duval X, Iung B, Klein I, et al. Effect of early cerebral magnetic resonance imaging on clinical decisions in infective endocarditis: a prospective study. *Ann Intern Med* 2010; 152: 497–504.
23. Snygg-Martin U, Gustafsson L, Rosengren L, et al. Cerebrovascular complications in patients with left-sided infective endocarditis are common: a prospective study using magnetic resonance imaging and neurochemical brain damage markers. *Clin Infect Dis* 2008; 47: 23–30.
24. Thuny F, Gaubert JY, Jacquier A, et al. Imaging investigations in infective endocarditis: Current approach and perspectives. *Arch Cardiovasc Dis* 2013; 106: 52–62.
25. Saby L, Le Dolley Y, Laas O, et al. Early diagnosis of abscess in aortic bioprosthetic valve by 18F-fluorodeoxyglucose positron emission tomography-computed tomography. *Circulation.* 2012; 126: e217–20.

26. Saby L, Le Dolley Y, Laas O, et al. Positron Emission Tomography/ Computed Tomography for Diagnosis of Prosthetic Valve Endocarditis: Increased Valvular 18F-Fluorodeoxyglucose Uptake as a Novel Major Criterion. *J Am Coll Cardiol* 2013; 61: 2374–82.

27. San Roman JA, Lopez J, Vilacosta I, et al. Prognostic stratification of patients with left-sided endocarditis determined at admission. *Am J Med* 2007; 120: 369 e 361–67.

28. Thuny F, Di Salvo G, Belliard O, et al. Risk of embolism and death in infective endocarditis: prognostic value of echocardiography: a prospective multicenter study. *Circulation* 2005; 112: 69–75.

29. Di Salvo G, Habib G, Pergola V, et al. Echocardiography predicts embolic events in infective endocarditis. *J Am Coll Cardiol* 2001; 37: 1069–76.

30. Steckelberg JM, Murphy JG, Ballard D, et al. Emboli in infective endocarditis: the prognostic value of echocardiography. *Ann Intern Med* 1991; 114: 635–40.

31. Vilacosta I, Graupner C, San Roman JA, et al. Risk of embolization after institution of antibiotic therapy for infective endocarditis. *J Am Coll Cardiol* 2002; 39: 1489–95.

32. Anguera I, Miro JM, Vilacosta I, et al. Aorto-cavitary fistulous tract formation in infective endocarditis: clinical and echocardiographic features of 76 cases and risk factors for mortality. *Eur Heart J* 2005; 26: 288–97.

33. Kang D-H, Kim Y-J, Kim S-H, et al. Early surgery versus conventional treatment for infective endocarditis. *N Engl J Med* 2012; 366: 2466–73.

34. Shapira Y, Weisenberg DE, Vaturi M, et al. The impact of intraoperative transesophageal echocardiography in infective endocarditis. *Isr Med Assoc J* 2007; 9: 299–302.

⊃ **For additional multimedia materials please visit the online version of the book (** ⌐ **http://www.esciacc.oxfordmedicine.com)**

SECTION IV

Coronary artery disease

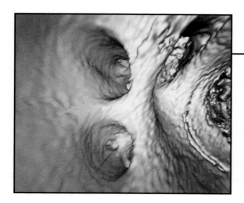

CHAPTER 18

Echocardiography and detection of coronary artery disease

Rosa Sicari

Contents

Pathophysiology of myocardial ischaemia

Myocardial ischaemia represents the final common pathway of different substrates that can be summarized into three main domains: epicardial coronary arteries, myocardium, and small coronary vessels. These three domains may overlap in the pathophysiology of myocardial ischaemia. Epicardial coronary artery lumen can be reduced and this reduction may be fixed or dynamic. Coronary flow reserve is the ability of the coronary arteriolar bed to dilate in response to increased metabolic demand. In normal conditions, arteriolar vasodilation can determine a 4–6-fold increment of coronary blood flow, leading to global increase in left ventricular contractility. A fixed stenosis reduces coronary flow reserve according to the scheme reported in ⮌ Fig. 18.1 [1]. Four different patterns can be recognized: (1) stenoses ranging between 0 and 40% identifying a haemodynamically silent zone, which does not affect coronary flow reserve; (2) stenoses ranging between 40 and 70% may reduce coronary flow reserve without reaching the threshold to induce ischaemia after an appropriate challenge; (3) stenoses between 75 and 90%, which progressively reduce coronary flow reserve, and create a transient imbalance between oxygen demand and supply; (4) stenoses >90%, which abolish coronary flow reserve and may reduce blood flow in resting conditions too. Dynamic stenoses can be triggered by three different mechanisms: increased tone at the level of an eccentric coronary plaque; complete vasospasm caused by local hyper-reactivity of the coronary smooth muscle cells, or intracoronary thrombosis. All these mechanisms coexist in variant angina and are detectable at resting echo, provided a flow reduction up to a certain threshold is reached. In the absence of atherosclerotic or obstructive coronary artery disease, coronary flow reserve can be reduced in microvascular disease (e.g. in syndrome X, arterial hypertension, diabetes, and/or left ventricular hypertrophy) [2, 3], which may per se reduce coronary flow reserve independently of microvascular damage [4–6]. In these conditions, angina with ST segment depression can occur with regional perfusion changes, typically in the absence of any regional wall motion abnormalities during stress [3, 7–9] (⮌ Fig. 18.2). Milder forms of reduction in regional coronary flow reserve and/or abnormal coronary microcirculatory function may occur in patients with angiographically normal coronary arteries and may give rise to a positive perfusion scan [4–6], or to a reduced perfusion limited to the sub-endocardial layer of the left ventricular wall [4]—of limited extent to reduce regional coronary flow reserve, but not severe enough and/or transmurally extended to give rise to transient wall motion abnormalities [3, 9]. In more advanced stages of reduction in coronary flow reserve, sub-endocardial underperfusion up to a threshold necessary to reach a critical ischaemic mass may evoke the transient dyssynergy, the prerequisite of stress echocardiography positivity by wall motion criteria. Myocardial ischaemia results in a typical 'cascade' of events in which the various markers are hierarchically ranked

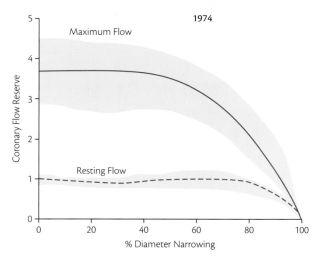

Fig. 18.1 Coronary blood flow curve (on the ordinate) for increasing levels of coronary stenosis (on the abscissa) experimentally obtained in resting conditions (lower curve) and at maximal post-ischaemic vasodilation (upper curve). Coronary reserve, i.e. the capacity of the coronary circulation to dilate following increased myocardial metabolic demands, is expressed as the difference between hyperaemic flow and the resting flow curve. For stenosis >70%, the reduction of coronary flow reserve is so severe to make the myocardium vulnerable to ischaemia.

Reprinted from the *American Journal of Cardiology*, 34:1, K.Lance Gould & Kirk Lipscomb, Effects of coronary stenoses on coronary flow reserve and resistance, 48–55, Copyright 1974, with permission from Elsevier.

in a well-defined time sequence [10]. Flow heterogeneity, especially between the sub-endocardial and sub-epicardial perfusion, is the forerunner of ischaemia, followed by metabolic changes, diastolic dysfunction, alteration in regional mechanical function and only at a later stage by electrocardiographic changes, global left ventricular dysfunction and pain. Transient regional systolic

dysfunction is the hallmark of myocardial ischaemia detectable by 2D-echocardiography.

Resting echocardiography to detect coronary artery disease

Myocardial ischaemia causes left ventricular regional dyssynergy (an early, sensitive, and specific marker of ischaemia) and global dysfunction (a late and non-sensitive sign).

To date, echocardiography has been the technique of choice for the assessment of regional ventricular function, both in resting conditions and even more so during stress, in spite of the dependence of echocardiographic imaging on the patient's acoustic window and on the experience of the cardiologist interpreting the study. The advantages of feasibility, safety, reliability, and unsurpassed temporal resolution allow the documentation under optimal conditions of a regional dysfunction, which can be extremely localized in space and transient in time.

The impairment of systolic function correlates with the severity of flow reduction. In fact, a 20% reduction in sub-endocardial flow produces 15–20% decrease in left ventricular wall thickening; a 50% reduction in sub-endocardial flow decreases regional wall thickening by about 40%; and when sub-endocardial flow is reduced by 80%, akinesia occurs. When the flow deficit is extended to the sub-epicardial layer, dyskinesia appears [11, 12] (⊃ Fig. 18.3). However, rest echocardiography suffers by being highly subjective and operator-dependent. Moreover, conventional echocardiographic assessment of contractile function is based on the measurement of the transmural thickening and does not provide information regarding the transmural distribution of contractile performance. The analysis of fibre thickening across the different layers of the myocardial wall is critical in order to differentiate the various

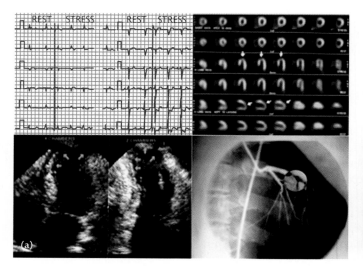

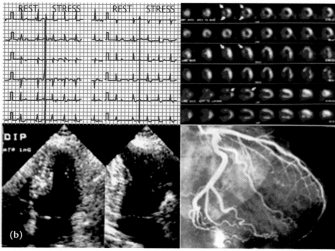

Fig. 18.2 (a) Positive ECG response (left upper panel), positive thallium scan (right upper panel), apical 4- and 2-chamber view of end-systolic frames at peak stress with apical akinesis (indicated by arrows, left lower panel) of a patient with significant left anterior descending coronary artery stenosis (right lower panel). (b) Positive ECG response (left upper panel), positive thallium scan (right upper panel), apical 4- and 2-chamber view of end-systolic frames at peak stress with normal left ventricular motion of a patient without significant coronary artery disease (right lower panel).

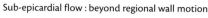

Sub-epicardial flow : beyond regional wall motion

Gallagher KP, Ross J Jr et al. Am J Physiol 1984

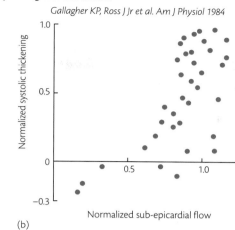

(a)

(b)

Fig. 18.3 The relationship between regional blood flow and systolic wall thickening in resting conscious dogs subjected to various degrees of circumflex coronary artery stenosis. Flow is expressed as a decimal fraction of that in a normal region of the ventricle, and percentage wall thickening (%WTh) is expressed as a fraction of the resting value prior to coronary stenosis. (a) Sub-endocardial blood flow vs. wall thickening, showing a nearly linear relationship (solid line). (b) Sub-epicardial blood flow vs. wall thickening, showing considerable scatter and no change in sub-epicardial flow until function is reduced by more than 50%.
Reproduced from Gallagher KP, Matsuzaki M, Koziol JA, Kemper WS, Ross J Jr. Regional myocardial perfusion and wall thickening during ischemia in conscious dogs. *American Journal of Physiology* 1984;247:H727-38.

- Lower LV volumes for any given pressure increase (*Sabbah, Marzilli. Am J Physiol* 1981)
- Possible anti-arrhythmic and anti-remodelling effect of sub-epicardium (*Kaul S. Circulation* 1995)

patterns of contractile abnormalities that may occur during acute or chronic (hibernation) myocardial ischaemia. Doppler tissue imaging (DTI) has been used to quantify the effects of ischaemia on myocardial function. In patients with chronic coronary artery obstruction, abnormalities of longitudinal shortening have been observed using DTI [13]. Experimental studies have shown that DTI-derived strain rate can be helpful in identifying and quantifying ischaemia-induced myocardial abnormalities. Unfortunately, clinical studies have not confirmed the clear advantage suggested by experimental studies and showed comparable accuracy of strain rate and tissue velocity imaging and expert reader eyeballing interpretation for diagnosis of coronary artery disease [14]. The major limitation of DTI-based strain imaging, is that peak amplitudes, and to some extent phase (timing), of velocity and strain variables are influenced by the angle of the incident beam with the myocardial wall. This restricts imaging to the apical views, wherein the operator attempts to align the myocardial wall parallel to the ultrasound beam; however, this is not always possible. The technique is heavily dependent on the sonographer's expertise, has a limited reproducibility even in expert hands, loses stability with high heart rates and degraded image quality, and is unsuitable to image apical segments (5 out of the total 17 of the left ventricle) [15]. 2D speckle-tracking echocardiography (STE)-derived strain has been validated experimentally with excellent results, especially for the sensitivity and reproducibility of longitudinal and circumferential strain [16, 17]. The accuracy of peak global longitudinal strain for the detection of the transmurality of a myocardial infarction was shown to closely correlate with the infarct mass, as assessed by cardiac MR [18]. In subjects with chest pain, 2D STE strain may allow detection of the earlier phases of the ischaemic response, not routinely visible on conventional 2D images. However, as stated in the ASE/EAE Consensus Statement on Methodology and Indications, currently, no new technology tool is recommended for the detection of acute, chronic and inducible ischaemia for clinical practice. The lack of clinical trials does not allow recommending specific parameters for diagnosing myocardial ischaemia at this time [19].

Exercise and pharmacological stress echo—the role of advanced echo modalities

The three most commonly used stressors are exercise, dobutamine, and dipyridamole. Exercise is the prototype of demand-driven ischaemic stress and the most widely used (⊃ Table 18.1). However, out of five patients, one cannot exercise, one exercises submaximally, and one has an uninterpretable ECG. Thus, the use of an exercise-independent approach allows diagnostic domain of a stress test laboratory to be expanded [20, 21]. Pharmacologic stressors minimize factors such as hyperventilation, tachycardia, hypercontraction of normal walls, and excessive chest wall movement, which render the ultrasonic examination difficult during exercise. All these factors degrade image quality and—in stress echo—worse image quality dramatically leads to higher interobserver variability and lower diagnostic accuracy (⊃ Fig. 18.4).

Dipyridamole (or adenosine) and dobutamine act on different receptor populations: dobutamine stimulates adrenoreceptors,

Table 18.1 Stress echo protocols

TEST	EQUIPMENT	PROTOCOLS
Exercise	Semi-supine bycicle ergometer	25 W × 2′ with incremental loading
Dobutamine	Infusion Pump	5 µg/kg/min 10–20–30–40 + atropine (0.25 × 4) up to 1 mg
Dipyridamole	Syringe	0.84 mg/kg in 6 min or 0.84 mg/kg in 10 min + atropine (0.25 × 4) up to 1 mg
Adenosine	Syringe	140 µg/kg/min in 6′
Pacing	External Pacing	From 100 bpm with increments of 10 beats/min up to target heart rate

Fig. 18.4 Stress echocardiography is a highly subjective technique as shown in this figure, assessing the diagnostic accuracy of six high-volume laboratories. However, the agreement between centres increases when image quality is high and clear-cut wall motion abnormalities are induced.

Reprinted from *Journal of the American College of Cardiology*, 27:2, Rainer Hoffmann et al, Analysis of interinstitutional observer agreement in interpretation of dobutamine stress echocardiograms, 330–36 Copyright 1996, with permission from Elseiver.

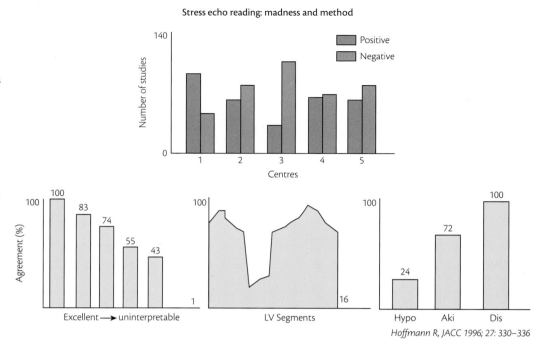

Hoffmann R, JACC 1996; 27: 330–336

while dipyridamole (which accumulates endogenous adenosine) stimulates adenosine receptors [22]. They induce ischaemia through different haemodynamic mechanisms: dobutamine primarily increases myocardial oxygen demand [23] and dipyridamole (or adenosine) mainly decreases sub-endocardial flow supply [11].

Diagnostic criteria

All stress echocardiographic diagnoses can be easily summarized into equations centred on regional wall function describing the fundamental response patterns as normal, ischaemic, viable, and necrotic myocardium (see ⊃ Table 18.2).

Diagnostic accuracy

In a recent meta-analysis of 55 studies with 3,714 patients, exercise, dobutamine, dipyridamole, and adenosine echocardiography showed a sensitivity, respectively, of 83%, 81%, 72%, and 79%, and a specificity of 84%, 84%, 95%, and 91% [24]. In another meta-analysis of 5 studies adopting state-of-the-art protocols for dipyridamole (fast or atropine-potentiated) and dobutamine (atropine-potentiated) tests, the two stresses had identical sensitivity (84%) and comparable specificity (92% vs. 87%) [25]. When compared to standard exercise electrocardiography, stress

echocardiography has a particularly impressive advantage in terms of specificity [26]. Compared to nuclear perfusion imaging, stress echocardiography at least has similar accuracy, with a moderate sensitivity gap that is more than balanced by a markedly higher specificity [24]. Familiarity with all forms of stress is an index of the quality of the echo lab. In this way, indications in the individual patient can be optimized, thereby avoiding the relative and absolute contraindications of each test (⊃ Tables 18.3 and 18.4). For instance, a patient with severe hypertension and/or a history of significant atrial or ventricular arrhythmias can more reasonably undergo the dipyridamole stress test, which, unlike dobutamine, has no arrhythmogenic or hypertensive effect. In contrast, a patient with severe conduction disturbances or advanced asthmatic disease should undergo the dobutamine stress

Table 18.3 Stress echocardiographic diagnostic criteria

Maximal Dose or Workload
Target Heart Rate
Echocardiographic Positivity
Chest Pain
ECG modification (ST Segment Shift > 2 mm)

Table 18.4 Submaximal non-diagnostic criteria for test interruption

Intolerable Symptoms
Hypertension: Systolic Blood Pressure >220 mmHg; Diastolic Blood Pressure > 120 mmHg
Hypotension (Absolute or Relative): Blood Pressure Fall > 30 mmHg
Supraventricular Arrhythmias: Tachycardia; Atrial Fibrillation
Ventricular Arrhythmias: Ventricular Tachycardia; Polymorphous PVCs

Table 18.2 Stress echocardiography in four equations

REST	+	STRESS	=	DIAGNOSIS
Normokinesis	+	Normo-Hyperkinesis	=	Normal
Normokinesis	+	Hypo, A, Dyskinesis	=	Ischaemia
Akinesis	+	Hypo, Normokinesis	=	Viable
A-, Dyskinesis	+	A-, Dyskinesis	=	Necrosis

Table 18.5 Indications to stress echocardiography

Diagnosis of CAD in patients in whom exercise ECG is contraindicated, not feasible, uninterpretable, non-diagnostic, or gives ambiguous results
Risk stratification in patients with established diagnosis
Pre-operative risk assessment (high-risk non emergent, poor exercise tolerance)
Evaluation after revascularization (not in the early post-procedure period, with change in symptoms)
Search for viability in patients with ischaemic cardiomyopathy eligible for revascularization
Coronary artery disease of unclear significance at angiography or computed tomography

test, since adenosine has a negative chronotropic and dromotropic effect, as well as a documented bronchoconstrictor activity. Patients either taking xanthine medication or under the effect of caffeine contained in drinks (tea, coffee, cola) should undergo the dobutamine test. Both dipyridamole and dobutamine have overall good tolerance and feasibility. The choice of one test over the other depends on patient characteristics, local drug cost, and the physician's preference. It is important for all stress echocardiography laboratories to become familiar with all stresses to achieve a flexible and versatile diagnostic approach that enables the best stress to be tailored to individual patient needs. Anti-anginal medical therapy (in particular, beta-blocking agents) significantly affects the diagnostic accuracy of all forms of stress; therefore, it is recommended, whenever possible, to withhold medical therapy at the time of testing to avoid a false-negative result (indications are reported in ⊃ Table 18.5; appropriateness criteria in ⊃ Table 18.6) [27].

Prognostic value of inducible myocardial ischaemia

The results of a large number of studies enrolling thousands of patients have demonstrated capability by exercise [28–30] or

pharmacological stress echocardiography [31, 32] to allow effective risk assessment in patients with known or suspected coronary artery disease. A normal stress echocardiogram yields an annual risk of 0.4–0.9% based on a total of 9,000 patients [33] the same as for a normal stress myocardial perfusion scan (⊃ Fig. 18.5). Thus, in patients with suspected coronary artery disease, a normal stress echocardiogram implies excellent prognosis and coronary angiography can safely be avoided. The positive and the negative responses can be further stratified with interactions with clinical parameters (diabetes, renal dysfunction, and therapy at the time of test), resting echo (global LV function), and additive stress echo parameters (LV cavity dilatation, CFR, and previous revascularization). The established prognostic stress echo parameters with their relative event rate are shown in ⊃ Tables 18.7 and 18.8, and ⊃ Figs 18.6 and 18.7.

Coronary flow reserve

In recent years the evaluation of coronary flow reserve by combining transthoracic Doppler assessment of coronary flow velocities

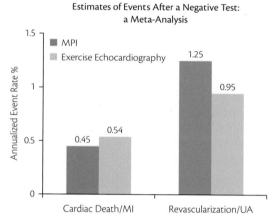

Fig. 18.5 In a meta-analysis stress echocardiography and perfusion nuclear techniques show similar prognostic power when the test is negative for inducible ischaemia.
Modified from [33].

Table 18.6 Appropriateness criteria and stress echo

Patients with	Appropriate	Uncertain	Inappropriate	Class
Uninterpretable ECG, inability to cycle, or submaximal uncertain exercise ECG	✓			I
Uncertain coronary stenosis significance	✓			I
Post-revascularization with symptom changes	✓			I
Before surgery, at high risk, with low exercise tolerance	✓			I
Viability in ischaemic cardiomyopathy	✓			I
Asymptomatic >5 years after CABG or >2 after PCI		✓		IIb
Asymptomatic, low risk			✓	III
Pre-op, intermediate risk surgery, good exercise tolerance			✓	III
Low pre-test probability, interpretable ECG, ability to exercise			✓	III
Asymptomatic <5 years after CABG or <2 after PCI			✓	III

Table 18.7 Risk stratification for a positive test

1-year Risk (hard events)	Intermediate (1–3% year)	High (>10% year)
Dose/workload	High	Low
Resting EF	>50%	<40%
Anti-ischaemic therapy	Off	On
Coronary territory	LCx/RCA	LAD
Peak WMSI	Low	High
Recovery	Fast	Slow
Positivity or baseline dyssynergy	Homozonal	Heterozonal
CFR	>2.0	<2.0

Table 18.8 Risk stratification for a negative test

1-year Risk (hard events)	Very Low (<0.5% year)	Low (1–3% year)
Stress	Maximal	Submaximal
Resting EF	>50%	<40%
Anti-ischaemic therapy	Off	On
CFR	>2.0	<2.0

with vasodilator stress has entered the echo lab as an effective modality for both diagnostic and prognostic purposes. The use of coronary flow reserve as a stand-alone diagnostic criterion suffers from two main limitations. In fact, only left anterior descending artery is sampled with a very high success rate (⊃ Fig. 18.8). Moreover, coronary flow reserve cannot distinguish between microvascular

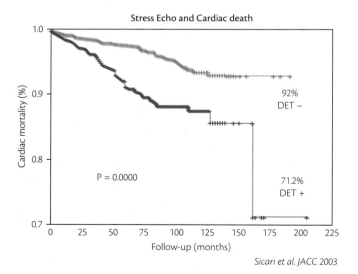

Sicari et al. JACC 2003

Fig. 18.6 Kaplan–Meier survival curves (considering cardiac death as an endpoint) in patients with presence (DET+) and absence (DET−) of myocardial ischaemia at pharmacological stress echocardiography. Survival is worse in patients with inducible ischaemia.
Reprinted from *Journal of the American College of Cardiology*, 41:4, Rosa Sicari et al, Stress echo results predict mortality: a large-scale multicenter prospective international study, 589–95, Copyright 2003 with permission from Elsevier.

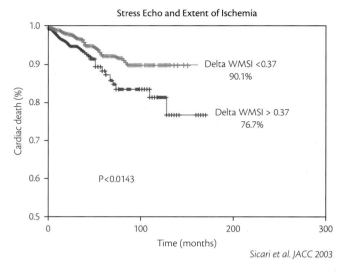

Sicari et al. JACC 2003

Fig. 18.7 Kaplan–Meier survival curves (considering death as an endpoint) in patients with a positive pharmacologic stress echo test separated on its turn on the extent of the inducible ischaemia identified by the delta WMSI set at 0.37. The survival is worse for larger variations of WMSI. Delta WMSI >0.37 vs. Delta WMSI <0.37.
Reprinted from *Journal of the American College of Cardiology*, 41:4, Rosa Sicari et al, Stress echo results predict mortality: a large-scale multicenter prospective international study, 589–95, Copyright 2003 with permission from Elsevier.

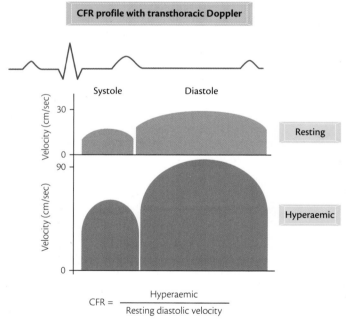

Fig. 18.8 Doppler spectra of coronary flow reserve during vasodilator stress testing.

and macrovascular coronary disease (⊃ Fig. 18.9). Therefore, it is much more interesting to assess the additional diagnostic value over conventional wall motion analysis. Coronary flow reserve on left anterior descending artery is a strong and independent indicator of mortality, conferring additional prognostic value over wall motion analysis in patients with known or suspected coronary

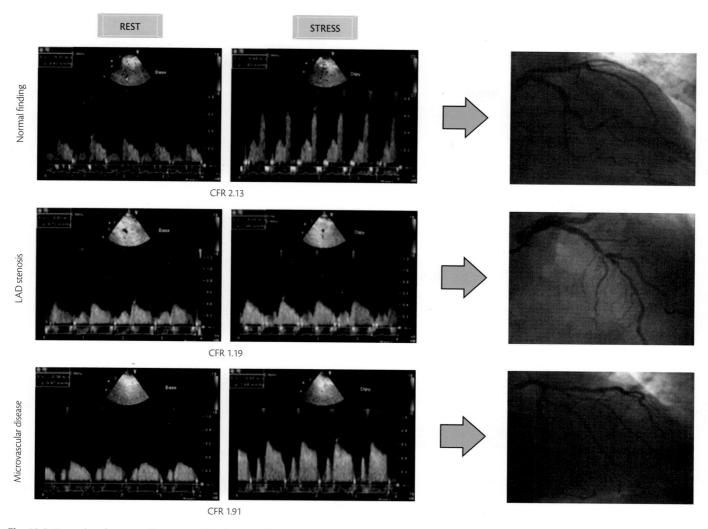

Fig. 18.9 Examples of coronary flow reserve (CFR) assessed by transthoracic Doppler of the mid-distal portion of left anterior descending artery. CFR is calculated as the ratio between peak diastolic coronary flow velocity at hyperaemia and its value in resting condition. The normal finding is characterized by CFR >2 associated with angiographically normal coronary arteries (upper row). In the presence of significant stenosis of the left anterior descending artery, CFR is <2 (second row). CFR can be <2 also in the presence of normal coronary anatomy, indicating underlying microvascular disease (third row).

artery disease. A negative result on stress echocardiography with a normal coronary flow reserve confers an annual risk of death <1% in both patient groups [34] (⮕ Fig. 18.10), and allows effective risk stratification in diabetic patients with unchanged wall motion during stress [35], and in patients with normal or near normal coronary arteries [36]. A coronary flow reserve <2.0 is an additional parameter of ischaemia severity in the risk stratification of the stress echocardiographic response, whereas patients with a negative test for wall motion criteria and coronary flow reserve >2.0 during dipyridamole stress echocardiography have a favourable outcome. Similar results have been obtained when perfusion imaging was added to wall motion analysis [37] (⮕ Fig. 18.11). Anti-ischaemic medication at the time of testing does not modulate the prognostic value of coronary flow reserve, which is per se a prognostic marker independent of therapy [38] (⮕ Fig. 18.12).

The search for a totally operator-independent quantitative tool for stress echocardiography is still on-going. The state-of-the art diagnosis of ischaemia in stress echocardiography remains the eyeballing interpretation of regional wall motion in black and white cine-loops. Myocardial contrast echocardiography (MCE) has undergone rapid development in the past 5 years. With the advent of newer-generation microbubbles, intravenous agents can now be used to both improve endocardial border delineation and, more importantly, detect myocardial perfusion. Along with the development of microbubbles, which consistently opacify the left heart from a venous injection, newer imaging modalities have evolved that permit the detection of myocardial perfusion abnormalities in real time, at frame rates that are greater than 25 Hz. In order to accurately detect wall motion abnormalities during stress echocardiography, a clear definition of endocardial borders is of particular importance. The approved indication for the use of contrast echocardiography currently lies in improving endocardial border delineation in patients in whom adequate imaging

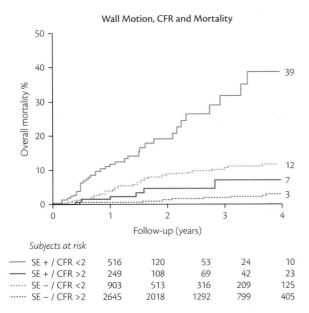

Fig. 18.10 Mortality rate for the study population separated on the basis of presence (+) or absence (−) of ischaemia at stress echocardiography (SE) and coronary flow reserve (CFR) on left anterior descending artery <2 or >2. Number of patients per year is shown.
Modified from [34].

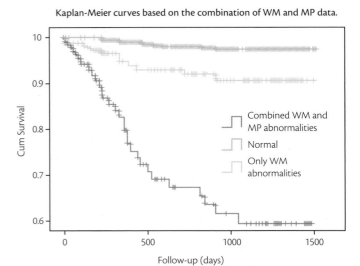

Gaibazzi N et al. Circulation 2012;126:1217–1224

Fig. 18.11 Kaplan–Meier curves based on the combination of WM and MP data. Differences between curves are statistically significant (P<0.001). WM indicates wall motion; MP, myocardial perfusion; Cum, cumulative.
Reproduced from Nicola Gaibazzi et al, Prognostic value of high-dose dipyridamole stress myocardial contrast perfusion echocardiography, Circulation, 126: 1217 Copyright 2012, with permission from Wolters Kluwer Health.

is difficult or suboptimal [39]. The EAE/ASE consensus document states that 3D stress transthoracic echocardiography holds promise for incorporation into clinical practice in the future. Its advantages are: (1) better visualization of the LV apex, which is frequently foreshortened on standard 2D apical images; (2) rapid acquisition of peak stress images before the heart declines in recovery; and (3) evaluation of multiple segments from different planes from a single dataset. Disadvantages include

lower spatial resolution and lower frame rates [40] (⮠ Fig. 18.13 and 18.14).

Competence

Interpretation of stress echocardiography requires extensive experience in echocardiography and should be performed only by physicians with specific training in the technique. The diagnostic accuracy of an experienced echocardiographer who is an absolute

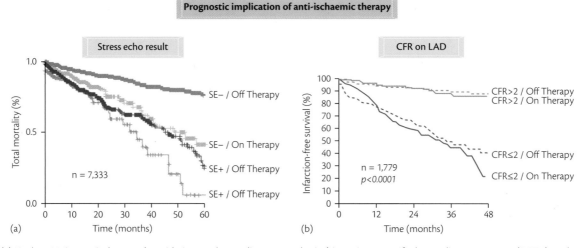

Fig. 18.12 (a) Kaplan–Meier survival curves (considering total mortality as an endpoint) in patients stratified according to presence (DET+) or absence (DET−) of myocardial ischaemia at pharmacological stress echocardiography on and off anti-anginal medical therapy. The best survival is observed in patients with no inducible ischaemia off therapy; the worst survival in patients with inducible ischaemia on therapy. (Positive DET vs. Negative DET off anti-anginal medical therapy, P<0.000; Postive DET vs. Negative DET on anti-anginal medical therapy, P<0.074). (b) Kaplan–Meier survival curves (considering hard events as an endpoint) in patients stratified according to normal (CFR>2) or abnormal (CFR<2) coronary flow reserve at Doppler echocardiography on and off anti-anginal medical therapy. Survival was comparable in patients with normal CFR on and off therapy and in patients with abnormal CFR on and off therapy.
Modified from [38].

Checklist to start: the human factor

	To start	To learn	To keep competence	Top level
Competence in resting TTE	√			
BLS and ALS certification	√			
Experience with exercise-ECG	√			
100 stresses under qualified supervision		√		
100 stress echo studies per year			√	
Familiarity with all stresses (exercise, vasodil, dob)				√
Mixed caseload (ischaemia, valvular, cardiomyopathy, CHD)				√
Appropriateness verification				√

Adapted from Sicari R et al, Stress echo EAE Recommendations, Eur Heart J, 2009

Fig. 18.13 Checklist to start stress echocardiography: the human factor. Source Data from R. Sicari et al, Stress echocardiography expert consensus statement: European Association of Echocardiography (EAE) (a registered branch of the ESC). *Eur J Echocardiogr* 2008; 9: 415–37 by permission of Oxford University Press.

Checklist to start: the technology factor

	Certainly helpful	Possibly helpful	Useless
Native second harmonic	◉		
Digital	◉		
Bed-ergometer for semisupine	◉		
MCE (≥ 2 difficult segments)	◉		
RT3D		○	
TDI, SRI, Backscatter			◉
MCE for perfusion			◉

EAE 2008 recommendations

Fig. 18.14 Checklist to start stress echocardiography: the technology factor. Source Data from R. Sicari et al, Stress echocardiography expert consensus statement: European Association of Echocardiography (EAE) (a registered branch of the ESC). *Eur J Echocardiogr* 2008; 9: 415–37 by permission of Oxford University Press.

beginner in stress echocardiography is more or less equivalent to that achieved by tossing a coin. However, 100 stress echocardiographic studies are more than adequate to build the individual learning curve and reach the plateau of diagnostic accuracy [41]. With stress echocardiography it is wise to test one's initial performance in patients who have recently undergone coronary angiography, and possibly with other imaging techniques using the same stress. After 15–30 days of exposure to a high-volume stress echocardiography lab, the physician should begin to accumulate his or her own experience with a stepwise approach, starting from more innocuous and simple stresses as vasodilator stress-testing and moving up to more technically demanding ones such as exercise. Diagnostic accuracy is not only a function of experience; for a given diagnostic accuracy every observer has his/her own sensitivity specificity curve: there are 'over-readers' (high sensitivity, low specificity) and 'under-readers' (low sensitivity, high specificity), depending on whether images are aggressively or conservatively interpreted as abnormal. Many studies are unquestionably negative or positive; still, there is a 'grey zone' of interpretable tests in which the visualization of some regions can be suboptimal and the cardiologist's level of experience in interpreting the test is critical for a correct reading. There are several ways to minimize this variability, representing the key factor that may ultimately determine the real impact of stress echocardiography in modern cardiological practice. These parameters are related to the physician interpreting the study, the technology used, the stress employed, and the patient under study. Variability will be substantially reduced if one agrees in advance not to consider minor degrees of hypokinesia, since mild hypokinesia is a normal variant under most stresses and a finding widely overlapping between normal and diseased population [42–44]. Also the inclusion among positivity criteria of isolated asynergy of basal-infero-lateral or basal-infero-septal segments will inflate variability. Finally, the single most important factor deflating variability is a dedicated course of training in a large volume stress echocardiography lab with exposure to joint reading [45] and *a priori* development of standardized [46] and conservative [47] reading criteria. Maintenance of competence requires at least 15 stress echo exams per month [27].

References

1. Gould KL, Lipscomb K. Effects of coronary stenoses on coronary flow reserve and resistance. *Am J Cardiol* 1974: 34: 48–55.

2. Picano E. *Stress Echocardiography*, 5th edn. Heidelberg: Springer-Verlag, 2009.

3. Palinkas A, Toth E, Amyot R, Rigo F, Venneri L, Picano E. The value of ECG and echocardiography during stress testing for identifying systemic endothelial dysfunction and epicardial artery stenosis. *Eur Heart J* 2002; 23: 1587–95.

4. Zeiher AM, Krause T, Schächinger V, Minners J, Moser E. Impaired endothelium-dependent vasodilation of coronary resistance vessels is associated with exercise-induced myocardial ischaemia. *Circulation* 1995; 91: 2345–52.

5. Panting JR, Gatehouse PD, Yang GZ, et al. Abnormal sub-endocardial perfusion in cardiac syndrome X detected by cardiovascular magnetic resonance imaging. *N Engl J Med* 2002; 346: 1948–53.

6. Lanza GA, Buffon A, Sestito A, et al. Relation between stress-induced myocardial perfusion defects on cardiovascular magnetic resonance and coronary microvascular dysfunction in patients with cardiac syndrome X. *J Am Coll Cardiol* 2008; 51: 466–72.

7. Picano E, Lattanzi F, Masini M, Distante A, L'Abbate A. Usefulness of a high-dose dipyridamole-echocardiography test for diagnosis of syndrome X. *Am J Cardiol* 1987; 60: 508–12.

8. Cannon RO 3rd, Bonow RO, Bacharach SL, et al. Left ventricular dysfunction in patients with angina pectoris, normal epicardial coronary

arteries, and abnormal vasodilator reserve. *Circulation* 1985; 71: 218–26.

9. Kaski JC, Crea F, Nihoyannopoulos P, Hackett D, Maseri A. Transient myocardial ischaemia during daily life in patients with syndrome X. *Am J Cardiol* 1986; 58: 1242–47.

10. Picano E. Dipyridamole-echocardiography test: historical background and physiologic basis. *Eur Heart J.* 1989; 10: 365–76.

11. Picano E. Stress echocardiography: from pathophysiological toy to diagnostic tool. Point of view. *Circulation* 1992; 85: 1604–12.

12. Gallagher KP, Matsuzaki M, Koziol JA, Kemper WS, Ross J Jr. Regional myocardial perfusion and wall thickening during ischaemia in conscious dogs. *Am J Physiol* 1984; 247: H727–38.

13. Bolognesi R, Tsialtas D, Barilli AL, et al. Detection of early abnormalities of left ventricular function by haemodynamic, echo-tissue Doppler imaging, and mitral Doppler flow techniques in patients with coronary artery disease and normal ejection fraction. *J Am Soc Echocardiogr* 2001; 14: 764–72.

14. Ingul CB, Stoylen A, Slordahl SA, Wiseth R, Burgess M, Marwick TH. Automated analysis of myocardial deformation at dobutamine stress echocardiography: an angiographic validation. *J Am Coll Cardiol* 2007; 49: 1651–59.

15. Helle-Valle T, Crosby J, Edvardsen T, et al. New noninvasive method for assessment of left ventricular rotation: speckle tracking echocardiography. *Circulation* 2005; 112: 3149–56.

16. Hoffmann R, Altiok E, Nowak B, et al. Strain rate measurement by doppler echocardiography allows improved assessment of myocardial viability inpatients with depressed left ventricular function. *J Am Coll Cardiol* 2002; 39: 443–49.

17. Amundsen BH, Helle-Valle T, Edvardsen T, et al. Noninvasive myocardial strain measurement by speckle tracking echocardiography: validation against sonomicrometry and tagged magnetic resonance imaging. *J Am Coll Cardiol* 2006; 47: 789–93.

18. Gjesdal O, Hopp E, Vartdal T, et al. Global longitudinal strain measured by two-dimensional speckle tracking echocardiography is closely related to myocardial infarct size in chronic ischaemic heart disease. *Clin Sci (Lond)* 2007; 113: 287–96.

19. Mor-Avi V, Lang RM, Badano LP, et al. Current and evolving echocardiographic techniques for the quantitative evaluation of cardiac mechanics: ASE/EAE consensus statement on methodology and indications endorsed by the Japanese Society of Echocardiography. *Eur J Echocardiogr* 2011; 12: 167–20.

20. Picano E, Lattanzi F, Masini M, Distante A, L'Abbate A. High dose dipyridamole echocardiography test in effort angina pectoris. *J Am Coll Cardiol* 1986; 8: 848–54.

21. Berthe C, Pierard LA, Hiernaux M, et al. Predicting the extent and location of coronary artery disease in acute myocardial infarction by echocardiography during dobutamine infusion. *Am J Cardiol* 1986; 58: 1167–72.

22. Mazeika P, Nihoyannopoulos P, Joshi J, Oakley CM. Evaluation of dipyridamole—Doppler echocardiography for detection of myocardial ischaemia and coronary artery disease. *Am J Cardiol* 1991; 68: 478–84.

23. Geleijnse ML, Fioretti PM, Roelandt JR. Methodology, feasibility, safety and diagnostic accuracy of dobutamine stress echocardiography. *J Am Coll Cardiol* 1997; 30: 595–606.

24. Heijenbrok-Kal MH, Fleischmann KE, Hunink MG. Stress echocardiography, stress single-photon-emission computed tomography and electron beam computed tomography for the assessment of coronary artery disease: a meta-analysis of diagnostic performance. *Am Heart J* 2007; 154: 415–23.

25. Picano E, Molinaro S, Pasanisi E. The diagnostic accuracy of pharmacological stress echocardiography for the assessment of coronary artery disease: a meta-analysis. *Cardiovasc Ultrasound* 2008; 6: 30.

26. Severi S, Picano E, Michelassi C, et al. Diagnostic and prognostic value of dipyridamole echocardiography in patients with suspected coronary artery disease. Comparison with exercise electrocardiography. *Circulation* 1994; 89: 1160–73.

27. Sicari R, Nihoyannopoulos P, Evangelista A, et al. Stress echocardiography expert consensus statement: European Association of Echocardiography (EAE) (a registered branch of the ESC). *Eur J Echocardiogr* 2008; 9: 415–37.

28. Marwick TH, Case C, Vasey C, Allen S, Short L, Thomas JD. Prediction of mortality by exercise echocardiography: a strategy for combination with the Duke treadmill score. *Circulation* 2001; 103: 2566–71.

29. Arruda-Olson AM, Juracan EM, Mahoney DW, McCully RB, Roger VL, Pellikka PA. Prognostic value of exercise echocardiography in 5,798 patients: is there a gender difference? *J Am Coll Cardiol* 2002; 39: 625–31.

30. Shaw LJ, Vasey C, Sawada S, Rimmerman C, Marwick TH. Impact of gender on risk stratification by exercise and dobutamine stress echocardiography: long-term mortality in 4234 women and 6898 men. *Eur Heart J* 2005; 26: 447–56.

31. Picano E, Severi S, Michelassi C, et al. Prognostic importance of dipyridamole-echocardiography test in coronary artery disease. *Circulation* 1989; 80: 450–9.

32. Sicari R, Pasanisi E, Venneri L, Landi P, Cortigiani L., Picano E. Stress echo results predict mortality: a large scale multicenter prospective international study. *J Am Coll Cardiol* 2003; 41: 589–95.

33. Metz LD, Beattie M, Hom R, Redberg RF, Grady D, Fleischmann KE. The prognostic value of normal exercise myocardial perfusion imaging and exercise echocardiography: a meta-analysis. *J Am Coll Cardiol* 2007; 49: 227–37.

34. Cortigiani L, Rigo F, Gherardi S, et al. Coronary flow reserve during dipyridamole stress echocardiography predicts mortality. *JACC Cardiovasc Imaging* 2012; 5: 1079–85.

35. Cortigiani L, Rigo F, Gherardi S, et al. Additional prognostic value of coronary flow reserve in diabetic and nondiabetic patients with negative dipyridamole stress echocardiography by wall motion criteria. *J Am Coll Cardiol* 2007; 50: 1354: 61.

36. Sicari R, Rigo F, Cortigiani L, Gherardi S, Galderisi M, Picano E. Long-term survival of patients with chest pain syndrome and angiographically normal or near normal coronary arteries: the additional prognostic value of coronary flow reserve. *Am J Cardiol* 2009; 103: 626–31.

37. Gaibazzi N, Reverberi C, Lorenzoni V, Molinaro S, Porter TR. Prognostic value of high-dose dipyridamole stress myocardial contrast perfusion echocardiography. *Circulation* 2012; 126: 1217–24.

38. Sicari R, Rigo F, Gherardi S, Galderisi M, Cortigiani L, Picano E. The prognostic value of Doppler echocardiographic-derived coronary flow reserve is not affected by concomitant anti-ischaemic therapy at the time of testing. *Am Heart J* 2008; 156: 573–9.

39. Crouse LJ, Cheirif J, Hanly DE, et al. Opacification and border delineation improvement in patients with suboptimal endocardial border definition in routine echocardiography: results of phase III Albunex multicenter trial. *J Am Coll Cardiol* 1993, 22: 1494–1500.

40. Lang RM, Badano LP, Tsang W, et al. American Society of Echocardiography; European Association of Echocardiography. EAE/ASE recommendations for image acquisition and display using three-dimensional echocardiography. *Eur Heart J Cardiovasc Imaging* 2012; 13: 1–46.

41. Picano E, Lattanzi F, Orlandini A, Marini C, L'Abbate A. Stress echocardiography and the human factor: the importance of being expert. *J Am Coll Cardiol* 1991; 17: 666–9.

42. Borges AC, Pingitore A, Cordovil A, Sicari R, Baumann G, Picano E. Heterogeneity of left ventricular regional wall thickening following dobutamine infusion in normal human subjects. *Eur Heart J* 1995; 16: 1726–30.

43. Carstensen S, Ali SM, Stensgaard-Hansen FV, et al. Dobutamine-atropine stress echocardiography in asymptomatic healthy individuals. The relativity of stress-induced hyperkinesia. *Circulation* 1995; 92: 3453–63.

44. Hoffmann R, Marwick TH, Poldermans D, et al. Refinements in stress echocardiographic techniques improve inter-institutional agreement in interpretation of dobutamine stress echocardiograms. *Eur Heart J* 2002; 23: 821–9.

45. Varga A, Picano E, Dodi C, Barbieri A, Pratali L, Gaddi O. Madness and method in stress echo reading. *Eur Heart J* 1999; 20: 1271–5.

46. Hoffmann R, Lethen H, Marwick T, et al. Standardized guidelines for the interpretation of dobutamine echocardiography reduce interinstitutional variance in interpretation. *Am J Cardiol* 1998; 82: 1520–24.

47. Imran MB, Palinkas A, Pasanisi EM, De Nes M, Picano E. Optimal reading criteria in stress echocardiography. *Am J Cardiol* 2002; 90: 44–445.

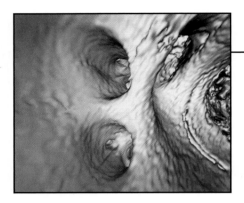

CHAPTER 19

Nuclear cardiology and detection of coronary artery disease

James Stirrup and S. Richard Underwood

Introduction

Experience with radionuclide assessments of myocardial perfusion can be measured over decades. Single-photon emission computed tomography (SPECT) myocardial perfusion scintigraphy (MPS) has been validated for the diagnosis and prognosis of cardiac disease and the technique is embedded in national and international guidelines. Positron emission tomography (PET) has been used to assess myocardial viability but it is now used increasingly to detect flow-limiting coronary artery disease (CAD). With alternative cardiac imaging techniques now available it is more important than ever to understand the principles, indications, and pitfalls of the options. No single technique provides a complete assessment of the heart; many provide complementary rather than equivalent information. In this chapter, the value of cardiac radionuclide imaging in stable CAD and acute coronary syndromes (ACS) is discussed, with a particular emphasis on the role of MPS, the most commonly used technique in nuclear cardiology.

Spectrum of coronary artery disease

CAD is characterized by the progressive development of atheromatous plaques within the intima of the coronary artery. Familiarity with the development and progression of atheroma is helpful in order to put the cardiac imaging techniques into context. Techniques concerned mainly with coronary artery anatomy, such as invasive coronary angiography (ICA) or computed tomography coronary angiography (CTCA), are well placed to detect atheromatous plaques causing minor luminal narrowing and beyond. However, these techniques, used in isolation, provide no assessment of the impact of these plaques on coronary flow or myocardial perfusion. The functional significance of a coronary artery stenosis is most often based on a visual estimate of its severity but this does not correlate well with its functional significance.

Ultimately, the choice of cardiac imaging test is determined by the clinical scenario. If the aim of imaging is to detect CAD of any type or severity, such as in a patient with a strong family history of premature CAD in whom the exclusion of CAD would be reassuring, then an anatomical test, such as CTCA, is indicated. However, the majority of patients present with symptoms of some kind and here it is coronary function that must be assessed.

The ischaemic cascade

Myocardial ischaemia is the result of oxygen demand exceeding its supply. This is usually due to impairment of myocardial perfusion, although excessive demand, such as in high-output

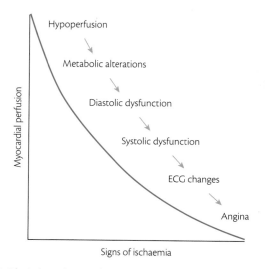

Fig. 19.1 The ischaemic cascade.

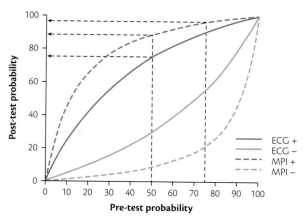

Fig. 19.2 Impact of pre-test probability on post-test likelihood of disease. In a patient with a 50% pre-test likelihood of coronary artery disease, positive stress electrocardiography renders the post-test likelihood around 75%. This is not sufficient to make the diagnosis with confidence. If the same patient goes on to have a positive myocardial perfusion scan (MPS), the probability is refined further to around 96%, which is sufficient to be confident of the diagnosis. If MPS had been performed as the initial test, pre-test likelihood would have been revised from 50% to around 90% based on a positive result, after which further testing would not be required. ECG + /−, stress electrocardiogram positive/negative; MPI + /−, myocardial perfusion imaging positive/negative.

heart failure or prolonged tachycardia, may have the same effect. Ischaemia leads to a cascade of effects on the cardiac myocyte, the manifestation of which depends on severity (◯ Fig. 19.1). The precursor to ischaemia is impaired myocardial perfusion, which, once sufficiently severe, leads to metabolic abnormalities such as switching of the primary myocardial energy source from fatty acids to glucose. It is only after alterations in myocardial metabolism that the cellular machinery within the cardiac myocyte becomes sufficiently deranged to cause abnormalities of first diastolic and then systolic left ventricular function. These changes lead to both electrical abnormalities, which may be seen on the surface electrocardiogram (ECG), and symptoms of chest pain. Functional imaging tests interrogate different parts of this cascade. As impairment of myocardial perfusion precedes both ischaemic wall motion and ECG abnormalities, MPS potentially provides the most sensitive technique.

Impact of pre-test likelihood of coronary artery disease on imaging strategy

When a patient presents with symptoms of possible coronary disease the decision to investigate, along with the appropriate choice of test, should be informed by the pre-test likelihood of significant CAD. It is helpful to consider the usefulness of any diagnostic test in Bayesian terms [1]. In summary, the post-test likelihood of having disease can be computed from the pre-test likelihood and the accuracy of the test (◯ Fig. 19.2). Here, an abnormal stress electrocardiogram (sECG) in a patient with a 50% pre-test likelihood of CAD generates a post-test likelihood of only 75%, which is not high enough to be sufficiently confident of the diagnosis and further testing might be required. If the same patient had abnormal MPS as the initial test, the post-test likelihood improves to 90%, allowing greater diagnostic certainty with a single test. Pre-test likelihood of significant CAD can be estimated by a number of nomograms. Among these, the Diamond and Forrester

predictive table integrates three clinical variables (quality of chest pain, gender, and age) to provide an estimate of the likelihood of angiographically significant coronary stenosis [2], although the approach is known to overestimate likelihood in a contemporary European population. It can be refined by incorporating other predictors, such as serum cholesterol, systolic blood pressure, and diabetes [3]. More recently, tables derived by Genders and colleagues [4] have been used and the methodology has been incorporated into ESC guidelines for the investigation of stable CAD [5]. Most predictors of pre-test likelihood are able to distinguish those at low and high likelihood of CAD but many remain classified as intermediate. In general terms, false-positive and false-negative results are more likely in patients at very low and very high pre-test likelihoods, respectively. Those at intermediate pre-test likelihood have the most to gain from further investigation as a positive or negative result allows revision of pre-test likelihood to either high or low post-test likelihood, respectively.

Methods of cardiac stress

Dynamic exercise

This is the preferred method of cardiac stress as it is the most physiological challenge of myocardial perfusion. Additionally, changes in haemodynamic and ECG variables during stress allow estimation of prognosis incremental to perfusion findings [6, 7]. However, exercise may be either difficult in those with limited mobility or contraindicated, such as in patients with severe left ventricular outflow tract obstruction or severe left main stem disease. Furthermore, certain conditions, such as left bundle branch block and permanent pacing, can be associated with stress-induced

Table 19.1 Characteristics of forms of stress commonly used for myocardial perfusion scintigraphy

	Exercise	Adenosine	Regadenoson	Dipyridamole	Dobutamine
Action	Reflex coronary vasodilatation in response to increased myocardial work	Direct non-selective adenosine receptor stimulation	Selective A2A adenosine receptor agonist	Endogenous adenosine reuptake inhibitor	Beta-adrenergic agonist
Half-life	–	10 s	Hyperaemia 2–5 min, side effects 15–30 min	40 min	2 min
Side effects	Tachyarrhythmia, hypotension	Bronchospasm, heart block	Headache, flushing, dyspnoea	Bronchospasm, heart block	Tachyarrhythmia, hypotension
Limitations	Limited mobility, severe 3-vessel disease, severe LVOTO	Persistent asthma, 2nd or 3rd degree heart block without PPM	2nd or 3rd degree heart block without PPM	Persistent asthma, 2nd or 3rd degree heart block without PPM	History of ventricular tachyarrhythmia, severe 3-vessel disease, severe LVOTO
Protocol	Dynamic exercise with 1–2 min increments up to maximum achievable	140 μg/kg/min	400 μg IV bolus over 10 s	140 μg/kg/min	5–40 μg/kg/min
Duration of stress	Terminate test and inject tracer once 85% target heart rate achieved or at peak exercise	6 min	~4 min	~20 min	Terminate infusion and inject tracer once 85% target heart rate achieved or after 3 min at 40 μg/kg/min
Radionuclide injection time		2–3 min after start of infusion	10–20 s after injection of regadenoson bolus	8 min after start of infusion	

PPM, permanent pacemaker; LVOTO, left ventricular outflow tract obstruction.

perfusion abnormalities at peak heart rates in the absence of obstructive coronary disease.

Pharmacological stress

Myocardial perfusion reserve can be assessed directly using coronary vasodilators such as adenosine, dipyridamole, and the adenosine A_{2A} receptor agonist, regadenoson (⊃ Table 19.1). Endogenous adenosine is the active agent in coronary autoregulation. When given in exogenous form, stimulation of adenosine A_2 receptors leads to coronary arteriolar dilatation and myocardial perfusion three to five times baseline levels. Dipyridamole causes the same effects, albeit indirectly through an increase in endogenous adenosine levels due to inhibition of local adenosine reuptake. Additional stimulation of A_1 receptors within the sinoatrial and atrioventricular nodes and in bronchial smooth muscle leads to heart block and bronchospasm, respectively, making the use of these agents in those with existing nodal disease or obstructive airways disease problematic. Selective stimulation of the A_{2A} receptor using regadenoson may mitigate some of these effects. An alternative in these patients is dobutamine, which is an α1, β1, and β2 adrenergic agonist that causes secondary coronary vasodilatation by increasing myocardial demand in a similar way to dynamic exercise. At higher doses, dobutamine causes direct coronary vasodilatation and can therefore be used to study perfusion heterogeneity even if target heart rate is not achieved.

Stable coronary artery disease

Diagnosis

Stable CAD is characterized by predictable central chest pain provoked by exertion and relieved by rest. Stable but progressive atherosclerosis causes reduction in myocardial perfusion reserve,

ultimately leading to myocardial ischaemia during periods of increased myocardial demand.

Stress electrocardiography (sECG) is commonly used to investigate chest pain because it is widely available, easy to administer, and it does not involves radiation exposure. sECG provides a more physiological evaluation of symptoms, exercise tolerance, haemodynamic response, and ECG changes during exercise that is usually equal to or greater than the normal level of exertion for the patient. However, in meta-analyses, the sensitivity and specificity of sECG is only 68% and 77%, respectively [8]. This means that its positive predictive value is poor [9], particularly in women [8]. Normal coronary angiography rates may be as high as 56% in women referred on the basis of the sECG alone [10]. Furthermore, sECG has limited value when exercise capacity is poor or in the presence of an abnormal resting ECG that precludes ST-segment assessment. These limitations have led to the suggestion that sECG fails to prevent downstream testing and can even lead to an increase in ICA [11].

MPS is ideally suited to the diagnosis of stable CAD because of its ability to detect, localize, and quantify impaired myocardial perfusion reserve, a phenomenon that occurs earlier than both wall motion and electrocardiographic abnormalities in the ischaemic cascade. Although differences exist in the physical properties, myocardial uptake and localization and elimination of the three SPECT MPS tracers available commercially, all have comparable accuracy for the detection of CAD [12]. Normal myocardial perfusion after stress (⊃ Fig. 19.3) indicates the absence of functionally significant CAD and is associated with a low likelihood (<1%) of future coronary events [13]. It should be noted that normal stress perfusion does not equal absence of CAD, as coronary atherosclerosis need not necessarily cause stenosis of sufficient severity to impair perfusion reserve (⊃ Fig. 19.4). However, such disease is unlikely to be the cause of exertional symptoms. Although normal perfusion

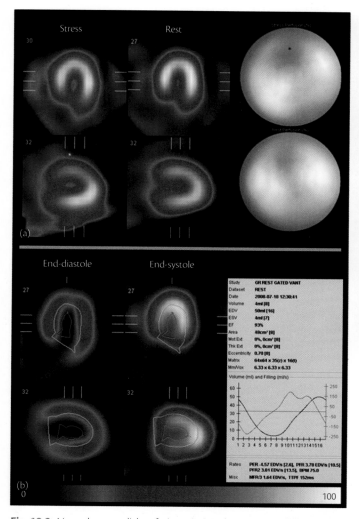

Fig. 19.3 Normal myocardial perfusion scintigraphy. A 70-year-old lady with diabetes, hyperlipidaemia, and hypertension presents to a rapid access chest pain clinic with atypical chest pain. Stress electrocardiography was equivocal and subsequent invasive coronary angiography showed 30% distal LAD and 50% mid-RCA stenoses. Stress-rest MPS (a) showed minor reduction in counts in the basal anterior wall (asterisks) consistent with breast attenuation artefact. Evaluation of raw data (Video 19.1a) demonstrates breast shadows. There is otherwise homogeneous myocardial tracer uptake during both stress and rest. ECG-gating of the resting tomograms (b, Video 19.1b) shows normal global and regional left ventricular function.

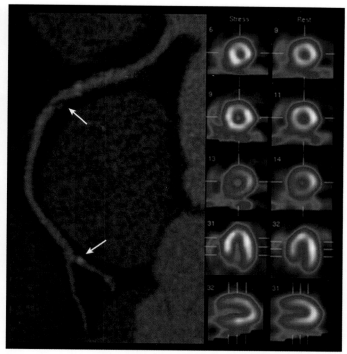

Fig. 19.4 Atheromatous plaques identified in the right coronary artery on computed tomography coronary angiography (arrows). These plaques are not of sufficient severity to cause abnormalities on myocardial perfusion scintigraphy.

carries a good prognosis, the prognostic importance of subclinical disease is still a matter of debate, especially in light of data derived from alternative techniques such as coronary calcium scoring.

MPS has a 15% greater median sensitivity for the detection of significant CAD on ICA than sECG [14]. In a recent meta-analysis, sensitivity and specificity were 85–90% and 70–75%, respectively, for the detection of angiographically significant CAD [15]. It should be reiterated that ICA is an anatomical rather than a functional technique and that 'significant' stenosis on ICA may be associated with normal perfusion reserve. Perfect agreement is therefore neither expected nor required. The specificity of MPS suffers from post-test referral bias in many studies and normalcy, the number of patients at low likelihood of coronary disease with normal MPS, is a better measure. Despite the various tracers and stress techniques available, MPS may be considered reasonably to be a single test, with a

sensitivity and normalcy as high as 90% and 89%, respectively, for the detection of functionally significant CAD [15]. The technique has slightly greater sensitivity but similar specificity to stress echocardiography [16] and magnetic resonance imaging [17]. However, unlike echocardiography, MPS does not suffer from operator dependence and the technique is more widely available than MRI.

The sensitivity and specificity of MPS is improved by ECG gating [18] and attenuation correction [19]. ECG gating provides information on global and regional ventricular function, which, aside from providing important prognostic information, aids in the distinction of artefact from true perfusion defect, thus improving specificity and normalcy. Fixed defects in the anterior and inferior walls, commonly due to breast and diaphragmatic attenuation in women and men, respectively, can be mistaken for myocardial infarction but for the fact that myocardial motion and thickening in these areas are normal on gated images. Similarly, attenuation correction recovers counts in these areas and further improves the recognition of artefact and hence diagnostic accuracy (Fig. 19.5).

The extent and depth of inducible perfusion abnormalities can provide diagnostic information and guide subsequent management (Figs 19.6–19.8). Ultimately, the clinician must decide whether to offer revascularization in addition to optimal medical management, and debate concerning the appropriateness of each in the management of CAD continues. Results from the COURAGE trial in particular suggest that, in patients with stable CAD and objective evidence of myocardial ischaemia, revascularization fails to reduce the risk of death, myocardial infarction, or other major cardiovascular events when added to optimal medical therapy [20]. Although sub-analysis suggests that the addition of PCI leads to

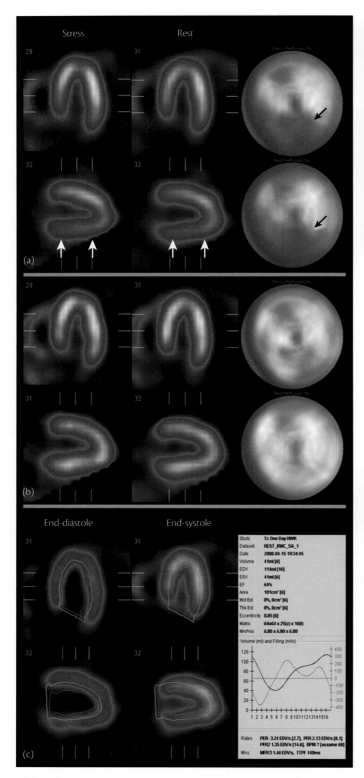

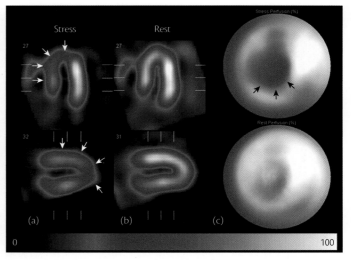

Fig. 19.6 Pure inducible ischaemia on stress (a) and rest (b) imaging and polar plots (c). A 62-year-old man with a family history of premature coronary artery disease and hyperlipidaemia presents to a chest pain clinic with typical angina. Stress electrocardiography showed no ECG changes, although the patient did get chest pain during Stage 4 of the Bruce protocol. On MPS, there is reduction of tracer uptake on stress imaging (arrows), severe at the apex and mild in the anterior wall, which returns to normal at rest.

greater reduction in ischaemia on MPS, the prognostic importance of this remains unclear [21]. Nonetheless, assessments of myocardial perfusion remain central to the management of stable CAD.

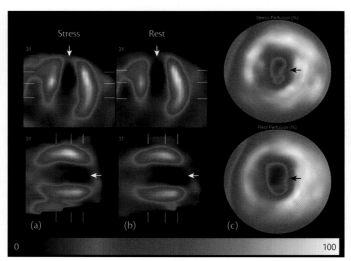

Fig. 19.7 Pure myocardial infarction on stress (a) and rest (b) imaging and polar plots (c). A 64-year-old man with previous myocardial infarction and two-vessel coronary artery bypass grafting is referred for pre-operative assessment prior to umbilical hernia surgery. Although suffering from occasional atypical chest pain, stable exertional breathlessness was the patient's main symptom. Evaluation of raw data (Video 19.3a) shows a dilated left ventricle with absent uptake at the apex. There is absent uptake at the apex on stress images that is unchanged at rest (arrows), indicating myocardial infarction without superimposed ischaemia. ECG-gating of the resting tomograms (Video 19.3b) confirms the dilated left ventricle. There is absent motion and thickening in the apex and apical anterior wall and moderate reduction in the adjacent apical parts of the anterior septum and the inferior wall. There is further reduced motion but preserved thickening in the remainder of the septum consistent with LBBB. The absence of inducible ischaemia indicates that the risk of peri-operative coronary events is not high.

Fig. 19.5 Diaphragmatic attenuation artefact. A 73-year-old man with hypertension and hyperlipidaemia presents with central chest pain unrelated to exertion and occasional palpitation. Uncorrected images (a) show mild reduction of counts in the whole inferior wall that is present in both stress and resting images. Evaluation of raw data (Video 19.2a) shows the presence of the diaphragm in the lateral projections. X-ray computed tomography attenuation correction (b) of the images recovers counts in the inferior wall to normal. Additionally, ECG-gating of the uncorrected images (c, Video 19.2b) demonstrates normal wall motion and thickening inferiorly despite the reduced counts. In this case, the clinical history, attenuation-corrected images and ECG-gating all point to diaphragmatic attenuation rather than partial thickness myocardial damage as a cause for the reduction in counts inferiorly.

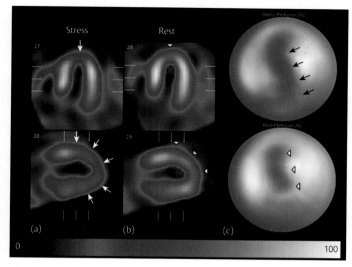

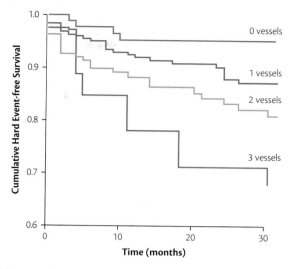

Fig. 19.8 Mixed inducible ischaemia and partial thickness myocardial infarction on stress (a) and rest (b) imaging and polar plots (c). A 45-year-old man with known previous myocardial infarction, right coronary artery stenting but untreated mid-left anterior descending artery occlusion presents with diminished exercise tolerance but no chest pain. There is moderate reduction of tracer uptake in the apex and apical anterior and inferior walls (arrows) on stress imaging. Images acquired at rest show improvement in these areas but the anterior wall and apex do not return to normal, indicating partial thickness myocardial damage (arrowheads). ECG-gating of the resting tomograms (📷 Video 19.4) shows mild reduction of wall motion and thickening in the apical anterior wall but normal regional function elsewhere.

Fig. 19.9 Cumulative hard event-free survival in patients with known or suspected CAD according to number of ischaemic vascular territories on ^{99m}Tc-MIBI MPS.

Reproduced from R. Stewart, C. Dickinson, I. Weissman, et al, Clinical outcome of patients evaluated with emergency centre myocardial perfusion SPET for unexplained chest pain, *Nuclear Medicine Communications*, 17:6, with permission from Wolters Kluwer Health.

Prognosis

The risk of future cardiac events, such as myocardial infarction (MI) or death, is a significant determinant of treatment type and intensity. A number of factors such as angina threshold, total ischaemic burden, extent of CAD, degree of LV dysfunction, presence of diabetes or other arterial disease, and other CAD risk factors contribute to the annual risk of cardiac events, which may be classified as low (<1%), intermediate (1–3%) or high (>3%) [21]. MPS has incremental prognostic value even when clinical history, sECG, and ICA are available [22].

The role of MPS in risk stratification and patient management has been validated extensively. Normal MPS is associated with a 0.7% mean annual risk of MI and cardiac death, which is similar to the general population [23]. This has important implications because a normal study generally renders further invasive investigation or treatment unnecessary. The annual risk quoted represents an average figure and a normal perfusion study should always be interpreted in the context of the individual patient. Patients with normal myocardial perfusion but significant ST-segment depression during adenosine stress are at increased risk of non-fatal MI, with an event rate of 7.6% compared with 0.5% in patients without such findings [24]. Specific groups, such as the elderly and those with diabetes or known CAD, have an annual event rate somewhat higher (1.4–1.8%) despite normal MPS. The 'warranty period' of normal MPS in this setting is around 2 years, depending upon risk factor control, after which repeat scanning may be necessary to redefine prognosis [25].

An abnormal scan confers a 7-fold increase in annual cardiac events compared with a normal study [22]. The likelihood of a cardiac event increases with the extent and severity of the inducible perfusion abnormalities (➲ Figs 19.9 and 19.10). Those with only mild inducible ischaemia have an annual event rate of around 3% rising to 7% in those with severe ischaemia (➲ Fig. 19.11) [13]. The presence of corollary markers of severe three-vessel disease, such as transient left ventricular dilatation or increased lung uptake of thallium-201, increases the event rate still further [26, 27]. On this basis, coronary revascularization is recommended on prognostic grounds if more than 10% of the left ventricular myocardium is ischaemic [28]. Patients with significant ischaemia and without extensive scar on MPS realize a survival benefit from early revascularization, whilst those with minimal ischaemia are better served by optimal medical therapy alone [29]. Whilst perfusion data are most useful in predicting the risk of ischaemic events, left ventricular function provides an independent estimate of the risk of cardiac death (➲ Fig. 19.10) [22].

MPS is not generally recommended to assess prognosis in asymptomatic individuals except in certain settings [30]. Coronary calcium scoring (CCS) using X-ray computed tomography identifies subclinical atherosclerosis and predicts the likelihood of coronary events [31]. Higher calcium scores are associated with increased likelihood of cardiac events even within individual Framingham risk groups [32]. This allows further risk stratification and definition of the appropriateness and intensity of medical treatment or the need for stress testing. Those with CCS≥400 have a high likelihood of at least one significant coronary artery stenosis; patients with diabetes or the metabolic syndrome may require a different CCS score threshold (100–400), as reversible perfusion defects may be seen in almost half of those with CCS>100 [33]. The current ESC position is that only asymptomatic type 2 diabetic patients without known CAD should be considered for coronary calcium imaging, with subsequent MPS for those with significant coronary calcium in order to identify subjects with a moderate to severe extent of ischaemia who are

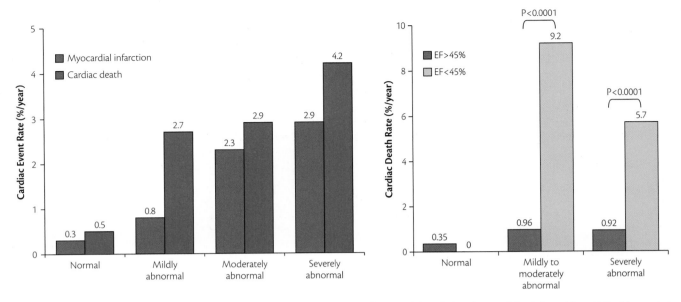

Fig. 19.10 (a) Rates of myocardial infarction and cardiac death according to severity of myocardial perfusion abnormalities. Adapted from [11] with permission. (b) Cardiac death rates in patients with differing severities of myocardial perfusion abnormalities, separated according to left ventricular ejection fraction (EF). Those with EF<45% are at a markedly higher risk of death compared with those with normal left ventricular function. Adapted from [68] with permission.

likely to benefit from revascularization (class IIa) [30]. CCS and MPS are synergistic in predicting short-term coronary events suggesting that CCS should be used routinely in asymptomatic diabetic adults to stratify risk more accurately [34]. However, those at high Framingham risk may derive greater benefit from direct

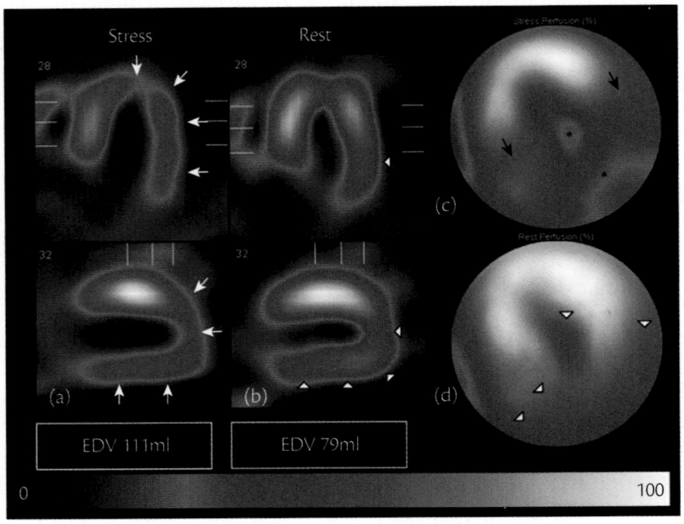

Fig. 19.11 Prognosis defined by extent and severity of inducible myocardial ischaemia. Stress imaging (a, c) demonstrates severe reduction of counts in the apex and the apical antero-septal region, the lateral wall, and adjacent inferolateral segments and moderate reduction inferiorly and infero-septally (arrows). Counts are poorest at the apex and infero-laterally (asterisks). Images at rest (b, d) show marked improvement in all areas, although the apex, inferior, and basal lateral and infero-lateral walls do not return to normal, indicating partial thickness myocardial damage (arrowheads). Of note, the end-diastolic volume after stress is significantly larger than at rest (111 ml vs. 79 ml; TID ratio 1.41). This transient left ventricular cavity dilatation is a marker of significant three vessel coronary disease. The total amount of ischaemia is extensive and severe, and the likelihood of future cardiac events is high. EDV, end-diastolic volume.

referral for MPS in order to quantify ischaemic burden [35]. MPS may also be considered a first-line test for first-degree relatives of patients with premature CAD (class IIb) [30].

Cost-effectiveness

By quantifying the presence, extent, and severity of inducible ischaemia, MPS allows either conservative or invasive management strategies to be recommended. Those with minor inducible ischaemia may be safely managed conservatively, suggesting that even a positive MPS need not lead to further investigation or invasive treatment. An investigation strategy involving MPS, therefore, ought to be more cost-effective than one based on either sECG alone or direct referral for ICA. This supposition is supported by assessments of cost-effectiveness in both Europe and the US. MPS is cost-effective in patients presenting with stable chest pain both at intermediate and high pre-test likelihood of CAD and with or without known CAD [36, 37]. In Europe strategies involving MPS are cheaper, have greater prognostic power at diagnosis and lead to lower normal ICA rates compared with strategies without MPS (⊃ Fig. 19.12) [38]. Where sECG is used as the initial test, MPS remains cost-effective for the further investigation of patients who remain at intermediate or greater likelihood of CAD [39, 40]. An MPS-led strategy reduces costs by 30–40% compared with an aggressive interventional strategy, presumably because of reduced use of downstream resources in those with normal scintigraphy [40]. This is particularly true in women, where stratification of patients to ICA based on MPS results leads to significant cost-savings, regardless of pre-test likelihood of disease [41]. In the UK, MPS performed after sECG results in a 20–25% reduction in unnecessary ICA and has equal diagnostic accuracy and cost for the identification of those requiring revascularization compared with direct referral for

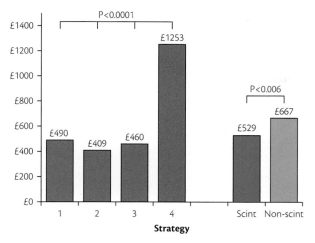

Fig. 19.12 Mean cost of diagnosis of coronary artery disease from the Economics of Myocardial Perfusion Imaging in Europe (EMPIRE) study. Four diagnostic strategies were employed: (1) stress electrocardiography (sECG) followed by invasive coronary angiography (ICA); (2) sECG followed by myocardial perfusion scintigraphy (MPS) followed by ICA; (3) MPS followed by ICA; (4) direct referral to ICA. The most cost-effective strategy involved referral of patients with positive or equivocal sECG to MPS with subsequent ICA only in those with evidence of inducible ischaemia. The mean cost of diagnosis was significantly lower in centres who were regular users of MPS (Scint) compared with those who referred infrequently (Non-scint).
Reprinted from *Journal of the American College of Cardiology*, 43:2, Rory Hachamovitch et al, Stress myocardial perfusion single-photon emission computed tomography is clinically effective and cost effective in risk stratification of patients with a high likelihood of coronary artery disease (CAD) but no known CAD, 200-208, Copyright 2004 with permission from Elsevier.

ICA [42]. For pre-operative assessment of patients with chronic stable angina, MPS allows more cost-effective assignment to ICA and revascularization or to medical therapy compared with other strategies [15].

Positron emission tomography

Although previously used mainly to assess myocardial viability, positron emission tomography (PET) is now more commonly used to assess myocardial perfusion and it is generally considered the non-invasive gold standard for this. Although cyclotron-produced radiotracers, such as ^{13}N-ammonia or ^{15}O-water, are regularly used, recent efforts have focused also on the use of rubidium-82. This tracer is produced by a generator, compares favourably with other PET tracers for measurements of myocardial perfusion and perfusion reserve [43], and is an attractive option for hospitals without easy access to a cyclotron. PET offers higher resolution images and provides quantification of perfusion in absolute terms (ml/g/min). PET may have better sensitivity and specificity than SPECT MPS for the detection of CAD, particularly where there is severe multi-vessel disease and in obese patients [44, 45].

Two meta-analyses with PET demonstrated 90–93% sensitivity and 81–88% specificity for CAD detection, superior to myocardial perfusion SPECT [46, 47]. Myocardial perfusion in absolute units measured by PET further improves diagnostic accuracy, especially in patients with multi-vessel disease, and can be used to monitor the effects of various therapies (⊃ Fig. 19.13) [48]. The method has also significant prognostic value [49, 50]. Despite demonstration of cost-effectiveness in high-throughput centres [51], the clinical utility of PET is still constrained by high upfront cost and low availability compared with SPECT.

Current guidelines

MPS is embedded in both European and US guidelines for the management of stable CAD (⊃ Tables 19.2 and 19.3) [5, 8, 28, 35, 52]. MPS, stress echocardiography, and stress cardiovascular magnetic resonance imaging (CMR) are considered equivalent tests

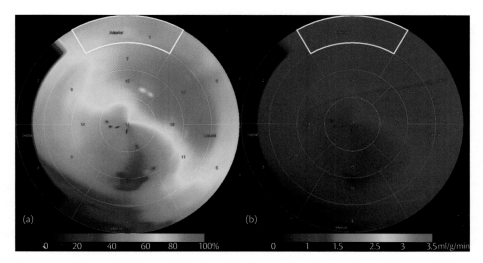

Fig. 19.13 Myocardial perfusion was evaluated with ^{15}O-water PET during adenosine stress in a 67-year-old man with angina. The images show polar maps of myocardial perfusion with normalization to maximum perfusion (a) or using an absolute scale from 0 to 3.5 ml/g/min (b). Relative perfusion appears abnormal within the RCA territory (70% of the maximum) but normal elsewhere (90% of maximum). Absolute perfusion is however abnormal in all three coronary territories (LAD 0.9, LCx 1.0 RCA 0.7 ml/g/min; normal value >2.5 ml/g/min). Coronary angiography showed severe proximal three vessel disease. The relative analysis did not miss the existence of CAD but it underestimated its severity.
Reproduced from *Journal of Nuclear Cardiology*, Vol 13 2006, 24–33, Diagnostic accuracy of rest/stress ECG-gated Rb-82 myocardial perfusion PET: Comparison with ECG-gated Tc-99m sestamibi SPECT, Timothy M. Bateman, with kind permission from Springer Science and Business Media.

Table 19.2 ESC recommendations for the performance of an exercise ECG for the initial diagnostic evaluation of possible stable CAD

Recommendations	Class	Level
Exercise ECG is recommended as the initial test for establishing a diagnosis of SCAD in patients with symptoms of angina and intermediate PTP of CAD (15–65%), free of anti-ischaemic drugs, unless they cannot exercise or display ECG changes which make the ECG non evaluable.	I	B
Stress imaging is recommended as the initial test option if local expertise and availability permit.	I	B
Exercise ECG should be considered in patients on treatment to evaluate control of symptoms and ischaemia.	IIa	C
Exercise ECG in patients with ≥0.1 mV ST-depression on resting ECG or taking digitalis is not recommended for diagnostic purposes.	III	C

SCAD, stable coronary artery disease, PTP, pre-test probability.

Table 19.4 Ranges from the literature for the sensitivity and specificity (%) for the detection of significant CAD defined by invasive coronary angiography

	Sensitivity	Specificity
Exercise ECG	45–50	85–90
Exercise echo	80–85	80–88
Exercise MPS	73–92	63–87
Dobutamine echo	79–83	82–86
Dobutamine MRI	79–88	81–91
Vasodilator echo	72–79	92–95
Vasodilator MPS	90–91	75–84
Vasodilator MRI	67–94	61–85
CTCA	95–99	64–83
Vasodilator PET	81–97	74–91

Adapted from [5]. ECG, electrocardiogram; echo, echocardiography; MPS, myocardial perfusion scintigraphy; MRI, magnetic resonance imaging.

for the assessment of myocardial perfusion, with availability and expertise defining the choice of technique (➲ Table 19.4). Wide availability, ease of administration, and prognostic value of exercise variables means that sECG remains the initial stress test in many centres and retains a class I indication in the US for symptomatic patients with a normal baseline ECG who can exercise [6]. However, functional testing for ischaemia offers superior diagnostic performance, particularly in women with at least intermediate likelihood of disease [5, 28]. MPS receives a class I indication for the evaluation of symptomatic patients with an intermediate pretest likelihood of obstructive coronary artery disease and should be the initial investigation in patients who are unlikely to exercise adequately or where resting ECG abnormalities, such as left bundle branch block, pre-excitation, left ventricular hypertrophy, or drug effects, are likely to render the sECG uninterpretable. For symptomatic female patients, the high false-positive rate of sECG argues even more strongly in favour of MPS as a first-line test, a strategy that receives a class IIa indication in current ESC guidelines [5].

Table 19.3 ESC recommendations for the performance of exercise or pharmacological functional imaging test for the initial diagnostic evaluation of possible stable CAD

Recommendations	Class	Level
An imaging stress test is recommended as the initial test for diagnosing SCAD if the PTP is between 66–85% or if LVEF is <50% in patients without typical angina.	I	B
An imaging stress test is recommended in patients with resting ECG abnormalities which prevent accurate interpretation of ECG changes during stress.	I	B
Exercise stress testing is recommended rather than pharmacologic testing whenever possible.	I	C
An imaging stress test should be considered in symptomatic patients with prior revascularization (PCI or CABG).	IIa	B
An imaging stress test should be considered to assess the functional severity of intermediate lesions on coronary arteriography.	IIa	B

SCAD, stable coronary artery disease, PTP, pre-test probability.

Patients with symptoms and low pre-test-likelihood of obstructive CAD usually require no further investigation, while those with symptoms and high pre-test-likelihood are usually better served by an invasive strategy; MPS is therefore not recommended in these patients (class III). It is similarly not recommended for screening asymptomatic patients (class III). As a secondary test, MPS should be performed when further information on myocardial perfusion or function is required to assist management decisions or to define prognosis (class I). In those with established but stable CAD, MPS is recommended for those in whom symptoms develop (or persist) after revascularization. PET receives a class IIa indication as a first-line test for the diagnosis of CAD but it is favoured as a secondary test in those in whom SPECT is equivocal (class I).

Future directions

Hybrid imaging (PET or SPECT with multi-detector X-ray CT) is conceptually attractive as it offers the possibility of assessing coronary function and anatomy at the same sitting [53]. The techniques are covered in a separate chapter of this textbook.

Acute coronary syndromes

Diagnosis

The acute coronary syndromes (ACS) comprise a spectrum from unstable angina, through non-ST-elevation myocardial infarction, to ST-elevation myocardial infarction (MI). The hallmark of acute coronary syndromes is atherosclerotic plaque rupture and intra-coronary thrombosis. In those with ST-elevation and chest pain, either immediate percutaneous coronary intervention or, if this is unavailable, thrombolysis is warranted. Patients without ST-elevation but with high-risk features may also require PCI. Patients who present with non-specific symptoms and equivocal electrocardiographic changes are a diagnostic challenge with many subsequently found to have non-cardiac chest pain.

Conversely, in some patients the diagnosis of MI may be missed with consequent increase in morbidity and mortality.

MPS has the same sensitivity for detection of acute MI as serial troponin analysis [54]. However, whilst cardiac biomarkers require 6–12 hours to attain sufficient negative predictive value, myocardial injury may be detected on acute resting MPS within 2 hours of chest pain, making it a more sensitive test at the time of presentation [55]. MPS is especially useful in those patients with an intermediate likelihood of CAD and chest pain in the absence of diagnostic ECG changes [35]. Abnormal resting MPS in this setting has a high sensitivity for acute infarction, particularly if it is associated with regional wall motion abnormalities on gated imaging [23]. Furthermore, because the technique provides information on both viability and regional myocardial blood flow at the time of injection, administration of tracer before and after thrombolysis or revascularization helps to define the extent of jeopardized myocardium and myocardial salvage. MPS is also useful after primary PCI to evaluate the functional significance and need for treatment of intermediate non-culprit coronary artery stenoses. Normal resting MPS excludes acute infarction and suggests that either sECG or stress MPS should be the next diagnostic step. If tracer injection occurs during chest pain, normal MPS rules out an acute coronary syndrome and allows the patient to be discharged. It is, therefore, especially useful in the management of patients with symptoms suggestive of ACS but without ECG changes [56].

Prognosis

Patients with acute coronary syndromes are often referred directly for invasive coronary angiography. However, patients with preserved LV function and without high-risk indicators may do at least equally well with a conservative approach. In the stable post-infarction period, intensive medical therapy alone is equally good at suppressing ischaemia compared with coronary revascularization and it is associated with a similar incidence of death and non-fatal MI at 1 year [57]. This suggests that in the absence of medical instability intensive medical therapy should be the primary treatment strategy. Cardiac catheterization can therefore be reserved for those with high-risk features or those who remain symptomatic despite optimal medical treatment.

The role of MPS in the early post-MI period is reflected in both European and American guidelines [23, 58–60]. The technique is helpful in those with atypical presentation and positive troponins because an abnormal scan is associated with a 7-fold increase in the risk of cardiac events at 6 months [61]. In patients without post-infarction angina, complex arrhythmias or congestive heart failure, early MPS using pharmacological stress is the test of choice for prognostic assessment. It is superior to sECG for risk stratification and can be performed safely 2–4 days after acute MI [62]. As well as quantifying myocardial ischaemia, MPS allows measurement of left ventricular ejection fraction (LVEF), an important prognostic predictor of cardiac death after MI [63]. Early MPS allows the prompt discharge of lower-risk patients and appropriate referral of those at higher risk, such as those with LVEF<35% or inducible ischaemia in >50% of the remaining viable myocardium, for invasive coronary angiography [64].

Cost-effectiveness

MPS is cost-effective in the assessment of acute chest pain. Although the initial costs are greater than strategies that involve assessment of the ECG, biomarkers, and potentially echocardiography, the downstream reduction in unnecessary treatment, hospital admission, and invasive coronary angiography leads to an overall reduction in cost. The use of normal resting MPS alone to exclude myocardial infarction in patients with non-diagnostic ECG changes cost-effectively reduces unnecessary admissions irrespective of gender, age, or risk factors for CAD [65]. When compared prospectively with usual care, acute resting MPS has no impact on the clinical decision-making in those with definitive acute cardiac ischaemia but reduces unnecessary admissions by up to 20% in those without [56]. This holds true even in patients with diabetes, a sub-population considered to have CAD-equivalent status [66]. Importantly, discharge of these patients is safe [67, 68]. When resting MPS is performed explicitly during an episode of chest pain, it allows more appropriate stratification to admission or discharge, and it reduces total admissions [69]. When used routinely in conjunction with early exercise testing in the emergency department, median costs are $1,843 (€1,400) lower and length of admission is shorter [70]. Studies of the cost-effectiveness of MPS in the acute setting largely originate from the US and it can be difficult to extrapolate this into other settings. Furthermore, the wider use of acute resting MPS in Europe is limited by local availability and experience. Nonetheless, the available evidence suggests that acute resting MPS offers a safe, rapid, and cost-effective strategy for the exclusion of coronary artery disease as a cause for acute chest pain when the ECG is non-diagnostic.

Guidelines

Resting MPS as an initial test in stabilized patients with acute coronary syndromes is discussed in European guidelines for ACS but it is not explicitly recommended [60]. Previous ESC Task Force guidance on the management of chest pain recommends MPS in patients with acute chest pain and equivocal clinical history, ECG, and cardiac biomarkers, where a low-risk study might prevent admission and unnecessary treatment [71]. Current ESC guidelines for non-ST elevation acute coronary syndromes incorporate outcome risk scoring (such as the GRACE or TIMI scores) and suggest that patients without recurrence of pain, normal ECG findings, negative troponin, and a low risk score should undergo non-invasive ischaemia testing before deciding on an invasive strategy (class I) [60]. Resting MPS is considered appropriate for the same patients in the US guidelines, while stress-rest MPS is considered appropriate for patients with possible ACS, absent ECG changes, and no more than borderline troponin elevations, regardless of TIMI risk score [58].

Both European and US guidelines acknowledge the role of MPS for risk stratification after acute myocardial infarction [58–60, 72]. In those admitted with NSTEMI, MPS is recommended to evaluate the presence, severity, and extent of inducible ischaemia either in patients with equivocal sECG, or who are unable to exercise or in women. The likelihood of future cardiac events is closely linked to the degree of abnormality and this has implications for subsequent management. After STEMI, MPS is recommended for the definition of infarct size and residual ischaemia to guide management and to assess prognosis. Those with high-risk features on MPS are candidates for revascularization, while those at low risk can be managed conservatively. MPS is also the initial test of choice to assess the functional significance of intermediate non-culprit coronary artery stenoses in patients who have already undergone ICA.

Future directions

In the future, diagnosis of patients with acute chest pain may be undertaken through assessment of myocardial metabolism. Under normal conditions, myocytes use fatty acids as the primary source of energy but during ischaemia cellular metabolism switches to glucose. After resolution of ischaemia there is a delay in the return of metabolism to normal (up to 24 hours) with continuation of glucose metabolism in preference to fatty acids. This is known as ischaemic memory; abnormal uptake of fatty acids during this time can be exploited by appropriately labelled radiotracers, the most common of which is iodine-123 beta-methyl-p-iodophenyl-pentadecanoic acid (BMIPP). Several studies have shown encouraging results and this could become an attractive option for assessment of patients whose ischaemic insult may have occurred hours before presentation.

Conclusion

MPS has proven value for the diagnosis and prognosis of both stable CAD and acute coronary syndromes, and is additionally safe and cost-effective in a wide variety of clinical settings. Experience with the technique can be measured over decades and there is a large amount of evidence to support its use. Although less widely available and relatively more expensive, PET may be used to detect obstructive coronary disease and it allows absolute quantification of myocardial perfusion. As with any test, appropriate referral depends upon local availability, pre-test likelihood of CAD, the suitability of the patient for different forms of cardiac stress, and an understanding of the answers that MPS can provide. When used appropriately, MPS continues to be a powerful tool for the investigation of CAD.

References

1. Goodman SN. Toward evidence-based medical statistics. 2: The Bayes factor. *Ann Intern Med* 1999; 130 (12): 1005–13.

2. Diamond GA, Forrester JS. Analysis of probability as an aid in the clinical diagnosis of coronary-artery disease. *N Engl J Med* 1979; 300 (24): 1350–8.

3. Wilson PW, D'Agostino RB, Levy D, Belanger AM, Silbershatz H, Kannel WB. Prediction of coronary heart disease using risk factor categories. *Circulation* 1998; 97 (18): 1837–47.

4. Genders TSS, Steyerberg EW, Alkadhi H, Leschka S, Desbiolles L, Nieman K, et al. A clinical prediction rule for the diagnosis of coronary artery disease: validation, updating, and extension. *Eur Heart J* 2011; 32 (11): 1316–30.

5. Montalescot G, Sechtem U, Achenbach S, et al. 2013 ESC guidelines on the management of stable coronary artery disease. *Eur Heart J* 2013; doi: 10.1093/eurheartj/eht296.

6. Fihn SD, Gardin JM, Abrams J, et al. 2012 ACCF/AHA/ACP/AATS/PCNA/SCAI/STS Guideline for the diagnosis and management of patients with stable ischemic heart disease: a report of the American College of Cardiology Foundation/American Heart Association Task Force on Practice Guidelines, and the American College of Physicians, American Association for Thoracic Surgery, Preventive Cardiovascular Nurses Association, Society for Cardiovascular Angiography and Interventions, and Society of Thoracic Surgeons. *J Am Coll Cardiol* 2012; 60 (24): e44–164.

7. Mark DB, Shaw L, Harrell FE, Jr, et al. Prognostic value of a treadmill exercise score in outpatients with suspected coronary artery disease. *N Engl J Med* 1991; 325 (12): 849–53.

8. Fox K, Garcia MA, Ardissino D, et al. Guidelines on the management of stable angina pectoris: executive summary: The Task Force on the Management of Stable Angina Pectoris of the European Society of Cardiology. *Eur Heart J* 2006; 27 (11): 1341–81.

9. Gershlick AH, de BM, Chambers J, et al. Role of non-invasive imaging in the management of coronary artery disease: an assessment of likely change over the next 10 years. A report from the British Cardiovascular Society Working Group. *Heart* 2007; 93 (4): 423–31.

10. Wong Y, Rodwell A, Dawkins S, Livesey SA, Simpson IA. Sex differences in investigation results and treatment in subjects referred for investigation of chest pain. *Heart* 2001; 85 (2): 149–52.

11. Marwick TH, Shaw L, Case C, Vasey C, Thomas JD. Clinical and economic impact of exercise electrocardiography and exercise echocardiography in clinical practice. *Eur Heart J* 2003; 24 (12): 1153–63.

12. Kapur A, Latus KA, Davies G, et al. A comparison of three radionuclide myocardial perfusion tracers in clinical practice: the ROBUST study. *Eur J Nucl Med Mol Imaging* 2002; 29 (12): 1608–16.

13. Hachamovitch R, Berman DS, Shaw LJ, et al. Incremental prognostic value of myocardial perfusion single photon emission computed tomography for the prediction of cardiac death: differential stratification for risk of cardiac death and myocardial infarction. *Circulation* 1998; 97 (6): 535–43.

14. Mowatt G, Vale L, Brazzelli M, et al. Systematic review of the effectiveness and cost-effectiveness, and economic evaluation, of myocardial perfusion scintigraphy for the diagnosis and management of angina and myocardial infarction. *Health Technol Assess* 2004; 8 (30): iii–207.

15. Underwood SR, Anagnostopoulos C, Cerqueira M, et al. Myocardial perfusion scintigraphy: the evidence. *Eur J Nucl Med Mol Imaging* 2004; 31 (2): 261–91.

16. Schuijf JD, Poldermans D, Shaw LJ, et al. Diagnostic and prognostic value of non-invasive imaging in known or suspected coronary artery disease. *Eur J Nucl Med Mol Imaging* 2006; 33 (1): 93–104.

17. Paetsch I, Jahnke C, Wahl A, et al. Comparison of dobutamine stress magnetic resonance, adenosine stress magnetic resonance, and adenosine stress magnetic resonance perfusion. *Circulation* 2004; 110 (7): 835–42.

18. Smanio PE, Watson DD, Segalla DL, Vinson EL, Smith WH, Beller GA. Value of gating of technetium-99m sestamibi single-photon

emission computed tomographic imaging. *J Am Coll Cardiol* 1997; 30 (7): 1687–92.

19. Garcia EV. SPECT attenuation correction: an essential tool to realize nuclear cardiology's manifest destiny. *J Nucl Cardiol* 2007; 14 (1): 16–24.

20. Boden WE, O'Rourke RA, Teo KK, et al. Optimal medical therapy with or without PCI for stable coronary disease. *N Engl J Med* 2007; 356 (15): 1503–16.

21. Shaw LJ, Berman DS, Maron DJ, et al. Optimal medical therapy with or without percutaneous coronary intervention to reduce ischemic burden: results from the Clinical Outcomes Utilizing Revascularization and Aggressive Drug Evaluation (COURAGE) trial nuclear substudy. *Circulation* 2008; 117 (10): 1283–91.

22. Marcassa C, Bax JJ, Bengel F, et al. Clinical value, cost-effectiveness, and safety of myocardial perfusion scintigraphy: a position statement. *Eur Heart J* 2008; 29 (4): 557–63.

23. Klocke FJ, Baird MG, Lorell BH, et al. ACC/AHA/ASNC guidelines for the clinical use of cardiac radionuclide imaging—executive summary: a report of the American College of Cardiology/American Heart Association Task Force on Practice Guidelines (ACC/AHA/ASNC Committee to Revise the 1995 Guidelines for the Clinical Use of Cardiac Radionuclide Imaging). *Circulation* 2003; 108 (11): 1404–18.

24. Abbott BG, Afshar M, Berger AK, Wackers FJ. Prognostic significance of ischemic electrocardiographic changes during adenosine infusion in patients with normal myocardial perfusion imaging. *J Nucl Cardiol* 2003; 10 (1): 9–16.

25. Hachamovitch R, Hayes S, Friedman JD, et al. Determinants of risk and its temporal variation in patients with normal stress myocardial perfusion scans: what is the warranty period of a normal scan? *J Am Coll Cardiol* 2003; 41 (8): 1329–40.

26. Abidov A, Bax JJ, Hayes SW, et al. Transient ischemic dilation ratio of the left ventricle is a significant predictor of future cardiac events in patients with otherwise normal myocardial perfusion SPECT. *J Am Coll Cardiol* 2003; 42 (10): 1818–25.

27. Gill JB, Ruddy TD, Newell JB, Finkelstein DM, Strauss HW, Boucher CA. Prognostic importance of thallium uptake by the lungs during exercise in coronary artery disease. *N Engl J Med* 1987; 317 (24): 1486–9.

28. Wijns W, Kolh P, Danchin N, et al. Guidelines on myocardial revascularization. *Eur Heart J* 2010; 31 (20): 2501–55.

29. Hachamovitch R, Rozanski A, Shaw LJ, et al. Impact of ischaemia and scar on the therapeutic benefit derived from myocardial revascularization vs. medical therapy among patients undergoing stress-rest myocardial perfusion scintigraphy. *Eur Heart J* 2011; 32 (8): 1012–24.

30. Perrone-Filardi P, Achenbach S, Mohlenkamp S, et al. Cardiac computed tomography and myocardial perfusion scintigraphy for risk stratification in asymptomatic individuals without known cardiovascular disease: a position statement of the Working Group on Nuclear Cardiology and Cardiac CT of the European Society of Cardiology. *Eur Heart J* 2011; 32 (16): 1986–93, 1993a, 1993b.

31. Shaw LJ, Raggi P, Schisterman E, Berman DS, Callister TQ. Prognostic value of cardiac risk factors and coronary artery calcium screening for all-cause mortality. *Radiology* 2003; 228 (3): 826–33.

32. Greenland P, LaBree L, Azen SP, Doherty TM, Detrano RC. Coronary artery calcium score combined with Framingham score for risk prediction in asymptomatic individuals. *JAMA* 2004; 291 (2): 210–5.

33. Anand DV, Lim E, Lahiri A, Bax JJ. The role of non-invasive imaging in the risk stratification of asymptomatic diabetic subjects. *Eur Heart J* 2006; 27 (8): 905–12.

34. Anand DV, Lim E, Hopkins D, et al. Risk stratification in uncomplicated type 2 diabetes: prospective evaluation of the combined use of coronary artery calcium imaging and selective myocardial perfusion scintigraphy. *Eur Heart J* 2006; 27 (6): 713–21.

35. Brindis RG, Douglas PS, Hendel RC, et al. ACCF/ASNC appropriateness criteria for single-photon emission computed tomography myocardial perfusion imaging (SPECT MPI): a report of the American College of Cardiology Foundation Quality Strategic Directions Committee Appropriateness Criteria Working Group and the American Society of Nuclear Cardiology endorsed by the American Heart Association. *J Am Coll Cardiol* 2005; 46(8):1587–605.

36. Hachamovitch R, Hayes SW, Friedman JD, Cohen I, Berman DS. Stress myocardial perfusion single-photon emission computed tomography is clinically effective and cost effective in risk stratification of patients with a high likelihood of coronary artery disease (CAD) but no known CAD. *J Am Coll Cardiol* 2004; 43(2): 200–8.

37. Berman DS, Hachamovitch R, Kiat H, et al. Incremental value of prognostic testing in patients with known or suspected ischemic heart disease: a basis for optimal utilization of exercise technetium-99m sestamibi myocardial perfusion single-photon emission computed tomography. *J Am Coll Cardiol* 1995; 26(3): 639–47.

38. Underwood SR, Godman B, Salyani S, Ogle JR, Ell PJ. Economics of myocardial perfusion imaging in Europe—the EMPIRE Study. *Eur Heart J* 1999; 20(2): 157–66.

39. Hachamovitch R, Berman DS, Kiat H, Cohen I, Friedman JD, Shaw LJ. Value of stress myocardial perfusion single photon emission computed tomography in patients with normal resting electrocardiograms: an evaluation of incremental prognostic value and cost-effectiveness. *Circulation* 2002; 105(7): 823–9.

40. Shaw LJ, Hachamovitch R, Berman DS, et al. The economic consequences of available diagnostic and prognostic strategies for the evaluation of stable angina patients: an observational assessment of the value of precatheterization ischemia. Economics of Noninvasive Diagnosis (END) Multicenter Study Group. *J Am Coll Cardiol* 1999; 33(3): 661–9.

41. Shaw LJ, Heller GV, Travin MI et al. Cost analysis of diagnostic testing for coronary artery disease in women with stable chest pain. Economics of Noninvasive Diagnosis (END) Study Group. *J Nucl Cardiol* 1999; 6(6): 559–69.

42. Sharples L, Hughes V, Crean A, et al. Cost-effectiveness of functional cardiac testing in the diagnosis and management of coronary artery disease: a randomised controlled trial. The CECaT trial. *Health Technol Assess* 2007; 11(49): iii–115.

43. Lortie M, Beanlands RS, Yoshinaga K, Klein R, Dasilva JN, Dekemp RA. Quantification of myocardial blood flow with 82Rb dynamic PET imaging. *Eur J Nucl Med Mol Imaging* 2007; 34(11): 1765–74.

44. Bateman TM, Heller GV, McGhie AI, et al. Diagnostic accuracy of rest/stress ECG-gated Rb-82 myocardial perfusion PET: comparison with ECG-gated Tc-99m sestamibi SPECT. *J Nucl Cardiol* 2006; 13(1): 24–33.

45. Nandalur KR, Dwamena BA, Choudhri AF, Nandalur SR, Reddy P, Carlos RC. Diagnostic performance of positron emission tomography in the detection of coronary artery disease: a meta-analysis. *Acad Radiol* 2008; 15(4): 444–51.

46. Mc Ardle BA, Dowsley TF, Dekemp RA, Wells GA, Beanlands RS. Does rubidium-82 PET have superior accuracy to SPECT perfusion imaging for the diagnosis of obstructive coronary disease?: A systematic review and meta-analysis. *J Am Coll Cardiol* 2012; 60(18): 1828–37.

47. Parker MW, Iskandar A, Limone B, et al. Diagnostic accuracy of cardiac positron emission tomography versus single photon emission computed tomography for coronary artery disease: a bivariate meta-analysis. *Circ Cardiovasc Imaging* 2012; 5(6): 700–7.

48. Saraste A, Kajander S, Han C, Nesterov SV, Knuuti J. PET: Is myocardial flow quantification a clinical reality? *J Nucl Cardiol* 2012; 19(5): 1044–59.

49. Dorbala S, Di Carli MF, Beanlands RS, et al. Prognostic value of stress myocardial perfusion positron emission tomography: results from a multicenter observational registry. *J Am Coll Cardiol* 2013; 61(2): 176–84.

50. Murthy VL, Naya M, Foster CR, et al. Association between coronary vascular dysfunction and cardiac mortality in patients with and without diabetes mellitus. *Circulation* 2012; 126(15): 1858–68.

51. Merhige ME, Breen WJ, Shelton V, Houston T, D'Arcy BJ, Perna AF. Impact of myocardial perfusion imaging with PET and ⁸²Rb on downstream invasive procedure utilization, costs, and outcomes in coronary disease management. *J Nucl Med* 2007; 48(7): 1069–76.

52. Patel MR, Dehmer GJ, Hirshfeld JW, Smith PK, Spertus JA. ACCF/SCAI/STS/AATS/AHA/ASNC/HFSA/SCCT 2012 Appropriate use criteria for coronary revascularization focused update: a report of the American College of Cardiology Foundation Appropriate Use Criteria Task Force, Society for Cardiovascular Angiography and Interventions, Society of Thoracic Surgeons, American Association for Thoracic Surgery, American Heart Association, American Society of Nuclear Cardiology, and the Society of Cardiovascular Computed Tomography. *J Am Coll Cardiol* 2012; 59(9): 857–81.

53. Flotats A, Knuuti J, Gutberlet M, et al. Hybrid cardiac imaging: SPECT/CT and PET/CT. A joint position statement by the European Association of Nuclear Medicine (EANM), the European Society of Cardiac Radiology (ESCR) and the European Council of Nuclear Cardiology (ECNC). *Eur J Nucl Med Mol Imaging* 2011; 38(1): 201–12.

54. Kontos MC, Jesse RL, Anderson FP, Schmidt KL, Ornato JP, Tatum JL. Comparison of myocardial perfusion imaging and cardiac troponin I in patients admitted to the emergency department with chest pain. *Circulation* 1999; 99(16): 2073–8.

55. Duca MD, Giri S, Wu AH, et al. Comparison of acute rest myocardial perfusion imaging and serum markers of myocardial injury in patients with chest pain syndromes. *J Nucl Cardiol* 1999; 6(6): 570–6.

56. Udelson JE, Beshansky JR, Ballin DS, et al. Myocardial perfusion imaging for evaluation and triage of patients with suspected acute cardiac ischemia: a randomized controlled trial. *JAMA* 2002; 288(21): 2693–700.

57. Mahmarian JJ, Dakik HA, Filipchuk NG, et al. An initial strategy of intensive medical therapy is comparable to that of coronary revascularization for suppression of scintigraphic ischemia in high-risk but stable survivors of acute myocardial infarction. *J Am Coll Cardiol* 2006; 48(12): 2458–67.

58. Hendel RC, Berman DS, Di Carli MF, et al. ACCF/ASNC/ACR/AHA/ASE/SCCT/SCMR/SNM 2009 appropriate use criteria for cardiac radionuclide imaging: a report of the American College of Cardiology Foundation Appropriate Use Criteria Task Force, the American Society of Nuclear Cardiology, the American College of Radiology, the American Heart Association, the American Society of Echocardiography, the Society of Cardiovascular Computed Tomography, the Society for Cardiovascular Magnetic Resonance, and the Society of Nuclear Medicine. *Circulation* 2009; 119(22): e561–87.

59. Steg PG, James SK, Atar D, et al. ESC Guidelines for the management of acute myocardial infarction in patients presenting with ST-segment elevation. *Eur Heart J* 2012; 33(20): 2569–619.

60. Hamm CW, Bassand JP, Agewall S, et al. ESC Guidelines for the management of acute coronary syndromes in patients presenting without persistent ST-segment elevation: The Task Force for the management of acute coronary syndromes (ACS) in patients presenting without persistent ST-segment elevation of the European Society of Cardiology (ESC). *Eur Heart J* 2011; 32(23): 2999–3054.

61. Dorbala S, Giugliano RP, Logsetty G, et al. Prognostic value of SPECT myocardial perfusion imaging in patients with elevated cardiac troponin I levels and atypical clinical presentation. *J Nucl Cardiol* 2007; 14(1): 53–8.

62. Brown KA, Heller GV, Landin RS, et al. Early dipyridamole (99m)Tc-sestamibi single photon emission computed tomographic imaging 2 to 4 days after acute myocardial infarction predicts in-hospital and postdischarge cardiac events: comparison with submaximal exercise imaging. *Circulation* 1999; 100(20): 2060–6.

63. Kroll D, Farah W, McKendall GR, Reinert SE, Johnson LL. Prognostic value of stress-gated Tc-99m sestamibi SPECT after acute myocardial infarction. *Am J Cardiol* 2001; 87(4): 381–6.

64. Van de WF, Ardissino D, Betriu A, et al. Management of acute myocardial infarction in patients presenting with ST-segment elevation. The Task Force on the Management of Acute Myocardial Infarction of the European Society of Cardiology. *Eur Heart J* 2003; 24(1): 28–66.

65. Heller GV, Stowers SA, Hendel RC, et al. Clinical value of acute rest technetium-99m tetrofosmin tomographic myocardial perfusion imaging in patients with acute chest pain and nondiagnostic electrocardiograms. *J Am Coll Cardiol* 1998; 31(5): 1011–7.

66. Kapetanopoulos A, Heller GV, Selker HP, et al. Acute resting myocardial perfusion imaging in patients with diabetes mellitus: results from the Emergency Room Assessment of Sestamibi for Evaluation of Chest Pain (ERASE Chest Pain) trial. *J Nucl Cardiol* 2004; 11(5): 570–7.

67. Stewart RE, Dickinson CZ, Weissman IA, O'Neill WW, Dworkin HJ, Juni JE. Clinical outcome of patients evaluated with emergency centre myocardial perfusion SPET for unexplained chest pain. *Nucl Med Commun* 1996; 17(6): 459–62.

68. Weissman IA, Dickinson CZ, Dworkin HJ, O'Neill WW, Juni JE. Cost-effectiveness of myocardial perfusion imaging with SPECT in the emergency department evaluation of patients with unexplained chest pain. *Radiology* 1996; 199(2): 353–7.

69. Knott JC, Baldey AC, Grigg LE, Cameron PA, Lichtenstein M, Better N. Impact of acute chest pain Tc-99m sestamibi myocardial perfusion imaging on clinical management. *J Nucl Cardiol* 2002; 9(3): 257–62.

70. Stowers SA, Eisenstein EL, Th Wackers FJ, et al. An economic analysis of an aggressive diagnostic strategy with single photon emission computed tomography myocardial perfusion imaging and early exercise stress testing in emergency department patients who present with chest pain but nondiagnostic electrocardiograms: results from a randomized trial. *Ann Emerg Med* 2000; 35(1): 17–25.

71. Erhardt L, Herlitz J, Bossaert L, et al. Task force on the management of chest pain. *Eur Heart J* 2002; 23(15): 1153–76.

72. O'Gara PT, Kushner FG, Ascheim DD, et al. 2013 ACCF/AHA guideline for the management of ST-elevation myocardial infarction: a report of the American College of Cardiology Foundation/American Heart Association Task Force on Practice Guidelines. *Circulation* 2013; 127(4): e362–425.

⟳ **For additional multimedia materials please visit the online version of the book (** http://www.esciacc.oxfordmedicine.com**)**

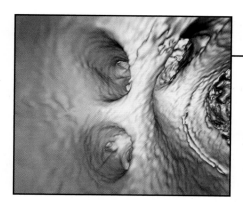

CHAPTER 20

MDCT and detection of coronary artery disease

Stephan Achenbach

Contents

Introduction

There are two possible approaches to imaging for coronary artery disease. One approach is to visualize the consequence of haemodynamically relevant coronary artery lesions, such as that done by stress echocardiography, stress magnetic resonance imaging, or nuclear medicine techniques ('functional imaging'). The alternative approach is to directly visualize the coronary arteries. Direct imaging of the coronary arteries requires a combination of high spatial resolution, high temporal resolution, and the ability to capture the entire complex course of the coronary artery tree. Of the non-invasive imaging techniques, multi-detector row computed tomography (MDCT) offers the best combination of these properties and, along with invasive coronary angiography, has become a clinically accepted diagnostic tool for direct coronary artery imaging. In selected patients, coronary CT angiography can identify and rule out coronary artery stenosis. However, the spatial and temporal resolution of CT imaging, even with the latest scanner generations, is not equal to invasive coronary angiography. Diagnostic accuracy is impaired when image quality is reduced and image quality, in turn, is influenced by a number of factors such as the patient's heart rate, body weight, ability to cooperate, and extent of coronary calcification. Therefore, the clinical utility of coronary CT angiography significantly depends on the patient to be investigated, on the specific clinical situation, and also on the local expertise regarding cardiac computed tomography. Thorough consideration of the advantages and disadvantages of CT angiography is therefore necessary when deliberating the use of CT imaging in the workup of patients with known or suspected coronary artery disease.

Direct visualization of the coronary arteries has the advantage that information about atherosclerotic plaque burden may be useful for risk stratification. In non-enhanced scans, coronary calcification is readily detectable and in contrast-enhanced coronary CT angiography datasets of high quality, coronary atherosclerotic plaques, including their calcified and non-calcified components, can be visualized. Both approaches have been shown to carry significant prognostic relevance.

This chapter will outline the strategies, limitations, and potential clinical applications, of CT imaging for coronary artery visualization, detection of coronary artery stenoses, and risk stratification.

Coronary CT angiography—stenosis detection

Imaging protocols

Multi-detector row computed tomography (MDCT) allows direct visualization of the coronary artery lumen. The method is referred to as 'coronary CT angiography'. To

Table 20.1 Prerequisites for the clinical use of coronary CT angiography

Institutional Characteristics
- Adequate hardware (usually at least 64-slice CT)
- Adequate expertise in image acquisition
- Adequate expertise in image interpretation
Patient Characteristics
- Ability to follow breath-hold commands and perform a breath-hold of approximately 10 s
- Regular heart rate (sinus rhythm) with a frequency, preferably < 65 beats/min, optimally < 60 beats/min
- Lack of pronounced obesity
- Ability to establish a sufficiently large peripheral venous access (cubital vein preferred)
- Absence of contraindications to radiation exposure and iodinated contrast media

achieve sufficient spatial and temporal resolution, high-end CT equipment and adequate imaging protocols must be used. Currently, 64-slice CT is considered the 'state of the art' for coronary artery imaging [1]. Newer technology, such as dual source CT and scanners with 256 or 320 detectors, provide further improved and more robust image quality.

There are some prerequisites that patients must fulfil to be suitable for coronary CT angiography (see ➲ Table 20.1). These include the ability to understand and follow breath-hold commands, since even slight respiratory motion during data acquisition will cause substantial artefacts. Of further importance is a regular and, preferably, low heart rate (optimally below 60 beats/min, even though this is not as strictly required for dual source CT) [2, 3]. Patients usually receive pre-medication with short-acting beta blockers to lower heart rate and nitrates are given to achieve coronary dilatation, which noticeably improves image quality. Iodine-based contrast agent is injected intravenously to achieve vascular enhancement during the scan. Typically, 40 to 100 ml of contrast agent is used. Data acquisition can follow various principles [1]. Retrospectively ECG-gated scans are acquired in 'spiral' mode (also called 'helical' mode) and usually provide for higher image quality, more flexibility to choose the cardiac phase during which images are reconstructed, as well as the ability to reconstruct 'functional' datasets throughout the cardiac cycle in order to assess wall motion.

Prospectively ECG-triggered axial scans are associated with substantially lower radiation exposure and, especially in patients with stable and low heart rates, are in many cases adequate to assess the coronary artery lumen. Less flexibility to reconstruct data at different time instants in the cardiac cycle, as well as greater susceptibility to artefacts caused by arrhythmia, sometimes impair image quality. However, in most adequately prepared patients, prospectively ECG-triggered axial acquisition can be used, so that it is the preferred image acquisition mode in many experienced centres.

Typical datasets for coronary artery visualization by CT consist of approximately 200 to 300 transaxial slices with a thickness of 0.5 mm to 0.75 mm (see Fig. 20.1). Data interpretation is based on interactive manipulation of these datasets using post-processing workstations. Useful post-processing tools include maximum intensity projections and multi-planar reconstructions. Three-dimensional renderings allow quite impressive visualization of the heart and coronary arteries, but they are not accurate for stenosis detection and play no role in data interpretation [4]. It is of importance that the reading physician must interactively manipulate the dataset, and integrate all information obtained by using the various post-processing techniques. Mere assessment of images pre-rendered by a technician or automated software is not adequate [5].

Accuracy

Under certain prerequisites, coronary CT angiography has high accuracy for the detection of coronary artery stenoses (see ➲ Figs 20.2–20.4). In addition to numerous small, single-centre studies, three multi-centre trials have assessed the accuracy of coronary CT angiography for the identification of coronary artery stenosis in comparison to invasive coronary angiography. Two trials performed in patients with suspected coronary artery disease, using 64-slice CT, have demonstrated sensitivities of 95–99% and specificities of 64–83%, as well as negative predictive values of 97–99% for the identification of individuals with at least one coronary artery stenosis [6, 7]. The positive predictive values were lower (64% and 86% in the trials cited), which is due to a tendency to overestimate stenosis degree in coronary CTA, as well as the fact that image artefacts often result in false-positive interpretations. As in any diagnostic test, there is a trade-off between sensitivity and specificity in coronary CT angiography: Most studies—and most clinical users—will aim to keep sensitivity high, at the cost of specificity. If, on the other hand, a high specificity is desired, sensitivity will suffer. In a multicentre study of 291 patients with 56% prevalence of coronary artery stenoses, as well as 20% of patients with previous myocardial infarction and 10% with prior revascularization, specificity was high (90%) and the positive predictive value was 91% [8]. However, this came at the cost of decreased sensitivity (85%) and negative predictive value (83%; see ➲ Table 20.2).

A large meta-analysis of 28 trials that compared coronary CT angiography to invasive coronary angiography for stenosis detection in a total of 3,764 patients yielded a patient-based sensitivity of 98% and specificity of 82% to identify individuals with at least one significant coronary artery stenosis. The negative predictive value was 99% and the positive predictive value was 75%. On an individual artery-based level, sensitivity was 91%, specificity 95%, negative predictive value 99%, and positive predictive value 69% [9] (see ➲ Table 20.3).

Accuracy values are not uniform across all patients. Several trials have demonstrated that high heart rates, obesity, and extensive calcification negatively influence accuracy [10–15]. Usually, degraded image will lead to false-positive rather than false-negative

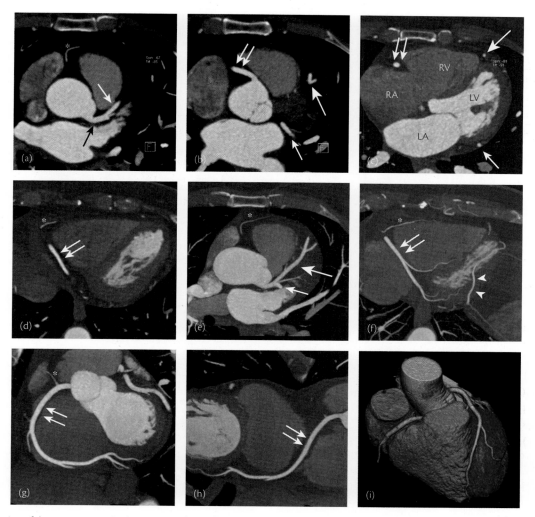

Fig. 20.1 Visualization of the coronary arteries in contrast-enhanced coronary CT angiography (dual-source CT). Spiral data acquisition with ECG-correlated tube current modulation and 100 kV tube current was used to reduce radiation exposure (here: 4.7 mSv). (a) Transaxial slice at the level of the left main coronary artery. The left main divides into the left anterior descending coronary artery (large arrow) and left circumflex coronary artery (small arrow). In addition, a very small intermediate branch is present. The asterisk (*) indicates a conus branch of the right coronary artery. (b) Transaxial slice at the level of the ostium of the right coronary artery (double arrows). In addition, cross-sections of the left anterior descending coronary artery (at a bifurcation with a diagonal branch, large arrow) and of the left circumflex coronary artery (small arrow) can be seen. (c) Transaxial slice at a mid-ventricular level. Cross-sections of the left anterior descending coronary artery (large arrow), obtuse marginal branch (small arrow, this branch is larger than the distal left circumflex) and right coronary artery (double arrows) can be seen. RA, right atrium; RV, right ventricle; LA, left atrium; LV, left ventricle. (d) Transaxial slice at the level of the distal right coronary artery (double arrows). The asterisk (*) indicates a small right ventricular branch. (e) Maximum intensity projection in transaxial orientation, showing the left main and the proximal to mid left anterior descending coronary artery. This image represents a 10-mm thick slice and therefore visualized longer segments of the coronary arteries. (Large arrow: left anterior descending coronary artery; small arrow: left circumflex coronary artery; asterisk: conus branch). (f) Maximum intensity projection in transaxial orientation, showing the distal right coronary artery (double arrows). The division of the right coronary artery into the posterior descending coronary artery and right posterolateral branch is visible. The asterisk (*) indicates a right ventricular branch. The arrowheads point at a vessel that is situated below the diaphragm. Because of the projectional nature of 'maximum intensity projections', the exact position cannot be discerned in this image. (g) Oblique maximum intensity projection, which shows almost the entire course of the right coronary artery (double arrows) in a single image. The asterisk (*) indicates the conus branch. (h) Curved multi-planar reconstruction of the right coronary artery (double arrows). These reconstructions allow visualization of the entire vessel course in a single image. (i) 3D rendering of the heart and coronary arteries. While visually appealing, 3D reconstructions are not helpful for the identification of stenoses.

findings [10] and specificity and positive predictive value will therefore be affected worst (see ⊃ Fig. 20.5).

Along with patient factors that influence image quality, the accuracy of coronary CT angiography depends on pre-test likelihood of disease [16]. In an analysis of 254 patients referred to invasive angiography and also studied by CT, it was demonstrated that coronary CT angiography performs best in patients with a low to intermediate clinical likelihood of coronary artery stenoses (negative predictive value: 100% in both groups), while accuracy is substantially lower in high-risk patients (see ⊃ Table 20.4) [16].

Overall, the good diagnostic performance of coronary CT angiography in patients who are not at high likelihood of having coronary artery stenoses, and especially the very high negative predictive value found for such patients, indicates that coronary

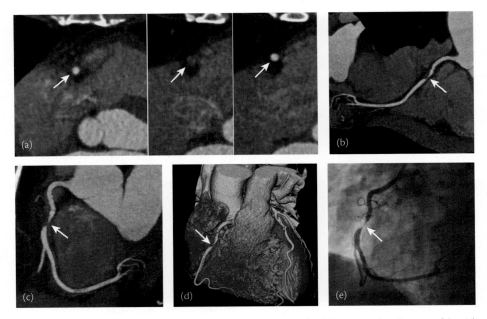

Fig. 20.2 Detection of a coronary artery stenosis in contrast-enhanced coronary CT angiography. (a) Cross-sectional images of the right coronary artery at three consecutive levels are shown (arrows). While the topmost image (left) shows a contrast-enhanced lumen, the next slice (middle) shows the vessel cross-section, but it is not enhanced by contrast. A few mm further distal (right), the lumen is again contrast-enhanced. (b) Maximum intensity projection in an oblique plane that shows a long segment of the right coronary artery. The stenosis is clearly visible (arrow). (c) Curved multi-planar reconstruction, which displays the right coronary artery along its centreline. Again, the short, concentric stenosis is clearly visible (arrow). (d) 3D reconstruction, also showing the stenosis of the right coronary artery (arrow). (e) Corresponding invasive coronary angiogram (arrow, stenosis).

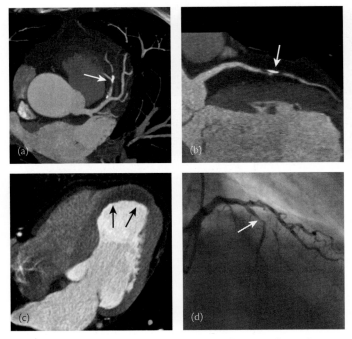

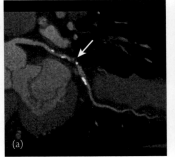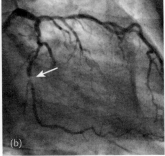

Fig. 20.3 Detection of a subtotal stenosis of the left anterior descending coronary artery. The vessel lumen is relatively small and there is some calcification. (a) Maximum intensity projection in a transaxial plane. The interruption of the contrast-enhanced lumen of the left anterior descending coronary artery is clearly seen (arrow). There is some calcium in the lesion. (b) Curved multi-planar reconstruction. The vessel is relatively small. The arrow points at the high grade stenosis. (c) A cross-section of the left ventricle shows thinning of the apical wall and a mural thrombus (arrows). Such morphologic information—along with detailed information on left ventricular function— can easily be obtained from coronary CT angiography datasets. (d) Invasive angiogram, which shows the subtotal lesion of the mid left anterior descending coronary artery (arrow), with very poor flow into the distal vessel segments.

Fig. 20.4 Visualization of the left circumflex coronary artery in a patient with diffuse, severe disease. Datasets of patients with severe atherosclerosis can be substantially more difficult to interpret as compared to patients who have less burden of disease. (a) Curved multi-planar reconstruction of the left main and left circumflex coronary artery, which shows multiple calcified plaques and several high grade luminal stenoses. (b) Corresponding invasive coronary angiogram.

CTA is a clinically useful tool in symptomatic patients who have a lower or intermediate likelihood of coronary artery disease, but require further workup to rule out significant coronary artery stenoses. A negative coronary CT angiography scan, if of high quality, will obviate the need for further testing. Indeed, several observational trials clearly demonstrated that symptomatic patients, when coronary CT angiography was negative, have an extremely favourable clinical outcome, even without further additional testing [17–21]. In one of these studies, 421 consecutive patients with chest pain and a positive SPECT myocardial perfusion scan indicating an intermediate degree of ischaemia were subjected to 64-slice coronary CT angiography. In 343 patients, CT permitted the need for invasive coronary angiography to be

Table 20.2 Multi-centre studies that investigated the accuracy of coronary artery stenosis detection by contrast-enhanced 64-slice coronary CT angiography in comparison to invasive coronary angiography

Author	Number of Sites	Number of patients	Prevalence of obstructive CAD*	Sensitivity	Specificity	Negative Predictive Value	Positive Predictive Value
Budoff [7]	16	230	25%	95 (85–99%)	83% (76–88%)	99% (96–100%)	64% (53–75%)
Meijboom [6]	3	360	68%	99% (98–100%)	64% (55–73%)	97% (94–100%)	86% (82–90%)
Miller [8]	9	291	56%	85% (79–90%)	90% (83–94%)	83% (75–89%)	91% (86–95%)

* Presence of at least one stenosis ≥50% diameter reduction.

Table 20.3 Results of a meta-analysis that investigated the accuracy of coronary artery stenosis detection by computed tomography angiography in comparison to invasive coronary angiography (modified from [9])

	Number of Trials	Sensitivity (95% CI)	Specificity (95% CI)	Negative Predictive Value (Range)	Positive Predictive Value (Range)
Per Patient Analysis	18	98.2% (97.4–98.8%)	81.6% (79.0%-84-0%)	99.0% (88–100%)	90.5% (75–100%)
Per Artery Analysis	17	94.9% (93.9–95.8%)	89.5% (88.8–90.2%)	99.0% (93–100%)	75.0% (53–95%)
Per Segment Analysis	17	91.3% (90.2–92.2%)	94% (93.7–94.2%)	99.0% (98–100%)	69.0% (44–86%)

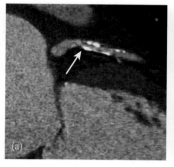 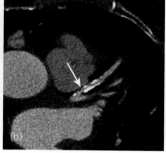 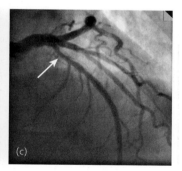

Fig. 20.5 Severe calcifications can impair evaluability of coronary CT angiography datasets. Substantially more frequently than causing false-negative findings, they tend to cause false-positive CT angiography results, such as in the case shown here. (a) Longitudinal multi-planar reconstruction showing the proximal left anterior descending coronary artery. A high grade stenosis seems to be present (arrow). Substantial calcifications can be seen. (b) The same lesion seen in an axial view. Again, a high grade luminal stenosis seems to be present (arrow). (c) Invasive angiography of the left anterior descending coronary artery shows severe atherosclerosis, but no high-grade stenosis. The arrow points at the site of the calcified lesion in CT.

Table 20.4 Diagnostic performance of 64-slice CT depending on the clinical pre-test likelihood of coronary artery disease in 254 patients (modified from [16])

Pre-test probability*	n	Sensitivity	Specificity	Pos. Pred. Value	Neg. Pred. Value
High	105	98%	74%	93%	89%
Intermediate	83	100%	84%	80%	100%
Low	66	100%	93%	75%	100%

* Estimated with the Duke clinical risk score.

ruled out and medical treatment was recommended. Over the course of the following 15 months, no infarct occurred, only 6 clinically driven coronary angiograms were performed, and only 1 revascularization occurred [17].

Similarly, Min et al. identified 1,647 individuals in whom coronary CT angiography was performed without previously known coronary artery disease [22]. The authors could show that the rate of downstream catheterization was substantially lower if CT was performed than in patients in whom stress myocardial perfusion imaging had been performed (1.7% vs. 9.6%), the rate of revascularization was 0.2% vs. 0.8%, but outcomes were not worse for CT angiography as the initial test, with a lower rate of hospitalization for CAD (0.7% vs. 1.1%) and a lower rate of angina (4.3% vs. 6.4%). Thus, sufficient data is available that indicates that it is indeed safe to forego further testing in chest pain patients if coronary CT angiography demonstrates the absence of coronary artery stenoses.

Acute chest pain

A clinical situation in which the use of a non-invasive imaging technology for rapidly and reliably ruling out coronary stenoses can be of tremendous clinical value is the setting of acute chest pain. This is especially the case if the ECG is normal and

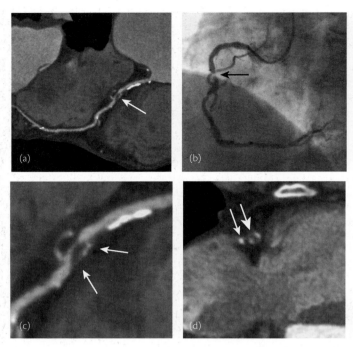

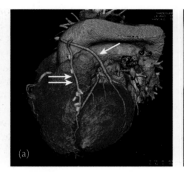

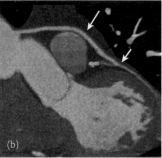

Fig. 20.7 CT visualization of bypass grafts. (a) 3D reconstruction in a patient with an internal mammary artery graft to the left anterior descending coronary artery (double arrows) and a vein graft from the aorta to a diagonal branch (large arrow). (b) Curved multi-planar reconstruction of the bypass graft to the diagonal branch, which shows the body of the bypass graft (large arrow), the coronary anastomosis (small arrow), and the distal lumen of the diagonal branch.

Fig. 20.6 Coronary CT angiography in a patient with acute chest pain. (a) Curved multi-planar reconstruction of the right coronary artery. Besides some calcification, a luminal stenosis of the proximal right coronary artery is visible (arrow). (b) Corresponding invasive coronary angiography (arrow, stenosis). (c) In CT angiography, the lesion of the right coronary artery shows some characteristics that are often observed in acute coronary syndromes. A typical finding is positive remodelling as seen in this enlarged view (arrows). (d) Another typical finding—but not observed in all cases—is ring-like enhancement (around a central thrombus, large arrow). The small arrow points at the cross-section of a side branch.

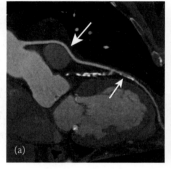

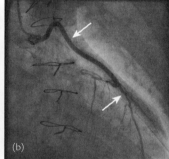

Fig. 20.8 Native coronary arteries in patients after bypass surgery are often severely calcified which makes their evaluation by CT angiography difficult. (a) Curved multi-planar reconstruction of a bypass graft to the left anterior descending coronary artery (large arrow). The bypass lumen is clearly visualized. However, there is substantial calcification of the distal left anterior descending coronary artery. Along with the small vessel lumen, this can cause problems with interpretation (small arrow). (b) Invasive coronary angiogram of the same patient, showing the bypass graft to the left anterior descending coronary artery and the distal vessel. No stenosis is present.

myocardial enzymes are not elevated, the likelihood of coronary artery disease is low, but the possibility of myocardial infarction requires a rapid and definite diagnosis. In this situation, the current ESC guidelines for the management of patients with acute coronary syndromes presenting without ST-segment elevation (non-ST-elevation ACS) state that the use of coronary CT angiography should be considered (class IIa indication for coronary CT angiography) [23]. This recommendation is based on numerous trials that have demonstrated that CT angiography is accurate and safe to stratify patients with acute chest pain and absence of ECG changes, as well as myocardial enzyme elevation [24] (see ⊃ Fig. 20.6), and that outcome is excellent if CT demonstrates the absence of coronary artery stenosis in acute chest pain patients [25–30]. A cost advantage of incorporating CT angiography in the workup of low-likelihood acute chest pain patients, as compared to the standard of care, has been demonstrated [27]. As for other applications, the coronary CT angiography should be considered in acute chest pain patients if patient characteristics promise full evaluability and high image quality.

Imaging of patients with bypass grafts and stents

Coronary CT angiography has substantial limitations in patients with previous coronary revascularization. In patients after

coronary artery bypass surgery, accuracy for the detection of bypass graft stenosis and occlusion is extremely high (see ⊃ Fig. 20.7) [31–36]. However, assessing the native coronary arteries can be extremely difficult because of their often small diameter and severe calcification (see ⊃ Fig. 20.8). Consequently, accuracy for detecting and ruling out stenoses in non-grafted and run-off vessels is substantially lower [32, 34]. A study performed by 64-slice CT found a sensitivity and specificity of only 86% and 76% for the detection of stenoses in the native coronary arteries of patients with bypass surgery [34]. A study performed by 320-slice CT demonstrated a sensitivity of 96% and specificity of 92% for bypass graft stenosis and occlusion, but an accuracy of only 89% in recipient vessels and 80% in non-grafted arteries [37].

Similarly, assessment of coronary artery stents is often unreliable. The dense metal of the stents can cause artefacts that impair evaluability. The ability to assess stents concerning in-stent restenosis depends on many factors that include the overall quality

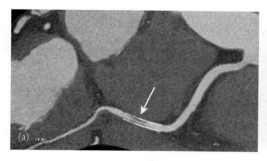

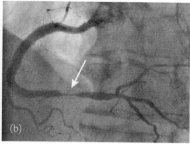

Fig. 20.9 Imaging of coronary artery stents by CT angiography. (a) Visualization of a stent implanted in the right coronary artery. No artefacts are present and the in-stent lumen can be assessed very clearly (arrow). A diffuse, high-grade in-stent stenosis is present. (b) Corresponding invasive coronary angiogram (arrow, in stent stenosis).

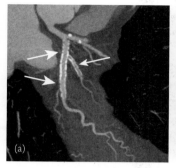

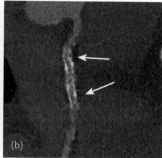

Fig. 20.10 Difficulties in stent assessment by coronary CT angiography. (a) The ability to visualize the stent lumen depends on stent diameter. While the lumen of a large stent (3.5 mm diameter) in the left circumflex coronary artery can be assessed (large arrows), the lumen of a smaller stent (2.5 mm diameter) in a side branch cannot be evaluated in CT angiography (small arrow). (b) Motion artefacts make the in-stent lumen even of larger stents impossible to interpret.

of the dataset, but very specifically also stent type and diameter [38–43] (see ⊃ Figs 20.9 and 20.10). Some recently published studies suggest that the analysis of large stents (for example, stents implanted in the left main coronary artery [39]) may be possible by CT. In some studies, sensitivities of up to 96% for the detection of in-stent restenosis have been reported, while sensitivity was only 33% in others [41–47]. In addition to the wide spread of reported results, the overall number of included stents was small in most trials and patients were typically heavily selected so that the results of single studies cannot be generalized. As an important clinical limitation, positive predictive values were low (46–94%). A meta-analysis reported that 20% of stents were unevaluable by CT, and sensitivity for stenosis detection was only 82% in evaluable stents [48]. With the exception of large stents (3.0 mm diameter or more) in locations very amenable to CT imaging (e.g. left main coronary artery), and if invasive coronary angiography is to be avoided, imaging of patients with previously implanted stents by coronary CT angiography should therefore not be routinely considered.

Coronary CTA and ischaemia

Coronary CTA, like invasive angiography, is a purely morphologic (anatomic) imaging modality and cannot demonstrate the functional relevance of stenoses (ischaemia). The correlation of CT results with the presence of ischaemia is low [49, 50]. Especially in the case of lesions with a borderline degree of stenosis, this may be a limitation. Not surprisingly, coronary CTA is a better

predictor of angiographic findings than testing for ischaemia [49, 51]. For example, an analysis of 114 patients with intermediate likelihood of coronary disease demonstrated that only 19 of 33 patients in whom stenoses were demonstrated by coronary CTA had ischaemia on SPECT myocardial perfusion imaging. On the other hand, 28 of the 33 patients had obstructive coronary artery lesions on invasive coronary angiography. However, all 25 patients who received invasive angiography, even though coronary CTA had ruled out the presence of obstructive stenosis, had, in fact, a 'negative' coronary angiogram [49]. Similarly, a comparison of SPECT and CT in 38 patients revealed that ruling out coronary artery stenoses by CTA had a negative predictive value of 94%, but detecting stenoses by CT had only a positive predictive value of 32% to predict ischaemia on myocardial perfusion imaging [51].

These results underscore that a 'negative' coronary CTA result is a reliable predictor to rule out the presence of coronary artery stenoses and the need for revascularization, and that it may therefore be used as a 'gatekeeper' to avoid invasive angiography. On the other hand, coronary CTA—like invasive angiography—should not be performed in an unselected patient population and not for 'screening' purposes. A positive CT scan taken by itself does not strongly predict the need for revascularization [52].

Several methods are under evaluation to improve the ability of coronary CT angiography to predict ischaemia. They include the combination with CT-based myocardial perfusion [53, 54] assessment and specific analysis methods, such as CT-based FFR [55], but they have not been sufficiently evaluated to play a significant role in clinical practice.

Imaging of coronary atherosclerotic plaque

Coronary calcification

Using cardiac CT, calcium deposits in the coronary arteries can be detected and quantified in low-radiation, non-enhanced image acquisition protocols (see ⊃ Fig. 20.11). Tissue within the vessel wall with a CT number of 130 HU or more is defined as 'calcified'. The so-called 'Agatston score', which takes into account the area and the CT density of calcified lesions, is most frequently used to quantify the amount of coronary calcium on CT. Other methods to quantify the amount of coronary calcium include the calcified volume and mass. In the general population, the coronary calcium score increases with age and, on average, is higher in

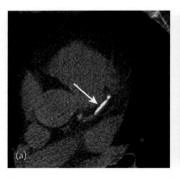
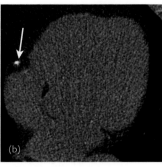

Fig. 20.11 Detection of coronary calcification by CT. (a) CT scans to detect coronary calcification are performed without contrast enhancement and with lower spatial resolution as compared to coronary CT angiography. Here, a calcification of the proximal left anterior descending coronary artery is visible (arrow). (b) Calcification of the right coronary artery (same patient as in Fig. 20.11a).

Table 20.5 Risk of coronary events (adjusted for risk factors) that was associated with an increasing 'Agatston score' in a population sample of 6,722 individuals without coronary artery disease at study entry, followed for a mean period of 3.8 years (modified from [63])

'Agatston Score'	Hazard Ratio (Major Coronary Events)	Number of Individuals	
		With Events	Total
0	1	8	3,409
1–100	3.89	25	1,728
101–300	7.08	24	752
≥301	6.84	32	833

men compared to women [56]. For the 'Agatston score', age- and gender-specific percentiles exist for various populations [56–58].

Coronary artery calcifications—with the possible exception of patients with renal failure [59] are always due to coronary atherosclerotic plaque. The amount of calcium roughly correlates to the overall plaque volume [60]. On the other hand, not every atherosclerotic coronary plaque is calcified and calcification is neither a sign of stability nor of instability of an individual plaque [61].

The correlation between calcium and stenosis is poor. While calcium is due to plaque, atherosclerotic lesions can be present even in the absence of calcium. Especially younger patients with more recent onset of symptoms may have significant coronary artery stenoses in complete absence of calcification [62]. The lack of calcium, therefore, in clinical practice does not reliably eliminate the possibility of coronary artery stenoses. On the other hand, it is also very important to note that even substantial amounts of coronary calcium are not necessarily associated with the presence of haemodynamically relevant luminal narrowing. Even very high calcium scores can be found in the absence of coronary stenoses. Therefore, the detection of coronary calcium, even in large amounts, should not prompt invasive coronary angiography in otherwise asymptomatic individuals.

Since the presence and amount of coronary artery calcium is tied to the presence and amount of coronary atherosclerotic plaque, and coronary artery disease events are typically caused by plaque rupture and erosion, coronary calcium is associated with individual coronary artery disease risk. In asymptomatic individuals, the absence of coronary calcium is associated with very low (<1% per year) risk of major cardiovascular events over the next 3 to 5 years, whereas an up to 11-fold relative risk increase of major cardiac events has been reported in asymptomatic subjects with extensive coronary artery calcification (63–67). Two of the most prominent prospective large-scale trials that have convincingly demonstrated that coronary calcium measurement by CT has incremental prognostic information beyond assessment of traditional risk factors are the Heinz Nixdorff Recall Study [67] and the MESA trial (see ⊃ Table 20.5) [57, 63]. Both have demonstrated that the presence of a certain amount of coronary artery calcium will reclassify individuals who seem to be at low or intermediate risk based on traditional risk factors to a high-risk category, and that this may mandate more intense risk factor modification. Furthermore, several studies have shown that coronary artery calcium allows better risk stratification than other novel markers of risk, such as C-reactive protein [68] or carotid intima-media-thickness [69].

Coronary artery calcium is progressive over time [70]. The amount of progression correlates to non-coronary atherosclerosis [71], is related to cardiovascular risk factors [72], and shows a genetic association [73]. One study has observed a higher coronary artery disease event rate in individuals who displayed more rapid progression of coronary artery calcium [74]. Trials that have evaluated the influence of lipid-lowering therapy on the progression of coronary artery calcium reported conflicting results [75–81]. In addition, inter-scan variability is high, especially for low scores, so that no sufficiently strong data would support the clinical use of repeated coronary calcium scans.

In summary, the predictive value of coronary artery calcium concerning the occurrence of future cardiovascular disease events in asymptomatic individuals is widely accepted [82–85]. A potential clinical role of coronary calcium for further risk stratification is assumed for patients who have an intermediate risk as assessed by traditional risk factors. In patients at high or very low risk, coronary calcium imaging will not be clinically reasonable, since the result is unlikely to influence treatment decisions ('… the current literature on coronary artery calcium does not provide support for the concept that high-risk asymptomatic individuals can safely be excluded from medical therapy for coronary heart disease even if coronary artery calcium score is 0' [83]). Unselected 'screening' or patient self-referral is uniformly not recommended [83, 1].

Plaque in coronary CT angiography

In datasets that are of high quality and free of artefact, coronary CT angiography allows visualization of non-stenotic coronary atherosclerotic plaque (see ⊃ Fig. 20.12 and 20.13). Given the fact that the vast majority of cardiac events are caused by plaque rupture, the detection and characterization not only of calcified, but also of non-calcified, plaque components is a promising tool for improved risk stratification. In comparison to intravascular ultrasound (IVUS), accuracy for detecting non-calcified plaque has been found to be approximately 80–90% [86–89], but these studies were performed in selected patients. With some limitations,

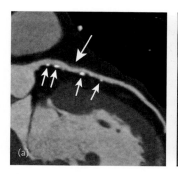
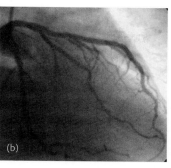

Fig. 20.12 Detection of non-stenotic plaque by contrast-enhanced CT angiography. (a) In this curved multi-planar reconstruction of the left main and left anterior descending coronary artery, several small coronary calcifications can be detected (small arrows) and, in addition, a larger non-calcified plaque is present. These atherosclerotic lesions do not cause a significant coronary artery stenosis. (b) Corresponding invasive coronary angiogram.

Table 20.6 Results of a follow-up study in 1059 patients over 27 months. The rate of acute coronary syndromes (ACS) during follow-up was substantially higher in patients with plaques that demonstrated positive remodelling and low CT attenuation (<30 HU) as compared to patients with plaque of other type or without plaque.

Finding at Baseline	Total Number of Patients	ACS during follow-up	No ACS during follow-up
Plaques with positive remodelling **and** CT attenuation <30 HU	45	10 (22%)	35 (78%)
Plaques with positive remodelling **or** CT attenuation <30 HU	27	1 (4%)	26 (96%)
Plaques with **neither** positive remodelling **nor** CT attenuation <30 HU	822	4 (0.5%)	816 (99%)
No plaque	167	0 (0%)	167 (100%)

Modified according to [100].

and again under the prerequisite of excellent image quality, plaque quantification and characterization is possible. On average, the CT attenuation within 'fibrous' plaques is higher than within 'lipid-rich' plaques (mean attenuation values of 91–116 HU versus 47–71 HU) [90–94]. However, the variability of density measurements within plaque types is large [93], and density measurements within plaque are heavily influenced by the contrast attenuation in the adjacent lumen [95]. Therefore, accurate classification of plaque composition by coronary CTA is currently not possible. On the other hand, some parameters that are more readily available from CT might contribute to the detection of 'vulnerable' plaques. They include the pattern of calcification, and the degree of arterial remodelling (see ⊃ Fig. 20.13) [96–99].

It has been shown that the characteristics that can be determined by CT in coronary atherosclerotic plaques, such as positive remodelling and low CT attenuation of the atherosclerotic material (below 30 HU), are associated with the occurrence of future acute coronary syndromes [100] (see ⊃ Table 20.6). However, the presence and extent of coronary atherosclerotic plaque seems to be a more robust marker of risk than individual plaque characteristics. Several studies, and data based on large registries, have been able to demonstrate a prognostic value of

atherosclerotic lesions detected by coronary CT angiography both in symptomatic and asymptomatic individuals. Min et al. demonstrated increased overall mortality in patients with atherosclerotic lesions in more than five coronary artery segments [101]. Ostrom et al. demonstrated increased mortality during long-term follow-up in patients with non-obstructive lesions in all three coronary arteries, or in patients who had obstructive lesions [102]. An analysis of a clinical registry including more than 23,000 patients confirmed the prognostic value of coronary CT angiography, where the presence of coronary stenoses, but also the presence of non-obstructive plaque, was associated with an increased risk of mortality [103]. However, the hazard ratio for non-obstructive plaque was relatively low (HR 1.6; 95% CI 1.2–2.2). Also, another analysis of the same registry was unable to demonstrate, for this mostly symptomatic patient group, an incremental prognostic value of contrast-enhanced coronary CT angiography over coronary artery calcium measurements [A33]. Therefore, coronary CT angiography for the

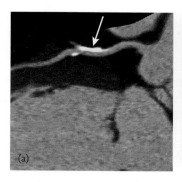
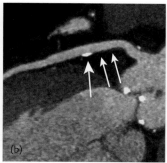
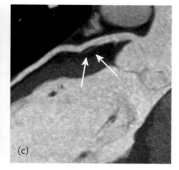

Fig. 20.13 Visualization of different plaque types by coronary CT angiography. (a) Completely calcified plaque of the proximal left anterior descending coronary artery (arrow). (b) Partly calcified plaque of the proximal left anterior descending coronary artery (large arrow: calcified plaque component; small arrows: non-calcified plaque component). (c) Completely non-calcified plaque of the proximal left anterior descending coronary artery (arrows). Pronounced positive remodelling is present.

identification of coronary atherosclerotic plaque is currently not recommended for risk assessment in asymptomatic individuals [1].

Coronary CT angiography and coronary calcium: guidelines and recommendations

Obviously, the possibility of performing non-invasive coronary angiography with CT is immensely attractive. While it can be very useful to rule out coronary artery stenosis and avoid further workup, including invasive coronary angiography in some patients, there is the potential of over-utilization and possibly using this imaging method in patient groups who ultimately will not benefit from the test. The availability of coronary CT angiography may create a 'new layer' of testing, which could be added to the currently available tools, without replacing other testing procedures or, in the worst case, even leading to additional, unnecessary downstream testing. Also, the accuracy and clinical utility of coronary CT angiography do depend on the expertise of the investigator. Due to the fact that coronary CT angiography stretches the available technology to the very limits of spatial and temporal resolution, this may potentially be more so than in the other, more established diagnostic imaging modalities that are used in cardiology. Finally, while there is rapidly accumulating evidence on accuracy, there is no data that links the use of CT angiography to improved outcomes. Consequently, official bodies and professional organizations have been reluctant to issue guidelines that would broadly support the use of CT imaging in the workup of coronary artery disease. The ESC will publish new guidelines on stable coronary artery disease in 2012 and they are expected to contain an endorsement of coronary CT angiography in specific situations. Besides that, the only official guideline of the European Society of Cardiology that endorses the utilization of coronary CT angiography is the guideline in the management of acute coronary syndromes in patients presenting without ST-segment elevation [23]. In these guidelines, the following is stated:

> Coronary CT angiography should be considered as an alternative to invasive angiography to exclude ACS when there is a low to intermediate likelihood of CAD and when troponin and ECG are inconclusive. (Class IIa, level of evidence B)

In a 'Scientific Statement' on non-invasive coronary artery imaging issued by the American Heart Association [104], the following comments are made regarding coronary CT angiography for the detection of coronary artery stenoses:

> Neither coronary CT angiography nor coronary MR angiography should be used to screen for coronary artery disease in patients who have no signs or symptoms suggestive of coronary artery disease. (Class III, level of evidence C)

> The potential benefit of non-invasive coronary angiography is likely to be greatest and is reasonable for symptomatic patients who are at intermediate risk for coronary artery disease after initial risk stratification, including patients with equivocal stress-test results (Class II, level of evidence B). Diagnostic accuracy favors coronary CT angiography over MR angiography for these patients. (Class I, level of evidence B)

A group of US-based professional societies (both cardiology and radiology) has jointly issued a statement of 'Appropriateness Criteria' for cardiac CT in the year 2010 (see ➲ Table 20.7). The document lists clinical situations in which coronary CT angiography could be applied, and rates them as inappropriate, appropriate, or uncertain [1]. Such situations include the use of CT coronary angiography to rule out coronary artery stenoses in patients who are symptomatic, but who have a non-interpretable or equivocal stress test, who are unable to exercise, or who have a non-interpretable ECG. Furthermore, the document considers the use of coronary CT angiography appropriate for patients with new onset heart failure and for patients who present with acute chest pain and an intermediate pre-test likelihood of coronary artery disease, but who have a normal ECG and absence of enzyme elevation (see ➲ Table 20.7) [1]. According to this document, coronary CT angiography can be appropriate to establish bypass patency and to assess left main coronary artery stents (even though there is a paucity of data to this effect). Finally, the use of CT angiography is considered 'appropriate' to evaluate patients with anomalous coronary arteries [1]. CT angiography for screening purposes is not endorsed.

Coronary artery calcium is included in European Prevention Guidelines [85]. They recognize that coronary artery calcium is a method to identify and quantify subclinical atherosclerosis, that 'many prospective studies have shown the prognostic relevance of the amount of coronary calcium'. And that the 'Agatston score is an independent risk marker regarding the extent of CHD and prognostic impact.' [85]. As a recommendation, the guidelines state that:

> Computed tomography for coronary calcium should be considered for cardiovascular risk assessment in asymptomatic adults at moderate risk. (Class IIa, level of evidence B)

Outlook

In spite of the impressive image quality—which continues to improve—coronary CT angiography does not constitute a general replacement for invasive, catheter-based diagnostic coronary angiography in the foreseeable future. Spatial and temporal resolutions are substantially lower than in invasive angiography. In addition, arrhythmias—most prominently atrial fibrillation—high heart rates, and inability to perform a sufficiently long breath-hold may preclude CT angiography in a significant number of patients who require a workup for coronary artery disease. Similarly, in patients with diffuse, severe disease, with substantial coronary artery calcification or with small coronary arteries (as often encountered, for example, in patients with diabetes), the spatial resolution of CT may not be high enough to allow reliable interpretation of the coronary system. For challenging cases like these, invasive angiography will remain the best diagnostic option. However, in many other situations, coronary CT angiography—if performed and interpreted with expertise—constitutes a reasonable tool to rule out coronary artery stenoses and avoid further testing.

Table 20.7 Appropriateness of coronary CT angiography in various clinical situations

Non-acute Symptoms Possibly Representing an Ischaemic Equivalent—No Stress Test Done	
ECG interpretable **and** able to exercise	
◆ Low pre-test likelihood (< 10%)	Uncertain
◆ Intermediate pre-test likelihood (10–90%)	**Appropriate**
◆ High pre-test likelihood (>90%)	Inappropriate
ECG uninterpretable **or** unable to exercise	
◆ Low pre-test likelihood	**Appropriate**
◆ Intermediate pre-test likelihood	**Appropriate**
◆ High pre-test likelihood	Uncertain
Non-acute Symptoms, Prior ECG Exercise Test	
Normal but continued symptoms	**Appropriate**
Abnormal	
◆ Low Duke Treadmill Score	Inappropriate
◆ Intermediate Duke Treadmill Score	**Appropriate**
◆ High Duke Treadmill Score	Inappropriate
Non-acute Symptoms, Prior Stress Imaging Procedure	
◆ Equivocal	**Appropriate**
◆ Mildly positive	Uncertain
◆ Moderately or severely positive	Inappropriate
◆ Discordant ECG exercise and stress imaging results	**Appropriate**
New or Worsening Symptoms with a Past Stress Imaging Study	
◆ Past study normal	**Appropriate**
◆ Past study abnormal	Uncertain
Acute Symptoms With Suspicion of ACS (Urgent Presentation)	
Definite MI	Inappropriate
Persistent ECG ST-segment elevation following exclusion of MI	Uncertain
Triple Rule Out for acute chest pain of uncertain cause (differential diagnosis includes pulmonary embolism, aortic dissection, and ACS)	Uncertain
Cardiac biomarkers normal or equivocal and ECG normal or uninterpretable	
◆ Low pre-test likelihood	**Appropriate**
◆ Intermediate pre-test likelihood	**Appropriate**
◆ High pre-test likelihood	Uncertain
Patient with Previous Revascularization by CABG	
◆ Patient symptomatic, assessment of bypass patency required	**Appropriate**
◆ Patient asymptomatic, surgery <5 years ago	Inappropriate
◆ Patient asymptomatic, surgery ≥5 years ago	Uncertain
Patient with Previous Revascularization by PCI	
◆ Patient symptomatic, stent < 3 mm	Inappropriate
◆ Patient symptomatic, stent ≥ 3 mm	Uncertain
◆ Asymptomatic, left main stent ≥ 3 mm	**Appropriate**
◆ Asymptomatic, other stents	Inappropriate

Modified according to [1].

References

1. Taylor AJ, Cerqueira M, Hodgson JM, et al. American College of Cardiology Foundation Appropriate Use Criteria Task Force; Society of Cardiovascular Computed Tomography; American College of Radiology; American Heart Association; American Society of Echocardiography; American Society of Nuclear Cardiology; North American Society for Cardiovascular Imaging; Society

for Cardiovascular Angiography and Interventions; Society for Cardiovascular Magnetic Resonance. ACCF/SCCT/ACR/AHA/ASE/ASNC/NASCI/SCAI/SCMR 2010 Appropriate Use Criteria for Cardiac Computed Tomography. A Report of the American College of Cardiology Foundation Appropriate Use Criteria Task Force, the Society of Cardiovascular Computed Tomography, the American College of Radiology, the American Heart Association, the American Society of Echocardiography, the American Society of Nuclear Cardiology, the North American Society for Cardiovascular Imaging, the Society for Cardiovascular Angiography and Interventions, and the Society for Cardiovascular Magnetic Resonance. *J Am Coll Cardiol* 2010; 56(22): 1864–94.

2. Achenbach S. Cardiac CT: state of the art for the detection of coronary arterial stenosis. *J Cardiovascular Computed Tomography* 2007; 1: 3–20.

3. Achenbach S, Ropers U, Kuettner A, et al. Randomized comparison of 64-slice single- and dual-source computed tomography for the detection of coronary artery disease. *J Am Coll Cardiol Img* 2008; 1: 177–86.

4. Ferencik M, Ropers D, Abbara S, et al. Diagnostic accuracy of image postprocessing methods for the detection of coronary artery stenoses by using multidetector CT. *Radiology* 2007; 243: 696–702.

5. Raff GL, Abidov A, Achenbach S, et al. Society of Cardiovascular Computed Tomography. SCCT guidelines for the interpretation and reporting of coronary computed tomographic angiography. *J Cardiovasc Comput Tomogr* 2009; 3: 122–36.

6. Meijboom WB, Meijs MF, Schuijf JD, et al.Diagnostic accuracy of 64-slice computed tomography coronary angiography: a prospective, multicentre, multivendor study. *J Am Coll Cardiol* 2008; 52: 2135–44.

7 Budoff MJ, Dowe D, Jollis JG, et al. Diagnostic performance of 64-multidetector-row coronary computed tomographic angiography for evaluation of coronary artery stenosis in individuals without known coronary artery disease. *J Am Coll Cardiol* 2008; 52: 1724–32.

8. Miller JM, Rochitte CE, Dewey M, et al. Diagnostic performance of coronary angiography by 64-row CT. *N Engl J Med* 2008; 359: 2324–36.

9. Paech DC, Weston AR. A systematic review of the clinical effectiveness of 64-slice or higher computed tomography angiography as an alternative to invasive coronary angiography in the investigation of suspected coronary artery disease. *BMC Cardiovasc Disord* 2011; 11: 32.

10. Hoffmann U, Moselewski F, Cury RC, et al. Predictive value of 16-slice multidetector spiral computed tomography to detect significant obstructive coronary artery disease in patients at high risk for coronary artery disease: patient-versus segment-based analysis. *Circulation* 2004; 110: 2638–43.

11. Gosthine S, Caussin C, Daoud B, et al. Non-invasive detection of coronary artery disease in patients with left bundle branch block using 64-slice computed tomography. *J Am Coll Cardiol* 2006; 48: 1929–34.

12. Budoff MJ, Dowe D, Jollis JG, et al. Diagnostic performance of 64-multidetector row coronary computed tomographic angiography for evaluation of coronary artery stenosis in individuals without known coronary artery disease: results from the prospective multicentre ACCURACY (Assessment by Coronary Computed Tomographic Angiography of Individuals Undergoing Invasive Coronary Angiography) trial. *J Am Coll Cardiol* 2008; 52: 1724–32.

13. Vanhoenacker PK, Heijenbrok-Kal MH, Van Heste R, et al. Diagnostic performance of multidetector CT angiography for assessment of coronary artery disease: meta-analysis. *Radiology* 2007; 244: 419–28.

14. Westwood ME, Raatz HD, Misso K, et al. Systematic review of the accuracy of dual-source cardiac CT for detection of arterial stenosis in difficult to image patient groups. *Radiology* 2013; 267 (2): 387–95.

15. Chen CC, Chen CC, Hsieh IC, et al. The effect of calcium score on the diagnostic accuracy of coronary computed tomography angiography. *Int J Cardiovasc Imaging* 2011; 27 Suppl 1: 37–42.

16. Meijboom WB, van Mieghem CA, Mollet NR, et al. 64-Slice computed tomography coronary angiography in patients with high, intermediate, or low pretest probability of significant coronary artery disease. *J Am Coll Cardiol* 2007; 50: 1469–75.

17. Danciu SC, Herrera CJ, Stecy PJ, Carell E, Saltiel F, Hines JL. Usefulness of multislice computed tomographic coronary angiography to identify patients with abnormal myocardial perfusion stress in whom diagnostic catheterization may be safely avoided. *Am J Cardiol* 2007; 100: 1605–8.

18. Gilard M, Le Gal, G, Cornily JC, et al. Midterm prognosis of patients with suspected coronary artery disease and normal multislice computed tomography findings. A prospective management outcome study. *Arch Intern Med* 2007; 165: 1686–89.

19. Lesser JR, Flygenring B, Knickelbine T, et al. Clinical utility of coronary CT angiography: coronary stenosis detection and prognosis in ambulatory patients. *Cath Cardiovasc Interv* 2007; 69: 64–72.

20. Chow BJ, Wells GA, Chen L, et al. Prognostic value of 64-slice cardiac computed tomography severity of coronary artery disease, coronary atherosclerosis, and left ventricular ejection fraction. *J Am Coll Cardiol* 2010; 55: 1017–28.

21. Hadamitzky M, Distler R, Meyer T, et al. Prognostic value of coronary computed tomographic angiography in comparison with calcium scoring and clinical risk scores. *Circ Cardiovasc Imaging* 2011; 4: 16–23.

22. Min JK, Kang N, Shaw LJ, et al. Costs and clinical outcomes after coronary multidetector CT angiography in patients without known coronary artery disease: comparison to myocardial perfusion SPECT. *Radiology* 2008; 249: 62–70.

23. Hamm CW, Bassand JP, Agewall S, et al.; ESC Committee for Practice Guidelines. ESC Guidelines for the management of acute coronary syndromes in patients presenting without persistent ST-segment elevation: The Task Force for the management of acute coronary syndromes (ACS) in patients presenting without persistent ST-segment elevation of the European Society of Cardiology (ESC). *Eur Heart J* 2011; 32(23): 2999–3054.

24. Meijboom WB, Mollet NR, Van Mieghem CA, et al. 64-slice computed tomography coronary angiography in patients with non-ST elevation acute coronary syndrome. *Heart* 2007; 93: 1386–92.

25. Hoffmann U, Nagurney JT, Moselewski F, et al. Coronary multidetector computed tomography in the assessment of patients with acute chest pain. *Circulation* 2006; 114: 2251–60.

26. Gallagher MJ, Ross MA, Raff GL, Goldstein JA, O'Neill WW, O'Neil B. The diagnostic accuracy of 64-slice computed tomography coronary angiography compared with stress nuclear imaging in emergency department low-risk chest pain patients. *Ann Emerg Med* 2007; 49: 125–36.

27. Goldstein JA, Gallagher MJ, O'Neill WW, Ross MA, O'Neil BJ, Raff GL. A randomized controlled trial of multi-slice coronary computed tomography for evaluation of acute chest pain. *J Am Coll Cardiol* 2007; 49: 863–71.

28. Coles DR, Wilde P, Oberhoff M, Rogers CA, Karsch KR, Baumbach A. Multislice computed tomography coronary angiography in patients admitted with a suspected acute coronary syndrome. *Int J Cardiovasc Imaging* 2007; 23: 603–14.

29. Litt HI, Gatsonis C, Snyder B, et al. CT angiography for safe discharge of patients with possible acute coronary syndromes. *N Engl J Med* 2012; 366: 1393–403.

30. Hoffmann U, Truong QA, Schoenfeld DA, et al.; ROMICAT-II Investigators. Coronary CT angiography versus standard evaluation in acute chest pain. *N Engl J Med* 2012; 367: 299–308.

31. Chiurlia E, Menozzi M, Ratti C, Romagnoli R, Modena MG. Follow-up of coronary artery bypass graft patency by multislice computed tomography. *Am J Cardiol* 2005; 95: 1094–97.

32. Salm LP, Bax JJ, Jukema JW, et al. Comprehensive assessment of patients after coronary artery bypass grafting by 16-detector-row computed tomography. *Am Heart J* 2005; 150: 775–81.

33. Anders K, Baum U, Schmid M, et al. Coronary artery bypass graft (CABG) patency: Assessment with high-resolution submillimeter 16-slice multidetector-row computed tomography (MDCT) versus coronary angiography. *Eur J Radiol* 2006; 57: 336–44.

34. Ropers D, Pohle FK, Kuettner A, et al. Diagnostic accuracy of non-invasive coronary angiography in patients after bypass surgery using 64-slice spiral computed tomography with 330-ms gantry rotation. *Circulation* 2006; 114: 2334–41.

35. Meyer TS, Martinoff S, Hadamitzky M, et al. Improved noninvasive assessment of coronary artery bypass grafts with 64-slice computed tomographic angiography in an unselected patient population. *J Am Coll Cardiol* 2007; 49: 946–50.

36. Feuchtner GM, Schachner T, Bonatti J, et al. Diagnostic performance of 64-slice computed tomography in evaluation of coronary artery bypass grafts. *AJR Am J Roentgenol* 2007; 189(3): 574–80.

37. de Graaf FR, van Velzen JE, Witkowska AJ, et al. Diagnostic performance of 320-slice multidetector computed tomography coronary angiography in patients after coronary artery bypass grafting. *Eur Radiol* 2011; 21(11): 2285–96.

38. Maintz D, Seifarth H, Raupach R, et al. 64-slice multidetector coronary CT angiography: in vitro evaluation of 68 different stents. *Eur Radiol* 2006; 16: 818–26.

39. Van Mieghem CA, Cademartiri F, Mollet NR, et al. Multislice spiral computed tomography for the evaluation of stent patency after left main coronary artery stenting: a comparison with conventional coronary angiography and intravascular ultrasound. *Circulation* 2006; 114: 645–53.

40. Rixe J, Achenbach S, Ropers D, et al. Assessment of coronary artery stent restenosis by 64-slice multi-detector computed tomography. *Eur Heart J* 2006; 27: 2567–72.

41. Oncel D, Oncel G, Karaca M. Coronary stent patency and in-stent restenosis: determination with 64-section multidetector CT coronary angiography—initial experience. *Radiology* 2007; 242: 403–9.

42. Ehara M, Kawai M, Surmely JF, et al. Diagnostic accuracy of coronary in-stent restenosis using 64-slice computed tomography. *J Am Coll Cardiol* 2007; 49: 951–59.

43. Cademartiri F, Schuijf JD, Pugliese F, et al. Usefulness of 64-slice multislice computed tomography coronary angiography to assess in-stent restenosis. *J Am Coll Cardiol* 2007; 49: 2204–10.

44. de Graaf FR, Schuijf JD, van Velzen JE, et al. Diagnostic accuracy of 320-row multidetector computed tomography coronary angiography to noninvasively assess in-stent restenosis. *Invest Radiol* 2010; 45(6): 331–40.

45. Wykrzykowska JJ, Arbab-Zadeh A, Godoy G, et al. Assessment of in-stent restenosis using 64-MDCT: analysis of the CORE-64 Multicentre International Trial. *AJR Am J Roentgenol* 2010; 194(1): 85–92.

46. Hecht HS, Zaric M, Jelnin V, Lubarsky L, Prakash M, Roubin G. Usefulness of 64-detector computed tomographic angiography for diagnosing in-stent restenosis in native coronary arteries. *Am J Cardiol*. 2008 101: 820–24.

47. Andreini D, Pontone G, Mushtaq S et al. Coronary in-stent restenosis: assessment with CT coronary angiography. *Radiology* 2012; 265: 410–17.

48. Vanhoenacker PK, Decramer I, Bladt O, et al. Multidetector computed tomography angiography for assessment of in-stent restenosis: meta-analysis of diagnostic performance. *BMC Med Imaging* 2008; 8: 14.

49. Schuijf JD, Wijns W, Jukema JW, et al. Relationship between noninvasive coronary angiography with multi-slice computed tomography and myocardial perfusion imaging. *J Am Coll Cardiol* 2006; 48: 2508–14.

50. Min JK, Shaw LJ, Berman DS. The present state of coronary computed tomography angiography a process in evolution. *J Am Coll Cardiol* 2010; 55: 957–65.

51. Hacker M, Jakobs T, Hack N, et al. Sixty-four slice spiral CT angiography does not predict the functional relevance of coronary artery stenoses in patients with stable angina. *Eur J Nucl Med Mol Imaging* 2007; 34: 4–10.

52. Berman DS, Hachamovitch R, Shaw LJ, et al. Roles of nuclear cardiology, cardiac computed tomography, and cardiac magnetic resonance: noninvasive risk stratification and a conceptual framework for the selection of noninvasive imaging tests in patients with known or suspected coronary artery disease. *J Nucl Med* 2006; 47: 1107–18.

53. Bamberg F, Becker A, Schwarz F, et al. Detection of haemodynamically significant coronary artery stenosis: incremental diagnostic value of dynamic CT-based myocardial perfusion imaging. *Radiology* 2011; 260(3): 689–98.

54. Tashakkor AY, Nicolaou S, Leipsic J, Mancini GB. The emerging role of cardiac computed tomography for the assessment of coronary perfusion: a systematic review and meta-analysis. *Can J Cardiol* 2012; 28: 413–22.

55. Taylor CA, Fonte TA, Min JK. Computational fluid dynamics applied to cardiac computed tomography for noninvasive quantification of fractional flow reserve: scientific basis. *J Am Coll Cardiol* 2013; 61(22): 2233–41.

56. Hoff JA, Chomka EV, Krainik AJ, Daviglus M, Rich S, Kondos GT. Age and gender distribution of coronary artery calcium deetected by electron beam tomography. *Am J Cardiol* 2001; 87: 1335–39.

57. McClelland RL, Chung H, Detrano R, Post W, Kronmal RA. Distribution of coronary artery calcium by race, gender, and age: results from the Multi-Ethnic Study of Atherosclerosis (MESA). *Circulation* 2006; 113: 30–37.

58. Schmermund A, Mohlenkamp S, Berenbein S, et al. Population-based assessment of subclinical coronary atherosclerosis using electron-beam computed tomography. *Atherosclerosis* 2006; 185: 117–82.

59. Amann K, Tyralla K, Gross ML, Eifert T, Adamczak M, Ritz E. Special characteristics of atherosclerosis in chronic renal failure. *Clin Nephrol* 2003; 60 Suppl 1: S13–21.

60. Rumberger JA, Simons DB, Fitzpatrick LA, Sheedy PF, Schwartz RS. Coronary artery calcium area by electron-beam computed tomography and coronary atherosclerotic plaque area. A histopathologic correlative study. *Circulation* 1995; 92: 2157–62.

61. Schmermund A, Erbel R. Unstable coronary plaque and its relation to coronary calcium. *Circulation* 2001; 104: 1682–87.

62. Marwan M, Ropers D, Pflederer T, Daniel WG, Achenbach S. Clinical characteristics of patients with obstructive coronary lesions in the absence of coronary calcification: an evaluation by coronary CT angiography. *Heart* 2009; 95: 1056–60.

63. Detrano R, Guerci AD, Carr JJ, et al. Coronary calcium as a predictor of coronary events in four racial or ethnic groups. *N Engl J Med* 2008; 358: 1336–45.

64. Sarwar A, Shaw LJ, Shapiro MD, et al. Diagnostic and prognostic value of absence of coronary artery calcification. *JACC Cardiovasc Imaging* 2009; 2: 675–88.

65. Taylor AJ, Bindeman J, Feuerstein I, Cao F, Brazaitis M, O'Malley PG. Coronary calcium independently predicts incident premature coronary heart disease over measured cardiovascular risk factors: mean three-year outcomes in the Prospective Army Coronary Calcium (PACC) project. *J Am Coll Cardiol* 2005; 46: 807–14.

66. Greenland P, LaBree L, Azen SP, Doherty TM, Detrano RC. Coronary artery calcium score combined with Framingham score for risk prediction in asymptomatic individuals. *JAMA* 2004; 291: 210–15.

67. Erbel R, Möhlenkamp S, Moebus S, et al.; Heinz Nixdorf Recall Study Investigative Group. Coronary risk stratification, discrimination, and reclassification improvement based on quantification of subclinical coronary atherosclerosis: the Heinz Nixdorf Recall study. *J Am Coll Cardiol* 2010 Oct 19; 56(17): 1397–406.

68. Park R, Detrano R, Xiang M, Fu P, Ibrahim Y, LaBree L, Azen S. Combined use of computed tomography coronary calcium scores and C-reactive protein levels in predicting cardiovascular events in nondiabetic individuals. *Circulation* 2002; 106: 2073–77.

69. Folsom AR, Kronmal RA, Detrano RC, et al. Coronary artery calcification compared with carotid intima-media thickness in the prediction of cardiovascular disease incidence: the Multi-Ethnic Study of Atherosclerosis (MESA). *Arch Intern Med* 2008; 168(12): 1333–9.

70. Schmermund A, Baumgart D, Möhlenkamp S, et al. Natural history and topographic pattern of progression of coronary calcification in symptomatic patients. *Arterioscler Thromb Vasc Biol* 2001; 21: 421.

71. Taylor AJ, Bindeman J, Le TP, et al. Progression of calcified coronary atherosclerosis: Relationship to coronary risk factors and carotid intima-media thickness. *Atherosclerosis* 2008; 197(1): 339–45.

72. Kronmal RA, McClelland RL, Detrano R et al. Risk factors for the progression of coronary artery calcification in asymptomatic subjects: results from the Multi-Ethnic Study of Atherosclerosis (MESA). *Circulation* 2007; 115: 2722–30.

73. Cassidy-Bushrow AE, Bielak LF, Sheedy PF 2nd, et al. Coronary artery calcification progression is heritable. *Circulation* 2007; 116: 25–31.

74. Raggi P, Callister TQ, Shaw LJ. Progression of coronary artery calcium and risk of first myocardial infarction in patients receiving cholesterol-lowering therapy. *Arterioscler Thromb Vasc Biol* 2004; 24: 1272–77.

75. Callister TQ, Raggi P, Cooil B, et al. Effect of HmG-CoA reductase inhibitors on coronary artery disease as assessed by electron-beam computed tomography. *N Engl J Med* 1998; 339: 1972.

76. Achenbach S, Ropers D, Pohle K, et al. Influence of lipid-lowering therapy on the progression of coronary artery calcification: a prospective evaluation. *Circulation* 2002; 106: 1077.

77. Budoff MJ, Lane KL, Bakhsheshi H, et al. Rates of progression of coronary calcium by electron beam tomography. *Am J Cardiol* 2000; 86: 8.

78. Raggi P, Davidson M, Callister TQ, et al. Aggressive versus moderate lipid-lowering therapy in hypercholesterolemic postmenopausal women: Beyond Endorsed Lipid Lowering with EBT Scanning (BELLES). *Circulation* 2005; 112: 563–71.

79. Schmermund A, Achenbach S, Budde T, et al. Effect of intensive versus standard lipid-lowering treatment with atorvastatin on the progression of calcified coronary atherosclerosis over 12 months: a multicentre, randomized, double-blind trial. *Circulation* 2006; 113: 427–37.

80. Arad Y, Spadaro LA, Roth M, et al. Treatment of asymptomatic adults with elevated coronary calcium scores with atorvastatin, vitamin C, and vitamin E: the St. Francis Heart Study randomized clinical trial. *J Am Coll Cardiol* 2005; 46: 166–72.

81. Terry JG, Carr JJ, Kouba EO, et al. Effect of simvastatin (80 mg) on coronary and abdominal aortic arterial calcium (from the coronary artery calcification treatment with zocor [CATZ] study). *Am J Cardiol* 2007; 99: 1714–17.

82. Budoff MJ, Achenbach S, Blumenthal RS, et al. Assessment of coronary artery disease by cardiac computed tomography: a scientific statement from the American Heart Association Committee on Cardiovascular Imaging and Intervention, Council on Cardiovascular Radiology and Intervention, and Committee on Cardiac Imaging, Council on Clinical Cardiology. *Circulation* 2006; 114: 1761–91.

83. Greenland P, Bonow RO, Brundage BH, et al. ACCF/AHA 2007 clinical expert consensus document on coronary artery calcium scoring by computed tomography in global cardiovascular risk assessment and in evaluation of patients with chest pain: a report of the American College of Cardiology Foundation Clinical Expert Consensus Task Force (ACCF/AHA Writing Committee to Update the 2000 Expert Consensus Document on Electron Beam Computed Tomography). *Circulation* 2007; 115: 402–26.

84. Schroeder S, Achenbach S, Bengel F, et al. Cardiac computed tomography: indications, applications, limitations, and training requirements: Report of a Writing Group deployed by the Working Group Nuclear Cardiology and Cardiac CT of the European Society of Cardiology and the European Council of Nuclear Cardiology. *Eur Heart J* 2008; 29: 531–56.

85. Perk J, De Backer G, Gohlke H, et al. European guidelines on cardiovascular disease prevention in clinical practice (version 2012). The Fifth Joint Task Force of the European Society of Cardiology and Other Societies on Cardiovascular Disease Prevention in Clinical Practice (constituted by representatives of nine societies and by invited experts). Developed with the special contribution of the European Association for Cardiovascular Prevention & Rehabilitation (EACPR). *Eur Heart J* 2012; 33: 1635–1701.

86. Gao D, Ning N, Guo Y, Ning W, Niu X, Yang J. Computed tomography for detecting coronary artery plaques: a meta-analysis. *Atherosclerosis* 2011; 219: 603–9.

87. Achenbach S, Moselewski F, Ropers D, et al. Detection of calcified and noncalcified coronary atherosclerotic plaque by contrast-enhanced, submillimeter multidetector spiral computed tomography: a segment-based comparison with intravascular ultrasound. *Circulation* 2004; 109: 14–17.

88. Leber AW, Knez A, Becker A, et al. Accuracy of multidetector spiral computed tomography in identifying and differentiating the composition of coronary atherosclerotic plaques: a comparative study with intracoronary ultrasound. *J Am Coll Cardiol* 2004; 43: 1241–47.

89. Leber AW, Becker A, Knez A, et al. Accuracy of 64-slice computed tomography to classify and quantify plaque volumes in the proximal coronary system: a comparative study using intravascular ultrasound. *J Am Coll Cardiol* 2006; 47: 672–27.

90. Schroeder S, Kopp AF, Baumbach A, et al. Noninvasive detection and evaluation of atherosclerotic coronary plaques with multislice computed tomography. *J Am Coll Cardiol* 2001; 37: 1430–35.

91. Caussin C, Ohanessian A, Ghostine S, et al. Characterization of vulnerable nonstenotic plaque with 16-slice computed tomography compared with intravascular ultrasound. *Am J Cardiol* 2004; 94: 99–100.

92. Carrascosa PM, Capunay CM, Garcia-Merletti P, Carrascosa J, Garcia MF. Characterization of coronary atherosclerotic plaques by multidetector computed tomography. *Am J Cardiol* 2006; 97: 598–602.

93. Pohle K, Achenbach S, MacNeill B, et al. Characterization of noncalcified coronary atherosclerotic plaque by multi-detector row CT: Comparison to IVUS. *Atherosclerosis* 2007; 190: 174–80.

94. Sun J, Zhang Z, Lu B, et al. Identification and quantification of coronary atherosclerotic plaques: a comparison of 64-MDCT and intravascular ultrasound. *AJR Am J Roentgenol* 2008; 190(3): 748–54.

95. Cademartiri F, Mollet NR, Runza G, et al. Influence of intracoronary attenuation on coronary plaque measurements using multislice computed tomography: observations in an ex vivo model of coronary computed tomography angiography. *Eur Radiol* 2005; 15: 1426–31.

96. Achenbach S, Ropers D, Hoffmann U, et al. Assessment of coronary remodeling in stenotic and nonstenotic coronary atherosclerotic lesions by multidetector spiral computed tomography. *J Am Coll Cardiol* 2004; 43: 842–47.

97. Moselewski F, Ropers D, Pohle K, et al. Comparison of measurement of cross-sectional coronary atherosclerotic plaque and vessel areas by 16-slice multidetector computed tomography versus intravascular ultrasound. *Am J Cardiol* 2004; 94: 1294–97.

98. Bruining N, Roelandt JR, Palumbo A, et al. Reproducible coronary plaque quantification by multislice computed tomography. *Catheter Cardiovasc Interv* 2007; 69: 857–65.

99. Gauss S, Achenbach S, Pflederer T, Schuhbäck A, Daniel WG, Marwan M. Assessment of coronary artery remodelling by dual-source CT: a head-to-head comparison with intravascular ultrasound. *Heart* 2011; 97(12): 991–97.

100. Motoyama S, Sarai M, Harigaya H, et al. Computed tomographic angiography characteristics of atherosclerotic plaques subsequently resulting in acute coronary syndrome. *J Am Coll Cardiol* 2009; 54: 49–57.

101. Min JK, Shaw LJ, Devereux RB, et al. Prognostic value of multidetector coronary computed tomographic angiography for prediction of all-cause mortality. *J Am Coll Cardiol* 2007; 50: 1161–70.

102. Ostrom MP, Gopal A, Ahmadi N, et al. Mortality incidence and the severity of coronary atherosclerosis assessed by computed tomography angiography. *J Am Coll Cardiol* 2008; 52: 1335–43.

103. Min JK, Dunning A, Lin FY, et al.; CONFIRM Investigators. Age- and sex-related differences in all-cause mortality risk based on coronary computed tomography angiography findings results from the International Multicentre CONFIRM (Coronary CT Angiography Evaluation for Clinical Outcomes: An International Multicentre Registry) of 23,854 patients without known coronary artery disease. *J Am Coll Cardiol* 2011; 58(8): 849–60.

104. Bluemke DA, Achenbach S, Budoff M, et al. Noninvasive coronary artery imaging: magnetic resonance angiography and multidetector computed tomography angiography: a scientific statement from the American Heart Association Committee on Cardiovascular Imaging and Intervention of the Council on Cardiovascular Radiology and Intervention, and the Councils on Clinical Cardiology and Cardiovascular Disease in the Young. *Circulation* 2008 118: 586–606.

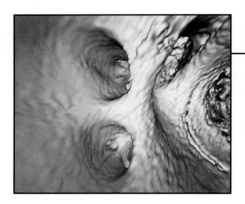

CHAPTER 21

CMR and detection of coronary artery disease

Eike Nagel, Juerg Schwitter, and Sven Plein

Contents

Introduction

Cardiovascular magnetic resonance (CMR) imaging has evolved from a niche-application to the centre of cardiovascular decision-making. Standardized CMR protocols have been defined and the availability of CMR is increasing in most healthcare systems. In parallel, the evidence for the use of CMR in a large variety of indications, including the diagnosis and assessment of coronary artery disease (CAD), has accumulated rapidly over the last years. This chapter will focus on the diagnosis of ischaemia with brief reference to viability assessment, which is covered in detail elsewhere. Coronary angiography by CMR will not be discussed in this chapter as it is only recommended for delineation of the course of coronary artery anomalies [1], while detection of coronary stenosis by non-invasive angiography is the domain of cardiac computed tomography.

Detection of ischaemia by CMR

CMR offers two principal methods for the detection of myocardial ischaemia. The first method, dobutamine-CMR, allows a direct assessment of ischaemia through the assessment of inducible wall motion abnormalities. The second method, myocardial perfusion CMR, relies on the detection of myocardial perfusion defects during vasodilator-induced hyperaemia. While both methods are used to detect flow-limiting coronary artery stenosis, they are based on fundamentally different concepts and therefore have different strengths and limitations. As described in the ischaemic cascade, a decrease in myocardial perfusion represents the first of several events in the progression of myocardial ischaemia, followed by metabolic changes, wall motion abnormalities, and eventually ECG changes and anginal pain. Perfusion imaging, therefore, detects the first pathological step in the ischaemic cascade making it theoretically the most sensitive method for the detection of flow-limiting coronary stenosis. Importantly, perfusion imaging can detect maldistribution of myocardial blood during vasodilator stress flow without necessarily provoking ischaemia, while wall motion abnormalities, as induced by dobutamine-stress, only occur in the presence of ischaemia. Consequently, wall motion abnormalities are less sensitive, but more specific for the detection of coronary artery stenosis than perfusion imaging [2]. On the other hand, wall motion imaging with CMR is technically less challenging than perfusion-CMR and may be superior in more complex patients, such as post-bypass surgery, after myocardial infarction, and in those with reduced coronary flow reserve due to microvascular disease. In practice, the choice of one method is, therefore, governed by patient-specific factors, as well as operator preference.

Indications for ischaemia detection by CMR

The main indication for the use of dobutamine or perfusion-CMR is the detection of significant CAD in patients with intermediate pre-test likelihood who are unable to exercise or whose ECG is not interpretable. US guidelines still focus primarily on stress echocardiography and SPECT for this patient group [3], despite the growing evidence for CMR and strong support in appropriateness scenarios [1]. Consequently, in the most recent ESC guidelines CMR, SPECT, and stress echo are ranked as interchangeable [4]. In patients with lower pre-test likelihood there is a tendency towards CT to exclude coronary artery disease. A further indication is the detection and quantification of ischaemia in patients with intermediate stenoses by luminography (CT or catheterization) [1]. Given that the severity of a luminal narrowing is only weakly related to the amount of blood flow reduction it causes, functional testing provides important additional information to luminography and has strong predictive value for future cardiac events. The results of the COURAGE and FAME trials have highlighted the importance of functional testing and further underline the need for adequate ischaemia testing to optimize outcome [5, 6]. Accordingly, only confirmed ischaemia is a Class 1A indication for revascularization [46]. Despite this evidence, such testing remains underused in clinical practice and only 45% of patients had ischaemia detection before interventions in the United States [7].

Dobutamine-CMR

Introduction

State-of-the-art scanners allow for rapid switching of the magnetic field resulting in very short measurement times. This allows us to perform high-resolution cine imaging of the heart at rest and under stress conditions up to heart rates of 200 beats per minute. Today's standard sequences (steady-state free-precession, SSFP) provide an excellent visualization of the endocardial border due to a high contrast between blood and myocardium without the need of contrast medium (CM) injection. Image quality is independent of limiting acquisition windows. While inadequate ECG triggering used to be a problem in some patients this has been solved for most scanners today. Image quality deteriorates with arrhythmias. In these patients real-time CMR can be used [8].

Stress agents

The limited space within the scanner necessitates the application of pharmacological stress agents (usually dobutamine) for the detection of inducible wall motion abnormalities. Pharmacological stress is a well-documented alternative stress method to ergometry and is superior in patients who are not able to exert themselves adequately. Even though vasodilator (adenosine/dipyridamole) stress has been suggested for the induction of ischaemic wall motion abnormalities, and considered interchangeable to dobutamine stress, a significantly lower diagnostic accuracy for the detection of epicardial coronary stenosis, both with CMR and echocardiography, has been reported for vasodilator versus dobutamine stress [2].

Dobutamine-CMR protocol

The pharmacological stress protocol for CMR follows the standard high-dose dobutamine/atropine regimen as used in stress echocardiography (Fig. 21.1). The myocardium is divided into 17 segments. At rest, each of these segments is visualized in two standard views (apical, mid and basal short-axis view, four-chamber, two-chamber and three-chamber view). Dobutamine is infused intravenously at 3-minute intervals at doses of 10, 20, 30, and 40 µg/kg/min and imaging is repeated in all views at each stress level. If target heart rate (age predicted sub-maximal heart rate (220 – age) × 0.85) is not reached at the maximal dobutamine dose, a maximal dose of 2 mg atropine is applied in 0.25 mg fractions and imaging is repeated once the required heart rate has been reached. Termination criteria are identical to those of dobutamine stress echocardiography [9, 10].

Safety of dobutamine-CMR

A report on the safety of high-dose dobutamine-CMR in 1,000 consecutive patients showed a safety profile similar to dobutamine stress echocardiography: one patient suffered sustained ventricular tachycardia with successful conversion; no cases of death or myocardial infarction occurred. The patients included into this study reflect current clinical practice with an intermediate pre-test likelihood and more than 50% positive findings [11].

Imaging technique

CMR cine imaging is usually performed with the patient in the supine position (Fig. 21.2). Surface coils with several elements (usually 4–8) are placed on the thorax for signal detection.

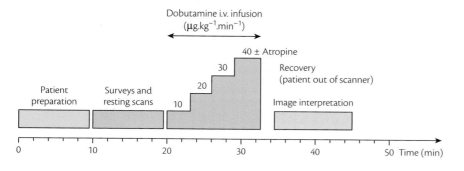

Fig. 21.1 Time sequence of high-dose dobutamine-atropine stress cardiovascular magnetic resonance.
Reproduced from Wahl A et al, Safety and feasibility of high-dose dobutamine-atropine stress cardiovascular magnetic resonance for diagnosis of myocardial ischaemia: Experience in 1000 consecutive cases. *Eur Heart J.* 2004; 25: 1230–6, by permission of Oxford University Press.

Routinely SSFP sequences in combination with parallel image acquisition and retrospective ECG gating are used. During an expiratory breath-hold of 4–6 s, a cine loop of >25 phases/cardiac cycle can be acquired up to heart rates of 200 beats per minute. The in-plane spatial resolution of MR cine scans is usually between 1.5–2 mm × 1.5–2 mm with a slice thickness of 8 mm.

Image display

During the pharmacological stress procedure the examiner evaluates the CMR cine images for the presence of new or worsening wall motion abnormalities. Cine images are displayed within 1 s after data acquisition and can be simultaneously transferred to an independent viewing station.

Diagnostic criteria

Standard assessment of wall motion and wall motion abnormalities is performed visually for all 17 segments using a synchronized display of the different dobutamine-dose levels at the same time (➲ Figs 21.3 and 21.4). First, image quality is graded as good, acceptable, or bad and the number of diagnostic segments is

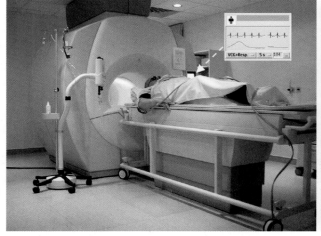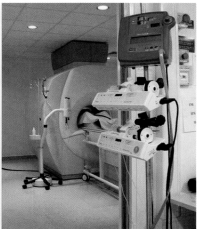

Fig. 21.2 Left panel: overview of the 1.5 T clinical whole body MR tomograph (ACS NT, Philips, Best, The Netherlands) used for the study. The inset shows vector-ECG and respiratory monitoring, which is displayed both at the scanner (arrow) and on the operator's console. Right panel: infusion pumps and blood-pressure monitoring system.
Reproduced from Wahl A et al, Safety and feasibility of high-dose dobutamine-atropine stress cardiovascular magnetic resonance for diagnosis of myocardial ischaemia: Experience in 1000 consecutive cases. *Eur Heart J*. 2004;25:1230–6, by permission of Oxford University Press.

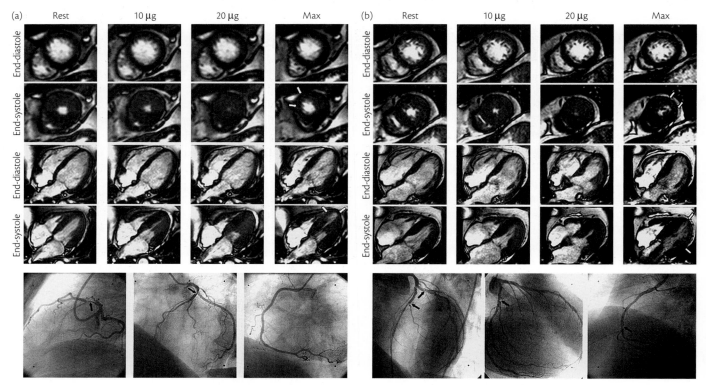

Fig. 21.3 (a) Cine images of the DSMR examination (apical short-axis and 4-chamber view) in a patient with single-vessel disease of the LAD. The four readers showed perfect agreement regarding newly developed wall motion abnormalities in the anterior and anteroseptal segment and the apex (segment 17). (b) Cine images of the DSMR examination (apical short-axis and 4-chamber view) in a patient with triple-vessel disease (significant stenoses of the first diagonal branch, proximal left circumflex, and distal RCA). The four readers detected newly developed wall motion abnormalities in the lateral wall (apical and equatorial segments). The development of a mitral regurgitation jet due to ischaemic papillary muscle dysfunction is depicted as well.
Paetsch I et al, Determination of interobserver variability for identifying inducible left ventricular wall motion abnormalities during dobutamine stress magnetic resonance imaging. *Eur Heart J* 2006; 27: 1459–64, by permission of Oxford University Press.

4-chamber

Mid-ventricular short-axis

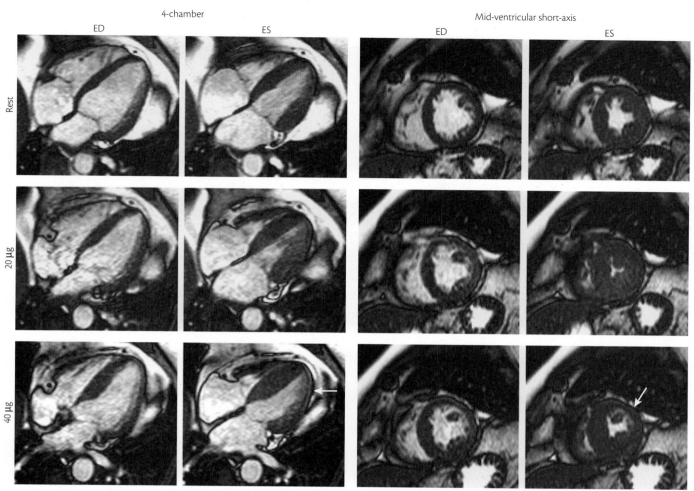

ED   ES   ED   ES

Rest

20 µg

40 µg

Fig. 21.4 Four-chamber and mid-ventricular short-axis views at rest, and at intermediate- and peak-dose dobutamine stress (steady-state free-precession technique). Both end-diastolic (ED) and end-systolic (ES) frames are shown. Note the development of mid-lateral akinesia (arrows) at peak dobutamine stress. In this patient, invasive coronary angiography demonstrated a left circumflex coronary artery stenosis.
Reproduced from Wahl A et al, Safety and feasibility of high-dose dobutamine-atropine stress cardiovascular magnetic resonance for diagnosis of myocardial ischaemia: Experience in 1000 consecutive cases. *Eur Heart J* 2004; 25: 1230–6, by permission of Oxford University Press.

reported. Segmental wall motion is classified as normokinetic, hypokinetic, akinetic, or dyskinetic and assigned one to four points. The sum of points is divided by the number of analysed segments and yields a wall motion score. Normal contraction results in a wall motion score of 1, a higher score is indicative of wall motion abnormalities. During dobutamine stress with increasing doses, a decrease or no change in wall motion or systolic wall thickening are regarded as pathological findings.

Diagnostic performance

In single-centre trials dobutamine-CMR has been shown to be superior to dobutamine stress echocardiography for the detection of inducible wall motion abnormalities in patients with suspected CAD [12], in patients with wall motion abnormalities at rest [13], and in patients not well suited for second harmonic echocardiography [14] ⊃ (Table 21.1). The superiority of dobutamine-CMR has been attributed primarily to the consistently high endocardial border visualization inherent to the CMR cine sequences, which is independent of limited acquisition windows, thereby allowing for the detection of subtle wall motion abnormalities. Thus, the gain in diagnostic accuracy is mainly seen in those patients with inadequate acoustic windows or limited echocardiographic image quality despite the use of second harmonic imaging [15]. No studies have compared dobutamine-CMR with contrast-echocardiography yet. The consistently high endocardial border visualization also leads to a high inter-observer reproducibility, as shown in a multi-centre read of 150 patients in 6 centres [16]. A meta-analysis of CMR for identifying coronary atherosclerosis showed a sensitivity of 83% with a specificity of 86% for all stressors—dobutamine, exercise (1 study only) or dipyridamole—as well as 85% sensitivity (95% CI 82–90%) and 86% specificity (95% CI 81–90%) for dobutamine and exercise only [17]. Diagnostic accuracy was found to be gender independent [18], even though responses of longitudinal function and aortic stiffness to dobutamine stress are different in men and women [19]. Diagnostic accuracy (and prognostic value) may be improved by the use of strain imaging (e.g. SENC)

Table 21.1 Diagnostic accuracy of dobutamine stress wall motion studies

Author	Year	Journal	#	characteristics	sens	spec	comment
Dobutamine stress							
Pennell et al. [74]	1992	AJC	25	Suspected CAD	91	100	non-breath-hold
van Rugge et al. [75]	1993	JACC	45	Suspected CAD	81	100	non-breath-hold
Baer et al. [76]	1994	Radiology	35	Known CAD	84	-	non-breath-hold
van Rugge et al. [77]	1994	Circulation	39	Suspected CAD	91	83	non-breath-hold
Hundley et al. [14]	1999	Circulation	41	Suspected CAD	83	83	poor acoustic windows on TTE
Nagel et al. [12]	1999	Circulation	172	Suspected CAD	86	86	superior to dobutamine stress echo
Schalla et al. [8]	2002	Radiology	220	Suspected CAD	81	83	real time imaging technique
Paetsch et al. [2]	2004	Circulation	79	Suspected or known CAD	89	81	superior to perfusion imaging
Wahl [13]	2004	Radiology	160	Wall motion abnormalities	89	84	patients with WMA at rest
Jahnke et al. [78]	2006	Radiology	40	Suspected or known CAD	89	75	4D single breath-hold technique
Paetsch et al. [16]	2006	EHJ	150	Suspected CAD	78	88	multi-centre read
Korosoglou [20]	2010	JACC CVI	80	Suspected or known CAD	98	91	by addition of SENC
Gebker et al. [79]	2012	Int J Cardiol	78	Suspected or known CAD	92	83	dobutamine stress perfusion
Gebker et al. [79]	2012	Int J Cardiol	78	Suspected or known CAD	81	87	wall motion

[20, 21] or feature tracking [22]. While adding perfusion to dobutamine wall motion assessment is possible, only high-resolution techniques seem to improve overall diagnostic accuracy due to a higher sensitivity [23].

Functional assessment of viable myocardium

In addition to the assessment of ischaemia, dobutamine-CMR offers the possibility to detect viable myocardium after myocardial infarction or in chronic CAD (hibernation). This information can be extracted from every dobutamine stress test and is based on the contractile response to low-dose dobutamine stimulation. Low-dose dobutamine stimulates recruitment of hibernating myocardium at a dose of 10–20 µg/kg/min. Thus, in areas with viable myocardium, typically a 'biphasic response' can be observed with a wall motion abnormality at rest, improvement at low dose, and deterioration at high-dose dobutamine. When low-dose dobutamine stimulation was compared with LGE-CMR for scar imaging, one study found that low-dose dobutamine is superior to scar imaging in predicting recovery of function after revascularization [24]. This observation was most pronounced in segments with non-transmural scar. As an explanation it was suggested that, even though scar imaging depicts the area of myocardial fibrosis, it does not assess the functional state of the surrounding (potentially viable) myocardium, and, thus, its capability for the prediction of functional recovery of non-transmurally scarred myocardium is limited. In contrast, Gutberlet et al. [25] found that LGE was a better predictor of recovery. For a detailed discussion of viability imaging we refer to a recent review article [26].

Prognostic value of dobutamine-CMR

Several single-centre studies have been presented on the prognostic value of dobutamine-CMR. Hundley et al. [27] found that the presence of inducible wall motion abnormalities during dobutamine-CMR identifies patients at risk of myocardial infarction and cardiac death independently of the presence of traditional risk factors for CAD. A low cardiac event rate was found in patients with negative dobutamine-CMR testing (2% over 2 years for patients with LVEF >40% and 0% over 2 years for patients with LVEF ≥60%). Jahnke et al. [28] reported a follow-up of 513 patients with known or suspected CAD for a median duration of 2.3 years. A normal dobutamine-CMR study resulted in a cumulative event rate (death or myocardial infarction) of 1.2%, 2.6%, and 3.3% in the first 3 years, whereas patients with an abnormal dobutamine-CMR had a significantly higher event rate (7.3%, 10.3%, and 18.8% in the first 3 years). More recently, Kelle et al. reported the outcomes of a bicentre cohort of 3,138 patients examined with dobutamine-CMR and followed over more than 3 years. They found a 0.6% annual event rate (myocardial infarction or cardiac death) in patients with a negative test. In patients with inducible wall motion abnormalities, prognosis was normalized by early revascularization (within 3 months of the stress test) [29].

Limitations

Dobutamine-CMR has several limitations, most of which are similar to dobutamine stress echocardiography:

- Since the test is stopped, whenever a diagnostic wall motion abnormality occurs, it is possible that only the haemodynamically leading stenosis is detected. Potentially, other stenoses, which cause significant ischaemia but to a lesser extent, might be overlooked.

- No quantification is performed and previous attempts to quantify regional wall motion have not been successful. One might draw conclusions on the severity of a stenosis from the stress level the wall motion abnormality occurs; however, since the haemodynamic response to the same dose of dobutamine is very different between different patients and even between two examinations of the same patient, this only provides a rough estimate.

◆ Up to now, no multi-centre studies on dobutamine-CMR have been performed. This might be less important for dobutamine-CMR than for other techniques, e.g. perfusion-CMR, since the data acquisition is highly standardized and robust, and the variability of data interpretation has been assessed in a multi-centre read with good inter-observer-variability. However, a multi-centre trial would enhance the evidence for this technique.

Conclusions

Dobutamine-CMR can be regarded as the imaging method of choice for ischaemia detection in patients with moderate or poor echocardiographic image quality. It provides prognostically relevant information and can be used for functional assessment of viable myocardium with low-dose dobutamine-CMR, in particular in non-transmural scar. This information on viability is readily at hand in all patients with resting wall motion abnormalities referred for ischaemia testing with dobutamine-CMR.

CMR and detection of coronary artery disease: perfusion-CMR

Introduction

While dobutamine-CMR directly visualizes functional consequences of ischaemia, i.e. impaired systolic thickening, perfusion-CMR utilizes a contrast medium (CM) to probe myocardial perfusion and myocardial perfusion reserve, usually during pharmacologically induced hyperaemia. The most commonly used perfusion-CMR method is T1-weighted, dynamic first-pass contrast enhanced imaging with a gadolinium-based CM. This method has been validated in preclinical studies and a large number of clinical single-centre [2, 30–36] and multi-centre studies [37–40], and has become an integral part of the work-up of patients with known or suspected CAD. Perfusion-CMR is typically combined with cine CMR imaging and scar imaging with late gadolinium enhancement (LGE) CMR for a comprehensive assessment of CAD [41–43]. When clinically indicated, viability assessment by low-dose dobutamine-CMR may be added.

This chapter will not address the perfusion techniques BOLD (blood-oxygen level dependent imaging) [44] and arterial spin labelling, which measure perfusion with endogenous contrast. These techniques typically provide a rather flat relationship between myocardial signal and perfusion, and appear therefore limited, at least with current approaches.

Perfusion-CMR techniques

In first-pass perfusion-CMR, the first passage of the CM through the myocardium is visualized and higher CM concentrations result in brighter signal intensities. To achieve this, a conventional Gd-based CM is injected into a brachial vein via a power injector

and simultaneously the CMR acquisition is started to acquire the perfusion data. Motion artefacts are minimized by ECG-triggering ('eliminates' cardiac contraction) and by breath-holding ('eliminates' respiratory motion). To detect haemodynamically relevant hypoperfusion, imaging is performed during hyperaemia, most commonly induced by an intravenous infusion of adenosine at a standard dose of 0.14 mg/kg/min over 3–5 min. Alternative vasodilators in current clinical use are dipyridamole and, more recently, regadenoson. A typical example of a perfusion-CMR study is given in ⊃ Fig. 21.5.

To obtain meaningful first-pass information, the LV myocardium must be covered with several short-axis slices every 1–2 heart beats, its spatial resolution must be adequate to differentiate transmural perfusion differences in the LV wall, and its sensitivity to the CM must yield a several-fold increase in signal vs. baseline during first-pass (recommended 250–300%) [30]. In the past, a large variety of technical approaches have been proposed but now significant consensus has been reached on the basic requirements for a perfusion-CMR pulse sequence [10]:

◆ Saturation–recovery technique (i.e. a 90° preparation pulse for each slice).

◆ Short read-out (≤150 ms).

◆ Coverage of the heart in at least 3 slices/every 1-2 heart beats.

◆ In-plane spatial resolution of <3 mm.

These requirements are typically met by fast-gradient echo-pulse sequences with hybrid-echoplanar read-outs, parallel imaging techniques, or, most recently, by a combination with temporo-spatial acceleration strategies [35, 45].

While induction of hyperaemia by adenosine is relatively straightforward and follows the well-established approach for single-photon emission computed tomography (SPECT), the determination of the optimum CM dose is more challenging. For an ideal CM, the degree of signal intensity change during a perfusion study should be directly proportional to myocardial blood flow. For current CM in use for perfusion-CMR, however, the relationship between myocardial perfusion and signal response in the tissue during CM first-pass is not linear and depends on a variety of factors, including the type of the CMR pulse sequence and the parameters selected, as well as the type and dose of CM. For visual analysis of perfusion-CMR studies, the CM dose should be as high as possible, but it is of particular importance to assure that the pulse sequence used is not susceptible to magnetic field inhomogeneities, which can be induced by high CM concentrations in the LV cavity during first-pass. Currently, doses of 0.075–0.10 mmol/kg are recommended for perfusion-CMR [10], but the use of higher doses of up to 0.15 mmol/kg have been shown to be feasible [38].

Perfusion-CMR protocols for the detection of CAD

All CMR perfusion protocols in CAD aim at the detection of inducible ischaemia. The detection of scar with LGE is usually added and scar tissue is not regarded as ischaemic, even if it

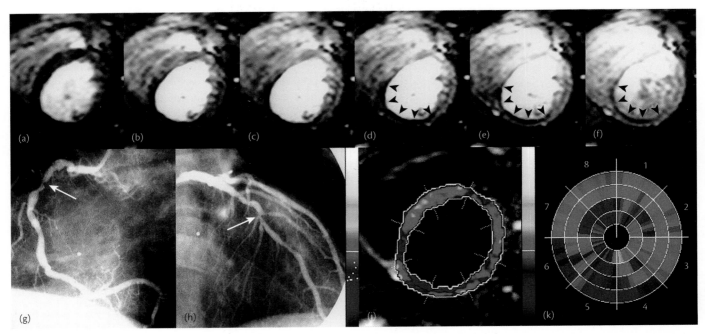

Fig. 21.5 In this patient with a stenosis in the right coronary artery (arrow in g), the transit of CM through the left ventricular myocardium during hyperaemia (time resolution, 4 slices every 1.2 s) demonstrates delayed wash-in in the sub-endocardium of sectors 4 through 6 (arrowheads in d through f). In the corresponding pixelwise parametric slope map (i), the perfusion deficit is demonstrated in blue while normal areas are encoded in red. In (k) a polar map represents perfusion in the sub-endocardium (with the apex located in the centre of the map and the anterior, lateral, inferior, and septal wall represented by sectors 1, 3, 5, and 6 through 8, respectively). The sub-endocardial perfusion deficit in the territory of the right coronary artery extends from base to apex, whereas the perfusion deficit in the anterior and septal wall (sectors 1, 7, and 8) extends from the mid-ventricular level to the apex (slices 3 and 4), in concordance with the stenosis in the mid-portion of the left anterior descending coronary artery (arrow in h).
Reproduced from J. Switter et al, Assessment of Myocardial Perfusion in Coronary Artery Disease by Magnetic Resonance: A Comparison With Positron Emission Tomography and Coronary Angiography, *Circulation*, 103:18, 2230-2235 with permission from Wolters Kluwer Health.

shows a perfusion defect during first-pass perfusion. In principle, detection of CAD can be achieved by a stress-only protocol. If a perfusion abnormality is present during hyperaemia, an LGE acquisition is added to differentiate whether the perfusion deficit is located in viable myocardium or in scar. Perfusion deficits found in viable myocardium are regarded as inducible ischaemia. If such areas represent a substantial amount of myocardium, invasive angiography and revascularization may be indicated [46] (➲ Fig. 21.6). This stress-only perfusion-CMR/LGE protocol matches the principle of the scintigraphic approach, where ischaemic territories are detected on the stress study and the rest injection study visualizes scar tissue through re-distribution of the radio-tracer. A more detailed description of these concepts is available elsewhere [47].

In clinical practice, rest perfusion is often added routinely to the CMR study in patients with CAD. The rest study is used to exclude artefacts, which are frequently found in both stress and rest images, and can thus be discriminated from inducible ischaemia, which occurs at stress only. A stress/rest protocol can also be used for the calculation of the myocardial perfusion reserve (MPR). This strategy follows the concept applied in PET imaging [48]. These various perfusion-CMR strategies (involving various pulse sequences, CM doses, protocols) have consequences with respect to the reading and analysis and post-processing of the data.

Reading and image display

The acquisition of adequate perfusion data requires a high-end scanner, operator skills, and patient cooperation with respect to both, the cessation of medication and caffeine intake, as well as breath-holding during first-pass. Consequently, before reading the perfusion data, images need to be checked for artefacts. The most common artefacts include motion during first-pass, extrasystoles or ECG mis-triggering during first-pass, ghosting, and wrap-around artefacts and can usually be readily identified by an experienced observer. Sub-endocardial dark-rim artefact, caused primarily by susceptibility effects, can be more challenging to differentiate from a true perfusion defect. However, this type of artefact is a consistent feature of the pulse sequence and CM strategy used and is not expected to differ substantially between patients. It can, therefore, be minimized by adequate tailoring of the pulse sequence, shimming of the magnet, and administration of a correct CM dose for the pulse sequence used. Dark-rim artefacts also typically occur *before* CM arrival in the myocardium, usually allowing differentiation from true perfusion defects. Even with an appropriate set-up, 6–15% of CMR perfusion studies have inadequate quality, as reported in large multi-centre trials [38, 47]. The influence of data quality on diagnostic performance is illustrated in ➲ Fig. 21.7.

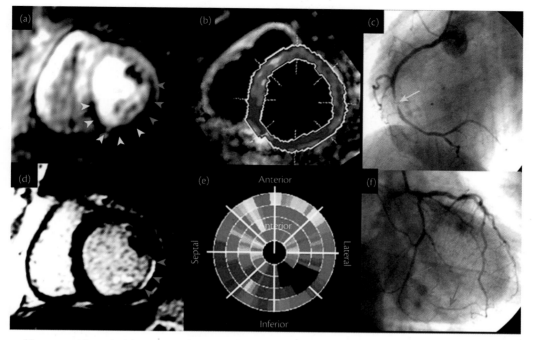

Fig. 21.6 In a 48-year-old woman with atypical chest pain and dyspnoea during exercise, a first-pass perfusion MR study (a) reveals a perfusion deficit in the sub-endocardial layer of the inferior wall extending into the basal portion of the septum and the lateral wall. A parametric map (b) demonstrates contrast medium wash-in kinetics for the slice shown in (a). On this parametric map, linear upslope data above/below the threshold (mean of controls minus 1.75 SD) are encoded in shades of red and blue, respectively. The sub-endocardial zone of hypoperfusion is also detected by the computer algorithm. Subsequent conventional X-ray coronary angiography confirmed stenosis of the right coronary artery (c). In the same patient delayed enhancement MR imaging (d) reveals a small sub-endocardial infarction in the lateral wall (bright zone), while viable myocardium appears dark. A polar map representation of perfusion is shown in (e) (with colour-encoding as given in b). In addition, the zone of infarction is depicted as black area in the lateral wall. Note that polar map representation of perfusion and viability/scar is given for the sub-endocardial layer (inner half of myocardial wall). In addition to the stenosis in the right coronary artery (c), conventional X-ray coronary angiography demonstrates an occluded branch of the circumflex coronary artery (arrows) with retrograde filling (f).
Reproduced from J. Switter et al, Assessment of Myocardial Perfusion in Coronary Artery Disease by Magnetic Resonance: A Comparison With Positron Emission Tomography and Coronary Angiography, *Circulation*, 103:18, 2230-2235 with permission from Wolters Kluwer Health.

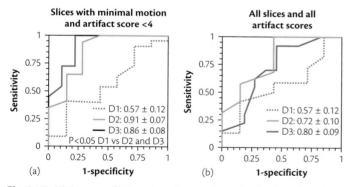

Fig. 21.7 ROC curves of MR upslope data are shown for the detection of coronary artery disease (≥50% diameter stenosis in ≥1 vessel by quantitative coronary angiography). MR upslope data from the sub-endocardial layer are highly reliable in the detection of disease when analysis is restricted to the 3 slices with minimal motion and the patients with adequate image quality. Numbers within the plots represent area under the ROC curve ± standard error for doses 1, 2, and 3 (= D1, D2, D3, respectively). AUC of dose 2 for the entire data (all slices, all quality scores, (b) was worst ($P < 0.05$ vs. dose 2 in (a)). A dose of 0.05 mmol/kg (= D1) performed inadequately in all analyses.
Reproduced from Giang TH et al, Detection of coronary artery disease by magnetic resonance myocardial perfusion imaging with various contrast medium doses: First European multi-centre experience. *Eur Heart J* 2004;25:1657–65 with permission from Oxford University Press.

In clinical practice, perfusion-CMR studies are usually analysed visually, by reviewing all available data (stress and rest and LGE) side-by-side, but other analysis methods are available. ⊃ Figure 21.8 shows the various levels for data analysis and it also addresses the issue of observer-interference with the data. Clearly, a fully automatic analysis is the ultimate aim, but for such analysis to be implemented in clinical routine, further improvement and standardization of perfusion-CMR techniques is required.

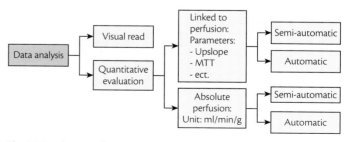

Fig. 21.8 Schematic for perfusion data analysis. MTT: mean transit time.

Diagnostic criteria

If image quality is adequate, perfusion abnormalities are typically evaluated in a 16-segment model of the LV (excluding the apical segment 17). In each segment the inflow of CM during hyperaemic conditions is assessed as reduced, if the signal at peak effect of the CM bolus is reduced (dark-grey) or delayed in the sub-endocardial layer in comparison to either the sub-epicardial layer of the same segment or in comparison to non-affected segments (in case of transmural perfusion deficits) [35, 40, 49, 50]. Additional criteria indicative for true hypoperfusion vs. artefacts are sub-endocardial signal reduction persisting longer than the CM first-pass through the LV cavity, signal reduction in several slices and neighbouring regions, and absence of breathing motion and triggering artefacts during CM first-pass [40, 49]. The perfusion defects should be described as sub-endocardial or transmural.

Perfusion abnormalities must be assessed in relation to the presence of scar tissue as detected by LGE. If hypoperfusion is detected in viable (LGE-negative) tissue, these segments will be reported as 'ischaemic' segments, whereas 'perfusion abnormalities' in scar (i.e. LGE-positive) tissue will be reported as scar tissue, and are not expected to benefit from revascularization. Since accumulation of CM in scarred tissue begins immediately after the contrast passage in the stress study, resting scans frequently do not show perfusion abnormalities in these segments.

When applying quantitative measures to detect ischaemia, a frequently used measure is the upslope of the signal–intensity–time profiles of the contrast passage [30, 31, 33, 36, 38]. This method has shown adequate reproducibility [38, 51] but thresholds depend on the perfusion method and contrast regime used. In one study, segmental upslope values of 1.75 standard deviations below the mean of healthy sub-endomyocardium yielded good sensitivities and specificities to detect ≥50% diameter coronary stenoses of 83–87% and 75–85%, respectively [36, 38]. Other parameters, such as time-to-peak, time-to-start, or peak signal intensity, are less robust and accurate, and should not be used [52]. Fully quantitative analysis methods, which estimate absolute myocardial blood flow in mg/ml/min are in development, but not currently used in clinical reporting.

Diagnostic performance

First-pass perfusion CMR imaging was validated in animal studies in the 1990s [53–55]. Soon thereafter, first single-centre studies in humans confirmed the feasibility of this approach in a clinical setting (⊃ Table 21.2 and ⊃ Fig. 21.9). With state-of-the-art techniques, detection of CAD (defined anatomically by QCA) is typically achieved with sensitivities and specificities ranging from 73% to 93%, and specificities ranging from 62% to 94%, as shown in ⊃ Table 21.2. A recent meta-analysis of perfusion CMR studies showed an average sensitivity of 89% and a specificity of 76% [56]. The largest single-centre study to date was reported by Greenwood and co-workers [50]. In this prospective study, 628 patients with suspected CAD underwent perfusion-CMR as part of a multi-parametric CMR study, gated-SPECT, and invasive coronary angiography. CMR in this study showed a sensitivity of 87% and a specificity of 83% to detect stenoses ≥50% on quantitative coronary angiography (QCA) with an AUC of 0.89 for all patients and 0.91 in the multi-vessel disease population. SPECT resulted in a sensitivity of 67%, specificity of 83% and AUC of 0.74. The multi-centre MR-IMPACT study involved 241 patients from 18 centres and all major CMR vendors closely matching the real clinical situation [40]. The study yielded an AUC of 0.86, a sensitivity of 85% (95% CI: 69–93%) and a specificity of 67% (95% CI: 35–89%) for the best dose applied in a subgroup of 42 patients. Importantly, perfusion-CMR in MR-IMPACT proved robust with a low exclusion rate of 2.2% and was safe with no major complications [40]. Subsequently, the larger MR-IMPACT II study of 465 patients was performed in 33 centres [57, 58]. At a single sensitivity/specificity point, CMR had a sensitivity of 67% and a specificity of 61% with an AUC of 0.75 for all patients and 0.80 in the multi-vessel disease population. SPECT resulted in a sensitivity of 59%, specificity of 72% and AUC of 0.65.

Prognostic value of perfusion-CMR

A normal perfusion-CMR test predicts a low event rate. The first study that reported outcome by perfusion-CMR showed

Table 21.2 Performance of perfusion-CMR (1.5 T systems)

	n	Protocol	CM (dose)	Acquisition	Analysis	Reference	AUC	Sens.	Spec.
Major Single Centre Studies *									
Schwitter et al. [36]	57	stress-only	Gd-DTPA-BMA	hybrid EP	upslope	QCA	0.91	87%	85%
vs. QCA		Dip	0.1 mmol/kg	same SR/slice	Sub-endo stress	≥50% stenosis			
vs. PET						13NH$_3$-PET	0.93	91%	94%
						CFR <1.7			
Nagel et al. [31]	84	stress-rest	Gd-DTPA	hybrid EP	upslope	QCA	0.93	88%	90%
		Adeno	0.025 mmol/kg	variable SR/slice	MPRI	≥75% area stenosis			
Paetsch et al. [2]	79	stress-rest	Gd-BOPTA	hybrid EP	visual	QCA	-	91%	62%
		Adeno	0.05 mmol/kg	same SR/slice	stress + rest	≥50% stenosis			

	n	Protocol	CM (dose)	Acquisition	Analysis	Reference	AUC	Sens.	Spec.
Gebker et al. [80]	40	stress-rest	Gd-DTPA	SSFP	visual	QCA	-	86%	78%
		Adeno	0.05 mmol/kg	k-t-Blast	stress-rest	≥50% stenosis			
					upslope		0.83	78%	71%
Ishida et al. [32]	104	stress-rest	Gd-DTPA	hybrid EP	visual	QCA	0.90	90%	85%
		Dip + handgrip	0.075 mmol/kg	same SR/slice	stress + rest	≥70% stenosis			
Sakuma et al. [81]	40	rest-stress	Gd-DTPA	fast-GRE	visual	QCA	0.85	70%	61%
		Dip	0.03 mmol/kg			≥70% stenosis			
Plein et al. [35]	54	stress-only	Gadobutrol	hybrid EP	visual	QCA	0.85	-	-
		Adeno	0.1 mmol/kg	k-t-Sense	stress	≥50% stenosis			
Plein et al. [33]	35	stress-only	Gadobutrol	hybrid EP	visual	QCA	0.80	-	-
		Adeno	0.1 mmol/kg	k-t-Sense	stress	≥50% stenosis			
Klem et al. [82] All females	92	stress-rest	Gadoversetamide	hybrid EP or	visual	QCA	0.91	84%	88%
		Adeno	0.065 mmol/kg	sense fast-GRE	stress + rest	≥70% stenosis			
				same SR/slice	plus LGE	≥50% for left main			
Merkle et al. [83]	256	stress-rest	Gd-DTPA	Sense SSFP	visual	QCA	-	91%	82%
		Adeno	0.1 mmol/kg	same SR/slice	stress + rest	≥50% stenosis			
Females	77						-	91%	91%
Males	179						-	91%	74%
Watkins et al. [84]	103	stress-rest	Gd-DTPA-BMA	fast-GRE	visual	FFR <075	-	91%	82%
		Adeno	0.1 mmol/kg	SR	stress + rest				
Bettencourt et al. [85]	103	stress-rest	Gadobutrol	fast-GRE	visual	FFR <0.75	-	93%	85%
		Adeno	0.07 mmol/kg	SR	stress + rest	FFR <0.80	-	89%	86%
					plus LGE				
Greenwood et al. [50]	628	stress-rest	Gd-DTPA	Sense fast-GRE	visual	QCA	0.84	82%	86%
		Adeno	0.05 mmol/kg	variable SR/slice	stress + rest	≥50% stenosis			
Multi-Centre Trials									
Wolff et al. [37] monitored	99 3 centres Single vendor	stress-rest Adeno	Gd-DTPA-BMA 0.15 mmol/kg	hybrid EP same SR/slice	visual stress + Rest	QCA ≥50% stenosis	0.83	-	-
Giang et al. [38] monitored	99 3 centres Single vendor	stress-only Adeno	Gd-DTPA-BMA 0.1 mmol/kg	hybrid EP same SR/slice	upslope subendo stress	QCA ≥50% stenosis	0.91	91%	78%
Kitagawa et al. [39]	50 3 centres Single vendor	stress-rest ATP	Gd-DTPA 0.05 mmol/kg	hybrid EP same SR/slice	visual stress + Rest	QCA ≥50% stenosis	0.88	86%	75%
Schwitter et al. [40] 'MR-IMPACT' monitored	228 18 centres Multi-vendor	stress-only Adeno	Gd-DTPA-BMA 0.1 mmol/kg	hybrid EP or fast-GRE same SR/slice	visual stress only	QCA ≥50% stenosis	0.86	85%	67%
Schwitter et al. [49, 57] 'MR-IMPACT II' monitored	425 33 centres Multi-vendor	stress-only Adeno	Gd-DTPA-BMA 0.075 mmol/kg	hybrid EP or fast-GRE same SR/slice	visual stress-only	QCA ≥50% stenosis	0.75	0.67	0.61

* Smaller single centre studies (*n*<35), studies using visual assessment of coronary stenosis degree, and studies with start of patient recruitment before 1995 (e.g. the WISE studies) and/or outdated sequences (e.g. inversion recovery) are not considered.

Monitored: trials were monitored by regulatory bodies (Food and Drug Administration (FDA) and European Medicines Agency (EMEA)).

Dip: dipyridamole: 0.56 mg/kg for 4 min; Adeno: adenosine: 0.14 mg/kg/min for 3 min; ATP: 0.14 mg/kg/min for 3 min; SR: saturation recovery preparation of magnetization; hybrid EP: hybrid echo-planar acquisition; fast-GRE: fast gradient-echo acquisition; QCA: quantitative coronary angiography; trans: full wall thickness considered in analysis; sub-endo: inner half of wall thickness considered for analysis; MPRI: myocardial perfusion reserve index; AUC: area under the receiver-operator characteristics curve.

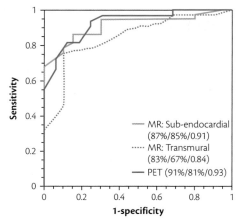

Fig. 21.9 ROC curves of MR upslope data are shown for the detection of coronary artery disease defined anatomically by quantitative coronary angiography (≥1 artery with ≥50% diameter stenosis; n = 57). MR upslope data, particularly from the sub-endocardial layer, are highly reliable in the detection of haemodynamically significant disease. In the detection of ≥50% diameter stenoses, the diagnostic performance of MR and PET are comparable. Numbers in parentheses represent sensitivity, specificity, and area under the ROC curve, respectively.

Reproduced from J. Switter et al, Assessment of Myocardial Perfusion in Coronary Artery Disease by Magnetic Resonance: A Comparison With Positron Emission Tomography and Coronary Angiography, *Circulation*, 103:18, 2230–5 with permission from Wolters Kluwer Health.

a rate of major adverse cardiac events (MACE) of 0.7% in the first year and 0.8%/year over a 3-year period after a normal test [28]. A similar prognostic value of a normal perfusion-CMR study was observed for men and women with annual MACE (death or new acute MI) of 0.3% and 1.1%, respectively, while ischaemia on perfusion-CMR carried a risk for MACE of 15.1% and 10.8%, respectively (difference between men and women not significant) [59]. In a large single-centre cohort, 1,152 patients with stable angina and known CAD (34% with a history of MI and 50% with a history of revascularizations) or with stable angina but without known CAD underwent perfusion-CMR for ischaemia detection [60]. MACE were as low as 1.0%/year in patients without ischaemia on perfusion-CMR over a follow-up period of 4.2 years, whereas MACE were 3.9%/year in patients positive on perfusion-CMR. Finally, in the European CMR registry, a network of 57 centres in 15 countries, a prospective protocol on the prognosis of ischaemia detection by CMR is ongoing. In an interim analysis of 1,706 cases with a completed follow-up of 1 year, MACE (all-cause death, non-fatal MI, and aborted sudden cardiac death) was 1%/year in patients with a normal CMR examination (= no ischaemia and no scar), whereas MACE was 2.5%/year (*P*<0.009) in patients with abnormal findings on either perfusion or LGE [61]. Thus, perfusion-CMR appears to be an excellent test to exclude prognostically relevant CAD.

Perfusion-CMR also confers prognostic information in the acute setting. In one study, a negative perfusion-CMR study showed a 100% sensitivity and a positive perfusion-CMR study a 91% specificity to predict future adverse cardiac events (= MI, death, CAD on invasive coronary angiography, pathological SPECT during a 1-year follow-up) [62].

The fact that perfusion-CMR performs similarly well as SPECT and that there is also prognostic value suggests that perfusion-CMR is now a valuable tool in the work-up of suspected CAD. Accordingly, CMR and, in particular, ischaemia detection by CMR, is recommended at the same level as other imaging techniques, such as stress-echo or stress SPECT, for the work-up of heart failure patients in the most recent guidelines of the European Society of Cardiology [63].

Cost-effectiveness of ischaemia detection by CMR

In a subset of patients in the European CMR registry, who underwent ischaemia testing by CMR, costs were calculated and compared with an invasive strategy to detect CAD. Of the 2,717 patients studied, 21% were positive for CAD (ischaemia and/or infarct scar), 73% negative, and 6% were uncertain and underwent additional testing. Compared with an invasive approach, the CMR strategy led to cost-savings in the public sectors of the German, United Kingdom, and Swiss healthcare systems of 50%, 25%, and 23%, respectively [64]. Another study assessed the cost-effectiveness of CMR in the emergency department and demonstrated cost-savings of approximately 35% over a 1-year follow-up when patients with suspected acute coronary syndrome (no ST elevations, normal initial troponin) were referred to CMR, compared with routine in-hospital work-up [65]. This cost-saving was obtained without a difference in clinical outcome in the two patient groups and was explained mainly by the facts that (1) hospitalization could be avoided in approximately 80% of the CMR group and (2) after discharge, i.e. during the 1-year follow-up, costs continued to decrease in the CMR group.

Limitations

A major limitation of CMR today remains its restricted availability. Along with this goes a heterogeneous and sometimes inadequate situation in Europe with regard to reimbursement of CMR studies. Recent and future evidence on cost-effectiveness of CMR should help to improve these financial aspects in the near future. In addition to these health-economical obstacles, CMR has a number of important contraindications, as given in ○ Table 21.3. These contraindications include many implantable devices. However, the first MR-compatible pacemaker obtained approval from the European Medicines Agency (EMEA) for marketing in December 2008. A recent multi-centre trial confirmed a high image quality of CMR studies in >95% of patients with implanted pacemakers [66]. It is expected that an increasing number of MR-compatible electronic devices, including ICDs, will be available in the near future.

Future developments

Perfusion-CMR is still a demanding technique, and with an increasing request for such studies, the need for well-trained cardiac

Table 21.3 Contraindications for CMR

Absolute contraindications:

- Active devices such as most pacemakers[1], ICDs, insulin pumps, and other electronic devices
- Metallic foreign bodies in the eyes, perform orbital x-ray in unclear cases

Relative contraindication

- Claustrophobia

MR-conditional

- Most of currently implanted stents, heart valves, sternum suture wires, cardiac closure and occluder devices, filters, embolization coils (at least up to 1.5T)
- MR-conditional pacemakers [86]

Contraindications for dobutamine-CMR

- Severe arterial hypertension (> 220/120 mmHg)
- Unstable angina pectoris
- Acute myocardial infarction
- Severe aortic stenosis (AVA <1cm²)
- Hypertrophic obstructive CMP
- Acute perimyocarditis or endocarditis
- Glaucoma

Contraindications for perfusion-CMR

- Contraindications for adenosine or dipyridamole infusion 2nd and 3rd degree AV-Block, trifascicular block, chronic obstructive pulmonary disease
- Allergy against vasodilator
- Allergy against contrast medium
- Contraindication for gadolinium-chelate contrast media²: Severe renal impairment (GFR <30ml/min/1.73m²). Relative contraindication: (GFR 30-60ml/min/1.73m²)

Adapted with permission from [68].

[1] MR-compatible pacemakers are in clinical use. Always check safety of a device on www.mr-safety-com

² Gd-chelates (primarily linear compounds) can cause nephrogenic systemic fibrosis (NSF) in patients with severe renal impairment. Approximately 335 cases of NSF were reported until Nov. 2009 out of a total of approximately 200 Mio. administrations. For more detailed information, also [68].

imagers will also increase and with it the need for ongoing standardization of training [67] and of CMR applications. Generally accepted protocols are available and will be updated as the technique progresses (⊃ Fig. 21.10) [10, 68]. Technically, recent years have seen a trend towards higher-resolution perfusion-CMR [35]. One study of 100 patients has suggested that high-resolution CMR may improve the overall diagnostic performance of the method further [69]. High-resolution perfusion-CMR may also prove beneficial for (semi)-automatic analysis of perfusion data, which would consequently improve post-processing reproducibility. First fully automated software approaches based on the transmural gradient are becoming available [70]. When exploiting the very fast temporo-spatial acceleration strategies that have also allowed high-resolution perfusion-CMR [35, 45], it has also become possible to acquire 3D perfusion data covering the entire heart at every heart beat. Methods for 3D perfusion-CMR have been proposed at 1.5T [71] and 3T [72] with promising initial results. Future multi-centre trials are warranted to evaluate the robustness of these accelerated 3D techniques and to show superiority with respect to diagnostic and prognostic performance versus 'conventional' 2D perfusion-CMR.

An increase in field strength by moving from 1.5T to 3T is accompanied by a better signal-to-noise ratio, which could be particularly useful for fast imaging, as needed for perfusion-CMR. However, the number of 3T CMR systems remains relatively low as shown in the European CMR registry data, where currently less than 6% of all CMR exams are performed on 3T systems [61]. Furthermore, perfusion-CMR at 1.5T is already very mature and it may be difficult to demonstrate a clinically significant improvement in diagnostic performance of CMR at 3T in adequately powered studies (see ⊃ Fig. 21.11) [35].

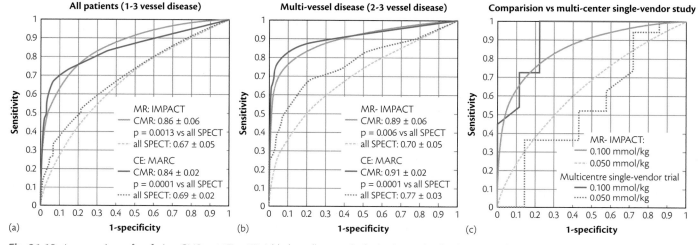

Comparison of perfusion-CMR vs single-photon emission computed tomography for the detection of coronary artery disease

All patients (1-3 vessel disease)

MR: IMPACT
— CMR: 0.86 ± 0.06
p = 0.0013 vs all SPECT
······ all SPECT: 0.67 ± 0.05
CE: MARC
— CMR: 0.84 ± 0.02
p = 0.0001 vs all SPECT
······ all SPECT: 0.69 ± 0.02

Multi-vessel disease (2-3 vessel disease)

MR- IMPACT
— CMR: 0.89 ± 0.06
p = 0.006 vs all SPECT
······ all SPECT: 0.70 ± 0.05
CE: MARC
— CMR: 0.91 ± 0.02
p = 0.0001 vs all SPECT
······ all SPECT: 0.77 ± 0.03

Comparison vs multi-center single-vendor study

MR- IMPACT:
— 0.100 mmol/kg
······ 0.050 mmol/kg
Multicentre single-vendor trial
— 0.100 mmol/kg
······ 0.050 mmol/kg

(a) 1-specificity   (b) 1-specificity   (c) 1-specificity

Fig. 21.10 A comparison of perfusion-CMR at 1.5T vs 3T yielded excellent results for both tests for the detection of coronary artery disease. With current techniques the perfusion data at 1.5T are of high quality, and the 3T approach yielded similar results (area under the ROC curve not different, a). In (b) an example is shown in a patient with perfusion deficits inferior and lateral, and a small deficit anterior. The coronary angiography confirmed a high grade stenosis in the LCX, occluded RCA, and several minor lesions in the LAD. Reproduced from [35] with kind permission from Radiology.

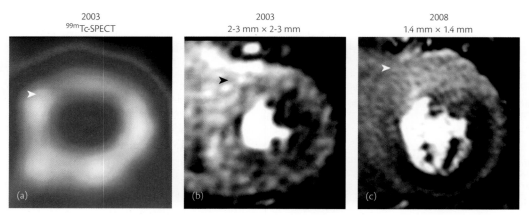

Fig. 21.11 Illustrates the impact of spatial resolution of perfusion data. A SPECT acquisition to the left (a) shows no clear perfusion deficit in this patient with a proven stenosis of >50% in the distal circumflex coronary artery. In the same patient, a perfusion-CMR study with higher in-plane spatial resolution (b) can resolve signal from the hypoperfused lateral wall and the anterior papillary muscle. The nominal resolution of perfusion-CMR is preserved due to elimination of cardiac and respiratory motion during acquisition (ECG-triggering and breath-holding). Newer perfusion-CMR techniques exploiting temporo-spatial correlations of data allow for high resolution imaging at 1.5T (c). This allows for excellent discrimination of intramural perfusion differences (patient in c is not the same as in a and b). The arrow head marks the anterior insertion of the right ventricular wall into the interventricular septum.
Reproduced from [35] with kind permission from the European Society of Cardiology and the American Society of Radiology, respectively.

Conclusions

Perfusion-CMR has matured to a reliable technique for the assessment of CAD. It detects and excludes CAD with a high diagnostic performance. There is also increasing evidence from single-centre studies and the European CMR registry for the high prognostic value of ischaemia detection by perfusion-CMR and a normal CMR study in patients with or without known CAD predicts a rate for MACE of 0.3–1%/year. In addition, European CMR registry data suggest substantial cost-savings when using CMR for the work-up of patients with suspected CAD. Since CMR lacks radiation exposure of patients, repetitive examinations can be safely performed, even in women of lower age. Accordingly, the evidence is now robust to recommend perfusion-CMR for the work-up of patients with suspected or known CAD, as well as for patients with heart failure, in particular when combined with an assessment of contractile function and viability.

References

1. Hendel RC, Patel MR, Kramer CM, et al. ACCF/ACR/SCCT/SCMR/ASNC/NASCI/SCAI/SIR 2006 appropriateness criteria for cardiac computed tomography and cardiac magnetic resonance imaging: a report of the American College of Cardiology Foundation Quality Strategic Directions Committee Appropriateness Criteria Working Group, American College of Radiology, Society of Cardiovascular Computed Tomography, Society for Cardiovascular Magnetic Resonance, American Society of Nuclear Cardiology, North American Society for Cardiac Imaging, Society for Cardiovascular Angiography and Interventions, and Society of Interventional Radiology. *J Am Coll Cardiol* 2006; 48: 1475–97.

2. Paetsch I, Jahnke C, Wahl A, et al. Comparison of dobutamine stress magnetic resonance, adenosine stress magnetic resonance, and adenosine stress magnetic resonance perfusion. *Circulation* 2004; 110: 835–42.

3. Fihn SD, Gardin JM, Abrams J, et al. ACCF/AHA/ACP/AATS/PCNA/SCAI/STS guideline for the diagnosis and management of patients with stable ischemic heart disease: A report of the American College of Cardiology Foundation/American Heart Association Task Force on Practice Guidelines, and the American College of Physicians, American Association for Thoracic Surgery, Preventive Cardiovascular Nurses Association, Society for Cardiovascular Angiography and Interventions, and Society of Thoracic Surgeons. *J Am Coll Cardiol* 2012; 60: e44–e164.

4. Montalescot G, Sechtem U, Achenbach S, et al. 2013 ESC guidelines on the management of stable coronary artery disease: The Task Force on the management of stable coronary artery disease of the European Society of Cardiology. *Eur Heart J* 2013; 34:2949–3003.

5. Boden WE, O'Rourke RA, Teo KK, et al; Group CTR. Optimal medical therapy with or without PCI for stable coronary disease. *N Engl J Med* 2007; 356: 1503–16.

6. Tonino PA, De Bruyne B, Pijls NH, et al; Investigators FS. Fractional flow reserve versus angiography for guiding percutaneous coronary intervention. *N Engl J Med* 2009; 360: 213–24.

7. Patel MR, Peterson ED, Dai D, et al. Low diagnostic yield of elective coronary angiography. *N Engl J Med* 2010; 362: 886–95.

8. Schalla S, Klein C, Paetsch I, et al. Real-time MR image acquisition during high-dose dobutamine hydrochloride stress for detecting left ventricular wall-motion abnormalities in patients with coronary arterial disease. *Radiology* 2002; 224: 845–51.

9. Nagel E, Lorenz C, Baer F, et al. Stress cardiovascular magnetic resonance: Consensus panel report. *J Cardiovasc Magn Reson* 2001; 3: 267–81.

10. Kramer CM, Barkhausen J, Flamm SD, et al. Society for Cardiovascular Magnetic Resonance Board of Trustees Task Force on Standardized Protocols. Standardized cardiovascular magnetic resonance (CMR) protocols 2013 update. *J Cardiovasc Magn Reson* 2013;15:91.

11. Wahl A, Paetsch I, Gollesch A, et al. Safety and feasibility of high-dose dobutamine-atropine stress cardiovascular magnetic resonance for diagnosis of myocardial ischaemia: Experience in 1000 consecutive cases. *Eur Heart J* 2004; 25: 1230–36.

12. Nagel E, Lehmkuhl HB, Bocksch W, et al. Noninvasive diagnosis of ischemia-induced wall motion abnormalities with the use of high-dose dobutamine stress MRI: comparison with dobutamine stress echocardiography. *Circulation* 1999; 99: 763–70.

13. Wahl A, Paetsch I, Roethemeyer S, Klein C, Fleck E, Nagel E. High-dose dobutamine-atropine stress cardiovascular MR imaging after coronary revascularization in patients with wall motion abnormalities at rest. *Radiology* 2004; 233: 210–16.

14. Hundley WG, Hamilton CA, Thomas MS, et al. Utility of fast cine magnetic resonance imaging and display for the detection of myocardial ischaemia in patients not well suited for second harmonic stress echocardiography. *Circulation* 1999; 100: 1697–1702.

15. Nagel E, Lehmkuhl HB, Klein C, et al. [Influence of image quality on the diagnostic accuracy of dobutamine stress magnetic resonance imaging in comparison with dobutamine stress echocardiography for the noninvasive detection of myocardial ischaemia]. *Z Kardiol* 1999; 88: 622–30.

16. Paetsch I, Jahnke C, Ferrari VA, et al. Determination of interobserver variability for identifying inducible left ventricular wall motion abnormalities during dobutamine stress magnetic resonance imaging. *Eur Heart J* 2006; 27: 1459–64.

17. Nandalur KR, Dwamena BA, Choudhri AF, Nandalur MR, Carlos RC. Diagnostic performance of stress cardiac magnetic resonance imaging in the detection of coronary artery disease: A meta-analysis. *J Am Coll Cardiol* 2007; 50: 1343–53.

18. Gebker R, Jahnke C, Hucko T, et al. Dobutamine stress magnetic resonance imaging for the detection of coronary artery disease in women. *Heart* 2010; 96: 616–20.

19. Puntmann VO, Nagel E, Hughes AD, et al. Gender-specific differences in myocardial deformation and aortic stiffness at rest and dobutamine stress. *Hypertension* 2012; 59: 712–18.

20. Korosoglou G, Lehrke S, Wochele A, et al. Strain-encoded CMR for the detection of inducible ischaemia during intermediate stress. *JACC Cardiovascular Imaging* 2010; 3: 361–71.

21. Korosoglou G, Gitsioudis G, Voss A, et al. Strain-encoded cardiac magnetic resonance during high-dose dobutamine stress testing for the estimation of cardiac outcomes: Comparison to clinical parameters and conventional wall motion readings. *J Am Coll Cardiol* 2011; 58: 1140–49.

22. Schuster A, Kutty S, Padiyath A, et al. Cardiovascular magnetic resonance myocardial feature tracking detects quantitative wall motion during dobutamine stress. *J Cardiovasc Magn Reson* 2011; 13: 58.

23. Gebker R, Jahnke C, Manka R, et al. High spatial resolution myocardial perfusion imaging during high dose dobutamine/atropine stress magnetic resonance using k-t sense. *Int J Cardiol* 2012; 158: 411–16.

24. Wellnhofer E, Olariu A, Klein C, et al. Magnetic resonance low-dose dobutamine test is superior to scar quantification for the prediction of functional recovery. *Circulation* 2004; 109: 2172–74.

25. Gutberlet M, Frohlich M, Mehl S, et al. Myocardial viability assessment in patients with highly impaired left ventricular function: Comparison of delayed enhancement, dobutamine stress MRI, end-diastolic wall thickness, and TL201-SPECT with functional recovery after revascularization. *Eur Radiol* 2005; 15: 872–80.

26. Schuster A, Morton G, Chiribiri A, et al. Imaging in the management of ischemic cardiomyopathy: special focus on magnetic resonance. *J Am Coll Cardiol* 2012;59(4):359–70.

27. Hundley WG, Morgan TM, Neagle CM, Hamilton CA, Rerkpattanapipat P, Link KM. Magnetic resonance imaging determination of cardiac prognosis. *Circulation* 2002; 106: 2328–33.

28. Jahnke C, Nagel E, Gebker R, et al. Prognostic value of cardiac magnetic resonance stress tests. Adenosine stress perfusion and dobutamine stress wall motion imaging. *Circulation* 2007; 115: 1769–76.

29. Kelle S, Nagel E, Voss A, et al. A bi-center cardiovascular magnetic resonance prognosis study focusing on dobutamine wall motion and late gadolinium enhancement in 3138 consecutive patients. *J Am Coll Cardiol* 2013; 61: 2310–12.

30. Bertschinger KM, Nanz D, Buechi M, et al. Magnetic resonance myocardial first-pass perfusion imaging: Parameter optimization for signal response and cardiac coverage. *J Magn Reson Imaging* 2001; 14: 556–62.

31. Nagel E, Klein C, Paetsch I, et al. Magnetic resonance perfusion measurements for the noninvasive detection of coronary artery disease. *Circulation* 2003; 108: 432–37.

32. Ishida N, Sakuma H, Motoyasu M, et al. Noninfarcted myocardium: Correlation between dynamic first-pass contrast-enhanced myocardial MR imaging and quantitative coronary angiography. *Radiology* 2003; 229: 209–16.

33. Plein S, Kozerke S, Suerder D, Luescher TF, Boesiger P, Schwitter J. High spatial resolution myocardial perfusion cardiac MR imaging for the detection of coronary artery disease. *Eur Heart J* 2008; 29: 2148–55.

34. Klem I, Heitner JF, Shah DJ, et al. Improved detection of coronary artery disease by stress perfusion cardiovascular magnetic resonance with the use of delayed enhancement infarction imaging. *J Am Coll Cardiol* 2006; 47: 1630–38.

35. Plein S, Schwitter J, Suerder D, Greenwood J, Boesiger P, Kozerke S. K-t sense-accelerated myocardial perfusion MR imaging at 3.0 tesla—comparison with 1.5 tesla. *Radiology* 2008; 249: 493–500.

36. Schwitter J, Nanz D, Kneifel S, et al. Assessment of myocardial perfusion in coronary artery disease by magnetic resonance: a comparison with positron emission tomography and coronary angiography. *Circulation* 2001; 103: 2230–35.

37. Wolff SD, Schwitter J, Coulden R, et al. Myocardial first-pass perfusion magnetic resonance imaging: a multicenter dose-ranging study. *Circulation* 2004; 110: 732–37.

38. Giang TH, Nanz D, Coulden R, et al. Detection of coronary artery disease by magnetic resonance myocardial perfusion imaging with various contrast medium doses: First European multi-centre experience. *Eur Heart J* 2004; 25: 1657–65.

39. Kitagawa K, Sakuma H, Nagata M, et al. Diagnostic accuracy of stress myocardial perfusion MRI and late gadolinium-enhanced MRI for detecting flow-limiting coronary artery disease: a multicenter study. *Eur Radiol* 2008; 18: 2808–16.

40. Schwitter J, Wacker C, van Rossum A, et al. MR-impact: comparison of perfusion-cardiac magnetic resonance with single-photon emission computed tomography for the detection of coronary artery disease in a multicentre, multivendor, randomized trial. *Eur Heart J* 2008; 29: 480–89.

41. Schwitter J, Saeed M, Wendland MF, et al. Influence of severity of myocardial injury on distribution of macromolecules: extravascular versus intravascular gadolinium-based magnetic resonance contrast agents. *J Am Coll Cardiol* 1997; 30: 1086–94.

42. Kim RJ, Wu E, Rafael A, et al. The use of contrast-enhanced magnetic resonance imaging to identify reversible myocardial dysfunction. *N Engl J Med* 2000; 343: 1445–53.

43. Klein C, Nekolla SG, Bengel FM, et al. Assessment of myocardial viability with contrast-enhanced magnetic resonance imaging: comparison with positron emission tomography. *Circulation* 2002; 105: 162–67.

44. Fieno DS, Shea SM, Li Y, Harris KR, Finn JP, Li D. Myocardial perfusion imaging based on the blood oxygen level-dependent effect using T2-prepared steady-state free-precession magnetic resonance imaging. *Circulation* 2004; 110: 1284–90.

45. Kellman P, Derbyshire JA, Agyeman KO, McVeigh ER, Arai AE. Extended coverage of first-pass perfusion imaging using slice-interleaved TSENSE. *Magn Reson Med* 2004; 51: 200–204.

46. Task Force on Myocardial Revascularization of the European Society of Cardiology, the European Association for Cardio-Thoracic Surgery, European Association for Percutaneous Cardiovascular Interventions; Wijns W, Kolh P, Danchin N, et al. Guidelines on myocardial revascularization. *Eur Heart J* 2010; 31: 2501–55.

47. Schwitter J. Myocardial perfusion imaging by cardiac magnetic resonance. *J Nuc Cardiol* 2006; 13: 841–54.

48. Schwaiger M. Myocardial perfusion imaging with PET. *J Nucl Med* 1994; 35: 693–98.

49. Schwitter J, Wacker C, Wilke N, et al; Investigators ftM-I. Superior diagnostic performance of perfusion-cardiovascular magnetic resonance versus SPECT to detect coronary artery disease: the secondary endpoints of the multicenter multivendor MR-impact II (magnetic resonance imaging for myocardial perfusion assessment in coronary artery disease trial). *J Cardiovascular Magnetic Resonance* 202; 14: 61.

50. Greenwood JP, Maredia N, Younger JF, et al. Cardiovascular magnetic resonance and single-photon emission computed tomography for diagnosis of coronary heart disease (CE-MARC): a prospective trial. *The Lancet* 2011; 379: 453–60.

51. Larghat AM, Maredia N, Biglands J, et al. Reproducibility of first-pass cardiovascular magnetic resonance myocardial perfusion. *J Magn Reson Imaging* 2013; 37: 865–74.

52. al-Saadi N, Gross M, Bornstedt A, et al. [Comparison of various parameters for determining an index of myocardial perfusion reserve in detecting coronary stenosis with cardiovascular magnetic resonance tomography]. *Z Kardiol* 2001; 90: 824–34.

53. Saeed M, Wendland MF, Sakuma H, et al. Coronary artery stenosis: detection with contrast-enhanced MR imaging in dogs. *Radiology* 1995; 196: 79–84.

54. Wilke N, Simm C, Zhang J, et al. Contrast-enhanced first pass myocardial perfusion imaging: Correlation between myocardial blood flow in dogs at rest and during hyperemia. *Magn Reson Med* 1993; 29: 485–97.

55. Schwitter J, Saeed M, Wendland MF, et al. Assessment of myocardial function and perfusion in a canine model of non-occlusive coronary artery stenosis using fast magnetic resonance imaging. *J Magn Reson Imaging* 1999; 9: 101–10.

56. Jaarsma C, Leiner T, Bekkers SC, et al. Diagnostic performance of noninvasive myocardial perfusion imaging using single-photon emission computed tomography, cardiac magnetic resonance, and positron emission tomography imaging for the detection of obstructive coronary artery disease: a meta-analysis. *J Am Coll Cardiol* 2012; 59: 1719–28.

57. Schwitter J, Wacker CM, Wilke N, et al; Investigators M-I. MR-impact II: magnetic resonance imaging for myocardial perfusion assessment in coronary artery disease trial: Perfusion-cardiac magnetic resonance vs. Single-photon emission computed tomography for the detection of coronary artery disease: a comparative multicentre, multivendor trial. *Eur Heart J* 2013; 34: 775–81.

58. Schwitter J, Wacker CM, Wilke N, et al; Investigators M-I. Superior diagnostic performance of perfusion-cardiovascular magnetic resonance versus SPECT to detect coronary artery disease: The secondary endpoints of the multicenter multivendor MR-impact ii (magnetic resonance imaging for myocardial perfusion assessment in coronary artery disease trial). *J Cardiovasc Magn Reson* 2012; 14: 61.

59. Coelho-Filho OR, Seabra LF, Mongeon F-P., et al. Stress myocardial perfusion imaging by CMR provides strong prognostic value to cardiac events regardless of patient's sex. *JACC: Cardiovascular Imaging* 2011; 4: 850–61.

60. Buckert D, Dewes P, Walcher T, Rottbauer W, Bernhardt P. Intermediate-term prognostic value of reversible perfusion deficit diagnosed by adenosine CMR: a prospective follow-up study in a consecutive patient population. *JACC: Cardiovascular Imaging* 2013; 6: 56–63.

61. Bruder O, Wagner A, Lombardi M, et al. European cardiovascular magnetic resonance (EUROCMR) registry—multi national results from 57 centers in 15 countries. *J Cardiovasc Magn Reson* 2013; 15: 9.

62. Ingkanisorn WP, Kwong RY, Bohme NS, et al. Prognosis of negative adenosine stress magnetic resonance in patients presenting to an emergency department with chest pain. *J Am Coll Cardiol* 2006; 47: 1427–32.

63. McMurray JJV, Adamopoulos S, Anker SD, et al; Guidelines ECfP, Reviewers D. ESC guidelines for the diagnosis and treatment of acute and chronic heart failure 2012: the Task Force for the Diagnosis and Treatment of Acute and Chronic Heart Failure 2012 of the European Society of Cardiology. Developed in collaboration with the Heart Failure Association (HFA) of the ESC. *Eur Heart J* 2012; 33: 1787–1847.

64. Moschetti K, Muzzarelli S, Pinget C, et al. Cost evaluation of cardiovascular magnetic resonance versus coronary angiography for the diagnostic work-up of coronary artery disease: application of the European cardiovascular magnetic resonance registry data to the German, United Kingdom, Swiss, and United States health care systems. *J Cardiovascular Magn Resonance* 2012; 14: 35.

65. Miller CD, Hwang W, Case D, et al. Stress CMR imaging observation unit in the emergency department reduces 1-year medical care costs in patients with acute chest pain: A randomized study for comparison with inpatient care. *JACC: Cardiovascular Imaging* 2011; 4: 862–70.

66. Schwitter J, Kanal E, Schmitt M, et al. Impact of the Advisa MRI™ pacing system on the diagnostic quality of cardiac MR images and contraction patterns of cardiac muscle during scans: Advisa MRI randomized clinical multicenter study results. *Heart Rhythm: the Official Journal of the Heart Rhythm Society* 2013;10(6):864–72.

67. Plein S, Schulz-Menger J, Almeida A, et al. Training and accreditation in cardiovascular magnetic resonance in Europe: A position statement of the working group on cardiovascular magnetic resonance of the European Society of Cardiology. *Eur Heart J* 2011; 32: 793–98.

68. Schwitter J *CMR Update*. Lausanne: Schwitter, J; 2012.

69. Motwani M, Maredia N, Fairbairn TA, et al. High-resolution versus standard-resolution cardiovascular MR myocardial perfusion imaging for the detection of coronary artery disease. *Circulation. Cardiovascular Imaging* 2012; 5: 306–13.

70. Chiribiri A, Hautvast GL, Lockie T, et al. Assessment of coronary artery stenosis severity and location: quantitative analysis of transmural perfusion gradients by high-resolution magnetic resonance versus fractional flow reserve. *JACC: Cardiovascular Imaging* 2013.

71. Manka R, Paetsch I, Kozerke S, et al. Whole-heart dynamic three-dimensional magnetic resonance perfusion imaging for the detection of coronary artery disease defined by fractional flow reserve: determination of volumetric myocardial ischaemic burden and coronary lesion location. *Eur Heart J* 2012; 33: 2016–24; 61: 2310-12..

72. Manka R, Jahnke C, Kozerke S, et al. Dynamic 3-dimensional stress cardiac magnetic resonance perfusion imaging: Detection of coronary artery disease and volumetry of myocardial hypoenhancement before and after coronary stenting. *J Am Coll Cardiol* 2011; 57: 437–44.

73. Fuster V, Corti R, Fayad ZA, Schwitter J, Badimon JJ. Integration of vascular biology and magnetic resonance imaging in the understanding of atherothrombosis and acute coronary syndromes. *J Thromb Haemost* 2003; 1: 1410–21.

74. Pennell DJ, Underwood SR, Manzara CC, Swanton RH, Walker JM, Ell PJ, Longmore DB. Magnetic resonance imaging during dobutamine stress in coronary artery disease. *Am J Cardiol* 1992; 70: 34–40.

75. van Rugge FP, van der Wall EE, de Roos A, Bruschke AV. Dobutamine stress magnetic resonance imaging for detection of coronary artery disease. *J Am Coll Cardiol* 1993; 22: 431–39.

76. Baer FM, Voth E, Theissen P, Schneider CA, Schicha H, Sechtem U. Coronary artery disease: findings with GRE MR imaging and tc-99m-methoxyisobutyl-isonitrile SPECT during simultaneous dobutamine stress. *Radiology* 1994; 193: 203–9.

77. van Rugge FP, van der Wall EE, Spanjersberg SJ, et al. Magnetic resonance imaging during dobutamine stress for detection and localization of coronary artery disease. Quantitative wall motion analysis using a modification of the centerline method. *Circulation* 1994; 90: 127–38.

78. Jahnke C, Paetsch I, Gebker R, Bornstedt A, Fleck E, Nagel E. Accelerated 4d dobutamine stress MR imaging with k-t blast: Feasibility and diagnostic performance. *Radiology* 2006; 241: 718–28.

79. Gebker R, Jahnke C, Manka R, et al. Additional value of myocardial perfusion imaging during dobutamine stress magnetic resonance for the assessment of coronary artery disease. *Circulation: Cardiovascular Imaging* 2008; 1: 122–30.

80. Gebker R, Jahnke C, Paetsch I, et al. MR myocardial perfusion imaging with k-space and time broad-use linear acquisition speed-up technique: feasibility study. *Radiology* 2007; 245: 863–71.

81. Sakuma H, Suzawa N, Ichikawa Y, et al. Diagnostic accuracy of stress first-pass contrast-enhanced myocardial perfusion MRI compared with stress myocardial perfusion scintigraphy. *Am J Roentgenol* 2005; 185: 95–102.

82. Klem I, Greulich S, Heitner JF, et al. Value of cardiovascular magnetic resonance stress perfusion testing for the detection of coronary artery disease in women. *JACC: Cardiovascular Imaging* 2008; 1: 436–45.

83. Watkins S, McGeoch R, Lyne J. Validation of magnetic resonance myocardial perfusion imaging with fractional flow reserve for the detection of significant coronary heart disease. *Circulation* 2009;120(22):2207–13.

84. Mikolyzk DK, Wei AS, Tonino P, et al. Effect of corticosteroids on the biomechanical strength of rat rotator cuff tendon. *The Journal of Bone and Joint Surgery* (American volume) 2009; 91: 1172–80.

85. Bettencourt N, Chiribiri A, Schuster A, et al. Cardiac magnetic resonance myocardial perfusion imaging for detection of functionally significant obstructive coronary artery disease: a prospective study. *Int J Cardiol* 2012.

86. Rod Gimbel J, Bello D, Schmitt M, et al; Advisa MRISSI. Randomized trial of pacemaker and lead system for safe scanning at 1.5 tesla. *Heart Rhythm* 2013; 10: 685–91.

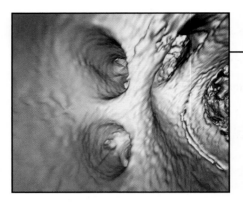

CHAPTER 22

Imaging the vulnerable atherosclerotic plaque

David Vancraeynest and Jean-Louis J. Vanoverschelde

Contents

Introduction: why image the vulnerable plaque?

Although atherosclerosis may cause stable angina, it is a relatively benign disease until it is complicated by thrombosis, usually triggered by the rupture or erosion of an atherosclerotic plaque. Thrombosis accounts for the mortality rate. Each year in Western countries, atherosclerotic diseases, including myocardial infarction (MI) [ST-elevation MI (STEMI) and non-STEMI], unstable angina, and stroke, are responsible for nearly half of all deaths and are among the leading causes of disability [1, 2]. Our ability to predict acute events is usually based on estimation of the 10-year probability (Framingham risk equation or the systematic coronary risk evaluation, known as the SCORE system) [3, 4], on coronary calcium scoring or the measurement of the carotid intima–media thickness by ultrasound, or on inflammatory biomarkers. The limitations of these approaches are well recognized. To refine risk assessment, clinicians frequently use stress testing or lumenography aiming to detect the significance or the severity of arterial stenoses. These tests allow only for the identification of obstructive, flow-limiting plaques. Because most events are caused by the rupture or erosion of non-haemodynamically significant plaques, which outnumber flow-limiting lesions [5], the predictive value of such testing is too low to be of any practical use for acute events on a per-patient basis. For this purpose, we must rely on imaging modalities that can assess the composition of the arterial wall and more precisely the presence (or absence) of features associated with subsequent risk of plaque rupture. Regarding non-invasive techniques for the assessment of plaque vulnerability, significant technical difficulties must be overcome before these can become useful clinical tools. This need is especially relevant for the interrogation of the coronary tree, mainly because of the small size and continuous movement of these imaging targets. By contrast, these techniques are already used successfully for carotid imaging.

The aim of this chapter is to summarize the current state of knowledge in this field and to give a description of the non-invasive techniques, their validation, their possible clinical usefulness, and their limitations in the search for the vulnerable plaque.

Features of vulnerable atherosclerotic plaques

Atherosclerosis is currently considered as a systemic, inflammatory disease of medium-sized and large arteries leading to multifocal thickening and plaque development [6, 7]. The disease is driven by LDL particles in excess, and plaques develop predominantly at sites of low shear stress [8]. Oxidative and enzymatic modifications of low density lipoprotein (LDL) particles induce endothelial cells to express leukocyte adhesion molecules (e.g. vascular cell adhesion molecule-1 or VCAM-1, selectins), which facilitate the recruitment of monocytes and T lymphocytes [7, 9] and initiate the inflammatory cascade. Monocytes differentiate into macrophages, which evolve into foam cells. During the progression of atherosclerosis, macrophages and smooth muscle cells undergo apoptosis [10]. The loss of smooth muscle cells and production of matrix metalloproteinases by activated leukocytes have detrimental consequences, leading to the formation of fragile and rupture-prone fibrous caps [11]. Neovascularization plays a part in atherosclerotic lesions and is probably a marker of ongoing disease activity and may thus characterize high-risk plaques. Hypoxia is the trigger of microvessel proliferation. These new microvessels, originating from adventitial vasa vasorum, are immature and leaky, resulting in local intraplaque haemorrhage [12]. The speed of progression of atherosclerosis varies greatly but generally takes years before becoming clinically evident [13]. Some lesions become obstructive and give 'stable' symptoms, while other plaques become vulnerable and cause acute thrombotic events.

There are two completely different morphological types of vulnerable plaques: the 'erosion-prone' plaque and the 'rupture-prone' plaque. The erosion-prone plaque is characterized by a lack of overlying endothelium. Eroded lesions are more common in young women and associated with smoking. These plaques usually contain fewer calcifications, less extensive neoangiogenesis, and less inflammation than rupture-prone plaques. On the other hand, they also commonly demonstrate more negative than positive remodelling and a greater proliferation of smooth muscle cells. These characteristics make them harder to detect than the rupture-prone plaque [14].

The rupture-prone plaque, usually referred to as a thin-cap fibroatheroma (TCFA), is the most common type of vulnerable plaque and accounts for more than two-thirds of coronary thrombosis. The morphological traits typically associated with rupture-prone plaques include a large eccentric necrotic core, a thin fibrous cap heavily infiltrated with macrophages and inflammatory cells, spotty calcifications, and vasa vasorum proliferation (➲ Fig. 22.1). All of these features are potential targets in the search for the vulnerable plaque [15]. Of note, none of these factors alone confers vulnerability, and they are also unrelated statistically. Vulnerability comes from a combination of several factors.

Necrotic core

Atherogenic lipoproteins that are retained within the intima in the first step of atherogenesis accumulate and form lipid pools, which will attract macrophages. These cells will devour lipids until they become foam cells and die from apoptosis and necrosis. The necrotic core is characterized by a semi-liquid destabilizing lipid-rich cavity containing cholesterol crystals [13, 14] and occupies approximately one quarter of the plaque area [16].

Expansive outward remodelling

One reason why vulnerable plaques are difficult to identify is that they do not cause luminal obstruction, even though they are generally large. Indeed, rupture-prone plaques appear typically to be non-obstructive because of compensatory expansive outward remodelling [17]. By contrast, stable plaques are more commonly associated with constrictive remodelling and cause luminal narrowing detectable by lumenography.

Fibrous cap thickness

The fibrous cap is the fibrocellular layer that separates the necrotic core from the lumen of the vessel. Cap thickness is the best discriminator of plaque type, typically measuring between 54 and 84 μm in TCFA [18]. Crystalline cholesterol is believed to induce plaque rupture by physical disruption of the fibrous cap covering atherosclerotic lesions [19]. When cholesterol crystallizes from a liquid to a solid state, it undergoes volume expansion, which can tear the plaque cap. Several agents (i.e. statins, aspirin, and ethanol) can dissolve cholesterol crystals and may exert their immediate benefits by this direct mechanism [20].

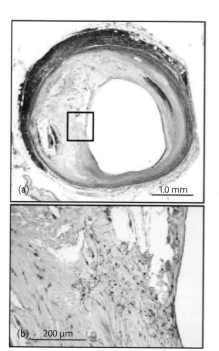

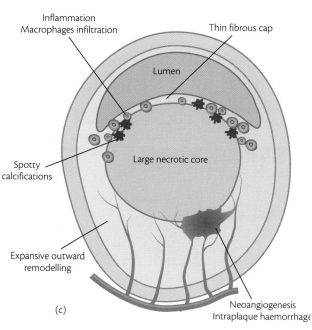

Fig. 22.1 (a) Representative images from a human case of sudden cardiac death of thin-cap fibroatheroma (or rupture-prone vulnerable plaque) and stained with Movat pentachrome. Prominent necrotic core with overlying thin fibrous cap. (b) Boxed area represents corresponding high-power view. Inflammation is seen at the shoulder regions of the intact fibrous cap. These features are typical of thin-cap fibroatheroma and represent higher risk for progression to clinical events. (c) Schematic representation of typical morphological traits associated with rupture-prone plaques [25]. Reproduced from AV Finn et al, Seeking Alternatives to Hard End Points: Is Imaging the Best APPROACH?, *Circulation*, 121:10, 1165–8 with permission from Wolters Kluwer Health.

Inflammation

The inflammatory nature of atherosclerosis is well established. Cholesterol crystals activate the NLRP3 inflammasome in phagocytes *in vitro* in a process that involves phago-lysosomal damage and acts as an endogenous danger signal [21]. The amount of inflammation varies, but vulnerable plaques are commonly more inflamed than those encountered in stable angina. Inflammatory cells, especially macrophages with a density of 14 ± 10%, usually infiltrate the fibrous cap [14]. Macrophages are thought to play a major role in the degradation of the cap by secreting proteolytic enzymes such as metalloproteinases and cysteine proteinases [7]. Nevertheless, at least two types of macrophages are observed in atherosclerotic plaques. The M1-macrophage, a.k.a., the 'bad one', is pro-inflammatory; the M2-macrophage, 'the good one', promotes anti-inflammatory activity [13].

Spotty calcifications

Another type of vulnerable lesion accounting for 2–7% of coronary events is characterized by the disruption of the cap and thrombi associated with eruptive, dense, calcific nodules [14, 22].

Neoangiogenesis and intraplaque haemorrhage

Plaque haemorrhage may play a crucial role in rapid progression of atherosclerosis. There are controversies about the mechanism by which intraplaque haemorrhage occurs [13]. Nevertheless, neoangiogenesis often develops at the base of plaques, leading to the formation of new microvessels originating from the vasa vasorum in the adventitia. They are leaky and fragile, giving rise to local extravasation of plasma proteins and erythrocytes [23]. By contributing to the deposition of free cholesterol, macrophage infiltration, and enlargement of the necrotic core, the accumulation of erythrocyte membranes within an atherosclerotic plaque may represent a potent atherogenic stimulus and a factor of vulnerability [24].

Computed tomography angiography

Over the past decades, technical improvements, including faster gantry rotation, increased number of detectors, decreased slice thickness, and use of dual X-ray sources, have considerably increased the temporal and the spatial resolution of computed tomography (CT) angiography (CTA). The entire heart can be visualized during a single breath-hold. Accordingly, CTA is commonly employed for excluding coronary artery disease. More interestingly, by virtue of its ability to measure local tissue attenuation, CTA allows better definition not only of the extent and significance of coronary artery disease, but also of plaque characteristics [15, 26, 27]. CTA can help to detect some of the features associated with plaque vulnerability, such as more positive remodelling, the presence of spotty calcifications, and a lower plaque density (<30 Hounsfield units) [28–31]. The presence of one of these features or the combination of many of them is significantly more frequent in culprit acute coronary syndrome (ACS) lesions. In the absence of all three features, the negative predictive value for a plaque being associated with an acute future event reaches 100% (30). CTA criteria for plaque vulnerability have been validated against histopathology in patients undergoing carotid endarterectomy [32]. Whenever identified in patients with atherosclerotic risk factors, these features have been shown to predict the occurrence of subsequent ACS. Motoyama et al. studied 1,059 patients who underwent CTA for suspected or known coronary artery disease. Plaques with both positive remodelling and low attenuation were identified in 45 patients; among these, 10 developed ACS [hazard ratio: 22.8, confidence interval (CI) = 6.9 – 75.2, P < 0.001] (⊃ Fig. 22.2) [33]. Undoubtedly, CTA is currently the first-line method in the search for vulnerable rupture-prone plaques. The reliable detection and classification that this technique potentially permits would help to identify patients who may benefit from invasive interrogation. Of

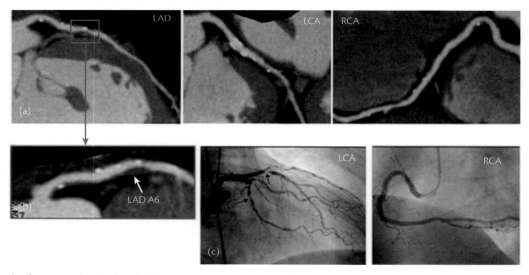

Fig. 22.2 An example of a patient who developed ACS 6 months after CTA. (a) Curved multi-planar reformation images of LAD, LCX, and RCA. (b) Positive remodelling, low-attenuation plaque and spotty calcification were detected in LAD#6 on coronary CT angiography. (c) ACS occurred 6 months after CT angiography, and LAD#6 was determined as the culprit lesion based on invasive coronary angiogram findings. LAD: left anterior descending; LCA: left coronary artery; LCX: left circumflex artery; RCA: right coronary artery.

Reprinted from Motoyama S et al, Computed tomographic angiography characteristics of atherosclerotic plaques subsequently resulting in acute coronary syndrome. *J Am Coll Cardiol.* 2009;54:49–57 with permission from Elsevier.

course, risk–benefit studies will be needed before CTA can be used for the detection and the longitudinal assessment of vulnerable plaques in patients because repeated radiation exposure remains an important and worrying limitation of X-ray imaging modalities. Another limitation of the technique is the wide overlap in Hounsfield unit values for lipid-rich vs. fibrous plaques. Finally, CTA cannot identify plaques with the strongest predictor of vulnerability, i.e. the thin fibrous cap, because current devices lack the spatial resolution to detect the thickness classically associated with TCFA (54–84 μm) [34].

CT has recently yielded promising data on molecular imaging of plaque inflammation. By use of newly designed iodine-based contrast agents (N1177) that selectively accumulate into activated macrophages, CT offers the opportunity to selectively detect plaques containing macrophages, i.e. vulnerable plaques. In a rabbit model of atherosclerosis, Hyafil et al. demonstrated that the signal obtained with CT correlated well with histopathology as well as with glucose uptake as measured by positron emission tomography (PET) [35, 36]. Gold-labelled high-density lipoprotein nanoparticles designed to target activated macrophages seem also to offer an interesting way to study inflammation in the plaque [37]. Although promising, these results need to be confirmed in patients.

Magnetic resonance imaging

Magnetic resonance imaging (MRI) allows evaluation of the biophysical response of tissues placed in a strong static magnetic field that are transiently exposed to electromagnetic radiofrequency pulses. By using different contrast weightings, MRI can now provide insights into the biological characteristics of the tissue of interest, such as its water, lipid, and fibrous content [38]. Accordingly, MRI can facilitate characterization of atherosclerotic plaque composition with more and more confidence. Because of their small dimensions and their continuous motion, coronary arteries are rather difficult to image. For this reason, most data on the detection of vulnerable plaques with MRI have been obtained in large and 'static' arteries, such as carotid arteries. Nevertheless, non-contrast T1-weighted imaging has recently provided encouraging data for the assessment of coronary plaque characterization in patients with coronary artery disease [39] (⊃ Fig. 22.3). Lipid and fibrotic plaque components have been accurately quantified on T2-weighted images in humans [40, 41]. The same imaging sequences have also been used to measure the fibrous cap thickness [42] and to identify fibrous cap ruptures [43] and intraplaque haemorrhages [44]. A good agreement between MRI and histopathology has been found for the identification of lipid-rich necrotic cores and intraplaque haemorrhages in human carotid plaques [40]. Furthermore, while these features correlated well with the clinical presentation (more frequent in patients experiencing minor stroke than in asymptomatic patients), they were found in a majority of arteries of <70% stenosis [45]. The reproducibility of MRI in identifying vulnerable plaques is relatively poor [46, 47], but this limitation can be overcome by using alternative imaging strategies, including diffusion-weighted imaging [48] and gadofluorine-enhanced imaging. Gadofluorine can be used either as a blood pool agent to detect plaque neovascularization [49] or as an extracellular matrix agent to enhance detection of lipid-rich plaques [50].

The fascinating development of targeted molecular imaging probes expands the potential contribution of MRI for the specific

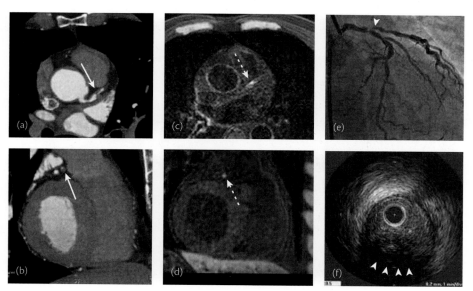

Fig. 22.3 Representative case of hyperintense plaque in the proximal left descending artery (LAD). A 60-year-old patient with a severe coronary stenosis in the proximal LAD is shown. Computed tomography angiography (a, horizontal; b, sagittal) demonstrates the low-density positive remodelling plaque (−32 Hounsfield units, remodelling index: 1.27) (arrow) with severe coronary stenosis in the proximal LAD. On the corresponding cardiac magnetic resonance (CMR) image (c, horizontal; d, sagittal), this low-density plaque was visualized as a 'hyperintense spot' (dashed arrow). On the coronary angiography, severe coronary stenosis was observed (e, arrowhead), and on IVUS examination (f), a positive remodelling plaque (remodelling index: 1.29) with ultrasound attenuation (arrowheads) was observed in the proximal LAD, corresponding with the plaque observed by both CTA and CMR.

Reprinted from *JACC: Cardiovascular Imaging*, 2:6, Tomohiro Kawasaki et al, Characterization of Hyperintense Plaque With Noncontrast T1-Weighted Cardiac Magnetic Resonance Coronary Plaque Imaging: Comparison With Multislice Computed Tomography and Intravascular Ultrasound, 720-728, copyright 2009 with permission from Elsevier.

characterization of the different plaque components. For instance, plaque inflammation can be targeted using ultrasmall superparamagnetic particles of iron oxide, which accumulate in plaque macrophages and lead to signal dropout [51–53]. The inflammatory state of the plaque can also be evaluated by targeting VCAM-1 [54], oxidation-specific epitopes [55, 56], and the oxidized LDL receptor LOX-1 [57]. MRI additionally allows plaque neoangiogenesis assessment by using $\alpha_v\beta_3$-integrin–targeted paramagnetic nanoparticles or a mimetic of RGD peptide grafted to gadolinium-DTPA [58, 59].

One of the striking advantages of MRI is its safety, which allows for repeated measurements and thus the longitudinal assessment of plaque progression or regression [60–62]. MRI is definitively a promising method for the simultaneous assessment of plaque morphology and composition. Furthermore, it could be used to calculate the mechanical stress within the plaque. This emerging application should better our understanding of the interaction among the stress within the plaque, the morphology of the plaque, and the risk of subsequent rupture [63].

Further technical improvements are needed, especially for the assessment of vulnerable plaques in the coronary tree. Finally, even though data exist on a very small sample of patients [64], the clinical value of MRI in predicting acute vascular events remains to be determined in large randomized trials.

Nuclear imaging

Thanks to their whole-body and targeted imaging capabilities, single photon emission computed tomography (SPECT) and PET offer the opportunity to specifically identify vulnerable plaque components along the entire length of the arterial tree. Because of its better spatial resolution (4–5 mm for PET vs. 1–1.6 cm for SPECT) and intrinsic ability to allow quantification of biological

processes in absolute terms, PET has been used in most of the studies on nuclear imaging of atherosclerosis [15, 65]. Co-registration with CT or MRI is needed to co-localize the nuclear tracer with anatomic structures [66].

^{18}F-labelled fluorodeoxyglucose (FDG) is currently the best-validated tracer for imaging of plaque inflammation. In metabolically active cells, such as activated macrophages, FDG competes with glucose to yield FDG-6-phosphate, which progressively accumulates in cells as the end product of the phosphorylation reaction. The intracellular accumulation of FDG-6-phosphate can then be imaged and quantified using PET. In animal models of atherosclerosis [67] and in humans with carotid plaques [68–70], areas of high ^{18}F-FDG uptake have been shown to co-localize with areas of macrophage accumulation (⊃ Fig. 22.4), irrespective of plaque size [68] or luminal narrowing [69]. The presence of high ^{18}F-FDG uptake is linked to circulating markers of inflammation such as matrix metalloproteinases [71, 72]. FDG-PET signal is a reproducible measure [73, 74] and like MRI varies in amplitude with therapeutic interventions, thus suggesting its potential role in treatment monitoring [75, 76]. FDG imaging of large artery inflammation is promising for the early identification of vulnerable plaques.

Nevertheless, imaging coronary artery plaques is clearly challenging for two main reasons. First, primarily because of the intense tracer uptake in the adjacent myocardium, adequate visualization of coronary plaque inflammation using FDG-PET will probably require suppression of the myocardial ^{18}F-FDG signal, for instance by use of low-carbohydrate, high-fat diets [77–79]. Second, coronary plaque imaging is hampered by respiratory and cardiac motion. Dual gating for both respiratory and cardiac motion will probably be mandatory to achieve adequate definition of coronary plaque. The value of FDG-PET for predicting an acute vascular event has not yet been evaluated prospectively. In retrospective analyses of cancer patients undergoing FDG-PET

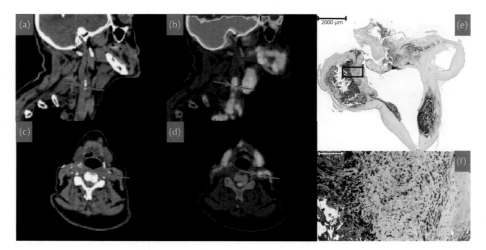

Fig. 22.4 This figure shows a high ^{18}F-FDG uptake in the left carotid bifurcation from a 68-year-old man who had experienced one episode of right-sided hemiparesis. Carotid ultrasound revealed the presence of a severe (>95%) left internal carotid artery stenosis. Moderate calcifications were demonstrated by CT at the level of the left proximal internal carotid artery (a, red arrows; CT image, sagittal plane; and c, CT image, axial plane) as well as high ^{18}F-FDG uptake (target-to-background ratio: 1.84) in the region of the carotid plaque by PET/CT (b, red arrows; co-registered PET/CT image, sagittal plane; and d, co-registered PET/CT image, axial plane). Carotid plaque specimen taken from the patient is shown in (e). The haematoxylin-stained histological specimen demonstrated a complex plaque with necrotic core and the CD68 staining (diaminobenzidine, in brown) demonstrated intense macrophage infiltration. The black box in (e) indicates the region corresponding to the high-powered CD68 stains (f).

imaging for staging of their neoplastic disease, increased ^{18}F-FDG uptake in large arteries was shown to predict subsequent acute ischaemic events [80]. It must also be mentioned that the underlying biological mechanism of FDG is not completely understood and that hypoxia may interfere with the FDG signal [34].

In addition to glucose uptake, numerous other metabolic and signalling pathways associated with plaque vulnerability have been targeted using nuclear imaging modalities. These include the oxidation and accumulation of LDL with [125]iodine-labelled oxidation-specific antibodies [81, 57]; matrix metalloproteinase activity using [99m]Technetium-labelled inhibitors [82]; macrophage apoptosis measurement using [99m]Technetium-labelled annexin-V [83–85]; inflammation measurement with 11C-PK11195, a selective ligand of the translocator protein that is expressed by activated macrophages [86]; monocyte recruitment with either [99m]Technetium-labelled monocyte chemotactic protein-1 [87] (known as MCP-1, a key player in the transendothelial migration of mononuclear cells) or the ^{18}F-labelled peptide, which can be internalized by endothelial cells through VCAM-1–mediated binding [88]; and finally, $\alpha_v\beta_3$-integrin–targeted PET using the tracer ^{18}F-galacto-RGD [89]. The preclinical results obtained with these tracers have to be confirmed in large human studies.

Although nuclear imaging is currently a leading modality for the detection of vulnerable plaques, repeated radiation exposure will probably limit its widespread use for longitudinal monitoring. Studies should thus probably concentrate not only on demonstrating the diagnostic and prognostic accuracy of these techniques but also on investigating their risk–benefit ratio.

Ultrasound imaging

Atherosclerotic plaques can be characterized by using ultrasound contrast agents (UCAs). However, regarding penetration and resolution, the use of this approach is confined to the carotid vasculature. UCAs consist of acoustically active microbubbles with a diameter of 3–4 μm. When insonated, these microbubbles expand and contract rhythmically, producing strong backscattered signals that can be detected by conventional ultrasound systems. Because UCAs are pure intravascular tracers (they behave like red blood cells), contrast-enhanced ultrasonography allows for the assessment of the blood volume contained in the microvasculature within the insonated region. This principle has been exploited to semi-quantitatively assess neovascularization in carotid plaques (⊃ Fig. 22.5).

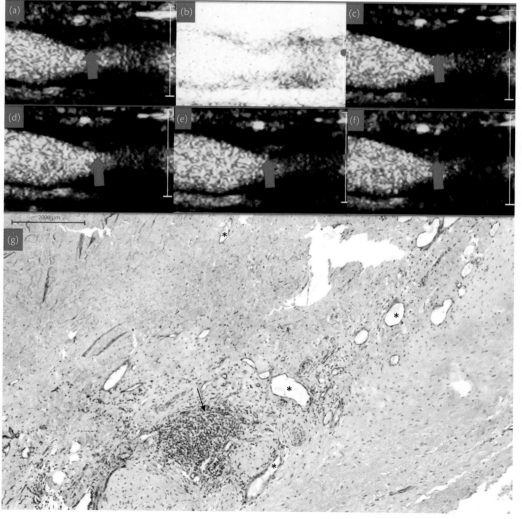

Fig. 22.5 This figure illustrates the presence of neovascularization (a–f) assessed by contrast-enhanced ultrasound imaging in a carotid atherosclerotic plaque of a 76-year-old patient scheduled for endarterectomy and the corresponding histopathology obtained on the surgical specimen (g). On the pre-flash image (a), contrast microbubbles (Sonovue, Bracco) are visualized into the plaque (red arrow). The microbubbles are destroyed by a high-energy (mechanical index: 1.0) ultrasound burst (b). The imaging frame immediately after the burst shows the complete disappearance of the microbubbles from the plaque (c, red arrow), and the progressive replenishment of the plaque by the microbubbles is clearly demonstrated after 1 s (d, red arrow), 3 s (e, red arrow), and 6 s (f, red arrow). This significant acoustic plaque enhancement over time suggests the presence of neovascularization into the plaque. Micrograph in (g) shows the presence of CD34 (Dako)-positive neovessels (diaminobenzidine, in brown, asterisk) co-existing with inflammatory infiltrates (black arrow) into the plaque (haematoxylin staining).

Significant acoustic plaque enhancement has been correlated with both histopathology [90, 91] and clinical presentation [92]. The lack of ionizing radiation is undoubtedly the best advantage of contrast-enhanced ultrasonography.

This approach also allows for molecular imaging using specific ligands, such as monoclonal antibodies, that are attached onto the microbubble's shell. Because microbubbles are constrained to the intravascular space, only molecular targets appearing on the endothelial surface can be imaged. When the targeted microbubbles stream through the capillary network, they are retained locally by the specific interaction between the antibody and the antigen of interest. The presence and extent of retention can then be assessed using ultrasound imaging, usually after subtraction of the signal emanating from the circulating microbubbles. This approach has been successfully tested in animal models of atherosclerosis by targeting VCAM-1 and P-selectin in aortic plaques [93–95]. The signal intensity obtained with this technique is dependent on the shear stress applied on the surface of the endothelium and could be a limitation. Up to now, molecular ultrasound imaging remains in the domain of preclinical research.

Current clinical use and future perspectives

Most of the features associated with plaque vulnerability are detectable by non-invasive modalities in humans (➲ Table 22.1), and this is especially true for carotid plaque imaging. However, it must be noted that several limitations restrict the clinical utility of most of the modalities in the search for the vulnerable coronary plaque (➲ Table 22.2). The small diameter of the coronary arteries and the cardiac and respiratory motion represent the main limitations of MRI while spatial resolution is the Achilles' heel of nuclear imaging techniques. CTA is the best-validated technique

Table 22.1 Detectability of features associated with vulnerable plaques by non-invasive imaging techniques

	Carotid arteries					Coronary arteries				
	CTA	**MRI**	**PET**	**SPECT**	**US**	**CT**	**MRI**	**PET**	**SPECT**	**US**
Cap thickness	–	+	–	–	–	–	–	–	–	–
Spotty calcifications	+	–	–	–	–	+	–	–	–	–
Positive remodelling	+	+	–	–	–	+	–	–	–	–
Necrotic core/tissue composition	+	+	–	–	–	+	+	–	–	–
Inflammation	+	+	+	+	+	–	–	–	–	–
Neoangiogenesis/ haemorrhage	–	+	+	–	+	–	–	–	–	–
CLINICAL STATUS	Yes Not for inflammation	Yes	Yes	No (limited data with annexin–V)	Yes for neovessels Not for molecular imaging	Yes	Yes	No	No	No

Legend: (+), detectable; (–), undetectable

Table 22.2 Technical characteristics and limitations restricting the clinical utility of non-invasive imaging modalities in the search for the vulnerable coronary plaque

	Energy	**Spatial resolution (mm)**	**Tissue penetration**	**Limitations**
CTA	X-rays	0.3	High	Radiation Use of contrast agents Overlap in the attenuation spectrum of lipid and fibrous plaque
MRI	Electromagnetic radiofrequency pulses	0.2	High	Cardiac motion Respiratory motion Spatial resolution
PET	Annihilation photons	4	High	Radiation Cardiac motion Respiratory motion Myocardial uptake of FDG Spatial resolution
SPECT	Gamma rays	10	High	Radiation Cardiac motion Respiratory motion Spatial resolution
US	Ultrasound waves	0.1	Low (<50 mm)	Spatial resolution Penetration

with the goal of identifying vulnerable coronary plaques, but ionizing radiation is a definite concern, especially if repeated or combined imaging (PET + CTA, SPECT + CTA) is needed. Finally, the poor penetration of high-frequency ultrasound waves will prevent contrast ultrasound imaging from becoming a useful modality for coronary imaging.

It is noteworthy that almost no modality can measure the cap thickness of the plaque, one of the best discriminators of plaque type [18]. This inability can be explained by the spatial resolution of the different techniques described in this chapter, which is largely higher than the cut-off value admitted to discriminate between a TCFA and a thick-cap fibrous atheroma.

Currently, there is little evidence proving that the presence of vulnerable plaques is associated with an increased risk of subsequent acute ischaemic events. Whether for carotid or coronary vascular events, very few studies have addressed the predictive accuracy of imaging techniques as the main endpoint (⊃ Table 22.3). Therefore, before these methods can be implemented into daily clinical routine, their diagnostic and predictive accuracy must be evaluated in large groups of patients, in multi-centre, randomized, controlled trials. Recent work has yielded important data on the predictive value of CTA [96], and ongoing studies are still underway [97].

We also need to learn which of the different features associated with vulnerability are clinically relevant to patient outcome. It is likely that more than one plaque feature will be needed to make a clinically useful assessment. In this regard, combined imaging will be necessary, and the safety of such an approach should be determined.

A series of other questions remain to be addressed. Studies will be needed to determine how the information provided by plaque imaging can be used. If the goal of imaging is to more precisely risk-stratify patients, imaging must prove superior over other means of risk stratification (e.g. Framingham risk score, hs-CRP, calcium score). If the goal of imaging is to detect rupture-prone plaques before they cause an acute ischaemic event, imaging must have a high positive predictive value so that individual rupture-prone lesions can be treated in a timely way. For this purpose, data on the natural history of these rupture-prone lesions, including their persistence or their spontaneous healing capabilities, will also be needed [15]. In other words, moving from 'diagnostic trial'

Table 22.3 Prediction of events by non-invasive imaging of vulnerable plaque

CTA	Prospective trial [33]: CT coronary angiography 1,059 patients 15 ACS Mean follow-up: 27 ± 10 months → Prediction of ACS: presence of positive remodelling and/or low-attenuation plaque; HR (hazard ratio): 22.8
MRI	Prospective trial [64]: Multicontrast-weighted carotid MRI 152 patients 12 carotid cerebrovascular events Mean follow-up: 38.2 months → Prediction of stroke: presence of a thin or ruptured fibrous cap; HR: 17.0
PET	Retrospective study [80]: 18F-FDG uptake in large arteries 932 patients (279 patients died from oncologic disease) 15 vascular events (stroke, MI, or revascularization) Median follow-up: 29 months → Kaplan–Meier curves for mean TBR (target-to-background ratio) showed a significantly inferior outcome for patients with a mean TBR > 1.7 ($P < 0.001$)
SPECT	No data
US	No data

to 'interventional trial' will be the next step. If the treatment of vulnerable plaques favourably modifies patient outcome, it is likely that vulnerable plaque imaging will not be an elusive goal. The target population who must benefit from imaging should also be better defined and the 'number needed to screen', as well as the risk–benefit ratio, must be determined in each category of risk and for each imaging modality. Finally, the question of how often testing must be repeated needs to be addressed. If repeated imaging is mandatory, safety will certainly become a major issue.

Plaque erosion, another type of vulnerable plaque, is not addressed in this chapter simply because none of the non-invasive imaging modalities enable its recognition. Although plaque erosion is not the most common cause of acute vascular events, it is not an infrequent cause (especially at the coronary level) [98]. This fact represents another limitation of non-invasive techniques in the goal of identifying vulnerable plaques.

References

1. Nichols M, Towsend N, Scarborough P, et al. *European Cardiovascular Disease Statistics*. Department of Public Health, University of Oxford.

2. Roger VL, Go AS, Lloyd-Jones DM, et al. Heart disease and stroke statistics 2012 Update. A report from the American Heart Association. *Circulation* 2012; 125: e2–220.

3. Anderson KM, Wilson PW, Odell PM, Kannel WB. An updated coronary risk profile. A statement for health professionals. *Circulation* 1991; 83: 356–62.

4. Conroy RM, Pyorala K, Fitzgerald AP, et al. Estimation of ten-year risk of fatal cardiovascular disease in Europe: the SCORE project. *Eur Heart J* 2003; 24: 987–1003.

5. Falk E, Shah PK, Fuster V. Coronary plaque disruption. *Circulation* 1995; 92: 657–71.

6. Libby P. Inflammation in atherosclerosis. *Nature* 2002; 420: 868–74.

7. Hansson GK. Inflammation, atherosclerosis and coronary artery disease. *N Engl J Med* 2005; 352: 1685–95.

8. Koskinas KC, Feldman CL, Chatzizisis YS, et al. Natural history of experimental coronary atherosclerosis and vascular remodeling in relation to endothelial shear stress: a serial, in vivo intravascular ultrasound study. *Circulation* 2010; 121: 2092–101.

9. Falk E. Pathogenesis of atherosclerosis. *J Am Coll Cardiol* 2006; 47: C7–12.

10. Littlewood TD, Bennett MR. Apoptotic cell death in atherosclerosis. *Curr Opin Lipidol* 2003; 14: 469–75.

11. Jones CB, Sane DC, Herrington DM. Matrix metalloproteinases: a review of their structure and role in acute coronary syndrome. *Cardiovasc Res* 2003; 59: 812–23.

12. Doyle B, Caplice N. Plaque neovascularization and antiangiogenic therapy for atherosclerosis. *J Am Coll Cardiol* 2007; 49: 2073–80.

13. Falk E, Nakano M, Bentzon JF, Finn AV, Virmani R. Update on acute coronary syndromes: the pathologists' view. *Eur Heart J* 2013; 34: 719–28.

14. Virmani R, Kolodgie FD, Burke AP, Farb A, Schwartz SM. Lessons from sudden coronary death. A comprehensive morphological classification scheme for atherosclerotic lesions. *Arterioscler Thromb Vasc Biol* 2000; 20: 1262–75.

15. Vancraeynest D, Pasquet A, Roelants V, Gerber BL, Vanoverschelde JL. Imaging the vulnerable plaque. *J Am Coll Cardiol* 2011; 57: 1961–79.

16. Virmani R, Burke AP, Farb A, Kolodgie FD. Pathology of the vulnerable plaque. *J Am Coll Cardiol* 2006; 47: C13–8.

17. Pasterkamp G, Galis ZS, de Kleijn PV. Expansive arterial remodeling: Location, Location, Location. *Arterioscler Thromb Vasc Biol* 2004; 24: 650–7.

18. Narula J, Nakano M, Virmani R, et al. Histopathologic characteristics of atherosclerotic coronary disease and implications of the findings for the invasive and non invasive detection of vulnerable plaques. *J Am Coll Cardiol* 2013; 61: 1041–51.

19. Grebe A, Latz E. Cholesterol crystals and inflammation. *Curr Rheumatol Rep* 2013; 15: 313.

20. Abela GS. Cholesterol crystals piercing the arterial plaque and intima trigger local and systemic inflammation. *J Clin Lipidol* 2010; 4: 156–64.

21. Duewell P, Kono H, Ravner KJ, et al. NLRP3 inflamasomes are required for atherogenesis and activated by cholesterol crystals that form early in disease. *Nature* 2010; 464: 1357–61.

22. Ehara S, Kobayashi Y, Yoshiyama M, Ueda M, Yoshikawa J. Coronary artery calcification revisited. *J Atheroscler Thromb* 2006; 13: 31–7.

23. Sluimer JC, Kolodgie FD, Bijnens APJJ, et al. Thin-walled microvessels in human coronary atherosclerotic plaques show incomplete endothelial junctions. Relevance of compromised structural integrity for intraplaque microvscular leakage. *J Am Coll Cardiol* 2009; 53: 1517–27.

24. Kolodgie FD, Gold HK, Burke AP, et al. Intraplaque hemorrhage and progression of coronary atheroma. *N Engl J Med* 2003; 349: 2316–25.

25. Finn AV, Chandrashekahr Y, Narula J. Seeking alternatives to hard end points: is imaging the best APPROACH? *Circulation* 2010; 121: 1165–8.

26. Motoyama S, Sarai M, Narula J, Ozaki Y. Coronary CT angiography and high-risk plaque morphology. *Cardiovasc Interv and Ther* 2013; 28: 1–8.

27. Schroeder S, Kopp AF, Baumbach A, et al. Non-invasive detection and evaluation of atherosclerotic coronary plaques with multislice computed tomography. *J Am Coll Cardiol* 2001; 37: 1430–5.

28. Leber AW, Knez A, Becker A, et al. Accuracy of multidetector spiral computed tomography in identifying and differentiating the composition of coronary atherosclerotic plaques: a comparative study with intracoronary ultrasound. *J Am Coll Cardiol* 2004; 43: 1241–7.

29. Hoffmann U, Moselewski F, Nieman K, et al. Non-invasive assessment of plaque morphology and composition in culprit and stable lesions in acute coronary syndrome and stable lesions in stable angina by multidetector computed tomography. *J Am Coll Cardiol* 2006; 47: 1655–62.

30. Motoyama S, Kondo T, Sarai M, et al. Multislice computed tomographic characteristics of coronary lesions in acute coronary syndromes. *J Am Coll Cardiol* 2007; 50: 319–26.

31. Kitagawa T, Yamamoto H, Horiguchi J, et al. Characterization of noncalcified coronary plaques and identification of culprit lesions in patients with acute coronary syndrome by 64-slice computed tomography. *JACC Cardiovasc Imaging* 2009; 2: 153–60.

32. de Weert TT, Ouhlous M, Meijering E, et al. In vivo characterization and quantification of atherosclerotic carotid plaque components with multidetector computed tomography and histopathological correlation. *Arterioscler Thromb Vasc Biol* 2006; 26: 2366–72.

33. Motoyama S, Sarai M, Harigaya H, et al. Computed tomographic angiography characteristics of atherosclerotic plaques subsequently resulting in acute coronary syndrome. *J Am Coll Cardiol* 2009; 54: 49–57.

34. Camici PG, Rimoldi OE, Gaemperli O, Libby P. Non-invasive anatomic and functional imaging of vascular inflammation and unstable plaque. *Eur Heart J* 2012; 33: 1309–17.

35. Hyafil F, Cornily JC, Feig JE, et al. Non-invasive detection of macrophages using a nanoparticulate contrast agent for computed tomography. *Nat Med* 2007; 13: 636–41.

36. Hyafil F, Cornily JC, Rudd JH, Machac J, Feldman LJ, Fayad ZA. Quantification of inflammation within rabbit atherosclerotic plaques using the macrophage-specific CT contrast agent N1177: a comparison with 18F-FDG PET/CT and histology. *J Nucl Med* 2009; 50: 959–65.

37. Cormode DP, Roessi E, Thran A, et al. Atherosclerotic plaque composition: Analysis with multicolor CT and targeted gold nanoparticles. *Radiology* 2010; 256: 774–82.

38. Wilensky RL, Song HK, Ferrari VA. Role of magnetic resonance and intravascular magnetic resonance in the detection of vulnerable plaques. *J Am Coll Cardiol* 2006; 47: C48–56.

39. Kawasaki T, Koga S, Koga N, et al. Characterization of hyperintense plaque with noncontrast T1-weighted cardiac magnetic resonance coronary plaque imaging. *JACC Cardiovasc Imaging* 2009; 2: 720–8.

40. Yuan C, Mitsumori LM, Ferguson MS, et al. In vivo accuracy of multispectral magnetic resonance imaging for identifying lipid-rich necrotic cores and intraplaque hemorrhage in advanced human carotid plaques. *Circulation* 2001; 104: 2051–6.

41. Cai JM, Hatsukami TS, Ferguson MS, Small R, Polissar NL, Yuan C. Classification of human carotid atherosclerosis lesions with in vivo multicontrast magnetic resonance imaging. *Circulation* 2002; 106: 1368–73.

42. Cai J, Hatsukami TS, Ferguson MS, et al. In vivo quantitative measurement of intact fibrous cap and lipid-rich necrotic core size in atherosclerotic carotid plaque. Comparison of high-resolution, contrast-enhanced magnetic resonance imaging and histology. *Circulation* 2005; 112: 3437–44.

43. Yuan C, Zhang SX, Polissar NL, et al. Identification of fibrous cap rupture with magnetic resonance imaging is highly associated with recent transient ischemic attack or stroke. *Circulation* 2002; 105: 181–5.

44. Chu B, Kampschulte A, Ferguson MS, et al. Hemorrhage in the atherosclerotic carotid plaque: a high-resolution MRI study. *Stroke* 2004; 35: 1079–84.

45. Lindsay AC, Biasiolli L, Lee JMS, et al. Plaque features associated with increased cerebral infarction after minor stroke and TIA. A prospective, case-control, 3-T carotid artery MR imaging study. *JACC Cardiovasc Imaging* 2012; 5: 388–96.

46. Touzé E, Toussaint JF, Coste J, et al. Reproducibility of high-resolution MRI for the identification and the quantification of carotid atherosclerotic plaque components. Consequences for prognosis studies and therapeutic trials. *Stroke* 2007; 38: 1812–9.

47. Kwee RM, van Engelshoven JM, Mess WH, et al Reproducibility of fibrous cap status assessment of carotid artery plaques by contrast-enhanced MRI. *Stroke* 2009; 40: 3017–21.

48. Qiao Y, Ronen I, Viereck J, Ruberg FL, Hamilton JA. Identification of atherosclerotic lipid deposits by diffusion-weighted imaging. *Arterioscler Thromb Vasc Biol* 2007; 27: 1440–6.

49. Sirol M, Moreno PR, Purushothaman KR, et al. Increased neovascularization in advanced lipid-rich atherosclerotic lesions detected by gadofluorine-M-enhanced MRI. Implications for plaque vulnerability. *Circ Cardiovasc Imaging* 2009; 2: 391–6.

50. Sirol M, Itskovich VV, Mani V, et al. Lipid-rich atherosclerotic plaques detected by gadofluorine-enhanced in vivo magnetic resonance imaging. *Circulation* 2004; 109: 2890–6.

51. Korosoglou, Weiss RG, Kedziorek DA, et al. Non-invasive detection of macrophage-rich atherosclerotic plaque in hyperlipidemic rabbits using « positive contrast » magnetic resonance imaging. *J Am Coll Cardiol* 2008; 52: 483–91.

52. Kooi ME, Cappendijk VC, Cleutjens KB, et al. Accumulation of ultrasmall superparamagnetic particles of iron oxide in human atherosclerotic plaques can be detected by in vivo magnetic resonance imaging. *Circulation* 2003; 107: 2453–8.

53. Tang TY, Howarth SP, Miller SR, et al. The ATHEROMA (atorvastatin therapy: effects on reduction of macrophages activity) study. Evaluation using ultrasmall superparamagnetic iron oxide-enhanced magnetic resonance imaging in carotid disease. *J Am Coll Cardiol* 2009; 53: 2039–50.

54. Nahrendorf M, Jaffer FA, Kelly KA, et al. Non-invasive vascular cell adhesion molecule-1 imaging identifies inflammatory activation of cells in atherosclerosis. *Circulation* 2006; 114: 1504–11.

55. Briley-Saebo KC, Shaw PX, Mulder WJ, et al. Targeted molecular probes for imaging atherosclerotic lesions with magnetic resonance using antibodies that recognize oxidation-specific epitopes. *Circulation* 2008; 117: 3206–15.

56. Briley-Saebo KC, Cho YS, Shaw PX, et al. Targeted iron oxide particles for in vivo magnetic resonance detection of atherosclerosis lesions with antibodies directed to oxidation-specific epitopes. *J Am Coll Cardiol* 2011; 57: 337–47.

57. Li D, Patel AR, Klibanov AL, et al. Molecular imaging of atherosclerosis plaques targeted to oxidized LDL receptor LOX-1 by SPECT/CT and magnetic resonance. *Circ Cardiovasc Imaging* 2010; 3: 464–72.

58. Winter PM, Morawski AM, Caruthers SD, et al. Molecular imaging of angiogenesis in early-stage atherosclerosis with $\alpha_v\beta_3$-integrin-tergeted nanoparticles. *Circulation* 2003; 108: 2270–4.

59. Burtea C, Laurent S, Murariu O, et al. Molecular imaging of $\alpha_v\beta_3$-integrin expression in atherosclerotic plaques with a mimetic of RGD peptide grafted to Gd-DTPA. *Cardiovasc Res* 2008; 78: 148–57.

60. Zhao XQ, Dong L, Hatsukami T, et al. MR imaging of carotid plaque composition during lipid-lowering therapy. *J Am Coll Cardiol* Img. 2011; 4: 977–86.

61. Sun J, Underhill HR, Hippe DS, Xue Y, Yuan C, Hatsukami TS. Sustained acceleration in carotid atherosclerotic plaque progression with intraplaque hemorrhage. *J Am Coll Cardiol Img* 2012; 5: 798–804.

62. Vucic E, Calcagno C, Dickson SD, et al. Regression of inflammation in atherosclerosis by the LXR agonist R211945. A non-invasive assessment and comparison with Atorvastatin. *J Am Coll Cardiol Img* 2012; 5: 819–28.

63. Tang D, Teng Z, Canton G, et al. Sites of rupture in human atherosclerotic carotid plaques are associated with high structural stresses: an in vivo MRI-based 3D fluid-structure interaction study. *Stroke* 2009; 40: 3258–63.

64. Takaya N, Yuan C, Chu B, et al. Association between carotid plaque characteristics and subsequent ischemic cerebrovascular events. A prospective assessment with MRI: initial results. *Stroke* 2006; 37: 818–23.

65. Davies JR, Rudd JHF, Weissberg PL, Narula J. Radionuclide imaging for the detection of inflammation in vulnerable plaques. *J Am Coll Cardiol* 2006; 47: C57–68.

66. Joshi FR, Lindsay AC, Obaid DR, Falk E, Rudd JHF. Non-invasive imaging of atherosclerosis. *Eur Heart J Cardiovasc Img* 2012; 13: 205–18.

67. Ogawa M, Ishino S, Mukai T, et al. ^{18}F-FDG accumulation in atherosclerotic plaques: immunohistochemical and PET imaging study. *J Nucl Med* 2004; 45: 1245–50.

68. Tawakol A, Migrino RQ, Bashian GG, et al. In vivo 18F-fluorodeoxyglucose positron emission tomography imaging provides a non-invasive measure of carotid plaque inflammation in patients. *J Am Coll Cardiol* 2006; 48: 1818–24.

69. Tahara N, Kai H, Nakaura H, et al. The prevalence of inflammation in carotid atherosclerosis: analysis with fluorodeoxyglucose-positron emission tomography. *Eur Heart J* 2007; 28: 2243–8.

70. Rudd JHF, Warburton EA, Fryer TD, et al. Imaging atherosclerotic plaque inflammation with [^{18}F]-Fluorodeoxyglucose positron emission tomography. *Circulation* 2002; 105: 2708–11.

71. Wu YW, Kao HL, Chen MF, et al. Characterization of plaques using 18F-FDG PET/CT in patients with carotid atherosclerosis and correlation with matrix metalloproteinase-1. *J Nucl Med* 2007; 48: 227–33.

72. Rudd JHF, Myers KS, Bansilal S, et al. Relationships among regional arterial inflammation, calcification, risk factors, and biomarkers. A prospective fluorodeoxyglucose positron-emission tomography/computed tomography imaging study. *Circ Cardiovasc Imaging* 2009; 2: 107–15.

73. Rudd JH, Myers KS, Bansilal S, et al. [18]Fluorodeoxyglucose positron emission tomography imaging of atherosclerotic plaque inflammation is highly reproducible. Implications for atherosclerosis therapy trials. *J Am Coll Cardiol* 2007; 50: 892–6.

74. Rudd JHF, Myers KS, Bansilal S, et al. Atherosclerosis inflammation imaging with 18F-FDG PET: carotid, iliac, and femoral uptake reproducibility, quantification methods, and recommendations. *J Nucl Med* 2008; 49: 871–8.

75. Ogawa M, Magata Y, Kato T, et al. Application of 18F-FDG PET for monitoring the therapeutic effect of anti-inflammatory drugs on stabilization of vulnerable atherosclerotic plaques. *J Nucl Med* 2006; 47: 1845–50.

76. Tahara N, Kai H, Ishibashi M, et al. Simvastatin attenuates plaque inflammation. Evaluation by fluorodeoxyglucose positron emission tomography. *J Am Coll Cardiol* 2006; 48: 1825–31.

77. Williams G, Kolodny GM. Suppression of myocardial 18F-FDG uptake by preparing patients with a high-fat, low-carbohydrate diet. *Am J Roentgen* 2008; 190: 151–6.

78. Wykrzykowska J, Lehman S, Williams G, et al. Imaging of inflamed and vulnerable plaque in coronary arteries with 18F-FDG PET/CT in patients with suppression of myocardial uptake using a low-carbohydrate, high fat preparation. *J Nucl Med* 2009; 50: 563–8.

79. Rogers IS, Nasir K, Figueroa AL, et al. Feasibility of FDG imaging of the coronary arteries. Comparison between acute coronary syndrome and stable angina. *J Am Coll Cardiol Img* 2010; 3: 388–97.

80. Rominger A, Saam T, Wolpers S, et al. 18F-FDG PET/CT identifies patients at risk for future vascular events in an otherwise asymptomatic cohort with neoplastic disease. *J Nucl Med* 2009; 50: 1611–20.

81. Torzewski M, Shaw PX, Han KR, et al. Reduced in vivo aortic uptake of radiolabeled oxidation-specific antibodies reflects changes in plaque composition consistent with plaque stabilization. *Arterioscler Thromb Vasc Biol* 2004; 24: 2307–12.

82. Fujimoto S, Hartung D, Ohshima S, et al. Molecular imaging of matrix metalloproteinase in atherosclerotic lesions. Resolution with dietary modification and statin therapy. *J Am Coll Cardiol* 2008; 52: 1847–57.

83. Kolodgie FD, Petrov A, Virmani R, et al. Targeting of apoptotic macrophages and experimental atheroma with radiolabeled annexin V. A technique with potential for non-invasive imaging of vulnerable plaque. *Circulation* 2003; 108: 3134–9.

84. Kietselaer BL, Reutelingsperger CP, Heidendal GA, et al. Non-invasive detection of plaque instability with use of radiolabeled annexin A5 in

patients with carotid-artery atherosclerosis. *N Engl J Med* 2004; 350: 1472–3.

85. Sarai M, Hartung D, Petrov A, et al. Broad and specific caspase inhibitor-induced acute repression of apoptosis in atherosclerotic lesions evaluated by radiolabeled annexin A5 imaging. *J Am Coll Cardiol* 2007; 50: 2305–12.

86. Gaemperli O, Shalhoub J, Owen DRJ, et al. Imaging intraplaque inflammation in carotid atherosclerosis with 11C-PK11195 positron emission tomography/computed tomography. *Eur Heart J* 2012; 33: 1902–10.

87. Hartung D, Petrov A, Haider N, et al. Radiolabeled monocyte chemotactic protein 1 for the detection of inflammation in experimental atherosclerosis. *J Nucl Med* 2007; 48: 1816–21.

88. Nahrendorf M, Keliher E, Panizzi P, et al. 18F-4V for PET-CT imaging of VCAM-1 expression in atherosclerosis. *JACC Cardiovasc Imaging* 2009; 2: 1213–22.

89. Laitinen I, Saraste A, Weidl E, et al. Evaluation of $\alpha_v\beta_3$ integrin-targeted positron emission tomography tracer 18F-galacto-RGD for imaging of vascular inflammation in atherosclerotic mice. *Circ Cardiovasc Imaging* 2009; 2: 331–8.

90. Shah F, Balan P, Weinberg M, et al. Contrast-enhanced ultrasound imaging of atherosclerotic carotid plaque neovascularization: a new surrogate marker of atherosclerosis? *Vasc Med* 2007; 12: 291–7.

91. Coli S, Magnoni M, Sangiorgi G, et al. Contrast-enhanced ultrasound imaging of intraplaque neovascularization in carotid arteries.

Correlation with histology and plaque echogenicity. *J Am Coll Cardiol* 2008; 52: 223–30.

92. Xiong L, Deng YB, Zhu Y, Liu YN, Bi XJ. Correlation of carotid plaque neovascularization detected by using contrast-enhanced US with clinical symptoms. *Radiology* 2009; 251: 583–9.

93. Kaufmann BA, Sanders JM, Davis C, et al. Molecular imaging of inflammation in atherosclerosis with targeted ultrasound detection of vascular cell adhesion molecule-1. *Circulation* 2007; 116: 276–84.

94. Kaufmann BA, Carr CL, Belcik, et al. Molecular imaging of the initial inflammatory response in atherosclerosis. Implications for early detection of disease. *Arterioscler Thromb Vasc Biol* 2010; 30: 54–9.

95. Hamilton AJ, Huang SL, Warnick D, et al. Intravascular ultrasound molecular imaging of atheroma components in vivo. *J Am Coll Cardiol* 2004; 43: 453–60.

96. Versteylen MO, Kietselaer BL, Dagnelie DC, et al. Additive value of semi-automated quantification of coronary artery disease using cardiac CT-angiography to predict for future acute coronary syndrome. *J Am Coll Cardiol* 2013; 61: 2296–305.

97. Muntendam P, McCall C, Sanz J, Falk E, Fuster V. The BioImage study: novel approaches to risk assessment in the primary prevention of atherosclerotic cardiovascular disease—study design and objectives. *Am Heart J* 2010; 160: 49–57.

98. Braunwald E. Coronary plaque erosion. Recognition and management. *JACC Cardiovasc Imaging* 2013; 6: 288–9.

SECTION V

Heart failure

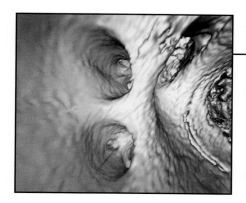

CHAPTER 23

Evaluation of left ventricular systolic function and mechanics

Rainer Hoffmann and Paolo Colonna

Parameters of systolic function

The severity of left ventricular (LV) systolic dysfunction is a strong predictor of clinical outcome for a wide range of cardiovascular diseases. Assessment of LV function is probably the most frequently requested indication to perform echocardiography and it is an integral part of cardiac magnetic resonance (CMR) and radionuclide studies. Visual estimates of global and regional function are supplemented by quantitative analysis of function. Left ventricular function is evaluated best from multiple tomographic planes, typically including parasternal long-axis, parasternal short-axis, apical four-chamber, apical two-chamber, and apical long-axis views. Systolic function relates to the function during the interval of the cardiac cycle lasting from mitral valve closure to aortic valve closure. Left ventricular diameters, as well as ejection fraction and related volumes, are the parameters normally determined to describe global LV function.

Left ventricular dimensions and volumes

The normal shape of the left ventricle is symmetric with two short axes of relatively similar length and a long axis from base to apex. Analysis of left ventricular dimensions should consider gender and body surface area of the patient [1].⊃ Table 23.1 displays normal values for LV dimensions, as well as volumes and function [1].

Global systolic function

The classic parameter of global LV systolic function is the ejection fraction (LVEF), calculated from the end-diastolic (LVEDV) and end-systolic (LVESV) volumes of the left ventricle (LVEF = [LVEDV – LVESV]/LVEDV). The volumes provide clues to increased LV preload (increased end-diastolic volume), as well as increased afterload or impaired myocardial contractility (increased end-systolic volume). Using 2D-echocardiography volumes should be calculated using the biplane discs' summation algorithm applied on the apical four- and two-chamber view. Monoplane discs' summation algorithm applied on the apical four-chamber view should not be used anymore or limited to normally shaped ventricles (normal subjects, pressure overload patients with normally sized ventricles) [1]. Typical difficulties in the analysis of these parameters using 2D-echocardiography relate to a foreshortened acquisition of the apical views and lack visualization of the true apex. This will result in underestimation of systolic and diastolic volumes, while the assessment of ejection fraction is less affected. 3D-echocardiography has been shown to result in significantly less underestimation of LV volumes and higher accuracy in the analysis of ejection fraction compared to measurements obtained by CMR [2]. Another difficulty of current 2D-echocardiographic techniques is potential impairment of endocardial contours' definition, in particular using apical views resulting in inaccuracies with regard to definition

Table 23.1 Normal values of the left ventricle

	Women	Men
LV diastol. diameter (cm)	3.9–5.3	4.2–5.9
LV diastol. diameter/BSA (cm/m²)	2.4–3.2	2.2–3.1
LV diastol. volume (ml)	56–104	67–155
LV diastol. volume/BSA (ml/m²)	35–75	35–75
LV systol. volume (ml)	19–49	22–58
LV systol. volume/BSA (ml/m²)	12–30	12–30
Ejection fraction (%)	>55	>55

of LV volumes. Administration of contrast agents may improve the accuracy in the analysis of LV volumes and ejection fraction [3].

Doppler echocardiography allows evaluation of global LV systolic function based on calculation of stroke volume and cardiac output. Using Doppler and 2D-echo data, stroke volume (SV) is calculated as LV outflow tract cross-sectional area (CSA) times the velocitytime integral of flow through that area (VTI): SV = CSA × VTI. However, the method is limited by potential inaccuracies related to the multiple required measurements.

Regional systolic function

Regional function abnormalities are most frequently due to coronary artery disease causing myocardial infarction, acute ischaemia, myocardial stunning, or hibernation. Dilative cardiomyopathy and myocarditis are less frequent causes. Regional LV function is normally evaluated considering a 16-segment model of the left ventricle (Fig. 23.1) as recommended by the American Society of Echocardiography, although a 17-segment model adding an apical segment has been suggested by the American Heart Association to homogenize with the myocardial scintigraphic perfusion analysis. Regional systolic function is characterized by wall

thickening and endocardial inward motion. In clinical practice, regional function is evaluated visually using a qualitative score ranging from:

- normokinesia: normal inward motion and normal thickening;
- hypokinesia: reduced but not absent inward motion and thickening;
- akinesia: absent inward motion and thickening; and
- dyskinesia: systolic outward motion of the ventricular wall.

Visual qualitative analysis of regional function on native 2D-echocardiography has been found to be observer-dependent with only moderate to fair inter-observer agreement. A special difficulty relates to segments with poor visibility in which there is pronounced uncertainty of the observers about the correct assessment of function. Application of left heart contrast agents enhances visibility of endocardial systolic motion and thereby improves accuracy of function analysis, as well as agreement between different observers on regional function analysis [4] (Fig. 23.2). Due to its superb image quality, CMR is known to allow high-quality assessment of LV function in almost all patients.

Several approaches for quantification of regional and global myocardial systolic function have been suggested. Myocardial deformation imaging based either on Doppler tissue velocity analysis or on speckle tracking within 2D- or 3D-echocardiograms are currently the preferred modalities for quantification using echocardiography [5, 6] (Fig. 23.3). The application of these techniques in clinical practice has been described in a recent ASE/EAE consensus statement [7]. Doppler tissue imaging analysis obtained from an apical view allows definition of peak systolic velocities in the longitudinal direction. These velocities are echo angle dependent, increase from apex to base and are affected by myocardial tethering. Deformation parameters obtained from speckle tracking echocardiography are not affected by these limitations. Speckle tracking echocardiography is based on tracking of speckles seen in grayscale B-mode images.

Fig. 23.1 16-segment-model of the left ventricle according to the American Society of Echocardiography. The perfusion areas of the LAD (left anterior descending artery) and the joint territory of the RCA (right coronary artery) and LCX (left circumflex artery) are indicated.

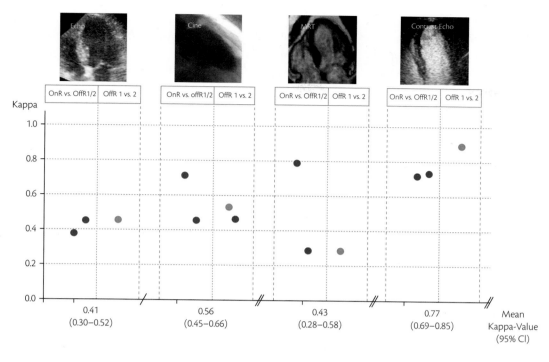

Fig. 23.2 Inter-observer agreement between three readers on cineventriculography, magnetic resonance imaging, echocardiography without and with contrast enhancement.

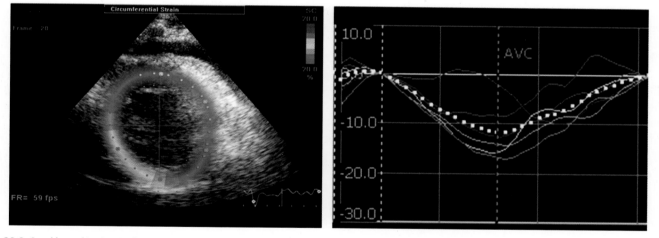

Fig. 23.3 Speckle tracking image showing circumferential strain of a patient with akinesia of the posterior wall.

Blocks of speckles can be tracked from frame to frame using block matching, and provide local displacement information, from which parameters of myocardial function, such as velocity, strain, and strain rate, can be derived. Quantification of strain and strain rate in any direction within the imaging plane is possible based on this technique. In particular, radial, circumferential, as well as longitudinal strain parameters can be derived based on parasternal short-axis and apical views. However, strain and strain-rate data obtained by speckle tracking echocardiography may be affected by artefacts and noise in particular in cases of limited image quality. Tagging, strain-encoded cardiac magnetic resonance (SENC), and the recently introduced feature tracking are modalities to quantify regional LV function based on CMR. Feature tracking is similar to speckle tracking echocardiography as it tracks image pixels from frame to frame.

An indication for regional function analysis has been the definition of intraventricular dyssynchrony in LV function affecting in particular patients with significantly impaired LV function and left bundle branch block. For this purpose myocardial strain or velocity curves obtained by deformation imaging or regional volume curves obtained by 3D-echocardiography are compared between different LV segments [8] (see also Chapter 30).

Other derived indexes of systolic function

In addition to conventional parameters to describe global LV function, several other indexes have been suggested recently:

◆ The longitudinal shortening of the left ventricle contributes significantly to the ejection. A high correlation between the long-axis extension of the mitral annulus motion determined in apical views and the ejection fraction could be proven.

◆ Myocardial deformation imaging has been used to define a parameter of global LV function called global strain. This parameter obtained by speckle tracking analysis within 2D-echocardiograms describes the degree of myocardial systolic shortening within all segments of an apical view. A high correlation has been shown for this parameter to the LV ejection fraction (➲ Fig. 23.3).

◆ Based on the analysis of a mitral insufficiency, continuous wave Doppler tracing the increase in early systolic pressure increase (dP/dt) can be calculated. Although this analysis is not based on the real LV pressure but a pressure difference between left ventricle and atrium, it provides a global parameter of LV contractility (normal >1000 mmHg/s). To determine this parameter the time interval between a regurgitant velocity of 1 m/s (equivalent to a ventriculo-atrial pressure difference of 4 mmHg) and 3 m/s (equivalent to a ventriculo-atrial pressure difference of 36 mmHg) is defined (➲ Fig. 23.4).

◆ The myocardial performance index (MPI or Tei-index) provides a parameter of systolic and diastolic function [9]. It is based on the analysis of the spectral Doppler mitral inflow and aortic outflow signal to determine the time interval between the end of mitral inflow from a first cardiac cycle and the start of mitral inflow from the next cardiac cyle (A) as well as the duration of the ejection period (B). The MPI is calculated as A – B/B (➲ Fig. 23.5). An alternative way to calculate the MPI is to use the spectral DTI at septal and/or lateral wall and measure the needed times in the usual way. This method allows the measurement of several parameters on the same cardiac cycle and to obtain these data also in patients with atrial fibrillation or irregular cardiac rhythm. Myocardial diseases prolong the isovolumetric contraction and relaxation time. As a consequence, the MPI, which is normally <0.49, increases.

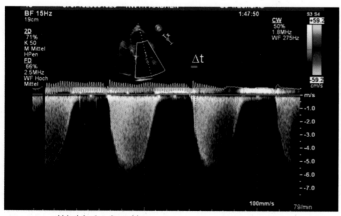

pLV-pLA t1 = 4 mmHg
pLV-pLA t2 = 36 mmHg
Δt = 60 msec
dp/dt = 36 – 4 mmHg/60ms
dp/dt = 533 mmHg/sec

Fig. 23.4 Calculation of left ventricular pressure rise dP/dt from the mitral regurgitant jet.

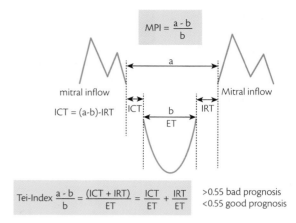

Fig. 23.5 Schematic drawing demonstrating the 'myocardial performance index' from mitral inflow and left ventricular outflow profile.

Imaging for diagnosis, guidance of treatment, and follow-up in heart failure

In clinical practice, cardiac imaging provides very important supplementary information to those obtained from the clinical scenario in guiding the therapeutic management of patients with congestive heart failure (CHF). Cardiac imaging allows the diagnosis of systolic and diastolic dysfunction, both in patients with overt heart failure and with asymptomatic LV dysfunction [12]. In the overt heart failure management, an individualized echocardiography guided strategy that monitors the haemodynamic profile is able to evaluate the therapeutic effects much better than a conventional clinically oriented strategy [13, 14]. When echocardiography has been used to guide pharmacologic therapy protocols in patients with heart failure and LV systolic dysfunction, mortality and hospitalization has been reduced. Besides overt heart failure, cardiac imaging (mostly echocardiography) was able to identify in the community a substantial number of subjects with asymptomatic LV dysfunction, mostly due to hypertensive cardiomyopathy and silent coronary artery disease [10, 11]. The CHF usually develops progressively, often beginning with asymptomatic LV dysfunction and culminates in the overt CHF with symptoms and signs from fluid overload and poor end-organ perfusion. The early identification of the subgroup of patients who may deteriorate is essential to establish the appropriate therapy [12, 13]. In patients identified to have asymptomatic LV dysfunction, a reduction of the progression rate to symptomatic heart failure with ACE inhibitors and beta blocker therapy has been demonstrated in large-scale clinical trials [12].

Furthermore, cardiac imaging can guide therapy also in patients with clinical syndrome of CHF and preserved systolic function, implying that abnormal LV diastolic function is the mechanism responsible for producing CHF symptoms. Recent guidelines recommend performing a cardiac imaging test (preferring echocardiography as screening test) in all patients with suspected CHF [12, 13]. In these patients cardiac imaging is essential in the diagnosis of heart failure with preserved EF and of its aetiology (ischaemia, remodelling, dyssynchrony, etc.).

Multiple pharmacologic and device-based treatment modalities have become available for treatment of patients with systolic LV dysfunction. To define the impact of specific new treatment modalities and to determine the spontaneous development of a disease process, as well as the efficacy of a selected treatment on LV function in individual patients, sequential studies are required. High reproducibility in the analysis of LV volumes and function is required for a reliable analysis of changes induced by treatment. The quality of repeated analysis of LV function is assessed either as intra- and inter-observer variability, which relates to the repeated measurement of a single dataset, or as test–retest reproducibility, which involves repetition of the entire acquisition and analysis. The different imaging techniques show varied potential for reproducibility, as well as in safety and costs.

Left ventricular systolic and diastolic volumes, as well as ejection fractions, are the conventional quantitative parameters to determine left ventricular function during follow-up studies. Subjective visual assessment of the LV ejection fraction is effective for single assessments but insufficiently reliable for sequential analysis. Conventional echocardiographic parameters based on 2D-echocardiography have also been shown to have limited test–retest reproducibility. Major limiting factors are poor image quality, geometric issues related to volume calculations, and the performance of off-axis cuts. In a study on 50 patients, test–retest correlation of LV ejection fraction was found to be only moderate (r = 0.66) using quantitative analysis based on 2D-echocardiography. In contrast, 3D-echocardiography has been proven to have high test–retest correlation (r = 0.92). Intra- and inter-observer variability of 3D-echocardiography derived LV volumes and ejection fractions have also been shown to be only in the range of 5.1–7.6%. Thus, using 3D-echocardiography intra- and inter-observer variability in the analysis of LV function can be similar to that obtained with CMR [15–17]. Newer parameters such as left atrial size and DTI parameters have also been described for serial clinical testing of LV function. However, they have demonstrated high variability. Thus, these parameters are not recommended for sequential LV assessment. Considering the high intra- and inter-observer agreement, as well as the low test–retest variation for 3D echocardiographic analysis of LV function parameters, 3D-echocardiography should be used as modality of choice if accurate echocardiographic analysis of LV function during follow-up studies is required.

Comparison of strengths and weaknesses of different modalities and techniques

When a clinician has to choose the best imaging technique to evaluate left and right ventricular function, he has to take into account the accuracy of different imaging techniques in calculating the exact function, the eventual presence of contraindications, and to balance the advantages and limitations in that particular subset of patients. The availability of a particular imaging technique is often the first reason for the selection, especially in patients with limited mobility, while the absence of ionizing radiation is important in young patients and in those who need frequent re-evaluations of ventricular function. The knowledge of all the characteristics, advantages, and limitations of different imaging techniques, summarized in ⊃ Table 23.2, have to guide the wise clinician to the right patient diagnostic management.

Echocardiography

Due to its portability and immediate availability, Doppler echocardiography is considered the technique of first choice (and very often the single one utilized) to assess regional and global LV function. Its features are also fundamental in all the uses in the emergency department and in the intensive care unit for ancillary anatomic information. This widespread use as initial imaging diagnostic test is indeed due to its capability for thoroughly detecting pathologies like ischaemic or non-ischaemic cardiomyopathies, valvular, pericardial, and other cardiac and extra-cardiac diseases. In a limited number of patients with unsatisfactory acoustic windows, the adoption of intravenous echo-contrast administration can improve the wall motion and volumes analysis. Echocardiography has the highest temporal resolution among imaging techniques and the spatial resolution is second only to last generation CMR scanners.

Echocardiography is quick and useful for estimation of RV function, although the 3D reconstruction of right ventricular volumes is still investigational. Conversely, the measurement of LV thickness and the calculation of LV mass are very precise with many confirmations in medical literature.

The calculation of the ejection fraction is accurate, especially when using echo-contrast and 3D-echocardiography, although it is highly operator-dependent and the automatic analysis of these parameters is still suboptimal. LV volumes determined by echocardiography are smaller than those obtained by CMR or cardiac computer tomography. In a recent meta-analysis, including 23 studies comparing 2D- and 3D-echocardiography with CMR, 3D-echocardiography was shown to result in a mean underestimation of LV ejection fraction of 0.6±11.8%, while LV end-diastolic volume was underestimated by 19±34 ml and LV end-systolic volume was underestimated by 10±30 ml. Considering 2D-echocardiography, the differences in the determined LV volumes to CMR were significantly larger [18]. Another study comparing echocardiography, CMR, and cardiac computer tomography on 36 patients demonstrated that 2D- and 3D-echocardiography based measurements of LV volumes are smaller than those obtained by CMR or those obtained by cardiac computer tomography [19], while there were no differences between CMR and cardiac computer tomography.

Cardiac magnetic resonance imaging (MRI)

CMR has become the clinical gold standard for quantification of left and right ventricular volumes and mass, thanks to its 3D

Table 23.2 Characteristics, advantages, and limitations of different imaging techniques to manage the diagnosis at best

	Echocardiography	Cardiac magnetic resonance	Nuclear radionuclide angiography (RNA)	Nuclear ECG-gated SPECT imaging
Operator skill (acquisition or evaluation)	Important in acquisition and evaluation	Important in evaluation	Mostly independent	Important in evaluation
Reproducibility	Dependent on acoustic window; excellent with contrast	Excellent in global function, good in regional	High	High
Spatial and temporal resolution	High	Highest spatial resolution	Intermediate	Limited with extensive perfusion defects
Perfusion	Investigational with contrast	Optimal resolution (also viability)	—	Largest data (also viability)
Regional systolic thickening	Largest data in literature	Includes different layers analysis (tagging)	—	Possible
Function during stress	Optimal	Optimal (expensive)	Feasible	Feasible
Diastolic dysfunction	Optimal	Untwisting study (tagging)	Quantitative LV filling	—
3D analysis	Novel technique	Optimal	No	—
Ancillary structural info	Excellent	Excellent	Limited	No
LV hypertrophy and mass	Very good	Excellent	No	No
RV function assessment	Good (estimate)	Optimal	Accurate (direct)	No
Safety (ionizing radiation/ contrast media)	Safe	Contrast (limited toxicity)	Ionizing radiation	Ionizing radiation
Portability and availability	Optimal	Limited	Limited	Limited
Cost	Lowest	High	Low	Low
Peculiar characteristics	Most useful and convenient as first/unique technique	Proximal coronary arteries visualization	Large literature data for function follow up	Simultaneous info on perfusion and function
Other limitations		Claustrophobia No metallic objects		

nature. The analysis of left and right ventricular regional function is very precise, due to the highest spatial resolution (➲ Fig. 23.6), the information on wall thickening, and the operator-independent imaging acquisition. However, the evaluation of the data obtained with CMR shows it to be operator-dependent and limitations in the inter-reader evaluation have been shown, perhaps due to the moving scanning plane (as stated in the previous paragraph).

CMR can supply information only partially achievable with novel echocardiographic techniques, such as the myocardial perfusion (obtained with gadolinium contrast) and the differential analysis of sub-endocardial, mid-wall, and sub-epicardial function (obtained with the tagging CMR). With high-speed CMR, it is possible to obtain anatomical information and myocardial perfusion at the same time.

Similarly to echocardiography, but with an increased spatial resolution, CMR supplies ancillary anatomic information on ventricles and other cardiac and paracardiac structures that can be fundamental for a complete clinical diagnosis.

An important advantage of this technique is its clinical safety, due to the absence of ionizing radiation and the use of gadolinium contrast agent, without renal toxicity. Several disadvantages limit its utilization in clinical practice. The cost of a CMR exam is high, the availability is limited and there is no portability of

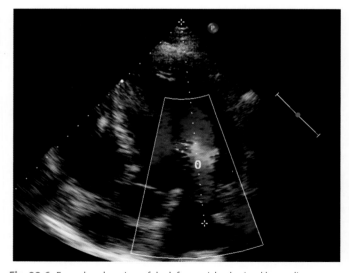

Fig. 23.6 Four-chamber view of the left ventricle obtained by cardiac magnetic resonance.

the equipment. Patients with pacemakers, implanted defibrillators, other devices and specific metal implants have to be excluded from the resonance analysis. In patients with impaired renal function, caution has to be considered with gadolinium contrast administration as nephrogenic systemic fibrosis may be a potential deleterious complication in these patients [20]. Patients with atrial fibrillation, as well as other cardiac arrhythmias, pose a challenge to the analysis of LV function using CMR. In the end, there is a small percentage of subjects suffering claustrophobia (especially during the pharmacologic stress test), which increases when analysing elderly and severely ill patients.

Nuclear techniques and regional function

The radionuclide angiography (RNA), also known as radionuclide ventriculography, can be performed by first-pass or by equilibrium-gated modalities (often referred to as MUGA scanning), obtaining similar results, but using different tracings and data acquisitions.

Both RNA techniques determine the changes in radionuclide counts in the left and right ventricles over the cardiac cycle, generating time–intensity curves. Ventricular volumes can then be obtained with the comparison of the counts described with the counts in a blood sample of known volume. Therefore, both quantitative ejection fraction and volumes obtained in this way are not affected by any assumption of ventricular geometry. An advantage of RNA techniques is its high accuracy and reproducibility in the analysis of LV volumes and ejection fraction. RNA techniques have therefore been applied in follow-up studies (e.g. analysis of chemotherapy toxicity, ventricular remodelling post-infarction, valvulopathy, etc.). Moreover, with RNA it is also possible to obtain the LV time–activity curve, representative of the volume changes along the cardiac cycle.

The major limitation of this technique is due to the lack of information on regional systolic thickening to supplement the regional wall motion and the lack of anatomic information supplementary to those on volumes and function.

The second nuclear method to evaluate ventricular function is the ECG-gated SPECT imaging, a recent and important evolution incorporated in the SPECT myocardial perfusion imaging, which enables the simultaneous analysis of LV function and perfusion. After a complex reconstruction, obtained with the gating of many cardiac cycles, the machine represents the LV wall in each frame and it is possible to analyse the global and regional wall motion, and to calculate end-systolic, end-diastolic volumes and ejection fraction. Thanks to the information supplied in the stress–rest myocardial perfusion imaging, this technique is complementary (but never primarily) utilized to detect regional and global LV function. Obviously, compared to CMR and echocardiography, the spatial and temporal resolution is suboptimal, as well as the lack of 3D information and the lack of diastolic data and of right ventricular function.

Both the nuclear techniques have the advantage of being mostly operator-independent. However, they share the disadvantages of the lack of portability of the machine and of patient exposure to ionizing radiation. Data obtained by nuclear techniques are not utilized for detection of LV hypertrophy and mass or other structural cardiac pathologies.

References

1. Lang R, Bierig M, Devereux R, et al. Recommendations for chamber quantification. A report from the American Society of Echocardiography's Nomenclature and Standards Committee, the Task Force on Chamber Quantification, and the European Association of Echocardiography. *Eur J Echocardiogr* 2006; 7: 79–108.

2. Kühl HP, Schreckenberg M, Rulands D, et al. High-resolution transthoracic real-time three-dimensional echocardiography: quantification of cardiac volumes and function using semi-automatic border detection and comparision with cardiac magnetic resonance imaging. *J Am Coll Cardiol* 2004; 43: 2083–90.

3. Hoffmann R, von Bardeleben S, ten Cate F, et al. Assessment of systolic left ventricular function: a multi-centre comparison of cineventriculography, cardiac magnetic resonance imaging, unenhanced and contrast-enhanced echocardiography. *Eur Heart J* 2005; 26: 607–16.

4. Hoffmann R, von Bardeleben S, Kasprzak JD, et al. Analysis of regional left ventricular function by cineventriculography, cardiac magnetic resonance imaging, and unenhanced and contrast-enhanced echocardiography: a multicenter comparison of methods. *J Am Coll Cardiol* 2006; 47: 121–8.

5. Urheim S, Edvardsen T, Torp H, Angelsen B, Smiseth OA. Myocardial strain by Doppler echocardiography: validation of a new method to quantify regional myocardial function. *Circulation* 2000; 102: 1158–64.

6. Amundsen BH, Helle-Valle T, Edvardsen T, et al. Noninvasive myocardial strain measurement by speckle tracking echocardiography: validation against sonomicrometry and tagged magnetic resonance imaging. *J Am Coll Cardiol* 2006; 47: 789–93.

7. Mor-Avi V, Lang RM, Badano LP, et al. Current and evolving echocardiographic techniques for the quantitative evaluation of cardiac mechanics: ASE/EAE consensus statement on methodology and indications. *J Am Soc Echocardiogr* 2011; 24: 277–313.

8. Becker M, Hoffmann R, Sasse A, et al. Long term benefit of cardiac resynchronization therapy is depending on the optimal lead position as defined by 3D-echocardiography. *Am J Cardiol* 2007; 100: 1671–6.

9. Tei C, Ling LH, Hodge DO, et al. New index of combined systolic and diastolic myocardial performance: a simple and reproducible measure of cardiac function—a study in normals and dilated cardiomyopathy. *J Cardiol* 1995; 26: 357–66.

10. Wang TJ, Evans JC, Benjamin EJ, et al. Natural history of asymptomatic left ventricular systolic dysfunction in the community. *Circulation* 2003; 108: 977–82.

11. Colonna P, Pinto FJ, Sorino M, Bovenzi F, D'Agostino C, de Luca I. The emerging role of echocardiography in the screening of patients at risk of heart failure. *Am J Cardiol* 2005; 96: 42L–51L.

12. McMurray JJV, Adamopoulos S, Anker SD, et al. ESC Guidelines for the diagnosis and treatment of acute and chronic heart failure. *Eur Heart J* 2012; 33; 1787–847.

13. Senni M, Rodeheffer RJ, Tribouilloy CM, et al. Use of echocardiography in the management of congestive heart failure in the community. *J Am Coll Cardiol* 1999; 33: 164–70.

14. Moreno R, Corros C, Zamorano J, Macaya C. Effect of intensive diuretic treatment over right ventricular behaviour: evidence provided from colour and pulsed-wave Doppler echocardiography. *Eur J Echocardiogr* 2003; 4(3): 226–8.

15. Soliman OII., Kirschbaum SW, van Dalen BM, et al. Accuracy and reproducibility of quantitation of left ventricular function by real-time three-dimensional echocardiography versus cardiac magnetic resonance. *Am J Cardiol* 2008; 102: 778–83.

16. Jenkins C, Bricknell K, Hanekom L, Marwick TH. Reproducibility and accuracy of echocardiographic measurements of left ventricular parameters using real-time three-dimensional echocardiography. *J Am Coll Cardiol* 2004; 44: 878–86.

17. Chuang ML, Hibberd MG, Salton CJ, et al. Importance of imaging method over imaging modality in noninvasive determination of left ventricular volumes and ejection fraction: Assessment by two- and three- dimensional echocardiography and magnetic resonance imaging. *J Am Coll Cardiol* 2000; 35: 477–84.

18. Dorosz JL, Lezotte DC, Weitzenkamp DA, Allen LA, Salcedo EE. Performance of 3-dimensional echocardiography in measuring left ventricular volumes and ejection fraction: a systematic review and meta-analysis. *J Am Coll Cardiol* 2012; 59(20): 1799–808.

19. Greupner J, Zimmermann E, Grohmann A, et al. Head-to-head comparison of left ventricular function assessment with 64-row computed tomography, biplane left cineventriculography, and both 2- and 3-dimensional transthoracic echocardiography: comparison with magnetic resonance imaging as the reference standard. *J Am Coll Cardiol* 2012; 59: 1897–907.

20. Thomsen HS, Morcos SK, Almén T, et al.; ESUR Contrast Medium Safety Committee. Nephrogenic systemic fibrosis and gadolinium-based contrast media: updated ESUR Contrast Medium Safety Committee guidelines. *Eur Radiol* 2013; 23: 307–18.

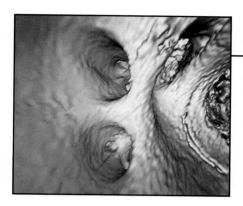

CHAPTER 24

Evaluation of diastolic LV function

Johan De Sutter and Jean-Louis J. Vanoverschelde

Contents

Introduction

Evaluation of diastolic left ventricular (LV) function is important for the diagnosis and management of all patients with heart failure, including those with a reduced LV ejection fraction (HFREF), as well as those with a preserved LVEF (HFPEF). In this chapter the pathophysiological basis of diastolic function will be discussed, as well as the principles of invasive and non-invasive evaluation of diastolic function and filling pressures. Also, newer echocardiographic and cardiac magnetic resonance techniques will be briefly explained, including myocardial deformation measurements during diastole, LV twist and untwisting, and evaluation of left atrial (LA) function. Finally, the clinical value of diastolic function parameters for diagnosis, prognosis, and therapy guidance in HFREF and HFPEF patients will be discussed.

Role of imaging for the evaluation of diastolic function

Pathophysiological basis of diastolic function

Because the main function of the heart is to ensure appropriate blood supply to the other organs, its pumping capacity, i.e. its ability to generate pressure and flow, has long been regarded as the most important component of its function. However, as with any pump, for the heart to efficiently propel blood into the circulation, its ability to fill swiftly at low filling pressures must be as efficient as its ejection performance. The maintenance of low filling pressures serves several purposes. First, it prevents excessive transudation at the capillary level, which would compromise oxygen diffusion, particularly in the lung. Second, it contributes to the generation of a pressure gradient necessary to drive flow across the capillary network. Last, it is essential to maintain coronary perfusion.

The ability of the LV to fill at low filling pressures is governed by its capacity to actively depressurize, a phenomenon referred to as diastolic relaxation, and subsequently to passively expand without an excessive increase in pressure, a feature referred to as ventricular stiffness [1].

Myocardial relaxation

Myocardial relaxation is an active process, caused by the release of elastic forces that have accumulated in the muscle as its structural elements were deformed during the preceding systole [2]. In the normal heart, during systole, the LV is contracted until its volume becomes smaller than its equilibrium volume, i.e. the volume at which filling pressures are exactly equal to zero [3]. As the contraction force dissipates, the release of these elastic forces allows the ventricle to expand until it reaches back its equilibrium volume. During early diastole,

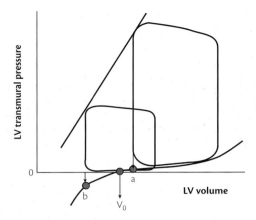

Fig. 24.1 Representative plots of two diastolic pressure–volume loops in a normally filling ventricle, superimposed on its passive pressure–volume relationship. When end-systolic volume (point b) becomes smaller than the equilibrium volume, V_0, the volume at which the transmural pressure of the fully relaxed LV is equal to zero, the ventricle generates a negative pressure which acts as the force driving early diastolic suction.

the LV thus acts as a suction pump, which generates a negative pressure and literally sucks the blood from the atrium [4–6]. Once the LV has reached its equilibrium volume, filling becomes entirely passive and solely dependent on atrial pressure and ventricular stiffness (see ⊃ Fig. 24.1). Twisting of the LV seems to play a key role in the storage of elastic forces during systole. Viewed from the apex, the apical portion of the LV normally twists counter-clockwise and the basal segment twists clockwise during systole, storing potential energy. Immediately after systolic contraction, the LV apex untwists, generating a pressure gradient between the apex and the base of the ventricle, which in turn acts as the suction force driving early diastolic filling [7, 8]. Besides the recoil forces, myocardial relaxation is also modulated by the rate of myofilaments inactivation, which is mostly dependent on calcium re-uptake by the sarcoplasmic reticulum, and by electro-mechanical non-informity [9].

Early diastolic relaxation and suction are critically important during exercise [10]. In normal individuals, the increase in cardiac output during dynamic exercise is largely brought about by a combined increase in heart rate and myocardial contractility. Despite large increases in heart rate, LV ejection times only decrease by 20–30%. By contrast, LV filling time shortens dramatically, falling to just above 100 ms at a rate of 150 beats/min. The maintenance of adequate LV filling, and hence stroke volume, under these conditions thus implies the ability to achieve mean filling rates during diastole that are far in excess of the ejection rates during systole. Greater systolic deformation and torsion, which allows end-systolic volume to decrease and hence elastic recoil to increase, are essential in this regard [11].

In patients with systolic heart failure, the LV usually does not twist appropriately and accordingly barely contracts beyond its equilibrium volume. Consequently, elastic energy is not stored to the same extent during systole and cannot be released as efficiently during early diastole [12]. As a consequence, LV filling becomes mostly inertial and dependent on venous pressure. When these pressures are low, the LV fills slowly in early diastole and most of its filling

depends on the increase in atrial pressure brought about by atrial contraction. At the opposite, when filling pressures are high, early diastolic filling increases and late diastolic filling decreases [13, 14].

Ventricular stiffness

Ventricular stiffness refers to the changes in end-diastolic LV pressure in relation to end-diastolic volume. Ventricular stiffness represents the resistance of the chamber to passive stretch. It is determined by the passive elastic properties of the myocardial muscle, which in turn depends on the amount of extracellular matrix collagen deposition and titin elastic properties. It is also influenced by ventricular interaction and by the pericardial constrain. Ventricular stiffness is usually characterized as the mono-exponential slope of the diastolic pressure–volume relation.

Invasive evaluation of diastolic function

Cardiac catheterization is the only technique that allows the direct measurement of LV diastolic pressures and the assessment of changes in the LV pressure–volume relationship. As they directly reflect the underlying physiology, parameters derived from cardiac catheterization often serve as a 'gold-standard' for the validation of non-invasive techniques.

The rate of isovolumic relaxation can be quantified by the instantaneous peak negative change in LV pressure (–dP/dt) and by the time constant of LV pressure decay (Tau). When diastolic relaxation is impaired, peak –dP/dt decreases and Tau increases.

The passive elastic properties are generally assessed from pressure–volume curves. Assessment of end-diastolic LV stiffness is cumbersome as it requires obtaining consecutive end-diastolic pressure volume data points under different loading conditions; for instance, during transient inferior vena cava occlusion. The passive elastic properties of the LV can then be quantified as β, the slope of the monoexponential end-diastolic pressure–volume relationship. As the LV becomes stiffer there is a greater change in pressure for an incremental change in volume and β increases.

Principles of non-invasive evaluation of diastolic function and filling pressures

Diastolic function is most commonly assessed by echocardiography, which has revolutionized our understanding and the clinical assessment of diastolic dysfunction. Nuclear imaging techniques, such as radionuclide angiography and single photon emission computed tomography (SPECT), can also provide information about diastolic function. Cardiac magnetic resonance (CMR) with its high spatial resolution, inherent 3D capabilities, and multitude of contrast mechanisms has the potential to provide unique information about diastolic performance.

Irrespective of the technique used, assessment of diastolic events relies on the study of instantaneous changes in LV volumes, segmental length, or a combination thereof. Non-invasive techniques thus mostly rely on the analysis of LV filling kinetics to evaluate 'diastolic function'. Unfortunately, normal LV filling depends not only on the diastolic properties of the chamber, i.e. relaxation and stiffness, but also, and probably even more so, on LA pressure [15].

Estimation of LV relaxation

Few parameters have been shown to correlate with invasive measures of LV relaxation, such as peak −dP/dt or Tau. These include the isovolumic relaxation time (IVRT), the calculation of Tau from the continuous wave (CW) Doppler signal of an aortic (AR) or a mitral regurgitant (MR) jet, the mitral annular early diastolic velocities, e' and the velocity of early diastolic flow propagation, Vp. More recently, global longitudinal strain during isovolumic relaxation and LV untwisting rates have also been used to estimate LV relaxation.

IVRT

Calculation of the IVRT is easy. It is best obtained by use of CW Doppler by placing the cursor in the LV outflow tract to simultaneously display the end of aortic ejection and the onset of mitral inflow (see ➲ Fig. 24.2). When LV relaxation is impaired, LV pressure falls slowly during the isovolumic relaxation period, delaying the opening of the mitral valve and thus prolonging IVRT [16]. Besides LV relaxation, IVRT is also influenced by the timing of mitral valve opening, which in turn is influenced by LA pressure. In clinical practice, the preload dependence of IVRT limits its usefulness as a measure of LV relaxation.

Indexes derived from AR or MR regurgitant jet

CW Doppler interrogation of the AR or MR jet allows the estimation of the instantaneous pressure gradient between the aorta and the LV during diastole, for AR jets, and between the LV and the LA during systole, for MR jets [17, 18]. Because both of these CW Doppler signals encompass the isovolumic relaxation period, to some extent, they permit assessment of the rate of LV depressurization. Experimental and clinical studies have demonstrated the feasibility of both methods. Since the fluctuation of aortic pressure is usually less than that in LA pressure during isovolumic relaxation, the AR method appears to provide an even more accurate estimate of the time constant compared with the MR method.

Mitral annular velocities

The velocity of mitral annular movement during early diastole, designated as e' velocity measured by Doppler tissue imaging (DTI) has been shown to correlate well with invasive measures of Tau [19, 20]. Although they are not entirely governed by relaxation, e' velocities are nonetheless frequently used to assess LV relaxation or to normalize preload dependent indexes, such the early transmitral filling velocity E, for relaxation.

PW Doppler DTI should be preferred over colour-coded DTI, as the latter lacks validation studies. Acquisition should be performed from the apical 4-chamber view, with the PW Doppler sample volume positioned at ±1 cm within the septal and lateral insertion sites of the mitral leaflets (see ➲ Fig. 24.3). The sample volume size should be adjusted to cover the longitudinal excursion of the mitral annulus during the cardiac cycle. Attention should be paid at gain settings, as annular velocities have high signal amplitude. The velocity scale should be set at ±20 cm/s, though lower settings may be necessary in patients with severe LV dysfunction. In those patients, the e' velocity should not be confused with isovolumic relaxation velocities. One should also carefully avoid angulation >20° between the ultrasound beam and the plane of cardiac motion. Finally, it is recommended to use the averaged of septal and lateral velocities.

Normal values of mitral annular velocities are influenced by age, similar to other indices of LV diastolic function. With age, e' velocity decreases, whereas a' velocity and the E/e' ratio increase [21]. Most patients with lateral e' <8.5 cm/s or septal e' <8 cm/s have impaired myocardial relaxation.

Early diastolic flow propagation

In the normal LV, the early filling wave propagates rapidly toward the apex and is driven by apical suction. In normal individuals, the forceful apical suction usually results in an almost instantaneous

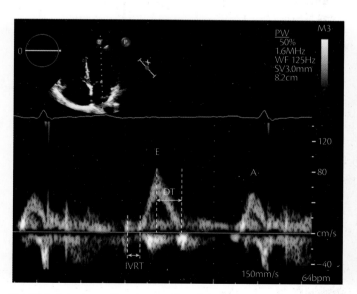

Fig. 24.2 Pulsed wave Doppler recording of the transmitral inflow obtained in a young individual with normal LV ejection fraction and relaxation. A: late filling velocity, DT: deceleration time, E: early filling velocity, IVRT: isovolumic relaxation time.

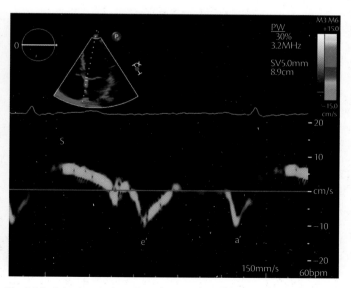

Fig. 24.3 Pulsed-wave tissue Doppler recording of the septal mitral annular velocities. a': late mitral annular velocity, e': early mitral annular velocity, s': systolic mitral annular velocity.

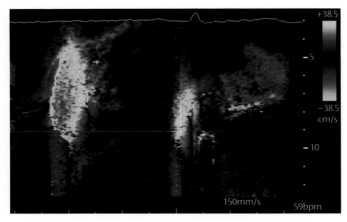

Fig. 24.4 Colour M-mode recording of the transmitral inflow illustrating the measurement of the velocity of inflow propagation, Vp.

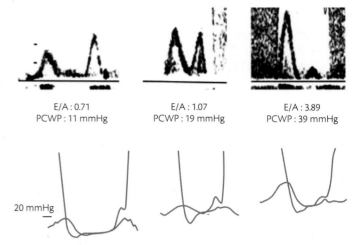

Fig. 24.5 Representative transmitral inflow velocities, together with the simultaneously measured high-fidelity LV pressure and pulmonary wedge pressure recordings in three patients with dilated cardiomyopathy.

filling of the apex. In patients with LV dysfunction, apical suction is reduced or absent, and early LV filling becomes solely inertial, resulting in the slowing down of early diastolic flow propagation. Good correlations have been reported between the velocity of early diastolic flow propagation, Vp, and Tau, both in normal and diseased LVs [22, 23].

The recommended approach for measuring early diastolic flow propagation is the slope method, because it is the least variable. Acquisition should be performed in the apical 4-chamber view, using a narrow colour flow sector. Gain should be adjusted to avoid noise. The M-mode scan line is then placed through the centre of the LV inflow. The colour scale should be adapted so that the central highest velocity jet is aliased. Vp is measured as the slope of the first aliasing velocity during early filling, measured from the mitral valve plane to ±4 cm distally into the LV cavity (see ◗ Fig. 24.4). Alternatively, the slope of the transition from no color to color can also be measured. Vp >50 cm/s is considered normal.

Estimation of LV stiffness

Thus far, there are no reliable non-invasive estimates of chamber stiffness. Surrogate measures include the deceleration time of early diastolic transmitral velocities [24, 25], the late diastolic velocity transit time [26], and the differences in duration between the transmitral A velocity and the pulmonary venous flow reversal [27].

Estimation of LV filling pressures

Numerous studies have demonstrated that the LV diastolic filling results from the complex interplay between LV relaxation, stiffness, and filling pressures [15]. Despite this complexity, the changes in the LV filling pattern induced by diseases of the heart are usually quite predictable [13]. Impairment of LV relaxation, in the presence of normal or low LA pressure produces characteristic changes in the LV filling dynamics, such as prolonged IVRT, reduced E velocity, and increased A velocity [13, 28]. Opposite changes are usually observed when elevated filling pressures

superimposed over impaired relaxation as a result of volume loading, new onset mitral regurgitation, or increased stiffness. Increasing LA pressure thus increases early filling velocities. It also results in shortening of the IVRT. At the same time, the atrial contribution to global LV filling diminishes, perhaps as a result of elevated LA afterload or systolic failure (see ◗ Fig. 24.5).

Because early filling velocities are equally dependent on LV relaxation and LA pressure, similar E velocities can be measured in young normal individuals and heart failure patients with combined slow relaxation and high LA pressures. Because E velocity is governed by both preload and relaxation, dividing E by an index of relaxation should provide information on preload. In daily clinical practice, two indices of LV relaxation have been used to normalize the E velocity and 'estimate' LV filling pressures: e' and Vp. Numerous studies have demonstrated that the ratios E/e' and E/Vp provide reasonably good estimates of LV filling pressures [29–31]. However, these indices should be used with caution in some patient populations, as will be delineated below [32].

New technologies in the assessment of diastolic function

New echocardiographic techniques

Several new parameters based on DTI and speckle tracking echocardiography (STE) have recently been introduced for the evaluation of regional and global LV diastolic function [33]. With these techniques, it is possible to measure global and regional myocardial velocity, displacement and deformation (strain and strain rate) [34, 35], mostly from apical LV views. Also evaluation of LV twisting and untwisting has become possible using DTI or STE from short-axis images of the LV [36, 37].

DTI measures velocities of myocardial tissue, which can be displayed as colour 2D images or as time versus distance or deformation (strain S and strain rate SR) curves. The advantage of DTI consists of its high temporal resolution if recordings are made with a high frame rate (>frames 100/s). The main disadvantage is its angle dependency.

STE is a technique that tracks very small myocardial structures ('speckles') from frame to frame in greyscale images. From these data myocardial velocities and deformation parameters can be derived. In contrast to DTI, it is not angle-dependent and lacks tethering and translational effects. It typically requires a frame rate of 40 to 80 frames/s.

These new techniques seem to be most attractive for clinical settings where the established Doppler echocardiographic methods may pose challenges. These include normal individuals and patients with mitral valve disease, heavy mitral annular calcifications, constrictive pericarditis, atrial fibrillation, left bundle branch block and severely dilated ventricles [33, 38]. The current limitations of these techniques include the need for high-quality signals, good myocardial visualization from the apical or short-axis views, experience in acquisition and analysis, and the longer time to measure strain, strain rate, twisting and untwisting.

Myocardial deformation measurements during diastole

During the IVRT interval, the mitral valve is closed and strain rate measurements during this period are therefore not affected by the transmitral pressure gradient. Also, in contrast to velocity measurement, SR measurements are not affected by mitral valve disease or mitral annulus calcifications. Therefore SR during IVRT (SR-IVR) is an attractive parameter for the evaluation of global LV relaxation (see ➲ Fig. 24.6). A good correlation between SR-IVR and the time constant of LV relation and –dP/dt has been documented and this relationship was not affected by changes in preload [39]. Also, the ratio of mitral E velocity to SR-IVR may be considered as an index of mean wedge pressure and was shown to be useful to identify patients with elevated filling pressures, particularly in patients with E/e' radio 8 to 15, normal EF, and regional dysfunction [39]. Similarly, Kasner et al. [40] performed a simultaneous

echocardiography-catheterization study in patients with HFNEF demonstrating the efficacy of diastolic SR indices and E/SR-IVR to detect LV diastolic dysfunction, but not a superiority compared with E/e'. Finally, in one larger study, SR-IVR ≤0.24 s⁻¹ was associated with incremental prognostic information in a cohort of 371 patients with acute-ST-elevated myocardial infarction [41]. Similarly to SR-IVR, global longitudinal strain and strain rate during peak mitral filling combined with the peak mitral E velocity has been assessed as a parameter of LV filling pressure [42]. It also showed a significant inverse correlation with mean wedge pressure and the time constant of LV relaxation but with a wide scatter that limits its clinical utility [42]. Also, no prognostic information is available yet for this parameter.

LV twist and untwisting

In a normal heart the apex of the LV twists counter-clockwise and the basal segments clockwise during systole. Torsion can be defined as the summation of these opposite rotations. The apical rotation normally exceeds the basal rotation and accounts for most of the observed twisting, a process that results in storing of potential energy. This stored energy is released in early diastole during untwisting. This process increases elastic recoil and the negative LA-LV pressure gradient that drives early passive filling [33, 43]. Twisting, torsion, and untwisting rate can be measured using DTI or STE from short-axis images of the LV or by CMR. These measurements are, however, complex and are currently mostly used for research on the pathophysiology of heart failure.

In patients with systolic heart failure, where myocardial dysfunction usually involves the mid-wall and sub-epicardial layers, circumferential strain and torsion are reduced. In contrast, HFPEF patients usually show a reduced sub-endocardial function with a resulting reduction in longitudinal and radial deformation but a preserved and even compensatory enhanced circumferential strain and torsion [44, 45]. The LV untwisting rate is dependent on the time

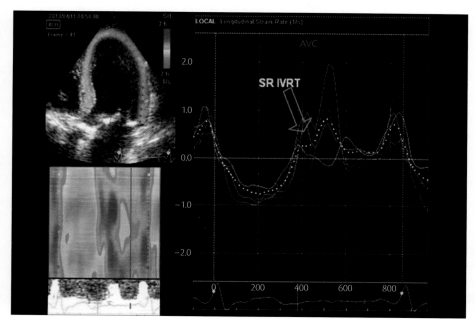

Fig. 24.6 Longitudinal strain rate measurements during systole and diastole in a heart failure patient with LV hypertrophy and a preserved LVEF of 60%, after stabilization with medical therapy. The strain rate value during isovolumic relaxation (SR-IVR, arrow) is slightly reduced (0.23 s⁻¹).

constant of LV relaxation but is also strongly influenced by loading conditions [46, 47]. Wang et al. [47] also showed that LV end-systolic volume is one the most important determinants of untwisting rate in patients with heart failure, irrespective of LV ejection fraction.

During exercise, there is an increase in both torsion and untwisting in the normal heart, which contributes significantly to LV filling. In patients with HFPEF, only a minimal increase of torsion and untwisting during exercise was documented, which might be an additional explanation of exercise intolerance in these patients [48].

Evaluation of LA function

Evaluation of LA volumes

An increase of LA volume may reflect chronic elevated filling pressures over time and is an important measurement of LV diastolic function in patients with heart failure [49]. It is now possible to measure maximal LA volumes with 3D-echocardiography [40]. Also, changes in LA volumes from mitral valve opening to its closure can be evaluated, although this can be technically challenging and may be easier to do with DTI or STE. It is important to realize, however, that an increase in LA volume can occur despite a normal diastolic function and filling pressures in the setting of, for example, intense sport activities, mitral valve disease, atrial fibrillation, and high output states.

Evaluation of LA strain by DTI and STE

LA strain can be measured by DTI or STE with sampling of several LA walls (varying between 2 and 12 segments). This allows evaluation of the different atrial functions: the LA reservoir function (measured by the maximal strain during LV systole), the LA conduit function (measured by the strain during early diastole) and the LA booster pump function (measured by the strain during atrial systole) [33]. Especially LA strain measured during LV systole appears to be a promising parameter for patients with heart failure. It relates significantly with LV end-diastolic pressure, especially in patients with reduced ejection fraction [50]. Also, it allows calculation of LA chamber stiffness by dividing LA pressure (wedge pressure or E/e') by LA strain measured during LV systole. This parameter relates well to pulmonary artery systolic pressure and may help to identify patients with HFPEF versus those with only diastolic dysfunction [51].

Cardiac magnetic resonance

Assessment of diastolic function is feasible with CMR with general principles similar to echocardiography. Although it is not frequently used in routine clinical practice, some unique features, such as CMR tagging and phosphorus-31 magnetic resonance spectroscopy, can be helpful in research settings to assess diastolic recoil properties and myocardial energy status.

Diastolic time–volume curves

The LV time–volume relationship represents relative volume changes throughout the cardiac cycle and may be used to evaluate LV filling, which is dependent on LV diastolic function [52]. This technique was first developed for SPECT images and later on for CMR. From the 3D volumetric data obtained with cine MR sequences of the LV short-axis, the endocardial borders are traced

phase by phase for each slice. This allows calculation of LV volume curves and LV filling rate during the cardiac cycle. Since it is time-consuming, it is rarely used in daily practice [53, 54].

Mitral inflow and pulmonary venous flow imaging

Similar to Doppler echocardiography, CMR contrast imaging can be used to evaluate the mitral inflow pattern (with E and A wave assessment) and the pulmonary venous flow pattern (with assessment of systolic flow, diastolic flow, and reversed flow at end-diastole due to atrial contraction) [54, 55]. Phase-contrast images are acquired with retrospective electrocardiogram gating covering the entire cardiac cycle (40–60 phases per cycle), usually using a velocity encoding of 90–150 cm/s for mitral inflow and 80–100 cm/s for pulmonary vein flow [52]. Also, it is possible to perform a Valsalva manoeuvre to reduce preload to unmask a pseudonormal filling pattern.

Myocardial tissue imaging

Myocardial tissue imaging may be used to evaluate mitral annular velocity (e'), similar to tissue Doppler imaging. It can be assessed by phase-contrast images using a velocity encoding of 20–30 cm/s [52]. Acquisition slices should be positioned parallel to the mitral annulus at two-thirds of the LV long-axis [56]. Similar to echocardiography, E/e' can be calculated with E/E' ≤8 usually predicting normal filling pressures and E/e' >15 elevated filling pressures. For intermediate E/e' values additional information obtained from pulmonary venous flow imaging or the Valsalva manoeuvre can be used to assess the filling status.

Myocardial tagging

CMR can label (or 'tag') the myocardium which allows easy visualization of systolic and diastolic myocardial deformations (strain, strain rate, torsion with twisting and untwisting). Especially, evaluation of LV torsion recovery and strain rate recovery that directly reflects the mechanisms of myocardial diastolic relaxation are interesting for research purposes [52, 57]. Although torsion is readily performed as part of any CMR examination, a variety of CMR imaging protocols can be used and there is a lack of standardization for methods to characterize the twisting motion of the LV [58]. Clearly more work needs to be done before these measurements can be introduced into a clinical setting.

^{31}P-MR spectroscopy

^{31}P-MR spectroscopy allows evaluation of the myocardial energy status. It is currently only available for research and measures the myocardial phosphocreatine/adenosine triphosphate ratio, which can be impaired in the presence of diastolic dysfunction [53].

Specific groups of patients

Heart failure patients with reduced ejection fraction (HFREF)

Diagnosis

In patients with systolic heart failure, the PW Doppler LV filling pattern correlates better with LV filling pressures, functional class, and prognosis than LVEF. In these patients, the mitral inflow pattern can be used to estimate LV filling pressures with reasonable accuracy.

As mentioned, normal LV filling consists in two distinct phases: an early diastolic filling phase, mostly driven by LV relaxation and LA pressure, and a late diastolic filling phase, related to atrial contraction and LV end-diastolic stiffness. In normal young individuals, the early diastolic E wave is usually higher than the late diastolic A wave, so that the E/A ratio is >1. Impaired LV relaxation, such as occurs with normal ageing, as well as in most patients with myocardial diseases, including LV hypertrophy, dilated cardiomyopathy, ischaemic heart disease, and asynchrony, alters the transmitral filling pattern in a characteristic and reproducible way. As long as LA pressure remains normal, impaired relaxation prolongs the IVRT and reduces the early diastolic pressure gradient between the LA and LV. Early diastolic filling and the E wave are consequently reduced. To some extent, late diastolic filling compensates for the decrease in early filling so that total filling volume remains unaffected. This first or 'early' stage of diastolic dysfunction, often referred to as stage I, is characterized by signs of altered relaxation. Patients presenting with this filling profile also display prominent systolic forward flow on pulmonary venous flow tracings. The duration of the late diastolic flow reversal is also similar to that of the A wave, so that the difference in duration between these two phenomena is negligible. When this pattern is observed in a patient with reduced LVEF, LV filling pressures are almost always normal.

When LV filling pressures are increased, the mitral valve opening pressure also increases. This causes the mitral valve to open sooner, which shortens the IVRT. Increases in LA pressure also increase the early diastolic pressure gradient between the LA and the LV, resulting in higher E velocities and filling volume. Because diseased ventricles are often stiffer than normal, the increase in early diastolic filling volume elevates mid-diastolic LV pressure, making it more difficult for LA contraction to contribute substantially to the final filling volume. At this stage, the patients usually manifest signs and symptoms of heart failure. Their transmitral filling profile closely resembles that of a normal young individual, and is therefore referred to as pseudonormal or normalized (⊃ Fig. 24.7). At this stage, which is named stage II diastolic dysfunction, assessment of LV filling pressures by use of the transmitral filling pattern alone requires caution, as it is frequently undistinguishable from a truly normal one. To differentiate between normal and pseudonormal filling patterns, one can simply rely on the pathological context of the patient. In patients with poorly contractile LVs but normal filling pressures, the 'normal' filling pattern should be stage I diastolic dysfunction. Accordingly, any other LV filling patterns should be considered as 'abnormal' and indicative of elevated filling pressures. In some patients, however, the context is not as self-explanatory as one would like and additional information is needed to further substantiate the pseudonormal origin of the filling pattern and the increase in filling pressures. One way to achieve this is to manipulate preload and observe the resulting changes in the transmitral filling profile. In daily clinical practice, this is best achieved using the Valsalva manoeuvre. During the strain phase of this manoeuvre, venous return dramatically decreases, which in turn reduces the LV filling pressures. In patients with stage II diastolic dysfunction, the Valsalva manoeuvre causes the E/A ratio to fall by >0.5 [59]. One can also normalize E velocities by an index related to LV relaxation such as the e' velocity, or the flow propagation velocity, Vp. An E/e' ratio >15 and E/Vp ratio >2.5 are strong arguments in favour of elevated filling pressures. Finally, one can also look at the pulmonary venous flow. With increasing filling pressures, the systolic forward flow (S) becomes less prominent, whereas the early diastolic forward flow (D) increases, so that the S/D ratio becomes <1 [60]. Also, the duration of the A wave decreases and becomes shorter than the late diastolic pulmonary venous flow reversal by >30 ms. It should be emphasized that use of these 'normalized' indices in isolation leaves quite a significant number of patients in a grey zone (between 8 and 15 for the E/e' ratio, and between 1.4 and 2.5 for the E/Vp ratio). This is the reason why the ASE and the EACVI strongly suggest using these indices in combination in order to better classify the patients.

When the underlying myocardial disease further progresses, the filling pattern becomes 'restrictive'. Restrictive physiology is characterized by further shortening of the IVRT, a marked increase in the amplitude of the E wave, together with a marked decrease in the amplitude of the A wave, so that the E/A ratio becomes >2, and a further shortening of the deceleration time of the E wave (⊃ Fig. 24.7). The duration of the A wave also shortens dramatically and diastolic filling usually stops before the next QRS complex. End-diastolic mitral regurgitation is not rare at this stage. The filling pattern seen in patients with such a restrictive physiology is referred to as stage III diastolic dysfunction.

From the description, it should be clear that changes in diastolic filling pressures, LV relaxation and stiffness result in predictable changes in the LV diastolic filling pattern. Using the diagnostic algorithm described, most patients with normal or elevated LV filling pressures can be identified. It is even possible to 'estimate' LA pressure or pulmonary capillary wedge pressure using the various indices described, alone or in combination. Although the accuracy of such an approach is not 100%, it can be used in daily clinical practice to risk stratify patients with heart failure and modulate the aggressiveness of the depletive treatment. In some patient populations, particularly those undergoing cardiac resynchronization therapy, the accuracy of these indexes have been questioned [32]. Indeed, in these patients, the correlation between the E/A ratio or the E/e' ratio and LV filling pressures has been shown to be less significant than in patients without CRT. Nonetheless, when used in combination, as recommended in the ASE and EACVI guidelines, these indices still allow estimation of LV filling pressures with reasonable accuracy and should therefore not be simply discarded [61].

Prognosis

Besides its ability to estimate LV filling pressures, echocardiographic measurements of diastolic function also provide important prognostic information. Numerous studies including meta-analyses [62] have demonstrated that in patients with reduced LVEF, parameters such as the E/A ratio [63], the deceleration of the E velocity [64] or the E/e' ratio [65, 66] provide incremental information to LVEF or wall motion score index. Although pulmonary

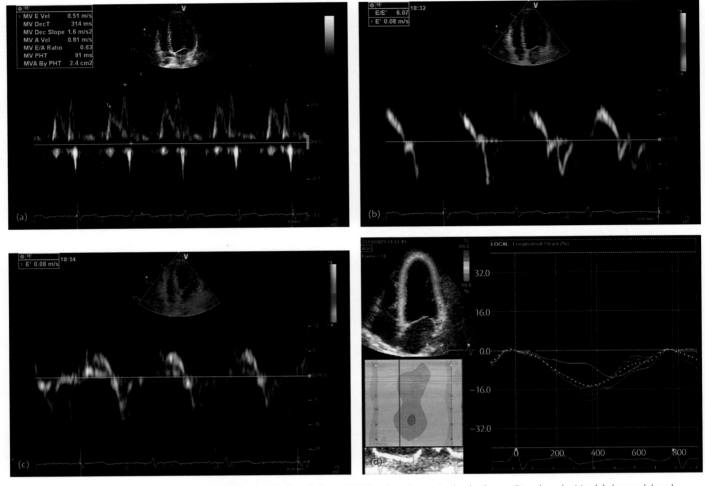

Fig. 24.7 Evaluation of diastolic function and global longitudinal strain in an HFPEF patient. Transmitral pulsed-wave Doppler velocities (a) show a delayed relaxation pattern with borderline e' values obtained by Doppler tissue imaging at the septal mitral annulus (b) and lateral mitral annulus (c), resulting in an E/e' value of 6. Global longitudinal systolic strain (GLS) measurements show however arguments for a mildly reduced systolic function (GLS value: −15%) (d).

venous velocities and Vp have not been studied as extensively, they seem to be predictive of clinical events as well.

Treatment follow-up

Because the LV filling pattern is intimately related to LV filling pressures, it can be affected by treatment. Several studies have demonstrated that diuretics, but also ACE inhibitors and beta blockers, improve the LV filling pattern and reduce the severity of diastolic dysfunction [67]. Interestingly, patients showing less restriction under treatment have a better long-term prognosis than those with persistent restrictive patterns [68]. These last patients probably have a more advanced disease stage and should probably be referred for heart transplantation or destination therapy sooner than those with reversible diastolic dysfunction.

Heart failure patients with preserved ejection fraction (HFPEF)

Diagnosis

Almost half of the patients with heart failure present with a preserved LVEF and show abnormalities of diastolic dysfunction, including increased diastolic LV stiffness and impaired relaxation,

resulting in abnormal LV filling [69]. These patients are usually elderly patients with predisposing factors for diastolic dysfunction such as hypertension, diabetes, atrial fibrillation, and obesity. Anatomically the hearts of patients are characterized by two important changes: (1) concentric LV hypertrophy in contrast to the eccentric changes and ventricular dilation in HFREF patients [70, 71] and (2) LA enlargement in response to elevations in LV filling pressure [72].

The most recent ESC guidelines on HFPEF [73] state that the diagnosis of HFPEF requires four conditions to be satisfied: (1) symptoms typical of HF, (2) signs typical of HF (which may not be present in the early stages of HFPEF and in patients treated with diuretics), (3) normal or only mildly reduced LVEF (typically LVEF ≥ 50%), in the absence of significant LV enlargement (end-diastolic volume ≤ 97 ml/m², end-systolic volume ≤ 49 ml/m²) and (4) relevant structural heart disease (concentric LV hypertrophy, LA enlargement) and/or diastolic dysfunction. Globally the diagnosis is more difficult than the diagnosis of HFREF because one should first exclude non-cardiac causes of the patient's symptoms (such as anaemia or chronic lung disease). Non-invasive imaging, and especially echocardiography, plays an important role in the evaluation of systolic and diastolic dysfunction but also in the identification of other conditions with predominant diastolic dysfunction that can lead to HFPEF, such as primary valve disease, pericardial disease, congenital defects, or pulmonary arterial hypertension. Importantly, the presence of both LA enlargement and concentric LV hypertrophy are readily assessed by 2D-echocardiography and corroborate the diagnosis of HFPEF. An LA volume more than 32 ml/m² is highly specific for diastolic dysfunction in the absence of valve disease or atrial fibrillation, and predicts elevated filling pressures and a worse clinical outcome when more than 34 ml/m² [72]. In patients with HFPEF concentric hypertrophy (increased mass and relative wall thickness), or remodelling (normal mass but increased relative wall thickness) can be observed [74]. Recently Ohtani et al. [75] showed that diastolic wall strain, defined as (posterior wall thickness at end-systole – posterior wall thickness at end-diastole)/posterior wall thickness at end-systole, might be used as a non-invasive index of diastolic stiffness and that a more advanced diastolic stiffness is associated with a worse outcome in HFPEF.

For the invasive diagnosis of diastolic dysfunction, the 2007 ESC consensus statement suggests four possible haemodynamic measurements: mean PCW >12 mmHg or LV end-diastolic pressure (EDP) >16 mmHg or τ >48 ms (parameter of impaired active relaxation) or b >0.27 (parameter of diastolic LV stiffness) [76]. These invasive measurements are rarely performed for the diagnosis of HFPEF in daily practice but may have a role in patients with unexplained dyspnoea. Penicka et al. [77], for example, showed that in 30 patients with LVEF >50% and unexplained dyspnoea, 66% of them had an LVEDP >16 mmHg indicating HFPEF, while only 25% of them fulfilled the echocardiographic criteria for HFPEF. For the non-invasive diagnosis of HFPEF, the 2007 ESC consensus statement [76] states that an E/e' ratio >15 (measured by DTI) is required. If the E/e' ratio is suggestive of diastolic LV dysfunction (15 >E/e' >8), additional non-invasive investigations are required for diagnostic evidence of diastolic LV dysfunction. These can consist of blood flow Doppler of the mitral valve (E/A ratio <0.5 and deceleration time >280 ms) or pulmonary veins (duration of reverse pulmonary vein atrial systole flow-duration of mitral valve atrial wave flow >30 ms), echo measures of LV mass index (>149 g/m² for men or >122 g/m² for women) or LA volume index (>40 ml/m²), electrocardiographic evidence of atrial fibrillation, or elevated plasma levels of natriuretic peptides. If plasma levels of natriuretic peptides are elevated, diagnostic evidence of diastolic LV dysfunction also requires additional non-invasive investigations such as E/e'>8, blood flow Doppler of mitral valve or pulmonary veins, echo measures of LV mass index or LA volume index, or electrocardiographic evidence of atrial fibrillation. The grading of the severity of diastolic dysfunction in HFPEF patients is similar to the grading in HFREF patients (⊃ Fig. 24.7). A comprehensive review of the techniques and the significance of echocardiographic diastolic parameters, as well as recommendations for nomenclature and reporting of diastolic data in patients with HFNEF, can be found in the most recent joint EACVI and ASE recommendation paper on the evaluation of LV diastolic function [74]. Additional validation of these guidelines for non-invasive diagnosis of HFPEF is however needed [78].

Finally, decreased longitudinal, radial, and circumferential systolic LV strains have been documented in HFPEF, supporting the hypothesis that LV systolic function is also impaired in these patients (see ⊃ Fig. 24.8) [79–81].

Diastolic stress test

Some patients with HFPEF develop mainly symptoms of dyspnoea during exertion and are asymptomatic at rest. This can be explained by the underlying diastolic dysfunction that causes an excessive rise in LV filling pressures that is needed to maintain adequate LV filling and stroke volume during exertion. Therefore, the evaluation of LV filling pressures by means of the E/e' ratio during exercise has been proposed as a potential echocardiographic marker to unmask diastolic dysfunction. In normal subjects the E and e' velocities increase proportionally and the E/e' ratio remains unchanged or is even reduced [82, 83]. In patients with impaired relaxation, however, the increase in e' with exercise is less pronounced than the E velocity increase and as a consequence the E/e' ratio increases. Additionally, mitral DT decreases slightly in normal individuals with exercise but shortens >50 ms in patients with a marked rise in filling pressures. Burgess et al. [84] showed that E/e' during exercise was significantly related to simultaneously invasively measured LV filling pressures. Also, Holland et al. [85] showed in a larger study that in patients with suspected HFPEF, almost 25% with an indeterminate resting E/e' ratio' between 8 and 15 (measured at the septal site) developed an E/e' ratio >13 during exercise, suggesting elevated filling pressures. However, conflicting results were reported by Maeder et al. [86] who could not document a relationship between the rise of PCWP and E/e' during exercise in HFPEF patients. Finally, Donal et al. [87] recently showed that in patients with HFPEF not only diastolic dysfunction may get worse during submaximal exercise, but also LV and RV longitudinal systolic function (assessed by STE). The exact place of the diastolic stress test in clinical practice is not determined yet.

Prognosis

Similar to patients with HFREF, several studies have assessed the prognostic value of the degree of diastolic dysfunction in the general population and in HFPEF patients. Halley et al. [88] recently showed, for example, that the presence of moderate and severe diastolic dysfunction had a significant impact on the long-term survival in a large outpatient population with normal LVEF. Importantly, it was also shown by Aljaroudi et al. [89] that in patients with normal baseline LVEF, worsening of diastolic dysfunction during follow-up is an independent predictor of mortality. In the CHARM Echocardiographic Substudy it was shown that in HF patients with LVEF ≥40%, the outcome (defined as risk of cardiovascular death or hospitalization) was significantly worse in patients with moderate or severe diastolic dysfunction as compared to patients with normal or only mild diastolic dysfunction [90]. E/e' >15, measured at the septal site, was also a predictor of outcome in HFPEF patients stabilized with medical therapy [91]. In contrast, Doppler echocardiographic measurements did not provide strong independent markers of prognosis in the I-PRESERVE study [92]. Similarly, LA size may be an independent predictor of mortality and cardiovascular events in HFPEF patients [93]

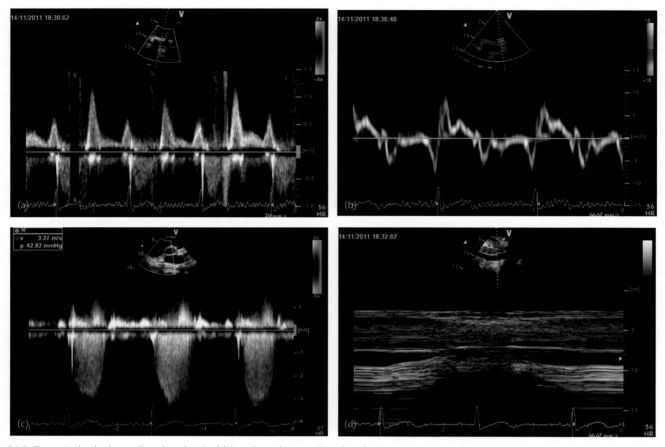

Fig. 24.8 Transmitral pulsed-wave Doppler velocities (a), lateral annular tissue Doppler velocities, tricuspid regurgitation continuous wave velocities (c) and M-mode through the vena cava inferior (d) of a 78-year old woman admitted with acute heart failure with an LVEF of 55%. The E/e' is 25 (obtained from a and b) and the systolic pulmonary artery pressure is calculated at 55 mmHg (obtained from c and d), indicating elevated left and right filling pressures.

although this not was confirmed in the CHARM Echocardiographic Substudy [90]. Finally, parameters of systolic dysfunction measured by DTI or STE may potentially predict outcome in these patients, but further studies are needed [94].

Treatment follow-up

The medical treatment of HFPEF patients remains controversial as, up to now, none of the standard medications for HFREF (including RAAS blockade, beta blockers, and aldosterone receptor antagonists) have shown a beneficial effect on mortality or morbidity in HFPEF patients [78, 95]. Also, the role of non-invasive imaging and echocardiography for treatment follow-up in these patients is not defined yet. Even the estimation and serial follow-up of LV filling pressures in HFPEF patients is challenging and not so clear as compared to patients with reduced EF. An average E/e' ≤8 usually identifies patients with normal filling pressures whereas a ratio ≥13 indicates an increase in LV filling pressures (see ⊃ Fig. 24.9). If the ratio is between 9 and 13, an Ar-A duration ≥30 ms, a change in E/A ratio with the Valsalva manoeuvre of ≥0.5, a maximal LA volume ≥34 ml/m², or pulmonary artery systolic pressure ≥35 mmHg (in the absence of pulmonary disease) can be used as indicators of increased LV filling pressures [74, 96]. Caution in applying this algorithm is, however, needed in different clinical scenarios, including elderly patients, hypertrophic

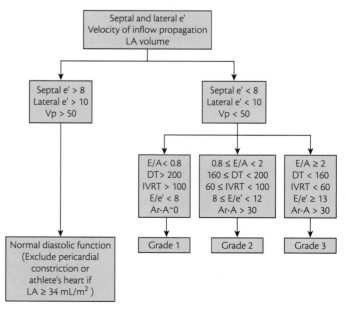

Fig. 24.9 Grading diastolic dysfunction in patients with heart failure (HFREF and HFPEF).

cardiomyopathy (with very low E' values), left bundle branch block, atrial fibrillation, a calcified mitral annulus (with high E values), and constrictive pericarditis [21, 74]. Also, different studies could not document a clear relationship between E/E' values and invasively assessed LV filling pressures at rest as well as during exercise or different loading conditions [86, 97]. This suggests that at least an approach with different clinical/echocardiographic parameters, as well as further validation studies, are needed.

Conclusions

The evaluation of diastolic function in patients with HFREF and HFPEF is important as it carries both diagnostic and prognostic information. In daily practice, this is most frequently done by standard echocardiographic techniques, including the evaluation of LV mass and LA volumes, as well as transmitral and pulmonary venous PW Doppler, CW Doppler for evaluation of the IVRT, and tissue Doppler imaging of the septal and lateral annular velocities. This permits grading the severity of diastolic dysfunction, which is related to outcome. These parameters may also be used to estimate LV filling pressures. The latter needs, however, further validation, especially in patients with HFPEF. Newer echocardiographic and cardiac magnetic resonance techniques, including myocardial deformation measurements during diastole, LV twist and untwisting, and parameters of LA function, are promising and will hopefully in the future help clinicians to make a more precise evaluation of diastolic function and filling pressures in heart failure patients.

References

1. Zile M, Baicu C, Gaasch W. Diastolic heart failure—abnormalities in active relaxation and passive stiffness of the left ventricle. *N Engl J Med* 2004; 350: 1953–59.
2. Caillet D, Crozatier B. Role of myocardial restoring forces in the determination of early diastolic peak velocity of fiber lengthening in the conscious dog. *Cardiovasc Res* 1982; 16: 107–12.
3. Yellin EL, Hori M, Yoran C, Sonnenblick EH, Gabbay S, Frater RWM. Left ventricular relaxation in the filling and non-filling intact canine heart. *Am J Physiol* 1986; 250: H620–29.
4. Hori M, Yellin EL, Sonnenblick EH. Left ventricular suction as a mechanism of ventricular filling. *Jap Circ J* 1982; 46: 124–29.
5. Robinson TF, Factor SM, Sonnenblick EH. The heart as a suction pump. *Sci Am* 1986; 254: 84–91.
6. Courtois M, Vered Z, Barzilai B, Ricciotti NA, Pérez JE, Ludbrook PA. The transmitral pressure-flow velocity relation: effect of abrupt preload reduction. *Circulation* 1988; 78: 1459–68.
7. Notomi Y, Popovic ZB, Yamada H, et al. Ventricular untwisting: a temporal link between left ventricular relaxation and suction. *Am J Physiol* 2008; 294: H505–13
8. Burns AT, La Gerche A, Prior DL, MacIsaac AI. Left ventricular untwisting is an important determinant of early diastolic function. *J Am Coll Cardiol Img* 2009; 2: 709–16.
9. Brutsaert DL, Rademakers F, Sys SU. The triple control of relaxation: Implications in cardiac diseases. *Circulation* 1984; 69: 190–96.
10. Vanoverschelde J-L, Essamri B, Vanbutsele R, et al. Contribution of left ventricular diastolic function to exercise capacity in normal subjects. *J Appl Physiol* 1993; 74: 2225–33.
11. Cheng CP, Igarashi Y, Little WC. Mechanism of augmented rate of left ventricular filling during exercise. *Circ Res* 1992; 70: 9–19.
12. Bertini M, Nucifora G, Marsan NA, et al. Left ventricular rotational mechanics in acute myocardial infarction and in chronic (ischemic and nonischemic) heart failure patients. *Am J Cardiol.* 2009; 103: 1506–12.
13. Appleton CP, Hatle LK, Popp RL. Relation of transmitral flow velocity patterns to left ventricular diastolic function: new insights from a combined hemodynamic and Doppler echocardiographic study. *J Am Coll Cardiol* 1988; 12: 426–40.
14. Vanoverschelde J-LJ, Raphaël D, Robert A, Cosyns J. Left ventricular filling in dilated cardiomyopathy: relation to functional class and hemodynamics. *J Am Coll Cardiol* 1990; 15: 1288–95.
15. Ishida Y, Meissner JS, Tsujioka K, et al. Left ventricular filling dynamics: influence of left ventricular relaxation and left atrial pressure. *Circulation* 1986; 74: 187–96.
16. Scalia GM, Greenberg NL, McCarthy PM, Thomas JD, Vandervoort PM. Noninvasive assessment of the ventricular relaxation time constant (tau) in humans by Doppler echocardiography. *Circulation* 1997; 95: 151–55.
17. Nishimura RA, Schwartz RS, Tajik AJ, Holmes DR Jr. Noninvasive measurement of rate of left ventricular relaxation by Doppler echocardiography: validation with simultaneous cardiac catheterization. *Circulation* 1993; 88: 146–55.
18. Yamamoto K, Masuyama T, Doi Y, et al. Noninvasive assessment of LV relaxation using continuous wave Doppler aortic regurgitant velocity curve: its comparative value to the mitral regurgitation method. *Circulation* 1995; 91: 192–200.
19. Nagueh S, Middleton K, Kopelen H, Zoghbi W, Quinones M. Doppler tissue imaging: a noninvasive technique for evaluation of left ventricular relaxation and estimation of filling pressures. *J Am Coll Cardiol* 1997; 30: 1527–33.
20. Sohn D, Chai I, Lee D. Assessment of mitral annulus velocity by Doppler tissue imaging in the evaluation of left ventricular diastolic function. *J Am Coll Cardiol* 1997; 30: 474–80.
21. De Sutter J, De Backer J, Van de Veire N, Velghe A, De Buyzere M, Gillebert TC. Effects of age, gender, and left ventricular mass on septal mitral annulus velocity (E') and the ratio of transmitral early peak velocity to e' (E/e'). *Am J Cardiol* 2005; 95: 1020–23.
22. Takatsuji H, Mikami T, Urasawa K, et al. A new approach for evaluation of left ventricular diastolic function: spatial and temporal analysis of left ventricular filling flow propagation by color M-mode Doppler echocardiography. *J Am Coll Cardiol* 1996; 27: 365–71.
23. Greenberg NL, Vandervoort PM, Firstenberg MS, Garcia MJ, Thomas JD. Estimation of diastolic intraventricular pressure gradients by Doppler M-mode echocardiography. *Am J Physiol* 2001; 280: H2507–15.
24. Little WC, Ohno M, Kitzman DW, Thomas JD, Cheng CP. Determination of left ventricular chamber stiffness from the time for deceleration of early left ventricular filling. *Circulation* 1995; 92: 1933–39.
25. Garcia MJ, Firstenberg MS, Greenberg NL, et al. Estimation of left ventricular operating stiffness from Doppler early filling deceleration time in humans. *Am J Physiol* 2001; 280: H554–61.
26. Pai RG, Suzuki M, Heywood T, Ferry DR, Shah PM. Mitral A velocity wave transit time to the outflow tract as a measure of left ventricular diastolic stiffness. Hemodynamic correlations in patients with coronary artery disease. *Circulation* 1994; 89: 553–57.

27. Rossvoll O, Hatle LK. Pulmonary venous flow velocities recorded by transthoracic Doppler ultrasound: relation to left ventricular diastolic pressures. *J Am Coll Cardiol* 1993; 21: 1687–96.
28. Vanoverschelde J-L., Essamri B, Michel X, et al. Hemodynamic and volume correlates of left ventricular diastolic relaxation and filling in patients with aortic stenosis. *J Am Coll Cardiol* 1992; 20: 813–21.
29. Nagueh SF, Mikati I, Kopelen HA, Middleton KJ, Quinones MA, Zoghbi WA. Doppler estimation of left ventricular filling pressure in sinus tachycardia. A new application of tissue Doppler imaging. *Circulation* 1998; 98: 1644–50.
30. Ommen SR, Nishimura RA, Appleton CP, et al. Clinical utility of Doppler echocardiography and tissue Doppler imaging in the estimation of left ventricular filling pressures: a comparative simultaneous Doppler-catheterization study. *Circulation* 2000; 102: 1788–94.
31. Garcia MJ, Ares MA, Asher C, Rodriguez L, Vandervoort P, Thomas JD. An index of early left ventricular filling that combined with pulsed Doppler peak E velocity may estimate capillary wedge pressure. *J Am Coll Cardiol* 1997; 29: 448–54.
32. Mullens W, Borowski A, RJ C, Thomas J, Tang W. Tissue Doppler imaging in the estimation of intracardiac filling pressure in decompensated patients with advanced systolic heart failure. *Circulation* 2009; 119: 62–70.
33. Oh J, Park S, Nagueh S. Established and novel applications of diastolic function assessment by echocardiography. *Circ Cardiovasc Imaging* 2011; 4: 444–55.
34. Edvardsen T, Gerber B, Garot J, et al. Quantitative assessment of intrinsic regional deformation by Doppler strain rate echocardiography in humans: validation against three-dimensional tagged magnetic resonance imaging. *Circulation* 2002; 106: 50–56.
35. Pirat B, Khoury D, Hartley C, et al. A novel feature-tracking echocardiographic method for the quantitation of regional myocardial function: validation in an animal model of ischemia-reperfusion. *J Am Coll Cardiol* 2008; 51: 651–59.
36. Notomi Y, Lysyanski P, Setser R, et al. Measurement of ventricular torsion by two-dimensional ultrasound speckle tracking imaging. *J Am Coll Cardiol* 2005; 45: 2034–41.
37 Notomi Y, Setser R, Shiota T, et al. Assessment of left ventricular torsional deformation by Doppler tissue imaging: validation study with tagged magnetic resonance imaging. *Circulation* 2005; 111: 1141–47.
38. Mullens W, Borowski A, Curten RJ, et al. Tissue Doppler imaging in the estimation of intracardiac filling pressure in decompensated patients with advance systolic heart failure. *Circulation* 2009; 119: 62–70.
39. Wang J, Khoury D, Thonan V, et al. Global diastolic strain rate for the assessment of left ventricular relaxation and filling pressures. *Circulation* 2007; 115: 1376–83.
40. Kasner M, Gaub R, Sinning D, et al. Global strain rate imaging for the estimation of diastolic function in HFNEF compared with pressure-volume analysis. *Eur J Echocardiogr* 2010; 11: 743–51.
41. Shanks M, Ng A, Van de Veire N, et al. Incremental prognostic value of novel left ventricular diastolic indexes for prediction of clinical outcome in patients with ST-elevation myocardial infarction. *Am J Cardiol* 2010; 105: 592–97.
42. Dokainish H, Sengupta R, Pillai M, et al. Usefulness of new diastolic strain and strain rate indexes for the estimation of left ventricular filling pressure. *Am J Cardiol* 2008; 101: 1504–9.
43. Notomi Y, Popovic ZB, Yamada H, et al. Ventricular untwisting: a temporal link between left ventricular relaxation and suction. *Am J Physiol Heart Circ Physiol* 2008; 294: H505–13.
44. Park S, Miyazaki C, Bruce C, et al. Left ventricular torsion by two-dimensional speckle tracking echocardiography in patients with diastolic dysfunction and normal ejection fraction. *J Am Soc Echocardiogr* 2008; 21: 1129–37.
45. Wang J, Khoury D, Yue Y, et al. Preserved left ventricular twist and circumferential deformation, but depressed longitudinal and radial deformation in patients with diastolic heart failure. *Eur Heart J* 2008; 29: 1283–9.
46. Dong S, Hees P, Siu C, et al. MRI assessment of LV relaxation by untwisting rate: a new isovolumic phase measure of tau. *Am J Physiol Heart Circ Physiol* 2001; 281: H2002–9.
47. Wang J, Khoury D, Yue Y, et al. Left ventricular untwisting rate by speckle tracking echocardiography. *Circulation* 2007; 116: 2580–86.
48. Tan Y, Wenzelburger F, Lee E, et al. The pathophysiology of heart failure with normal ejection fraction: exercise echocardiography reveals complex abnormalities of both systolic and diastolic ventricular function, involving torsion, untwist and longitudinal motion. *J Am Coll Cardiol* 2009; 54: 36–46.
49. Abhayaratna WP, Seward JB, Appleton CP, et al. Left atrial size: physiologic determinants and clinical applications. *J Am Coll Cardiol* 2006; 47: 2357–63.
50. Wakami K, Ohte N, Asada K, et al. Correlation between left ventricular end-diastolic pressure and peak left atrial strain during left ventricular systole. *J Am Soc Echocardiogr* 2009; 22: 847–51.
51. Kurt M, Wang J, Torre-Amione G, et al. Left atrial function in diastolic heart failure. *Circ Cardiovasc Imaging* 2009; 2: 10–15.
52. Duarte R, Fernandez-Perez G, Bettencourt N, et al. Assessment of left ventricular diastolic function with cardiovascular MRI: what radiologist should know. *Diagn Interv Radiol* 2012; 18: 446–53.
53. Rathi VK, Biederman RW. Expanding role of cardiovascular magnetic resonance in left and right ventricular diastolic function. *Heart Fail Clin* 2009; 5: 421–35.
54. Caudron J, Fares J, Bauer F, et al. Evaluation of left ventricular diastolic function with cardiac MR imaging. *Radiographics* 2011; 31: 239–59.
55. Paelinck BP, Lamb HJ, Bax JJ, et al. Assessment of diastolic function by cardiovascular magnetic resonance. *Am Heart J* 2002; 144: 198–205.
56. Paelinck BP, de Roos A, Bax JJ, et al. Feasibility of tissue magnetic resonance imaging: a pilot study in comparison with tissue Doppler imaging and invasive measurements. *J Am Coll Cardiol* 2005; 45: 1109–16.
57. Rathi VK, Doyle M, Yamrozik J, et al. Routine evaluation of left ventricular diastolic function by cardiovascular magnetic resonance: a practical approach. *J Cardiovasc Magn Reson* 2008; 10: 36.
58. Young AA, Cowan BR. Evaluation of left ventricular torsion by cardiovascular magnetic resonance. *J Cardiovasc Magn Reson* 2012; 14: 49.
59. Hurrell D, Nishimura RA, Ilstrup DM, Appleton CP. Utility of preload alteration in assessment of left ventricular filling pressure by Doppler echocardiography: a simultaneous catheterization and Doppler echocardiographic study. *J Am Coll Cardiol* 1997; 30: 459–67.
60. Rossvoll O, Hatle LK. Pulmonary venous flow velocities recorded by transthoracic Doppler ultrasound: relation to left ventricular diastolic pressures. *J Am Coll Cardiol* 1993; 21: 1687–96.
61. Nagueh SF, Bhatt R, Vivo RP, et al. Echocardiographic evaluation of hemodynamics in patients with decompensated systolic heart failure. *Circ Cardiovasc Imaging* 2011; 4: 220–27.
62. Somaratne JB, Whalley GA, Gamble GD, Doughty RN. Restrictive filling pattern is a powerful predictor of heart failure events post acute myocardial infarction and in established heart failure: a literature-based meta-analysis. *J Card Fail* 2007; 13: 346–52.
63. Pinamonti B, Di Lenarda A, Sinagra G, Camerini F; Heart Muscle Disease Study Group. Restrictive left ventricular filling pattern in dilated cardiomyopathy assessed by Doppler echocardiography: clinical, echocardiographic and hemodynamic correlations and prognostic implications. *J Am Coll Cardiol* 1993; 22: 808–15.
64. Lapu-Bula R, Robert A, De Kock M, et al. Risk stratification in patients with dilated cardiomyopathy: contribution of Doppler-derived left ventricular filling. *Am J Cardiol* 1998; 82: 772–85.

65. Wang M, Yip G, Yu CM, et al. Independent and incremental prognostic value of early mitral annulus velocity in patients with impaired left ventricular systolic function. *J Am Coll Cardiol* 2005; 45: 272–77.

66. Hillis GS, Moller JE, Pellikka PA, et al. Noninvasive estimation of left ventricular filling pressure by E/e' is a powerful predictor of survival after acute myocardial infarction. *J Am Coll Cardiol* 2004; 43: 360–67.

67. Traversi E, Pozzoli M, Cioffi G, et al. Mitral flow velocity changes after 6 months of optimized therapy provide important hemodynamic and prognostic information in patients with chronic heart failure. *Am Heart J* 1996; 132: 809–19.

68. Pinamonti B, Zecchin M, Di Lenarda A, Gregori D, Sinagra G, Camerini F. Persistence of restrictive left ventricular filling pattern in dilated cardiomyopathy: an ominous prognostic sign. *J Am Coll Cardiol* 1997; 29: 604–12.

69. Hayley BD, Burwash IG. Heart failure with normal ejection fraction: role of echocardiography. *Curr Opin Cardiol* 2012; 27: 169–80.

70. Van Heerebeek L, Borbély A, Niessen HW, et al. Myocardial structure and function differ in systolic and diastolic heart failure. *Circulation* 2006; 113: 1966–73.

71. Wood P, Piran S, Liu PP. Diastolic heart failure: progress, treatment challenges, and prevention. *Can J Cardiol* 2011; 27: 302–10.

72. Abhayaratna WP, Seward JB, Appleton CP et al. Left atrial size: physiologic determinants and clinical applications. *J Am Coll Cardiol* 2006; 47: 2357–63.

73. McMuray J, Adamopoulos S, Anker S, et al. ESC guidelines for the diagnosis and treatment of acute and chronic heart failure 2012. The task force for the diagnosis and treatment of acute and chronic heart failure 2012 of the European Society of Cardiology; Developed in collaboration with the Heart Failure Association of the ESC. *Eur Heart J* 2012; 33: 1787–1847.

74. Nagueh SH, Appleton CP, Gillebert TC, et al. Recommendations for the evaluation of left ventricular diastolic dysfunction by echocardiography. *J Am Soc Echocard* 2009; 22: 107–33.

75. Ohtani T, Mohammed SF, Yamamoto K, et al. Diastolic stiffness as assessed by diastolic wall strain is associated with adverse remodeling and poor outcomes in heart failure with preserved ejection fraction. *Eur Heart J* 2012; 33: 1742–49.

76. Paulus WJ, Tschope C, Sanderson JE, et al. How to diagnose diastolic heart failure: a consensus statement on the diagnosis of heart failure with normal left ventricular ejection fraction by the Heart Failure and Echocardiography Associations of the European Society of Cardiology. *Eur Heart J* 2007; 28: 2539–50.

77. Penicka M, Bartunek J, Trakalova H, et al. Heart failure with preserved ejection fraction in outpatients with unexplained dyspnea. A pressure-volume loop analysis. *J Am Coll Cardiol* 2010; 55: 1701–10.

78. Borlaug B, Paulus J. Heart failure with preserved ejection fraction: pathophysiology, diagnosis and treatment. *Eur Heart J* 2011; 32; 670–79.

79. Yip GW, Zhan Q, Jie M, et al. Resting global and regional left ventricular contractility in patients with heart failure and normal ejection fraction: insights from speckle tracking echocardiography. *Heart* 2011; 97: 287–94.

80. Carluccio E, Biagioli P, Alunni G, et al. Advantages of deformation indices over systolic velocities in assessment of longitudinal systolic function in patients with heart failure and normal ejection fraction. *Eur J Heart Fail* 2011; 13: 292–302.

81. Morris DA, Gailani M, Vaz Pérez A, et al. Right ventricular myocardial systolic and diastolic dysfunction in heart failure with normal left ventricular ejection fraction. *J Am Soc Echocardiogr* 2011; 24: 886–97.

82. Ha JW, Lulic F, Bailey KR, et al. Effects of treadmill exercise on mitral inflow and annular velocities in healthy adults. *Am J Cardiol* 2003; 91: 114–5.

83. Ha JW, Oh JK, Pellikka PA, et al. Diastolic stress echocardiography: a novel noninvasive diagnostic test for diastolic dysfunction using supine bicycle exercise Doppler echocardiography. *J Am Soc Echocardiogr* 2005; 18: 63–8.

84. Burgess MI, Jenkins C, Sharman JE, et al. Diastolic stress echocardiography: hemodynamic validation and clinical significance of estimation of ventricular filling pressure with exercise. *J Am Coll Cardiol* 2006; 47: 1891–900.

85. Holland DJ, Prasad SB, Marwick TH. Contribution of exercise echocardiography to the diagnosis of heart failure with preserved ejection fraction (HFpEF). *Heart* 2010; 96: 1024–8.

86. Maeder MT, Thompson BR, Brunner-La Rocaa HP, et al. Hemodynamic basis of exercise limitation in patients with heart failure and normal ejection fraction. *J Am Coll Cardiol* 2010; 56: 855–63.

87. Donal E, Thebault C, Lund LH, et al. Heart Failure with a preserved ejection fraction additive value of an exercise echocardiography. *Eur Heart J Cardiovasc Imag* 2012; 13: 656–65.

88. Halley CM, Houghtaling Pl, Khalil MK, et al. Mortality rate in patients with diastolic dysfunction on long-term survival in a large outpatient population with normal LVEF. *Arch Intern Med* 2011; 171: 1082–87.

89. Aljaroudi W, Alraies C, Halley C, et al. Impact of progression of diastolic dysfunction on mortality in patients with normal ejection fraction. *Circulation* 2012; 125: 782–88.

90. Persson H, Lonn E, Edner M, et al. Diastolic dysfunction in heart failure with preserved systolic function: need for objective evidence: results from the CHARM Echocardiographic Substudy—CHARMES. *J Am Coll Cardiol* 2007; 49: 687–94.

91. Okura H, Kubo T, Asawa K, et al. Elevated E/E' predicts prognosis in congestive heart failure patients with preserved systolic function. *Circ J* 2009; 73: 86–91.

92. Zile MR, Gottdiener JS, Hetzel SJ, et al; I-PRESERVE Investigators. Prevalence and significance of alterations in cardiac structure and function in patients with heart failure and a preserved ejection fraction. *Circulation* 2011; 124: 2491–2501.

93. Rossi A, Cicoira M, Florea VG, et al. Chronic heart failure with preserved left ventricular ejection fraction: diagnostic and prognostic value of left atrial size. *Int J Cardiol* 2006; 110: 386–92.

94. Shin HW, Kim H, Son J, et al. Tissue Doppler imaging as a prognostic marker for cardiovascular events in heart failure with preserved ejection fraction and atrial fibrillation. *J Am Soc Echocardiogr* 2010; 23: 755–61.

95. Cleland JG, Pellicori P. Defining diastolic heart failure and identifying effective therapies. *JAMA* 2013; 309: 825–26.

96. Dokainish H, Nguyen JS, Sengputa R, et al. Do additional echocardiographic variables increase the accurary of E/e' for predicting left ventricular filling pressure in normal ejection fraction? An echocardiographic and invasive hemodynamic study. *J Am Soc Echocardiogr* 2010; 23: 156–61.

97. Bhella PS, Pacini EL, Prasad A, et al. Echocardiographic indices do not reliably track changes in left-sided filling pressure in healthy subjects or patients with heart failure with preserved ejection fraction. *Circ Cardiovasc Imaging* 2011; 4: 482–89.

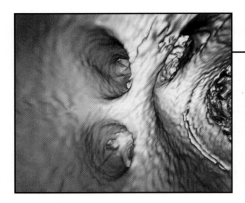

CHAPTER 25

Evaluation of right ventricular function

Luc A. Pierard and Raluca E. Dulgheru

Introduction

The right ventricle frequently remains the 'forgotten chamber of the heart'. A correct and attentive evaluation of RV morphology and function is, however, mandatory in each patient, as this might be the key in making the diagnosis and predicting outcome in pathologies such as heart failure [1], RV myocardial infarction [2], pulmonary hypertension [3, 4], or congenital heart disease [5]. Unfortunately, in many clinical conditions, assessment of the RV is not carried out, in part because the RV is considered difficult to assess by imaging techniques, because we are lacking a structured algorithm for assessing RV function with echocardiography and because the normal reference values regarding right heart size and function are rather scarce and sometimes discordant between different publications.

Because of its non-invasive nature, wide availability, and repeatability, echocardiography is still the first-line imaging technique used to assess RV morphology and function. Although sometimes challenging, because of the complex geometry of the RV, poor delineation of endocardial borders, retrosternal position of the RV, which limits the acoustic window, transthoracic echocardiography is, in the right hands, a powerful diagnostic tool. The recent advances in 3D-echocardiography helped ultrasonic techniques overcome the limitations related to the complex shape of the RV. Cardiac magnetic resonance (CMR) is the current 'gold-standard' for RV morphology and function evaluation [6], with some limitations related to availability, costs, and presence of patient-related contraindications. However, several studies validated 3D-echocardiography against CMR in RV evaluation, and the increasing availability of 3D-echocardiography in the clinical setting makes 3D-echocardiography a promising tool for the systematic evaluation of RV function and morphology [7]. Cardiac computed tomography (CT) adds important information in RV function evaluation where ultrasound techniques and CMR are limited.

Because echocardiography is still the first-line technique used in clinical practice in patients with suspected right heart disease, this chapter will focus on describing RV evaluation by conventional 2D-echocardiography, deformation imaging, and 3D-echocardiography. The advantages and clinical utility of CMR and cardiac CT will be discussed.

Overview of the RV anatomy

The RV has a median position in the chest, immediately behind the sternum. It is the most anterior chamber of the heart, in front of, and slightly lateral to the right of the left ventricle (LV). Its position makes it hardly accessible to transthoracic echocardiography (TTE). Even with transoesophageal echocardiography (TOE), imaging of the RV might be sometimes sub-optimal, as the RV is hiding in front of the LV, and away from the transducer. CT and CMR are less limited by near-field resolution and are better than echocardiography in imaging of the RV, especially the RV anterior wall [8].

The shape of the RV cannot be fitted to any simple geometrical model. This is why 2D-imaging techniques do not offer adequate quantification of RV volumes, as opposed to LV volumes and ejection fraction. Again, CMR and CT can overcome these limitations related to the complex 3D geometry of the RV. In an oversimplified 2D manner, the RV has a triangular appearance in the sagittal plane and a crescent shape in the coronal plane [8]. The normal RV is a 'three compartment' structure consisting of: (1) an inlet part (tricuspid annulus, leaflets, chordae, papillary muscles); (2) the trabeculated apical myocardium; and (3) the RV outflow tract (RVOT)/ RV infundibulum, which corresponds to the smooth myocardial outflow region [9]. The RV can be additionally divided into anterior, lateral, and inferior walls, and basal, mid, and apical segments.

The normal RV wraps around the LV and does not form the cardiac apex. The inter-ventricular septum is a 'shared' wall between the two ventricles (controversies remaining whether to consider it or not as part of the RV when assessing RV function with deformation imaging) and forms a convex arch towards the right under normal loading conditions. The normal RV is thin walled (3–5 mm, in diastole) and sometimes difficult to differentiate from adjacent structures. It has coarse trabeculations in its apical part, which complicates endocardial border detection, even when using high spatial resolution techniques, such as CMR. Both of these traits make the computation of RV volume and mass difficult and highly operator dependent, irrespective of the imaging modality.

Histologically, the RV is built up from multiple muscle layers that form a 3D framework [10]. Within this framework two distinct patterns of arrangement can be identified: fibres oriented predominately in the *circumferential* direction (parallel to the AV groove) and forming the *superficial layer* of the RV wall, and fibres located profoundly—*inner layer*—and having a more *longitudinal* direction (base to apex) [10]. In a normal RV, longitudinal fibres are better represented, while in a hypertrophied RV, fibres oriented in the circumferential direction seem to be more numerous, especially in the RVOT [11].

This arrangement of muscle fibres within the RV wall contributes to the movement of the RV free wall towards the septum (which makes the RV function like bellows) and to the base to apex movement of the free wall (which gives a piston-like function) [12]. Additionally, owing to the pattern of electrical activation in the RV, there is a sequential contraction of the RV free wall from the apex to the RV outflow tract that generates a peristaltic motion of the RV free wall and facilitates blood flow into the pulmonary artery [13].

Of note, the superficial fibres of the RV turn obliquely toward the cardiac apex and continue into the superficial layer of fibres of the LV. This binds the ventricles together and represents one of the components of inter-ventricular dependence, together with the sharing of the inter-ventricular septum, and the pericardial sac by the two ventricles [14]. It also explains the RV free wall traction exerted by LV contraction and the fact that both ventricles function as a single unit.

Longitudinal shortening is more pronounced than circumferential shortening in the normal RV, while rotation and torsion are negligible [11].

Overview of RV physiology and function

The RV is a high-volume low-pressure pump [14]. Thin walled and with a muscular mass of only 25% of the LV mass, the RV pumps, into the pulmonary vasculature, the same stroke volume as the LV, using only 25% of the stroke work used by the LV. It does so because it is coupled with a low impedance highly compliant vascular bed [9]. The lower impact of the reflected waves from a normal pulmonary arterial bed on the RV accounts also for the lower afterload of the RV as compared to the LV [14]. RV systolic function results from the complex interplay of RV contractility, RV preload and afterload. It can also be influenced by ventricular interdependence, heart rhythm, and synchronicity of ventricular contraction [9].

RV afterload is the load that the RV has to overcome during ejection. In clinical practice, the most frequently assessed index of RV afterload is pulmonary vascular resistance, although far from being the perfect estimate of RV afterload. Other factors, such as the complex haemodynamic of the pulmonary arterial bed, with forward and reflected arterial waves, also play an important role in defining RV afterload, as for the LV and the systemic circulation.

RV preload is the load present before contraction. RV works according to a force–interval relationship, generating a higher stroke volume after a longer filling period [15]. According to the Frank–Starling law, an increase in RV preload, within physiologic limits, increases myocardial contraction. However, an excessive RV volume loading in a failing RV might be haemodynamically unfavourable from two standpoints: (1) the range of the Frank–Starling mechanism might be overcome and further increase in RV preload will alter RV contractility, and (2) shifting of the interventricular septum towards the left might compress the LV and alter its performance [16].

Pathophysiology of the RV: volume overload vs. pressure overload

RV tolerates well an increase in preload (such as acute or chronic volume overload state), but is highly sensitive to any increase in afterload (such as acute or chronic pressure overload state) [17]. An acute increase in afterload, as in pulmonary embolism, can lead to acute RV failure because the thin-walled RV has few compensatory mechanisms to cope with this condition. The RV rapidly dilates, aiming to increase contractility, but from a certain point, RV dilation goes beyond the boundaries of the Frank–Starling law, leading to acute RV failure. Excessive RV dilatation is also responsible for alteration of LV filling, through inter-ventricular dependence. Chronic increase in RV afterload leads to RV hypertrophy, a compensatory mechanism aiming to reduce systolic wall stress. The hypertrophied RV can tolerate a progressive increase in pulmonary artery pressure without a decrease in stroke volume. When adequate stroke volume can no longer be sustained, RV dilatation ensues as a compensatory mechanism. If RV pressure overload persists and all compensatory mechanisms have been overcome, RV failure ensues.

This high susceptibility to increased afterload seems to be the usual pattern of behaviour of the RV facing the pulmonary vascular bed. In contrast, in patients with a systemic RV (such as in ventricular inversion or in patients with complete transposition of the great arteries and a Mustard or Senning atrial baffle) the RV is able to cope with high afterload for long periods of time, and RV dysfunction ensues late during life [5]. The explanation for such a behaviour seems to be related to the fact that the systemic RV is trained to work against a high resistance vascular bed from the foetal life and never loses this ability. It never gets to work under the low resistance pulmonary bed, it does not undergo a reverse remodelling, its walls never become thin, and the RV remains capable of facing very high afterload without failing, as it did during foetal life [18].

In contrast to chronic pressure load, chronic RV volume load is very well tolerated for longer periods of time. In chronic volume overload, the RV dilates and progressively hypertrophies, while RV systolic function is maintained [5]. Ultimately, long-standing high volume overload may lead to RV systolic dysfunction.

This basic knowledge of RV pathophysiology is necessary in order to correctly interpret echocardiographic, CT, or CMR findings in a patient with suspected right heart disease.

A moderately dilated RV with no RV hypertrophy and signs of RV systolic dysfunction must evoke RV infarction or pulmonary embolism, especially when estimated pulmonary systolic pressures is not very high (<55–60 mmHg; the failing RV is not able to generate high trans-tricuspid gradients). Absence of inferior wall motion abnormalities during rest echocardiography in such patients, will be in favour of pulmonary embolism and rapid confirmation of diagnosis can be made with angio CT. Presence of secondary tricuspid regurgitation related to papillary muscle dysfunction and presence of inferior wall motion abnormalities will be in favour of RV infarction.

The presence of RV hypertrophy usually suggests a chronic pathology involving the RV. A hypertrophied and dilated RV, together with a septal flattening persistent both in diastole and systole, suggests chronic pressure overload of the RV, such as in pulmonary stenosis or pulmonary hypertension. Signs of RV dysfunction in this setting, especially if associated with sudden changes in symptoms, must intrigue the investigator to search for concomitant pulmonary embolism or RV infarction before concluding RV failure as the natural course of chronic PAH. Exclusion of RV infarction can be made by searching for wall motion abnormalities of the inferior LV wall, as isolated RV infarction is extremely rare.

A severely dilated RV in the presence of RV hypertrophy, preserved RV systolic function, and diastolic septal flattening suggest chronic RV volume overload. Absence of significant tricuspid or pulmonary regurgitation should prompt the search for a left-to-right shunt, such as an atrial septal defect (ASD) or arteriovenous fistula.

With imaging techniques, the distinction between volume and pressure overload of the RV may be easily made by looking at the pattern of septal movement throughout the cardiac cycle [19]. In the absence of tricuspid regurgitation, echocardiography is not useful for estimation of pulmonary artery pressures, but septal flattening, both during diastole and systole, is indicative of significant chronic pulmonary hypertension. Such a patient should be referred for RV catheterization and measurement of pulmonary artery pressures. Absence of tricuspid regurgitation jet, needed to derive systolic pulmonary artery pressure, does not exclude pulmonary hypertension, and an attentive search for RV hypertrophy, as an indirect sign of RV pressure overload, is important. Absence of RV hypertrophy, dilation, or RV systolic dysfunction would be in favour of normal pulmonary artery pressure.

Pathologies that might lead to RV dysfunction

The main pathologies involving the RV and leading to RV failure are summarized in ➲ Table 25.1.

Assessment of RV morphology

Often, a change in RV geometry and/or volume might be the first sign of RV involvement in a pathological state. A minimal evaluation of RV geometry should include: (1) assessment of RV linear dimensions and volumes, and (2) assessment of RV wall thickness.

Scanning of RV wall for morphological changes should also be part of a routine echocardiographic evaluation. Unfortunately,

Table 25.1 Main pathologies involving the RV and leading to RV failure

Intrinsic myocardial diseases involving the RV
Arrhythmogenic RV dysplasia
Takotsubo cardiomyopathy
Amyloidosis with RV involvement
Myocarditis
RV myocardial infarction and ischaemia
Pressure overload states
Chronic pulmonary hypertension of different aetiologies according to Dana Point Classification
Acute pulmonary hypertension—pulmonary embolism
RV outflow tract obstruction and pulmonary/supra-pulmonary valve stenosis
Systemic right ventricle (TGA after Senning or Mustard atrial switch procedure, ventricular inversion)
Volume overload states
Severe tricuspid regurgitation (organic or functional)
Severe pulmonary regurgitation
Atrial septal defects
Anomalous pulmonary venous return
Coronary artery fistula to RA/arterio-venous fistula with high debit
High volume states (sepsis, chronic severe anaemia, etc.)

RV, right ventricle; TGA, transposition of great arteries; RA, right atrium.

tissue characterization is suboptimal with 2D-echocardiography. Flagrant abnormalities, such as RV free wall aneurysms or thin and akinetic segments, can be detected with 2D-echocardiography. However, subtle changes in RV wall structure might be undetected, and the role of CMR in such cases, as well as in measuring RV volumes, is indisputable.

The available views to assess RV geometry and function by TTE are summarized in ⊃ Table 25.2.

Owing to the complex geometry of the RV, no single image plane can provide enough information to adequately evaluate RV geometry and function. Careful scanning of the RV in all views should be performed, because each view might add complementary information to the test.

The simplest method used in clinical practice to screen for RV dilatation is the measurement of RV areas (RV end-diastolic and end-systolic area) and linear dimensions (RV basal and mid-cavity diameters, RVOT proximal and distal diameters) using single tomographic echocardiographic planes [6]. Planimetered RV area and RV basal diameter measured at end-diastole in normal RV showed a satisfactory correlation with end-diastolic RV volumes

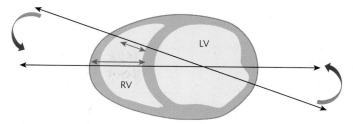

Fig. 25.1 Diagram showing that by a simple rotation of the probe anticlockwise from (red arrows) the apical 4-chamber view, the measured RV diameter can change significantly. Light red arrow is the diameter obtained without careful rotation of the probe, much smaller as compared to the correct RV diameter (green arrow). RV, right ventricle; LV, left ventricle.

[20, 21], but these correlations worsen with increased preload [22] or afterload [23], making them less accurate in dilated RVs [6]. Mild to moderate RV enlargement might pass undetected if only RV linear dimensions are used to screen for RV dilatation. Part of this lack of sensitivity of linear dimensions to detect RV enlargement, can be explained by the lack of fixed reference points in 2D - TTE when assessing the RV. The complex 3D geometry of the RV accounts for the rest. By a simple rotation of the probe clockwise or anticlockwise from the apical 4-chamber view, the basal and mid-cavity diameters of the RV change, so that dilatation of the RV might be easily missed. It is thus important to adjust the apical 4-chamber view, by rotation of the probe, while positioning the probe over the cardiac apex to avoid foreshortening, to get the maximal RV diameter (⊃ Fig. 25.1). From this view, RV linear dimensions are evaluated at end-diastole (⊃ Fig. 25.2a). At end-diastole, an RV basal diameter >42 mm, a mid-cavity RV diameter >35 mm, or an apex-to-base length >86 mm, indicate RV enlargement [6].

Measurement of the RVOT is also part of the routine evaluation of RV geometry. RVOT diameter measurement is performed at the level of sub-pulmonary infundibulum (proximal RVOT) and pulmonary valve (distal RVOT), from the parasternal long - (⊃ Fig. 25.3a) and short-axis views (⊃ Fig. 25.3b). Proximal RVOT can be measured in PLAX and PSAX views, from the anterior aortic wall to the RV free wall above the aortic valve (⊃ Fig. 25.3a–c). Distal RVOT linear dimension can be measured from PSAX view just proximal to pulmonary valve leaflets (⊃ Fig. 25.3c), the latter being preferred for calculation of RV stroke volume, regurgitant fraction or Qp/Qs ratio, because is the most reproducible. The upper reference limit for PSAX distal RVOT linear dimension is 27 mm [6].

Measurement of RV wall thickness is also important for disclosure of RV pathology. The normal RV has a wall thickness <5 mm, as measured from the sub-costal or PLAX views (⊃ Fig. 25.4) [24]. RV hypertrophies in response to chronic pressure or volume overload states. RV thinning is rarely the result of a myocardial infarction. Uhl's anomaly or arrhythmogenic RV cardiomyopathy are rare conditions associated with RV wall thinning.

Severely dilated or hypertrophied RV is usually hard to miss in a routine echocardiogram, and the diagnosis is made 'at a glance', just by a qualitative evaluation. A quick comparison of the basal diameters of each ventricle can confirm the eyeball evaluation of RV dilatation. A non-dilated RV has a basal diameter smaller than the LV, provided that the LV is not dilated (⊃ Fig. 25.2b) [25].

Table 25.2 Acoustic windows for transthoracic echocardiography evaluation of the RV

Acoustic window	Target measurement
Parasternal long-axis (PTLX)	RVOT proximal diameter RVOT wall thickness
Modified parasternal long-axis (long-axis of RV inflow)	Tricuspid valve anatomy and function Trans-tricuspid systolic gradient for sPAP estimation
Parasternal short-axis (PTSAX) view at the level of the great arteries	RVOT proximal diameter RVOT distal diameter Pulmonary artery morphology and function Trans-pulmonary artery flow (PW Doppler) Pulmonary regurgitation flow (CW Doppler) Trans-tricuspid systolic gradient for sPAP estimation
Parasternal short-axis (PTSAX) view (slightly upper from papillary muscle level)	LV eccentricity index
Apical 4-chamber view—focused on the RV	RV basal and mid cavity diameters RV base-to-apex diameter RV end-diastolic and end-systolic area FAC TAPSE Peak s' wave velocity of the tricuspid annulus Global and regional RV systolic strain Tricuspid valve morphology and function Trans-tricuspid systolic gradient for sPAP estimation
Subcostal view	RV free wall thickness Tricuspid valve morphology and function Trans-tricuspid systolic gradient for sPAP estimation IVC diameter and diameter variation with respiration

RV, right ventricle; RVOT, right ventricular outflow tract; sPAP, systolic pulmonary artery pressure; LV, left ventricle; FAC, fractional area change; TAPSE, tricuspid annular plane excursion; IVC, inferior vena cava.

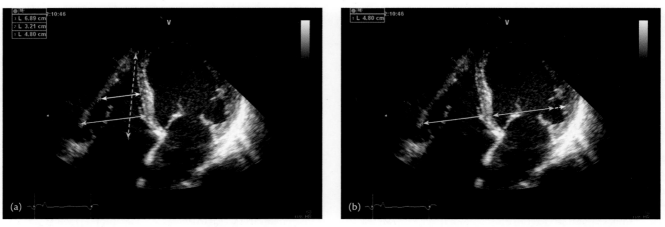

Fig. 25.2 (a) RV linear dimensions in a patient with a dilated RV. RV basal diameter yellow arrow; RV mid cavity diameter white arrow; RV base-to-apex diameter dashed arrow. (b) Note that even if RV is clearly enlarged, as assessed by RV basal diameter (yellow flash), relative comparison with LV basal diameter is misleading as LV is dilated. The yellow arrows have the same length, representing RV basal diameter; dashed white arrow represents the difference of LV to RV diameter.

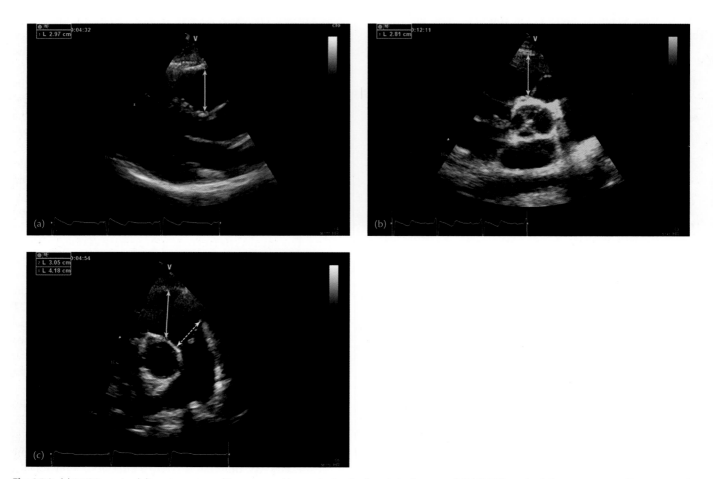

Fig. 25.3 (a) RVOT proximal diameter measured in parasternal long-axis view, in diastole (yellow arrow). (b) RVOT proximal diameter measured in parasternal short-axis view, in diastole, and showing RVOT dilatation. (c) RVOT proximal (yellow arrow) and distal diameter (white dashed arrow) measured in parasternal short-axis view, in end-diastole, and showing RVOT dilatation.

Another qualitative assessment of RV enlargement, although not validated, is the eyeball detection of the 'apex-forming' ventricle (➲ Fig. 25.5a and b). When RV enlarges, the cardiac apex becomes round because the RV becomes the 'apex-forming' ventricle by pushing the LV posterior and to the left (➲ Fig. 25.5b).

Another qualitative assessment of RV involvement in a pathological state is the evaluation of inter-ventricular septal geometry. Whenever the RV is submitted to pressure or volume overload, its normal crescent shape is lost and the inter-ventricular septum flattens. The pattern of septal movement in systole and diastole can help

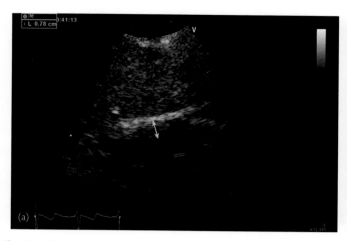

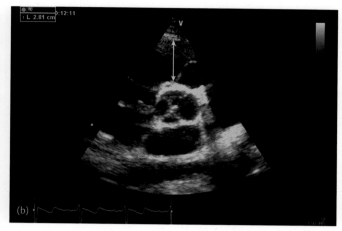

Fig. 25.4 Zoomed mode from the subcostal view with RV wall thickness measurement (yellow arrow). RV hypertrophy confirmed in a patient with chronic pulmonary hypertension.

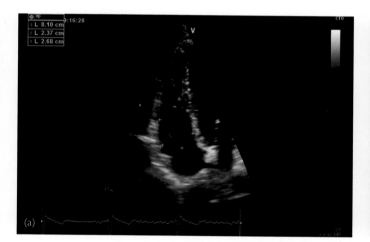

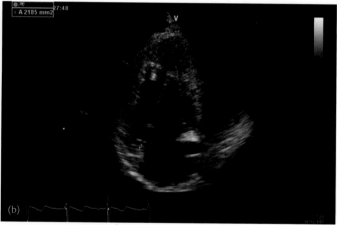

Fig. 25.5 (a) RV focused apical 4-chamber view in a patient without RV dilatation. The RV is not the 'apex-forming' ventricle. (b) RV focused apical 4-chamber view in a patient with RV dilatation. The RV is the 'apex-forming' ventricle, pushing aside the LV.

distinguish between volume and pressure overload states (➲ Fig. 25.6) [19]. In purely volume overload states (such as in severe pulmonary or tricuspid regurgitation, unrestrictive atrial septal defect) the septum flattens in diastole because the RV end-diastolic pressure is increased and pushes against the inter-ventricular septum. In systole, the LV systolic pressure remains higher then RV systolic pressure and the septum regains its normal configuration. In pressure overload states, the flattening of the inter-ventricular septum persists during both systole and diastole (➲ Fig. 25.7). Although easy to memorize if explained this way, the dynamics of septal motion in pressure or volume overload states is much more complex, and not entirely explained by the trans-septal pressure gradient [26]. Interested readers can be referred to other publications on this topic [27, 28].

The LV eccentricity index, the ratio of the LV antero-posterior to septo-lateral diameters in short-axis view, measured just slightly upper from the papillary muscles, is one of the parameters that can detect changes in RV shape, providing quantitative assessment of septal flattening. In normal states, the LV eccentricity index is 1, both in systole and diastole. A value higher than 1 at end-diastole indicates a change in RV shape due to volume overload (➲ Fig. 25.6c and d). A value higher than 1

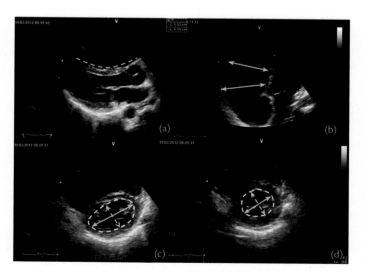

Fig. 25.6 Pattern of septal motion in a patient without tricuspid valve (surgically excised after tricuspid endocarditis) and severe volume overload of the RV. Marked RV enlargement (b) and a flattened inter-ventricular septum in diastole (a and c), but normal septal configuration at end-systole (d).

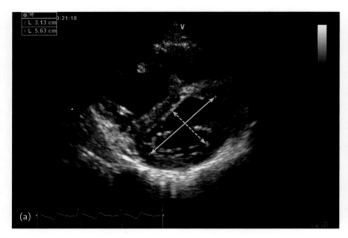
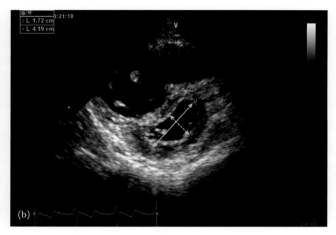

Fig. 25.7 (a) Septal shape in end-diastole in a patient with RV pressure overload. LV eccentricity index at end-diastole >1. (b) Septal shape in end-systole in a patient with RV pressure overload. LV eccentricity index at end-systole >1.

persisting through end-systole indicates a change in RV shape due to pressure overload (⮌ Fig. 25.7) [19]. Additionally, a high LV eccentricity index is an important echocardiographic predictor of mortality in patients with pulmonary artery hypertension (PAH) [3]. When measuring the LV eccentricity index, care must be taken to obtain a correct PSAX image (avoid oblique cutting planes) and to make the measurements just slightly upper from the papillary muscles in order to get the best endocardial detection [19].

RV geometry (⮌ Table 25.3) assessment based only on RV linear dimension might lead to under-detection of mild or moderate RV enlargement. In doubtful cases, calculation of RV volumes with CMR or 3D-echocardiography is recommended [6].

Assessment of RV systolic function

An ideal index of RV contractility should be independent of preload and afterload changes [29]. Most investigators consider RV elastance (the slope that unifies all points of end-systolic pressure-volume loops corresponding to different loading states) a good estimate of RV contractility [30]. A normal RV elastance was defined by Dell'Italia et al. to be around 1.3±0.84 mmHg/ml [30]. Unfortunately, this parameter requires invasive measurements and cannot be routinely measured in clinical practice.

With imaging techniques, all non-invasive and usually widely available, all parameters of RV systolic function are highly dependent on preload and afterload. This should always be taken into account when assessing RV function by imaging techniques.

Fractional area change

The fractional area change is the percentage of change in RV chamber area during the cardiac cycle measured in apical 4-chamber view. RV chamber area at end-diastole and end-systole are obtained by carefully tracing RV endocardial border from the tricuspid annulus, along the RV free wall, to the RV apex and back to the tricuspid annulus along the inter-ventricular septum.

Trabeculations and tricuspid leaflets are enclosed within the area (⮌ Fig. 25.8). Fractional area change correlates with RVEF measured by CMR [22, 31] and is an independent predictor of mortality, heart failure, and sudden death after myocardial infarction [32] or pulmonary embolism [33]. It is easy to perform and can be included systematically in each echocardiographic evaluation of RV function. The lower reference value for fractional area change for normal RV systolic function is 35% [6].

RV myocardial performance index (MPI)

RV myocardial performance index (MPI), also known as the Tei index, is defined as the ratio of isovolumic time intervals to RV ejection time. It is considered an estimate of global RV function because it also takes into consideration the isovolumic relaxation period of the RV. With increase in RV pressure and volume, and with RV systolic dysfunction, the isovolumic periods of the RV lengthen. Thus, the longer the isovolumic phases, the higher the RV MPI. There are two modalities to calculate RV MPI, and *the cut-off values established for each modality are not interchangeable.* The first one uses PW or CW in the RV inflow tract to calculate the tricuspid valve opening–closure time, and PW Doppler in the RVOT to calculate RV ejection time. In the tricuspid valve opening–closure time interval, the isovolumic periods and RV ejection time are confined. The duration of time intervals is identified by recording the time between the onset and cessation of blood flow. The Tei index is calculated as the ratio between the differences of the two intervals to RV ejection time. Presence of tricuspid regurgitation flow is not required for Tei index calculation. In this case, PW at the RV inflow, with measurement of time from the end of the A wave to the beginning of the E wave, is sufficient. Care must be taken to increase sample volume, but lower wall filters, to have a good detection of flow, and to perform measurements on tracings with similar R–R intervals in order to minimize errors. The normal value for this index is 0.28±0.04, with an upper reference limit of 0.40 [6].

The second method to calculate RV MPI is the tissue Doppler method. With this method, all time intervals are measured from a

Table 25.3 Summary of reference values for different indices of RV geometry and function in 2D- and 3D-echocardiography

Variable	Abnormal value	Limitations	Figure
RV geometry			
RV basal diameter, mm	>42	Correct measurement depends on probe rotation	⊃ Figs 25.2, 25.3
RV mid cavity diameter, mm	>35	Correct measurement depends on probe rotation, no fixed reference point available to minimize inter-observer variability	⊃ Fig. 25.2
RV base-to-apex diameter, mm	>86	Difficulty in detecting the apical point of this diameter Correct measurement depends on probe rotation	⊃ Fig. 25.2
RVOT proximal diameter, mm (PSLA)	>33	Correct measurement depends on probe angulation and rotation	⊃ Fig. 25.3a
RVOT distal diameter, mm	>27	Difficult delineation of endocardial border due to near field artefacts	⊃ Fig. 25.3c
RV free wall thickness, mm (subcostal or PSLA view)	>5	Difficult delineation of endocardial border due to trabeculations	⊃ Fig. 25.4
LV eccentricity index	>1	Off axis image planes results in biased values	⊃ Figs 25.6, 25.7
RV systolic function			
FAC,%	<35	Difficult delineation of endocardial border, especially in end-systole and at apical level	⊃ Fig. 25.8
Pulsed Doppler RV MPI	>0.40	Different cardiac cycle needed for measurement Pseudonormal values in severe RV dysfunction	
Tissue Doppler MPI	>0.55		⊃ Fig. 25.9
TAPSE, mm	<16	Depend on good alignment with RV free wall	⊃ Fig. 25.10
Peak s' wave velocity of the tricuspid annulus, cm/s	<10	Depend on good alignment with RV free wall	⊃ Fig. 25.12
Peak systolic longitudinal strain of the RV free wall, %	No defined reference value	Depend on good image quality, sometimes suboptimal due to lower lateral resolution	⊃ Fig. 25.11f ⊃ Fig. 25.13
3D RV EF, %	<44	Highly dependent of image quality Difficult endocardial border delineation, especially in the apical region, in end-systole	⊃ Fig. 25.14
RV diastolic dysfunction			
E/A	>0.8	Dependent on correct alignment of PW sample volume with RV inflow	
E/e'	>6	Dependent on correct alignment of PW sample volume with the RV free wall	

RV, right ventricle; RVOT, right ventricular outflow tract; PSLA, parasternal long-axis; LV, left ventricle; FAC, fractional area change; MPI, myocardial performance index; TAPSE, tricuspid annular plane systolic excursion; EF, ejection fraction; E, peak early diastolic velocity at the level of RV inflow; E', peak early diastolic velocity by PW TDI at the level of the tricuspid annulus.

single beat, by interrogating the velocity of the tricuspid annulus (⊃ Fig. 25.9). This method is much easier to perform, avoids errors related to R–R interval variability but has a different cut-off value. The upper reference limit for this method is 0.55 [6].

RV MPI is not a load independent index [34, 35]. Pseudonormal values of RV MPI might be obtained in cases of acute or severe RV dysfunction, such as RV infarction. In such cases, RV diastolic pressure increases and the isovolumic relaxation time shortens due to rapid equalization of pressure between RV and RA. The shortening of the IVRT accounts for deceptively low RV MPI in spite of severe RV dysfunction [35]. This also occurs in cases with increased RA pressure, which can mask RV dysfunction if judged only by RV MPI.

RV dP/dt

RV dP/dt, the rate in pressure rise of the RV in systole, can be used as an estimate of RV systolic function. RV dP/dt can be calculated from the descending slope of the tricuspid regurgitation CW Doppler signal [36]. The time for the TR velocity to increase from 0.5 m/s to 2 m/s is calculated. This represents the time necessary for the RV to increase the systolic pressure by 15 mmHg. To calculate RV dP/dt, 15 mmHg is divided by the time necessary to attain this change in pressure. A value <400 mmHg/s is considered a sign of RV systolic dysfunction [6]. However, this echocardiographic parameter is not well validated and is highly dependent on loading conditions.

Tricuspid annular plane systolic excursion (TAPSE)

TAPSE (tricuspid annular plane systolic excursion) is a reflection of the RV longitudinal function because it reflects the amount of displacement of the tricuspid annulus towards the apex, in the longitudinal plane, from end-diastole to end-systole [21]. TAPSE is measured from the standard 4-chamber apical view by placing the

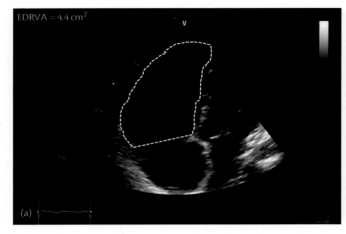

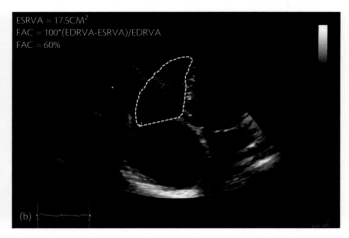

Fig. 25.8 (a) End-diastolic RV area measured in RV focused 4-chamber view in a patient with a severely dilated RV due to severe volume overload. This patient has no tricuspid valve and careful tracing of the RV endocardial border is made, starting from the tricuspid annulus plane, toward the RV apex and down to the septal aspect of the tricuspid annulus plane. (b) End-systolic RV area measurement. Normal RV systolic function as assessed by FAC (FAC=60%) in spite of severe volume overload and RV chambers dilatation. EDRVA, end-diastolic RV area; ESRVA, end-systolic RV area; FAC, fractional area change.

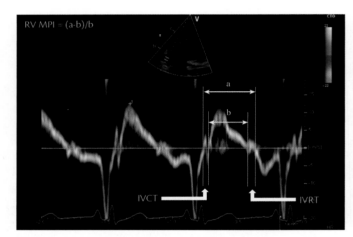

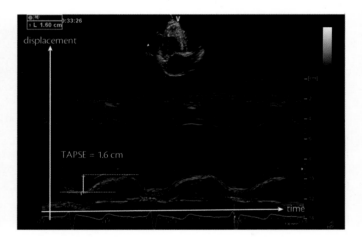

Fig. 25.9 RV myocardial performance index (RV MPI) by TDI method. With this method, the lateral tricuspid annulus is interrogated by pulsed Doppler from the apical 4-chamber view, and RV isovolumic intervals (IVCT+IVRT) and RV ejection time are calculated. Time interval 'b' represents RV ejection time. Isovolumic time intervals (IVCT+IVRT) are measured by subtracting time interval 'b' from time interval 'a', as shown in the figure. The RV MPI is the ratio between the RV isovolumic intervals and the RV ejection time. IVCT-isovolumic contraction time. IVRT, isovolumic relaxation time.

Fig. 25.10 Tricuspid plane annular excursion (TAPSE) measurement in a patient with RV chronic pressure overload, showing borderline RV systolic function, a value below this limit being considered pathological (yellow line). On the x axis time is represented, while on the y axis, displacement is represented.

M-mode cursor through the tricuspid annulus (◑ Fig. 25.10). Care must be taken in order to align the cursor as parallel as possible to the RV free wall. Lowering the gain enables a good detection of the annulus excursion, avoiding confusion with adjacent atrial or RV free wall. The simplicity of the concept and measurement makes TAPSE one of the parameters easily applicable in clinical practice [6]. It was validated against radionuclide derived RVEF [21] and showed prognostic information in several diseases involving the RV [37, 38]. TAPSE should be reported in each echocardiographic protocol. A value less than 16 mm is considered as abnormal [6].

Normal RV systolic function is highly dependent on longitudinal shortening. The greater the descent of the tricuspid annular plane, the better the RV systolic function. However, the contribution of inter-ventricular septum [39] and RVOT contraction [40] to RV systolic function, disregarded by TAPSE, is not negligible, especially

in the setting of a longitudinal RV systolic dysfunction. Because TAPSE looks at the displacement of only one point (the tricuspid annulus), in relation to a fixed, extra-cardiac reference point (the ultrasound probe) it can be influenced by the overall movement of the heart [41], especially in cases with high mobility of the heart, such as after pericardiotomy, and in the presence of pericardial effusion (◑ Fig. 25.11). Care should be taken when interpreting TAPSE after open heart surgery, because decrease in TAPSE does not always represent RV systolic dysfunction and proved to diminish at the time of pericardial incision [42]. In the presence of pericardial effusion, because of the overall motion of the heart in the pericardial sac, TAPSE might be deceivingly normal, in spite of RV systolic dysfunction. Heart size also influences tricuspid annular displacement [43], smaller hearts showing higher displacement. TAPSE is load-dependent and angle-dependent. It may be influenced by LV systolic performance due to inter-ventricular interdependence [44]. TAPSE infers that the displacement of the basal segment of the RV free wall

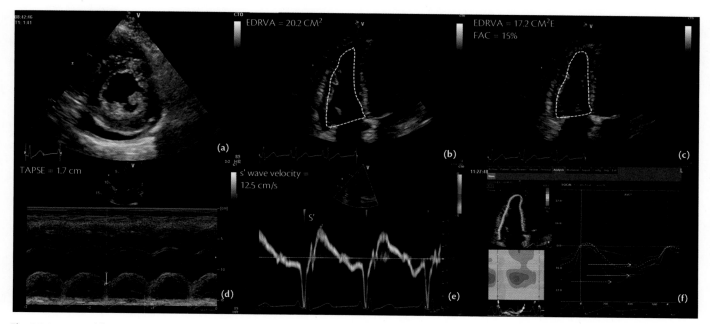

Fig. 25.11 TAPSE (d) and S' wave velocity's dependency (e) on tethering from adjacent segments in a patient with severe RV dysfunction (FAC=15%, b, c) and depressed longitudinal systolic strain of the mid and basal segments of the RV free wall (f). Strain analysis by speckle tracking shows diminished longitudinal systolic strain in the mid (white arrow, f) and basal segments (yellow arrow, f) of the RV free wall. RV systolic dysfunction is confirmed by measurement of FAC. TAPSE and S' wave velocity have normal values because of the passive traction exerted by the left ventricle and apical segment of the RV free wall (showing normal longitudinal systolic strain, dashed arrow, f). Presence of pericardial effusion (a) contributes to the falsely normal TAPSE and S' wave velocity values. EDRVA, end diastolic RV area; ESRVA, end systolic RV area; FAC, fractional area change; TAPSE, tricuspid plane annular excursion.

is representative for the function of a complex 3D structure, such as the RV. Thus, it has a low sensitivity to detect RV dysfunction [45].

Its prognostic importance in patients with chronic heart failure has recently been reinforced. A TAPSE ≤14 mm and an estimated systolic pulmonary pressure ≥40 mmHg were able to indicate patients with dismal prognosis [46].

TDI-derived measurements

TDI can also be used to evaluate regional and longitudinal RV systolic function. Peak systolic annular velocities have been validated as a measure of systolic function [47], being related to acceleration, which is a direct measure of force, and thus, to contractility. Peak systolic tissue Doppler velocity of the tricuspid annulus (s') can be used as an estimate of RV longitudinal function [48]. Like TAPSE, it does not take into account RVOT contraction and septal contribution to RV ejection, and is a measurement of regional RV longitudinal function. Additionally, peak S' wave velocity can be affected by overall motion of the heart and tethering by adjacent myocardial segments (➲ Fig. 25.11). It is important to acknowledge that with TDI techniques, two distinct estimates of RV longitudinal systolic function can be assessed: peak systolic tricuspid annular velocity (➲ Fig. 25.12a) and peak systolic velocities of the RV basal wall (➲ Fig. 25.12b). The former is obtained by interrogation of tricuspid annulus using PW tissue Doppler, the latter using colour-coded TDI of the basal RV free wall in apical 4-chamber view. Colour-coded tissue Doppler imaging of the RV free wall enables off line measurement of the systolic velocities of the basal RV free wall but gives the mean myocardial velocities of that region of interest. These two values, one obtained by spectral

Doppler at tricuspid annulus and one derived for colour-coded DTI in the basal segment of the RV free wall, are not interchangeable. The latter is about 20–25% lower [49]. Peak systolic tricuspid annular velocity can be also derived from colour-coded DTI. The same observation can be made: values obtained by colour-coded DTI are lower than those obtained by PW DTI. Both techniques, being Doppler derived, are angle-dependent. Thus, a good alignment of the Doppler interrogation line with the region of interest is mandatory to obtain peak velocities. For the PW DTI, the sample volume must be kept at the level of the tricuspid annulus throughout systole. This is particularly difficult in dilated RV. For colour-coded DTI, care must be taken to acquire images at a higher frame rate (>150 frames per second) to avoid underestimation of velocities related to poor temporal resolution. As opposed to PW DTI, colour-coded DTI has the advantage that sample volume can be set to follow closely myocardial motion throughout systole, and that off line analysis enables comparisons of deformation parameters (velocity and regional strain) during the same cardiac cycle, in three distinct RV free wall segments: apical, mid and basal. Such analysis in normal subjects, has shown that there is a systolic velocity gradient between basal and apical segments of the RV free wall, with basal segments having higher velocities (➲ Fig. 25.12b) [49]. This can be explained by the tethering exerted by the more apical segments on the basal segment. A peak s' wave velocity by PW measured at the level of the tricuspid annulus <10 cm/s is considered a sign of RV systolic dysfunction, especially when found in a young subject [6]. Colour-coded DTI is not routinely used in clinical practice and cut-off values for prediction of RV dysfunction are less well defined.

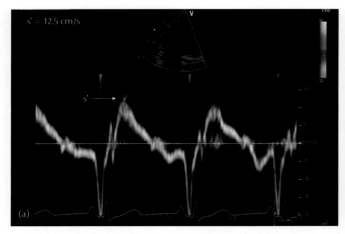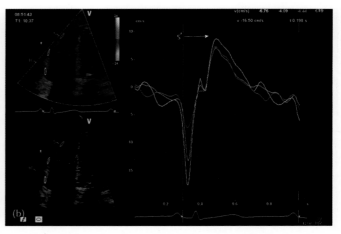

Fig. 25.12 (a) Peak systolic wave velocity (S') at the level of the lateral tricuspid wall, from the apical 4-chamber view by TDI. (b) Peak systolic velocities of the RV basal wall (yellow tracing), of the mid (green tracing) and apical segment (red tracing) of the RV free wall by colour coded TDI. The sample volume can be set to track frame by frame the RV free wall during the cardiac cycle and can be aligned with the RV free wall. Peak systolic velocity at the basal segment (yellow tracing) is higher than at the apical (red tracing) and mid segments (green tracing). This base-to-apex velocity gradient is normally found in the RV free wall and is due to tethering effect. However, in this patient there is severe mid and basal RV systolic dysfunction and mid segment velocity is equal with apical segment velocity, which means there is virtually no contraction of the mid segment. S', peak systolic wave velocity.

Strain and strain rate

Strain is defined as percentage change in myocardial deformation and strain rate as the speed of deformation of myocardial segments. None of strain or strain rate derived parameters represents pure myocardial contractility, and none of them is load-independent [50]. However, RV systolic strain and strain rate are validated indices of RV systolic function. RV strain values are reduced in patients with pulmonary artery hypertension [51], after tetralogy of Fallot (TOF) repair [52], and systemic RV [53].

Systolic strain and strain rate of the RV are size-independent estimates of contraction, as opposed to tricuspid and RV free wall velocities and TAPSE. They also have the advantage of overcoming some of the limitations related to tethering and passive motion of the RV free wall. Peak systolic strain and strain rate, as estimates of RV systolic function, can be derived from two different datasets: TDI and greyscale images. One-dimensional strain/strain rate

of the RV, usually longitudinal strain and strain rate, are acquired using TDI (⊃ Fig. 25.13a) or speckle tracking (⊃ Fig. 25.13b) in the apical 4-chamber view. Careful alignment of the RV free wall with the Doppler scan lines is necessary to avoid underestimation related to angle dependency with the TDI method. The speckle tracking based modality to derive strain and strain rate is angle-independent, but much more dependent on good image quality. Frame by frame tracking of speckles from greyscale images, throughout the entire cardiac cycle, allows calculation of strain and strain rate of each myocardial segment in longitudinal, radial, and circumferential direction. Measurement of RV radial and circumferential strain is less well validated. However, measurement of RV longitudinal strain has gathered valuable information regarding RV performance in patients with PAH [54, 55], amyloidosis [56], arrhythmogenic RV cardiomyopathy [57], and complex congenital heart diseases [53]. Some investigators have reported also, in normal subjects, an apex to base strain gradient, with higher systolic

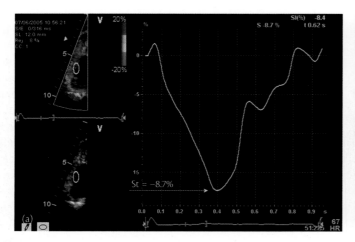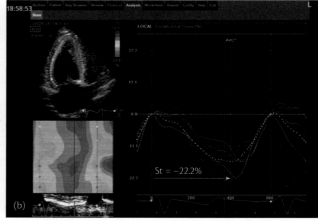

Fig. 25.13 (a) Peak longitudinal systolic strain (St) at the level of the mid segment of RV free wall by TDI. (b) Global peak longitudinal systolic strain (dashed tracing) and peak longitudinal strain of each segment of the RV free wall and inter-ventricular septum, by speckle tracking. The arrow designates peak longitudinal systolic strain of the basal segment of the RV free wall, with a value of −22.2%.

strain at the apex and lower strain in the basal segments of the RV free wall [58]. As opposed to normal subjects, in patients with PAH, systolic strain was higher in basal segments [58].

In patients with arrhythmogenic RV cardiomyopathy [59] regional deformation parameters (strain and strain rate) were able to detect early subclinical RV systolic dysfunction where conventional 2D measures failed. One recent study aimed to detect RV subclinical involvement in patients with amyloidosis by looking at TAPSE and systolic strain of the basal segment of RV wall [56]. These parameters were successful in detecting abnormal RV systolic function in patients with amyloidosis as compared to normal subjects, despite normal standard 2D measurements [56]. Thus, regional deformation parameters might be used to detect early changes in RV systolic function. However, due to the lack of cut-off values and inter-vendor differences in the algorithm of analysis, regional deformation parameters are not yet ready for clinical application.

RV ejection fraction

CMR is the most accurate method for measurement of RVEF. Radionuclide-derived RVEF can also be used for this purpose, but with lower clinical value in regards to patient follow-up. Reference values for RVEF are different between the two methods. According to Lorenz et al. the normal value for RVEF derived from CMR is 61±7%, ranging from 47% to 76% [60]. The lower limit of radionuclide-derived RVEF ranges from 40% to 45% [61]. Simpson's rule and the area–length method applied in 2D-TTE do not correlate well with CMR or radionuclide-derived RVEF. This method is not recommended in clinical practice for estimation of RV systolic performance. As compared with 2D-echocardiography,

3D-echocardiography shows better correlation with CMR, with less underestimation of RV end-diastolic and end-systolic 3D volumes, and also higher reproducibility [62]. However, 3D-echocardiography derived RV volumes are slightly smaller than ones derived by CMR. The lower reference limit for 3D-echocardiography RVEF is 44% [6], while upper limits for RV end-diastolic and end-systolic volumes is 89 ml/m^2 and 45 ml/m^2, respectively [6]. However, in clinical practice, difficulties related to delineation of the anterior RV wall and identification of the infundibular plane make the evaluation of RVEF still challenging (➲ Fig. 25.14).

RV diastolic function evaluation

Available data regarding RV diastolic function are scarce, although many of the right-sided heart diseases are associated with a certain degree of RV diastolic dysfunction. One of the most clinically relevant pathologies leading to marked RV dysfunction is acute RV myocardial infarction. The parameters used in clinical practice to asses RV diastolic dysfunction are very similar with those used for LV diastolic dysfunction evaluation: E wave velocity over A wave velocity ratio at the level at RV inflow (tricuspid E/A), E wave deceleration time, the ratio of E wave velocity over e' velocity measured by PW DTI at the level of the tricuspid annulus (tricuspid E/e'), RV isovolumic relaxation time, right atrial (RA) enlargement and RA pressure estimated from the IVC diameter. Routinely, in clinical practice, a quick evaluation of RV diastolic function can be made by the assessment of tricuspid E/A and E/e'. A tricuspid E/A ratio >2.1 and a tricuspid E/e'ratio >6 suggest RV restrictive filling, thus, severe RV diastolic dysfunction

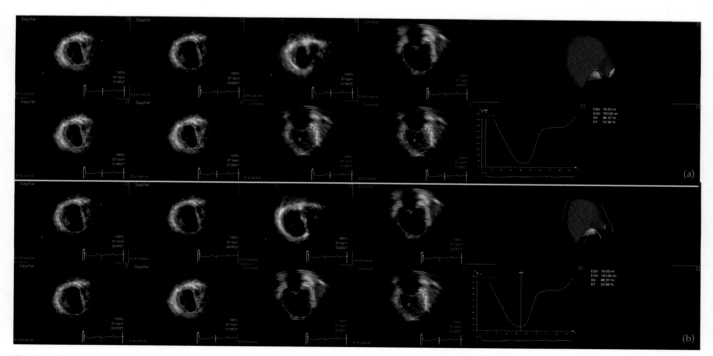

Fig. 25.14 RV volumes and RV EF evaluation with 3D-TTE in a patient with atrioventricular canal defect and Eisenmenger physiology. Evaluation of end-diastolic volumes (a) and end-systolic volumes (b) and RV ejection fraction in a full-volume single beat acquisition.

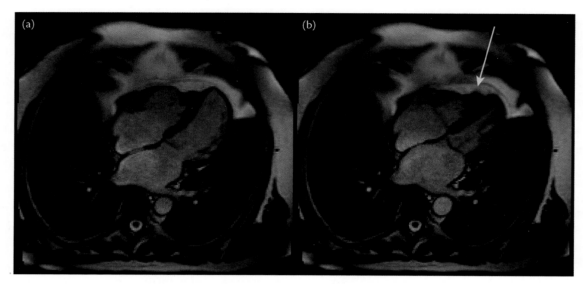

Fig. 25.15 CMR evaluation in a patient with right ventricular arrhythmogenic dysplasia showing localized wall motion abnormality. In systole (b), as compared to diastole (a), a small segment of the RV free wall does not contract (yellow arrow).

[6]. Careful alignment with RV inflow, measurement at held end-expiration and increased sample volume are necessary to obtain an accurate E/A measurement. Careful alignment with the RV free wall and high frame rate (>150 FPS) are necessary to obtain a correct e' wave velocity. A dilated IVC with no respiratory variation in the absence of significant tricuspid regurgitation and in the presence of a dilated RA are also indirect signs of severe RV diastolic dysfunction.

Cardiac magnetic resonance (CMR)

Cardiac magnetic resonance is, in clinical practice, the second-line modality for RV evaluation. Echocardiography is still the first-line imaging technique because of the accessibility and rapidity of evaluation. However, often, for a comprehensive RV morphological and functional evaluation, both techniques are necessary. CMR can offer valuable information that other techniques are not able to provide, and confirm diagnostic hypotheses evoked in each individual patient on the basis of echocardiography. CMR has the advantage of being able to provide information on RV tissue structure, which is invaluable in patients with arrhythmogenic RV dysplasia (ARVD) [63], metabolic storage disease [64], or infiltrative disease [65]. Late gadolinium enhancement (LGE) CMR studies are able to detect intra-myocardial fibrosis, scars, and fibro-fatty infiltration. However, the detection of such structural changes may be sometimes difficult due to reduced thickness of RV wall and vicinity of extra-pericardial fat tissue. Presence of myocardial fibrosis, as detected by LGE, in patients with systemic RV was related to age, RV dysfunction, QRS width, and clinical events, and seemed to provide prognostic information in such patients [66]. In TOF patients, RV LGE was significantly associated with clinical arrhythmias [67].

The most accurate assessment of RV volumes and function available to date is, undoubtedly, offered by CMR. CMR has high reproducibility with a low inter-observer variability (around 7% for end-diastolic RV volumes and RVEF and 14% for end-systolic volumes) [68]. Hot spots in CMR assessment of RV volumes and ejection fraction remain the correct identification of the tricuspid and pulmonary valve planes, correct delineation of endocardial border in the heavily trabeculated apical segments and correct definition of RV apex.

RV dilatation is an important criterion in the definition of ARVD (⊃ Fig. 25.15). RV dilatation is confirmed or excluded by CMR volume measurement. An indexed RV end-diastolic volume above 110 ml/m^2 in men and above 100 ml/m^2 in women, as measured by CMR, is one of the diagnostic criteria [63].

Timing of pulmonary valve replacement, in patients after TOF repair, might be decided according to the severity of RV dilatation, as assessed by CMR (⊃ Fig. 25.16). An indexed RV end-diastolic volume >150–170 ml/m^2 seems to be able to predict the absence of RV reversed remodelling after pulmonary valve replacement in such patients [69]. Furthermore, follow-up of RV remodelling in these patients is best appreciated by CMR volume assessment.

Besides such valuable information regarding RV morphology and RV global function, cine CMR can offer information regarding regional RV function at rest or during pharmacological stress testing [70].

Conclusion

RV function can be accurately assessed with the help of different imaging modalities, in spite of its complex shape and lower accessibility to echocardiographic evaluation. In clinical practice, its initial evaluation usually starts with a comprehensive transthoracic echocardiography and can be carried on, depending on initial findings, with complementary imaging techniques, such as 3D-TTE/TOE, deformation imaging, CMR of cardiac CT. With TTE, a structured algorithm, based on the most validated parameters

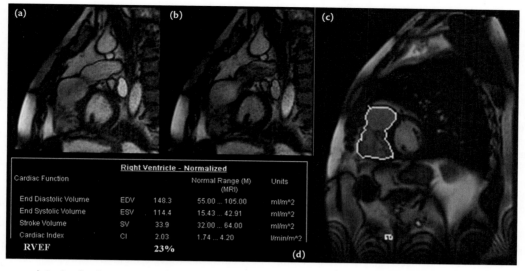

Fig. 25.16 RV volumes and ejection fraction assessment, by CMR, in a patient with repaired tetralogy of Fallot. Cine CMR study shows the presence of a persistent pulmonary regurgitation in diastole (a). A turbulent jet in the pulmonary artery can be seen in systole (b), due both to pulmonary stenosis and a high flow volume across the pulmonary valve. The RV is dilated and RVEF is calculated, by serial tracing of the endocardial border, around 23% (c and d).

and permanently modulated by the clinical question to be answered, can provide reliable information regarding RV function. To date, 2D-TTE and CMR are the most validated techniques, having robust reference values for different parameters of RV function. It is hoped that, both deformation imaging and 3D-TTE will soon gather enough evidence, form larger studies, to provide normal reference values and be routinely implemented in clinical practice.

References

1. Di Salvo T, Mathier M, Semigran M, et al. Preserved right ventricular ejection fraction predicts exercise capacity and survival in advanced heart failure. *J Am Coll Cardiol* 1995; 25: 1143–53.
2. Mehta S, Eikelboom J, Natarajan M, et al. Impact of right ventricular involvement on mortality and morbidity in patients with inferior myocardial infarction. *J Am Coll Cardiol* 2001; 37: 37–43.
3. Raymond R, Hinderliter A, Willis P, et al. Echocardiographic predictors of adverse outcomes in primary pulmonary hypertension. *J Am Coll Cardiol* 2002; 39: 1214–19.
4. Yeo T, Dujardin K, Tei C, et al. Value of a Doppler-derived index combining systolic and diastolic time intervals in predicting outcome in primary pulmonary hypertension. *Am J Cardiol* 1998; 81: 1157–61.
5. Davlouros P, Niwa K, Webb G, et al. The right ventricle in congenital heart disease. *Heart* 2006; 92 Suppl 1: i27–38.
6. Rudski L, Lai W, Afilalo J, et al. Guidelines for the echocardiographic assessment of the right heart in adults: a report from the American Society of Echocardiography endorsed by the European Association of Echocardiography, a registered branch of the European Society of Cardiology, and the Canadian Society of Echocardiography. *J Am Soc Echocardiogr* 2010; 23: 685.
7. Niemann P, Pinho L, Balbach T, et al. Anatomically oriented right ventricular volume measurements with dynamic three-dimensional echocardiography validated by 3-Tesla magnetic resonance imaging. *J Am Coll Cardiol* 2007; 50: 1668–76.
8. Mertens L, Friedberg M. Imaging the right ventricle—current state of the art. *Nat Rev Cardiol* 2010; 7: 551–63.
9. Haddad F, Hunt S, Rosenthal D, et al. Right ventricular function in cardiovascular disease, part I: Anatomy, physiology, aging, and functional assessment of the right ventricle. *Circulation* 2008; 117: 1436–48.
10. Ho S, Nihoyannopoulos P. Anatomy, echocardiography, and normal right ventricular dimensions. *Heart* 2006; 92 Suppl 1: i2–13.
11. Pettersen E, Helle-Valle T, Edvardsen T, et al. Contraction pattern of the systemic right ventricle shift from longitudinal to circumferential shortening and absent global ventricular torsion. *J Am Coll Cardiol* 2007; 49: 2450–56.
12. Haber I, Metaxas D, Geva T, et al. Three-dimensional systolic kinematics of the right ventricle. *Am J Physiol Heart Circ Physiol* 2005; 289: h1826–33.
13. Meier G, Bove A, Santamore W, et al. Contractile function in canine right ventricle. *Am J Physiol* 1980; 239: h794–804.
14. Dell'Italia L. The right ventricle: anatomy, physiology, and clinical importance. *Curr Probl Cardiol* 1991; 16: 653–720.
15. Dell'Italia L. Mechanism of postextrasystolic potentiation in the right ventricle. *Am J Cardiol* 1990; 65: 736–41.
16. Chin K, Kim N, Rubin L. The right ventricle in pulmonary hypertension. *Coron Artery Dis* 2005; 16: 13–18.
17. Sheehan F, Redington A. The right ventricle: anatomy, physiology and clinical imaging. *Heart* 2008; 94: 1510–15.
18. Hopkins W. Right ventricular performance in congenital heart disease: a physiologic and pathophysiologic perspective. *Cardiol Clin* 2012; 30: 205–18.
19. Ryan T, Petrovic O, Dillon J, et al. An echocardiographic index for separation of right ventricular volume and pressure overload. *J Am Coll Cardiol* 1985; 5: 918–27.
20. Watanabe T, Katsume H, Matsukubo H, et al. Estimation of right ventricular volume with two dimensional echocardiography. *Am J Cardiol* 1982; 49: 1946–53.
21. Kaul S, Tei C, Hopkins J, et al. Assessment of right ventricular function using two-dimensional echocardiography. *Am Heart J* 1984; 107: 526–31.

22. Lai W, Gauvreau K, Rivera E, et al. Accuracy of guideline recommendations for two-dimensional quantification of the right ventricle by echocardiography. *Int J Cardiovasc Imaging* 2008; 24: 691–98.

23. Karunanithi M, Feneley M. Limitations of unidimensional indexes of right ventricular contractile function in conscious dogs. *J Thorac Cardiovasc Surg* 2000; 120: 302–12.

24. Prakash R. Determination of right ventricular wall thickness in systole and diastole. Echocardiographic and necropsy correlation in 32 patients. *Br Heart J* 1978; 40: 1257–61.

25. Lang R, Bierig M, Devereux R, et al. Recommendations for chamber quantification: a report from the American Society of Echocardiography's Guidelines and Standards Committee and the Chamber Quantification Writing Group, developed in conjunction with the European Association of Echocardiography, a branch of the European Society of Cardiology. *J Am Soc Echocardiogr* 2005; 18: 1440–63.

26. Piene H, Myhre E. Position of inter-ventricular septum during heart cycle in anesthetized dogs. *Am J Physiol* 1991; 260: h158–64.

27. Tanaka H, Tei C, Nakao S, et al. Diastolic bulging of the inter-ventricular septum toward the left ventricle. An echocardiographic manifestation of negative inter-ventricular pressure gradient between left and right ventricles during diastole. *Circulation* 1980; 62: 558–63.

28. Shimada R, Takeshita A, Nakamura M. Noninvasive assessment of right ventricular systolic pressure in atrial septal defect: analysis of the end-systolic configuration of the ventricular septum by two-dimensional echocardiography. *Am J Cardiol* 1984; 53: 1117–23.

29. Carabello B. Evolution of the study of left ventricular function: everything old is new again. *Circulation* 2002; 105: 2701–3.

30. Dell'Italia L, Walsh R. Application of a time varying elastance model to right ventricular performance in man. *Cardiovasc Res* 1988; 22: 864–74.

31. Anavekar N, Gerson D, Skali H, et al. Two-dimensional assessment of right ventricular function: an echocardiographic-MRI correlative study. *Echocardiography* 2007; 24: 452–56.

32. Anavekar N, Skali H, Bourgoun M, et al. Usefulness of right ventricular fractional area change to predict death, heart failure, and stroke following myocardial infarction (from the VALIANT ECHO Study). *Am J Cardiol* 2008; 101: 607–12.

33. Nass N, McConnell M, Goldhaber S, et al. Recovery of regional right ventricular function after thrombolysis for pulmonary embolism. *Am J Cardiol* 1999; 83: 804–6.

34. Blanchard D, Malouf P, Gurudevan S, et al. Utility of right ventricular Tei index in the noninvasive evaluation of chronic thromboembolic pulmonary hypertension before and after pulmonary thromboendarterectomy. *JACC Cardiovasc Imaging* 2009; 2: 143–49.

35. Yoshifuku S, Otsuji Y, Takasaki K, et al. Pseudonormalized Doppler total ejection isovolume (Tei) index in patients with right ventricular acute myocardial infarction. *Am J Cardiol* 2003; 91: 527–31.

36. Anconina J, Danchin N, Selton-Suty C, et al. Measurement of right ventricular dP/dt. A simultaneous/comparative hemodynamic and Doppler echocardiographic study. *Arch Mal Cœur Vaiss* 1992; 85: 1317–21.

37. Forfia P, Fisher M, Mathai S, et al. Tricuspid annular displacement predicts survival in pulmonary hypertension. *Am J Respir Crit Care Med* 2006; 174: 1034–41.

38. Engstrom A, Vis M, Bouma B, et al. Right ventricular dysfunction is an independent predictor for mortality in ST-elevation myocardial infarction patients presenting with cardiogenic shock on admission. *Eur J Heart Fail* 2010; 12: 276–82.

39. Klima U, Guerrero J, Vlahakes G. Contribution of the inter-ventricular septum to maximal right ventricular function. *Eur J Cardiothoracic Surg* 1998; 14: 250–55.

40. Morcos P, Vick G, Sahn D, et al. Correlation of right ventricular ejection fraction and tricuspid annular plane systolic excursion in tetralogy of Fallot by magnetic resonance imaging. *Int J Cardiovasc Imaging* 2009; 25: 263–70.

41. Giusca S, Dambrauskaite V, Scheurwegs C, et al. Deformation imaging describes right ventricular function better than longitudinal displacement of the tricuspid ring. *Heart* 2010; 96: 281–88.

42. Unsworth B, Casula R, Kyriacou A, et al. The right ventricular annular velocity reduction caused by coronary artery bypass graft surgery occurs at the moment of pericardial incision. *Am Heart J* 2010; 159: 314–22.

43. Koestenberger M, Ravekes W, Everett A, et al. Right ventricular function in infants, children and adolescents: reference values of the tricuspid annular plane systolic excursion (TAPSE) in 640 healthy patients and calculation of z score values. *J Am Soc Echocardiogr* 2009; 22: 715–19.

44. Popescu B, Antonini-Canterin F, Temporelli P, et al. Right ventricular functional recovery after acute myocardial infarction: relation with left ventricular function and inter-ventricular septum motion. GISSI-3 echo substudy. *Heart* 2005; 91: 484–88.

45. Tamborini G, Pepi M, Galli C, et al. Feasibility and accuracy of a routine echocardiographic assessment of right ventricular function. *Int J Cardiol* 2007; 115: 86–89.

46. Ghio S, Temporelli P, Klersy C, et al. Prognostic relevance of a non-invasive evaluation of right ventricular function and pulmonary artery pressure in patients with chronic heart failure. *Eur J Heart Fail* 2013; 15: 408–14.

47. Gulati V, Katz W, Follansbee W, et al. Mitral annular descent velocity by tissue Doppler echocardiography as an index of global left ventricular function. *Am J Cardiol* 1996; 77: 979–84.

48. Lindqvist P, Waldenstrom A, Henein M, et al. Regional and global right ventricular function in healthy individuals aged 20–90 years: a pulsed Doppler tissue imaging study: Umea General Population Heart Study. *Echocardiography* 2005; 22: 305–14.

49. Kukulski T, Hubbert L, Arnold M, et al. Normal regional right ventricular function and its change with age: a Doppler myocardial imaging study. *J Am Soc Echocardiogr* 2000; 13: 194–204.

50. Becker M, Kramann R, Dohmen G, et al. Impact of left ventricular loading conditions on myocardial deformation parameters: analysis of early and late changes of myocardial deformation parameters after aortic valve replacement. *J Am Soc Echocardiogr* 2007; 20: 681–89.

51. Puwanant S, Park M, Popovi-ç Z, et al. Ventricular geometry, strain, and rotational mechanics in pulmonary hypertension. *Circulation* 2010; 121: 259–66.

52. Weidemann F, Eyskens B, Mertens L, et al. Quantification of regional right and left ventricular function by ultrasonic strain rate and strain indexes after surgical repair of tetralogy of Fallot. *Am J Cardiol* 2002; 90: 133–38.

53. Bos J, Hagler D, Silvilairat S, et al. Right ventricular function in asymptomatic individuals with a systemic right ventricle. *J Am Soc Echocardiogr* 2006; 19: 1033–37.

54. Dambrauskaite V, Herbots L, Claus P, et al. Differential changes in regional right ventricular function before and after a bilateral lung transplantation: an ultrasonic strain and strain rate study. *J Am Soc Echocardiogr* 2003; 16: 432–36.

55. Borges A, Knebel F, Eddicks S, et al. Right ventricular function assessed by two-dimensional strain and tissue Doppler echocardiography in patients with pulmonary arterial hypertension and effect of vasodilator therapy. *Am J Cardiol* 2006; 98: 530–34.

56. Bellavia D, Pellikka P, Dispenzieri A, et al. Comparison of right ventricular longitudinal strain imaging, tricuspid annular plane systolic excursion, and cardiac biomarkers for early diagnosis of cardiac involvement and risk stratification in primary systematic (AL) amyloidosis: a 5-year cohort study. *Eur Heart J Cardiovasc Imaging* 2012; 13: 680–89.

57. Teske A, Cox M, Te Riele A, et al. Early detection of regional functional abnormalities in asymptomatic ARVD/C gene carriers. *J Am Soc Echocardiogr* 2012; 25: 997–1006.

58. Lopez-Candales A, Rajagopalan N, Gulyasy B, et al. Differential strain and velocity generation along the right ventricular free wall in pulmonary hypertension. *Can J Cardiol* 2009; 25: e 73–7.

59. Prakasa K, Wang J, Tandri H, et al. Utility of tissue Doppler and strain echocardiography in arrhythmogenic right ventricular dysplasia/cardiomyopathy. *Am J Cardiol* 2007; 100: 507–12.

60. Lorenz C, Walker E, Morgan V, et al. Normal human right and left ventricular mass, systolic function, and gender differences by cine magnetic resonance imaging. *J Cardiovasc Magn Reson* 1999; 1: 7–21.

61. Jain D, Zaret B. Assessment of right ventricular function. Role of nuclear imaging techniques. *Cardiology Clinics* 1992; 10: 23–39.

62. Gopal A, Chukwu E, Iwuchukwu C, et al. Normal values of right ventricular size and function by real-time 3-dimensional echocardiography: comparison with cardiac magnetic resonance imaging. *J Am Soc Echocardiogr* 2007; 20: 445–55.

63. Marcus F, McKenna W, Sherrill D, et al. Diagnosis of arrhythmogenic right ventricular cardiomyopathy/dysplasia: proposed modification of the Task Force Criteria. *Eur Heart J* 2010; 31: 806–14.

64. Mahrholdt H, Wagner A, Judd R, et al. Delayed enhancement cardiovascular magnetic resonance assessment of non-ischaemic cardiomyopathies. *Eur Heart J* 2005; 26: 1461–74.

65. Marcu C, Beek A, Van Rossum A. Cardiovascular magnetic resonance imaging for the assessment of right heart involvement in cardiac and pulmonary disease. *Heart Lung Circ* 2006; 15: 362–70.

66. Babu-Narayan S, Goktekin O, Moon J, et al. Late gadolinium enhancement cardiovascular magnetic resonance of the systemic right ventricle in adults with previous atrial redirection surgery for transposition of the great arteries. *Circulation* 2005; 111: 2091–98.

67. Babu-Narayan S, Kilner P, Li W, et al. Ventricular fibrosis suggested by cardiovascular magnetic resonance in adults with repaired tetralogy of Fallot and its relationship to adverse markers of clinical outcome. *Circulation* 2006; 113: 405–13.

68. Sarikouch S, Peters B, Gutberlet M, et al. Sex-specific pediatric percentiles for ventricular size and mass as reference values for cardiac MRI: assessment by steady-state free-precession and phase-contrast MRI flow. *Circ Cardiovasc Imaging* 2010; 3: 65–76.

69. Oosterhof T, van Straten A, Vliegen H, et al. Preoperative thresholds for pulmonary valve replacement in patients with corrected tetralogy of Fallot using cardiovascular magnetic resonance. *Circulation* 2007; 116: 545–51.

70. Robbers-Visser Dl, Luijnenburg S, van den Berg J, et al. Stress imaging in congenital cardiac disease. *Cardiol Young* 2009; 19: 552–62.

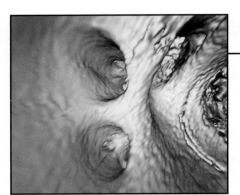

CHAPTER 26

Echocardiography to assess viability

Roxy Senior, Nuno Cortez Dias, Benoy N. Shah, and Fausto J Pinto

Contents

Introduction

The prevalence of heart failure (HF) is increasing worldwide mainly as the result of coronary artery disease (CAD), responsible for almost two-thirds of cases of left ventricular (LV) dysfunction. Established treatment options for ischaemic HF include medical therapy, revascularization, and cardiac transplantation. Cardiac resynchronization therapy (CRT) has been recently introduced as a treatment modality of HF, but other treatment strategies remain investigational [1]. Despite significant therapeutic advances, the outcome of medical therapy in severe HF is poor [2–3]. A large body of evidence from retrospective trials suggested that revascularization was superior to optimal medical therapy in patients with a significant amount of myocardial viability. This practice has been challenged by the recent results of the STICH trial, which suggested both lack of mortality benefit from revascularization and also from viability testing [4–5]. However, despite the STICH results, which will be discussed, there are specific subsets of patients where viability testing is useful because of the potential benefits of revascularization.

Dysfunctional myocardium in coronary artery disease

Systolic LV dysfunction due to CAD is the complex result of necrosis and scarring, but also of functional and morphological adaptive abnormalities of the viable myocardium. Preservation of myocardial viability refers to the tissue capacity for survival. Although viable myocardium encompasses normally contracting and hypocontractile tissue, the term 'viability' has been used interchangeably with 'contractile recovery'. So, in the setting of chronic LV dysfunction, this definition usually refers to the downregulation of contractile function in surviving myocardium in response to periodic or sustained reduction in coronary blood flow, which may be potentially reversed if normal blood flow is restored.

Viable myocardium exists as a spectrum, from complete transmural infarction with no viability, to transmural hibernation or stunning with potential of full recovery. Moreover, patients can have various mixtures of stunned, hibernating, ischaemic, and fibrotic myocardium, in a variety of arrangements. As roughly 40% of myocardial segments with resting wall motion abnormalities after acute myocardial infarction (AMI) have viable tissue that may recover contractile function if revascularized, detection of viable myocardium is clinically relevant.

Myocardial stunning describes the post-ischaemic metabolic and contractile compromise in viable myocardium after a transient coronary occlusion (e.g. post-successful reperfusion in AMI). In stunned myocardium, blood flow has been restored but contraction has not returned to baseline. The pathogenesis likely involves oxygen free radicals, calcium overload, and structural changes in collagen fibres of myocytes–myocyte struts. Dysfunction might persist from hours to weeks, but generally improves with time. An exception is repetitive stunning, defined as repeated episodes of ischaemia producing prolonged post-ischaemic contractile dysfunction [6], which is similar to hibernation in that revascularization has the potential to improve contractile function.

Myocardial hibernation is a chronic state of contractile dysfunction at rest in non-infarcted myocardium as the result of persistently reduced blood flow, which has the potential to improve function after restoration of myocardial blood supply. Observations suggest that hibernation may be a temporal progression of chronic repetitive stunning, with an initial state of near-normal blood flow but reduced flow reserve, leading finally to decreased resting flow. The term 'jeopardized myocardium' has been proposed to include the entire spectrum from repetitive stunning to hibernation. The deprived hibernating myocytes spend energy to preserve cellular integrity at the expense of contractile function. Biopsy studies demonstrated that hibernating myocardium (HM) develops histological changes of cellular de-differentiation and an embryonic phenotype, including expression of foetal isoforms of structural proteins, disorganization of the cytoskeleton, depletion of myofilaments, loss of sarcoplasmic reticulum and T tubules, leading finally to progressive apoptosis and interstitial fibrosis [6]. The improvement of myocardial oxygen supply/demand relationship with revascularization and/or medical therapy alone leads to functional recovery of HM. However, the ability to recover systolic function after intervention depends on the severity of structural abnormalities (i.e. the correction of cellular changes and the amount of tissue fibrosis) [7]. These observations, and evidence that apoptosis is important in hibernation, underscore the importance of early revascularization in this dynamic transition from reversible to irreversible contractile dysfunction [6, 8].

Theoretically, hibernation and stunning are different pathophysiologic states but, practically, they are often indistinct, appear to co-exist in varying degrees in the same patient or myocardial region, and represent a continuum of the same process [9]. However, the timing of functional recovery after revascularization appears to differ between stunned and hibernating myocardium. Stunned myocardium recovery appears to be early after revascularization and more complete, while recovery of HM is late and often incomplete [8].

Revascularization in ischaemic cardiomyopathy (ICM)

Until recently, clinical management decisions were based largely on surgical studies performed nearly two decades ago, because of a paucity of data from contemporary therapy. A meta-analysis comprising 24 studies reported patient survival using thallium SPECT ($n = 6$), fluorodeoxyglucose (FDG) PET ($n = 11$) or dobutamine stress echocardiography ($n = 8$) to assess HM [10]. A strong association between presence of HM and improved survival after revascularization was noted. In patients with HM, revascularization was associated with an 80% reduction in annual mortality compared with OMT (16% vs. 3.2%) whereas, in those without HM, there was no difference in outcome irrespective of management strategy. (⊃ Fig. 26.1). As a result, thereafter some even questioned if it would be ethical to randomize ICM patients to medical therapy in future studies [11]. Although these and other

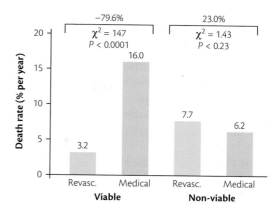

Fig. 26.1 Mortality rates for patients with and without myocardial viability treated by revascularization and medical therapy or only medical therapy. Patients with viability treated by revascularization benefited from a 79.6% reduction in mortality (P<0.0001). In patients without myocardial viability, there was no significant difference in mortality with revascularization versus medical therapy.

Reprinted from *Journal of the American College of Cardiology*, 39:7, Kevin Allman et al, Myocardial viability testing and impact of revascularization on prognosis in patients with coronary artery disease and left ventricular dysfunction: a meta-analysis, Copyright 2002 with permission from Elsevier.

smaller studies, overall, favoured surgery over medical therapy, important limitations include lack of randomized trials, the selection bias for revascularization, inadequate medical therapy in both medical and surgical groups, outdated surgical techniques [12], and small number of patients (particularly with predominant HF symptoms).

Therefore, a trial addressing the concerns raised was needed and the STICH trial was thus formulated. The trial had a complex design and aimed to answer three issues: first, the added value of revascularization over OMT (hypothesis 1), second, the benefit of adding surgical ventricular reconstruction (SVR) to CABG (hypothesis 2), and third, the impact of determining myocardial viability prior to revascularization. In short, the trial did not find revascularization superior to OMT nor found benefit for the use of viability testing in guiding management decisions or influencing mortality outcome. However, there were several key factors that may have influenced the trial results. First, the STICH trial was a study in CAD patients with LV dysfunction and angina rather than patients with heart failure syndrome per se, since presence of clinical HF was not necessary for trial enrolment. Second, many cardiologists already had preconceptions about the 'correct' management of such patients and were reticent to put their patients forward for randomization, which introduced a selection bias. Third, the cross-over rate between groups was 17% for patients assigned to OMT who underwent CABG and 9% of patients randomized to CABG never underwent surgery. Therefore, although the intention-to-treat analysis did not demonstrate a beneficial impact of revascularization, the as-treated analysis *did* show significant benefit for CABG over OMT alone (P<0.001). The viability sub-study, similarly, had severe limitations. Approximately only 50% who were randomized underwent non-invasive tests and the majority had severely dilated ventricles, a group unlikely to benefit from revascularization. Only 19% demonstrated non-viable myocardium.

Based upon the discussion, and consistent with the ESC 2010 guidelines on myocardial revascularization [13], an algorithm for integrating non-invasive imaging into contemporary ICM management was recently suggested (see ⊃ Fig. 26.2) [14]. The current role of viability testing remains the prediction of potential functional and clinical improvement in patients with impaired LV EF, thereby facilitating a better estimate of the potential benefit of revascularization therapy, versus its risks.

Assessment of myocardial viability

A number of non-invasive imaging procedures have been developed to evaluate myocardial viability and to identify markers of

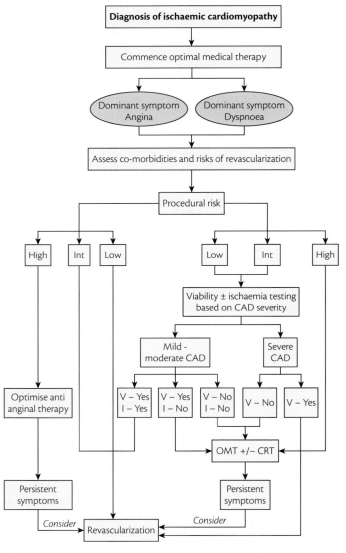

Fig. 26.2 Algorithm suggesting how to integrate viability (V) and ischaemia (I) testing into clinical practice. Patients with predominant angina are on the left side, those with predominant dyspnoea on the right side. In dyspnoiec patients at high risk of revascularization, but who remain symptomatic despite OMT +/− CRT, viability testing should also be performed before deciding on revascularization.

Reproduced from B. Shah et al, *European Heart Journal*, The hibernating myocardium: current concepts, diagnostic dilemmas, and clinical challenges in the post-STICH era, 34:18, copyright 2013 by permission of Oxford University Press.

functional recovery, including dobutamine stress echocardiography (DSE), myocardial contrast echocardiography (MCE), single-photon emission computed tomography (SPECT), positron emission tomography (PET), and cardiovascular magnetic resonance (CMR).

The currently available imaging techniques assess distinct characteristics of viable and dysfunctional myocardium, having different limitations and diagnostic accuracy. Comparison of the clinical utility of each in the assessment of myocardial viability is currently limited by the lack of randomized prospective trials. Besides, there is uncertainty about the best criterion to determine the clinical benefit of the assessment of myocardial viability, by which they should be compared. Several studies evaluated their accuracy for prediction of segmental improvement, but of greater clinical relevance is the global LV functional recovery after revascularization. Theoretically, the best method should be the one with the optimal sensitivity (Sn) and specificity (Sp) for detection of viability. However, since the amount of HM is the critical determinant of global functional recovery, even methods of moderately high Sn may eventually identify those patients with great benefit. The precise extent of viability necessary to predict benefit from revascularization is unclear and may vary in different clinical circumstances. Most studies suggested that a substantial amount of viable myocardium (at least 20—30% of LV mass) is required for the improvement of LVEF. Hence, both identification and quantification of the extent of viable myocardium are required for a careful selection of patients who have a higher likelihood of benefit from revascularization.

However, several authors showed that survival rates after coronary artery bypass surgery were similar whether or not function improved after intervention, suggesting that relevant clinical benefits may occur even without LVEF recovery. Preservation of small viable areas may improve clinical outcome by reducing the risk of subsequent ischaemic events, improving LV remodelling processes, preventing additional LV dilatation, promoting electrical stability, and eventually improving symptoms and functional capacity. So, large-scale prospective head-to-head comparisons of the available imaging modalities are needed to determine their independent value for detection of viable myocardium and to evaluate their accuracy in predicting patient response to therapy, regarding LV function recovery, symptoms and survival. ⊃ Table 26.1 summarizes the sensitivity and specificity of various non-invasive techniques for the prediction of regional recovery of function after revascularization [14].

Since the use of a single viability test may not be optimal, the value of sequential multi-modality imaging should be also evaluated. Multi-modality imaging approach may theoretically enhance the prediction of functional recovery after revascularization in selected patients with ischaemic LV dysfunction.

Rest echocardiography

The resting echocardiographic examination is the single most useful test in the assessment of heart failure since structural

Table 26.1 Comparison of the various imaging techniques for detecting viable myocardium

Technique	No. of Studies	No. of Patients	Mean EF (%)	Sensitivity (%)	Specificity (%)
Dobutamine Echocardiography—TOTAL	**41**	**1,421**	**25–48**	**80**	**78**
Low-dose DbE	33	1,121	25–48	79	78
High-dose DbE	8	290	29–38	83	79
Myocardial contrast echocardiography—TOTAL	**10**	**268**	**29–38**	**87**	**50**
Thallium scintigraphy—TOTAL	**40**	**1,119**	**23–45**	**87**	**54**
Tl-201 rest-redistribution	28	776	23–45	87	56
Tl-201 re-injection	12	343	31-49	87	50
Technetium scintigraphy—TOTAL	**25**	**721**	**23–54**	**83**	**65**
Without nitrates protocol	17	516	23–52	83	57
With nitrates protocol	8	205	35–54	81	69
Positron Emission Tomography—TOTAL	**24**	**756**	**23–53**	**92**	**63**
Cardiovascular Magnetic Resonance—TOTAL	**14**	**450**	**24–53**	**80**	**70**
Low-dose dobutamine protocol	9	272	24–53	74	82
Late gadolinium enhancement protocol	5	178	32–52	84	63

abnormalities, systolic dysfunction, diastolic dysfunction or a combination of these abnormalities needs to be confirmed for the diagnosis of heart failure. Moreover, resting echocardiography provides valuable information that may guide the choice of imaging technique to use and assist in its interpretation. If there is adequate image quality, allowing full visualization of endocardial border and wall thickening in all myocardial segments, DSE may be the test of choice. If the acoustic window is insufficient to provide a high degree of diagnostic certainty, despite contrast enhancement, another imaging approach should be used. Moreover, the wall motion score and LV ejection fraction (LVEF) at rest differently affects accuracy of the several imaging methods used to assess viability. Severe dysfunction at rest reduces the predictive accuracy of stress tests (either DSE or dobutamine-CMR), and in such patients delayed-enhancement CMR may be preferable.

The assessment of LV end-diastolic wall thickness can be used to obtain an initial evaluation of myocardial viability: thinned (<6mm) and hyper-echoic myocardial segments typically reflect scar tissue and have particularly low probability of improvement in function, while dysfunctional segments with preserved wall thickness (≥6mm) may be viable. The involvement of >4 ventricular wall segments by scarring is associated with low probability of global functional recovery after revascularization. Furthermore, the degree of LV remodelling and dilatation may be an additional guide to predict functional recovery post revascularization. The likelihood of significant recovery of global LV function is inversely related to ventricular volume. End-diastolic volume >220ml is unlikely to show significant functional recovery, as the likelihood of significant scar tissue is high in the severely remodelled LV.

Until recently, resting echocardiography was considered of limited utility in discriminating viable from non-viable myocardium. However, myocardial velocity assessment with tissue Doppler imaging (TDI) and speckle tracking-derived parameters may unmask viable myocardium. TDI allows accurate assessment of regional myocardial function during all phases of the cardiac

cycle. Experimental and clinical studies showed that TDI-derived analysis of ejection systolic velocities, strain and strain rate allows accurate definition of transmurality of myocardial infarction. TDI-based longitudinal strain and strain rate are reduced in segments with sub-endocardial scarring, although the relationship is nonlinear since sub-endocardium governs transmural contraction and longitudinal function. However, angle dependency (incapacity to assess shortening or thickening whenever the principal vector of contraction is not aligned with the ultrasound beam) significantly impairs their accuracy. Other TDI-derived parameters may be useful to assess myocardial viability, particularly the detection of myocardial positive pre-ejection velocity occurring during isovolumic contraction.

Penicka and co-workers [15] demonstrated high accuracy of TDI-derived myocardial positive pre-ejection velocity qualitatively assessed by pulsed TDI to predict recovery of contractile function in patients with chronic CAD, wall motion abnormalities, and global systolic dysfunction submitted to revascularization. The presence of positive pre-ejection velocity predicted improvement of regional function after revascularization (Sn: 93%; Sp: 77%), and the presence of positive pre-ejection velocity in ≥5 dysfunctional segments had a high accuracy to predict moderate (Sn: 92%; Sp: 79%) and marked (Sn: 93%; Sp: 60%) recovery of global systolic function. Moreover, in another group of similar but non-revascularized patients, Penicka and co-workers showed a good agreement between positive pre-ejection velocity and detection of viable myocardium at DSE, FDG-PET, and DE-CMR. However, the incremental value of positive pre-ejection velocity over reference techniques in the evaluation of myocardial viability was not assessed.

Speckle tracking echocardiography is a new technique that tracks frame-to-frame movement of natural acoustic markers, or speckles, identified on standard 2-dimensional ultrasound tissue images. Local 2-dimensional tissue velocities are derived from spatial and temporal data of each speckle. Myocardial strain

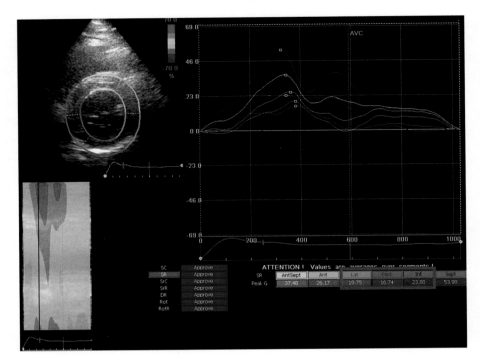

Fig. 26.3 Short-axis radial strain images in a patient with previous history of postero-lateral acute myocardial infarction, showing a low peak systolic radial strain of the posterior, inferior and lateral segments.

can be assessed from temporal differences in mutual distance of neighbouring speckles, allowing the evaluation of circumferential, radial and longitudinal strain. Recently, Becker and co-workers [16] showed that myocardial deformation imaging in rest based on speckle tracking allows the assessment of transmurality since radial and circumferential strain impairment is proportional to the transmural scarring extent. Moreover, they also found that peak systolic radial strain identifies reversible myocardial dysfunction and predicts regional and global functional recovery at 9±2 months follow-up. Segments with functional recovery had significantly higher baseline peak systolic radial and circumferential strain values and a peak systolic strain >17.2% predicted segmental functional recovery (Sn: 70.2%; Sp: 85.1%). Besides, a positive correlation was found between the number of segments with a peak systolic strain >17.2% and LVEF improvement after surgical or percutaneous coronary revascularization. Moreover, the predictive value was similar to that achieved by contrast-enhanced CMR (➲ Fig. 26.3) [16].

Myocardial contrast echocardiography (MCE)

MCE is a technique that uses acoustically active gas-filled microbubbles during echocardiography. These microbubbles remain exclusively within the intravascular space, and their presence within any myocardial territory denotes the status of microvascular perfusion within that region. The volume of blood present in the entire coronary circulation (arteries, arterioles, capillaries, venules, and veins) is approximately 12 ml/100 g of cardiac muscle; approximately one-third of this is present within the myocardium itself, and is termed 'myocardial blood volume' [17]. The predominant

(90%) component of the myocardial blood volume resides within the capillaries. Myocardial contrast intensity reflects the concentration of microbubbles within the myocardium. When a steady state of microbubble concentration has been achieved in the myocardium, during a continuous infusion of contrast, the observed signal intensity denotes the capillary blood volume [18–20]. Any alteration of signal intensity in this situation thus occurs principally as a result of a change in the capillary blood volume. Furthermore, it has been shown that after the destruction of microbubbles in the myocardium with high energy ultrasound, myocardial contrast replenishment, both during low and high power imaging, reflects myocardial blood velocity [20]. The product of these two components (myocardial blood volume and red cell velocity) denotes myocardial blood flow at the tissue level [20, 21]. MCE can thus detect capillary blood volume, and, by virtue of its temporal resolution, can also assess myocardial blood flow.

Myocardial contrast echocardiography for the detection of myocardial viability

Assessment of myocardial viability is based on the assumption that myocardial viability necessitates a preserved microvasculature, which can be assessed by MCE. With its excellent spatial resolution (<3 mm axially), MCE can accurately depict the presence of microvascular integrity. Kloner et al. showed that with myocardial infarction, myocyte loss was associated with a loss of microvasculature [22]. Therefore, absence of myocardial contrast enhancement on MCE should define regions that lack myocardial viability. In ICM patients undergoing coronary artery bypass grafting, Shimoni et al. [23], in an important study, demonstrated an excellent correlation between contrast signal intensity and capillary density obtained from myocardial biopsies of the same region. Moreover, contrast signal intensity was inversely related to the extent of fibrosis. Peak contrast signal intensity after microbubble destruction denotes capillary volume, which in turn is a measure of myocardial viability. Peak contrast intensity obtained in this manner has also been shown to correlate with the extent and severity of myocardial necrosis, as assessed by gadolinium-enhanced CMR imaging 7 days after AMI in a study by Janardhanan et al. [24] (⭕ Figs 26.4 and 26.5). Both studies evaluated the usefulness of

peak contrast intensity as a measure of myocardial viability. Once the contrast agent has reached a steady state, during continuous intravenous infusion, high-energy impulses are used to achieve microbubble destruction within the myocardium. The replenishment of contrast can then be visualized using either high-power (mechanical index 0.9–1.0) or low-power (mechanical index 0.1–0.2) techniques. Myocardial replenishment is then observed over

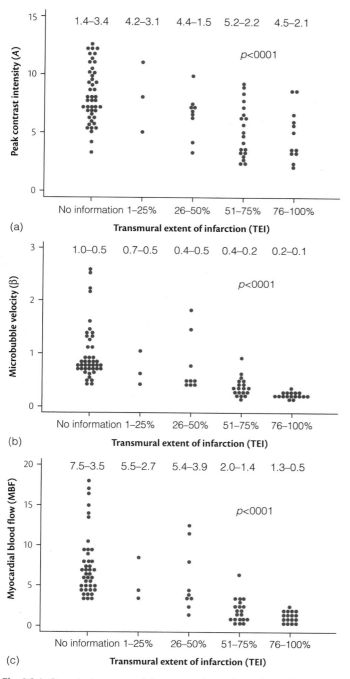

Fig. 26.4 Quantitative myocardial contrast echocardiography in relation to transmural extent of infarction (TEI) in dysynergic segments: (a) peak contrast intensity; (b) microbubble velocity; (c) myocardial blood flow.
Reproduced from Janardhanan R, Moon JC, Pennell DJ, Senior R. Myocardial contrast echocardiography accurately reflects transmurality of myocardial necrosis and predicts contractile reserve after acute myocardial infarction. *Am Heart J* 2005; 149(2): 355–62 with permission from Elsevier.

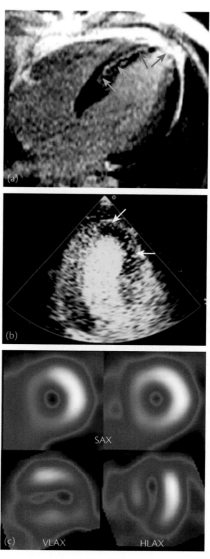

Fig. 26.5 Images from a 62-year-old patient who presented with an anterior myocardial infarction. (a) CMR demonstrates a full thickness apical infarct (red arrows), which extends to the mid-septum with less than 100% but greater than 50% myocardial wall involvement (blue arrows), again implying low likelihood of viability. (b) The MCE apical 3-chamber view demonstrates not only an absence of contrast uptake at the apex but also severely reduced opacification extending to the mid septum. (c) Although the SPECT images clearly demonstrate an apical full thickness infarct, they only show a mild reduction in tracer uptake in the septum as demonstrated in the mid-apical short-axis view implying ≤50% TEI with significant viability in the infarct related territory.
Reprinted from *Am J Cardiol* 2006; 97(12):1718–21. Hayat SA, Janardhanan R, Moon JC et al. Comparison between myocardial contrast echocardiography and single-photon emission computed tomography for predicting transmurality of acute myocardial infarction.

10–15 cardiac cycles; fully replenished myocardium, which is of homogenous contrast intensity, indicates the presence of myocardial viability. Normal contrast intensity by qualitative MCE has been shown to have a predictive value of almost 90% for the presence of contractile reserve, whereas the absence of contrast enhancement predicts a lack of contractile reserve in approximately 90% of cases [24].

The concept underlying this is that in a low-flow state, such as occurs after AMI, myocardial blood flow in the infarcted muscle is reduced either because of severe flow-limiting stenosis, capillary plugging, or an occluded infarct-related artery (IRA), with the myocardium being supplied by collateral blood flow. In a novel study by Coggins et al., using an experimental model, they showed that after occlusion, infarct size was best determined when contrast replenishment is observed 15 s after a destructive impulse [25]. In other words, collateral blood flow, which is usually low, maintains myocardial viability despite an occluded IRA. This was also shown in a human study in which Swinburn et al. [26] studied 96 patients after AMI. MCE was performed 3–5 days after AMI; the authors found that the absence of homogenous contrast replenishment within 10 s of myocardial microbubble destruction resulted in the non-recovery of these segments in 84% of cases (⊃ Fig. 26.6).

Detection of myocardial viability after acute myocardial infarction

A number of studies have demonstrated the important role MCE plays in assessing viability and predicting the recovery of regional and global systolic function post-AMI. It was noted that patients with a patent IRA and good contrast opacification demonstrated an improvement in contractile function compared with those patients with a poor or absent contrast opacification one month after AMI. Such studies have established the importance of an intact microvasculature after AMI, as assessed by MCE, to predict myocardial viability. In post-AMI patients treated with thrombolysis, Jeetley et al. [27] demonstrated that the extent and severity of contrast perfusion defects predicted adverse LV remodelling. Low-dose DSE is widely used to assess myocardial viability. Senior and Swinburn specifically addressed the incremental value of MCE, demonstrating that the presence of contrast enhancement, even in segments that lacked contractile response during dobutamine, resulted in an improvement in regional function compared with those with no contrast enhancement [28]. This is probably because after thrombolysis a significant number of patients demonstrate residual IRA stenosis, which prevents the occurrence of contractile response in viable segments. As MCE is performed at rest, the uptake of contrast is unaffected in these patients.

Hickman et al. [29] compared MCE with SPECT for evaluating myocardial viability in post-AMI patients treated with thrombolysis. In this study of 56 patients, they found that 90% of segments showing homogenous contrast opacification on MCE demonstrated viability, whereas only 45% demonstrating normal radionuclide tracer uptake showed viability. Conversely, 85% of segments without contrast opacification on MCE did not show recovery of function; however, 25% of patients subsequently demonstrated

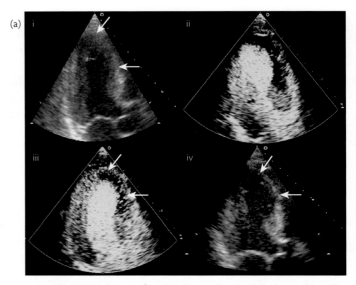

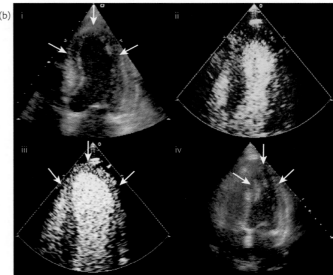

Fig. 26.6 (a) End-systolic frames of the apical 3-chamber view showing: (i) akinetic mid-anterior septum and apex (arrows); (ii) complete destruction of myocardial contrast immediately after a high mechanical index pulse on MCE; (iii) lack of contrast opacification of the dysynergic segments, even at 15 cycles (arrows); (iv) lack of functional recovery at 12 weeks despite revascularization (arrows). (b) End-systolic frames of the apical 4-chamber view showing: (i) akinetic mid-septum, apex, and mid-lateral segments (arrows); (ii) complete destruction of myocardial contrast immediately after a high mechanical index pulse on MCE; (iii) homogenous contrast opacification of the dysynergic segments by 15 cardiac cycles (arrows); (iv) functional recovery at 12 weeks after revascularization (arrows).
Reprinted from *Journal of the American College of Cardiology*, 38:1, J Swinburn et al, Intravenous myocardial contrast echocardiography predicts recovery of dysynergic myocardium early after acute myocardial infarction, Copyright 2001 with permission from Elsevier.

recovery of function despite a severe reduction in tracer uptake on SPECT. This is probably because SPECT has a lower spatial and temporal resolution compared to MCE (⊃ Fig. 26.5).

Several MCE studies have demonstrated high Sn (75–90%) but poorer Sp (50–60%) in identifying the recovery of contractile function after AMI. The majority of the studies consisted of patients studied early after reperfusion and only assessed at rest. The combination of reactive hyperaemia, dynamic changes in the microcirculation early after AMI, and the fact that myocardial infarction involving more than 20% of the sub-endocardium can render the myocardium akinetic despite significant epicardial and mid-myocardial viability [30], tend to make MCE less specific for the detection of myocardial viability, if viability is defined in terms of the recovery of systolic function. Technical factors such as the inability to distinguish microbubble signature from the underlying tissue can also contribute to the low Sp of MCE. Recent studies have, however, shown that assessing patients 3–5 days after AMI using background subtraction techniques, either on-line (low-power or high-power imaging) or off-line, considerably improved the Sp (75–80%) and positive predictive value (75–80%) of MCE [31, 32]. The study by Main et al. [32] is an important paper that demonstrates the impact of technological advances in imaging techniques on the accuracy of MCE in identifying stunning and in the prediction of recovery of function after myocardial infarction.

Recent data indicated that the extent and severity of contrast perfusion defect after AMI predicted mortality and combined mortality re-infarction independent of clinical factors, ECG parameters, cardiac biomarkers, and resting LVEF [33] (⊃ Fig. 26.7).

Detection of myocardial viability in chronic coronary artery disease

In the first human study to use quantitative MCE for the detection of HM in chronic ischaemic LV dysfunction, Shimoni et al. [34] studied 20 ICM patients, who underwent MCE, DSE, and rest-distribution thallium-201 scintigraphy 1–5 days before bypass surgery. They found that the Sn of quantitative resting MCE for predicting the recovery of function was 90% and was similar to thallium-201 scintigraphy (92%) and superior to DSE (80%); the Sp was higher than for thallium-201 and also for DSE (63, 45, and 54%, respectively; $P<0.05$). Hickman et al. showed that the superior predictive value of contrast intensity compared to contractile reserve detected by DSE is because, in HM, contractile reserve is very low and therefore, the myocardium is unable to mount a contractile response while MCE relies on resting parameters only

(35). Better spatial and temporal resolution of MCE compared to SPECT also translated to better predictive value for outcome (36). Hummel et al. [37] demonstrated the application of viability assessment by MCE in patients with ICM undergoing CRT. The authors found that perfusion score index (PSI) based on a visual assessment of contrast opacification correlated with an acute improvement in EF ($P = 0.003$), stroke volume ($P = 0.02$) and end systolic volume ($P = 0.05$). In a multivariate regression model, PSI provided incremental predictive value to the degree of dyssynchrony, measured by TDI, for predicting an improvement in the LVEF. At 6 months, PSI remained positively correlated with an improvement in ventricular performance and with a reduction in LV end-diastolic volume. Furthermore, patients with a higher PSI subsequently tended to have a lower New York Heart Association class, a better 6-minute walking distance, an improved quality-of-life score, and fewer hospital admissions for HF after CRT. In summary, MCE is reliable for the detection of myocardial viability after AMI and chronic HF. However, more outcome data is required to establish this technique as a robust marker of myocardial viability.

Stress echocardiography

Stress echocardiography is based on evaluation of contractile reserve, a characteristic feature of viable myocardium, which may be elicited by catecholamine stimulation. The underlying principle is that adrenoceptor stimulation by dobutamine will augment function before ischaemia is engendered by increased myocardial work and metabolic demands. Typically, primarily inotropic response occurs at low doses and tachycardia—potentially eliciting ischaemia—usually only develops at higher doses.

Conventional DSE involves various stages of either low- or high-dose protocols, with increments from 5 to 40 µg/kg/min, with each stage lasting 3 or 5 minutes. Some advocate using an even lower starting dose of 2.5 µg/kg/min, since in patients with critical coronary stenosis, myocardial ischaemia may be elicited with doses as low as 5 µg/kg/min. Infusions of low-dose dobutamine (5–10 µg/kg/min) increase contractility in dysfunctional but viable myocardium, usually without significant tachycardia.

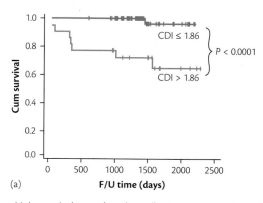
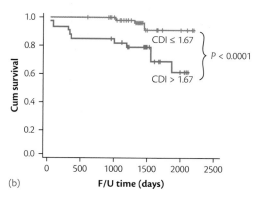

Fig. 26.7 (a) Kaplan–Meier survival curve (unadjusted) using a contrast defect index (CDI) cut-off of 1.86 for the prediction of cardiac death. (b) Kaplan–Meier survival curve using a CDI cut-off of 1.67 for the prediction of cardiac death or non-fatal AMI.
Reprinted from *Journal of the American College of Cardiology*, 50:4, G. Dwivedi et al, Prognostic value of myocardial viability detected by myocardial contrast echocardiography early after acute myocardial infarction, Copyright 2007 with permission from Elsevier.

A combination of low and high (≥20 µg/kg/min) doses has been shown to provide the greatest diagnostic information and accuracy for prediction of functional recovery after revascularization. This is ascribed to the ability of high-dose dobutamine infusion to recognize ischaemia with higher accuracy. Echocardiographic images are acquired at each stage to determine new wall motion abnormalities, worsening of pre-existing wall motion abnormalities, or enhanced wall motion. Clear endocardial definition is crucial for optimal regional function evaluation, which is performed using a five-point wall motion scoring system (1 = normokinesis; 2 = mild hypokinesis; 3 = moderate or severe hypokinesis; 4 = akinesis; and 5 = dyskinesis) for the 16- or 17-segment model of the LV. As with conventional echocardiography, patient-dependent factors, such as obesity and lung disease, may lead to poor acoustic windows and reduce diagnostic accuracy. In those patients, ultrasound contrast agents may be used during DSE to improve endocardial border detection. Moreover, evaluation of wall motion abnormalities may be challenging in patients with previous myocardial infarction, in whom passive tethering motion is a confounding variable. Finally, signal dropout can cause sub-optimal images, leading to misdiagnosis in some patients.

During dobutamine infusion, there are four possible responses of regions with abnormal resting function: (1) biphasic response—at low levels of dobutamine stimulation, systolic wall thickening increases and starts earlier, improving contractile function, but at higher levels the increase in myocardial demand cannot be matched by further increases in blood flow, leading to ischaemia and systolic function deterioration; (2) sustained functional improvement at low doses that persisted or further improved until peak dose; (3) worsening of resting wall motion during dobutamine infusion without any improvement; and (4) no change in function. The stress echocardiographic sign of myocardial viability is a stress-induced improvement of contractile function during low levels of stress in a region that is abnormal at rest. However, the pattern of response is predictive of post-revascularization functional improvement. A biphasic response (⊃ Fig. 26.8), indicating that the tissue is not only viable but also supplied by a stenosed artery, has greatest predictive accuracy for recovery—in a recent study, 72% of segments with biphasic response recovered function. A uni-phasic response with sustained improvement has limited Sp to predict functional recovery since augmentation alone may occur not only with non-jeopardized myocardium (stunned) but also in areas of non-transmural infarction without hibernating myocardium (sub-endocardial scar) or in remodelled myocardium. Finally, about 20–25% of viable segments do not improve functionally during inotropic stimulation since they have an almost exhausted blood flow reserve and extensive structural abnormalities. However, those viable segments without improvement with dobutamine stimulation usually do not recover contractile function after revascularization.

From experienced laboratories, DSE using visual wall motion assessment demonstrated a mean Sn of 85% and Sp of 79% in regional functional recovery prediction [38]. Identification of contractile reserve by DSE is highly specific, but may lack Sn, since some myocardial segments without inotropic reserve may demonstrate recovery of function following revascularization. Moreover, due to the subjectivity of visual wall-motion interpretation, DSE is an experience-dependent technique with a degree of inter- and intra-observer variability. However, in clinical setting, diagnostic accuracy of DSE is generally adequate for prediction of regional recovery after revascularization.

In addition, various studies demonstrated that LVEF improved only in patients with substantial viability on DSE. A linear relation was present between the number of viable segments and the likelihood of recovery of overall LV function after revascularization,

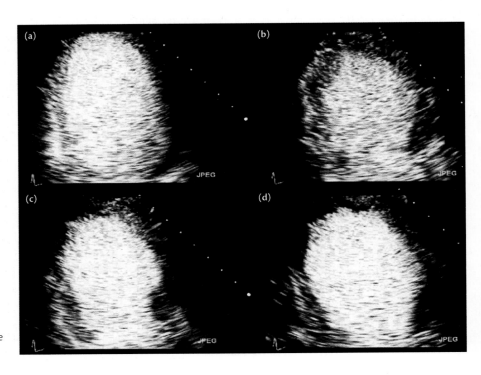

Fig. 26.8 Quad-screen still image from apical 2-chamber view during contrast-enhanced dobutamine stress echocardiography. Rest (a), low-dose (b), mid-dose (c), and peak-dose (d) images are shown, with reduction in LV cavity size at low and mid-dose dobutamine, compared to rest, but with subsequent clear cavity dilation at peak stress, indicating both viability and inducible ischaemia (the biphasic response).

and the identification of ≥4 viable segments accurately predicted LVEF improvement (e.g. ≥5%) after revascularization (Sn: 86%; Sp: 90%), improvement in heart failure symptoms and reduction of event-rate [38].

Alternative protocols for echocardiographic assessment of myocardial viability include dipyridamole, low-level exercise, and more recently, levosimendan. Exercise induces catecholamine stimulation but the early development of tachycardia may provoke ischaemia and mask the inotropic response. Dipyridamole stress has been used for myocardial viability assessment, mainly in continental Europe, but the pathophysiology of dipyridamole response is less clear. Dipyridamole induces endogenous adenosine accumulation. It has been proposed that the stimulation of adenosine receptors, which induces regional vasodilatation, may cause an increase in tissue turgor and produce a reflex increase of regional function. Exercise, dobutamine, and dipyridamole show similar diagnostic accuracy in the induction of ischaemia. However, DSE is the most extensively studied and the most widely used test for the assessment of myocardial viability.

Recently, Cianfrocca and co-workers [39] compared the accuracy of levosimendan stress echocardiography with conventional DSE. Levosimendan enhances cardiac contractility via Ca^{2+} sensitization without increasing myocardial oxygen consumption, and induces vasodilatation through the activation of adenosine triphosphate-sensitive potassium channels. They found that levosimendan was more reliable than dobutamine in predicting reversible dysfunction, having higher Sn (75% vs. 59%; $P = 0.026$) and similar Sp (80%). Of note, a further improvement for prediction of functional recovery was found when wall motion response during levosimendan stress echocardiography was complemented by measurement of peak systolic strain rate based in TDI (Sn: 93%).

Similarly, Karagiannis and co-workers [40] proved the additional value of evaluating the recovery phase of DSE after acute beta-blocker administration, identifying some additional ischaemic segments otherwise classified as normal. Dobutamine stimulates β1, β2, and α1-adrenergic receptors. Acute beta-blockade at the peak dose of DSE leaves unopposed α1-adrenergic vasoconstriction, reducing the coronary flow reserve, which can paradoxically enhance the ischaemic response in the recovery phase. This method applied to DSE increased Sn for viability estimation from 72% to 85% ($P<0.001$), while Sp remained unchanged (78%). However, some concerns remain regarding the potential risk of myocardial infarction and arrhythmias induced by acute beta-blockade, which should be further addressed in larger trials.

The state-of-the art diagnosis of ischaemia and myocardial viability in DSE remains the quantitative analysis of regional wall motion. The major potential drawback for use of this index is semi-quantitative assessment of wall motion, which is limited by subjectivity and technical challenges. Inter- and intra-observer wall motion score variability is even greater in those patients with previous myocardial infarction due to pre-existing wall motion abnormalities and intra-ventricular conduction defects. In the last few years, quantitative parameters have been studied to provide objective and reproducible information on global and regional wall function during stress. The most important methods

aimed to improve DSE diagnostic accuracy and to reduce its operator dependency are: (1) automatic contour techniques, including acoustic quantification and colour kinesis; and (2) tissue Doppler myocardial velocity derived parameters. In this context, myocardial tissue velocity, strain and strain rate evaluated by TDI have emerged as promising echocardiographic tools for quantitative assessment of regional ventricular function. Ventricular systole is a complex three-dimensional deformation process, in which the apex stays relatively stationary, while the base of the heart is moving downward, making a global twist, and resulting in longitudinal and circumferential shortening, as well as radial thickening. TDI measures low-frequency, high-amplitude signals of myocardial tissue motion allowing the assessment of myocardial velocities. However, myocardial velocity profiles are unable to discriminate passive motion from active deformation. During the pre-ejection period, the LV does not change in shape and the tethering effect is thus minimized. Aggeli and co-workers [41] showed that pre-ejection longitudinal tissue velocity change and peak systolic longitudinal velocity change, assessed by pulsed-wave TDI during low-dose dobutamine, are reliable parameters of myocardial viability, since their increase during the stress test strongly predicts recovery after revascularization. However, evaluation of myocardial velocities by pulsed-wave TDI during DSE is a time-consuming technique without proven incremental value, thus being impracticable in everyday practice at present.

The post-processing of colour-coded tissue Doppler data allows quantification of myocardial deformation by measuring strain and strain rate. These new TDI-derived techniques assess velocity gradients between different points in space allowing the evaluation of active contraction of a given segment, independent of local tethering of the neighbouring regions. Strain and strain rate reflect, respectively, the percentage of deformation and intrinsic rate of deformation of the analysed myocardial segment. These parameters are less dependent on image quality and less subjective than the visual assessment of endocardial border motion. During DSE, circumferential strain and strain rate are significantly lower in segments with myocardial infarction, compared to both sub-endocardial infarcts and normal myocardium, thus assessing the degree of transmurality. Hanekom and co-workers [42] demonstrated that the assessment of strain rate imaging as an adjunct to routine visual wall-motion scoring during conventional DSE provides incremental value to predict regional and global functional recovery following revascularization, increasing Sn from 73 to 83% compared with visual assessment alone, without affecting the Sp. A strain rate increment of 0.25/s during DSE was the optimal cut-off for functional recovery prediction (Sn 80%; Sp 75%). Further experimental and clinical studies have validated strain rate imaging for the assessment of myocardial viability and suggested that strain rate is a better quantitative parameter for the prediction of functional recovery compared to strain (⊃ Fig. 26.9). However, SRI is limited by signal noise, low reproducibility, and angle dependence, making the TDI evaluation of apical myocardial segments unreliable.

Cianfrocca and co-workers [39] compared the accuracy of two different pharmacological stress protocols, full-dose dobutamine and levosimendan, with and without combination of strain rate

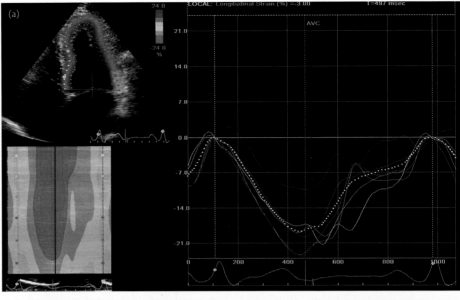

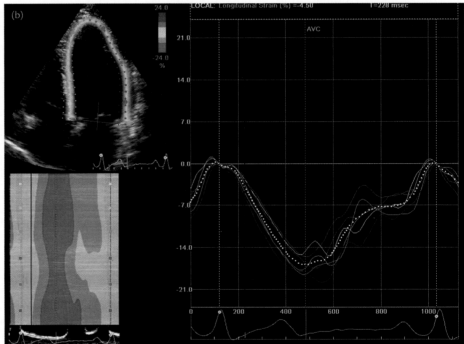

Fig. 26.9 Example of strain curves at rest (a) and with low-dose dobutamine (b) in a patient with previous lateral acute myocardial infarction, showing improvement in the basal lateral segment demonstrating the presence of a viable segment.

analysis to the conventional subjective wall motion evaluation. As discussed, the levosimendan stress protocol was more reliable than dobutamine in predicting reversible dysfunction. Moreover, peak strain rate assessment was superior to wall motion analysis in detecting inotropic recruitment during pharmacological stress testing, with either dobutamine or levosimendan. Besides, an increment in peak strain rate greater than −0.29s⁻¹ after levosimendan had the highest Sp (93%) for predicting segmental function recovery after revascularization.

Recent advances in this technology raised the prospect that SRI may become a routinely employed modality for quantitative assessment of viability during DSE. However, it should be noted that strain rate analysis is time-consuming, requiring 15 to 25 minutes

of additional analysis. Finally, technological advances in transducer and computer technology led to introduction of real-time 3D-echocardiography during stress but no data currently show the additional value of this technique over conventional DSE.

Comparison with other modalities

Single-photon emission computed tomography (SPECT)

Among the radionuclide imaging techniques available to assess myocardial viability, the most commonly used is SPECT, whether using thallium-201 or Tc-99m sestamibi. There are several SPECT protocols to evaluate myocardial viability, in stress and/or rest, which include imaging from 8 to 72 h after stress injection, reinjection of tracer at rest on the same day as the stress injection, a resting injection on a separate day, or adjuncts such as nitrates.

Thallium-201 is a potassium analogue that is actively transported through the intact cell membrane of the myocyte. Thus, the initial uptake of thallium is determined by myocardial perfusion (either during stress or at rest) and is unaffected by hypoxia, hibernation, or stunning, unless myocardial infarction is present. Conversely, delayed retention in the redistribution phase is dependent on cell membrane integrity, being flow-independent. Thus, areas without thallium uptake in early rest image that fill-in in the redistribution phase represent hibernating myocardium, whereas fixed defects represent scars. Several protocols have been proposed with thallium-201, the most frequently used being rest-redistribution and stress-redistribution-reinjection. The former assesses myocardial viability alone and the latter assesses myocardial ischaemia and viability, being the recommended SPECT imaging modality. Both protocols have high Sn for predicting regional function recovery after revascularization (86%), but a relatively low Sp (50%) [38].

Myocardial uptake and retention of technetium-99m sestamibi/tetrofosmin is dependent on regional perfusion and requires mitochondrial membrane integrity, thus reflecting myocardial viability. Technetium-SPECT has also high Sn (79%) but a relatively low Sp (58%) for the prediction of post-revascularization improvement of regional ventricular function [38]. Nitrates administration increases antegrade and collateral blood flow to areas of reduced resting perfusion and therefore improves tracer delivery (either thallium or sestamibi) to viable regions of the myocardium. So, nitrate-enhanced rest perfusion imaging and gated SPECT has higher accuracy for detection of myocardial viability.

SPECT, either with thallium or technetium tracers, is more sensitive for detecting recoverable myocardium than DSE. Effectively, Baumgartner and co-workers [43] showed that the minimum critical mass of viable myocardium needed for the detection by DSE is higher than that required by thallium-SPECT or FDG–PET. By histological examination of 12 hearts of patients with CAD and severely reduced ventricular function referred for cardiac transplantation and previously submitted to the various imaging procedures, it was found that segments with <25% viable myocytes showed echocardiographic evidence of viability in only 19% of cases, compared with 33% for fluorodeoxyglucose-PET and 38% for thallium-SPECT. However, DSE is more specific for predicting functional improvement after revascularization since the small amounts of viable tissue additionally recognized by nuclear modalities are frequently unable to contribute to regional function recovery.

Finally, the integrated biological risk–benefit balance of the examination method should be taken into account whenever SPECT is considered. Current protection standards and practices are based on the premise that ionizing radiation can result in serious detrimental health effects. These include long-term development of cancer and genetic damage. At a patient level, the effective dose of a single nuclear stress imaging ranges from 10 to 27 mSv, which is equivalent to the exposure to 500 chest X-rays (sestamibi-SPECT) or 1,200 chest X-rays (thallium-SPECT). Since in practical terms SPECT and DSE accuracies are relatively similar, DSE should be preferred due to lower cost, wider availability, absence of environmental impact, and lack of biological effects justified by its radiation-free nature.

Positron emission tomography (PET)

PET allows the evaluation of myocardial viability by qualitative and quantitative assessment of myocardial function, perfusion, and metabolism. The assessment of function identifies regions with contractile dysfunction, which potentially may be viable myocardium. For assessment of perfusion, several tracers are available, including N-13 ammonia, O-15 labelled water, and rubidium-82. For assessment of metabolism, F-18-fluorodeoxyglucose (FDG) is the most extensively used tracer due to the central role of glucose metabolism in myocardial ischaemic areas, particularly if given under conditions that encourage glucose metabolism, such as oral glucose load, nicotinic acid or insulin and glucose infusion. The viable tissue is metabolically active, having preserved or increased glucose consumption, whereas scarred tissue is metabolically inactive. FDG and ammonia studies have been combined to achieve the maximum accuracy for detection of viability. Normal tissue shows normal function, perfusion, and metabolism. Stunned myocardium shows diminished function but relatively normal perfusion and metabolism. HM can be identified by reduced perfusion with preserved or increased metabolism (metabolism–perfusion mismatch). Conversely, scar tissue has reduced function, perfusion, and metabolism (metabolism-perfusion match).

Several non-randomized retrospective studies showed that FDG-PET predicts recovery of regional function after revascularization with high Sn (71–100%) but a relatively low Sp (33–91%) [38]. PET systems have generally better Sn and spatial resolution than SPECT systems and provide more accurate attenuation correction. When compared to DSE, FDG-PET has higher Sn, identifying uptake of the tracer in 30 to 50% of presumably non-viable segments. However, the identification of islets of viable myocytes in segments without contractile reserve does not necessarily result in regional recovery, explaining why Sp of FDG-PET is lower than DSE. Furthermore, since PET demands significant exposure to radiation without relevant additional benefit, alternative imaging methods without biological adverse effects should be preferred.

Cardiovascular magnetic resonance (CMR)

CMR is a rapidly emerging non-invasive imaging technique, providing information on cardiac anatomy, function, and perfusion with excellent spatial resolution in any desired plane and without radiation. CMR consists of several techniques that can be performed separately or in various combinations during a patient examination. The two most important CMR techniques to assess myocardial viability are delayed enhancement CMR (DE-CMR) and dobutamine-CMR.

DE-CMR is a newly established technique to detect areas of acute or chronic infarct, which manifests as bright regions in inversion recovery images acquired 5–20 min after the intravenous administration of an extracellular gadolinium-based contrast agent. In the setting of AMI, the contrast agent passively diffuses into the intracellular space due to the loss of membrane integrity of necrotic cells, resulting in an increased tissue level contrast concentration and therefore for hyper-enhancement of the affected areas. In chronic infarcts, the increased interstitial space between collagen fibres and the delayed washout due to reduced capillary density accounts for contrast enhancement in the scar tissue. So, in chronic CAD, hyper-enhanced areas correspond to fibrotic tissue within the myocardial wall, often referred to as transmural extent of infarction (TEI). Conversely, viable myocardium, either stunned or hibernating, has a normal distribution volume of the contrast medium and so retention of contrast does not occur. Due to its superior special resolution, DE-CMR has the unique ability to assess small volumes of irreversibly injured myocardium, as low as 2 g, and to measure the transmural extent of myocardial infarction.

DE-CMR has been extensively validated in animal models of ischaemic injury, as well as in a variety of patient cohorts. Clinical studies demonstrated that DE-CMR is effective in identifying the presence, location, and transmural extent of myocardial scarring, and a strong correlation has been found between DE-CMR, thallium-SPECT, and FDG-PET. Moreover, the TEI on a segmental basis is useful for the prediction of improvement in contractile function after revascularization in CAD patients. Regional wall motion improvement can be expected in dysfunctional segments with <50% TEI, with the chance of functional improvement lower in those segments with higher TEI. Besides, unlike stress tests (either DSE or dobutamine CMR), which appear to have reduced accuracy if more severe dysfunction is present, DE-CMR seems to have greater accuracy in those segments with the most severe dysfunction. Historical studies suggest that DE-CMR may have higher Sn (≈90%) but lower Sp (≈50%), which is mainly due to the variable functional recovery in myocardial segments with 25–75% hyper-enhancement. Importantly, the cut-off value of TEI used, directly influences the technique's accuracy. As the cut-off value for TEI increases, the sensitivity for predicting recovery falls but specificity rises. For example, >75% TEI has a 100% negative predictive value for functional recovery after revascularization [44]. However, in patients with <75% TEI, the additional assessment of contractile reserve by Db-CMR improves predictive accuracy over LGE imaging alone [45].

Dobutamine-CMR assesses contractile reserve during low dose dobutamine stress testing. Similar to echocardiography, CMR allows visualization of regional wall motion and systolic wall thickening but is characterized by superior endocardial border definition. Regional function is qualitatively assessed as normal, hypokinetic, akinetic, or dyskinetic. The improvement of contractile function during low-dose dobutamine stress is indicative of myocardial viability. The majority of studies suggest that dobutamine-CMR has a relatively modest Sn but high Sp for prediction of regional recovery after revascularization, ranging from 50 to 90% and 73 to 94%, respectively.

The diagnostic performance of dobutamine-CMR is comparable to DSE and superior in patients with poor acoustic windows. Moreover, DE-CMR appears to have a greater accuracy than dobutamine-CMR, even in segments with severe dysfunction, does not require pharmacological test, is technically easier, as well as less observer-dependent for interpretation. Thus, DE-CMR will probably become the routine procedure for CMR assessment of myocardial viability. However, in those patients with multiple segments having intermediate transmurality (25–75%), complementary use of DE-CMR and dobutamine-CMR may be the optimal CMR strategy for predicting post-revascularization functional recovery.

When compared with DSE, disadvantages of CMR (either DE-CMR or dobutamine-CMR) include higher costs, lower availability, need for multiple breath-holding sequences during acquisition, lower temporal resolution, poor images with irregular rhythms, and is unemployable in patients with implanted metallic devices. However, due to the absence of ionizing radiation, CMR is an excellent option when stress echocardiography is inconclusive or not feasible.

Multi-slice computed tomography (MSCT)

Advances in multi-detector computed tomography, particularly with the introduction of ECG-gated multi-slice spiral computed tomography (MSCT) have radically changed the role of computed tomography in cardiac imaging. MSCT assessment of myocardial morphology, myocardial perfusion imaging, and delayed myocardial contrast enhancement were introduced, with the latter evolving as the key concept of MSCT viability imaging.

On delayed enhanced MSCT, myocardial infarction shows increased attenuation values when compared with healthy myocardium, which is explained by a combination of delayed wash-in and wash-out contrast kinetics and an increased volume of distribution of the contrast in the expanded interstitial compartment of the fibrous scar.

Several studies in animals, as well as in patients, proved the reliability of enhanced MSCT to detect and characterize scar tissue. The majority of these clinical studies evaluated the accuracy of MSCT in detecting viable segments as identified by DSE, SPECT, or CMR, in patients with previous myocardial infarction (1–6 months). Chiou and co-workers [46] recently showed that increasing segmental extent of MSCT late-enhancement is associated with an increase in segments classified as non-viable by both SPECT and DSE, and that the concordance between MSCT and DSE reached 91.1% when the segmental extent was >75%.

Cardiac MSCT is a promising non-invasive imaging technique that offers a better spatial resolution than CMR. However, it is coupled with a relevant radiation exposure, which seriously limits its clinical application. Moreover, MSCT usefulness for predicting contractile function recovery after revascularization in patients with chronic CAD was never evaluated.

Is it important to demonstrate ischaemia beyond viability?

This issue was addressed in a recent review article on HM [14]. The authors concluded that demonstration of myocardial ischaemia is important only in those with mild–moderate CAD but in those with severe CAD, defined as >70% CAD in three major vessels with at least one occluded artery, myocardial viability assessment only is sufficient (see ⊃ Fig. 26.2). The premise for such a strategy is that LV dysfunction may occur due to cardiomyopathy or sub-endocardial infarction and CAD may be a bystander condition especially if it is mild-moderate. Hence, mere demonstration of myocardial viability may not translate into improved LV function after intervention for ischaemia. However, demonstration of significant ischaemia may translate into improvement of outcome after intervention.

Future perspectives

Molecular imaging is a new and promising area of research. It aims to develop techniques applicable to echocardiography, CT or CMR, enabling the assessment of physiological and metabolic processes with these diagnostic modalities. In a simplistic view, molecular imaging will enable the study of physiological processes that are currently assessed only by PET/SPECT, without the drawbacks of the nuclear techniques and with higher spatial resolution. As an example, ligands or antibodies can be attached to the surface of contrast echocardiography microbubbles, resulting in their binding to specific epitopes up-regulated on the endothelial surface.

Molecular imaging is still predominantly in the preclinical research phase. Recent studies in animal models have presented particularly promising results for ultrasound detection of arteriogenesis (desintegrins conjugated with microbubbles), severity and extent of post-ischaemic inflammation (phosphatidylserine incorporated into microbubbles), or remote ischaemic areas (P-selectins attached to microbubbles) [47].

Integrated imaging in clinical practice

DSE, SPECT, DE-CMR, dobutamine-CMR, and MCE proved useful for detecting myocardial viability and predicting overall LV function recovery, HF symptom reduction, and clinical outcome improvement in retrospective non-randomized studies. The absence of randomized clinical trials for head-to-head comparison of those imaging modalities limits the choice of the optimal diagnostic strategy and one should exercise some care in their application to patient management. Nonetheless, considering diagnostic accuracy, availability, and risk of adverse effects, a pragmatic approach may be proposed—see ⊃ Table 26.2 and ⊃ Fig. 26.10.

The assessment of myocardial viability should start with a resting echocardiographic study, evaluating the wall thickening in all segments, severity of wall motion abnormalities, and LVEF. In those patients with sub-optimal acoustic windows, ultrasound

Table 26.2 Criteria indicating low probability of improvement with revascularization in patients with global LV dysfunction and multi-vessel disease

≥4 major criteria
3 major plus 1 minor
2 major plus 2 minor
Major Criteria
LV wall thickness ≤5 to 6 mm
No response to low-dose DSE
SPECT negative for viability
>50% of wall thickness hyper-enhancement in DE-CMR
PET negative for hibernating myocardium
No myocardial enhancement on MCE
Minor Criteria
LVEF ≤20%
LV volumes: 1 or more of the following:
By angiography: LVEDVI ≥200 ml/m² and/or LVESVI ≥120 ml/m²
By echocardiography: LVEDVI ≥170 ml/m² and/or LVESVI ≥90 ml/m²
Echocardiographic dimension: LVEDDI ≥5.5 cm²/m²

Adapted from [48].
LVEDVI, left ventricle end-diastolic volume/index; LVEDDI, left ventricle end-diastolic dimension/index; LVESVI, left ventricle end-systolic volume/index.

contrast should be given in order to improve endocardial border delineation and thus allow assessment of regional and global systolic function. Very severe LV dysfunction at rest (e.g. EF <20%) reduces the predictive accuracy of DSE, since the contractile response to dobutamine may be absent despite preserved myocardial viability. Thus, in patients with preserved or minimally reduced LV wall thickness and with severe LV dysfunction at rest, assessment of resting myocardial perfusion by MCE is recommended.

In patients with inadequate acoustic windows despite use of contrast, alternative imaging modalities such as SPECT, PET, and DE-CMR should be employed. DE-CMR may be a preferred alternative due to its radiation-free nature and good diagnostic accuracy. In those patients with multiple segments having intermediate TEI (25–75%), complementary use of DE-CMR and dobutamine-CMR may be relevant. MCE may also be a reasonable alternative

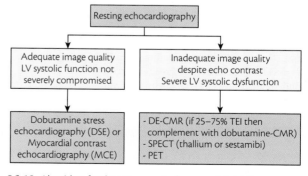

Fig. 26.10 Algorithm for the assessment of myocardial viability.

but larger outcome data are required. SPECT is a well-established modality, readily available, and with proven usefulness. However, it entails significant exposure to radiation, which can result in detrimental health effects. Thus, it is likely that the growth of MRI and MCE in the coming years may make them the preferred diagnostic modalities for patients who cannot be adequately assessed by DSE. The choice of diagnostic modality will, to a great extent, depend on the expertise of the medical centre.

References

1. Melo LG, Pachori AS, Kong D, et al. Molecular and cell-based therapies for protection, rescue, and repair of ischaemic myocardium: reasons for cautious optimism. *Circulation* 2004; 109(20): 2386–93.
2. Bax JJ, van der Wall EE, Harbinson M. Radionuclide techniques for the assessment of myocardial viability and hibernation. *Heart* 2004; 90(Suppl 5): v26–33.
3. Cleland JG, Pennell DJ, Ray SG, et al. Myocardial viability as a determinant of the ejection fraction response to carvedilol in patients with heart failure (CHRISTMAS trial): randomized controlled trial. *Lancet* 2003; 362(9377): 14–21.
4. Velazquez EJ, Lee KL, Deja MA, et al. Coronary-artery bypass surgery in patients with left ventricular dysfunction. *New Engl J Med* 2011; 364(17): 1607–16.
5. Bonow RO, Maurer G, Lee KL, et al. Myocardial viability and survival in ischaemic left ventricular dysfunction. *New Engl J Med* 2011; 364(17): 1617–25.
6. Dispersyn GD, Borgers M, Flameng W. Apoptosis in chronic hibernating myocardium: sleeping to death? *Cardiovasc Res* 2000; 45(3): 696–703.
7. Bax JJ, Visser FC, Poldermans D, et al. Time course of functional recovery of stunned and hibernating segments after surgical revascularization. *Circulation* 2001; 104(12 Suppl 1): I314–318.
8. Beanlands RS, Hendry PJ, Masters RG, deKemp RA, Woodend K, Ruddy TD. Delay in revascularization is associated with increased mortality rate in patients with severe left ventricular dysfunction and viable myocardium on fluorine 18-fluorodeoxyglucose positron emission tomography imaging. *Circulation* 1998; 98(19 Suppl): II51–56.
9. Senior R, Lahiri A. Dobutamine echocardiography predicts functional outcome after revascularization in patients with dysfunctional myocardium irrespective of the perfusion pattern on resting thallium-201 imaging. *Heart* 1999; 82(6): 668–73.
10. Allman KC, Shaw LJ, Hachamovitch R, Udelson JE. Myocardial viability testing and impact of revascularization on prognosis in patients with coronary artery disease and left ventricular dysfunction: a meta-analysis. *J Am Coll Cardiol* 2002; 39(7): 1151–58.
11. Lytle BW. The role of coronary revascularization in the treatment of ischaemic cardiomyopathy. *Ann Thorac Surg* 2003; 75(6 Suppl): S2–5.
12. Krishnamani R, El-Zaru M, DeNofrio D. Contemporary medical, surgical, and device therapies for end-stage heart failure. *Current Treatment Options in Cardiovascular Medicine* 2003; 5(6): 487–99.
13. Wijns W, Kolh P, Danchin N, et al. Guidelines on myocardial revascularization. *Eur Heart J* 2010; 31(20): 2501–55.
14. Shah BN, Khattar RS, Senior R. The hibernating myocardium: current concepts, diagnostic dilemmas, and clinical challenges in the post-STICH era. *Eur Heart J* 2013; in press.
15. Penicka M, Tousek P, De Bruyne B, et al. Myocardial positive pre-ejection velocity accurately detects presence of viable myocardium, predicts recovery of left ventricular function and bears a prognostic value after surgical revascularization. *Eur Heart J* 2007; 28(11): 1366–73.
16. Becker M, Lenzen A, Ocklenburg C, et al. Myocardial deformation imaging based on ultrasonic pixel tracking to identify reversible myocardial dysfunction. *J Am Coll Cardiol* 2008; 51(15): 1473–81.
17. Kaul S, Jayaweera AR. Coronary and myocardial blood volumes: noninvasive tools to assess the coronary microcirculation? *Circulation* 1997; 96(3): 719–24.
18. Linka AZ, Sklenar J, Wei K, Jayaweera AR, Skyba DM, Kaul S. Assessment of transmural distribution of myocardial perfusion with contrast echocardiography. *Circulation* 1998; 98(18): 1912–20.
19. Wei K, Jayaweera AR, Firoozan S, Linka A, Skyba DM, Kaul S. Basis for detection of stenosis using venous administration of microbubbles during myocardial contrast echocardiography: bolus or continuous infusion? *J Am Coll Cardiol* 1998; 32(1): 252–60.
20. Wei K, Jayaweera AR, Firoozan S, Linka A, Skyba DM, Kaul S. Quantification of myocardial blood flow with ultrasound-induced destruction of microbubbles administered as a constant venous infusion. *Circulation* 1998; 97(5): 473–83.
21. Cobb FR, Bache RJ, Rivas F, Greenfield JC, Jr. Local effects of acute cellular injury on regional myocardial blood flow. *J Clin Invest* 1976; 57(5): 1359–68.
22. Kloner RA, Rude RE, Carlson N, Maroko PR, DeBoer LW, Braunwald E. Ultrastructural evidence of microvascular damage and myocardial cell injury after coronary artery occlusion: which comes first? *Circulation* 1980; 62(5): 945–52.
23. Shimoni S, Frangogiannis NG, Aggeli CJ, et al. Microvascular structural correlates of myocardial contrast echocardiography in patients with coronary artery disease and left ventricular dysfunction: implications for the assessment of myocardial hibernation. *Circulation* 2002; 106(8): 950–56.
24. Janardhanan R, Moon JC, Pennell DJ, Senior R. Myocardial contrast echocardiography accurately reflects transmurality of myocardial necrosis and predicts contractile reserve after acute myocardial infarction. *Am Heart J* 2005; 149(2): 355–62.
25. Coggins MP, Sklenar J, Le DE, Wei K, Lindner JR, Kaul S. Noninvasive prediction of ultimate infarct size at the time of acute coronary occlusion based on the extent and magnitude of collateral-derived myocardial blood flow. *Circulation* 2001; 104(20): 2471–77.
26. Swinburn JM, Lahiri A, Senior R. Intravenous myocardial contrast echocardiography predicts recovery of dysynergic myocardium early after acute myocardial infarction. *J Am Coll Cardiol* 2001; 38(1): 19–25.
27. Jeetley P, Swinburn J, Hickman M, Bellenger NG, Pennell DJ, Senior R. Myocardial contrast echocardiography predicts left ventricular remodelling after acute myocardial infarction. *J Am Soc Echocardiogr* 2004; 17(10): 1030–36.
28. Senior R, Swinburn JM. Incremental value of myocardial contrast echocardiography for the prediction of recovery of function in dobutamine nonresponsive myocardium early after acute myocardial infarction. *Am J Cardiol* 2003; 91(4): 397–402.
29. Hickman M, Janardhanan R, Dwivedi G, Burden L, Senior R. Clinical significance of perfusion techniques utilising different physiological mechanisms to detect myocardial viability: a comparative study with myocardial contrast echocardiography and single photon emission computed tomography. *Int J Cardiol* 2007; 114(1): 139–40.
30. Myers JH, Stirling MC, Choy M, Buda AJ, Gallagher KP. Direct measurement of inner and outer wall thickening dynamics with epicardial echocardiography. *Circulation* 1986; 74(1): 164–72.

31. Swinburn JM, Senior R. Real time contrast echocardiography—a new bedside technique to predict contractile reserve early after acute myocardial infarction. *Eur J Echocardiogr* 2002; 3(2): 95–99.

32. Main ML, Magalski A, Chee NK, Coen MM, Skolnick DG, Good TH. Full-motion pulse inversion power Doppler contrast echocardiography differentiates stunning from necrosis and predicts recovery of left ventricular function after acute myocardial infarction. *J Am Coll Cardiol* 2001; 38(5): 1390–94.

33. Dwivedi G, Janardhanan R, Hayat SA, Swinburn JM, Senior R. Prognostic value of myocardial viability detected by myocardial contrast echocardiography early after acute myocardial infarction. *J Am Coll Cardiol* 2007; 50(4): 327–34.

34. Shimoni S, Frangogiannis NG, Aggeli CJ, et al. Identification of hibernating myocardium with quantitative intravenous myocardial contrast echocardiography: comparison with dobutamine echocardiography and thallium-201 scintigraphy. *Circulation* 2003; 107(4): 538–44.

35. Hickman M, Chelliah R, Burden L, Senior R. Resting myocardial blood flow, coronary flow reserve, and contractile reserve in hibernating myocardium: implications for using resting myocardial contrast echocardiography vs. dobutamine echocardiography for the detection of hibernating myocardium. *Eur J Echocardiogr* 2010; 11(9): 756–62.

36. Chelliah RK, Hickman M, Kinsey C, Burden L, Senior R. Myocardial contrast echocardiography versus single photon emission computed tomography for assessment of hibernating myocardium in ischaemic cardiomyopathy: preliminary qualitative and quantitative results. *J Am Soc Echocardiogr* 2010; 23(8): 840–47.

37. Hummel JP, Lindner JR, Belcik JT, et al. Extent of myocardial viability predicts response to biventricular pacing in ischaemic cardiomyopathy. *Heart Rhythm* 2005; 2(11): 1211–17.

38. Rizzello V, Poldermans D, Bax JJ. Assessment of myocardial viability in chronic ischaemic heart disease: current status. *Q J Nucl Med Mol Imaging* 2005; 49(1): 81–96.

39. Cianfrocca C, Pelliccia F, Pasceri V et al. Strain rate analysis and levosimendan improve detection of myocardial viability by dobutamine echocardiography in patients with post-infarction left ventricular dysfunction: a pilot study. *J Am Soc Echocardiogr* 2008; 21(9): 1068–74.

40. Karagiannis SE, Feringa HH, Bax JJ, et al. Myocardial viability estimation during the recovery phase of stress echocardiography after acute beta-blocker administration. *Eur J Heart Fail* 2007; 9(4): 403–8.

41. Aggeli C, Giannopoulos G, Roussakis G, et al. Pre-ejection tissue-Doppler velocity changes during low dose dobutamine stress predict segmental myocardial viability. *Hellenic J Cardiol* 2007; 48(1): 23–29.

42. Hanekom L, Jenkins C, Jeffries L, et al. Incremental value of strain rate analysis as an adjunct to wall-motion scoring for assessment of myocardial viability by dobutamine echocardiography: a follow-up study after revascularization. *Circulation* 2005; 112(25): 3892–3900.

43. Baumgartner H, Porenta G, Lau YK, et al. Assessment of myocardial viability by dobutamine echocardiography, positron emission tomography and thallium-201 SPECT: correlation with histopathology in explanted hearts. *J Am Coll Cardiol* 1998; 32(6): 1701–8.

44. Kim RJ, Wu E, Rafael A, et al. The use of contrast-enhanced magnetic resonance imaging to identify reversible myocardial dysfunction. *N Engl J Med* 2000; 343(20): 1445–53.

45. Wellnhofer E, Olariu A, Klein C, et al. Magnetic resonance low-dose dobutamine test is superior to SCAR quantification for the prediction of functional recovery. *Circulation* 2004; 109(18): 2172–74.

46. Chiou KR, Liu CP, Peng NJ, et al. Identification and viability assessment of infarcted myocardium with late enhancement multidetector computed tomography: comparison with thallium single photon emission computed tomography and echocardiography. *Am Heart J* 2008; 155(4): 738–45.

47. Villanueva FS, Lu E, Bowry S, et al. Myocardial ischaemic memory imaging with molecular echocardiography. *Circulation* 2007; 115(3): 345–52.

48. Rahimtoola SH, Dilsizian V, Kramer CM, Marwick TH, Vanoverschelde JL. Chronic ischaemic left ventricular dysfunction: from pathophysiology to imaging and its integration into clinical practice. *JACC Cardiovasc Imaging* 2008; 1(4): 536–55.

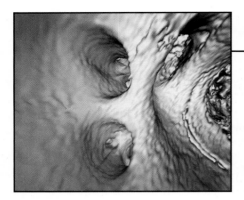

CHAPTER 27

Nuclear imaging and multi-detector computed tomography to assess viability

Pasquale Perrone-Filardi and Bernhard L. Gerber

Contents

Introduction

The concept of '*myocardial viability*' was established in the early 1970s when several clinical studies reported the observation that areas of dysfunctional myocardium at rest partially or completely recovered contraction following coronary revascularization. These observations led to the innovative conclusion that lack of contraction of the myocardium does not necessarily indicate irreversible myocyte damage due to myocardial necrosis but may be a reversible phenomenon exhibiting recovery of function upon revascularization. This new pathophysiological condition was conceptualized later on by Rahimtoola and termed *hibernating myocardium* [1]. Almost in parallel with the recognition of hibernation, the identification of *stunned myocardium,* a distinct pathophysiological phenomenon leading to transient and spontaneously reversible regional contractile dysfunction immediately following an acute ischaemic insult, was also gaining growing clinical relevance as it was repeatedly demonstrated in several clinical conditions spanning from chronic stable coronary artery disease to acute coronary syndromes [2]. Thus, the three distinct pathophysiological conditions listed in ⮩ Table 27.1 are possibly responsible for LV dysfunction in patients with ischaemic cardiomyopathy. For clinical purposes the concept of *viable myocardium* refers to the potential recovery of regional myocardial contractile function at rest independently on its pathophysiological substrate. Although useful and simple for clinicians, the introduction of such a broad clinical definition of viability reflects the difficulty of characterizing the substrate of regional contractile dysfunction in humans, which is very rarely sustained by a unique condition but is more often the sum of admixture of viable dysfunctional (either stunning or hibernating), necrotic, and normal myocardium. The original concept of hibernation has also been challenged in several aspects since the evidence of reduced blood flow yielded conflicting results in human studies [3], and the possibility that the phenomenon could also be due to repetitive episodes of stunning due to reduced coronary flow reserve has been postulated. In addition, the postulate of preserved, albeit transient, contractile reserve despite reduced blood flow has also been questioned, as it was demonstrated that contractile reserve is abolished in metabolically viable myocardium where coronary reserve is severely reduced or absent [4], which explains the reduced sensitivity for predicting functional recovery of techniques that evaluate contractile reserve in dysfunctional myocardium supplied by occluded coronary vessels [5]. Finally, more recent histopathologic studies have demonstrated progressive ultrastructural changes in hibernating myocardium characterized by

Table 27.1 Pathophysiology of left ventricular regional contractile dysfunction

Condition	Resting Perfusion	Metabolic Activity	Contractile Reserve	Recovery
Stunning	Normal	Enhanced	++	++
Hibernation	Reduced	Enhanced	+/−	+/−
Scar	Reduced	Absent	—	—

an embryonic phenotype and apoptotic damage [6], challenging the concept of a long-term smart adaptation to chronic hypoperfusion and emphasizing the need for prompt revascularization to prevent irreversible impairment of the contractile machinery and obtain recovery of function. Experimental data further challenged the benign conception of hibernation demonstrating a propensity for fatal arrhythmias in animals with pure hibernation, despite lack of necrosis, providing a potential explanation for the negative prognosis of patients with evidence of viable myocardium undergoing medical therapy [7].

Clinical outcomes and the 'gold standard' of viability

From a histopathologic and pathophysiological point of view, myocardial viability is the *absence of myocardial necrosis*; however, from a clinical point of view, and when assessing the value of tests for identification of myocardial viability, several targets for assessing myocardial viability may be considered (⊃ Table 27.2).

Traditionally, the concept of viability refers to the identification *of reversible regional dysfunction* after revascularization, and all techniques so far evaluated for the identification of viable myocardium in humans have been tested against this end-point. Besides improving function, other outcomes for defining benefit from therapy can be evaluated. Revascularization of viable myocardium may also have a significant favourable effect on left ventricular volumes and thus remodelling, even without improving, ejection fraction. Increased LV end-diastolic and, in particular, end-systolic volumes are powerful predictors of mortality in patients with LV dysfunction, which are independent of EF [8]. Yet this end-point has never been adopted to test the accuracy of techniques assessing viability, although extent of viable myocardium directly correlates with the degree of LV remodelling and can predict reverse LV remodelling, i.e. reduction of end-systolic and end-diastolic LV volumes, after revascularization [9]. Also, in

Table 27.2 Favourable effects of revascularization of viable myocardium

- ◆ Recovery of resting ejection fraction
- ◆ Recovery of diastolic function
- ◆ Prevention of inducible ischaemia
- ◆ Prevention/stabilization of adverse remodelling
- ◆ Prevention of ventricular arrhythmias

patients with severe LV dysfunction undergoing resynchronization therapy, it has been reported that 6-months' reduction of LV end-systolic volumes predicts short-term survival improvement, suggesting that changes in LV volumes could represent a valuable surrogate end-point to predict the effects of therapies on prognosis. Interestingly, similar data are not available for EF at rest. From the patients' point of view, another important parameter to consider might be improvement of functional status and, in particular, of heart failure symptoms. This parameter can be assessed either subjectively (NYHA class) or objectively (maximal VO2 or 6 minutes' walking test), but has only very infrequently been evaluated.

A final important endpoint is improvement of survival. Although it would be intuitive to suspect that the beneficial effects of revascularization on LV ejection fraction (EF) and reverse remodelling might translate into improved outcomes in patients with depressed LV function [10], the benefit of revascularization in the setting of myocardial viability on survival remains debated. Indeed, in chronic ischaemic heart disease, three prospective randomized trials, the PET and recovery following revascularization (PARR-2) trial [11], the heart failure revascularization (HEART) trial [12], and, most importantly, the surgical treatment for ischaemic heart failure (STICH) trial [13], failed to demonstrate a clear survival benefit of revascularization in the setting of viable myocardium over optimal medical treatment alone. Yet because each of these trials had significant methodological limitations, considerable debate remains as to how these results should be interpreted [14, 15]. Also, these data conflict with meta-analysis pooling data from single-centre retrospective studies (⊃ Figs 27.1 and 27.2) [16], which suggested that the presence of viable myocardium represents an independent unfavourable determinant of survival in patients with ischaemic LV dysfunction. In fact, it may be questioned whether the randomized survival trials may have failed to adequately address the issue of survival benefit in viable myocardium by presenting a strong selection bias. Also,

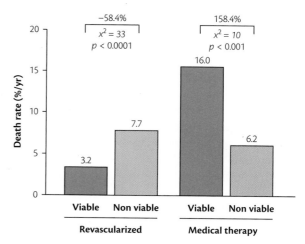

Fig. 27.1 Death rates for patients with ischaemic LV dysfunction undergoing medial therapy or revascularization, subgrouped according to the presence of viable or non-viable myocardium. Revascularization of patients with viability is associated with a 79% yearly difference in mortality.
Source data from Perrone-Filardi P, Pinto FJ. Looking for myocardial viability after a STICH trial: not enough to close the door. *J Nucl Med* 2012; 53:349–52.

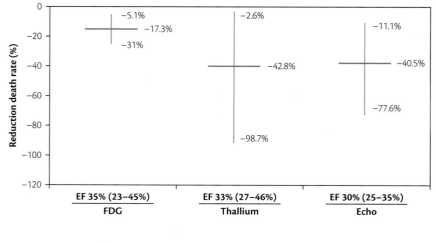

Fig. 27.2 Decrease in mortality in patients with ischaemic LV dysfunction undergoing revascularization and with evidence of viability evaluated by PET FDG, Tl SPECT, or dobutamine echocardiography. Data shown as mean value with 95% confidence limits. No measurable difference in test performance was observed.
Source data from Perrone-Filardi P, Pinto FJ. Looking for myocardial viability after a STICH trial: not enough to close the door. *J Nucl Med* 2012; 53:349–52.

there remains the question of the magnitude of myocardial viability needed to obtain benefit. MRI data suggest [17] that even small areas of viable myocardium, although not large enough to impact global LV function, may represent territories of electrical instability potentially accounting for the development of malignant arrhythmias. Presence of intra-myocardial scarring has clearly been demonstrated to be a remarkably powerful predictor of events, superior to ejection fraction alone, also in the setting of acute myocardial infarction, and in non-ischaemic dilated and hypertrophic cardiomyopathies, as well as in valvular heart disease.

Therefore, evaluation of myocardial viability by cardiac imaging, despite the somewhat deceiving results on survival, still plays an important role in the post-STICH era. It enables the clinician to predict the potential benefit vs. risk of revascularization in individual patients with ischaemic left ventricular (LV) dysfunction. It may also be used to guide response to treatments other than revascularization. In particular, several studies demonstrated that CRT response is directly affected by the amount of myocardial viability, and, in particular, scar tissue in the posterolateral wall predicts absence of CRT response [18]. Finally, infarct imaging and viability testing allows the clinician to understand the underlying nature of the cardiac dysfunction; for instance, to identify post-myocardial stunning or to diagnose stress cardiomyopathy (Takutsubo) or conditions such as myocarditis, dilated cardiomyopathy from acute or chronic coronary infarction, and therefore to adequately treat the underlying condition of LV dysfunction in patients. Therefore, even in the post-STICH area, viability testing remains clinically very important and continues to be largely requested for diagnostic purposes, for prognostication and treatment selection of patients with LV dysfunction.

Imaging techniques to assess viability

⮞ Table 27.3 summarizes currently available imaging techniques for evaluating non-invasive myocardial viability in patients with ischaemic cardiomyopathy. As it appears from the grouping of different modalities, there are three distinct pathophysiological approaches to distinguish viable from non-viable dysfunctional myocardium. One is represented by the demonstration of

Table 27.3 Current non-invasive techniques for assessing myocardial viability

Assessment of perfusion and metabolism
◆ Positron emission tomography
◆ Single-photon emission computed tomography
◆ Contrast echocardiography
Assessment of systolic function and contractile reserve
◆ Dobutamine echocardiography
◆ Dobutamine magnetic resonance imaging
◆ Dobutamine gated single-photon emission computer tomography
◆ Doppler tissue imaging
Imaging of necrotic myocardium
◆ Magnetic resonance delayed enhancement imaging
◆ Multi-slice computed tomography delayed enhancement imaging

membrane cell and mitochondrial integrity within areas of dysfunction. Nuclear techniques, including PET and SPECT, are used for this purpose, since uptake of perfusion and metabolic nuclear tracers indicate presence of viable myocytes. The second approach relies on the documentation of contractile reserve within areas of dysfunction and is based on the imaging of dysfunctional myocardium using echocardiography or MRI during stimulation with dobutamine, an inotropic synthetic agent. Finally, the third approach is more recent and relies on the direct documentation of necrotic myocardium by MRI and, more recently, by MDCT. As is evident from ⮞ Table 27.3, it has to be noted that, due to recent technical progress, each imaging technique has the potential to assess more than one aspect of viability, on a regional as well as global basis, during the same study. In addition, comparison between different techniques has been made more reliable by the recommended use of a standard segmentation of the left ventricle (⮞ Fig. 27.3) [19].

PET and SPECT represent the most used nuclear techniques for viability assessment, both relying on the documentation of cell integrity using metabolic or perfusion tracers, or their combination. Commonly used perfusion and metabolic tracers are listed in ⮞ Table 27.4 and their mechanism of action is reported in ⮞ Fig. 27.4.

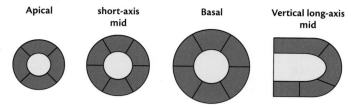

Fig. 27.3 Segmentation of the left ventricle for cardiac imaging analysis recommended by the principal cardiac and nuclear medicine associations. The left ventricle is divided in 17 myocardial segments derived from three short-axis planes (basal, mid-ventricular, and apical) with an additional apical segment from either long-horizontal or long-vertical axis.
Reprinted with permission. *Circulation* 2002;105:539–542, Copyright 2002 American Heart Association, Inc.

Table 27.4 Perfusion and metabolic radionuclide tracers employed for clinical use

- ◆ **SPECT perfusion tracers**
  - [201]thallium
  - [99m]technetium sestamibi
  - [99m]technetium tetrofosmin
- ◆ **PET perfusion tracers**
  - ^{15}O-water
  - ^{13}N-ammonia
  - [82]Rb-rubidium
- ◆ **PET metabolic tracers**
  - ^{18}F-fluorodeoxyglucose (glucose metabolism)
  - ^{11}C-acetate (oxygen metabolism)
  - ^{11}C-palmitate (fatty acids metabolism)

PET

PET has not only been a valuable technique for clinical detection of myocardial viability. By allowing to quantitatively measure physiological parameters, such as absolute myocardial perfusion (using ^{13}N-ammonia and ^{15}O-water), oxidative (using ^{11}C-acetate) and glucose metabolism (using [18]Fluoro-deoxyglucose) (FDG) in dysfunctional myocardium, the technique has also provided important insights into the pathophysiology of dysfunctional hibernating myocardium [20, 21].

Insights into the pathophysiology of hibernating myocardium and principles of detection of viability by PET imaging

Quantitative measurements of myocardial blood flow, using ^{13}N-ammonia and ^{15}O-water PET, challenged the initial hypothesis that hibernating myocardium might result from a chronic state of resting myocardial hypoperfusion due to (sub)-occlusion of an epicardial coronary artery. In fact, both in patients with a pure

state of collateral-dependent dysfunctional hibernating myocardium without necrosis, and in infarcted dysfunctional myocardium recovering function after revascularization, measurements of absolute resting myocardial perfusion using PET were found to be normal or near normal [20]. This suggested that in order to avoid irreversible myocardial necrosis, resting perfusion in hibernating myocardium must be maintained close to normal. Measurements of maximal absolute myocardial blood flow reserve in dysfunctional myocardium using PET demonstrated reduced flow reserve, indicating a potential role for repeated stress-induced ischaemia and post-ischaemic stunning in the genesis of chronic myocardial hibernation [22]. Recently developed animal models mimicking human hibernation [7] have shed a new light on both the mechanisms and the temporal progression of reversible ischaemic dysfunction. These studies suggest that development of chronic myocardial hibernation is a progressive phenomenon. During the first weeks after the onset of dysfunction, endocardial blood

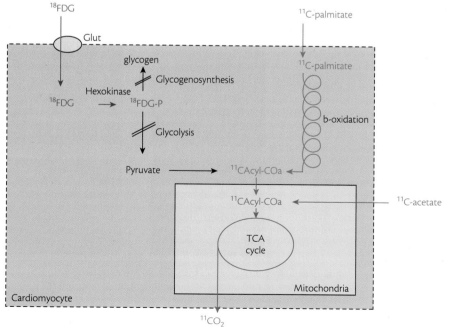

Fig. 27.4 Mechanism of action of different metabolic PET tracers.

flow must remain normal or only marginally decreased, otherwise myocardial necrosis will occur. At that point in time, repetitive episodes of myocardial stunning were suggested as being the most likely mechanism for inducing dysfunction, an hypothesis that is further supported by the strong relation existing between the reduction in sub-endocardial flow reserve and the severity of dysfunction. With time, and presumably also due to progression in the physiological significance of the underlying coronary stenosis, some of the dysfunctional segments, which appeared 'chronically stunned' on early examination, eventually develop morphological abnormalities, such as reduction of myocardial contractile proteins. It is currently believed that these alterations, which occur in the transition from repeated stunning to chronic hibernations, reduce metabolic demand of oxygen and myocardial perfusion [23]. It is noteworthy that the transition from chronic stunning to chronic hibernation only occurs for threshold reductions in myocardial flow reserve. The critical nature of coronary flow reserve reduction required to produce hibernating myocardium possibly explains why not all studies have demonstrated a progression to hibernating myocardium distal to a chronic stenosis.

Studies of myocardial glucose metabolism using FDG PET have also been important for our understanding of myocardial hibernation. The normal myocardium can use a variety of substrates for metabolism, depending on dietary conditions. Under fasting conditions, when plasma insulin and glucose levels are low, free fatty acids are the preferred substrates of the myocardium. In the fed state, when plasma glucose and insulin levels are high, glucose becomes the preferred substrate of the myocardium. Dysfunctional hibernating myocardium was found to have higher uptake rates of FDG than normal myocardium, especially under fasting conditions. Initially this was interpreted as indicating a shift from normal metabolism to anaerobic glycolysis in hibernating myocardium surviving under conditions of chronic low flow ischaemia. This view was, however, challenged by studies demonstrating maintained overall oxidative metabolism using ^{11}C-acetate in human hibernating myocardium, as well as by biopsies of human hibernating myocardium demonstrating increased rather than decreased glycogen storage. Experimental studies in animals demonstrated that the repeated aggression of ischaemia and reperfusion in the hibernating myocardium induces a series of changes in gene and protein expression. Among these are changes in membrane glucose transporters, with a shift from Glut 4 (insulin-dependent) to Glut 1 (insulin non-dependent) transport molecules. It is believed that this increase of Glut 1 transporters allows higher inflow of FDG under low insulin (fasting) conditions into the hibernating myocardium, compared to the normal myocardium, explaining the higher uptake of FDG in dysfunctional hibernating myocardium under fasting conditions [21].

Clinical assessment of myocardial viability using PET

The typical assessment of myocardial viability using PET relies on a combination of semiquantitative assessment of myocardial perfusion using an extractable perfusion tracer (either ^{13}N-ammonia or ^{82}Rubidium) and glucose extraction using FDG (⊃ Fig. 27.5). Diagnosis of myocardial viability is based on the comparison of

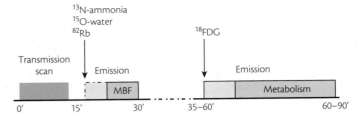

Fig. 27.5 Typical study protocol for ^{13}N-ammonia FDG PET viability study. First, a transmission scan is performed to allow correction of emission studies for attenuation. Myocardial perfusion is assessed using ^{13}N-ammonia. After decrease of radioactivity, glucose metabolism is assessed after injection of FDG. To allow better image quality, FDG imaging is best performed either during euglycaemic glucose clamp or after oral administration of nicotinic acid.

relative ^{13}N-ammonia and FDG uptake in the dysfunctional area relative to remote normally contracting myocardium. Three different ^{13}N-ammonia FDG patterns have been described in dysfunctional myocardium and related to recovery of myocardial function (⊃ Fig. 27.6):

1. Normal perfusion and FDG uptake. As discussed previously, the preservation of perfusion and glucose metabolism in dysfunctional myocardium is indicative of maintained myocyte viability.

2. Reduced perfusion with concomitant reduced or absence of FDG uptake (perfusion-metabolism match) pattern. Such severe reduction of perfusion and metabolism are incompatible with myocardial survival and are thus indicative of myocellular death and absence of viability.

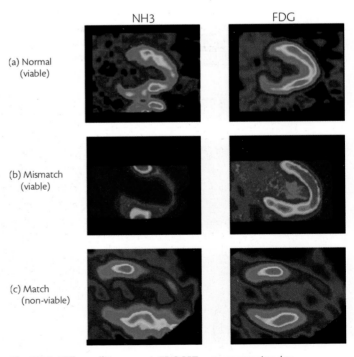

Fig. 27.6 Different ^{13}N-ammonia FDG PET patterns associated to dysfunctional myocardium. (a) Normal perfusion and metabolism. (b) Perfusion metabolism mismatch pattern, i.e. reduced ^{13}N-ammonia uptake and increased/maintained FDG uptake. (c) Perfusion metabolism match pattern, i.e. reduced ^{13}N-ammonia uptake and proportionally reduced FDG uptake.

3. Reduced perfusion with increased FDG uptake (perfusion-metabolism mismatch pattern). This pattern is observed mainly if studies are performed under post-prandial conditions or after glucose load, since under such conditions with high plasma insulin glucose uptake in normal myocardium is enhanced. As previously discussed, the increased FDG uptake translates to maintained metabolic viability and preferential use of glucose rather than free fatty acids as metabolic substrate in dysfunctional stunned and hibernating myocardium.

Initially, PET studies were performed either after overnight fasting conditions or after an oral glucose load. This approach resulted, however, in poor image quality in diabetic patients and in patients with insulin resistance. Therefore, it is currently proposed to perform studies during hyperinsulinaemic euglycaemic glucose clamp or after administration of nicotinic acid, which blocks lipid utilization by the heart. This approach improves image quality, but somewhat reduces the incidence and magnitude of mismatch pattern vs. normal FDG uptake in dysfunctional segments by the fact that normal myocardium also presents high FDG uptake during insulin stimulation.

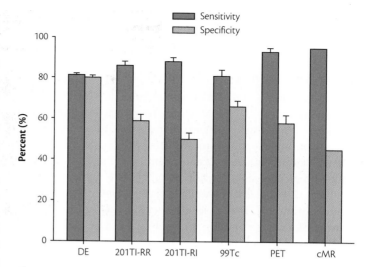

Fig. 27.7 Diagnostic accuracy of nuclear imaging techniques compared to dobutamine echocardiography and MRI. RI, reinjection.
Source data from Shen YT, Vatner SF. Mechanism of impaired myocardial function during progressive coronary stenosis in conscious pigs. *Circ Res* 1995; 76: 479–88.

Clinical value of ¹³N-ammonia FDG PET

Several studies have evaluated the diagnostic accuracy of ¹³N-ammonia FDG PET for predicting recovery of regional dysfunction after revascularization. According to a meta-analysis [24] for predicting recovery of regional dysfunction, combined information on perfusion and FDG uptake had a mean sensitivity of 88% and mean specificity of 74%, respectively (⊃ Table 27.5 and ⊃ Fig. 27.7). Recovery of global EF after revascularization is clinically more relevant than recovery of regional function but has been addressed in fewer studies. In a multi-centre study involving six European countries [25], sensitivity of PET during glucose clamp to predict significant (>5%) increase of EF was high (79%) but specificity was low (55%). Bax et al. [26] suggested that critical amounts of at least four dysfunctional segments with viability needs to be present to obtain a significant improvement of LV EF (>5%) after revascularization. Other studies indicated

a direct relationship between the number of dysfunctional viable segments by PET and the magnitude of recovery of EF after revascularization [27].

Several studies have examined the value of detection of viability by ¹³N-ammonia FDG PET for predicting prognosis in patients with poor LV function in relation to medical or surgical treatment. Pooled analysis of these studies [16] demonstrated improved survival for patients with dysfunctional viable myocardium undergoing revascularization rather than medical treatment (⊃ Fig. 27.2). The major limitation of these studies was, however, their observational retrospective non-randomized design. So far there is only one study [11] that in a randomized design assessed whether PET assisted management of patients with LV dysfunction affects outcome. Unfortunately, this study did not demonstrate a significant reduction in cardiac events in patients with LV dysfunction and suspected coronary disease for FDG PET-assisted management versus standard evaluation. This was probably related to the fact that revascularization management was not always dictated by PET findings. However, in the subgroup of patients managed according to PET findings, significant benefits were observed. Ongoing trials will allow assessment of the value of viability testing on survival in patients randomized to revascularization vs. medical treatment.

PET strengths and weaknesses

As opposed to other techniques, PET has significant strengths. Its major advantage is the ability to correct for attenuation of photons and to quantify perfusion and metabolism in absolute terms, making it an ideal tool to study the pathophysiology of dysfunctional myocardium. Also, as opposed to traditional nuclear imaging techniques, PET has higher image quality and higher spatial resolution not hampered by attenuation effects. Therefore, it has higher diagnostic accuracy than traditional nuclear imaging

Table 27.5 Accuracy of nuclear techniques to predict recovery of regional contractile function in patients with left ventricular dysfunction

Technique	Sensitivity (%)	Specificity (%)	PPA (%)	NPA (%)
Positron emission tomography				
◆ Mismatch	93	58	71	86
²⁰¹Thallium				
◆ Reinjection	86	50	57	83
◆ Rest-redistribution	88	59	69	80
⁹⁹Technetium sestamibi	81	66	71	77
Dobutamine echocardiography	81	80	77	85

techniques. The major limitation of PET is its higher cost relative to isotope production.

SPECT

201Thallium (Tl) imaging

Tl is a potassium analogue that was first used for the evaluation of viability with SPECT. It is actively transported by the Na+/K+ ATPase pump through an intact cell membrane of the myocardial cells and its initial uptake is mostly dependent on perfusion level, whereas late accumulation is dependent on cell integrity. At variance with more recent 99mtechnetium (Tc) tracers, uptake of Tl is not irreversible but is influenced by gradient concentration across the cell membrane. The consequence of this characteristic is that it greatly influences imaging protocols and the interpretation is that collected images always represent uptake at the time of image acquisition and not at the time of injection, as is the case for Tc agents. Therefore, areas of dysfunctional hypoperfused yet viable myocardium, where uptake of Tl is initially reduced compared to normally perfused myocardium, may show enhanced uptake at later imaging (usually at least 3 to 4 hours following initial administration) due to slow accumulation of Tl with partial or complete disappearance of the initial perfusion defect. This phenomenon, pertaining only to Tl, is termed *redistribution* and represents the basis for viability evaluation using this tracer. The two most used protocols to evaluate viability are represented by stress-redistribution-reinjection and rest-redistribution imaging.

Stress-redistribution-reinjection

With this protocol, images are acquired immediately after pharmacologic or physical stress and again after 3–4 hours. If in this last set of images, persistent fixed and severe defects are observed, a second dose of Tl is administered and a third set of images acquired immediately thereafter. This approach was developed from the observation that with fixed defects at 3–4 hours, redistribution may not necessarily represent necrotic myocardium, as they frequently show preserved metabolic activity by PET or residual contraction with potential for recovery of function following revascularization [28] (⮞ Fig. 27.8). The identification of viability using this protocol is based on the demonstration of significant redistribution (usually an increase of at least 10% from initial uptake) or on the presence of at least >50% of maximal tracer uptake in a dysfunctional segment.

Data from 11 studies enrolling 301 patients using this protocol reported high sensitivity (weighted mean 86%, range 33–100%) but reduced specificity (weighted mean 50%, range 16–80%) (⮞ Table 27.5 and ⮞ Fig. 27.7), indicating an overestimation of functional recovery in a substantial number of dysfunctional segments. Similarly, high sensitivity but suboptimal specificity has been reported when improvement of global EF was considered [24]. However, the advantage of this approach is that it takes into account also the presence of inducible ischaemia that is an additional determinant of prognosis representing a clinically relevant aspect for therapeutic management. As for PET, the prognostic independent role of this imaging approach has been reported in clinical studies [16] (⮞ Fig. 27.2).

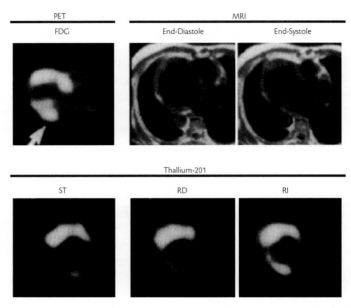

Fig. 27.8 Abnormal myocardial region (arrow) with reduced FDG activity by PET, normal end-diastolic wall thickness and presence of systolic thickening by MRI. SPECT images demonstrate a corresponding fixed defect on stress and redistribution images that improves after reinjection.
Reproduced from Beanlands RS, Ruddy TD, Dekemp RA, et al. Positron emission tomography and recovery following revascularization (PARR-1): the importance of scar and the development of a prediction rule for the degree of recovery of left ventricular function, *Journal of the American College of Cardiology*, 40:10, 2002, with permission from Elsevier.

Rest-redistribution

Using this approach Tl is injected at rest and images are acquired immediately thereafter and following 3–4 hours of redistribution. Therefore, inducible ischaemia is not evaluated. Viability is defined when a dysfunctional segment shows significant redistribution (>10% increase in Tl uptake) or a relative uptake >50% of maximal activity. With these criteria, mean sensitivity for prediction of regional functional recovery averaged 88% (range 44–100%) and mean specificity was 59% (range 22–92%) in a pooled analysis of 22 studies reporting 557 patients [24] (⮞ Table 27.5 and ⮞ Fig. 27.7). Acquiring a third late set of images 24 hours after injection to allow a prolonged redistribution time and fill-in of severely hypoperfused myocardium did not prove to be of incremental usefulness for predicting recovery of regional function [29]. The value of this protocol imaging to predict changes in global EF has been investigated in few clinical studies reporting high sensitivity but suboptimal specificity. The prognostic value of resting Tl imaging was tested in small clinical studies in which both the amount of viable myocardium and that of necrotic myocardium were identified to influence mortality and morbidity in patients with ischaemic LV dysfunction [16].

Tc-labelled agent

Two compounds, i.e. Tc-sestamibi and Tc-tetrafosmin, are currently used for clinical purposes, although only the former has been adequately tested for viability evaluation. At variance with Tl, Tc agents are trapped almost irreversibly in mitochondria after intravenous injection and flow-dependent distribution to myocardial cells, and they do not undergo a clinically significant redistribution process. Therefore, the images reflect the uptake of the tracer at the time of injection and not at the time of acquisition, as it is for Tl. When only viability needs to be evaluated, a single set of images is sufficient, usually obtained after sublingual nitrate administration to maximally enhance uptake in hypoperfused myocardium, whereas for a more comprehensive evaluation of viability and ischaemia, two set of images, and, therefore, two separate injections of the tracer, are needed: one during maximal physical or pharmacologic stress and a second one at rest or after nitrate administration. The criterion for defining viability is represented by a relative uptake >50% of maximal tracer activity in a dysfunctional segment. Pooled analysis of 13 studies using this approach and enrolling 308 patients reported average sensitivity of 79% (range 62–100%) and average specificity of 58% (range 30–86%), similar to other nuclear techniques using Tl [24] (⟳ Table 27.5 and ⟳ Fig. 27.7). Seven studies (reporting 180 patients) in whom tracer uptake was maximized with nitrate administration reported a sensitivity of 86% and increased specificity of 83% to predict regional functional improvement [24].

An additional relevant advantage, deriving from favourable physical properties of these agents, is represented by the opportunity to acquire ECG-gated images, which allow the evaluation of regional and global function, in particular regional wall thickening, end-systolic and end-diastolic volumes, and LV EF. Thus, gated Tc SPECT is also suitable for dobutamine studies assessing, at the same time, global and regional contractile reserve and perfusion reserve. The accuracy of this approach to predict recovery of global LV function has been only evaluated in a small, single-centre study reporting a promising 79% sensitivity and 78% specificity [24]. As for Tc-tetrofosmin, that was less investigated than Tc-sestamibi; available studies reported a good agreement between the two tracers with similar accuracy for prediction of functional recovery after revascularization [24].

MDCT

Principles of detection of myocardial viability by MDCT

Although it is possible to sometimes identify chronic myocardial infarcts on non-enhanced MDCT scans, as areas with regional thinning, hypo-enhancement (corresponding to replacement of myocardium by fatty tissue), or calcification [30], reliable identification of myocardial viability by MDCT requires contrast enhanced imaging. The ability of contrast enhanced computed tomography to detect myocardial infarction and thus myocardial viability was demonstrated in experimental animal models more than 30 years ago. However, the poor image quality of single-slice computed tomography without cardiac gating resulted in numerous artefacts and prohibited clinical use for *in vivo* cardiac imaging at that time and the technique was only recently matured to clinical use in humans with the advent of fast spiral MDCT imaging systems, which allows fast ECG-gated cardiac imaging without motion artefacts. The principles underlying detection of myocardial viability by MDCT resemble very closely those of MRI. As a matter of fact, although iodinated contrast agents employed for MDCT imaging have completely different molecular structure than gadolinium-DTPA based contrast agents employed for MRI, they have surprisingly very similar molecular weight and extravascular distribution volume. Therefore, they present similar kinetics in acutely and chronically infarcted myocardium as gadolinium-DTPA [31]. Thus contrast-enhanced MRI, characterizes myocardium by MDCT with different contrast enhancement patterns, depending on the time when imaging is performed with respect to contrast injection. On images performed immediately after contrast injection, the distribution of contrast agent in the myocardium reflects blood volume and myocardial perfusion [32]. Similar to Gd-contrast enhanced MR, such early imaging may reveal resting perfusion defects in acute myocardial infarcts. These areas, which typically are found in the sub-endocardial core of these acutely infarcted regions, correspond histologically to areas of microvascular obstruction (the no-reflow phenomenon). They represent, therefore, only a part of the total infarcted area. When infarcts become chronic, these areas of no-reflow disappear. They are thus a hallmark of acute infarcts.

Also similar to the behaviour of Gd-DTPA, on images performed at later time (5–10 minutes) after contrast injection, the iodinated contrast agent equilibrates between blood and the extravascular space. Late MDCT imaging will, similar to late gadolinium enhanced MRI, demonstrate higher relative signal intensity in areas where distribution volume of contrast in increased as compared to normal myocardium. In areas of acute myocardial infarction, this occurs because sarcolemmal membranes have been disrupted, allowing accessibility of contrast agent into intracellular space. In chronic infarcts this occurs because myocardium has been replaced by scar tissue (⟳ Fig. 27.9). Late enhancement

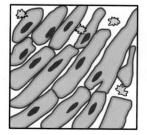

Normal myocardium

Extravascular volume ±20%

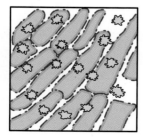

Acute infarct
Rupture of membranes

Extravascular volume ±100%

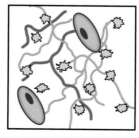

Chronic infarct
Fibrotic scar tissue

Extravascular volume 50–70%

Fig. 27.9 Principles underlying MDCT contrast enhancement on late imaging. Iodinated contrast agents (star) have extravascular distribution volume. At equilibrium, in normal myocardium the distribution volume is relatively small (approximately 20% of total cardiac volume). In acute myocardial infarct, due to rupture of cell membranes, distribution volume increases to almost the entire myocardial volume. In chronic infarcts, muscle is replaced by fibrous scar tissue. This tissue has large amounts of extravascular proteins, such as collagen and elastin, and low concentrations of cells. Therefore the distribution volume of the iodinated contrast agent is also increased.

is thus a non-specific hallmark of increased distribution volume of the contrast agent in myocardium, and may thus indicate acute, as well as chronic, infarcts or any process in which myocardium is replaced by areas of regional fibrosis, or deposition of extravascular proteins, such as amyloid. As for MRI, this late-enhancement occurs in disease-specific locations, i.e. ischaemic patterns of late-enhancement are typically sub-endocardial or transmural, while non-ischaemic patterns are more usually focal and mid-ventricular or sub-epicardial [33].

The major advantage of MDCT over other techniques is the ability to combine coronary imaging with viability imaging in a single comprehensive exam [34, 35]. Therefore, a typical imaging protocol for assessment of myocardial viability by MDCT will consist of imaging at least two time points (⊃ Fig. 27.10). Early images of the myocardium are typically obtained simultaneously with imaging of coronary arteries immediately after bolus injection of contrast. Acquisitions for coronary imaging and perfusion imaging can be performed using prospective gating to reduce radiation dose. Information on myocardial function can also be obtained at the same time point but requires retrospectively gated acquisition, with higher radiation burden. Late images are obtained by performing a second CT acquisition several minutes post-injection, either making use of the contrast injected from coronary imaging or with additional contrast given. According to experimental studies that evaluated the time course of MDCT enhancement in infarcts, late hyper-enhancement appears to be feasible at any time point between 4 and 24 minutes after contrast injection, but the optimal time varied between studies and appears to depend on the contrast agent. Typically, it is performed approximately 10 minutes post-contrast injection. Unlike contrast MR, MDCT has not the ability to null signal in normal myocardium through inversion recovery techniques. Therefore, distinction between infarcted and normal myocardium is less distinct. To enhance signal strength of late-enhancement, it is generally necessary to infuse a larger dose of contrast than required for coronary imaging alone (i.e. typical protocols used a total dose 120–140 cc). This dose can be given either as a larger bolus during coronary imaging or by giving an additional slow infusion of contrast after the coronary imaging acquisition. It is also possible to obtain late images making use of iodinated contrast media injected for other purposes. For instance, late MDCT infarct imaging can be performed immediately after angioplasty of acute infarcts, to reveal size of infarcted areas, using simply the contrast media injected in the haemodynamic laboratory [36]. To reduce radiation dose exposure and to increase contrast to noise, late imaging is typically performed with lower tube voltage (80–90 kV) and preferably with prospective ECG triggering. To maximize image contrast, images can be acquired with larger collimation, thicker slices, and softer reconstruction filters than coronary imaging.

Clinical results using MDCT

Several studies have compared infarct imaging by MDCT to histology and to gadolinium-enhanced MRI, both in experimental animal models and in humans. In animals [37] the location and size of early defects by MDCT were found to correlate closely to histological measurements of no-reflow area, while size of LE was found to correlate closely to areas of myocardial necrosis at histology. In humans the location and extent of contrast enhancement patterns by MDCT corresponded closely to those detected by contrast-enhanced MRI patterns (⊃ Fig. 27.11) and there is excellent correlation between measurements of infarct size by both modalities. Also moderate correlation between delayed MDCT and FDG PET imaging [38] has been reported. Several clinical studies demonstrated the ability of late MDCT imaging to predict functional recovery of post-ischaemic myocardium and LV remodelling after acute myocardial infarction [29, 39]. Also it was recently shown in a series of 102 patients with first acute MI, that viability imaging by MDCT immediately after successful PCI can predict risk of cardiac death or hospitalization for heart failure [40] (⊃ Fig. 27.13). So far no study has been performed to evaluate the value of MDCT to predict recovery of dysfunction in chronic contractile dysfunction. However, the technique combining coronary and LE MDCT imaging has been shown be useful to differentiate ischaemic vs. non-ischaemic aetiology of heart failure [41]. Indeed similar to MRI, MDCT may reveal atypical mid-ventricular or epicardial late-enhancement patterns in dilated cardiomyopathy, or other diseases, such as acute myocarditis, cardiac sarcoidosis, hypertrophic cardiomyopathy or Chagas disease, which may be useful to identify these entities.

MDCT strengths and weaknesses

MDCT has some unique advantages over other viability techniques: The most important advantage of the technique is that it

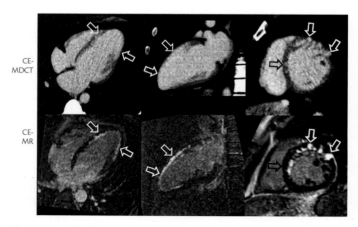

Fig. 27.11 Examples of late MDCT and corresponding ce MRI images in a patient with acute myocardial infarction 25 days earlier. ce, contrast enhanced. Bernhard L. Gerber et al, Characterization of acute and chronic myocardial infarcts by multidetector computed tomography: comparison with contrast-enhanced magnetic resonance, *Circulation*, 113:6, 823–33 with permission from Wolters Kluwer.

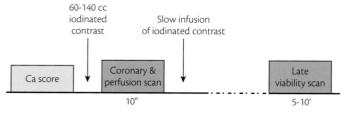

Fig. 27.10 Typical study protocols for assessment of myocardial viability by MDCT.

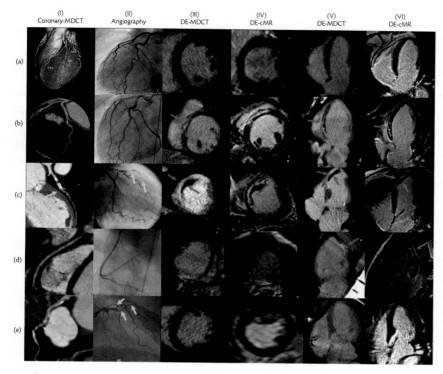

(I) Coronary-MDCT   (II) Angiography   (III) DE-MDCT   (IV) DE-cMR   (V) DE-MDCT   (VI) DE-cMR

(a)
(b)
(c)
(d)
(e)

Fig. 27.12 Example of combined coronary (panel I) and late MDCT (panels III and V) to differentiate aetiology of heart failure in five representative patients and their correlations to coronary anatomy (panel II) and LE-MRI (panels IV and VI). (a) No coronary artery disease and absence of LE. (b) No coronary artery disease and mid-ventricular LE. (c) Occlusion of the proximal left descending coronary artery (yellow arrow) with transmural LE in the apex, septum, and antero-septal region (red arrows) and mural thrombus (green arrows). (d) Absence of coronary artery disease with transmural inferior necrosis. (e) Proximal and mid left descending coronary artery and 1st diagonal stenosis (yellow arrows) without LE. LE: late enhancement. Reproduced from e Polain de Waroux JB et, Combined coronary and late-enhanced multidetector-computed tomography for delineation of the etiology of left ventricular dysfunction: comparison with coronary angiography and contrast-enhanced cardiac magnetic resonance imaging, *European Heart Journal*, 2008; 29:2544–51 by permission of Oxford University Press.

allows the combination of assessment of myocardial viability with non-invasive coronary (and eventually functional) imaging in a single test (Fig. 27.12 and Table 27.6). Also, viability assessment by MDCT can be performed in patients with devices contraindicating MRI (such as non-compatible pacemakers, CRT or ICD devices), and can be a valuable alternative to MRI in such patients. Additionally, viability assessment by MDCT is substantially faster (10 minutes) than by MRI (30 minutes), or by SPECT and PET (1–2 hours) and MDCT may be more available and less technically demanding than PET and MRI.

MDCT viability imaging has, however, also some significant limitations: The single most important limitation is that while the

quality of early images of MDCT is comparable to that of MRI with extremely high spatial resolution allowing visualization of discrete sub-endocardial perfusion defects, the quality of late images by MDCT remains inferior to that of contrast-enhanced MRI images. Differentiation of soft tissue contrast might be increased with dual-energy MDCT. An additional limitation is that LE MDCT imaging causes extra radiation dose exposure in addition to that related to non-invasive coronary imaging. There is concern whether MDCT-induced radiation exposure may contribute to increased lifelong risk of cancer [42]. The advent of a new generation of MDCT scanners with faster rotation times, higher number (128–320) of detector rows, and new acquisition protocols (reduction of tube voltage,

Table 27.6 Differentiation of different myocardial diseases by MDCT

Condition	Unenhanced Images	Early Contrast-enhanced Images				Late Contrast-enhanced Images
		Coronary Arteries	Myocardial Thickness	Myocardial Motion	Myocardial Perfusion	
Normal myocardium	Normal	Normal or non-occlusive stenosis	Normal	Normal	Normal	No DE
Acute Infarct (non-viable)	Normal	Occlusive stenosis if not reperfused	Normal	Focal akinesia	Sub-endocardial perfusion defects	Sub-endocardial or transmural DE
Chronic Infarct (non-viable)	Hypo-enhanced areas or calcification	Occlusive stenosis	Regional thinning	Regional akinesia	Normal	Sub-endocardial or transmural DE
Viable myocardium (chronic hibernating or acutely stunned)	Normal	Non-occlusive stenosis	Normal	Regional hypo or akinesia	Normal	No DE
Non-ischaemic cardiomyopathy	Normal	Normal	Diffuse thinning	Diffuse hypokinesia	No perfusion defect	No DE or sub-epicardial DE

Modified from [35].

prospective ECG gating acquisitions, or dual-source high-pitch acquisition) has, however, allowed significant reduction of radiation doses, and viability acquisition has been shown to be feasible with doses as low as 0.89 mSv for DE-MDCT alone or 2.3 mSv for a comprehensive protocol combining coronary imaging, functional, and viability imaging [43]. This radiation dose exposure is comparable or even lower than that of nuclear imaging techniques (SPECT and PET) used for viability imaging. Also, if concerns about radiation dose may certainly be appropriate in asymptomatic young patients undergoing MDCT for screening purposes, the risk of radiation-induced cancer is probably negligible when balanced to disease-related prognosis in patients with low EF (up to 50% mortality at 5 years) requiring viability testing. A more important limitation to the use of MDCT for viability, is probably the requirement to inject large doses of iodinated contrast agents to obtain adequate image quality, exposing these patients to the risk of aggravating renal function, especially given the high presence of comorbidities such as diabetes or pre-existing renal function impairment in such patients with heart failure.

PET-CT/SPECT-CT fusion and hybrid imaging

In recent years attempts have been made to combine nuclear and computed tomography (CT) imaging. Details on fusion and hybrid imaging are discussed in other chapters. Hybrid imaging allows registering information of coronary anatomy and regional contractile function obtained from CT with myocardial perfusion or metabolism by SPECT or PET (⊃ Fig. 27.13). Combining CT with SPECT imaging allows for a reliable CT-based attenuation correction of SPECT imaging, thereby minimizing attenuation artefacts. Because of their recent introduction, the value of these techniques for assessment of myocardial viability, as compared to conventional SPECT or PET imaging, has not yet extensively been studied, but in theory these approaches might be better suited to define the localization and size of the dysfunctional area with respect to the location of coronary obstruction.

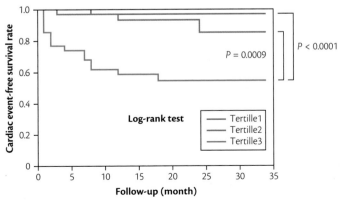

Fig. 27.13 Incidence of cardiac events (death or hospitalization for heart failure) defined by tertiles of myocardial contrast delayed enhancement (DE) size.
Reproduced from Sato, A, et al, Prognostic value of myocardial contrast delayed enhancement with 64-slice multidetector computed tomography after acute myocardial infarction, *Journal of American College of Cardiology*, 59:8 2012, with permission from Elsevier.

Which is the optimal test for assessment of myocardial viability? Comparison of techniques

Several studies have compared the diagnostic accuracy of SPECT and PET for detection of myocardial viability vs. other imaging techniques. Results have been summarized in a meta-analysis [23]. No significant differences between Tl and Tc SPECT tracers was reported, yet Tc tracers allow better image quality than Tl with reduced radiation exposure. PET appears to have higher sensitivity for detection of myocardial viability than SPECT, but similar suboptimal specificity. Pooled analysis suggests furthermore that nuclear imaging techniques (SPECT and PET) have higher sensitivity and negative predictive values, but lower specificity and positive predictive value than dobutamine echocardiography. More recently, LE MRI was found to have similar good diagnostic performance as PET and SPECT. The major advantage of MRI is higher spatial resolution, allowing differentiation of sub-endocardial vs. transmural scars. Furthermore, MRI benefits from greater availability, less cost, and faster imaging than PET, without radiation exposure. Therefore, MRI has challenged PET as the gold-standard for assessment of myocardial viability in clinical practice. However, in clinical practice, PET and MRI appear to perform similarly well for detection of myocardial viability.

As opposed to predicting functional outcome, for predicting improvement of survival, all imaging techniques, i.e. dobutamine echo, MRI, SPECT, and PET, appear to have similar high values (⊃ Fig. 27.2) [15]. However, only head to head comparisons of SPECT and dobutamine echocardiography, but not of other techniques, were reported for this purpose. Also, only one of the studies was performed in a prospective randomized design. Obviously, the decision about which test to choose for assessment of myocardial viability in an individual patient will depend on several factors. The decision must be individually targeted to the patient and will not only depend on diagnostic performance of the test, but also on patients' preferences, potential contraindications, availability, and local experience with different techniques, as well as with concomitant medical therapy and coronary anatomy [7].

Conclusions

Both SPECT and PET are established and well-validated techniques for assessment of myocardial viability. PET offers higher image quality and diagnostic accuracy than SPECT, but it is more costly and less available. MDCT viability imaging has recently been introduced and could be an interesting alternative to MRI or nuclear imaging. Hybrid SPECT/CT and PET/CT imaging offer new opportunities of integrating coronary anatomy and function with myocardial perfusion and metabolism in a single exam, and might improve the ability of nuclear imaging techniques to characterize the areas of dysfunction in chronic coronary artery disease. However, it is still too early to predict whether these appealing technical advances in cardiac imaging will translate into more accurate decision-making processes for individual patients. At this time no optimal imaging technique exists that can accurately describe the very complex pathophysiological substrate that often determines LV dysfunction and the potential for its reversibility. As a consequence, decisions about revascularization of patients with ischaemic LV dysfunction remains challenging in most cases, requiring integration of different imaging modalities with clinical and anatomic factors.

References

1. Rahimtoola SH. The hibernating myocardium. *Am Heart J* 1989; 117: 211–21.

2. Heyndrickx GR, Millard RW, McRitchie RJ, Maroko PR, Vatner SF. Regional myocardial functional and electrophysiological alterations after brief coronary artery occlusion in conscious dogs. *J Clin Invest* 1975; 56: 978–85.

3. Vanoverschelde JL, Wijns W, Borgers M, et al. Chronic myocardial hibernation in humans. From bedside to bench. *Circulation* 1997; 95: 1961–71.

4. Lee HH, Dávila-Román VG, Ludbrook PA, et al. Dependency of contractile reserve on myocardial blood flow. Implications for the assessment of myocardial viability with dobutamine stress echo. *Circulation* 1997; 96: 2884–91.

5. Piscione F, Perrone-Filardi P, De LG, et al. Low dose dobutamine echocardiography for predicting functional recovery after coronary revascularisation. *Heart* 2001; 86: 679–86.

6. Elsasser A, Schlepper M, Klovekorn WP, et al. Hibernating myocardium: an incomplete adaptation to ischaemia. *Circulation* 1997; 96: 2920–31.

7. Canty JM, Jr, Suzuki G, Banas MD, Verheyen F, Borgers M, Fallavollita JA. Hibernating myocardium: chronically adapted to ischaemia but vulnerable to sudden death. *Circ Res* 2004; 94: 1142–9.

8. White HD, Norris RM, Brown MA, Brandt PWT, Whitlock RML, Wild CJ. Left ventricular end-systolic volume as the major determinant of survival after recovery from myocardial infarction. *Circulation* 1987; 76: 44–51.

9. Carluccio E, Biagioli P, Alunni G, et al. Patients with hibernating myocardium show altered left ventricular volumes and shape, which revert after revascularization: evidence that dyssynergy might directly induce cardiac remodeling. *J Am Coll Cardiol* 2006; 47: 969–77.

10. Samady H, Elefteriades JA, Abbott BG, Mattera JA, McPherson CA, Wackers FJ. Failure to improve left ventricular function after coronary revascularization for ischaemic cardiomyopathy is not associated with worse outcome. *Circulation* 1999; 100: 1298–304.

11. Beanlands RS, Nichol G, Huszti E, et al. F-18-fluorodeoxyglucose positron emission tomography imaging-assisted management of patients with severe left ventricular dysfunction and suspected coronary disease: a randomized, controlled trial (PARR-2). *J Am Coll Cardiol* 2007; 50: 2002–12.

12. Cleland JG, Calvert M, Freemantle N, et al. The Heart Failure Revascularisation Trial (HEART). *Eur J Heart Fail* 2011; 13: 227–33.

13. Bonow RO, Maurer G, Lee KL, et al. Myocardial viability and survival in ischaemic left ventricular dysfunction. *N Engl J Med* 2011; 364: 1617–25.

14. Shah BN, Khattar RS, Senior R. The hibernating myocardium: current concepts, diagnostic dilemmas, and clinical challenges in the post-STICH era. *Eur Heart J* 2013.

15. Perrone-Filardi P, Pinto FJ. Looking for myocardial viability after a STICH trial: not enough to close the door. *J Nucl Med* 2012; 53: 349–52.

16. Allman KC, Shaw LJ, Hachamovitch R, Udelson JE. Myocardial viability testing and impact of revascularization on prognosis in patients with coronary artery disease and left ventricular dysfunction: a meta-analysis. *J Am Coll Cardiol* 2002; 39: 1151–8.

17. Schmidt A, Azevedo CF, Cheng A, et al. Infarct tissue heterogeneity by magnetic resonance imaging identifies enhanced cardiac arrhythmia susceptibility in patients with left ventricular dysfunction. *Circulation* 2007; 115: 2006–14.

18. Bleeker GB, Kaandorp TA, Lamb HJ, et al. Effect of posterolateral scar tissue on clinical and echocardiographic improvement after cardiac resynchronization therapy. *Circulation* 2006; 113: 969–76.

19. Cerqueira MD, Weissman NJ, Dilsizian V, et al. Standardized myocardial segmentation and nomenclature for tomographic imaging of the heart. A statement for healthcare professionals from the Cardiac Imaging Committee of the Council on Clinical Cardiology of the American Heart Association. *Circulation* 2002; 105: 539–42.

20. Gerber BL, Vanoverschelde JL, Bol A, et al. Myocardial blood flow, glucose uptake, and recruitment of inotropic reserve in chronic left ventricular ischaemic dysfunction. Implications for the pathophysiology of chronic myocardial hibernation. *Circulation* 1996; 94: 651–9.

21. Canty JM, Jr, Fallavollita JA. Hibernating myocardium. *J Nucl Cardiol* 2005; 12: 104–19.

22. Vanoverschelde JL, Wijns W, Depre C, et al. Mechanisms of chronic regional postischaemic dysfunction in humans. New insights from the study of noninfarcted collateral-dependent myocardium. *Circulation* 1993; 87: 1513–23.

23. Shen YT, Vatner SF. Mechanism of impaired myocardial function during progressive coronary stenosis in conscious pigs. *Circ Res* 1995; 76: 479–88.

24. Bax JJ, Poldermans D, Elhendy A, Boersma E, Rahimtoola SH. Sensitivity, specificity, and predictive accuracies of various noninvasive techniques for detecting hibernating myocardium. *Curr Probl Cardiol* 2001; 26: 141–86.

25. Gerber BL, Ordoubadi FF, Wijns W, et al. Positron emission tomography using(18)F-fluoro-deoxyglucose and euglycaemic hyperinsulinaemic glucose clamp: optimal criteria for the prediction of recovery of post-ischaemic left ventricular dysfunction. Results from the European Community Concerted Action Multicenter study on use of (18)F-fluoro-deoxyglucose Positron Emission Tomography for the Detection of Myocardial Viability. *Eur Heart J* JID—8006263 2001; 22: 1691–701.

26. Bax JJ, Visser FC, Poldermans D, et al. Relationship between preoperative viability and postoperative improvement in LVEF and heart failure symptoms. *J Nucl Med* 2001; 42: 79–86.

27. Beanlands RS, Ruddy TD, Dekemp RA, et al. Positron emission tomography and recovery following revascularization (PARR-1): the importance of scar and the development of a prediction rule for the degree of recovery of left ventricular function. *J Am Coll Cardiol* 2002; 40: 1735–43.

28. Perrone-Filardi P, Bacharach SL, Dilsizian V, Maurea S, Frank JA, Bonow RO. Regional left ventricular wall thickening. Relation to regional uptake of 18fluorodeoxyglucose and 201Tl in patients with chronic coronary artery disease and left ventricular dysfunction. *Circulation* 1992; 86: 1125–37.

29. Perrone-Filardi P, Pace L, Prastaro M, et al. Assessment of myocardial viability in patients with chronic coronary artery disease. Rest-4-hour-24hour 201 thallium tomography versus dobutamine echocardiography. *Circulation* 1996; 94: 2712–9.

30. Gupta M, Kadakia J, Hacioglu Y, et al. Non-contrast cardiac computed tomography can accurately detect chronic myocardial infarction: Validation study. *J Nucl Cardiol* 2011; 18: 96–103.

31. Gerber BL, Belge B, Legros GJ, et al. Characterization of acute and chronic myocardial infarcts by multi-detector computed tomography: comparison with contrast-enhanced magnetic resonance. *Circulation* 2006; 113: 823–33.

32. George RT, Silva C, Cordeiro MA, et al. Multi-detector computed tomography myocardial perfusion imaging during adenosine stress. *J Am Coll Cardiol* 2006; 48: 153–60.

33. Mahrholdt H, Wagner A, Judd RM, Sechtem U, Kim RJ. Delayed enhancement cardiovascular magnetic resonance assessment of non-ischaemic cardiomyopathies. *Eur Heart J* 2005; 26: 1461–74.

34. Schuleri KH, George RT, Lardo AC. Applications of cardiac multi-detector CT beyond coronary angiography. *Nat Rev Cardiol* 2009; 6: 699–710.

35. Tsai IC, Lee WL, Tsao CR, et al. Comprehensive evaluation of ischaemic heart disease using MDCT. *AJR Am J Roentgenol* 2008; 191: 64–72.

36. Habis M, Capderou A, Ghostine S, et al. Acute myocardial infarction early viability assessment by 64-slice computed tomography immediately after coronary angiography comparison with low-dose dobutamine echocardiography. *J Am Coll Cardiol* 2007; 49: 1178–85.

37. Lardo AC, Cordeiro MA, Silva C, et al. Contrast-enhanced multi-detector computed tomography viability imaging after myocardial infarction: characterization of myocyte death, microvascular obstruction, and chronic scar. *Circulation* 2006; 113: 394–404.

38. Dwivedi G, Al-Shehri H, Dekemp RA, et al. Scar imaging using multislice computed tomography versus metabolic imaging by F-18 FDG positron emission tomography: A pilot study. *Int J Cardiol* 2012.

39. Sato A, Hiroe M, Nozato T, et al. Early validation study of 64-slice multi-detector computed tomography for the assessment of myocardial viability and the prediction of left ventricular remodelling after acute myocardial infarction. *Eur Heart J* 2008; 29: 490–8.

40. Sato A, Nozato T, Hikita H, et al. Prognostic value of myocardial contrast delayed enhancement with 64-slice multi-detector computed tomography after acute myocardial infarction. *J Am Coll Cardiol* 2012; 59: 730–8.

41. le Polain de Waroux JB, Pouleur AC, et al. Combined coronary and late-enhanced multi-detector-computed tomography for delineation of the etiology of left ventricular dysfunction: comparison with coronary angiography and contrast-enhanced cardiac magnetic resonance imaging. *Eur Heart J* 2008; 29: 2544–51.

42. Einstein AJ, Henzlova MJ, Rajagopalan S. Estimating risk of cancer associated with radiation exposure from 64-slice computed tomography coronary angiography. *JAMA* 2007; 298: 317–23.

43. Williams MC, Cruden NL, Uren NG, Newby DE. A low-dose comprehensive cardiac CT protocol assessing anatomy, function, perfusion, and viability. *Cardiovasc Comput Tomogr* 2013; 7: 69–72.

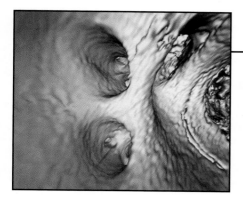

CHAPTER 28

Heart failure—CMR to assess viability

John-Paul Carpenter, Dudley J. Pennell, and Sanjay K. Prasad

Contents

Heart failure and coronary disease

Coronary artery disease is the most common underlying cause of myocardial dysfunction, accounting for at least 50% of all cases of heart failure [1]. Following myocardial infarction, remodelling may occur due to abnormal loading conditions, not just in the infarcted segments but also in the surrounding areas of myocardium. This may lead to dilatation of the ventricle with an alteration in shape to a more spherical, less efficient pump, with an adverse effect on contractile function (◐ Fig. 28.1). Revascularization can improve function and outcome but it is important to be able to distinguish viable and hibernating myocardium from non-viable scar to target patients appropriately for intervention to achieve a positive risk/benefit ratio.

Viability and hibernation

Before considering revascularization of a coronary artery territory subtended by a diseased or occluded epicardial coronary artery, it is essential to know if the underlying myocardial tissue is viable. Viable and hibernating myocardium can be characterized as dysfunctional myocardium with limited or no scarring, which has evidence of preserved, but down-regulated metabolic activity in the presence of impaired coronary blood supply during stress, and which has the potential for functional recovery following successful revascularization. The concept of hibernation was initially proposed by Rahimtoola [2]. There has been much debate about whether hibernating myocardium has normal resting blood flow and oxygen consumption. Current data indicate that myocardial perfusion is significantly impaired during stress in comparison to normally perfused myocardium (reduced or

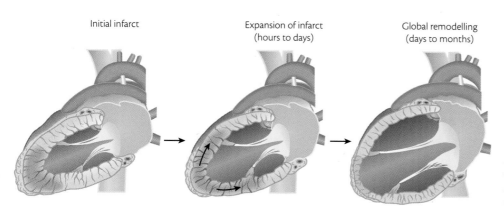

Initial infarct

Expansion of infarct (hours to days)

Global remodelling (days to months)

Fig. 28.1 Ventricular remodelling after acute infarction. At the time of an acute myocardial infarction, there is no clinically significant change in overall ventricular geometry. Within hours to days, the area of myocardium affected by the infarction begins to expand and become thinner. Within days to months, global remodelling can occur, resulting in wall thinning, overall ventricular dilatation, decreased systolic function, mitral valve dysfunction and the formation of an aneurysm.
Reproduced from [41].

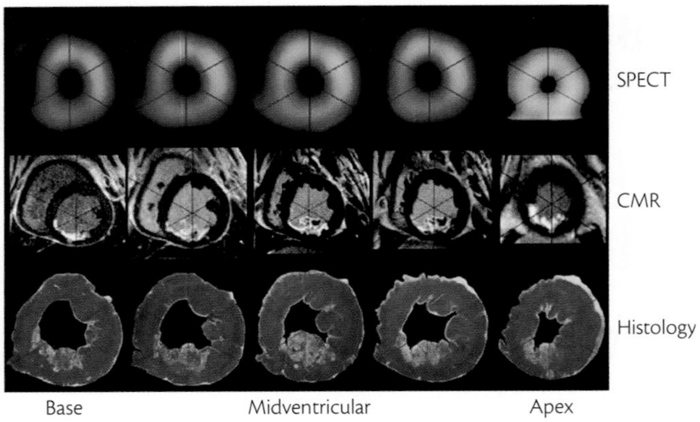

Fig. 28.2 Comparison of SPECT images in a canine model of infarction (top row), delayed enhancement CMR images (middle row), and histological slides stained for infarction using TTC (bottom row). Sub-endocardial infarcts that are detected by CMR and confirmed by tissue staining are missed by SPECT due to its inferior resolution.

Reprinted from *The Lancet*, 361, Wagner A, Marholdt H, Holly TA et al, Contrast-enhanced MRI and routine single photon emission computed tomography (SPECT) perfusion imaging for detection of subendocardial myocardial infarcts: an imaging study, 374–9, Copyright 2003 with permission from Elsevier.

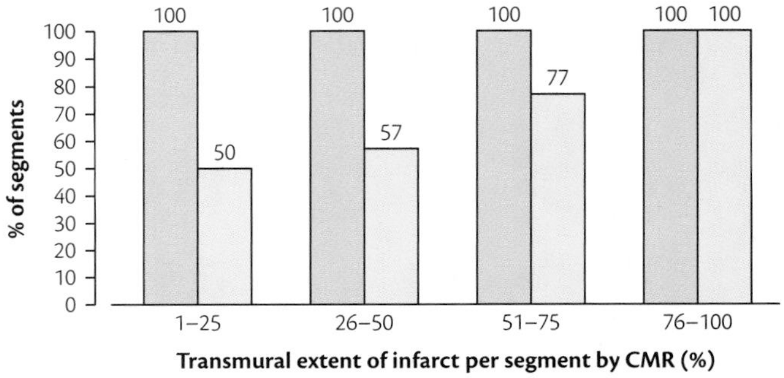

Fig. 28.3 Patient data. Comparison of infarcts detected by SPECT (pink bars) against those detected by CMR delayed enhancement (green bars). For segments in which the transmural extent of infarction is less than 75% by CMR, the number of segments not detected by SPECT increases as the transmural extent of infarction decreases.

Reprinted from *The Lancet*, 361, Wagner A, Marholdt H, Holly TA et al, Contrast-enhanced MRI and routine single photon emission computed tomography (SPECT) perfusion imaging for detection of subendocardial myocardial infarcts: an imaging study, 374–9, Copyright 2003 with permission from Elsevier.

abolished coronary flow reserve), but that resting myocardial perfusion is normal or near normal. Resting perfusion to hibernating areas may be mildly reduced as a direct consequence of reduced demand, because non-contractile myocardium has a lower oxygen (and therefore perfusion) requirement. However, there is no clinical evidence of a major reduction in perfusion to the level that is required in animal models to produce akinesia. Hibernation is distinct from myocardial stunning, which is transient, post-ischaemic myocardial dysfunction; however, the physiological induction of hibernation may result from repeated episodes of stunning due to reduced myocardial perfusion reserve. Hibernation can only be confirmed retrospectively once revascularization has been successful and objective evidence of contractile improvement is seen.

The current options available for clinical viability testing include [^{18}F] fluorodeoxyglucose positron emission tomography (FDG-PET), single photon emission computed tomography (SPECT) with an injectable myocardial perfusion tracer, dobutamine stress echocardiography (DSE), or cardiovascular magnetic resonance (CMR). Each technique has its strengths and weaknesses. The main strength of CMR is the combination of accurate assessment of function, regional wall motion, scar detection, as well as perfusion in a single study. CMR is the only technique with sufficiently high resolution to determine the transmurality of infarction, and detect small sub-endocardial infarcts that are missed by SPECT (➲ Figs 28.2 and 28.3).

Improvement in LV function and prognosis following revascularization

Recovery of contractile function in patients with left ventricular dysfunction due to chronic ischaemic heart disease occurs in some, but not all, patients who undergo revascularization. The recovery in function is not immediate but follows a progressive course over the weeks and months following the procedure. Recovery appears to be faster in stunned myocardium than in hibernating myocardium, which can take longer (up to 14 months) to recover function [3]. It is frequently observed that those with the most severely impaired ventricular function gain important functional recovery and therefore these patients may especially benefit from revascularization (➲ Fig. 28.4).

A meta-analysis of 24 studies looking at the impact of revascularization on prognosis in patients with coronary artery disease and LV dysfunction showed a strong association between myocardial viability on non-invasive testing and improved survival; however, these were not randomized trials, and none of the studies included CMR assessment [4]. In patients with evidence of viability, there was a 76% reduction in annual mortality in

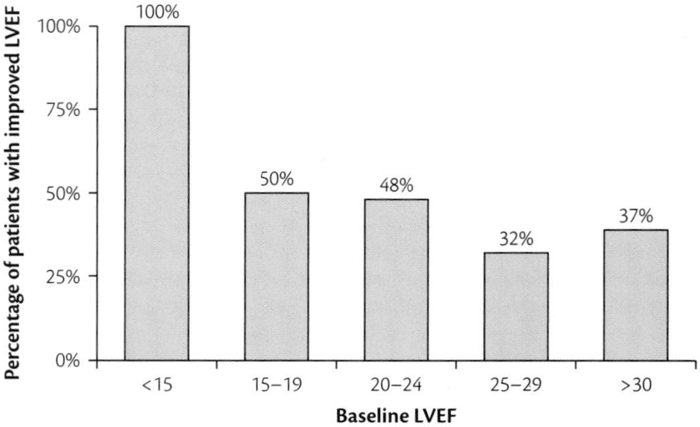

Fig. 28.4 Improvement in global LV ejection fraction (EF) by ≥5% after revascularization was observed more frequently in patients with the lowest baseline LVEF.

Reprinted from the *Journal of the American College of Cardiology*, 93:1, Schinkel AFL, Poldermans D, Vanoverschelde JLJ et al. Incidence of recovery of contractile function following revascularisation in patients with ischemic left ventricular dysfunction, 14-17, Copyright 2004 with permission from Elsevier.

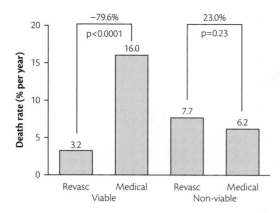

Fig. 28.5 Death rates for patients with and without evidence of myocardial viability treated by revascularization or medical therapy. There is a 79.6% relative reduction in mortality for patients with viability treated by revascularization. In patients without evidence of viability, there was no significant difference in mortality.
Reprinted from the *Journal of the American College of Cardiology*, 39:7, Allman KC, Shaw LJ, Hachamovitch R et al. Myocardial viability testing and impact of revascularisation on prognosis in patients with coronary artery disease and left ventricular dysfunction: a meta-analysis, 228–36, with permission for Elsevier.

those who underwent revascularization compared with medical therapy. There was also a direct relationship between the severity of LV dysfunction and the magnitude of benefit from revascularization. In contrast, absence of viability was associated with no significant difference in outcomes (⊃ Fig. 28.5). The recent Surgical Treatment for Ischemic Heart Failure (STICH) viability trial assessed myocardial viability using single-photon emission computed tomography (SPECT) myocardial perfusion imaging, dobutamine stress echo, or both [5]. The presence of viability did not predict a survival advantage in patients undergoing bypass surgery in comparison to medical management; however, there has been debate as to whether CMR assessment of viability would have led to a different conclusion.

CMR assessment of ventricular function, regional wall motion and valves

Baseline steady-state free precession (SSFP) cine images of the left ventricle provide the current 'gold-standard' for measurement of volumes and function, and these allow an excellent appreciation of regional function and systolic thickening. Regional function at rest can, however, be misleading for assessment of infarction. Contraction may appear normal even in infarcted myocardium with ~50% transmural extent of infarction [6]. This may either represent true contraction or artefact because of tethering to normally functioning neighbouring segments or through-plane motion giving the appearance of wall thickening. These effects can result in an underestimation of infarct size and, therefore, wall motion at rest cannot be relied upon in isolation to exclude myocardial infarction.

CMR assessment of LV function can also provide information regarding the risks associated with bypass surgery. Patients with very poor systolic function are known to be at higher peri-operative risk of death and those with severe LV dilatation (end-systolic volume ≥140ml) are less likely to show improvement in LV ejection fraction, despite evidence of viability [7]. The presence of mitral regurgitation (due to annular dilatation or restriction of the posterior leaflet) helps to guide surgical management. CMR accurately delineates the size and extent of LV aneurysms (⊃ Fig. 28.6), although ventricular reconstructive surgery remains controversial [8]. Additional findings (such as ventricular thrombus) may also be identified (⊃ Fig. 28.7).

Wall thickness

End-diastolic wall thickness has been used as a surrogate marker for the assessment of viability and can predict recovery of myocardial function. Echocardiographic studies have suggested that dysfunctional myocardial segments with end-diastolic wall thickness of less than 6mm are significantly scarred and show little improvement with revascularization. The remodelling that occurs in the first weeks following myocardial infarction leads to wall thinning in regions with significant degree of transmurality of infarction and scar with compensatory hypertrophy of other areas of the ventricle. Even with better treatment of acute myocardial infarction, the use of ACE inhibitors, statins, and beta blockers, remodelling is still frequently seen, albeit to a lesser extent than before.

Early CMR trials examined end-diastolic wall thickness to assess whether this was related to the presence of viability in thinned, akinetic areas of myocardium. Baer et al. compared CMR to both FDG-PET and SPECT [9, 10]. An end-diastolic wall thickness of <5.5 mm was taken as the cut-off for identifying non-viable myocardium based on the normal range of wall thickness in healthy volunteers (5.5mm = mean normal wall thickness minus 2.5 standard deviations). This correlated well with technetium SPECT perfusion defects and autopsy specimens of hearts with full thickness infarcts, which showed that regions with transmural scar measured <6 mm. When compared with FDG-PET, regions were graded as viable if [¹⁸F] fluorodeoxyglucose uptake was ≥50% of the maximum uptake in a viable region of myocardial infarction with normal wall motion. Using these criteria, there was an 83% agreement between the CMR measurement of wall thickness and viability on FDG-PET. End-diastolic wall thickness of >5.5cm was found to have 72% sensitivity, 89% specificity, and 91% positive predictive value for residual metabolic activity.

In a prospective study using CMR before and after bypass surgery, segments that remained akinetic after revascularization had a significantly lower end-diastolic wall thickness than those that showed an improved systolic wall thickening (6.0 +/- 3.1 mm versus 9.8 +/- 2.6 mm, *P*<0.001). Segments with end-diastolic wall thickness <5.5mm were highly unlikely to show functional improvement at follow-up (negative predictive value of 90.4%). Baer et al. concluded that the presence of significantly reduced end-diastolic wall

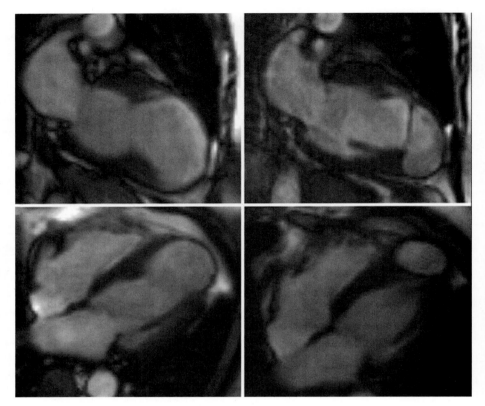

Fig. 28.6 The Dor procedure can be used to reconstruct the ventricular geometry. Pre-operatively, there was a large antero-apical aneurysm following anterior myocardial infarction (left upper and lower panels). At operation, a purse string suture was inserted between the muscular and fibrotic zones of the infarct and the resulting oval defect was closed with a patch of collagen-impregnated Dacron. The residual left ventricular wall was closed over this patch. The aneurysmal part of the ventricle is therefore excluded and will eventually thrombose (right upper and lower panels). 🎥 Video 28.1 shows the improvement in ejection fraction.

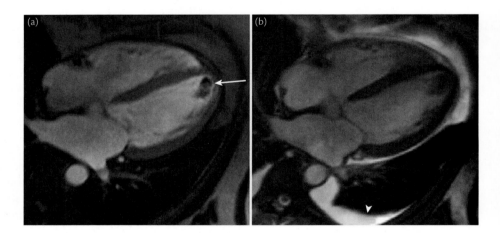

Fig. 28.7 Apical left ventricular thrombus. (a) Thrombus appears as a dark filling defect in the early phase after gadolinium injection (white arrow). (b) Still image from SSFP cine (see 🎥 Video 28.2). There is also a pleural effusion (arrowhead).

thickness reliably indicated irreversible myocardial damage and that dobutamine stress CMR could be restricted to those who had preserved LV end-diastolic wall thickness [11]. It was felt that if the myocardium was thin, this essentially excluded the presence of a clinically relevant residual amount of viable myocardium. However, other data indicate that end-diastolic wall thickness may not be sufficient on its own to predict metabolic activity measured by FDG-PET in patients with ischaemic cardiomyopathy [12].

Reliance on wall thickness alone as a measure of viability is therefore suboptimal and it has since been demonstrated that improvement in function can occur even in the presence of severe wall thinning, which itself can thicken after revascularization in a poorly understood process of reverse remodelling (see ➲ Fig. 28.17). The poor predictive value with respect to functional recovery may result because wall thickness cannot assess the degree of transmurality of infarction that corresponds to the degree of scarring. A more recent study combining end-diastolic wall thickness with measurement of late gadolinium enhancement has confirmed that while wall thickness is an independent predictor of functional recovery, combination with other techniques of viability assessment adds incremental value (➲ Fig. 28.8) [13]. The development of the late enhancement technique has shown that areas less than 5 mm thick (which would have previously been considered dead) can still sometimes have the potential for functional recovery. In

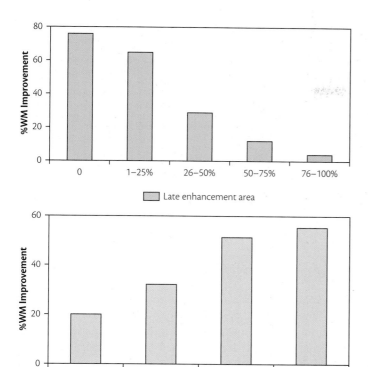

Fig. 28.8 The relationship between CMR markers of viability and recovery of left ventricular function after coronary artery bypass surgery. The degree of recovery declines with increasing transmurality of late gadolinium enhancement (LGE) (upper panel) and decreasing end-diastolic wall thickness (lower panel).
Reproduced from Krittayaphong R, Laksanabunsong P, Maneesai A et al. Comparison of cardiovascular magnetic resonance of late gadolinium enhancement and diastolic wall thickness to predict recovery of left ventricular function after coronary artery bypass. J Cardiovasc Magn Reson 2008;10:41, with permission from BioMed Central Ltd.

patients with coronary artery disease and regional wall thinning, a limited scar burden (late enhancement ≤50% of total extent) predicts not only improved contractility but also resolution of wall thinning after revascularization [14].

Dobutamine stress CMR

The evaluation of contractile reserve is another option for assessment of viability (◗ Fig. 28.9). Gradient-echo cine sequences generate excellent blood pool-myocardial definition and this can be exploited for the assessment of wall thickening in response to low dose dobutamine stress (with doses of 5 to 10 µg/kg/min). Segmental analysis is used to assess contractile reserve, which simulates the effect of revascularization. During low-dose dobutamine infusion, systolic wall thickening increases in viable myocardium but not in irreversibly scarred areas. If contractile reserve can be elicited, the myocardium is more likely to improve after revascularization. With high-dose dobutamine infusion (20 to 40 µg/kg/min), the presence of inducible wall motion abnormalities using cine CMR provides additional accurate information regarding the presence of ischaemia and prognosis [15].

The use of dobutamine stress CMR to assess patients with coronary artery disease was first described in 1992 [16]. Baer et al. subsequently demonstrated that an inotropic response to dobutamine was present in akinetic segments that were ischaemic but remained viable (when compared to FDG-PET) and that this response was a better predictor of viability than end-diastolic wall thickness. When combined with wall thickness measurements, response to dobutamine predicted viability with a sensitivity of 88%, specificity of 87%, and positive predictive accuracy of 92%. Dobutamine-induced systolic thickening also proved a better predictor of LV functional recovery than end-diastolic wall thickness [11]. They further investigated this dobutamine-induced contractile reserve in 103 patients with previous myocardial infarction before and after successful revascularization using transoesophageal echo and CMR. Patients had a mean LV ejection fraction of 38.7 +/− 12.5% and, while there was no statistical difference between the two techniques, dobutamine CMR gave a positive predictive accuracy of 92% and negative predictive accuracy of 85%, predicting an overall increase of 13 +/−7% in predominantly viable regions compared to only 2 +/−7% in regions graded as scar [17]. Sandstede et al. also tested the diagnostic value of dobutamine CMR for predicting

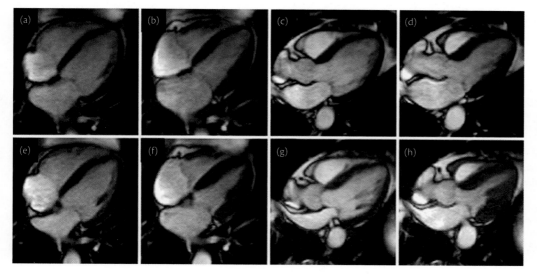

Fig. 28.9 Response to low-dose dobutamine stress. The top row of images shows a 4-chamber view (a and b) and LV outflow tract view (c and d) at end-diastole and end-systole with resting anteroseptal wall hypokinesia and reduced wall thickening. With low-dose dobutamine infusion (10 µg/kg/min), there is evidence of contractile reserve with improvement in regional function and increased wall thickening (e to h). See Videos 28.3–28.6.

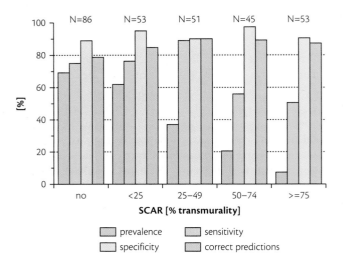

Fig. 28.10 Dobutamine stress CMR and transmurality of scar. Prevalence of functional recovery, sensitivity, specificity, and correct predictions by dobutamine CMR are grouped with respect to degree of transmurality. There is high specificity irrespective of the extent of scar but sensitivity of dobutamine CMR declines with more than 50% scar.
Reproduced from Wellnhofer E et al, Magnetic resonance low-dose dobutamine test is superior to scar quantification for the prediction of functional recovery, *Circulation*, 109:18, 2004, with permission from Wolters Kluwer.

recovery of regional myocardial contractility after revascularization. On a per-segment analysis, they reported 61% sensitivity, 90% specificity, and 87% positive predictive value for recovery of function, but if a patient-based analysis was performed, this was improved to 76% sensitivity with 100% specificity and positive predictive value [18]. Despite these encouraging results, the inotropic response to dobutamine depends on the presence of viable myocardium that has not undergone severe ultrastructural change with myofibrillar degeneration, which would prevent contractile improvement with inotropic stimulation. The technique is more sensitive for lesser grades of transmural infarction (➲ Fig. 28.10) [19].

Developments in quantification of wall motion assessment

Tagging, coupled with 3D strain analysis, allows quantitative assessment of regional myocardial contractility and, although still predominantly a research tool, it has promise in detection of viability using dobutamine stress. Tagging may improve sensitivity for the detection of viability because true myocardial contraction is assessed rather than wall motion, with its inherent limitations. Specialized post-processing analysis software is available, and advanced techniques have made tagging much more approachable for clinical use (➲ Fig. 28.11). These include harmonic phase (HARP) tagging and DENSE imaging (Displacement Encoding with Stimulated Echoes). CMR feature-tracking can also be used to assess myocardial strain and provide quantitative viability assessment in conjunction with low-dose dobutamine stress [20]. Newer techniques (such as CMR diffusion tensor imaging) may also help provide a better understanding of myocardial structure, function, and viability [21].

Late gadolinium enhancement

An alternative approach to the assessment of viability is the accurate delineation of infarcted from normal myocardium using gadolinium chelates. Following a bolus injection via a peripheral vein, these contrast agents are distributed in the extracellular space, altering the relaxation properties of the tissues by predominantly shortening the T1 recovery time. Gadolinium chelates do not enter cells with an intact cell membrane, but in areas of non-viable tissue, they exhibit delayed wash-in, wash-out kinetics and an increased volume of distribution. In normal myocardium, wash-in and wash-out rates are rapid. This means that late after injection, once gadolinium has mainly washed out of viable myocardium, the concentration remains increased in both acutely and chronically infarcted regions [22].

In acute infarction, the disruption of myocyte sarcomere integrity and cell membrane rupture allows gadolinium to enter the previously intracellular space. In chronic infarct tissue, replacement fibrosis causes an increase in the interstitial space and hence the volume of distribution of gadolinium. Therefore, depending on the dose of gadolinium given, approximately 5 to 15 minutes after initial injection a time window exists where the concentration of gadolinium in infarcted tissue is higher than the surrounding normal, viable myocardium (➲ Fig. 28.12).

This results in higher signal on T1-weighted MR sequences, and is best visualized using inversion recovery imaging

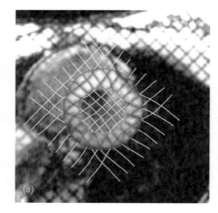
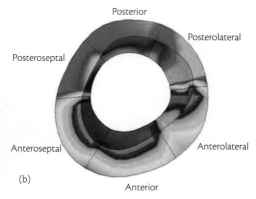

Fig. 28.11 Regional strain analysis using myocardial tagging. (a) Short-axis image at end-systole demonstrating myocardial borders and computer-assisted tag line representation. (b) Colour contour map of calculated circumferential strain. Areas in red indicate reduced contraction in this example from a patient with a large inferoposterior infarct.
Reproduced from Wellnhofer E et al, Magnetic resonance low-dose dobutamine test is superior to scar quantification for the prediction of functional recovery, *Circulation*, 109:18, 2004, with permission from Wolters Kluwer.

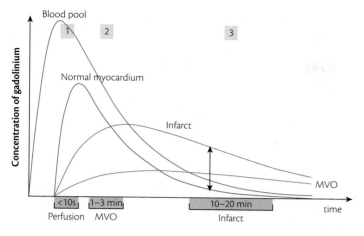

Fig. 28.12 Representation of the kinetics of gadolinium concentration following a bolus intravenous injection. The wash-in and wash-out is slower in infarcted tissue (blue line) than normal myocardium (green line) and results in a concentration difference (arrowed line), which is exploited for delayed enhancement imaging. Perfusion images are acquired during the first-pass phase (1). Early phase images allow the detection of microvascular obstruction (MVO) or ventricular thrombus (2). Delayed enhancement images are obtained in the late phase (3).

techniques. These sequences rely on imaging the heart at the precise moment that the T1 recovery of normal myocardium passes through the point of zero signal following an inversion pulse (a technique known as nulling of the normal myocardium). This creates intense signal contrast between normal and infarcted myocardium (➲ Fig. 28.13) and created the aphorism 'Bright is Dead', although this is now known to be an oversimplification, especially in other conditions such as cardiomyopathy. The strongly T1-weighted images allow differentiation between injured and normal regions of myocardium with up to 500% difference in

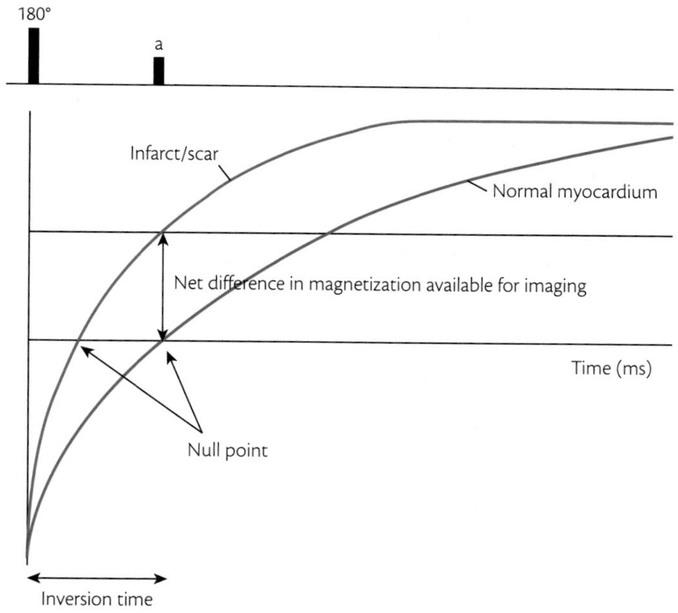

signal intensity and high resolution, such that transmural depiction of viability is now possible [23]. Images have an in-plane resolution of 1.5–2 mm, which approximates to 1 g of tissue. This late gadolinium enhancement technique has been shown to correlate very accurately with the area of infarction and quantitative analysis software can be used to estimate the volume of infarcted tissue (➲ Fig. 28.14).

The use of late gadolinium enhancement to identify infarcted myocardium

As proof of concept, Kim et al. described the ligation of the left anterior descending or circumflex artery in a canine model causing acute myocardial infarction [22]. The area of late enhancement revealed a high correlation with the infarct distribution when the *ex vivo* hearts were stained with 2,3,5 triphenyltetrazolium chloride (TTC). The TTC stain forms a red precipitate in areas of viable myocardium but necrotic areas fail to stain. In areas of myocardium subtended by coronary arteries where only transient ischaemia was induced, there was no evidence of infarction by either CMR or tissue staining. The spatial extent of enhancement is near identical to the spatial extent of infarction at every stage of healing. Injection of fluorescent microparticles during coronary artery occlusion confirms that the ischaemic area at risk can be reliably distinguished from the infarct zone as detected by late enhancement (➲ Fig. 28.15). In addition, areas of enhancement, representing sub-endocardial or transmural infarction have significantly altered electro-mechanical properties when assessed using endocardial voltage mapping. Klein et al. investigated 31 patients with poor LV systolic function secondary to ischaemic heart disease using late gadolinium enhancement CMR and FDG-PET. There was close agreement (r = 0.91, P<0.0001) between techniques but importantly, 11% of the segments that were defined as viable according to PET criteria had evidence of late enhancement on CMR. This is likely to be the result of the superior resolution of CMR [24].

Fig. 28.13 Inversion recovery. The T1 relaxation curves for normal myocardium (green) and infarct (red) are shown. The longitudinal relaxation time, T1, is shortened by gadolinium chelates. Due to a higher concentration of gadolinium in infarct tissue, the T1 will be shorter than normal myocardium. A 180° prepulse will result in a T1-weighted image which will accentuate the contrast between normal myocardium (dark) and scar (bright). Contrast will be greatest if images are acquired at the correct inversion time when normal myocardium is passing through the null point.

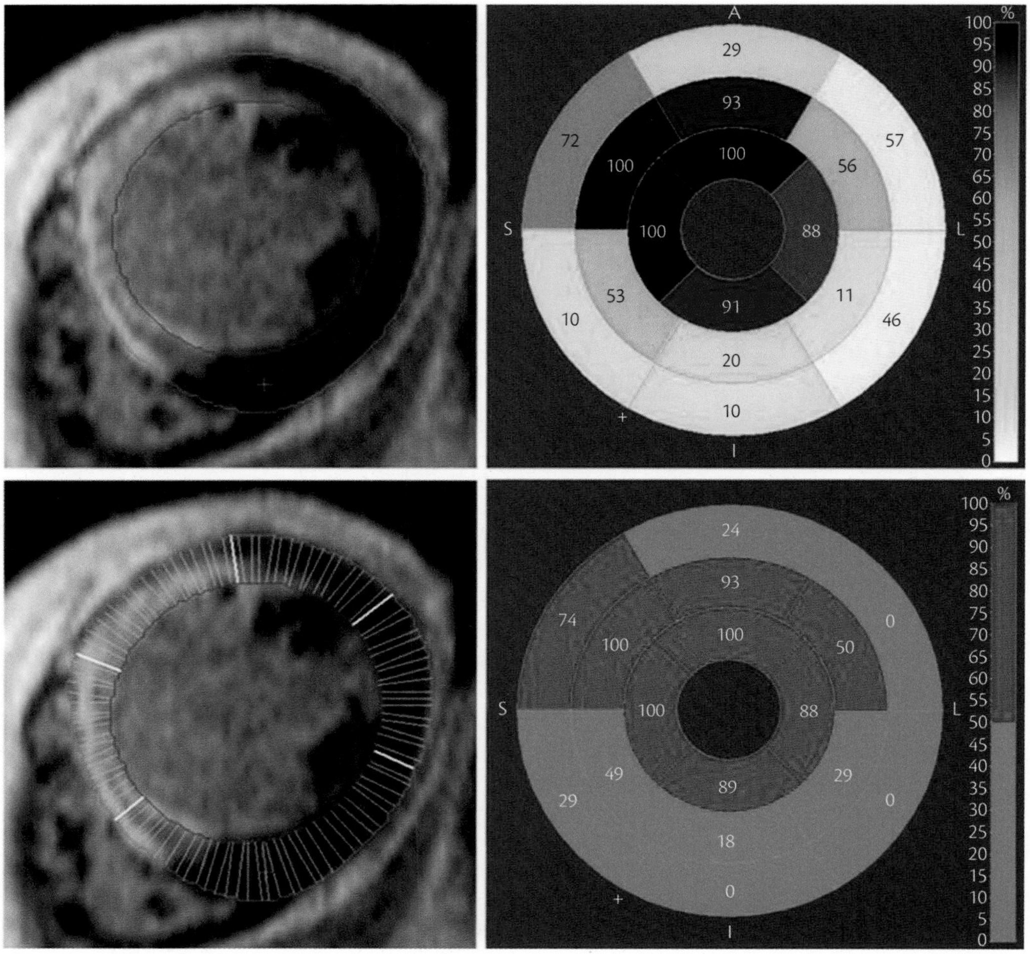

Fig. 28.14 Quantitative analysis of infarct volume. This example shows an anteroseptal myocardial infarction. Top left: Thresholding delineates enhanced areas of scar (pink shading). Top right: 16 segment model bull's eye plot depicting transmurality of scar in each segment (no scar = 0%, white; transmural scar = 100%, black). Bottom left: Radial chords superimposed on the image allow measurement of degree of transmurality of infarct. Bottom right: Bull's eye viability plot. The threshold for viability is set at 50%. Any areas over 50% transmural scar are graded as non-viable (red). LV mass = 259 g. Calculated scar tissue volume = 115 ml (46%).
Analysis performed with QMassMR (Medis Medical Imaging Systems B.V, Leiden, The Netherlands).

Use of late gadolinium enhancement to assess recovery after revascularization

When correlated with coronary angiographic data, nearly all patients with confirmed myocardial infarction have the hallmark finding of sub-endocardial or transmural late enhancement in the relevant corresponding coronary artery territory. In patients with heart failure due to ischaemic heart disease, there is almost always evidence of sub-endocardial or transmural enhancement; however, in cases of dilated cardiomyopathy, there is usually either no enhancement or a diffuse mid-wall pattern of enhancement, which does not follow coronary artery territory. Having said this, up to 13% of patients with a diagnostic label of presumed idiopathic dilated cardiomyopathy have a pattern of enhancement that identifies ischaemic heart disease as the underlying cause for the LV dysfunction [25]. The pattern of enhancement is therefore extremely useful in determining the underlying aetiology of left ventricular impairment, differentiating those with coronary artery disease from cardiomyopathy, in which revascularization would not result in an improvement in LV function.

In animal models and human studies, myocardial salvage with recovery in function following acute infarction has been shown to be inversely related to the degree of transmurality of enhancement. In a canine model of acute infarction, myocardial segments with less than 25% enhancement at day 3 post-MI showed 87% spontaneous recovery by 1 month, but if there was complete transmural enhancement, no recovery was seen [26]. In patients undergoing successful reperfusion therapy for acute MI, either with primary percutaneous coronary intervention or thrombolysis, the degree of improvement is inversely related to the transmurality of enhancement. The best predictor of improvement in segmental function at 2–3 months following acute infarction has been shown to be late enhancement of less than 25% of the LV wall thickness [27]. Patients who undergo primary percutaneous coronary intervention to treat acute MI also have greater predicted recovery of myocardial contraction with lesser degrees of enhancement.

In chronic heart failure, the likelihood of functional improvement with revascularization had been previously described in histological studies looking at degree of fibrosis in needle biopsy specimens taken at the time of surgery. Viable areas of myocardium showed a lower degree of fibrosis, which in turn was an independent predictor of functional recovery. As the extent of late gadolinium enhancement accurately mirrors infarcted tissue, researchers went on to investigate whether this technique could predict recovery of function following revascularization. In a landmark study, Kim et al. prospectively studied patients with

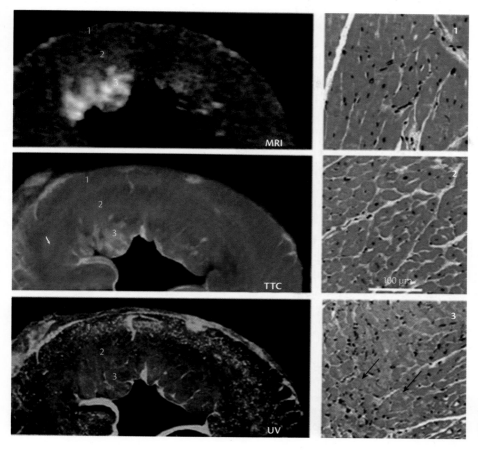

Fig. 28.15 Comparison of delayed enhancement (left upper panel), TTC staining (left middle panel), and the myocardium at risk (region without green fluorescent microparticles, left lower panel) in a dog with a 1-day-old reperfused infarction. Light microscopy views of region 1 (not at risk, not infarcted), region 2 (at risk but not infarcted), and region 3 (infarcted) are shown on the right panels. Arrows point to contraction bands. This shows that the area of delayed enhancement correlates exactly with the area of infarction.

Reprinted from *Journal of the American College of Cardiology*, 36:6, Fieno DS, Kim RJ, Chen EL et al. Contrast-enhanced magnetic resonance imaging of myocardium at risk, Copyright 2000, 1985-91, with permission from Elsevier.

established myocardial dysfunction and chronic coronary artery disease to assess the likelihood of recovery of akinetic or dysfunctional myocardial segments following revascularization. This study demonstrated that, in the context of chronic infarction, the likelihood of functional recovery with successful surgical or percutaneous revascularization declined with increasing transmurality of enhancement, such that patients with 50% or less transmural gadolinium enhancement showed a good degree of recovery, whereas those with 75% had far less, and those with 100% virtually no response (Fig. 28.16) [28]. Similar studies have since replicated these findings. It is clear that improvement in myocardial function is highly likely if there is less than 25% transmurality of enhancement and very unlikely if there is more than 75% enhancement. Between these two extremes, there is a grey zone with variable recovery, but even up to 75% enhancement, there is evidence of some improvement in function with revascularization and some groups therefore recommend dobutamine CMR for this cohort. The absence of late gadolinium enhancement (even in thinned myocardial wall segments that were previously felt to be scarred and unlikely to respond) is strongly associated with improvement in contractility and functional recovery after revascularization (Fig. 28.17) [14]. It is therefore very important to offer the correct treatment to patients who are likely to benefit as, without revascularization, the presence of dysfunctional but viable myocardium by late enhancement is an independent predictor of mortality in patients with ischaemic LV dysfunction [29]. In addition to recovery in LV systolic function, both viability (assessed by

total scar burden) and end-systolic volume index are independent predictors of survival following revascularization—better survival is associated with lower volumes and less scar [30].

Interestingly, the response to beta blockade in patients with impaired LV function as a result of coronary artery disease can also be predicted by the extent of gadolinium enhancement. Improvement in contractile function with carvedilol or metoprolol is inversely related to the transmurality of enhancement [31]. Infarct size, measured by CMR, may also be of prognostic significance following myocardial infarction—those with large amounts of scar being more likely to have inducible monomorphic ventricular tachycardia and hence a higher theoretical risk of sudden arrhythmic death [32]. Kwong et al. looked at late gadolinium enhancement in elderly patients with suspected coronary disease but no known myocardial infarction and found that the degree of late enhancement predicted worse event-free survival [33]. It is interesting to note that the greater the number of viable myocardial segments, the more likely the patient is to improve global LV systolic function following revascularization [34].

The thickness of the residual epicardial rim of viable tissue overlying an infarct is another way of predicting recovery. Kneusel et al. compared CMR with FDG-PET and showed that viable myocardial segments on CMR correlated well with FDG uptake. The segments with a viable rim of greater than 4.5 mm were found to have FDG uptake of greater than or equal to 50% (a positive predictor of recovery). These thick, metabolically active segments had a high likelihood of recovery (85%) following revascularization,

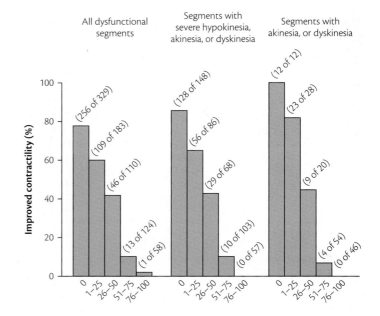

Fig. 28.16 Relationship between the transmural extent of hyper-enhancement before revascularization and the likelihood of increased contractility after revascularization. Data are shown for all dysfunctional segments and separately for the segments with at least severe hypokinesia and segments with akinesia or dyskinesia. There was an inverse relation between the transmural extent of hyper-enhancement and the likelihood of improvement in contractility.
Reproduced from [28].

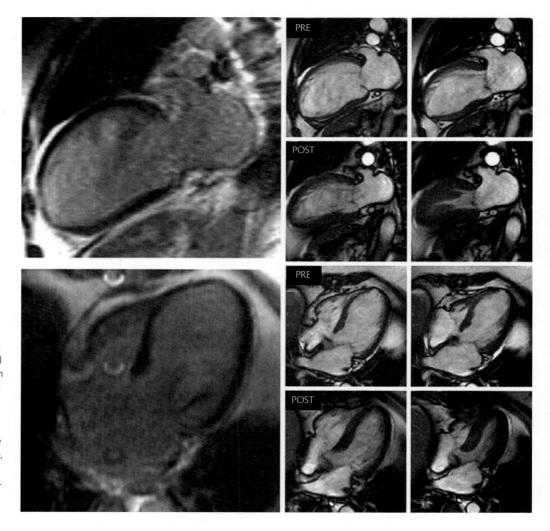

Fig. 28.17 Marked recovery of function following revascularization in an 81-year-old lady with severe left main stem disease and an occluded right coronary artery. The upper left panel shows the vertical long axis late gadolinium enhancement image next to the systolic and diastolic frames before (PRE) and after (POST) revascularization. The lower left panel shows the 4-chamber late gadolinium enhancement image next to diastolic and systolic frames before and after revascularization. On these late gadolinium images, there was no detectable enhancement and despite the severely dilated, thinned ventricle, there was remarkable recovery following successful revascularization. See Videos 28.7 and 28.8.
Reproduced from [46].

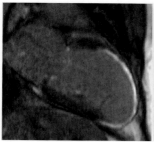
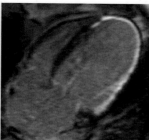
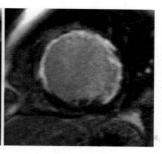

Fig. 28.18 Extensive myocardial infarction involving the anteroseptal wall, anterior wall, lateral wall and apex. There is at least 75% transmurality. The corresponding Video clip shows extensive wall motion abnormality with dyskinetic anterior wall and akinetic septum. The likelihood of recovery of function in this situation is low. See ▣ Video 28.9.

whereas segments that had a thin viable rim of tissue (albeit metabolically active) were less likely to recover (36%). In contrast, only 13% of thin, non-viable segments improved (⊃ Fig. 28.18) [35].

With direct measurements of infarction, it is important to note that the results apply mainly to chronic infarction (i.e. months after the acute event). The relative thickness of the infarct and the epicardial rim varies with time after acute myocardial infarction, due to infarct resorption and hypertrophy of the epicardium. Even without revascularization, the thickness of the viable epicardial rim is a predictor of improvement in myocardial contractility between the acute convalescent phase (within the first week) and the chronic state following the infarct a few months later.

Microvascular obstruction

The presence of microvascular obstruction (demonstrated by a region of dense signal void at the endocardial surface of the ventricle surrounded by gadolinium-enhanced myocardial tissue) signifies a poorer likelihood of recovery of ventricular function following an acute myocardial infarction [36].

Practical aspects of late gadolinium enhancement imaging

Timing of image acquisition

One of the pitfalls to be aware of is the problem of imaging too early after gadolinium injection. It has been confirmed that imaging at 5–30 minutes after injection gives the best diagnostic correlation between the presence of transmural enhancement and

non-viable myocardium that is unlikely to show functional improvement [37]. If images are acquired too early with very short inversion times, the intermediate wash-in kinetics in viable peri-infarct border zones will give rise to enhancement, and the delayed contrast kinetics in the core of an infarct may mean that this area is relatively hypointense. As a result, infarct size may be wrongly estimated.

Optimizing inversion time

The optimal inversion time (TI) must be chosen to allow the best contrast enhancement of the infarcted region with nulling of normal, viable ventricular myocardium [23]. As the concentration of gadolinium in normal myocardium is constantly changing due to the dynamic nature of wash-in/wash-out kinetics, the T1 will lengthen with time and therefore the TI needs to be progressively lengthened throughout the scan to ensure that normal, viable myocardium is nulled. If the TI is too short or too long, normal myocardium will appear grey rather than black, which can lead to poor discrimination of infarcted tissue from normal myocardium (⊃ Fig. 28.19). Many centres use a 'TI scout' sequence, which acquires a preliminary set of images with a range of inversion times, allowing the best value to be chosen. With experience, it is usually possible to predict the inversion time needed (bearing in mind that inversion times will vary with different gadolinium chelates). A typical range of values starting from 260 ms up to about 400 ms may be needed. Newer phase-sensitive inversion recovery (PSIR) sequences (⊃ Fig. 28.20) are less dependent on choice of correct inversion time, have less background noise, and give an improved contrast-to-noise ratio between areas of high signal intensity (such as infarct tissue) and low signal intensity (such as normal myocardium which is nulled) [38].

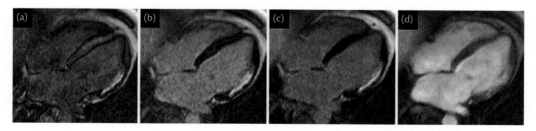

Fig. 28.19 The effect of inversion time on nulling of normal myocardium. (a) With the inversion time set too low, there is high signal both from normal myocardium and the lateral wall infarct. (b) Inversion time is still too low. (c) Correctly adjusted inversion time gives good differentiation between normal and enhanced myocardium. (d) When the inversion time is too high, there is once again high signal in both infarct tissue and normal myocardium.

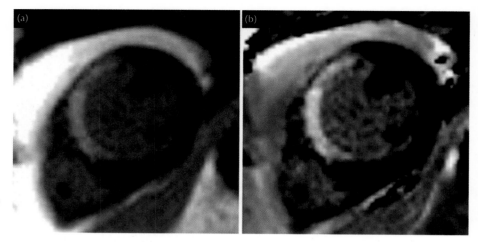

Fig. 28.20 The phase-sensitive inversion-recovery sequence generates two sets of images, the magnitude image (a) and the phase image (b), both of which need to be correctly windowed to visualise areas of enhancement such as this transmural anteroseptal infarct.

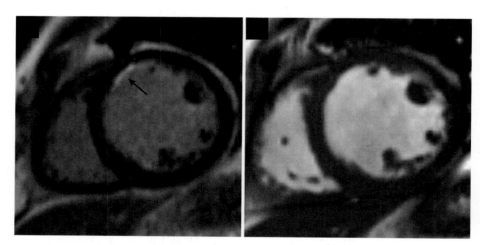

Fig. 28.21 Sub-endocardial infarction. (a) The inversion-recovery T1-weighted image following gadolinium shows a limited area of sub-endocardial enhancement. (b) Comparison with the identical slice SSFP cine allows accurate measurement of the extent of transmurality (graded as 25–50% enhancement) in the severely hypokinetic anteroseptal wall. See 🎥 Video 28.10.

Comparison with cine images

It is often very useful to compare late gadolinium images with a cine at the same slice position. The nature of balanced steady-state, free precession (SSFP) cine sequences gives very good blood/myocardial contrast, which allows the measurement of the thickness of corresponding wall segments, as well as assessing regional function, including wall thickening (➲ Fig. 28.21). This is important when assessing hibernation, which by definition only occurs in segments that have resting contractile dysfunction.

Artefact or true enhancement?

Artefacts can be a problem when deciding whether there is evidence of late enhancement or not. Artefacts due to high signal from the chest wall, fat, or cerebrospinal fluid occur only in the phase encode direction. Saturation bands applied over areas of high signal will help but if artefacts are projected onto the myocardium, it can be difficult to see if there is true enhancement. Acquiring images in two, orthogonal phase-swapped sets will mean that any artefact seen will be in a different position in each series (➲ Fig. 28.22).

Assessment of viability using magnetic resonance spectroscopy

Myocardial cells require adenosine triphosphate (ATP) and phosphocreatine (PCr) for their energy supply. Alterations in myocardial high-energy phosphate metabolism are present in patients with coronary artery disease and heart failure, and this can be directly observed using magnetic resonance spectroscopy (MRS). Phosphorous (^{31}P) MRS can directly measure ATP and PCr to allow assessment of the energetic state of the heart. Neubauer et al. demonstrated that PCr/ATP ratio correlated well with the severity of heart failure in the context of LAD stenosis and chronic myocardial infarction [39]. Although it has a potential use in the assessment of viability, MR spectroscopy remains challenging due to the inherently low signal-to-noise ratio, as well as cardiac and respiratory motion. It requires a different radiofrequency (RF) coil from that used for conventional proton imaging, presents technical difficulties, and scan times are long. As a result, this technique has excellent research application but has not found routine clinical use, although it may become more useful with higher field strength systems at 3 Tesla.

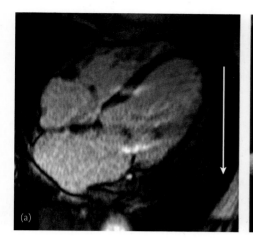
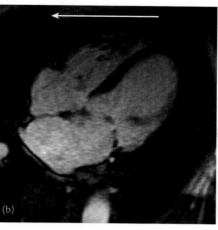

Fig. 28.22 Differentiating artefacts from true enhancement. (a) Artefact from the anterior chest wall is superimposed on the septum in the 4-chamber view. (b) If the phase-encode direction is changed, the area of high signal in the septum is no longer visible and it becomes clear that this was artefact. The white arrow shows the phase-encode direction.

Table 28.1 Sensitivity and specificity of different CMR techniques (based on weighted mean values from pooled CMR trials)

	No. of patients	Sensitivity (%)	95% CI	99% CI	Specificity (%)	95% CI	99% CI
End-diastolic wall thickness	100	95	91–99	90–100	41	31–50	28–53
Dobutamine stress	259	73	68–78	66–80	83	78–87	77–89
Late gadolinium enhancement	132	95	91–99	90–100	45	37–54	34–56

Reproduced from [47].

Magnetic resonance protocols for the investigation of myocardial viability

A combination of CMR techniques can be used to assess viability in order to give the optimal prediction for recovery of function (⊃ Table 28.1). All patients should undergo a standard protocol, including cine imaging, for volumes and function, and, unless there are contraindications, late gadolinium enhancement should be performed. Selected patients may then require dobutamine stress CMR for further evaluation (⊃ Fig. 28.23). This could be applied to those in whom the late enhancement CMR is not conclusive. Some groups recommend that this is used for patients with predominantly 25–50% transmural infarction.

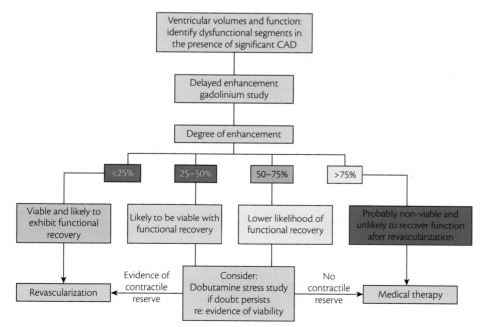

Fig. 28.23 Suggested protocol for the use of CMR to assess viability in ischaemic LV dysfunction. CAD, coronary artery disease.

Failure of recovery following revascularization and peri-procedural infarcts

Despite the best available evidence of viability, some myocardial segments do not recover function when revascularized. The reasons for this are not always clear but possible factors include myocardial damage at the time of surgery or incomplete revascularization. The presence of extensive ventricular remodelling, especially in those with dilated ventricles and end-systolic volume of ≥140ml, may also be a factor. Approximately 38% of patients who have coronary artery bypass surgery and 28% of those undergoing percutaneous coronary intervention have evidence of new areas of late enhancement secondary to peri-procedural myocardial necrosis. Areas of new enhancement following PCI or surgery will worsen outcome and this may also be the cause of non-recovery in functional status after revascularization [40]. The presence of new areas of late enhancement following the procedure is a negative predictor for improvement in global LV ejection fraction and volumes. This highlights the need for myocardial protection and optimal technique during these procedures.

Conclusion

In conclusion, CMR is a valuable tool in the assessment of myocardial viability in heart failure. It is becoming more widely available and has several major areas of strength. There is excellent spatial resolution and it is highly reproducible for measurement of LV volumes and function, allowing serial evaluation of ventricular remodelling together with assessment of regional function. The transmural extent of infarction can be assessed, quantification of the total infarct burden can be performed, and presence of microvascular obstruction identified. Dobutamine stress also allows assessment of contractile reserve. CMR not only allows assessment of likelihood of functional recovery, but also provides important prognostic information relating to survival following revascularization.

References

1. Fox KF, Cowie MR, Wood DA, et al. Coronary artery disease as the cause of incident heart failure in the population. *Eur Heart J* 2001; 22: 228–36.
2. Rahimtoola SH. The hibernating myocardium. *Eur Heart J* 1989; 117(1): 211–21.
3. Bax JJ, Visser FC, Poldermans D, et al. Time course of functional recovery of stunned and hibernating segments after surgical revascularization. *Circulation* 2001; 104(Suppl I): I314–8.
4. Allman KC, Shaw LJ, Hachamovitch R, et al. Myocardial viability testing and impact of revascularization on prognosis in patients with coronary artery disease and left ventricular dysfunction: a meta-analysis. *J Am Coll Cardiol* 2002; 39: 1151–1158.
5. Bonow RO, Maurer G, Lee KL, et al. Myocardial viability and survival in ischemic left ventricular dysfunction. *N Engl J Med* 2011 Apr 28; 364(17): 1617–25.
6. Marholdt H, Wagner A, Parker M, et al. Relationship of contractile function to transmural extent of infarction in patients with chronic coronary artery disease. *J Am Coll Cardiol* 2003; 42: 505–12.
7. Schinkel AF, Poldermans D, Rizzello V, et al. Why do patients with ischemic cardiomyopathy and a substantial amount of viable myocardium not always recover in function after revascularization? *J Thorac Cardiovasc Surg* 2004; 127: 385–90.
8. Jones RH, Velazquez EJ, Michler RE, et al. Coronary bypass surgery with or without surgical ventricular reconstruction. *N Engl J Med* 2009 Apr 23; 360(17): 1705–17.
9. Baer FM, Voth E, Schneider CA, et al. Comparison of low-dose dobutamine-gradient-echo magnetic resonance imaging and positron emission tomography with [18F] fluorodeoxyglucose in patients with chronic coronary artery disease. *Circulation* 1995; 91: 1006–15.
10. Baer FM, Smolarz K, Jungehulsing M, et al. Chronic myocardial infarction: assessment of morphology, function, and perfusion by gradient echo magnetic resonance imaging and 99mTc-methoxyisobutyl-isonitrile SPECT. *Eur Heart J* 1992; 123: 636–45.
11. Baer FM, Theissen P, Schneider CA, et al. Dobutamine magnetic resonance imaging predicts contractile recovery of chronically dysfunctional myocardium after successful revascularization. *J Am Coll Cardiol* 1998; 31: 1040–48.
12. Perrone-Filardi P, Bacharach SL, Dilsizian V, et al. Metabolic evidence of viable myocardium in regions with reduced wall thickness and absent wall thickening in patients with chronic ischemic left ventricular dysfunction. *J Am Coll Cardiol* 1992; 20: 161–68.
13. Krittayaphong R, Laksanabunsong P, Maneesai A, et al. Comparison of cardiovascular magnetic resonance of late gadolinium enhancement and diastolic wall thickness to predict recovery of left ventricular function after coronary artery bypass. *J Cardiovasc Magn Reson* 2008; 10: 41.
14. Shah DJ, Kim HW, James O, et al. Prevalence of regional myocardial thinning and relationship with myocardial scarring in patients with coronary artery disease. *JAMA* 2013; 309(9): 909–18.
15. Jahnke C, Nagel E, Gebker R, et al. Prognostic value of cardiac magnetic resonance stress tests. Adenosine stress perfusion and dobutamine stress wall motion imaging. *Circulation* 2007; 115: 1769–76.
16. Pennell DJ, Underwood SR, Manzara CC, et al. Magnetic resonance imaging during dobutamine stress in coronary artery disease. *Am J Cardiol* 1992; 70: 34–40.
17. Baer FM, Theissen P, Crnac J, et al. Head to head comparison of dobutamine-transoesophageal echocardiography and dobutamine-magnetic resonance imaging for the prediction of left ventricular functional recovery in patients with chronic coronary artery disease. *Eur Heart J* 2000; 21: 981–91.
18. Sandstede JJW, Bertsch G, Beer M, et al. Detection of myocardial viability by low-dose dobutamine cine MR imaging. *Magn Reson Imaging* 1999; 17: 1437–43.
19. Wellnhofer E, Olariu A, Klein C, et al. Magnetic resonance low-dose dobutamine test is superior to scar quantification for the prediction of functional recovery. *Circulation* 2004; 109: 2172–74.
20. Schuster A, Paul M, Bettencourt N, et al. Cardiovascular magnetic resonance myocardial feature tracking for quantitative viability assessment in ischemic cardiomyopathy. *Int J Cardiol* 2011.
21. Mekkaoui C, Huang S, Chen HH, et al. Fiber architecture in remodeled myocardium revealed with a quantitative diffusion CMR

tractography framework and histological validation. *J Cardiovasc Magn Reson* 2012; 14: 70.

22. Kim RJ, Fieno DS, Parrish TB, et al. Relationship of MRI delayed contrast enhancement to irreversible injury, infarct age, and contractile function. *Circulation* 1999; 100: 1992–2002.

23. Simonetti OP, Kim RJ, Fieno DS, et al. An improved MR imaging technique for the visualization of myocardial infarction. *Radiology* 2001; 218: 215–23.

24. Klein C, Nekolla SG, Bengel FM, et al. Assessment of myocardial viability with contrast-enhanced magnetic resonance imaging: comparison with positron emission tomography. *Circulation* 2002; 105: 162–67.

25. McCrohon JA, Moon JCC, Prasad SK, et al. Differentiation of heart failure related to dilated cardiomyopathy and coronary artery disease using gadolinium-enhanced cardiovascular magnetic resonance. *Circulation* 2003; 108: 54–49.

26. Hillenbrand HB, Kim RJ, Parker MA, et al. Early assessment of myocardial salvage by contrast-enhanced magnetic resonance imaging. *Circulation* 2000; 102: 1678–683.

27. Choi KM, Kim RJ, Gubernikoff G, et al. Transmural extent of myocardial infarction predicts long-term improvement in contractile function. *Circulation* 2001; 104: 1101–107.

28. Kim RJ, Wu E, Rafael A, et al. The use of contrast-enhanced magnetic resonance imaging to identify reversible myocardial dysfunction. *N Engl J Med* 2000; 343: 1445–53.

29. Gerber BL, Rousseau MF, Ahn SA, et al. Prognostic value of myocardial viability by delayed-enhanced magnetic resonance in patients with coronary artery disease and low ejection fraction: impact of revascularization therapy. *J Am Coll Cardiol* 2012; 59(9): 825–35.

30. Kwon DH, Hachamovitch R, Popovic ZB, et al. Survival in patients with severe ischemic cardiomyopathy undergoing revascularization versus medical therapy: association with end-systolic volume and viability. *Circulation* 2012; 126(11 Suppl 1): S3–8.

31. Bello D, Shah DJ, Farah GM, et al. Gadolinium cardiovascular magnetic resonance predicts reversible myocardial dysfunction and remodeling in patients with heart failure undergoing beta-blocker therapy. *Circulation* 2003; 108: 1945–53.

32. Bello D, Fieno DS, Kim RJ, et al. Infarct morphology identifies patients with substrate for sustained ventricular tachycardia. *J Am Coll Cardiol* 2005; 45: 1104–8.

33. Kwong RY, Chan AK, Brown KA, et al. Impact of unrecognized myocardial scar detected by cardiac magnetic resonance imaging on event-free survival in patients presenting with signs or symptoms of coronary artery disease. *Circulation* 2006; 113: 2733–43.

34. Pegg TJ, Selvanayagam JB, Jennifer J, et al. Prediction of global left ventricular functional recovery in patients with heart failure undergoing surgical revascularization, based on late gadolinium enhancement cardiovascular magnetic resonance. *J Cardiovasc Magn Reson* 2010; 12: 56.

35. Kneusel PR, Nanz D, Wyss C, et al. Characterization of dysfunctional myocardium by positron emission tomography and magnetic resonance: relation to functional outcome after revascularization. *Circulation* 2003; 108: 1095–100.

36. Wu KC. CMR of microvascular obstruction and hemorrhage in myocardial infarction. *J Cardiovasc Magn Reson* 2012; 14: 68.

37. Wagner A, Marholdt H, Thomson L, et al. Effects of time, dose, and inversion time for acute myocardial infarct size measurements based on magnetic resonance imaging-delayed contrast enhancement. *J Am Coll Cardiol* 2006; 47: 2027–33.

38. Kellmann P, Arai AE, McVeigh ER, et al. Phase-sensitive inversion recovery for detecting myocardial infarction using gadolinium-delayed hyperenhancement. *Magn Reson Med* 2002; 47: 372–83.

39. Neubauer S, Krahe T, Schindler R, et al. 31P magnetic-resonance spectroscopy in dilated cardiomyopathy and coronary artery disease. Altered cardiac high-energy phosphate metabolism in heart failure. *Circulation* 1992; 86: 1810–18.

40. Bondarenko O, Beek AM, Nijveldt R, et al. Functional outcome after revascularization in patients with chronic ischemic heart disease: a quantitative late gadolinium enhancement CMR study evaluating transmural scar extent, wall thickness and periprocedural necrosis. *J Cardiovasc Magn Reson* 2007; 9: 815–21.

41. Jessup M and Brozena S. Heart failure. *N Engl J Med* 2003; 348: 2007–18.

42. Wagner A, Marholdt H, Holly TA, et al. Contrast-enhanced MRI and routine single photon emission computed tomography (SPECT) perfusion imaging for detection of subendocardial myocardial infarcts: an imaging study. *Lancet* 2003; 361: 374–79.

43. Schinkel AFL, Poldermans D, Vanoverschelde JLJ, et al. Incidence of recovery of contractile function following revascularization in patients with ischemic left ventricular dysfunction. *Am J Cardiol* 2004; 93: 14–17.

44. Bree D, Wollmuth JR, Cupps BP, et al. Low-dose dobutamine tissue-tagged magnetic resonance imaging with 3-dimensional strain analysis allows assessment of myocardial viability in patients with ischemic cardiomyopathy. *Circulation* 2006; 114: I-33–I-36.

45. Fieno DS, Kim RJ, Chen EL, et al. Contrast-enhanced magnetic resonance imaging of myocardium at risk. *J Am Coll Cardiol* 2000: 36; 1985–991.

46. John AS, Dreyfus GD, Pennell DJ. Reversible wall thinning in hibernation predicted by cardiovascular magnetic resonance. *Circulation* 2005; 11: e24–e25.

47. Kaandorp TAM, Lamb HJ, van der Wall EE, et al. Cardiovascular MR to assess myocardial viability in chronic ischaemic LV dysfunction. *Heart* 2005; 91: 1359–365.

⊃ **For additional multimedia materials please visit the online version of the book (⏏ http://www.esciacc.oxfordmedicine.com)**

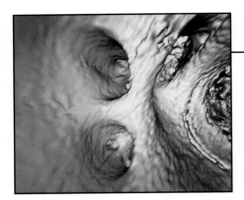

CHAPTER 29

Imaging cardiac innervation

Albert Flotats and Ignasi Carrió

Contents

Introduction

The cardiac autonomic nervous system is crucial for maintaining haemodynamic and electrophysiological stability to changing demands through two efferent components, with complementary and opposing effects on cardiac inotropy and chronotropy: the sympathetic (stimulatory) and parasympathetic (inhibitory) nervous systems.

There is increasing evidence showing that imaging the cardiac autonomic nervous system can evaluate patients with different cardiac disturbances, being especially useful in heart failure (HF), where it has an independent prognostic value and provides a potential tool for improving patient management. Excellent reviews on cardiac autonomic imaging with SPECT and PET tracers have been recently published [1–5]. This chapter updates the subject with inclusion of novel data, highlighting the use of innervation imaging for monitoring therapy in patients with HF.

Different radiotracers have been developed for the assessment of pre- and postsynaptic receptors of the cardiac autonomic nervous system, either for SPECT (and planar imaging) and PET, with sufficient sensitivity to assess processes that take place at picomolar concentrations in the human heart. PET offers higher resolution allowing for improved regional analysis, kinetic modelling, and quantification.

Most autonomic radiotracers under investigation target postganglionic presynaptic neurons, although there is ongoing work on PET tracers that bind to other neurotransmitter receptors. ^{123}I-metaiodobenzylguanidine (^{123}I-mIBG) is the most used tracer for cardiac innervation imaging. Cardiac ^{123}I-mIBG uptake and retention is reflected, with good reliability [6, 7], by the heart to mediastinum ratio (HMR) at early (15 minutes) and late (4 hours) planar images and the wash-out rate (WR) between them. The late HMR reflects the relative distribution of sympathetic nerve terminals, offering the global information about neuronal function resulting from uptake, storage and release (see ⊃ Fig. 29.1). The WR is an index of the sympathetic tone [1, 2, 4]. Recently development of different methods to derive quantitative parameters for SPECT images have been proposed [8, 9]. ^{11}C-Hydroxyephedrine (^{11}C-HED) is the most used PET tracer for cardiac sympathetic imaging. ^{11}C-HED uptake is commonly quantified by the retention index, a ratio of activity in the myocardium in the final image of a 40- or 60-minute dynamic sequence to the integral of the image-derived arterial blood time activity curve. WR of ^{11}C-HED has been suggested to reflect sympathetic neuronal activity.

Currently, there is interest in developing analogues of mIBG labelled with ^{18}F to take advantage of the higher spatial resolution of PET. ^{18}F-LMI1195 (N-[3-bromo-4-(3-[^{18}F] fluoro-propoxy)-benzyl]-guanidine) was designed as a benzylguanidine analogue and is in phase-1 trials [10]. Initial animal kinetic and imaging studies with ^{18}F-4-fluoro-m-hydroxyphenethylguanidine (^{18}F-4F-MHPG) suggest that it may allow for more accurate quantification of regional cardiac sympathetic nerve density than is currently possible with existing imaging agents [11].

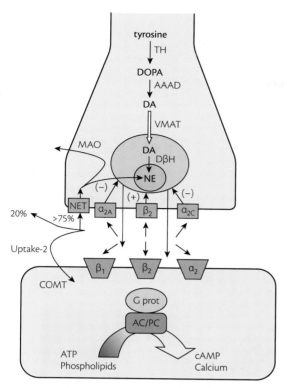

Fig. 29.1 Diagram of the sympathetic neurotransmission. Norepinephrine (NE), the major sympathetic neurotransmitter, is synthesized in the presynaptic nerve terminal by the conversion of tyrosine to dihydroxyphenylalanine (DOPA) by tyrosine hydroxylase (TH). Aromatic L-amino acid decarboxylase (AAAD) then converts DOPA to dopamine (DA), which is transported into storage vesicles through vesicular monoamine transporter (VMAT). Once inside these vesicles, DA is transformed to NE by dopamine-β-hydroxylase (DβH). On nerve firing, NE is released into the synaptic cleft by exocytosis of vesicles stimulating pre-and-postsynaptic adrenoceptors. Symbols (+) and (−) indicate positive and negative feedback mechanisms that affect NE exocytosis. Interaction of stimulated adrenoceptors with GTP-associated regulatory proteins (G prot) leads to stimulation of adenyl cyclase (AC) or phospholipase C (PC), resulting in increase of cAMP and calcium, which in turn results in activation of different protein kinases. The resultant protein phosphorylation modifies the activity of enzymes and the function of other proteins, leading to the cellular response. The most important mechanism for the termination of NE action in the synaptic cleft is active reuptake into the neuron through the NE uptake-1 transporter (NET), while some NE diffuses into the plasma and very little is transported into myocardium through uptake-2, where it is metabolized by catecholamine-O-methyl-transferase (COMT). ^{123}I-mIBG undergoes the same uptake, storage and release mechanisms of NE in the sympathetic nerves, but it is neither metabolized nor interacts with adrenoceptors, thus providing a marker for sympathetic nerve activity.
Springer and *Journal of Nuclear Cardiology*, 11:5, 2004, 587–602, 2. Flotats A, Carrió I. Cardiac neurotransmission SPECT imaging, With kind permission from Springer Science and Business Media.

Imaging cardiac innervation in coronary artery disease (CAD)

The sympathetic nervous tissue is more sensitive to ischaemia than the myocardial tissue. ^{123}I-mIBG uptake is significantly reduced in areas of myocardial infarction (MI) and adjacent non-infarcted regions, as well as in areas with acute and chronic ischaemia

(see ⮞ Fig. 29.2). Reinnervation late after MI in peri-infarct regions has been demonstrated by reappearance of ^{123}I-mIBG uptake, which may be in part responsible for the improvement of function. It is likely that ischaemia induces damage to sympathetic neurons, which may take a long time to regenerate resulting in decreased ^{123}I-mIBG uptake. This characteristic may be important in the pathophysiology of HF and arrhythmias [12] and offers potential for ^{123}I-mIBG imaging at rest for the detection of sporadic transient ischaemic attacks, such as those of vasospastic angina, and for the evaluation of the area at risk in the subacute phase of acute coronary syndromes by revealing more extensive defects than myocardial perfusion imaging at rest, as well as a marker of reversible ischaemia in patients with contraindications for stress myocardial perfusion imaging [2].

Recently Katsikis et al. [13] reported a transient increase in ^{123}I-mIBG SPECT defect score after one week of CABG intervention in patients with CAD, which reversed after 6 months of follow-up and was associated with adverse events related to arrhythmia and myocardial dysfunction during this period. It is possible that peri-procedural effects during CABG and/or direct nerve injury would be associated with clinically important but reversible reduction in cardiac sympathetic nerve function.

Imaging cardiac innervation in arrhythmogenesis

Sudden cardiac death (SCD) occurs mainly among subjects with no previous cardiovascular history, which highlights the need of tools to identify patients at risk. Heterogeneity of sympathetic innervation in response to injury is highly arrhythmogenic. Sequential changes consisting of nerve degeneration followed by neurilemma cell proliferation and axonal regeneration have been described in different altered states of the myocardium [14]. The coexistence of denervated and hyperinnervated areas in the diseased myocardium could result in increased electrophysiological heterogeneity during sympathetic activation, leading to ventricular arrhythmia and SCD [14]. On the other hand, adrenergic denervation of viable myocardium may also result in denervation supersensitivity, with exaggerated response of myocardium to sympathetic stimulation and increased vulnerability to ventricular arrhythmias (see ⮞ Fig. 29.2) [12].

Impaired cardiac adrenergic imaging has been described in patients with idiopathic ventricular fibrillation, long-QT and Brugada syndromes, and arrhythmogenic right ventricular cardiomyopathy, as well as in most of the disorders that result in LV dysfunction and potentially lethal ventricular arrhythmias [2].

Recently, Akutsu et al. [15] in a study of ^{123}I-mIBG imaging in 98 patients with paroxysmal atrial fibrillation (AF), with no structural heart disease, preserved LV systolic function, and no symptoms of HF, reported that a low late HMR was a powerful independent predictor of the development of permanent AF and HF plus permanent AF.

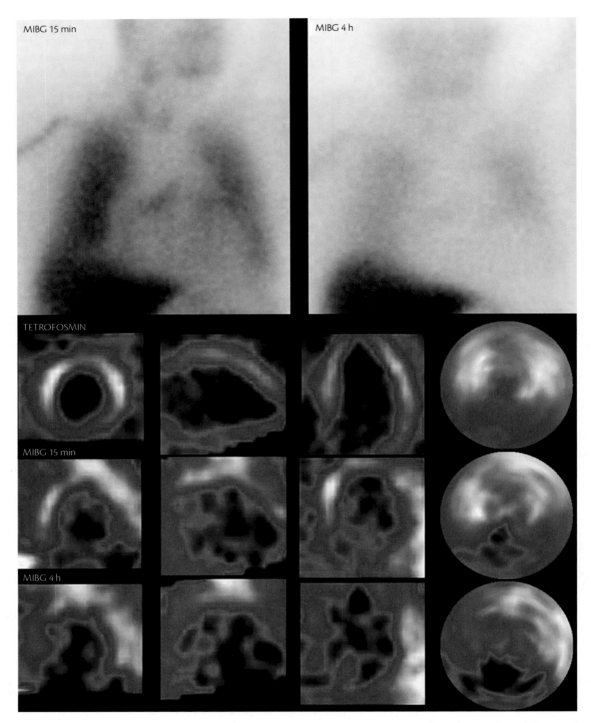

Fig. 29.2 High risk myocardial ^{123}I-mIBG imaging of a 64-year-old male with dilated cardiomyopathy and heart failure (NYHA class III, left ventricular ejection fraction 15%). The patient had history of coronary artery disease with inferior myocardial infarction, arterial and pulmonary hypertension, type 2 diabetes mellitus, and mitral and aortic valve replacement. At the top of the figure, early (15 minutes) and late (4 h) planar ^{123}I-mIBG images show impaired sympathetic innervation with severely decreased myocardial ^{123}I-mIBG uptake, which is more pronounced in the late image (early and late heart to mediastinum ratios are 1.39 and 1.08, respectively; wash-out rate is 45). The bottom of the figure shows the reconstructed slices at mid-left ventricle and polar maps of ^{99m}Tc-tetrofosmin SPECT myocardial perfusion imaging at rest (in the upper row) and early and late ^{123}I-mIBG SPECT innervation imaging (in the two lower rows). Note that myocardial innervation is more impaired than myocardial perfusion.

Imaging cardiac innervation in heart failure

Activation of endogenous neurohormonal systems plays an important role in the pathophysiology of HF [16, 17]. The hyperadrenergic state present in HF results in downregulation and uncoupling of cardiac β-adrenergic receptors, which contribute to progressive impairment of LV systolic function by altering postsynaptic signal transduction. Increased sympathetic tone in HF is associated to disease progression, prognosis, and risk of SCD [18].

Several studies have shown reduced cardiac ^{123}I-mIBG uptake and increased WR in different cardiomyopathies, which could reflect the contribution of the altered cardiac sympathetic nervous function to the development of the myocardial disorder [2].

Assessment of prognosis

Long-term prognosis of patients with HF remains poor, with a 5-year mortality rate of 59% for men and 45% for women [19]. Furthermore, prognosis in HF can be determined reliably only in populations and not in individuals. To improve survival, adequate risk stratification is needed.

Impaired cardiac adrenergic innervation, as assessed by radionuclide imaging, is strongly related to mortality in patients with HF independent of its cause [1–5].

Verberne et al. [20] in a meta-analysis that included a total of 1,755 patients reported that decreased late HMR and increased WR were significantly associated with a higher incidence of cardiac events, and with both cardiac death and cardiac events (cardiac death, MI, transplant, HF hospitalization), respectively.

The prospective, multi-centre, international trial AdreView Myocardial Imaging for Risk Evaluation in Heart Failure (ADMIRE-HF) [21], which included 961 patients with New York Heart Association functional class (NYHA) II-III and LV ejection fraction (LVEF) ≤35% for a 17-month follow-up, showed that a late HMR <1.6 more than doubled (from 15% to 37%) the incidence of worsening NYHA class, life-threatening arrhythmias, and cardiac death (see ⊃ Fig. 29.3). Late HMR ≥1.6 had a composite hazard ratio of 0.40 (P<0.001) and was a predictor of cardiac and all-cause deaths independent of clinical and image variables such as age, NYHA functional class, LVEF, and brain natriuretic peptide (BNP) at multivariate analysis. These results confirmed the high negative predictive value of a preserved late HMR with respect to cardiac death or cumulative arrhythmic events from previous studies in less consistent populations and that ^{123}I-mIBG cardiac imaging in otherwise high-risk HF patients can identify a significantly large subgroup being in fact at low risk.

Ketchum et al. [22], in a substudy with complete 2-year follow-up survival analysis of the ADMIRE-HF patients, showed that late HMR treated as a continuous variable for risk assessment, rather than dichotomized at 1.60 as in the primary analyses, added meaningful prognostic information when combined with the modified Seattle Heart Failure Model (SHFM-D, an algorithm of routinely collected demographic, imaging, laboratory, and therapeutic

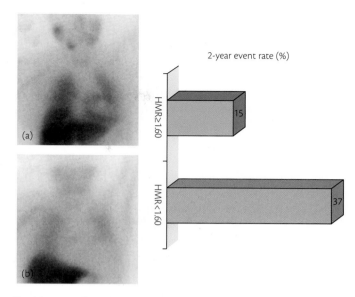

Fig. 29.3 Data from the ADMIRE-HF trial showed a 2-year event probability (worsening NYHA class, life-threatening arrhythmias, and cardiac death) of 15% for patients with late HMR ≥1.60 (a) as compared to a value of 37% for patients with late HMR <1.6 (b). HMR, heart to mediastinum ratio.
Data source from [21]. Jacobson AF, Senior R, Cerqueira MD, Wong ND, Thomas GS, Lopez VA, et al. Myocardial iodine-123 meta-iodobenzylguanidine imaging and cardiac events in heart failure. Results of the prospective ADMIRE-HF (AdreView Myocardial Imaging for Risk Evaluation in Heart Failure) study. J Am Coll Cardiol 2010;55:2212–21.

parameters that determine the likely 1–5 year mortality). Net reclassification improvement for such a combination was 22.7%, with 14.9% of patients who died reclassified into a higher risk category and 7.9% of patients who survived reclassified into a lower risk category. In another subanalysis of the ADMIRE-HF trial, Shah et al. [23] reported that ^{123}I-mIBG imaging had the same predictive prognostic value across the LVEF spectrum. In this study, LVEF was available for core lab recalculation in 901 patients. At all levels of LVEF (range 20–58%, mean 34±7%), a late HMR of <1.6 was associated with a higher risk of death or potentially lethal arrhythmic event and of the composite of cardiovascular death, arrhythmic event, and HF progression. Comparing subjects with LVEF ≤35% and >35%, there was no evidence of effect modification of LVEF on the risk associated with low HMR for death or arrhythmic event. For such endpoints, late HMR improved the risk discrimination beyond clinical and biomarker data among both LVEF groups, highlighting the prognostic value of ^{123}I-mIBG imaging.

Recently, Doi et al. [24] in a follow up study of 60.5 months among 468 HF patients with LVEF<50% reported that late HMR, haemoglobin, and estimated glomerular filtration rate (GFR) were independently and synergistically associated with increased cardiac mortality, together with NYHA class, with hazard ratios of 0.215, 0.821, and 0.984, respectively. Receiver-operating-characteristic analysis determined the thresholds for identifying patients at increased risk for cardiac death to be 1.57 for late HMR, 11.9 g/dl for haemoglobin, and 46.4 ml/min/1.73 m² for estimated GFR. The combination of the four independent predictors significantly improved the prognostic power.

Monitoring therapy

As clinical status and/or LV function improve in response to conventional medical treatment for HF, there is a parallel improvement in cardiac sympathetic nerve function as assessed by radionuclide imaging [1–5], supporting the concept that a restoration of cardiac neuronal uptake of NE is one of the beneficial effects of such treatment.

Kasama et al. [25] analysed the usefulness of serial ^{123}I-mIBG scanning for prognostication in 208 stable HF patients. The variation in the WR between the sequential ^{123}I-mIBG scans was the only independent predictor of cardiac death, which raises the possibility that patients showing worsening of cardiac sympathetic imaging on serial studies would need additional or alternate therapies (e.g. device therapy and cardiac transplantation) to improve outcome. Likewise, ^{123}I-mIBG imaging could provide a method to determine, in patients who do not tolerate full proven therapeutic doses, which drug and dose are indicated.

Device therapy

Prevention of sudden death is an important target in HF since about 50% of mortality occurs suddenly and unexpectedly, especially in patients with milder symptoms. Mainly, mortality is related to ventricular arrhythmias. Implantable cardioverter-defibrillators (ICD) reduce mortality in survivors of cardiac arrest and in patients with sustained symptomatic ventricular arrhythmias. Therefore, an ICD is recommended in the secondary prevention of such patients, irrespective of LVEF, with good functional status and a life-expectancy of >1 year [26]. An ICD is also recommended in the primary prevention of patients with symptomatic HF and good functional status (NYHA class II-III), a life-expectancy of >1 year, and LVEF ≤35% despite ≥3 months of optimal pharmacological treatment [26]. In these last patients, recommendations derive largely from four large randomized trials from which LVEF ≤30–35% became a principal variable for deciding who should receive a device [27–30]. However, >50% of HF patients who die suddenly have an LVEF>30% [31]. Other, different, independent univariate predictors of SCD have been identified (low NYHA class, unsustained VT, and inducibility of VT in electrophysiological testing—EPS), but their positive predictive value is low, thus better individual risk assessment is needed to select patients with HF who are candidates for ICD placement, most of all considering that the cost for a device is about €20,000 (not including ICD follow-up costs).

Despite the fact that techniques such as analysis of heart rate variability (HRV) and measurement of baroreflex sensitivity have shown an association between cardiac autonomic innervation abnormalities and SCD [32], their use in clinical practice is not clear.

In a phase-2, open-label, multi-centre study among 50 patients with LV dysfunction and previous MI, Bax et al. [33] found that late ^{123}I-mIBG SPECT defect score was the only variable that showed a significant difference between patients with and without positive EPS. A defect score of ≥37 yielded a sensitivity of 77% and specificity of 75% for predicting EPS results. Tamaki et al. [34]

prospectively compared the predictive value of ^{123}I-mIBG imaging for SCD with that of the signal-averaged ECG, HRV, and QT dispersion in 106 patients with chronic stable HF (LVEF <40%). After a follow-up of 65±31 months, only WR and LVEF were significantly and independently associated with SCD. In addition, the ADMIRE-HF trial showed that arrhythmia was significantly more common in patients with late HMR <1.60 than in patients with higher values (10.4% vs. 3.5%) [21].

Other studies have shown the usefulness of ^{123}I-mIBG cardiac imaging to predict ventricular arrhythmia in patients receiving an ICD. Nishisato et al. [35] reported that patients with a late HMR ≤1.9 and a tetrofosmin summed score ≥12 had a significantly greater ICD discharge rate than did those who had a late HMR >1.90 and a summed score <12 (94% vs. 18%) (see ⊃ Fig. 29.4). The former combination was associated with a hazard ratio of 3.8, and resulted in an independent and better predictor than age, sex, signal-averaged ECG, BNP, medications, inducible arrhythmias, and LVEF in predicting ICD shocks or cardiac death. In addition, in a study among 116 HF patients, Boogers et al. [36] reported that late ^{123}I-mIBG SPECT summed defect score was an independent predictor for both arrhythmias causing appropriate ICD therapy, as well as the composite of appropriate ICD therapy or cardiac deaths in patients referred for ICD therapy. During a mean follow-up of 23±15 months, appropriate ICD therapy was documented in 24 (21%) patients and appropriate ICD therapy or cardiac death in 32 (28%) patients. Patients with a large defect score (>26) showed significantly more appropriate ICD therapy (52% vs. 5%) and appropriate ICD therapy or cardiac death (57% vs. 10%) than patients with a small defect score (≤26) at 3-year follow-up (see ⊃ Fig. 29.5). Remarkably, only two (3%) patients

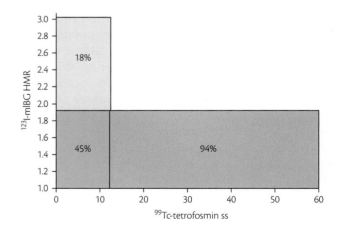

Fig. 29.4 Receiver operating-characteristic analysis of cut-off values of late HMR and tetrofosmin summed score identified three significant different implantable cardioverter-defibrillator (ICD) discharge rates among 60 patients referred for ICD therapy. The ICD discharge rate was of 94% for the 18 patients who had a late HMR ≤1.9 and a tetrofosmin summed score ≥12 (blue area); it was of 45% for the 20 patients who had a late HMR ≤1.9 and a tetrofosmin summed score <12 (green area); and it was of 18% for the 22 patients who had a late HMR >1.90 and a tetrofosmin summed score < 12 (yellow area). HMR, heart to mediastinum ratio.
Modified from [35].

Patients with HF referred for ICD therapy

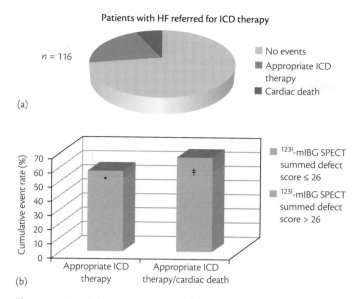

n = 116

- No events
- Appropriate ICD therapy
- Cardiac death

(a)

(b)

Fig. 29.5 ^{123}I-mIBG imaging for heart failure risk stratification. During a mean follow-up of 23±15 months, (a) appropriate ICD therapy was documented in 24 (21%) patients and appropriate ICD therapy or cardiac death in 32 (28%) patients. (b) Late ^{123}I-mIBG SPECT summed defect score was an independent predictor for both end points: patients with a large defect showed significantly more appropriate ICD therapy and appropriate ICD therapy or cardiac death than patients with a small defect. ICD, implantable cardioverter-defibrillator. *, ‡ *P*< 0.01.

Data source from 36. Boogers MJ, Borleffs CJ, Henneman MM, van Bommel RJ, van Ramshorst J, Boersma E, et al. Cardiac sympathetic denervation assessed with 123-iodine metaiodobenzylguanidine imaging predicts ventricular arrhythmias in implantable cardioverter-defibrillator patients. *J Am Coll Cardiol* 2010;55:2769–77.

with a small defect score received appropriate ICD therapy vs. 22 (40%) patients with a large defect score. Furthermore, the risk for appropriate ICD therapy was 13 times higher in patients with a large defect score as compared with patients with a small defect score; besides, in patients with a large defect score, the risk for appropriate ICD therapy or cardiac death was 8 times higher than in patients with a small defect score.

Recently, Marshall et al. [37] followed up 27 patients with HF referred for ICD implantation for a median of 16 months. Patients who experienced a significant arrhythmic event (37%) had lower early and late HMR and higher SPECT defect score and mismatch perfusion-innervation score than those with no events. Optimal thresholds for predicting arrhythmia were <1.94 for early HMR

(sensitivity 70%, specificity 88%); <1.54 for late HMR (sensitivity 60%, specificity 88%); and SPECT defect score ≥31 (sensitivity 78%, specificity 77%). Despite all this evidence, no single measurement provides sufficient reassurance to obviate device implantation if otherwise indicated by current guidelines. This is so because medical–legal consequences may arise if a patient meeting guidelines does not receive an ICD based on ^{123}I-mIBG imaging and subsequently suffers an SCD. Further studies are needed to define which parameter (HMR, WR, or SPECT defect score, and respective cut-off values) will be more effective for risk stratification.

Although current guidelines include specific recommendations for the use of cardiac resynchronization therapy (CRT) in patients with HF [26] there is less consensus about its use in HF patients with right bundle branch block or inter-ventricular conduction delay and those in atrial fibrillation. Another area of debate is what to do in HF patients without an indication for CRT who need a conventional pacemaker. The possibility that patients with a QRS duration of <120 ms may have 'mechanical dyssynchrony' (detectable by imaging) and might benefit from CRT is another area of research interest but remains to be proven. CRT has been shown to have a favourable effect on cardiac sympathetic innervation, as reflected by improved ^{123}I-mIBG uptake, which supports the potential value of cardiac innervation imaging in the assessment of the efficacy of CRT in patients with HF [38–40]. Furthermore, decreased late HMR has been associated with poor response to CRT (see ⊃ Fig. 29.6) [41, 42]. Recently, Tanaka et al. [43] found that HF patients with dyssynchrony had significantly less cardiac sympathetic activity than those without dyssynchrony, despite having similar LVEF. Dyssynchrony and late HMR ≥1.6 were associated with a high frequency of response to CRT and favourable long-term outcome over 3 years, thus highlighting the potential value of ^{123}I-mIBG cardiac imaging for predicting the response to CRT (see ⊃ Fig. 29.7).

In selected patients presenting with end-stage HF, ventricular assist devices for mechanical circulatory support may be used as a 'bridge to decision' or longer term [26]. Drakos et al. [44] reported that LV assist device therapy produces clinical, functional, and haemodynamic improvements accompanied by improvements in ^{123}I-mIBG imaging, which might be relevant, particularly for recipients of ventricular assist devices whose native cardiac function

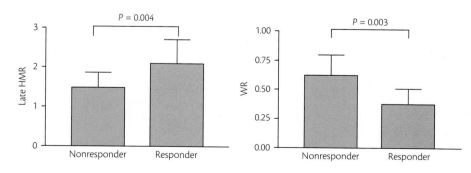

Fig. 29.6 Graphs showing baseline values for late HMR and WR (mean±SD) in 45 patients with heart failure who received cardiac resynchronization therapy (CRT). Responders (22 patients) had a significantly higher late HMR (2.11 vs. 1.48) and lower WR (37% vs. 62%) than non-responders (23 patients). HMR, heart to mediastinum ratio; WR, wash-out rate. Reproduced from Yong-Mei Cha et al, Cardiac sympathetic reserve and response to cardiac resynchronization therapy, *Circulation: Heart Failure*, 4:3 2011, 339–44, with permission from Wolters Kluwer.

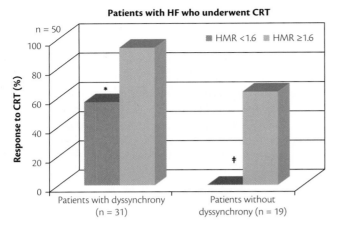

Fig. 29.7 Relationship between response rate to CRT and combined assessment of LV mechanical dyssynchrony and late HMR. Patients with dyssynchrony and HMR ≥1.6 had the highest frequency of LV functional improvement. Contrarily, patients without dyssynchrony and HMR <1.6 had the lowest frequency of LV functional improvement. CRT, cardiac resynchronization therapy; HMR, heart to mediastinum ratio; LV, left ventricular. *, ‡ P = 0.03. Modified from [43].

is difficult to evaluate. Moreover, improvement in ^{123}I-mIBG imaging together with sustained myocardial functional recovery could potentially identify responders to mechanical circulatory support who might become candidates for explantation of the device. Further studies are needed to determine if patients with severe HF and a poor vs. favourable cardiac adrenergic imaging to maximal medical therapy have a more favourable outcome with ventricular assist devices compared to continued medical therapy alone.

Imaging cardiac innervation in dysautonomias

Cardiac ^{123}I-mIBG uptake may be impaired in some patients with disorders of the central and peripheral nervous system associated with autonomic dysfunction.

Diabetes mellitus

Diabetes and prolonged hyperglycaemia are associated with terminal autonomic neuropathy, which in its turn is associated with orthostatic hypotension, resting tachycardia, exercise intolerance, derangement in myocardial blood flow regulation, LV dysfunction, and silent myocardial ischaemia/infarction, resulting in higher susceptibility to cardiac death [45].

Association of reduced ^{123}I-mIBG uptake and autonomic dysfunction has been reported to correlate with increased mortality in diabetics. In addition, cardiac ^{123}I-mIBG imaging appears to be more sensitive than autonomic nervous function tests for the detection of dysautonomia, particularly in the early stages of diabetes. Moreover, the impairment of cardiac sympathetic innervation by means of ^{123}I-mIBG imaging has been shown to correlate with abnormal response to exercise, and may contribute to LV dysfunction before the appearance of irreversible damage and overt HF or CAD in epicardial arteries.

Recently, another substudy of the ADMIRE-HF trial showed that diabetics have lower late HMR than non-diabetic counterparts, which is associated with a greater incidence of cardiac events and HF progression [46]. Further studies are needed to establish if cardiac innervation imaging in diabetics can effectively detect higher risk than is clinically apparent.

Conclusions

Imaging cardiac innervation has provided significant understanding of sympathetic innervation of the heart and its functional role in physiologic and pathophysiologic states, identifying the consequences of presynaptic sympathetic denervation in CAD, arrhythmogenesis, and HF, with high prognostic value, providing a potential tool for improving patient management. Future of cardiac neurotransmission imaging includes the development of tracers for the postsynaptic sympathetic system and for the parasympathetic system, the combination of different tracers for detailed insight into the pathobiology or biology of cardiac innervation, and the establishment of quantitative measures for global and regional innervation [47].

References

1. Carrió I. Cardiac neurotransmission imaging. *J Nucl Med* 2001; 42: 1062–76.
2. Flotats A, Carrió I. Cardiac neurotransmission SPECT imaging. *J Nucl Cardiol* 2004; 11: 587–602.
3. Bengel FM, Schwaiger M. Assessment of cardiac sympathetic neuronal function using PET imaging. *J Nucl Cardiol* 2004; 11: 603–16.
4. Travin MI. Cardiac autonomic imaging with SPECT tracers. *J Nucl Cardiol* 2013; 20: 128–43.
5. Thackeray JT, Bengel FM. Assessment of cardiac autonomic neuronal function using PET imaging. *J Nucl Cardiol* 2013; 20: 150–65.
6. Veltman CE, Boogers MJ, Meinardi JE, et al. Reproducibility of planar ^{123}I-meta-iodobenzylguanidine (mIBG) myocardial scintigraphy in patients with heart failure. *Eur J Nucl Med Mol Imaging* 2012; 39: 1599–608.
7. Jacobson AF, Matsuoka DT. Influence of myocardial region of interest definition on quantitative analysis of planar ^{123}I-mIBG images. *Eur J Nucl Med Mol Imaging* 2013; 40: 558–64.
8. Chen JI, Folks RD, Verdes L, Manatunga DN, Jacobson AF, Garcia EV. Quantitative I-123 mIBG SPECT in differentiating abnormal and normal mIBG myocardial uptake. *J Nucl Cardiol* 2012; 19: 92–9.
9. van der Veen BJ, Al Younis I, de Roos A, Stokkel MPM. Assessment of global cardiac I-123 mIBG uptake and washout using volumetric quantification of SPECT acquisitions. *J Nucl Cardiol* 2012; 19: 4; 752–62.

10. Yu M, Bozek J, Lamoy M, et al. Evaluation of LMI1195, a novel 18F-labeled cardiac neuronal PET imaging agent, in cells and animal models. *Circ Cardiovasc Imaging* 2011; 4: 435–43.

11. Jang KS, Jung YW, Sherman PS, Quesada CA, Gu G, Raffel DM. Synthesis and bioevaluation of [(18)F]4-fluoro-m-hydroxyphenethyl-guanidine ([(18)F]4F-MHPG): A novel radiotracer for quantitative PET studies of cardiac sympathetic innervation. *Bioorg Med Chem Lett* 2013 pii: S0960-894X(13)00139-X. doi: 10.1016/j.bmcl.2013.01.106 [Epub ahead of print].

12. Fallavollita JA, CantyJr JM. Dysinnervated but viable myocardium in ischaemic heart disease. *J Nucl Cardiol* 2010; 17: 1107–15.

13. Katsikis A, Ekonomopoulos G, Papaioannou S, Kouzoumi A, Koutelou M. Reversible reduction of cardiac sympathetic innervation after coronary artery bypass graft surgery: an observational study using serial iodine 123-labeled meta-iodobenzyl-guanidine (mIBG) imaging. *J Thorac Cardiovasc Surg* 2012; 144: 210–6.

14. Chen LS, Zhou S, Fishbein MC, Chen PS. New perspectives on the role of autonomic nervous system in the genesis of arrhythmias. *J Cardiovasc Electrophysiol* 2007; 18: 123–7.

15. Akutsu Y, Kaneko K, Kodama Y, et al. Iodine-123mIBG imaging for predicting the development of atrial fibrillation. *J Am Coll Cardiol Imaging* 2011; 4: 78–86.

16. Ungerer M, Bohm M, Elce J, Erdmann E, Lohse MJ. Altered expression of beta-adrenergic receptor kinase and beta-adrenergic receptors in the failing human heart. *Circulation* 1993; 87: 454–63.

17. Henderson EB, Kahn JK, Corbett JR, et al. Abnormal I-123-mIBG myocardial wash-out and distribution may reflect myocardial adrenergic derangement in patients with congestive cardiomyopathy. *Circulation* 1988; 78: 1192–9.

18. Cohn JN, Levine TB, Olivari MT, et al. Plasma norepinephrine as a guide to prognosis in patients with chronic congestive heart failure. *N Engl J Med* 1984; 311: 819–23.

19. Levy D, Kenchaiah S, Larson MG, Benjamin EJ, Kupka MJ, Ho KK, et al. Long-term trends in the incidence of and survival with heart failure. *N Engl J Med* 2002; 347: 1397–402.

20. Verberne HJ, Brewster LM, Somsen GA, van Eck-Smit BL. Prognostic value of myocardial 123I-metaiodobenzylguanidine (mIBG) parameters in patients with heart failure: A systematic review. *Eur Heart J* 2008; 29: 1147–59.

21. Jacobson AF, Senior R, Cerqueira MD, et al. Myocardial iodine-123 meta-iodobenzylguanidine imaging and cardiac events in heart failure. Results of the prospective ADMIRE-HF (AdreView Myocardial Imaging for Risk Evaluation in Heart Failure) study. *J Am Coll Cardiol* 2010; 55: 2212–21.

22. Ketchum ES, Jacobson AF, Caldwell JH, et al. Selective improvement in Seattle Heart Failure Model risk stratification using iodine-123 meta-iodobenzylguanidine imaging. *J Nucl Cardiol* 2012; 19: 1007–16.

23. Shah AM, Bourgoun M, Narula J, Jacobson AF, Solomon SD. Influence of ejection fraction on the prognostic value of sympathetic innervation imaging with iodine-123 mIBG in heart failure. *JACC Cardiovasc Imaging* 2012; 5: 1139–46.

24. Doi T, Nakata T, Hashimoto A, et al. Cardiac mortality assessment improved by evaluation of cardiac sympathetic nerve activity in combination with hemoglobin and kidney function in chronic heart failure patients. *J Nucl Med* 2012; 53: 731–40.

25. Kasama S, Toyama T, Sumino H, et al. Prognostic value of serial cardiac mIBG imaging in patients with stabilized chronic heart failure and reduced left ventricular ejection fraction. *J Nucl Med* 2008; 49: 907–14.

26. McMurray JJ, Adamopoulos S, Anker SD, et al. ESC Committee for Practice Guidelines. ESC Guidelines for the diagnosis and treatment of acute and chronic heart failure 2012: The Task Force for the Diagnosis and Treatment of Acute and Chronic Heart Failure 2012 of the European Society of Cardiology. Developed in collaboration with the Heart Failure Association (HFA) of the ESC. *Eur Heart J* 2012; 33: 1787–847.

27. Moss AJ, Hall WJ, Cannom DS, et al. Improved survival with an implanted defibrillator in patients with coronary disease at high risk for ventricular arrhythmia. Multicenter Automatic Defibrillator Implantation Trial Investigators. *N Engl J Med* 1996; 335: 1933–40.

28. Hohnloser SH, Connolly SJ, Kuck KH, Dorian P, Fain E, Hampton JR, et al. The defibrillator in acute myocardial infarction trial (DINAMIT): study protocol. *Am Heart J* 2000; 140: 735–9.

29. Kadish A, Dyer A, Daubert JP, et al. Prophylactic defibrillator implantation in patients with nonischaemic dilated cardiomyopathy. *N Engl J Med* 2004; 350: 2151–8.

30. Bardy GH, Lee KL, Mark DB, et al. Amiodarone or an implantable cardioverter-defibrillator for congestive heart failure. *N Engl J Med* 2005; 352: 225–37.

31. Kelesidis I, Travin MI. Use of cardiac radionuclide imaging to identify patients at risk for arrhythmic sudden cardiac death. *J Nucl Cardiol* 2012; 19: 142–52.

32. Barron HV, Viskin S. Autonomic markers and prediction of cardiac death after myocardial infarction. *Lancet* 1998; 351: 461–2.

33. Bax JJ, Kraft O, Buxton AE, et al. 123I-mIBG Scintigraphy to predict inducibility of ventricular arrhythmias on cardiac electrophysiology testing: a prospective multicenter pilot study. *Circ Cardiovasc Imaging* 2008; 1: 131–40.

34. Tamaki S, Yamada T, Okuyama Y, et al. Cardiac iodine-123 meta-iodobenzylguanidine imaging predicts sudden cardiac death independently of left ventricular ejection fraction in patients with chronic heart failure and left ventricular systolic dysfunction: results from a comparative study with signal-averaged electrocardiogram, heart rate variability, and QT dispersion. *J Am Coll Cardiol* 2009; 53: 426–35.

35. Nishisato K, Hashimoto A, Nakata T, Doi T, Yamamoto H, Nagahara D, et al. Impaired cardiac sympathetic innervation and myocardial perfusion are related to lethal arrhythmia: quantification of cardiac tracers in patients with ICDs. *J Nucl Med* 2010; 51: 1241–9.

36. Boogers MJ, Borleffs CJ, Henneman MM, et al. Cardiac sympathetic denervation assessed with 123-iodine metaiodobenzylguanidine imaging predicts ventricular arrhythmias in implantable cardioverter-defibrillator patients. *J Am Coll Cardiol* 2010; 55: 2769–77.

37. Marshall A, Cheetham A, George RS, Mason M, Kelion AD. Cardiac iodine-123 metaiodobenzylguanidine imaging predicts ventricular arrhythmia in heart failure patients receiving an implantable cardioverter-defibrillator for primary prevention. *Heart* 2012; 98: 1359–65.

38. Higuchi K, Toyama T, Tada H, Naito S, Ohshima S, Kurabayashi M. Usefulness of biventricular pacing to improve cardiac symptoms, exercise capacity and sympathetic nerve activity in patients with moderate to severe chronic heart failure. *Circ J* 2006; 70: 703–9.

39. Burri H, Sunthorn H, Somsen A, et al. Improvement in cardiac sympathetic nerve activity in responders to resynchronization therapy. *Europace* 2008; 10: 374–8.

40. Shinohara T, Takahashi N, Saito S, et al. Effect of cardiac resynchronization therapy on cardiac sympathetic nervous dysfunction and serum C-reactive protein level. *Pacing Clin Electrophysiol* 2011; 34: 1225–30.

41. Nishioka SA, Martinelli Filho M, Brandão SC, et al. Cardiac sympathetic activity pre and post resynchronization therapy evaluated by 123I-mIBG myocardial scintigraphy. *J Nucl Cardiol* 2007; 14: 852–9.

42. Cha YM, Chareonthaitawee P, Dong YX, et al. Cardiac sympathetic reserve and response to cardiac resynchronization therapy. *Circ Heart Fail* 2011; 4: 339–44.

43. Tanaka H, Tatsumi K, Fujiwara S, et al. Effect of left ventricular dyssynchrony on cardiac sympathetic activity in heart failure patients with wide QRS duration. *Circ J* 2012; 76: 382–9.

44. Drakos SG, Athanasoulis T, Malliaras KG, et al. Myocardial sympathetic innervation and long-term left ventricular mechanical unloading. *J Am Coll Cardiol Imaging* 2010; 3: 64–70.

44. Flotats A, Carrió I. The role of nuclear medicine technique in evaluating electrophysiology in diabetic hearts especially with 123I-mIBG cardiac SPECT imaging. *Minerva Endocrinol* 2009; 34: 263–71.

46. Gerson MC, Caldwell JH, Ananthasubramaniam K, et al. Influence of diabetes mellitus on prognostic utility of imaging of myocardial sympathetic innervation in heart failure patients. *Circ Cardiovasc Imaging* 2011; 4: 87–93.

47. Bengel FM. Imaging targets of the sympathetic nervous system of the heart: translational considerations. *J Nucl Med* 2011; 52: 1167–70.

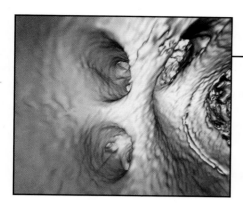

CHAPTER 30

Cardiac resynchronization therapy: selection of candidates

Victoria Delgado and Jeroen J. Bax

Contents

Introduction

Heart failure is a major public-health problem with a prevalence of 1–2% of the adult population in developed countries [1, 2]. Cardiac resynchronization therapy (CRT) is an established therapy for patients with heart failure who remain symptomatic despite optimal medical treatment. The first randomized trials in the early 1990s showed the benefit of CRT in heart failure patients with New York Heart Association (NYHA) class III–IV, left ventricular ejection fraction (LVEF) <35% and wide QRS complex (>120 ms) [3–8]. Subsequently, the efficacy of CRT in patients with mild heart failure (NYHA class I–II) was shown [9–11], although data in patients with NYHA class I are limited. In addition, subsequent sub-analyses and one meta-analysis have demonstrated the efficacy of CRT in reducing all-cause mortality and heart failure hospitalizations in patients with complete left bundle branch block (LBBB) morphology, but not in patients with non-LBBB patterns [12]. Similarly, a meta-analysis with 6,501 patients demonstrated that CRT reduced all-cause mortality and heart failure hospitalizations in patients with QRS duration ≥150 ms (hazard ratio: 0.58, 95% confidence interval 0.50–0.68; P<0.001), but not in patients with QRS duration <150 ms (hazard ratio: 0.95, 95% confidence interval 0.83–1.10; $P = 0.51$) [13]. Finally, the majority of patients included in randomized controlled trials were in sinus rhythm and only 1% of patients had atrial fibrillation. Therefore, current guidelines limit a class IA indication for CRT to patients with NYHA II–IV heart failure symptoms, despite optimal medical treatment, who have sinus rhythm, QRS with LBBB morphology, and ≥150 ms duration and LVEF<35% [14, 15].

An important question remains the prediction of response to CRT, since 30–40% of patients do not respond to the therapy [16]. A related problem is that the definition of response to CRT is not clear, and echocardiographic response (frequently defined as LV reverse remodelling) occurs less often than clinical response (e.g. improvement in NYHA class or 6-minute walk distance) [17, 18]. It has, however, been shown that a reduction in LV end-systolic volume was associated with better long-term outcome than clinical response [19].

Identification of patients who will benefit from CRT remains challenging. Several studies have shown that LV dyssynchrony, the extent and location of myocardial scar, and the position of the LV pacing lead are independent determinants of CRT response and were associated with improved long-term outcome after CRT [20–23]. The variable response to heart failure therapies, particularly to CRT, underscores the need of a personalized approach targeting the underlying pathophysiological mechanisms related to CRT response. In this regard, non-invasive cardiac imaging provides detailed structural and functional information, which may improve selection of patients with high likelihood of CRT response. Multimodality imaging permits accurate assessment of LV volumes and

LVEF, LV mechanics and dyssynchrony, but also myocardial scar and venous anatomy can be visualized.

This chapter reviews the current applications of multimodality imaging in the selection of CRT candidates.

Imaging LV dyssynchrony

Heart failure is frequently associated with impaired electromechanical coupling including prolonged atrioventricular, inter-ventricular, and intra-ventricular conduction (➲ Fig. 30.1) [24]. Prolonged atrioventricular conduction leads to impaired LV diastolic filling and reduced LV preload and stroke volume. Prolonged inter-ventricular and intra-ventricular conduction cause regional mechanical contraction delay leading to reduced LV systolic function, adverse remodelling and development of functional mitral regurgitation. CRT optimizes LV diastolic filling and stroke volume by resynchronizing the atrioventricular, the inter-ventricular, and the intra-ventricular (LV) contractions. Particularly, presence of significant inter-ventricular and intra-ventricular dyssynchrony, as assessed with imaging techniques, has been associated with

improved long-term outcome of patients undergoing CRT implantation (➲ Table 30.1) [21, 25–28].

Atrioventricular dyssynchrony

Prolonged atrioventricular conduction can be assessed with pulsed wave Doppler echocardiographic recordings of the mitral valve inflow: fusion of the early (E) and late (A) diastolic waves can be observed leading to a reduced LV filling time relative to the cardiac cycle length (➲ Fig. 30.2a). An LV filling time <40% of the total cardiac length denotes significant atrioventricular dyssynchrony [6].

Inter-ventricular dyssynchrony

The time difference between right ventricular and LV ejection defines inter-ventricular mechanical dyssynchrony. The CARE-HF trial considered this measurement as one of the inclusion criteria for patients with QRS duration between 120 and 149 ms [7]. Using pulsed wave Doppler echocardiography at the level of the pulmonic valve and LV outflow tract, the time elapsed between the onset of the pulmonic and aortic flow can be calculated (➲ Fig. 30.2b). A time delay >40 ms indicates significant inter-ventricular mechanical delay.

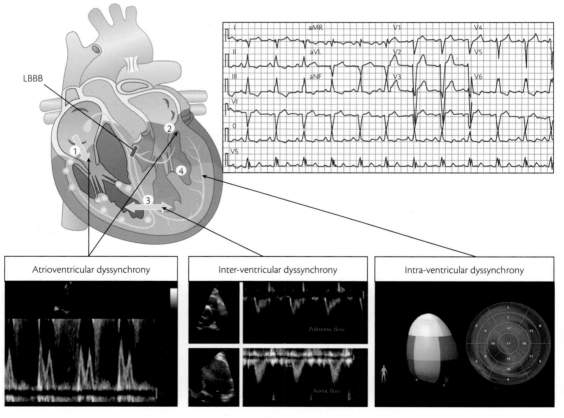

Fig. 30.1 Cardiac dyssynchrony. Different types of cardiac dyssynchrony can be assessed in patients with heart failure. A prolonged atrioventricular conduction reflected on the ECG by a PR interval >200 ms can be visualized on transmitral flow from pulsed wave Doppler recordings, showing a fusion of the E and A waves, with a reduced left ventricular filling time (<40% of the cardiac cycle). Left bundle branch block (LBBB) will cause inter-ventricular dyssynchrony that can be assessed with echocardiography measuring the time delay between the right and left ventricular ejection on pulsed wave Doppler recordings of right and left ventricular outflow tracts. Finally, prolonged intra-ventricular conduction can be also reflected by a wide QRS complex and can be assessed with several LV dyssynchrony parameters derived from non-invasive imaging.

Reprinted from *The Lancet*, 378:9792, Holzmeister J et al, Implantable cardioverter defibrillators and cardiac resynchronisation therapy, 722–30, Copyright 2011, with permission from Elsevier.

Table 30.1 Relation between cardiac dyssynchrony and long-term prognosis of patients treated with cardiac resynchronization therapy

First Author	Patients, n	Follow-up, months	Cardiac dyssynchrony parameter	Endpoint	Hazard ratio (95% confidence interval)
Richardson et al. [26]	813	29.4	IVMD ≥49.2 ms	All-cause mortality of hospitalization for heart failure	0.50 (0.36–0.70)
Wiesbauer et al. [27]	200	10	IVMD ≥60 ms	All-cause mortality	0.21 (0.07–0.6)
Zhang et al. [28]	239	37±20	TDI maximal opposing delay ≥65 ms	All-cause mortality	0.46 (0.27–0.79)
Delgado et al. [25]	397	21	Radial strain speckle tracking anteroseptal to posterior delay ≥130 ms	All-cause mortality	0.995 (0.992–0.998)
Gorcsan et al. [21]	210	48	Standard deviation of time to peak systolic velocity of 12 segments ≥32 ms Radial strain speckle tracking anteroseptal to posterior delay ≥130 ms	Freedom from death, transplant or LVAD	2.21 (1.35–4.79) 2.13 (1.38–4.46)

Abbreviations: IVMD, inter-ventricular mechanical dyssynchrony; LVAD: left ventricular assistance device; TDI: tissue Doppler imaging.

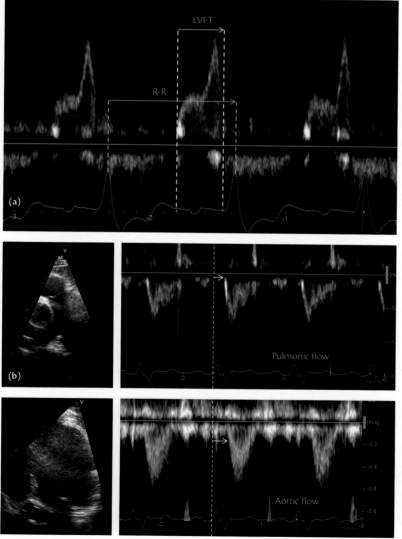

Fig. 30.2 Assessment of atrioventricular and inter-ventricular dyssynchrony with pulsed wave Doppler echocardiography. (a) An example of transmitral flow assessed by pulsed wave Doppler of a patient with atrioventricular dyssynchrony measured as the ratio between left ventricular filling time (onset of the E wave and end of A wave) and the R–R interval <40%. (b) An example of a patient with inter-ventricular dyssynchrony measured as the time difference between onset of right ventricular ejection (time from QRS onset to pulmonic flow onset) and onset of left ventricular ejection (time from QRS onset to aortic flow onset) >40 ms. LVFT, left ventricular filling time.

LV dyssynchrony, echocardiographic techniques

Echocardiography has provided numerous LV dyssynchrony indices. A comprehensive overview of the different echocardiographic techniques and their proposed cut-off values, used to indicate significant LV dyssynchrony, are provided in ⊃ Table 30.2. Patients with LBBB typically exhibit a delay in contraction between the septum and posterior wall on M-mode echocardiography, and a time difference ≥130 ms predicted CRT response with a sensitivity and specificity of 100% and 63%, respectively [29]. In patients with previous infarction however, this approach may not be feasible [30].

Table 30.2 Echocardiographic indices of LV dyssynchrony

Echocardiographic technique	LV dyssynchrony parameter cut-off value
M-mode 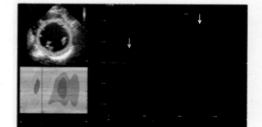	Septal-to-posterior wall motion delay ≥130 ms
Tissue Doppler imaging	Maximum delay between 4 opposing walls (septal, lateral, anterior and inferior) ≥65 ms Standard deviation of time to peak systolic velocity of 12 mid and basal LV segments; ≥34.4 ms
Tissue Doppler derived strain	Time to peak radial strain between anteroseptal and posterior wall ≥130 ms
Speckle tracking	Radial strain: anteroseptal-to-posterior wall delay ≥130 ms Longitudinal strain: systolic delay index ≥25% Septal systolic rebound stretch ≥4.7%

Echocardiographic technique	LV dyssynchrony parameter cut-off value
3-dimensional echocardiography 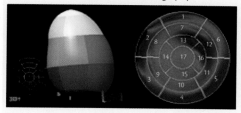	Standard deviation of time to minimum volume of 16 or 17 subvolumes ≥9.8%
Triplane tissue synchronization imaging 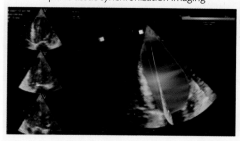	Standard deviation of time to peak systolic velocity of 12 segments ≥33ms

Tissue Doppler imaging (TDI) permits assessment of regional myocardial velocities, and the delay in activation/displacement between two or more opposing LV segments provides another measurement of dyssynchrony. Different models have been proposed, including 2, 4, or 12 myocardial segments, to assess LV dyssynchrony [31, 32]. Assessment of myocardial velocity or displacement is affected by translational artefacts and tethering effects from surrounding segments. TDI-derived strain (rate) may overcome this limitation, since it permits differentiation between passive motion and active deformation. A time delay ≥130 ms between peak radial strain of the anteroseptal and posterior segments (on the mid-ventricular LV short-axis view) was associated with improvement in LVEF after CRT [33]. TDI-derived velocity or strain are limited to the basal and mid-ventricular segments, since the angle insonation dependency precludes assessment of the apical segments.

Despite the promising results in single-centre trials, the multi-centre PROSPECT (prediction of response to CRT) trial (which included 498 CRT candidates) revealed only modest accuracy of the echocardiographic dyssynchrony indices to predict CRT response [34]. This finding may partially be related to patient selection but also to technical issues, including limited reproducibility of measurements. More robust dyssynchrony techniques have been developed subsequently, including 2-dimensional (2D) speckle tracking strain assessment and 3-dimensional (3D) echocardiography.

The introduction of 2D speckle tracking echocardiography has realized multidirectional angle-independent strain assessment of all LV segments. A time difference ≥130 ms of peak radial strain (thickening) between the anteroseptal and posterior walls was predictive of CRT response (sensitivity 83%, specificity 80%) and, more importantly, was related to improved long-term prognosis [25, 35]. Furthermore, assessment of LV longitudinal strain with speckle tracking provided the so-called strain delay index, which combines LV dyssynchrony and mechanical efficiency [36]. In addition, evaluation of abnormal septal myocardial stretching

during systole with longitudinal strain speckle tracking echocardiography (septal systolic rebound stretch index) has been proposed as a novel index of mechanical dyscoordination [37, 38]. This index is quantified as the amount of septal systolic stretch occurring after initial shortening and patients with favourable CRT response showed 2.5 times higher septal systolic rebound stretch compared to non-responders ($2.8\pm1.7\%$ versus $7.1\pm3.1\%$, $P<0.001$) [38].

The other important technical innovation is the use of 3D-echocardiography for LV dyssynchrony assessment. The available 3D techniques employ TDI or speckle tracking. These techniques provide graphic displays with colour-coding to indicate segmental times to mechanical activation (either velocity or strain) (⊃ Fig. 30.3) [39, 40]. A different 3D approach relies on the assessment of segmental times to minimum volume, and the dispersion of times in a 16- or 17-segment model provides the systolic dyssynchrony index (⊃ Fig. 30.4). From a pooled analysis including 600 patients undergoing CRT, a systolic dyssynchrony index of 9.8% yielded a sensitivity of 93% with a specificity of 75% to predict CRT response [41]. The 3D techniques facilitate visualization of the site of latest mechanical activation or latest ventricular emptying (minimal volume).

LV dyssynchrony, non-echocardiographic techniques

Various MRI approaches have been introduced for the detection of LV dyssynchrony (⊃ Table 30.3). Velocity-encoded MRI permits similarly to echocardiographic TDI, assessment of timing of segmental peak systolic velocities, and the time difference between peak systolic velocity of the basal septum and lateral wall provides a measure of LV dyssynchrony [42]. Head-to-head comparison between velocity-encoded MRI and echocardiographic TDI demonstrated good agreement for LV dyssynchrony assessment.

A second approach utilizes cine steady-state free precession (SSFP) sequences, encompassing the left ventricle from the apex to

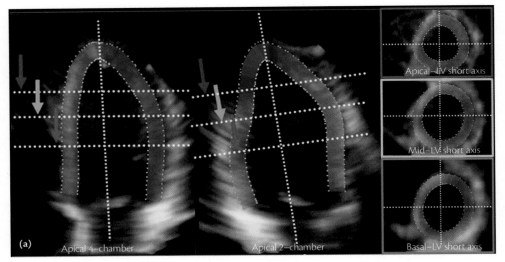

Fig. 30.3 LV dyssynchrony assessment with 3-dimensional speckle tracking echocardiography. (a) From a 3D full volume acquisition of the left ventricle, the apical 4- and 2-chamber views and three sequential short-axis views (apical—blue arrow and panel; mid-ventricular—yellow arrow and panel; and basal—purple arrow and panel) are displayed. The endocardial region of interest is counter-clockwise traced in the apical views and the software automatically traces a region of interest that includes the entire myocardial thickness in all views and divides the left ventricle into 16 segments. (b) A colour-coded 3D reconstructed model of the LV with the 16 segments; the polar maps are provided demonstrating the dyssynchronous contraction of the left ventricle with the posterior wall as the most delayed region. The time to radial strain curves permit the measurement of the standard deviation of time to peak radial strain of the 16 segments and time difference between the earliest and the latest activated segments (white arrow). Reprinted from the *American Journal of Cardiology*, 105:2, Hidekazu Tanaka et al, Usefulness of three-dimensional speckle tracking strain to quantify dyssynchrony and the site of latest mechanical activation, 235–42, Copyright 2010 with permission from Elsevier.

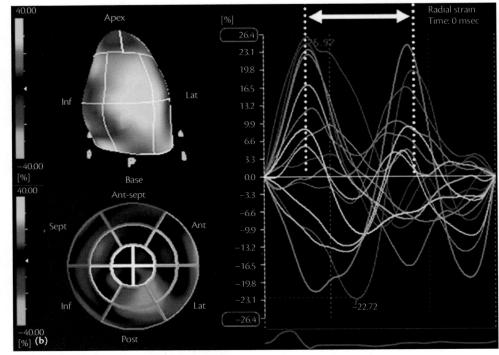

Fig. 30.4 Real-time 3-dimensional echocardiography: volumetric assessment of LV dyssynchrony. (a) The example of synchronous LV contraction assessed with real-time 3D-echocardiography. From a 3D full volume of the left ventricle, the time dispersion to minimum regional volume of 16 segments is calculated. The graph shows the time-volume curves of the 16 segments providing a systolic dyssynchrony index (SDI) of 2.2%. (b) The example of dyssynchronous LV contraction with an SDI of 13.4%.

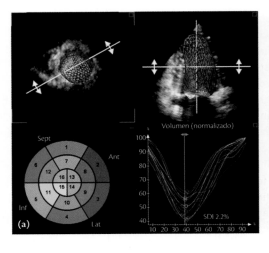

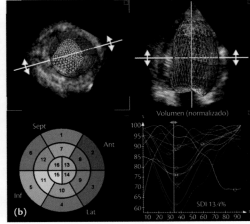

Table 30.3 Magnetic resonance imaging techniques to assess LV dyssynchrony

MRI technique		LV dyssynchrony parameter
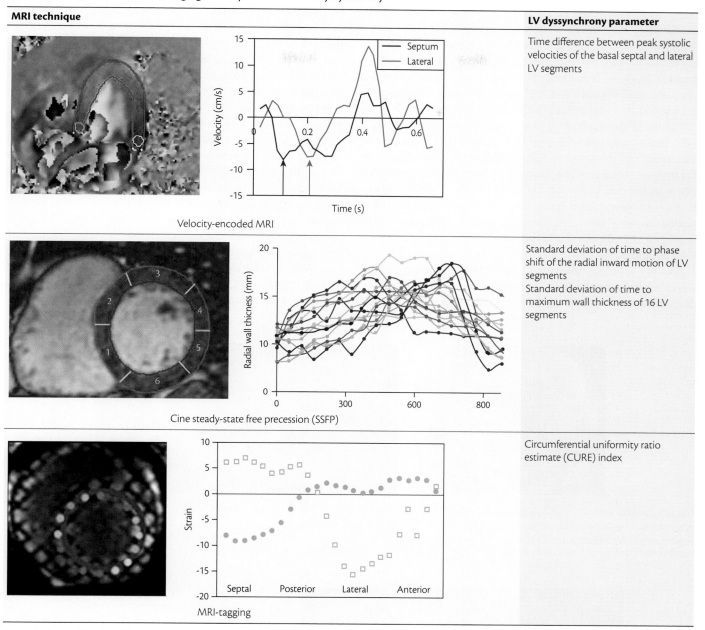		Time difference between peak systolic velocities of the basal septal and lateral LV segments
Velocity-encoded MRI		
Cine steady-state free precession (SSFP)		Standard deviation of time to phase shift of the radial inward motion of LV segments Standard deviation of time to maximum wall thickness of 16 LV segments
MRI-tagging		Circumferential uniformity ratio estimate (CURE) index

Adapted with permission from Westenberg et al. [42], Marsan et al. [44], and Bilchick et al. [45].
Abbreviations: LV: left ventricular; MRI: magnetic resonance imaging.

the mitral annulus; sequential LV short-axis slices are reconstructed and radial wall motion is analysed for the different segments of each short-axis slice along 20–40 phases of the R–R interval [43, 44]. The standard deviation of all segmental phase shifts of the radial inward motion, provides the tissue synchronization index [43]. In a similar manner, LV dyssynchrony can be also quantified by calculation of the standard deviation of time to maximum wall thickness in 16 myocardial segments [44].

A third approach employs MRI tagging from which LV circumferential shortening can be evaluated on LV short-axis acquisitions and the time dispersion to segmental peak circumferential shortening can be derived. The circumferential uniformity ratio

estimate (CURE) is an LV dyssynchrony index derived from the measurement of circumferential strain in 24 segments of 3 evenly spaced LV short-axis slices and its value ranges from 0 (pure dyssynchronous) to 1 (perfectly synchronous) [45]. In 20 heart failure patients, a CURE cut-off value >0.75 predicts CRT response with a sensitivity and specificity of 100% and 71%, respectively [45].

LV dyssynchrony assessment using nuclear imaging techniques has also proven to be accurate in the identification of patients who will benefit from CRT [46, 47]. LV contraction patterns can be assessed with gated blood-pool ventriculography and gated blood-pool single photon emission computed tomography (SPECT). From myocardial perfusion SPECT data, the amplitude (reflecting systolic wall thickening) and phase (reflecting onset of mechanical contraction) can be calculated from the LV short-axis images and the phase standard deviation and the histogram bandwidth can be derived providing measures of LV dyssynchrony (⊃ Fig. 30.5). Prediction of CRT response has been demonstrated using a cut-off value of ≥19.6° for phase standard deviation and ≥72° for histogram bandwidth, yielding a sensitivity and specificity of 83% and 81%, respectively [46].

Finally, LV dyssynchrony can also be determined from MDCT [48]. In 38 patients undergoing ECG-gated MDCT, the time to maximum wall thickness, maximum wall motion, and minimum volume were measured in sequential LV short-axis images at 10% phase increments of the cardiac cycle (⊃ Fig. 30.6). Clear differences in these dyssynchrony parameters were observed when healthy controls were compared with heart failure patients; the feasibility to predict CRT response with MDCT, however, has not been demonstrated yet.

Another approach integrated non-invasive electrophysiological epicardial imaging and CT, enabling reconstruction of cardiac activation maps with high spatial resolution during a single heartbeat [49, 50]. This 'electrocardiographic imaging' is based on acquisition of body surface potentials at 1-ms intervals during the cardiac cycle using a 224-electrode vest and a multichannel mapping system. With the use of thoracic CT, the epicardial geometry and the body surface electrode positions are obtained. These data are fused with the electrocardiographic imaging algorithms to obtain epicardial potentials, electrograms, and activation sequences (isochrones) (⊃ Fig. 30.7). From the isochrone maps, lines or regions of conduction block and sites of latest activation can be localized and time activation differences between the right and left ventricle (so-called ventricular electrical uncoupling index) can be assessed. Recently, Ploux et al. demonstrated that patients with LBBB QRS morphology had longer ventricular electrical uncoupling times than patients with non-specific intra-ventricular conduction disturbance (75±12 ms vs. 40±22 ms, P<0.001). Similarly, CRT responders had longer ventricular electrical uncoupling times than non-responders (72±16 ms vs. 38±23 ms, P<0.001) [51]. A ventricular electrical uncoupling index >50 ms predicted clinical response to CRT with a sensitivity and specificity of 90% and 82%, respectively, regardless of the QRS morphology [51].

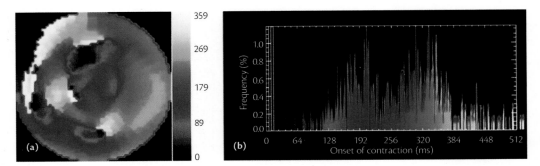

Fig. 30.5 Assessment of LV dyssynchrony with gated myocardial perfusion SPECT. Example of a patient with significant LV dyssynchrony as quantified with the phase standard deviation, presented graphically as a polar map (left), and the bandwidth histogram (right).
Reprinted from the *Journal of the American College of Cardiology*, 49:16, Maureen Henneman et al, Phase analysis of gated myocardial perfusion single-photon emission computed tomography compared with tissue doppler imaging for the assessment of left ventricular dyssynchrony, 1708–14 Copyright 2007 with permission from Elsevier.

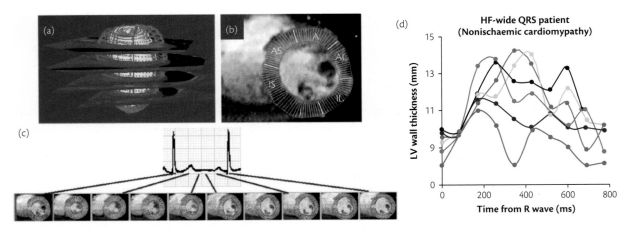

Fig. 30.6 Multi-detector row computed tomography to assess LV dyssynchrony. From the 3D full-volume reconstruction of the left ventricle (a) sequential short-axis images are obtained (b) and evaluated along 10% phase increments of the cardiac cycle (c). The time to maximal wall thickness can be displayed in a graph for each segment of the short-axis image and the time dispersion can be calculated as LV dyssynchrony index (d).
Reprinted from *JACC: Cardiovascular Imaging*, 1:6, Quynh Truong et al, Quantitative analysis of intraventricular dyssynchrony using wall thickness by multidetector computed tomography, 772–81, Copyright 2008 with permission from Elsevier.

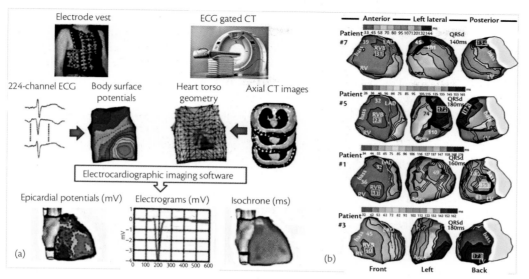

Fig. 30.7 Electrocardiographic imaging for LV dyssynchrony assessment. (a) The data acquisition process using an electrode vest with 224-channel ECG and the ECG-gated computed tomography. From the electrode vest, body surface potentials are obtained and merging with the axial computed tomography data renders a meshed heart-torso geometry. With the electrocardiographic imaging software, epicardial potentials, electrograms and isochrones are obtained. (b) Provides the epicardial isochrones maps of four patients with LBBB QRS morphology and various QRS durations. The epicardial surfaces of the right and left ventricles are displayed in three views: anterior, left lateral, and posterior. The left anterior descending coronary artery is displayed. The grey area indicates the atrioventricular valvular plane. All the epicardial isochrones maps show an early activation of the right ventricle followed by a more delayed activation of the left ventricle. The black lines indicate line/region of conduction block.

Reprinted by permission from Macmillan Publishers Ltd: *Nature Medicine*, Charulatha Ramanathan et al, Noninvasive electrocardiographic imaging for cardiac electrophysiology and arrhythmia, 10:4, Copyright 2004. Adapted with permission [49, 50].

Site of latest activation and cardiac venous anatomy: implications for LV lead implantation

Stable LV lead placement in one of the tributaries of the coronary sinus with good capture thresholds and without phrenic nerve stimulation, can be challenging. Anatomical variants of the coronary sinus ostium, pronounced Thebesian or Vieussens' valves may be important hurdles to cannulate the coronary sinus or to advance the wires through the distal vessels. Moreover, in patients with ischaemic cardiomyopathy, areas with previous infarction may contain fewer veins; particularly the left marginal

vein is less frequently present in patients with ischaemic cardiomyopathy or in patients with lateral infarction [52]. Therefore, accurate knowledge of the cardiac venous anatomy is important, and invasive venography is used during CRT implantation. Frontal or right anterior oblique projections visualize the distribution of veins in the basal, mid-ventricular, and apical regions, whereas the left anterior oblique projection visualizes anterior, postero lateral, or inferior veins (⊃ Fig. 30.8). Alternatively, MDCT also provides high-spatial resolution images of the cardiac venous anatomy (⊃ Fig. 30.9), and also MRI has been used for this purpose [53]. Non-invasive assessment of venous anatomy prior to CRT implantation may help to decide whether transvenous LV lead implantation is feasible or that a minimally

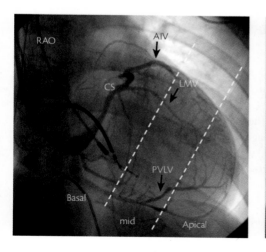

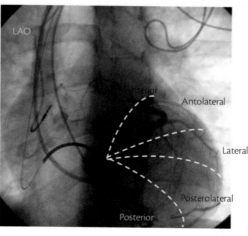

Fig. 30.8 Invasive venous angiography during CRT implantation. In the right anterior oblique projection, the tributaries of the coronary sinus can be visualized on the long-axis view of the left ventricle (arrows) and the position of the LV lead can be divided into basal, mid-ventricular and apical regions. In the left anterior oblique projection the short-axis view of the left ventricle is displayed and the position of the LV lead can be classified into anterior, anterolateral, lateral, posterolateral and posterior. AIV, anterior inter-ventricular vein; CS, coronary sinus; PVLV, posterior vein of the left ventricle.

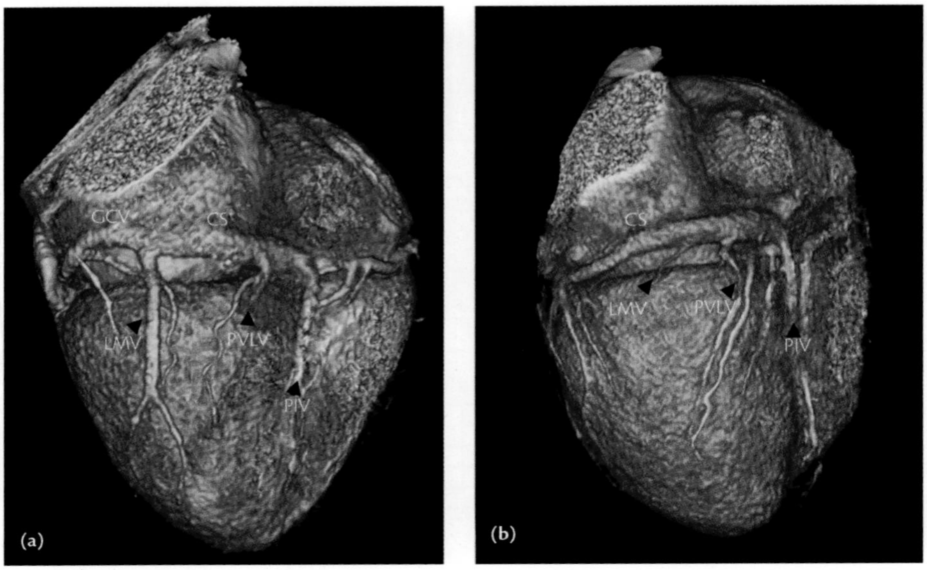

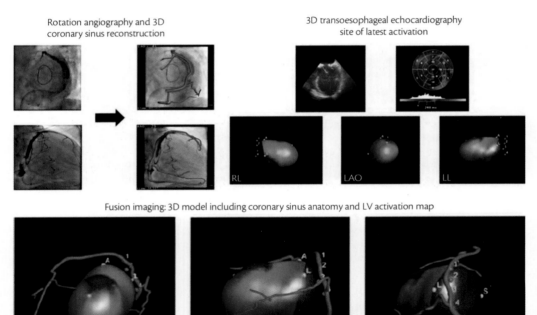

Fig. 30.9 MDCT for assessment of the cardiac venous anatomy. (a) Obtained from a patient with non-ischaemic cardiomyopathy. The first tributary is the posterior inter-ventricular vein (PIV) that runs through the inter-ventricular sulcus. Subsequently, a small posterior vein of the left ventricle (PVLV) can be visualized followed by a well-developed left marginal vein (LMV) suitable for LV lead implantation. Afterwards, the coronary sinus is followed by the great cardiac vein (GCV). (b) Example of a patient with prior posterolateral myocardial infarction. Note the absence of a suitable LMV and the presence of a small PVLV.

Rotation angiography and 3D coronary sinus reconstruction

3D transoesophageal echocardiography site of latest activation

Fig. 30.10 Fusion imaging to guide LV lead implantation. Using rotation angiography a 3D model of the coronary sinus and tributaries is created. In addition, LV mechanical activation is evaluated with 3D transoesophageal echocardiography providing an LV 3D full volume and activation map. The sites of latest activation are colour-coded in red, while the earliest activated segments are colour-coded in blue. The 3D model of the coronary sinus is then overlaid onto the LV 3D activation map allowing for identification of a suitable coronary sinus tributary in the LV areas with latest activation.
Reproduced from Michael Doring et al, Individually tailored left ventricular lead placement: lessons from multimodality integration between three-dimensional echocardiography and coronary sinus angiogram, *Europace*, 15:5 Copyright 2013, by permission of Oxford University Press.

Fusion imaging: 3D model including coronary sinus anatomy and LV activation map

invasive epicardial approach is preferred. Ideally, fusion of 3D maps of venous anatomy and sites of latest mechanical activation may provide a roadmap to decide on the feasibility of transvenous LV lead positioning (➲ Fig. 30.10) [54].

Assessment of myocardial scar prior to CRT implantation

The majority of patients referred for CRT have ischaemic heart failure and previous myocardial infarction(s) [55]. In general, patients with ischaemic heart failure respond less well to CRT as compared to patients with non-ischaemic cardiomyopathy [56], which was recently confirmed by sub-analyses from the CARE-HF and MADIT-CRT trials [20, 57]. The lesser response is most likely related to the presence, location, and extent of scar tissue. Bleeker and colleagues have shown that patients with scar tissue in the postero lateral wall (where the LV pacing lead was positioned) had a low response rate to CRT (14%) [58].

Furthermore, several studies have shown that the extent and transmurality of LV scar is an important determinant of (non-) response to CRT [44, 59, 60]. Accordingly, extensive scar tissue in the LV may be a contraindication to CRT; this, however, remains to be determined in a randomized, controlled trial.

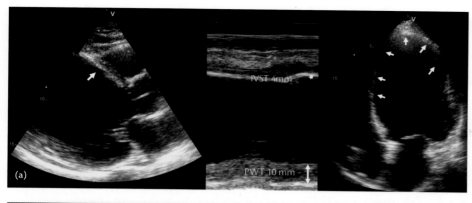

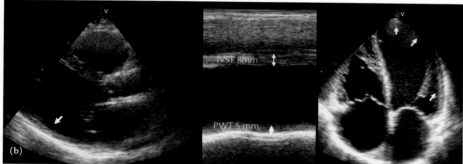

Fig. 30.11 2D-echocardiography to assess myocardial viability. Regions with an end-diastolic wall thickness <6 mm most likely represent scar tissue. (a) Example of a patient with ischaemic heart failure. The parasternal long-axis view shows a bright, thinned anteroseptal wall (arrow) with preserved wall thickness of the posterior wall. The M-mode recordings indicate that the anteroseptal has a thickness of 4 mm, whereas the posterior wall measures 10 mm. The apical 4-chamber view shows the mid-septal segment and the apical region with an end-diastolic wall thickness <6 mm (arrows). (b) Example of patient with a history of inferoposterolateral myocardial infarction. Note the 5-mm thickness of the akinetic posterior wall on the parasternal long-axis view (arrow), which is confirmed on the M-mode recording. The apical 4-chamber view shows a thinned lateral wall (arrows).

Different imaging modalities can detect myocardial scar and viability in CRT candidates. Thinned myocardium on 2D-echocardiography, with an end-diastolic wall thickness <6 mm, is likely to contain transmural scar tissue (⊃ Fig. 30.11) [61]. In segments with preserved LV end-diastolic wall thickness ≥6 mm, it is important to demonstrate contractile reserve (using low-dose dobutamine echocardiography) in order to predict response to CRT [62]. Alternatively, contrast echocardiography can be used to demonstrate or exclude scar tissue (⊃ Fig. 30.12) [63], and the presence of LV segments with scar tissue on contrast echocardiography was associated with lesser improvement in LVEF at follow-up [64].

Nuclear imaging can also be used to assess scar tissue and viable myocardium; both perfusion tracers and F18-fluorodeoxyglucose

have been used for this purpose. Perfusion defects at rest on single photon emission computed tomography (SPECT) or positron emission tomography (PET) indicate the presence of scar tissue (⊃ Fig. 30.13). Based on the number of segments with abnormal perfusion, and the severity of the perfusion defects, a summed score is derived, reflecting the LV total scar burden. In 190 patients with ischaemic heart failure referred for CRT implantation, Adelstein and co-workers demonstrated that a low scar burden was associated with improvement in LVEF at follow-up and superior long-term outcome, as compared to patients with a high scar burden [59].

The preferred technique is contrast-enhanced MRI, which has the highest spatial resolution, permitting differentiation

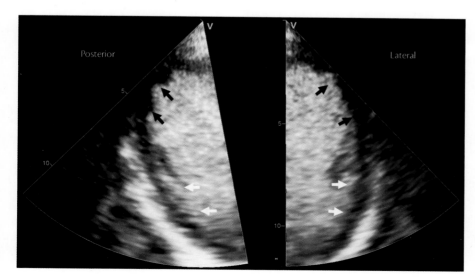

Fig. 30.12 Myocardial contrast echocardiography to assess myocardial viability. With the infusion of echocardiographic contrast agents and application of ultrasound pulses, the integrity of the myocardial capillaries can be evaluated. Areas with scar will appear as perfusion defects (black arrows) whereas viable myocardium will appear bright with intact perfusion (white arrows).

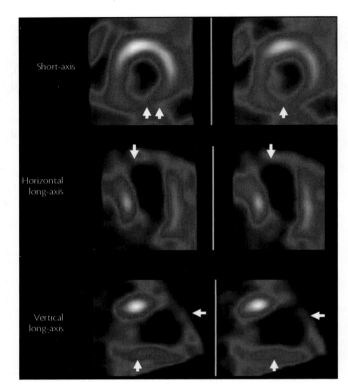

Fig. 30.13 Single photon emission computed tomography to assess myocardial scar. Rest technetium-99m tetrofosmin SPECT images of a heart failure patient undergoing CRT implantation. The short-axis, horizontal and vertical long-axes are presented, showing a large perfusion defect in the posterior, inferior, mid-anterior, and apical regions (arrows).

between transmural and non-transmural scar tissue. The gadolinium contrast agent is trapped in the extracellular matrix, which is larger in scarred regions. Myocardial scar is shown as hyper-enhanced (white) areas and the percentage of hyper-enhancement relative to the wall thickness defines the scar transmurality (⊃ Fig. 30.14). Segments with >75% scar are considered non-viable [65]. The impact of transmural scar at the region targeted by the LV lead on CRT response and clinical outcome was assessed in 209 patients treated with CRT who underwent contrast-enhanced MRI [66]. The clinical response rate to CRT was significantly lower among patients with an LV lead placed in areas with transmural scar as compared to patients without transmural scar (44% vs. 77%, P<0.001) [66]. In addition, patients with an LV lead placed in areas with transmural scar had a significantly increased risk of cardiovascular death and heart failure hospitalizations at follow-up (hazard ratio 5.57, 95% confidence interval 3.4–9.14; P<0.001) [66].

Future directions: integrative evaluation of pathophysiological determinants of CRT outcomes

Current criteria to select patients for CRT (NYHA class, LVEF, QRS duration and morphology) have shown modest accuracy to identify the patients who will benefit from this therapy. Personalized medicine with an integrative evaluation of all pathophysiological

Fig. 30.14 Delayed contrast-enhanced MRI to assess myocardial scar. (a and b) Example of a patient with prior inferoposterior myocardial infarction. On the 4-chamber view (a) the arrows indicate sub-endocardial scar in the basal septum and lateral segments. On the short-axis view (b) the arrows indicate the presence of a transmural scar in the posterior wall. (c and d) Example of a patient with ischaemic cardiomyopathy and extensive apical transmural scar on the 4-chamber view (c) that spreads toward the septum and lateral segments. On the short-axis view, the arrows indicate a large area of transmural scar. Only the posterior and inferior segments contain viable myocardium.

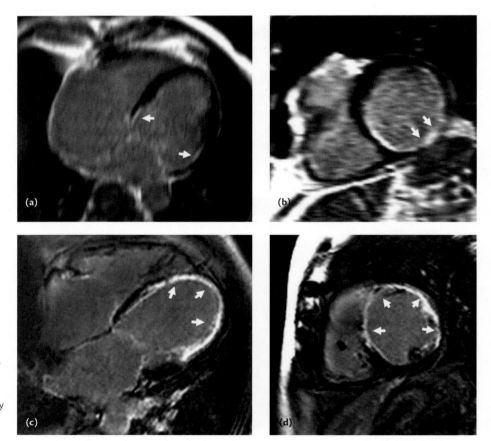

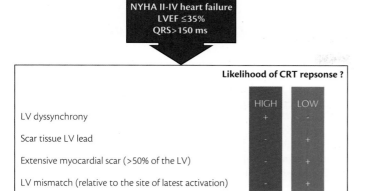

Fig. 30.15 Integrative evaluation of heart failure patients who are candidates to CRT: LV dyssynchrony, myocardial scar and region of latest activation. LV, left ventricular; LVEF, left ventricular ejection fraction; NYHA, New York Heart Association.

Reprinted from the *Journal of the American College of Cardiology* 53:21, Jeroen Bax et al, Echocardiography and noninvasive imaging in cardiac resynchronization therapy: results of the PROSPECT (Predictors of Response to Cardiac Resynchronization Therapy) study in perspective, 1933–43, with permission from Elsevier.

determinants of response to CRT may help to further improve the therapeutic outcomes. ◔ Figure 30.15 illustrates the likelihood of favourable response to CRT based on an ideal integrative approach of patients with heart failure who fulfil current criteria for CRT. Patients with significant LV dyssynchrony, no or minimal myocardial scar tissue (particularly in the LV segments targeted by the LV lead), and with an LV placed at the site of latest activation would have high probability of benefiting from CRT. In contrast, patients with synchronous LV contraction, extensive myocardial scar (or transmural scar in the segments where the LV lead is positioned), or an LV lead position far from the site of latest activation (LV lead mismatch) would have low probability of response to CRT.

There is increasing evidence, that implantation of the LV lead according to an integrative evaluation of LV dyssynchrony, site of latest activation and location, and extent of myocardial scar is associated with increased rates of response and improved long-term survival [22, 25, 67]. Selection of the appropriate imaging technique to evaluate these parameters will depend on the availability and expertise of the centre and the presence/absence of specific characteristics of the patients. Echocardiography will remain the first-choice imaging technique to evaluate CRT candidates. Current echocardiographic technologies permit accurate assessment of LV dyssynchrony and identification of the site of latest mechanical activation. This information can then be combined with the venous anatomy and the presence, transmural extent and location of scar tissue. The venous anatomy can be obtained with MDCT or MRI, and the scar assessment can be performed with contrast-enhanced MRI.

Recent work has demonstrated the potential of specific imaging software that allows for segmentation of MRI data displaying the cardiac veins in relation to the location of transmural scar (◔ Fig. 30.16) [68]. Future studies will determine the precise role of non-invasive imaging in the selection of patients who are candidates for this therapy.

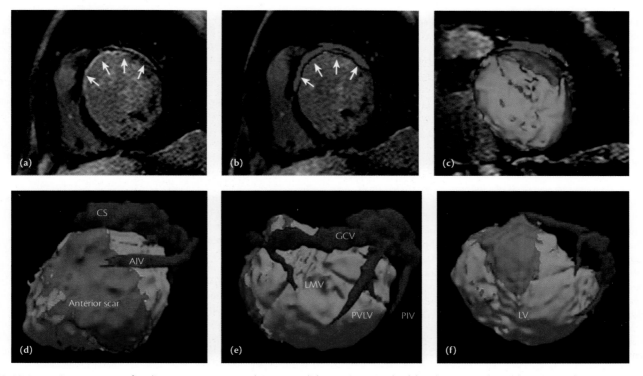

Fig. 30.16 Integrative assessment of cardiac venous anatomy and LV myocardial scar using MRI. The delayed contrast-enhanced MRI image shows an anterior transmural myocardial scar (a, arrows). Using specific software, the anterior myocardial scar is segmented (b, arrows) and colour-coded in red whereas the viable myocardium is colour-coded in green (c). By superimposition of the segmented cardiac veins (colour-coded in blue) onto the segmented LV volume, the spatial relationship of the coronary sinus tributaries with the transmural scar can be assessed (d–f). AIV, anterior inter-ventricular vein; CS, coronary sinus; GCV, great cardiac vein; LMV, left marginal vein; LV, left ventricle; PIV, posterior inter-ventricular vein; PVLV, posterior vein of the left ventricle. Reproduced with permission from [68].

References

1. Go AS, Mozaffarian D, Roger VL, et al. Heart disease and stroke statistics—2013 update: a report from the American Heart Association. *Circulation* 2013; 127: e6–245.

2. Mosterd A, Hoes AW. Clinical epidemiology of heart failure. *Heart* 2007; 93: 1137–46.

3. Abraham WT, Hayes DL. Cardiac resynchronization therapy for heart failure. *Circulation* 2003; 108: 2596–603.

4. Auricchio A, Stellbrink C, Block M, et al. Effect of pacing chamber and atrioventricular delay on acute systolic function of paced patients with congestive heart failure. The Pacing Therapies for Congestive Heart Failure Study Group. The Guidant Congestive Heart Failure Research Group. *Circulation* 1999; 99: 2993–3001.

5. Bristow MR, Saxon LA, Boehmer J, et al. Cardiac-resynchronization therapy with or without an implantable defibrillator in advanced chronic heart failure. *N Engl J Med* 2004; 350: 2140–50.

6. Cazeau S, Leclercq C, Lavergne T, et al. Effects of multisite biventricular pacing in patients with heart failure and intra-ventricular conduction delay. *N Engl J Med* 2001; 344: 873–80.

7. Cleland JG, Daubert JC, Erdmann E, et al. The effect of cardiac resynchronization on morbidity and mortality in heart failure. *N Engl J Med* 2005; 352: 1539–49.

8. Linde C, Leclercq C, Rex S, Garrigue S, et al. Long-term benefits of biventricular pacing in congestive heart failure: results from the MUltisite STimulation in Cardiomyopathy (MUSTIC) study. *J Am Coll Cardiol* 2002; 40: 111–8.

9. Linde C, Abraham WT, Gold MR, St John SM, Ghio S, Daubert C. Randomized trial of cardiac resynchronization in mildly symptomatic heart failure patients and in asymptomatic patients with left ventricular dysfunction and previous heart failure symptoms. *J Am Coll Cardiol* 2008; 52: 1834–43.

10. Moss AJ, Hall WJ, Cannom DS, et al. Cardiac-resynchronization therapy for the prevention of heart-failure events. *N Engl J Med* 2009; 361: 1329–38.

11. Tang AS, Wells GA, Talajic M, et al. Cardiac-resynchronization therapy for mild-to-moderate heart failure. *N Engl J Med* 2010; 363: 2385–95.

12. Sipahi I, Chou JC, Hyden M, Rowland DY, Simon DI, Fang JC. Effect of QRS morphology on clinical event reduction with cardiac resynchronization therapy: meta-analysis of randomized controlled trials. *Am Heart J* 2012; 163: 260–7.

13. Sipahi I, Carrigan TP, Rowland DY, Stambler BS, Fang JC. Impact of QRS duration on clinical event reduction with cardiac resynchronization therapy: meta-analysis of randomized controlled trials. *Arch Intern Med* 2011; 171: 1454–62.

14. Brignole M, Auricchio A, Baron-Esquivias G, et al. 2013 ESC Guidelines on cardiac pacing and cardiac resynchronization therapy: The Task Force on cardiac pacing and resynchronization therapy of the European Society of Cardiology (ESC). Developed in collaboration with the European Heart Rhythm Association (EHRA). *Eur Heart J* 2013; 34: 2281–329.

15. Epstein AE, DiMarco JP, Ellenbogen KA, et al. 2012 ACCF/AHA/HRS focused update incorporated into the ACCF/AHA/HRS 2008 guidelines for device-based therapy of cardiac rhythm abnormalities: a report of the American College of Cardiology Foundation/American Heart Association Task Force on Practice Guidelines and the Heart Rhythm Society. *Circulation* 2013; 127: e283–352.

16. Bax JJ, Gorcsan J, III. Echocardiography and noninvasive imaging in cardiac resynchronization therapy: results of the PROSPECT (Predictors of Response to Cardiac Resynchronization Therapy) study in perspective. *J Am Coll Cardiol* 2009; 53: 1933–43.

17. Auger D, Van Bommel RJ, Bertini M, et al. Prevalence and characteristics of patients with clinical improvement but not significant left ventricular reverse remodeling after cardiac resynchronization therapy. *Am Heart J* 2010; 160: 737–43.

18. Fornwalt BK, Sprague WW, Bedell P, et al. Agreement is poor among current criteria used to define response to cardiac resynchronization therapy. *Circulation* 2010; 11; 121: 1985–91.

19. Bertini M, Hoke U, Van Bommel RJ, et al. Impact of clinical and echocardiographic response to cardiac resynchronization therapy on long-term survival. *Eur Heart J Cardiovasc Imaging* 2013; 14: 774–81.

20. Goldenberg I, Moss AJ, Hall WJ, et al. Predictors of response to cardiac resynchronization therapy in the Multicenter Automatic Defibrillator Implantation Trial With Cardiac Resynchronization Therapy (MADIT-CRT). *Circulation* 2011; 124: 1527–36.

21. Gorcsan J, III, Oyenuga O, Habib PJ, et al. Relationship of echocardiographic dyssynchrony to long-term survival after cardiac resynchronization therapy. *Circulation* 2010; 122: 1910–8.

22. Khan FZ, Virdee MS, Palmer CR, et al. Targeted left ventricular lead placement to guide cardiac resynchronization therapy: the TARGET study: a randomized, controlled trial. *J Am Coll Cardiol* 2012; 59: 1509–18.

23. Shanks M, Delgado V, Ng AC, et al. Clinical and echocardiographic predictors of nonresponse to cardiac resynchronization therapy. *Am Heart J* 2011; 161: 552–7.

24. Holzmeister J, Leclercq C. Implantable cardioverter defibrillators and cardiac resynchronisation therapy. *Lancet* 2011; 378: 722–30.

25. Delgado V, Van Bommel RJ, Bertini M, et al. Relative merits of left ventricular dyssynchrony, left ventricular lead position, and myocardial scar to predict long-term survival of ischaemic heart failure patients undergoing cardiac resynchronization therapy. *Circulation* 2011; 123: 70–8.

26. Richardson M, Freemantle N, Calvert MJ, Cleland JG, Tavazzi L. Predictors and treatment response with cardiac resynchronization therapy in patients with heart failure characterized by dyssynchrony: a pre-defined analysis from the CARE-HF trial. *Eur Heart J* 2007; 28: 1827–34.

27. Wiesbauer F, Baytaroglu C, Azar D, et al. Echo Doppler parameters predict response to cardiac resynchronization therapy. *Eur J Clin Invest* 2009; 39: 1–10.

28. Zhang Q, van BR, Fung JW, et al. Tissue Doppler velocity is superior to strain imaging in predicting long-term cardiovascular events after cardiac resynchronization therapy. *Heart* 2009; 95: 1085–90.

29. Pitzalis MV, Iacoviello M, Romito R, et al. Ventricular asynchrony predicts a better outcome in patients with chronic heart failure receiving cardiac resynchronization therapy. *J Am Coll Cardiol* 2005; 45: 65–9.

30. Marcus GM, Rose E, Viloria EM, Schafer J, De MT, Saxon LA, Foster E. Septal to posterior wall motion delay fails to predict reverse remodeling or clinical improvement in patients undergoing cardiac resynchronization therapy. *J Am Coll Cardiol* 2005; 46: 2208–14.

31. Bax JJ, Bleeker GB, Marwick TH, et al. Left ventricular dyssynchrony predicts response and prognosis after cardiac resynchronization therapy. *J Am Coll Cardiol* 2004; 44: 1834–40.

32. Yu CM, Fung JW, Zhang Q, et al. Tissue Doppler imaging is superior to strain rate imaging and postsystolic shortening on the prediction of reverse remodeling in both ischaemic and nonischemic heart failure after cardiac resynchronization therapy. *Circulation* 2004; 110: 66–73.

33. Dohi K, Suffoletto MS, Schwartzman D, Ganz L, Pinsky MR, Gorcsan J, III. Utility of echocardiographic radial strain imaging to quantify left ventricular dyssynchrony and predict acute response to cardiac resynchronization therapy. *Am J Cardiol* 2005; 96: 112–6.

34. Chung ES, Leon AR, Tavazzi L, et al. Results of the Predictors of Response to CRT (PROSPECT) trial. *Circulation* 2008; 117: 2608–16.

35. Delgado V, Ypenburg C, Van Bommel RJ, et al. Assessment of left ventricular dyssynchrony by speckle tracking strain imaging comparison between longitudinal, circumferential, and radial strain in cardiac resynchronization therapy. *J Am Coll Cardiol* 2008; 51: 1944–52.

36. Lim P, Buakhamsri A, Popovic ZB, et al. Longitudinal strain delay index by speckle tracking imaging: a new marker of response to cardiac resynchronization therapy. *Circulation* 2008; 118: 1130–7.

37. Lumens J, Leenders GE, Cramer MJ, et al. Mechanistic evaluation of echocardiographic dyssynchrony indices: patient data combined with multiscale computer simulations. *Circ Cardiovasc Imaging* 2012; 5: 491–9.

38. De Boeck BW, Teske AJ, Meine M, et al. Septal rebound stretch reflects the functional substrate to cardiac resynchronization therapy and predicts volumetric and neurohormonal response. *Eur J Heart Fail* 2009; 11: 863–71.

39. Gorcsan J, III, Tanaka H. Echocardiographic assessment of myocardial strain. *J Am Coll Cardiol* 2011; 58: 1401–13.

40. Tanaka H, Hara H, Saba S, Gorcsan J, III. Usefulness of three-dimensional speckle tracking strain to quantify dyssynchrony and the site of latest mechanical activation. *Am J Cardiol* 2010; 105: 235–42.

41. Kleijn SA, Aly MF, Knol DL, et al. A meta-analysis of left ventricular dyssynchrony assessment and prediction of response to cardiac resynchronization therapy by three-dimensional echocardiography. *Eur Heart J Cardiovasc Imaging* 2012; 13: 763–75.

42. Westenberg JJ, Lamb HJ, van der Geest RJ, et al. Assessment of left ventricular dyssynchrony in patients with conduction delay and idiopathic dilated cardiomyopathy: head-to-head comparison between tissue doppler imaging and velocity-encoded magnetic resonance imaging. *J Am Coll Cardiol* 2006; 47: 2042–8.

43. Chalil S, Stegemann B, Muhyaldeen S, et al. Intra-ventricular dyssynchrony predicts mortality and morbidity after cardiac resynchronization therapy: a study using cardiovascular magnetic resonance tissue synchronization imaging. *J Am Coll Cardiol* 2007; 50: 243–52.

44. Marsan NA, Westenberg JJ, Ypenburg C, et al. Magnetic resonance imaging and response to cardiac resynchronization therapy: relative merits of left ventricular dyssynchrony and scar tissue. *Eur Heart J* 2009; 30: 2360–7.

45. Bilchick KC, Dimaano V, Wu KC, et al. Cardiac magnetic resonance assessment of dyssynchrony and myocardial scar predicts function class improvement following cardiac resynchronization therapy. *JACC Cardiovasc Imaging* 2008; 1: 561–8.

46. Boogers MM, Van Kriekinge SD, Henneman MM, et al. Quantitative gated SPECT-derived phase analysis on gated myocardial perfusion SPECT detects left ventricular dyssynchrony and predicts response to cardiac resynchronization therapy. *J Nucl Med* 2009; 50: 718–25.

47. Henneman MM, Chen J, Ypenburg C, et al. Phase analysis of gated myocardial perfusion single-photon emission computed tomography compared with tissue Doppler imaging for the assessment of left ventricular dyssynchrony. *J Am Coll Cardiol* 2007; 49: 1708–14.

48. Truong QA, Singh JP, Cannon CP, et al. Quantitative analysis of intra-ventricular dyssynchrony using wall thickness by multidetector computed tomography. *JACC Cardiovasc Imaging* 2008; 1: 772–81.

49. Jia P, Ramanathan C, Ghanem RN, Ryu K, Varma N, Rudy Y. Electrocardiographic imaging of cardiac resynchronization therapy in heart failure: observation of variable electrophysiologic responses. *Heart Rhythm* 2006; 3: 296–310.

50. Ramanathan C, Ghanem RN, Jia P, Ryu K, Rudy Y. Noninvasive electrocardiographic imaging for cardiac electrophysiology and arrhythmia. *Nat Med* 2004; 10: 422–8.

51. Ploux S, Lumens J, Whinnett Z, et al. Noninvasive electrocardiographic mapping to improve patient selection for cardiac resynchronization therapy: Beyond QRS duration and left bundle-branch block morphology. *J Am Coll Cardiol* 2013; 61: 2435–43.

52. van de Veire NR, Schuijf JD, De Sutter J, et al. Non-invasive visualization of the cardiac venous system in coronary artery disease patients using 64-slice computed tomography. *J Am Coll Cardiol* 2006; 48: 1832–8.

53. Chiribiri A, Kelle S, Gotze S, et al. Visualization of the cardiac venous system using cardiac magnetic resonance. *Am J Cardiol* 2008; 101: 407–12.

54. Doring M, Braunschweig F, Eitel C, et al. Individually tailored left ventricular lead placement: lessons from multimodality integration between three-dimensional echocardiography and coronary sinus angiogram. *Europace* 2013; 15: 718–27.

55. Al-Majed NS, McAlister FA, Bakal JA, Ezekowitz JA. Meta-analysis: cardiac resynchronization therapy for patients with less symptomatic heart failure. *Ann Intern Med* 2011; 154: 401–12.

56. Bilchick KC, Kamath S, DiMarco JP, Stukenborg GJ. Bundle-branch block morphology and other predictors of outcome after cardiac resynchronization therapy in Medicare patients. *Circulation* 2010; 122: 2022–30.

57. Wikstrom G, Blomstrom-Lundqvist C, Andren B, et al. The effects of aetiology on outcome in patients treated with cardiac resynchronization therapy in the CARE-HF trial. *Eur Heart J* 2009; 30: 782–8.

58. Bleeker GB, Kaandorp TA, Lamb HJ, et al. Effect of posterolateral scar tissue on clinical and echocardiographic improvement after cardiac resynchronization therapy. *Circulation* 2006; 113: 969–76.

59. Adelstein EC, Tanaka H, Soman P, et al. Impact of scar burden by single-photon emission computed tomography myocardial perfusion imaging on patient outcomes following cardiac resynchronization therapy. *Eur Heart J* 2011; 32: 93–103.

60. Ypenburg C, Roes SD, Bleeker GB, et al. Effect of total scar burden on contrast-enhanced magnetic resonance imaging on response to cardiac resynchronization therapy. *Am J Cardiol* 2007; 99: 657–60.

61. Schinkel AF, Bax JJ, Boersma E, et al. Assessment of residual myocardial viability in regions with chronic electrocardiographic Q-wave infarction. *Am Heart J* 2002; 144: 865–9.

62. Ypenburg C, Sieders A, Bleeker GB, et al. Myocardial contractile reserve predicts improvement in left ventricular function after cardiac resynchronization therapy. *Am Heart J* 2007; 154: 1160–5.

63. Porter TR, Xie F. Myocardial perfusion imaging with contrast ultrasound. *JACC Cardiovasc Imaging* 2010; 3: 176–87.

64. Hummel JP, Lindner JR, Belcik JT, et al. Extent of myocardial viability predicts response to biventricular pacing in ischaemic cardiomyopathy. *Heart Rhythm* 2005; 2: 1211–7.

65. Kim RJ, Wu E, Rafael A, et al. The use of contrast-enhanced magnetic resonance imaging to identify reversible myocardial dysfunction. *N Engl J Med* 2000; 343: 1445–53.

66. Leyva F, Foley PW, Chalil S, et al. Cardiac resynchronization therapy guided by late gadolinium-enhancement cardiovascular magnetic resonance. *J Cardiovasc Magn Reson* 2011; 13: 29.

67. Saba S, Marek J, Schwartzman D, et al. Echocardiography-guided left ventricular lead placement for cardiac resynchronization therapy: results of the speckle tracking assisted resynchronization therapy for electrode region (STARTER) trial. *Circ Heart Fail* 2013; 6: 427–34.

68. Duckett SG, Ginks M, Knowles BR, et al. A novel cardiac MRI protocol to guide successful cardiac resynchronization therapy implantation. *Circ Heart Fail* 2010; 3: e18–21.

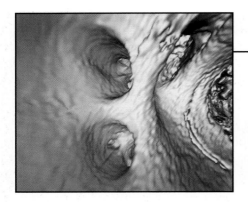

CHAPTER 31

Cardiac resynchronization therapy: optimization and follow-up

Marta Sitges and Genevieve Derumeaux

Contents

Introduction

While the role of cardiac imaging in the selection of candidates for cardiac resynchronization therapy remains controversial, it is well established that imaging is essential to evaluate response to the therapy. Also, echocardiography is often used to optimize device programming. In the present chapter, the role of cardiac imaging in optimizing the programming of cardiac resynchronization therapy (CRT) devices, as well as the usefulness in the follow-up of patients treated with CRT, will be discussed.

CRT optimization

Rationale for optimizing the programming of the device

In patients with heart failure, the presence of a prolonged atrio-ventricular (AV) interval is not unusual. Also, left bundle branch block (LBBB) is present in up to one-third of these patients. Both prolonged AV interval and LBBB result in delayed ejection and consequently, in shortened diastolic time (⮞ Fig. 31.1). This leads to shortened filling time, decreased preload, and the consequent decrease in stroke volume. Restoring adequate AV interval and intra-ventricular conduction delays results in a longer filling time and an increased preload. However, excessively short AV delays may result in early closure of the mitral valve impeding

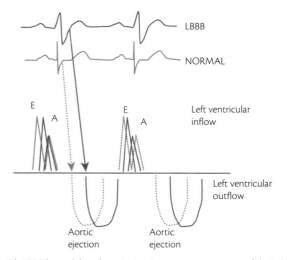

Fig. 31.1 Patients with LBBB have delayed aortic ejection as a consequence of their delayed conduction and mechanical contraction. Delayed aortic ejection results in shortened diastolic time which in turn causes fusion of the E and A wave of the left ventricular filling flow.

the whole contribution of the atrial contraction to left ventricular filling (A-wave truncation). Consequently, finding the optimum AV delay that yields the longest diastolic filling time without truncating the atrial contribution to ventricular filling is of most interest.

On the other hand, optimization of the inter-ventricular (VV) delay may be justified according to several issues. First, a good ventricular synchronization may explain why patients in atrial fibrillation also benefit from CRT and not only because of the benefit on diastolic filling due to optimized AV intervals. Additionally, the epicardial position of the lead implies that transmural activation, usually lasting for 30 ms, should be taken into account when considering time delays between both ventricles. Finally, delayed ventricular segments may be located at different sites of the left ventricle due to underlying myocardial scars or different conduction abnormalities; consequently, dyssynchrony may be corrected by different device programmings.

How to optimize the programming of CRT devices with imaging

Optimization of the AV delay

Echocardiography has typically been used for optimizing the AV interval to obtain the greatest diastolic filling time and the optimum haemodynamic effect; however, there are also other methods based on invasive approaches (assessment of dP/dt and cardiac output with catheters at the time of the implantation) and non-invasive approaches such as impedance cardiography, intra-cardiac electrograms, endocardial acceleration detected by a micro-accelerometer, or algorithms based on electric intervals detected by the device. The big advantage of these latter ones is that they are incorporated in the device, can be performed automatically and continuously, allowing for adaptive optimization of the AV interval according to physical activity or heart rate. The limitation is that these methodologies are not well validated and are limited to each vendor's device. Based on the experience demonstrating the benefits of AV interval optimization in dual-chamber pacing, most of the large clinical trials proving the clinical benefit of CRT, such as the Multi-centre InSync Randomized Clinical Evaluation (MIRACLE) [1] or the Cardiac Resynchronization—Heart Failure (CARE-HF) [2] trials have performed AV optimization with echocardiography. Accordingly, AV optimization using echocardiography has been recommended [3].

The most used echocardiographic method to optimize the AV delay is the iterative method. By the use of pulsed wave (PW) Doppler of the left ventricular inflow, diastolic filling time is measured from the onset of the E wave to the end of the A wave. The AV delay is reduced by 10–20 ms until the longest diastolic filling time is obtained without interrupting the A wave (⊃ Fig. 31.2). Another approach, derived from dual-chamber pacing in patients with AV block and not validated in CRT, is the Ritter's method. This calculates the optimum AV interval by calculations derived from a setting with a very long AV delay and another one with a very short AV delay. For each AV delay, the time from QRS onset to the end of the A wave is determined and the optimum AV delay is calculated by a formula:

AVopt = AVlong – (QAshort-QAlong).

This optimum AV corresponds in fact to the longest diastolic filling time without interrupting the A wave resulting in similar AV delays to those obtained by the iterative method but in a shorter procedure.

Another approach to optimize the AV delay with echocardiography has been proposed by determining the maximum mitral

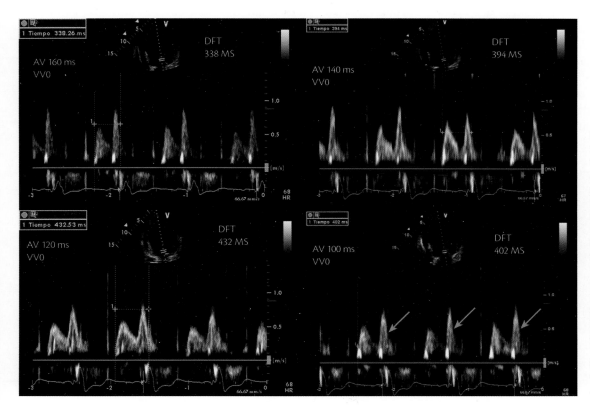

Fig. 31.2 Optimization of the AV interval according to the iterative method: the AV interval is progressively reduced at 20-ms intervals trying to obtain the largest diastolic filling time and consequently, the largest left ventricular filling. As the AV interval decreases, the diastolic filling time increases until the A wave is early interrupted (green arrows). Accordingly, the optimum AV interval selected in this patient was 120 ms, which yielded the largest diastolic filling time without interrupting the A wave.

inflow or the aortic velocity time integral, both as surrogates of the left ventricular cardiac output. In one study, including 30 patients [4], the optimization of the AV delay with these four echocardiographic methods was compared to invasive dP/dt. The optimum AV delay invasively determined was largely concordant with the one determined by the maximum mitral velocity time integral (97%), while there was no agreement with the AV delay determined by Ritter's method. Agreement of dP/dt with the iterative method and the aortic velocity time integral was modest (67% and 43%, respectively).

The AV delay has been also optimized by echocardiography with similar iterative methods that aim to obtain the largest cardiac output as determined by the left ventricular outflow tract velocity time integral (as a surrogate of cardiac output) or the Doppler-derived left ventricular dP/dt, as well as the myocardial performance index (Tei index). Again, the widespread use and, especially, the validation and utility of the methodologies among CRT patients remain uncertain.

Optimization of the VV delay

The VV delay can be optimized by determining invasive left ventricular dP/dt or cardiac output, by the surface ECG or by a variety of device-based algorithms or intra-cardiac electrograms. Echocardiography has also been used to optimize the VV delay either by empirically assessing the VV delay that yields the largest cardiac output or the best left ventricular synchrony. The most commonly used echocardiographic method for VV delay optimization is the evaluation of cardiac output determined by the left ventricular outflow tract velocity time integral. Several VV delays are programmed at 20-ms intervals and the effect on cardiac output is tested (⊃ Fig. 31.3). Few authors have also used tissue Doppler imaging to evaluate left ventricular synchrony and optimize the VV delay, by testing the effect of several VV intervals on left ventricular dyssynchrony on tissue displacement or strain rate traces of opposite myocardial walls (⊃ Fig. 31.4, 📷 Video 31.1). A small study has reported good agreement between optimization of the VV interval according to either left ventricular outflow tract velocity time integral or intra-ventricular dyssynchrony, indicating that the best intra-ventricular synchrony results in the best haemodynamics [5].

Impact of optimization of CRT programming

Acute effect of optimization of the programming of CRT devices

Several groups have reported the beneficial acute effect of optimization of the CRT programming on haemodynamics and left ventricular dyssynchrony, either by invasive or non-invasive methods. Early on the clinical application of CRT, Auricchio et al. [6] already demonstrated an acute incremental benefit on cardiac output and pulse aortic pressure by small changes in the AV delay. Similarly, an optimized VV delay has resulted in larger dP/dt (up to 8% increase), particularly by pre-activation of the left ventricle (%) [7]. When the VV delay has been optimized with echocardiography, mainly by using an iterative method to reach the largest aortic or left ventricular outflow tract velocity time integral, an additional 5-point increase in left ventricular ejection fraction and a 20% increase in cardiac output have been reported [8–11]. On the other hand, selecting a non-optimal VV delay may have a deleterious impact, reducing cardiac output by even more than 25% [8, 11].

Effect of optimization of the programming of CRT devices on clinical outcomes

Despite compelling evidence that AV and VV delay optimization may have an acute haemodynamic beneficial effect, scarce evidence supports the clinical impact of such an optimization.

Few studies have evaluated the impact of optimizing the AV interval by echocardiography on clinical outcomes. Most of them were carried among patients with dual-chamber pacemakers without heart failure and none demonstrated an improvement on clinical outcomes; techniques used to optimize the delay and outcome definition were also different between studies. Among CRT patients, few studies have used optimization only of the AV interval and evaluated the clinical evolution. One study reported on the optimization of the AV delay by maximizing the left ventricular outflow tract velocity time integral in 33 patients, which resulted in improvements in functional capacity and plasma levels of BNP [12]; however, this effect could have resulted simply

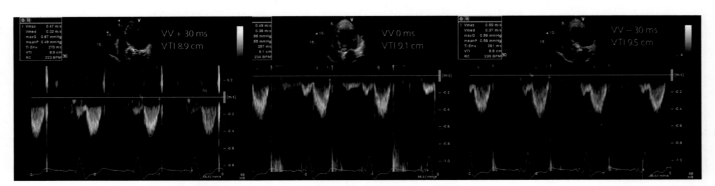

Fig. 31.3 Optimization of the VV interval according to the iterative method using left ventricular outflow tract velocity time integral: the VV interval is tested to obtain the largest velocity time integral. In this patient, despite variation was not large, optimum VV was set at −30 ms (left ventricular pre-activation at 30 ms) as this yielded the largest velocity time integral.

VV –30 ms   VV 0 ms   VV +30 ms

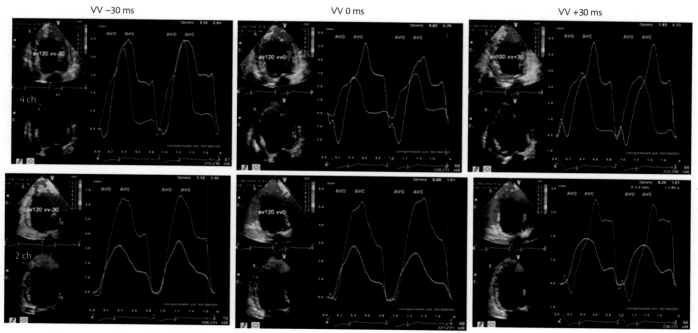

Fig. 31.4, 📹 Video 31.1 Optimization of the VV interval according to the iterative method using left ventricular dyssynchrony: the superposition of the displacement of two opposing walls is evaluated both in the 4- and 2-chamber apical views with tissue Doppler imaging. The superposition and the amount of displacement were maximal with the setting of a VV interval of –30 ms, especially present and evident in the traces from the 4-chamber view. In the 2-chamber images, there are no significant changes among the different VV intervals. These images come from the same patient shown in Fig. 31.3. The selected optimum VV interval was the same either by the velocity time integral or dyssynchrony assessment. Quantitative and semiqualitative analysis of intra-ventricular dyssynchrony or quantification of aortic velocity time integral provided useful information to select the optimum VV interval. Importantly, no clear decision for optimal timing of VV interval could be determined when it was taken based only on visual assessment of left ventricular motion (see 📹 Video 31.1); there was a slight improvement with a little more synchronic motion in the VV 0 ms and VV –30 ms loops as compared to that without CRT (OFF) and in VV + 30 ms; no significant difference in visually estimated ventricular motion and synchrony could be observed between VV 0 ms and –30 ms.

from CRT and the lack of a control group precludes conclusions regarding the effect of AV delay optimization alone. Sawhney et al. [13] compared AV delay optimization by echocardiography (iterative method using aortic velocity time integral) to an empirical AV delay set at 120 ms in a randomized study of 40 patients with CRT, finding an improvement in quality of life and NYHA functional class. Morales et al. [14] evaluated 41 CRT patients who were randomized to receive an empirical AV delay of 120 ms or to optimize their AV delay with echo Doppler-derived *dP/dt*. At 6 months follow-up, left ventricular ejection fraction was significantly higher and NYHA functional class significantly lower in the AV-optimized group.

Regarding the clinical impact of VV interval optimization, reports have also been scarce. Mortensen et al. [11] reported the acute beneficial effects on haemodynamics of VV delay optimization with echocardiography (left ventricular outflow tract velocity time integral), but they were unable to show any additional clinical improvement in the optimized group as compared to conventional simultaneous biventricular pacing at 3 months follow-up. In another study [15], the 6-month clinical outcome of 359 patients included in the InSync III Study who received VV delay optimization with echocardiography (iterative method using the left ventricular outflow tract velocity time integral) were compared against the outcome of the patients included in the MIRACLE study

(without VV optimization). All patients received AV delay optimization with echocardiography. There was an incremental benefit on the 6-minute walking distance (median increase in the InSync 38% versus 15% in the MIRACLE, *P* < 0.0001) while no differences in quality of life or NYHA functional class could be demonstrated.

The first randomized study trying to demonstrate the beneficial clinical effect of VV delay optimization has been the Resynchronization for the HaemodYnamic Treatment for Heart failure Management II Implantable Cardioverter Defibrillator (RHYTHM II ICD) [16], which included 121 patients with CRT. AV delay was optimized in all patients. VV delay was optimized only in randomly assigned patients using echocardiography (with the maximum aortic velocity time integral). Similarly to previous findings, VV optimization conferred no benefit in 6-minute walking distance, quality of life, NYHA functional class, or hospital admissions. More recently, another randomized double-blinded study [17], including 238 CRT patients, showed only modest benefit on a composite clinical endpoint with optimized sequential VV stimulation, as compared to simultaneous biventricular pacing; VV delay optimization was performed according to dyssynchrony indices derived from M-mode echocardiography. The results of these echocardiography-based optimization studies are in keeping with the observations found in another trial that used a device-based algorithm to optimize the VV delay [18]; in this study, sequential pacing was equivalent but not superior, to simultaneous biventricular pacing for the composite end-point of peak oxygen consumption and left ventricular end-systolic dimension. A larger impact of VV optimization has been described in ischaemic heart failure patients, as compared to non-ischaemic patients [19].

Finally, the effect of optimizing both the AV and the VV delay was studied in a single-centre study comparing two historical cohorts of CRT patients [5]: the first 50 patients with an empirical AV delay set at 120 ms and simultaneous biventricular pacing, and the next 51 patients undergoing a standardized systematic echocardiographic optimization of the AV and VV intervals. Once the optimum AV delay was chosen (iterative method), the VV interval was optimized and selected as the one that resulted in larger superposition of the systolic displacement of two opposing ventricular walls with the use of tissue Doppler imaging (i.e. less dyssynchrony) (⊃ Fig. 31.4). Patients undergoing optimization increased in 6-minute walking distance and left ventricular cardiac output at 6 months follow-up; however, there were no differences in NYHA functional class, quality of life, left ventricular ejection fraction and dimensions and, more importantly, in the rates of cardiac death or heart transplantation.

More recently, several studies have compared the outcomes of optimizing the programming of CRT by echocardiography or other methods (intra-cardiac devices or device algorithms) with controversial results. Kamdar et al. [20] already showed a poor agreement between optimal AV and VV delays determined by echocardiography or a device algorithm (QuickOpt™), with echocardiographic optimization yielding a superior haemodynamic acute outcome. On the other hand, in a small study, optimization of CRT by an intra-cardiac electrogram-based algorithm or by echocardiography resulted in a similar exercise capacity [21]. The largest compelling evidence on CRT optimization was provided by the SmartDelay Determined AV Optimization: A Comparison to Other AV Delay Methods Used in Cardiac Resynchronization Therapy (SMART-AV) Trial [22]. In this study, 980 CRT patients were randomized to a fixed empirical AV delay (120 ms), an echocardiographically optimized AV delay, or to AV delay optimized with an electrogram-based algorithm (SmartDelay). Left ventricular reverse remodelling was evaluated at 6 months follow-up showing that neither SmartDelay nor echocardiography was superior to a fixed AV delay of 120 ms. Additionally, the Frequent Optimization Study Using the QuickOpt Method (FREEDOM) trial [17] evaluated the impact of frequent optimization of the AV and VV delays using an algorithm based on the intra-cardiac electrogram (as compared to empiric device programming or echocardiographic optimization on clinical heart failure) among 1,500 CRT patients; there was no significant difference in a clinical composite endpoint regardless of optimization.

Current perspective: limitations and unresolved issues

Many questions remain unanswered regarding optimization of the programming of CRT devices. Methodology is not completely standardized, although most groups use the iterative method for optimization of the AV and the VV delay, trying to obtain the largest diastolic filling time without truncating the A wave and the largest aortic velocity time integral.

However, little is known about the interaction (and sequence) between programming of the AV and VV delays. Most authors have reported a stepwise optimization usually starting with the AV and finishing with the VV; the impact of optimizing the VV first and then the AV delay is unknown.

Also, the equivalence between different methods is far from being established, especially regarding the programming of the AV delay. Another matter of controversy is the stability of the programming of the delay through follow-up when reverse ventricular remodelling develops and potentially impacts on AV and VV delays. Should therefore, the AV and VV delays periodically be optimized and if so, how frequently?

Finally, the cost-efficacy of programming the device with imaging has to be taken into consideration. According to the time and resource consumption of the optimization procedure, routine empirical programming has been proposed leaving optimization for selected non-responder patients.

As most of the major clinical trials demonstrating the beneficial effect of CRT have employed AV optimization, previous recommendations were to routinely optimize AV delay with echocardiography with the Ritter's or the iterative method without any consensus on VV delay optimization. However, after the results of more recent studies, including the SMART-AV and the FREEDOM trials, latest recommendations from the EHRA/HRS [23] state that AV or VV delay optimization may be considered only in selected patients, although their role in improving response has not been proven. Indeed, in clinical practice, AV and VV optimization is not performed in a high proportion of patients in line with a sub-analysis of data from the FREEDOM trial [24]. A recent study showed that individual optimization of the delays yielded additional acute haemodynamic effect in only 23–45% of CRT patients [25]. Therefore, the most extended belief is that complex, echocardiography-based optimization of the programming should only be applied to non-responders, while easy, widely available programmes that are incorporated in the device systems should be used for the vast majority of CRT patients to allow adequate AV and VV programmings at rest and during exercise. However, their potential to improve response in all CRT patients remains to be proved.

Follow-up of patients treated with CRT

Reversing left ventricular remodelling in heart failure

The deleterious action of incoordination on myocardial contractility and geometry has been extensively considered with the development of non-invasive cardiac imaging and has gained interest as the basis of effect of the resynchronization therapy. In heart disease, both intra- and inter-ventricular asynchronous activation has marked adverse consequence on ventricular pump function leading to prolonged contraction, reduced ejection time, delayed and prolonged relaxation, reduced diastolic filling time, and mitral regurgitation [26]. The overall result is left ventricular remodelling, which is a dynamic process characterized by a progressive chamber dilatation, a distortion of cavity shape towards sphericity, a disruption of the mitral valve geometry with tenting and occurrence of mitral regurgitation, and deterioration in contractile function that culminates in heart failure [27–29]. The left ventricular remodelling process is the final common pathway for all of the causes of heart failure and portends a poor prognosis. CRT can improve most of these deleterious effects. The two primary targets of CRT are modifying the pattern of left ventricular activation, and the delay between atrial and ventricular systole. Synchrony of contraction is important because it results in more effective and energetically efficient ejection. Indeed, the clinical success of CRT attests to the importance of dyssynchrony in the pathophysiology of heart failure.

Cardiac imaging techniques play a key role in the diagnosis of reverse remodelling and especially echocardiography, which is easily applied in the follow-up of these patients. Currently used MRI systems still have the limitation on their application among patients with pacemakers.

Evidence for reverse remodelling from randomized controlled trials of CRT

CRT often results in reverse remodelling where left ventricular size and function progressively improved over time (⊃ Fig. 31.5, 📷 Video 31.2). This is a CRT-dependent, dynamic process where subsequent cessation of CRT results in progressive deterioration in left ventricular function toward baseline values. The effects of CRT on reverse ventricular remodelling are additive and to a larger degree than those observed with medical therapy.

The MIRACLE study [1] demonstrated significant reductions in left ventricular end-diastolic and end-systolic volumes at 3 and 6 months in the CRT group compared with the control group (inactive pacing), in which no change was observed from baseline values. In addition, left ventricular mass also significantly decreased, whereas left ventricular contractile function increased in the CRT group but not in the control group. These beneficial effects on left ventricular remodelling were sustained after 2 year follow-up.

The MUltisite STimulation In Cardiomyopathy (MUSTIC) trial [30] also showed sustained reduction in left ventricular size measured by echocardiography at 1 year in a small cohort of patients. The Cardiac Resynchronization—Heart Failure (CARE-HF trial) [2], was the first to demonstrate conclusively that CRT alone can reduce mortality, presumably by favourable effects on left ventricular function. In addition, reverse left ventricular remodelling was assessed at 3 and 18 months, showing a significant and sustained increase in left ventricular ejection fraction (+3.7% and +6.9%, respectively) associated with a decrease in left ventricular end-systolic volume index (–18.2 ml/m² and –26 ml/m², respectively) and in mitral regurgitation area.

More recently, several studies have shown the benefit of CRT in less severe heart failure with evidence of progressive reverse remodelling. The REsynchronization reVErses Remodeling in Systolic left vEntricular dysfunction (REVERSE) study [31] was the first to show that the benefit in terms of recovery of left ventricular function, and in morbidity and mortality, was similar among these patients as compared to that observed in patients with more severe heart failure. The REVERSE study enrolled 684 patients with NYHA functional class I or II, in sinus rhythm, with QRS duration ≥120 ms, and left ventricular ejection fraction ≤40%. The left ventricular end-systolic volume index improved (–18.4±29.5 ml/m²) in the CRT-ON group (n = 324) compared with the CRT-OFF group (–1.3±23.4 ml/m²; n = 163; P<0.0001 versus CRT-ON), especially (three times greater) in the patients

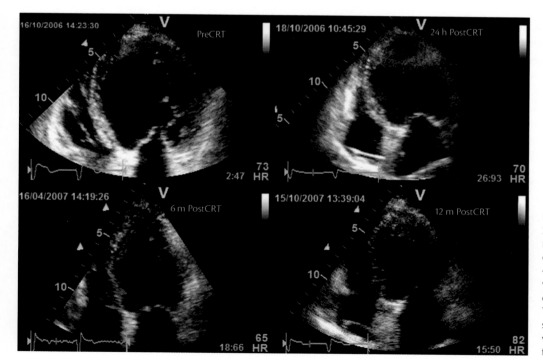

Fig. 31.5, 📷 Video 31.2 Progressive left ventricular reverse remodelling in a patient effectively treated with CRT: 4-chamber apical view of the left ventricle at baseline and after CRT at different time points during 1 year. The reduction in the left ventricular size can be progressively observed as well as the improvement in systolic function.

with non-ischaemic cardiomyopathy. Left ventricular ejection fraction also improved significantly with active CRT but not in the CRT-OFF group. By comparison with the most recent heart failure trials and actual clinical practice, the pharmacological management in the REVERSE trial was optimal. This result suggests that CRT produces significant additive effects on ventricular remodelling that occur in addition to heart failure drug therapy.

Similarly, the Multi-centre Automatic Defibrillator Implantation Trial With Cardiac Resynchronization Therapy (MADIT-CRT) [32] and the Resynchronization/Defibrillation for Ambulatory Heart Failure (RAFT) [33] trials also demonstrated reductions in left ventricular volumes and increase in ejection fraction among patients with NYHA functional class I–II with CRT. Subsequent analysis of MADIT-CRT showed that CRT-ICD therapy also resulted in a significant improvement in both left ventricular dyssynchrony and contractile function measured by global longitudinal strain at 1 year and improvement in dyssynchrony and contractile function were associated with better clinical outcomes [34]. The occurrence of ventricular reverse remodelling with CRT has been also described in patients with atrial fibrillation undergoing CRT [35], with similar reductions in left ventricular end-systolic volume and increase in ejection fraction between patients with atrial fibrillation and sinus rhythm.

Real-time three-dimensional echocardiography has been also used to describe reverse remodelling after CRT. Marsan et al. [36] reported a good inter- and intra-observer agreement for the assessment of left ventricular end-systolic volume and left ventricular ejection fraction evaluation post CRT implantation.

⊃ Figure 31.6 summarizes the main results regarding left ventricular reverse remodelling after CRT, showing the changes in left ventricular end-systolic volume, end-diastolic volume, and ejection fraction reported in some of the largest randomized controlled trials.

Recent studies have also pointed out a subgroup of patients identified as 'super-responders'. Those patients improved dramatically after CRT with almost complete symptomatic recovery and marked reverse remodelling, suggesting some kind of 'heart failure remission phase' (⊃ Fig. 31.7, 🎥 Video 31.3). In an observational longitudinal study recruiting 520 patients, Gasparini et al. [37] observed 16 remissions per 100 person-years, usually reached within the first 2 years of CRT. The most powerful predictors of heart failure remission included a baseline left ventricular ejection fraction of 30–35%, a baseline left ventricular end-diastolic volume of 180 ml, and non-ischaemic heart failure. The concomitance of all three factors was strongly predictive of heart failure remission [37]. In another prospective observational study [38] conducted in 84 consecutive patients, 13% of patients treated with CRT for severe, chronic heart failure showed a dramatic improvement in ejection fraction (>50%) and were considered as 'hyper-responders'. This improvement was mainly related to the aetiology of the underlying heart disease, as all hyper-responders had non-ischaemic dilated cardiomyopathy.

In a recent multi-centric French study (Marseille, Bordeaux, Rennes) [39], 186 patients were investigated before and 6 months after CRT by 2-dimensional strain. Super-responders were defined as a reduction of end-systolic volume of at least 15% and an ejection fraction >50%, and were compared to normal responder patients (reduction of end-systolic volume of at least 15% but an ejection fraction <50%). CRT super-responders were observed in 9% of the population and were associated with less depressed left ventricular function as determined by strain analysis (global longitudinal strain: –12.8±3% versus –9±2.6%, P<0.001). Global longitudinal strain obtained by receiver operator characteristic curves was identified as the best parameter for predicting super-response with a cut-off value of –11% (sensitivity 80%, specificity 87%, area under curve 0.89, P<0.002) and was confirmed as an independent predictor by the logistic regression (RR: 21.3, P<0.0001).

Conversely, a subgroup of patients do not present reverse remodelling after CRT in a proportion around 50%. Cardiac imaging in any of its modalities allows for identification of these non-responder patients in serial follow-up. Factors related to the absence of reverse remodelling have been lack of resynchronization [40], extensive scar [41, 42], and advanced stage of myocardial dysfunction [43].

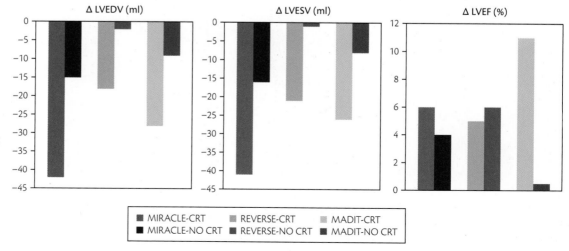

Fig. 31.6 Graphs showing overall decrease in left ventricular end-diastolic volume (LVEDV), end-systolic volume (LVESV) and ejection fraction (LVEF) in three landmark CRT randomized studies in the CRT and in the non-CRT groups: MIRACLE [28], REVERSE [31], and MADIT CRT [32].

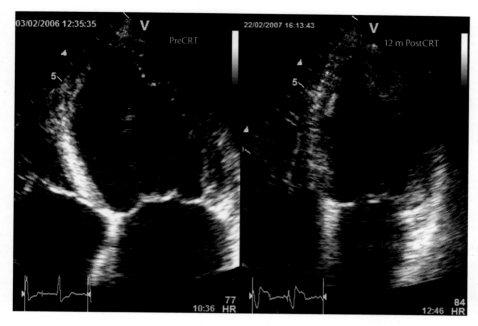

Fig. 31.7 and ▦ Video 31.3 An example of a patient who showed a super-response to CRT with normalization of left ventricular volumes and ejection fraction. The image shows a 4-chamber apical view of the left ventricle before and 12 months after CRT.

Effects of CRT on mitral regurgitation

Reduction of mitral regurgitation is one of the most immediate and often substantial effects of CRT and reduction in mitral regurgitation by CRT is associated with an improved outcome. CRT can reduce mitral regurgitation by improved temporal coordination of mechanical activation of the papillary muscles acutely and by later improvements in left ventricular size and geometry from reverse remodelling [44] (➲ Fig. 31.8, ▦ Videos 31.4–31.6). Indeed, there is some evidence that the decrease in the severity of mitral regurgitation precedes the reduction in left ventricular volumes and the associated changes in left ventricular and mitral valve architecture [29]. Breithardt et al. [45] used the proximal isovelocity surface area method during both pacing-off and CRT in the first week after CRT to report a significantly reduced regurgitant volume and effective regurgitant orifice area with CRT. Kanzaki et al. [46] associated reductions in MR after CRT with acute improvements in the timing of mechanical activation of the papillary muscle sites, using mechanical strain activation mapping.

In addition, the progressive reduction in left ventricular volumes and architecture with CRT are associated with restoration of mitral valvular geometry towards normal. In the MIRACLE study, the severity of mitral regurgitation had decreased significantly with CRT at 3 months, and this improvement was maintained at 6 and 12 months, particularly in non-ischaemic patients. In contrast, no change was observed in the control group [27].

Effects of CRT on left ventricular diastolic function and right ventricular function

The effect of CRT on left ventricular diastolic function has been more scarcely described; some studies with long term follow-up report increases in diastolic filling time and decreases in E wave velocity and E/é ratio indicating improvements in filling pressures mainly in responder patients [47, 48]. Malagoli et al. [49] also showed a decrease in left atrial volume and an improvement in left atrial emptying after 6 months of CRT.

Reports on the effects of CRT on right ventricular function are scarce and the benefical effects are related to left ventricular reverse remodelling. D'Andrea et al. [50] demonstrated, in responders to CRT, a significant improvement in right ventricular peak systolic strain and global longitudinal strain. Conversely, in non-responders to CRT improvement in right ventricular function was not observed.

Predictors of left ventricular reverse remodelling with CRT

The clinical response to CRT is variable and, so far, its prediction from baseline variables has met with limited success. Left ventricular reverse remodelling does not occur in all patients (➲ Figs 30.9 and 30.10, ▦ Videos 31.7–31.10). Between two-thirds and three-quarters of patients exhibit reverse left ventricular remodelling with CRT. There is no current consensus on baseline clinical data that may predict optimal left ventricular reverse remodelling after CRT. Among the number of possible mechanisms that have been proposed, the absence of mechanical left ventricular dyssynchrony, the advanced and irreversible left ventricular dysfunction, and the suboptimal placement of the leads are the most likely causes. Small, non-randomized studies have generated interest in markers of mechanical intra-ventricular dyssynchrony to predict reverse remodelling as extensively discussed in the previous chapter. Conversely, the identification of non-responders is also crucial since non-responders represent approximately 30% of CRT patients and CRT is an invasive treatment with potential complications.

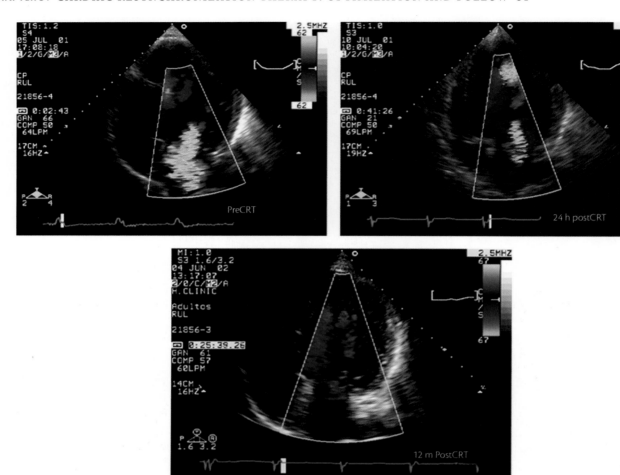

Fig. 31.8 and ▣ Videos 31.4–31.6 An example of a patient who showed a progressive reduction in mitral regurgitation. The image shows a 4-chamber apical view with colour-Doppler of the mitral valve and the left ventricle before (▣ Video 31.4), 24 hours after (▣ Video 31.5) and 12 months (▣ Video 31.6) after CRT. A significant reduction in mitral regurgitation can be observed immediately after the activation of CRT. At 12 months follow-up, mitral regurgitation has virtually disappeared.

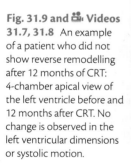

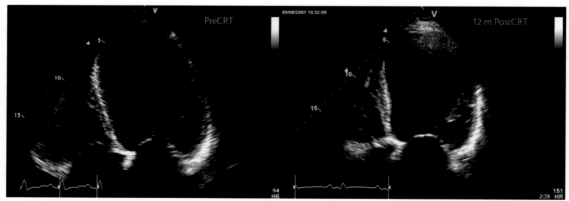

Fig. 31.9 and ▣ Videos 31.7, 31.8 An example of a patient who did not show reverse remodelling after 12 months of CRT: 4-chamber apical view of the left ventricle before and 12 months after CRT. No change is observed in the left ventricular dimensions or systolic motion.

Clinical response and reverse remodelling

In general terms, the clinical response to CRT is greater (up to 70% of patients in most studies) than the remodelling response (up to 50% as described by most groups). Consequently, there is a correlation between remodelling and clinical response in some patients, while others may show paradoxical responses [51, 52].

In the MIRACLE trial, change in left ventricular end-diastolic volume and NYHA class correlated weakly and reverse left ventricular remodelling was greater in patients with non-ischaemic cardiomyopathy, whereas clinical outcomes improved irrespective of heart failure aetiology [27]. The paradox between the effects of CRT on left ventricular function and outcome in patients

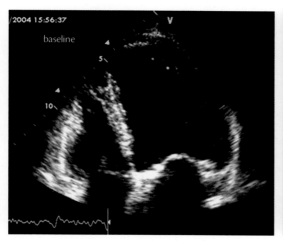
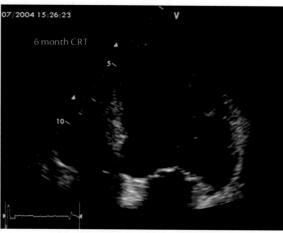

Fig. 31.10 and 📹 **Videos 31.9, 31.10** An example of a patient who showed reverse remodelling after 6 months of CRT: 4-chamber apical view of the left ventricle before and 6 months after CRT. A significant reduction in the left ventricular size and an improvement in the systolic function (particularly at the septum) can be observed.

with ischaemic heart disease suggests that only some of the benefit of CRT is mediated by improving ventricular function. CRT reduces the risk of sudden cardiac death and it is possible that CRT suppresses arrhythmias directly or by even small improvements in cardiac function. Vidal et al. [52] also found a significant correlation between left ventricular ejection fraction improvement and the change in 6 minute walking distance at 12 months follow-up post CRT.

Yu et al. [53] showed in 141 patients who received CRT, that patients who decreased left ventricular end-systolic volume by at least 10% at 3–6 months had a more favourable long-term clinical outcome, including lower all-cause mortality (7% versus 31%), cardiovascular mortality (2% versus 24%), and heart failure events (12% versus 33%; all P<0.005). Finally, Ypenburg et al. [54] studied 302 patients who were categorized according to left ventricular end-systolic volume reduction after 6 months

of CRT; and importantly, an inverse relation between the extent of left ventricular reverse remodelling and outcome was noted.

Conclusion

The use of echocardiography has been demonstrated for the optimization of AV and VV intervals acutely after CRT. Quick and personalized methods to continuously optimize CRT programming are available, but further studies are needed to clarify the precise value of (echocardiographic) CRT programming at longer term follow-up.

Cardiac imaging is also essential in the follow-up of patients treated with CRT, since it provides objective evidence on the effect of the therapy, namely reverse left ventricular remodelling, reduction of mitral regurgitation and improvement of right ventricular function.

References

1. Abraham WT, Fisher WG, Smith AL, et al. Cardiac resynchronization in chronic heart failure. *N Engl J Med* 2002; 346(24): 1845–53.
2. Cleland JGF, Daubert J-C, Erdmann E, et al. The effect of cardiac resynchronization on morbidity and mortality in heart failure. *N Engl J Med* 2005; 352(15): 1539–49.
3. Gorcsan J, III, Abraham T, Agler DA, et al. Echocardiography for cardiac resynchronization therapy: recommendations for performance and reporting—a report from the American Society of Echocardiography Dyssynchrony Writing Group endorsed by the Heart Rhythm Society. *J Am Soc Echocardiogr* 2008; 21(3): 191–213.
4. Jansen AH, Bracke FA, van Dantzig JM, et al. Correlation of echo-Doppler optimization of atrioventricular delay in cardiac resynchronization therapy with invasive haemodynamics in patients with heart failure secondary to ischaemic or idiopathic dilated cardiomyopathy. *Am J Cardiol* 2006; 97(4): 552–7.
5. Vidal B, Sitges M, Marigliano A, et al. Optimizing the programation of cardiac resynchronization therapy devices in patients with heart failure and left bundle branch block. *Am J Cardiol* 2007; 100(6): 1002–6.
6. Auricchio A, Stellbrink C, Block M, et al. Effect of pacing chamber and atrioventricular delay on acute systolic function of paced patients

with congestive heart failure. The Pacing Therapies for Congestive Heart Failure Study Group. The Guidant Congestive Heart Failure Research Group. *Circulation* 1999; 99(23): 2993–3001.
7. Perego GB, Chianca R, Facchini M, et al. Simultaneous vs. sequential biventricular pacing in dilated cardiomyopathy: an acute haemodynamic study. *Eur J Heart Fail* 2003; 5(3): 305–13.
8. Sogaard P, Egeblad H, Pedersen AK, et al. Sequential versus simultaneous biventricular resynchronization for severe heart failure: evaluation by tissue Doppler imaging. *Circulation* 2002; 106(16): 2078–84.
9. Leon AR BS, Liang CS, Abraham WT, Chinchoy E, Hill MRS; US InSync III Investigators and Coordinators. Interventricular delay increases stroke volume in cardiac resynchronization patients. *Eur Heart J* 2002; 23(Abstr Suppl): 529.
10. Bordachar P, Lafitte S, Reuter S, et al. Echocardiographic parameters of ventricular dyssynchrony validation in patients with heart failure using sequential biventricular pacing. *J Am Coll Cardiol* 2004; 44(11): 2157–65.
11. Mortensen PT, Sogaard P, Mansour H, et al. Sequential biventricular pacing: evaluation of safety and efficacy. *Pacing Clin Electrophysiol* 2004; 27(3): 339–45.

12. Hardt SE, Yazdi SH, Bauer A, et al. Immediate and chronic effects of AV-delay optimization in patients with cardiac resynchronization therapy. *Int J Cardiol* 2007; 115(3): 318–25.

13. Sawhney NS, Waggoner AD, Garhwal S, Chawla MK, Osborn J, Faddis MN. Randomized prospective trial of atrioventricular delay programming for cardiac resynchronization therapy. *Heart Rhythm* 2004; 1(5): 562–7.

14. Morales MA, Startari U, Panchetti L, Rossi A, Piacenti M. Atrioventricular delay optimization by doppler-derived left ventricular dP/dt improves 6-month outcome of resynchronized patients. *Pacing Clin Electrophysiol* 2006; 29(6): 564–8.

15. Leon AR, Abraham WT, Brozena S, et al. Cardiac resynchronization with sequential biventricular pacing for the treatment of moderate-to-severe heart failure. *J Am Coll Cardiol* 2005; 46(12): 2298–304.

16. Boriani G, Muller CP, Seidl KH, et al. Randomized comparison of simultaneous biventricular stimulation versus optimized interventricular delay in cardiac resynchronization therapy. The Resynchronization for the Haemodynamic Treatment for Heart Failure Management II Implantable Cardioverter Defibrillator (RHYTHM II ICD) study. *Am Heart J* 2006; 151(5): 1050–8.

17. Abraham WT, Leon AR, St John Sutton MG, et al. Randomized controlled trial comparing simultaneous versus optimized sequential interventricular stimulation during cardiac resynchronization therapy. *Am Heart J* 2012; 164(5): 735–41.

18. Rao RK, Kumar UN, Schafer J, Viloria E, De Lurgio D, Foster E. Reduced ventricular volumes and improved systolic function with cardiac resynchronization therapy: a randomized trial comparing simultaneous biventricular pacing, sequential biventricular pacing, and left ventricular pacing. *Circulation* 2007; 115(16): 2136–44.

19. Marsan NA, Bleeker GB, Van Bommel RJ, et al. Cardiac resynchronization therapy in patients with ischaemic versus non-ischaemic heart failure: Differential effect of optimizing interventricular pacing interval. *Am Heart J* 2009; 158(5): 769–76.

20. Kamdar R, Frain E, Warburton F, et al. A prospective comparison of echocardiography and device algorithms for atrioventricular and interventricular interval optimization in cardiac resynchronization therapy. *Europace* 2010; 12(1): 84–91.

21. Jensen CJ, Liadski A, Bell M, et al. Echocardiography versus intracardiac electrocardiography-based optimization for cardiac resynchronization therapy: a comparative clinical long-term trial. *Herz* 2011; 36(7): 592–9.

22. Ellenbogen KA, Gold MR, Meyer TE, et al. Primary results from the SmartDelay determined AV optimization: a comparison to other AV delay methods used in cardiac resynchronization therapy (SMART-AV) trial: a randomized trial comparing empirical, echocardiography-guided, and algorithmic atrioventricular delay programming in cardiac resynchronization therapy. *Circulation* 2010; 122(25): 2660–8.

23. Daubert JC, Saxon L, Adamson PB, et al. 2012 EHRA/HRS expert consensus statement on cardiac resynchronization therapy in heart failure: implant and follow-up recommendations and management. *Europace* 2012; 14(9): 1236–86.

24. Gras D, Gupta MS, Boulogne E, Guzzo L, Abraham WT. Optimization of AV and VV delays in the real-world CRT patient population: an international survey on current clinical practice. *Pacing Clin Electrophysiol* 2009; 32(Suppl 1): S236–9.

25. Bogaard MD, Meine M, Tuinenburg AE, Maskara B, Loh P, Doevendans PA. Cardiac resynchronization therapy beyond nominal settings: who needs individual programming of the atrioventricular and interventricular delay? *Europace* 2012; 14(12): 1746–53.

26. Leclercq C, Kass DA. Retiming the failing heart: principles and current clinical status of cardiac resynchronization. *J Am Coll Cardiol* 2002; 39(2): 194–201.

27. Sutton MG, Plappert T, Hilpisch KE, Abraham WT, Hayes DL, Chinchoy E. Sustained reverse left ventricular structural remodeling with cardiac resynchronization at one year is a function of etiology: quantitative Doppler echocardiographic evidence from the Multicenter InSync Randomized Clinical Evaluation (MIRACLE). *Circulation* 2006; 113(2): 266–72.

28. Sutton MS, Keane MG. Reverse remodelling in heart failure with cardiac resynchronisation therapy. *Heart* 2007; 93(2): 167–71.

29. Yu CM, Chau E, Sanderson JE, et al. Tissue Doppler echocardiographic evidence of reverse remodeling and improved synchronicity by simultaneously delaying regional contraction after biventricular pacing therapy in heart failure. *Circulation* 2002; 105(4): 438–45.

30. Linde C, Leclercq C, Rex S, et al. Long-term benefits of biventricular pacing in congestive heart failure: results from the MUltisite STimulation in cardiomyopathy (MUSTIC) study. *J Am Coll Cardiol* 2002; 40(1): 111–8.

31. Linde C, Abraham WT, Gold MR, St John Sutton M, Ghio S, Daubert C. Randomized trial of cardiac resynchronization in mildly symptomatic heart failure patients and in asymptomatic patients with left ventricular dysfunction and previous heart failure symptoms. *J Am Coll Cardiol* 2008; 52(23): 1834–43.

32. Moss AJ, Hall WJ, Cannom DS, et al. Cardiac-resynchronization therapy for the prevention of heart-failure events. *N Engl J Med* 2009; 361(14): 1329–38.

33. Tang AS, Wells GA, Talajic M, et al. Cardiac-resynchronization therapy for mild-to-moderate heart failure. *N Engl J Med* 2010; 363(25): 2385–95.

34. Pouleur AC, Knappe D, Shah AM, et al. Relationship between improvement in left ventricular dyssynchrony and contractile function and clinical outcome with cardiac resynchronization therapy: the MADIT-CRT trial. *Eur Heart J* 2011; 32(14): 1720–9.

35. Tolosana JM, Arnau AM, Madrid AH, et al. Cardiac resynchronization therapy in patients with permanent atrial fibrillation. Is it mandatory to ablate the atrioventricular junction to obtain a good response? *Eur J Heart Fail* 2012; 14(6): 635–41.

36. Marsan NA, Bleeker GB, Ypenburg C, et al. Real-time three-dimensional echocardiography as a novel approach to assess left ventricular and left atrium reverse remodeling and to predict response to cardiac resynchronization therapy. *Heart Rhythm* 2008; 5(9): 1257–64.

37. Gasparini M, Regoli F, Ceriotti C, et al. Remission of left ventricular systolic dysfunction and of heart failure symptoms after cardiac resynchronization therapy: temporal pattern and clinical predictors. *Am Heart J* 2008; 155(3): 507–14.

38. Castellant P, Fatemi M, Bertault-Valls V, Etienne Y, Blanc JJ. Cardiac resynchronization therapy: 'nonresponders' and 'hyperresponders'. *Heart Rhythm* 2008; 5(2): 193–7.

39. Reant P, Zaroui A, Donal E, et al. Identification and characterization of super-responders after cardiac resynchronization therapy. *Am J Cardiol* 2010; 105: 1327–35.

40. Bleeker GB, Mollema SA, Holman ER, et al. Left ventricular resynchronization is mandatory for response to cardiac resynchronization therapy: analysis in patients with echocardiographic evidence of left ventricular dyssynchrony at baseline. *Circulation* 2007; 116(13): 1440–8.

41. Ypenburg C, Roes SD, Bleeker GB, et al. Effect of total scar burden on contrast-enhanced magnetic resonance imaging on response to cardiac resynchronization therapy. *Am J Cardiol* 2007; 99(5): 657–60.

42. Ypenburg C, Sieders A, Bleeker GB, et al. Myocardial contractile reserve predicts improvement in left ventricular function after cardiac resynchronization therapy. *Am Heart J* 2007; 154(6): 1160–5.

43. Vidal B, Delgado V, Mont L, et al. Decreased likelihood of response to cardiac resynchronization in patients with severe heart failure. *Eur J Heart Fail* 2010; 12(3): 283–7.

44. Sitges M, Vidal B, Delgado V, et al. Long-term effect of cardiac resynchronization therapy on functional mitral valve regurgitation. *Am J Cardiol* 2009; 104(3): 383–8.

45. Breithardt OA, Sinha AM, Schwammenthal E, et al. Acute effects of cardiac resynchronization therapy on functional mitral regurgitation in advanced systolic heart failure. *J Am Coll Cardiol* 2003; 41(5): 765–70.

46. Kanzaki H, Bazaz R, Schwartzman D, Dohi K, Sade LE, Gorcsan J, III. A mechanism for immediate reduction in mitral regurgitation after cardiac resynchronization therapy: insights from mechanical activation strain mapping. *J Am Coll Cardiol* 2004; 44(8): 1619–25.

47. Aksoy H, Okutucu S, Kaya EB, et al. Clinical and echocardiographic correlates of improvement in left ventricular diastolic function after cardiac resynchronization therapy. *Europace* 2010; 12(9): 1256–61.

48. Waggoner AD, Faddis MN, Gleva MJ, de las Fuentes L, Davila-Roman VG. Improvements in left ventricular diastolic function after cardiac resynchronization therapy are coupled to response in systolic performance. *J Am Coll Cardiol* 2005; 46(12): 2244–9.

49. Malagoli A, Rossi L, Franchi F, et al. Effect of cardiac resynchronization therapy on left atrial reverse remodeling: Role of echocardiographic AV delay optimization. *Int J Cardiol* 2012.

50. D'Andrea A, Salerno G, Scarafile R, et al. Right ventricular myocardial function in patients with either idiopathic or ischaemic dilated cardiomyopathy without clinical sign of right heart failure: effects of cardiac resynchronization therapy. *Pacing Clin Electrophysiol* 2009; 32(8): 1017–29.

51. Bleeker GB, Bax JJ, Fung JW, et al. Clinical versus echocardiographic parameters to assess response to cardiac resynchronization therapy. *Am J Cardiol* 2006; 97(2): 260–3.

52. Vidal B, Sitges M, Marigliano A, et al. Relation of response to cardiac resynchronization therapy to left ventricular reverse remodeling. *Am J Cardiol* 2006; 97(6): 876–81.

53. Yu CM, Bleeker GB, Fung JW, et al. Left ventricular reverse remodeling but not clinical improvement predicts long-term survival after cardiac resynchronization therapy. *Circulation* 2005; 112(11): 1580–6.

54. Ypenburg C, van Bommel RJ, Borleffs CJ, et al. Long-term prognosis after cardiac resynchronization therapy is related to the extent of left ventricular reverse remodeling at midterm follow-up. *J Am Coll Cardiol* 2009; 53(6): 483–90.

⊃ **For additional multimedia materials please visit the online version of the book (⌁ http://www.esciacc.oxfordmedicine.com)**

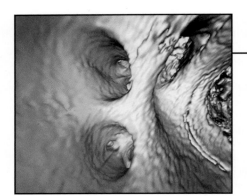

CHAPTER 32

Echocardiography for advanced extracorporeal support

Susanna Price and Jean-Luc Canivet

Introduction

Extracorporeal support became a reality with the discovery of heparin a century ago, however it was not until the mid-twentieth century before its clinical application became routine [1]. Since this time, the use of extracorporeal therapies has gradually emerged as a plausible option for advanced cardiac and/or respiratory support in the critically ill patient. Echocardiography has a vital role in its successful implementation, extending beyond diagnosis to excluding contraindications, confirming/guiding correct cannula placement, ensuring the goals of support are met, detecting complications, assessing tolerance to assistance, and in weaning from mechanical circulatory support.

Indications for extracorporeal support

Extracorporeal support may be indicated in cardiac and/or respiratory failure. Most frequently this is temporary, used as a bridge to recovery, transplantation, or decision regarding further intervention [2]. In a very small number of patients, extracorporeal cardiac support may be used as destination therapy. Common indications for requirement of circulatory support include cardiogenic shock and refractory low cardiac output (CI <2.2L/min/m²) and hypotension (SBP <90 mmHg), despite adequate intravascular volume and high-dose inotropic agents, inability to wean from cardiopulmonary bypass post-cardiotomy, primary graft failure after heart/heart-lung transplantation, severe myocardial depression of sepsis, drug toxicity, myocarditis, and post-cardiac arrest [3–6]. The use of extracorporeal support for severe acute respiratory failure (SARF) has recently expanded with the development of miniaturized devices for CO_2 removal, and also with the H1N1 pandemic [7, 8]. The types of advanced mechanical circulatory and respiratory support commonly used are shown in ⊃ Table 32.1. Clinical indications relating to the timing of ventricular assist and extracorporeal membrane oxygenation (ECMO) are found in the respective national and international registries, in addition to published guidelines [2, 3, 5, 9].

Diagnosis

Echocardiographic imaging in the critically ill, in particular where advanced extracorporeal support is potentially indicated, can be challenging. Diagnostic 2D-TTE images are unobtainable in up to 30% of the general ICU patient population, rising to 85% in patients with SARF (⊃ Fig. 32.1). Where TOE is performed, the coagulation status of the patient should be known, and, if required and acceptable, any coagulopathy corrected prior to the study.

Table 32.1 Types of advanced mechanical circulatory and respiratory support

Cardiac support required	Respiratory support required		
	Oxygenation	CO$_2$ removal	Nil respiratory support
Right heart	VA ECMO	VA ECMO	RVAD/VA ECMO/ Impella RD
Left heart	VA ECMO	–	LVAD/VA ECMO/ Tandem heart/LV Impella
Biventricular	VA ECMO	–	BiVAD/VA ECMO
Nil	VV ECMO	(AV)ECCO(2)R	–

CO$_2$, carbon dioxide; VA ECMO, veno-arterial extracorporeal membrane oxygenation; VV ECMO, veno-venous extracorporeal membrane oxygenation; (AV)ECCO(2)R, arterio-venous extracorporeal carbon dioxide removal; RVAD, right ventricular assist device; LVAD, left ventricular assist device; BiVAD, biventricular ventricular assist device.

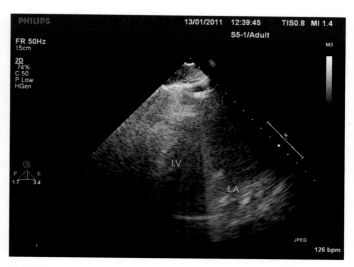

Fig. 32.1 Transthoracic echo, parasternal long axis view in a patient with severe acute respiratory failure with poor windows due to lung interstitial oedema. LA, left atrium; LV, left ventricle.

Oropharyngeal bleeding can be life-threatening in patients fully anticoagulated on ECMO, and generally oesophageal intubation using direct laryngoscopy is recommended. Echocardiographic diagnosis in patients being considered for advanced extracorporeal support has three main components:

◆ Excluding important underlying potentially treatable pathology.

◆ Determining the requirement for right ventricular (RV) and/or left ventricular (LV) support, and the level of support required, and assessing the ability of the right and left ventricles to support the extracorporeal circuit.

◆ Exclusion of cardiovascular contraindications to initiation of support.

Exclusion of relevant underlying pathology

Extracorporeal support is not a treatment per se, but rather a supportive therapy whilst awaiting resolution of the underlying pathological process. Where this remains undiagnosed and untreated, patient prognosis is poor. Thus a comprehensive echocardiographic examination must be undertaken in patients referred for cardiac and/or respiratory support, and where a potentially treatable cause is found, appropriate intervention undertaken. This applies equally for patients referred for respiratory support, as interstitial oedema due to diffuse acute lung injury may be radiographically indistinguishable from that due to elevated left atrial pressure [10]. An example is shown in ➲ Fig. 32.2a, b, and c.

Diagnosing requirement for support and ability of the heart to support the circuit

The types of systems used are predominantly determined by the failing organ(s), and the level of support required, i.e. respiratory and/or cardiac failure (➲ Tables 32.1 and 32.2). Determining the requirement for support is clinical, however, once this decision is made, echocardiography becomes pivotal to guide the type and configuration used. In every case each side of the heart must be assessed whilst considering the existing level of inotropic and respiratory support, and anticipating the additional circulatory load of

any extracorporeal circuit. A further challenge in extracorporeal cardiac support is to anticipate the effect of the additional forward stroke volume delivered to the apparently non-affected ventricle, as a significant increase may reveal covert ventricular failure. Some commonly used types of support, together with their related flows are shown in ➲ Table 32.2. Different configurations are thus determined by the type and level of assist required, and defined additionally by the position of the inflow (ventricular/atrial/peripheral) and return (atrial/aorta/pulmonary artery/peripheral) cannulae. The site and mechanism of cannulation in turn depends not only on the patient pathology, but also local expertise.

Echocardiographic contraindications to extracorporeal support

There are a number of absolute and relative contraindications to extracorporeal support, some of which can be detected using echocardiography (➲ Table 32.3). Additional contraindications may exist that relate to the specific device, for example AS and the Impella [11].

Extracorporeal respiratory support

In its most extreme form, SARF may make oxygenation by ventilation alone impossible, mandating extracorporeal support with ECMO (➲ Fig. 32.3). In other circumstances only CO$_2$ removal is required. Both situations require adequate RV function to tolerate the addition of a significant circulatory shunt; however, the clinical status of such patients makes a universal definition of what constitutes 'adequate' for all patients impossible. Thus RV function must be interpreted on an individual basis and in the context of the level of inotropic support, degree of hypoxaemia and/or hypercarbia (increase PVR), ventilatory pressures required, and degree of hypotension in the context of any pulmonary hypertension. In addition to the standard assessment of RV function

Fig. 32.2 (a) Chest radiograph and CT thorax of a patient referred to a national centre with severe acute respiratory failure for veno-venous extracorporeal membrane oxygenation, demonstrating bilateral diffuse pulmonary infiltrates. (b) CW Doppler transthoracic echocardiography of transmitral filling in a patient with severe acute respiratory failure referred for veno-venous extracorporeal membrane oxygenation, demonstrating high forward velocities (arrowed). (c) Two-dimensional transoesophageal echocardiogram in a patient with severe acute respiratory failure referred for veno-venous extracorporeal membrane oxygenation, demonstrating flail posterior mitral valve leaflet (arrowed) and severe mitral regurgitation (broken arrow) on colour Doppler. LA, left atrium; LV, left ventricle.

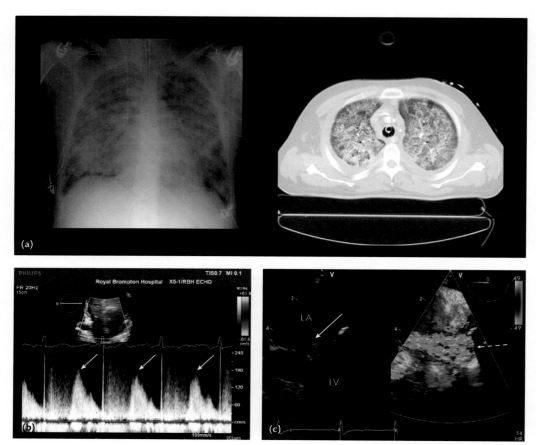

Table 32.2 Flow rates associated with some types of extracorporeal support

Device	Flow (l/min)	Comments
Impella	≤2.5 or 5.0	Percutaneous positioning across AV (left heart) Surgical RA–PA insertion (right heart)
Tandem heart	≤4.0	Catheter insertion with trans-septal puncture
Centrifugal	≤9.0–10.0	Relatively rapid insertion
Centrifugal VA ECMO	≤9.0	Surgical or percutaneous
Centrifugal VV ECMO	≤3.0	Surgical or percutaneous
Extracorporeal AV CO_2 removal	≤1.0–1.8	Percutaneous femoral

AV, aortic valve; RA, right atrium; PA, pulmonary artery; VA ECMO, veno-arterial extracorporal membrane oxygenation; VV ECMO, veno-venous extracorporeal membrane oxygenation; (AV)ECCO(2)R, arterio-venous extracorporeal carbon dioxide removal. For all devices, a significant limit to the amount of flow deliverable is cannula dimension.

Table 32.3 Echocardiographic contraindications to extracorporeal support

Absolute contraindications to VA ECMO/LVAD	Absolute contraindications to VV ECMO
Unrepaired aortic dissection Severe aortic regurgitation Unrepaired coarctation of the aorta	Severe ventricular dysfunction Severe pulmonary hypertension

Relative contraindications to VA ECMO/LVAD	Relative contraindications to VV ECMO
Severe aortic atheroma Abdominal/thoracic aneurysm with intraluminal thrombus	Large PFO/ASD TV pathology (TS/TVR)

VA ECMO, veno-arterial extracorporeal membrane oxygenation; LVAD, left ventricular assist device; VV ECMO, veno-venous extracorporeal membrane oxygenation; PFO, patent foramen ovale; ASD, atrial septal defect; TV, tricuspid valve; TS, tricuspid stenosis; TVR, tricuspid valve replacement.

VV ECMO

Current commonly used adult VV ECMO systems generally use a dual-lumen cannula, with blood drawn from the SVC and IVC pumped through an oxygenator, then returned to the mid-RA directed towards the TV (⊃ Fig. 32.4). Echocardiography is used to confirm and/or guide correct cannula placement (⊃ Figs 32.4 and 32.5) [13]. The distal part of the IVC cannula should ideally have its cannula inlet distal to the suprahepatic vein, and a suprahepatic diameter of >10 mm, thus avoiding venous obstruction. The SVC inlet should be just proximal to SVC/RA junction, with no SVC obstruction. There should be no

and pulmonary circulation, evidence of RV restriction should be sought and any intra-cardiac shunt assessed with respect to its size and direction, if necessary using contrast [12]. When the right heart is judged on echocardiography to be significantly impaired, full cardio-respiratory support with VA ECMO may be indicated; however, achieving normoxia may result in rapid resolution of RV dysfunction.

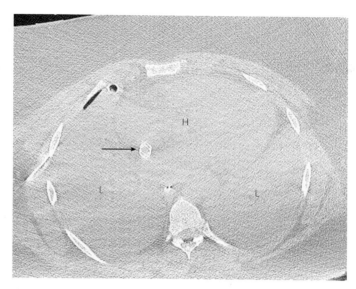

Fig. 32.3 Transversal CT thorax in a patient with severe H1N1 influenza referred for veno-venous extracorporeal membrane oxygenation (VV ECMO). There is no airspace shadowing in the lungs (L) and the patient is unventilatable. Treatment has been started with VV ECMO, and the cannula can be seen clearly in the right atrium (arrowed). H, heart.

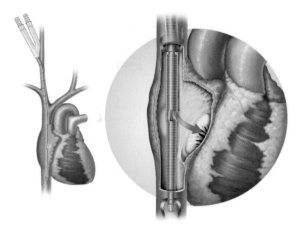

Fig. 32.4 Dual-lumen cannula for internal jugular vein catheterisation in order to deliver veno-venous extracorporeal membrane oxygenation (VV ECMO). The inlets to the cannula (removing deoxygenated blood, shown as blue arrows) are in the superior and inferior cavae, and the returning oxygenated blood (arrowed in red) is directed towards the tricuspid valve orifice. (*Source:* http://www.avalonlabs.com).

kinking of the cannula in the RA, and the return jet should be directed away from the cavae and inter-atrial septum, towards the TV inlet. A daily focused TTE confirms there has been no superior/inferior migration or rotation of the cannula, no deterioration of RV function, and no significant change in the presence/direction of any intra-cardiac shunt (which may be dynamic). Additional studies are indicated where a complication of ECMO is suspected (see Complications of extracorporeal support). Where single-lumen cannulae are used, the distance between the inlet and outlet should be monitored in order to prevent recirculation.

When interpreting ventricular function in any patient on VV ECMO the flow rates should be routinely recorded as, although when a greater proportion of the venous return is aspirated and better oxygenation achieved, this may be at the expense of progressive RV failure. Further, the LV may fail if RV function is very good when the venous return is significantly increased. Finally, where the circulation is hyperdynamic and ventricular function good, treatment for inadequate oxygenation may be to use beta blockade in order to reduce the cardiac output. Thus balancing biventricular function, inotropy, and oxygenation requires a level of expertise, and collaboration between echocardiographer and intensivist. Where cardiorespiratory stability is not achievable, VA ECMO may be required.

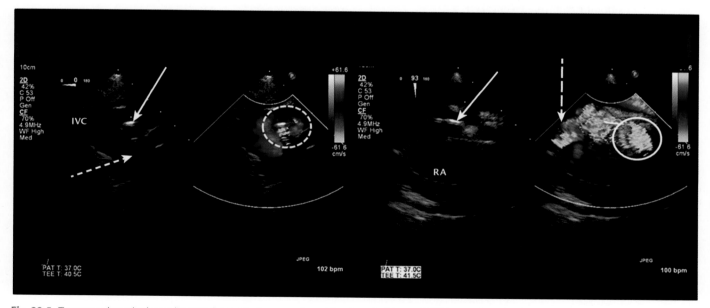

Fig. 32.5 Transoesophageal echocardiogram demonstrating cannula position for a dual-lumen ECMO cannula. In the figure on the left, the cannula (solid arrow) is seen passing into the inferior vena cava (IVC), close to the suprahepatic vein (dashed arrow), with the inlet (dashed circle) away in the centre of the IVC. In the figure on the right, the cannula is seen crossing the right atrium (solid arrow) with the inlet (circled) at the SVC: RA junction, and the return jet (broken arrow) directed towards the tricuspid valve and away from the inter-atrial septum.

Extracorporeal cardiac support

A range of devices for mechanical circulatory support are available (⊃ Table 32.2). These are defined by the type (left/right/biventricular), duration (short/intermediate/long term), mechanics (continuous flow/volume displacement), and implantation approach (percutaneous/surgical/combination). Where severe respiratory failure co-exists, extracorporeal oxygenation will additionally be required (⊃ Table 32.1). Support may be instituted as a bridge to recovery, transplantation, or decision [2]. Knowledge of different devices is mandatory prior to attempting to use echocardiography to guide their use, as for each, specific considerations exist. All echocardiographic studies performed on support should have pump speed, ventilator settings (if relevant), level of vasoactive support and haemodynamics recorded.

Impella

This axial pump may be used to provide short-term (5–10 days depending upon the device) partial assistance to either left or right heart. For LV support, the device is usually inserted percutaneously, positioned across the aortic valve into the cavity of the LV [14, 15]. The procedure is performed with echocardiographic guidance to monitor catheter progression across the aortic valve, ensure there is no disruption/distortion of the mitral subvalvar apparatus and no increase in mitral regurgitation. Correct positioning is confirmed by demonstration of inlet flow in the LV (no more than 40 mm below the aortic valve), and return flow approximately 10 mm above the aortic valve (⊃ Fig. 32.6). As the LV is decompressed, its dimensions should decrease in parallel, with a reduction in any previously documented mitral regurgitation. Right heart support using the Impella RD (either RA–PA, or retrograde insertion from PV to RV) demands surgical insertion, with correct positioning confirmed using TOE.

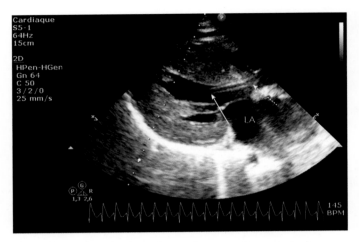

Fig. 32.6 Transthoracic echocardiogram (parasternal long-axis view) demonstrating correct placement of the Impella in a patient with hypertrophic cardiomyopathy. The inlet portion of the cannula can be seen in the left ventricle (solid arrow) below the aortic valve, approximately 3cm below the aortic valve (broken arrow). LA, left atrium.

VA ECMO

VA ECMO is indicated for the short-term assistance of either or both ventricles, with/without associated respiratory failure. It can be used as a bridge to recovery, or to improve organ function prior to longer term VAD insertion. Cannulation may be peripheral or central, draining blood from the RA and pumping it through an oxygenator to be returned to either the ascending (central) or descending (peripheral) aorta. In addition to diagnosis of the underlying condition and exclusion of contraindications (⊃ Table 32.3), echocardiographic findings may also influence the choice of central vs. peripheral cannulation. Thus in the presence of very severe LV failure, the delivery of oxygenated blood to the descending aorta can increase LV afterload, resulting in worsening pulmonary congestion. If AR co-exists, in the absence of AV opening (⊃ Fig. 32.7),

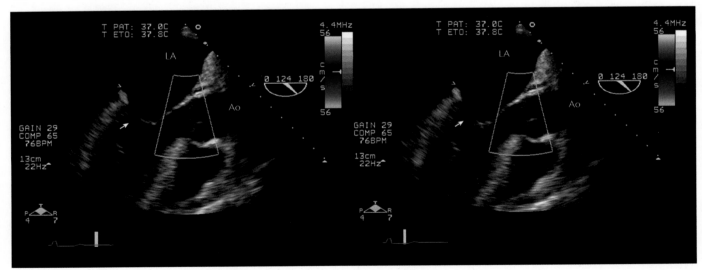

Fig. 32.7 Transoesophageal echocardiogram (mid-oesophageal left ventricular outflow tract view) in a patient with severe pulmonary oedema despite veno-arterial extracorporeal membrane oxygenation for cardiac support. On the left is a diastolic frame, with the aortic valve closed and mitral valve open (arrowed). On the right is a systolic frame. The aortic valve remains closed, and there is persistent (systolic) opening of the mitral valve (arrowed). This demonstrates inappropriate left ventricular offloading. LA, left atrium; Ao, ascending aorta.

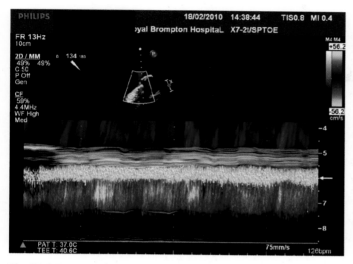

Fig. 32.8 Transoesophageal echocardiogram in a patient on veno-arterial extracorporeal membrane oxygenation for cardiac support post-aortic valve replacement. Colour M-mode across the aortic valve shows continuous aortic regurgitation, with no aortic valve opening.

AR becomes continuous (Fig. 32.8), and may become progressively more severe, and worsen LV dilatation (Fig. 32.9). One potential option is to introduce a minimal level of inotropic support in order to achieve some degree of LV ejection and AV systolic opening (monitored by echocardiography). Where this is not possible measurement of the pressure difference between the ascending aorta and LV indicates a potentially very high LV diastolic pressure (Fig. 32.10). In this setting, insertion of an 'LV vent' may be required. Here, central cannulation provides the opportunity for optimizing offloading with the additional potential to directly

insert an 'LV vent' (Fig. 32.11). Although mild secondary MR may improve with VA ECMO when the LV is adequately offloaded, more severe MR in the presence of very severe LV dysfunction may result in LV dilatation and the aortic valve may not open. This can result in thrombosis in the ascending aorta, LV and pulmonary veins (Fig. 32.12). Venting (centrally or via percutaneous balloon atrial septostomy) has been reported in this situation [16, 17].

Intra-procedurally TOE is used to confirm inlet and outlet cannulae positions, specifically confirming avoidance of the cannulae impacting on any cardiac/extra-cardiac structure, no kinking/distortion of the cannula, and avoidance of suprahepatic vein cannulation/obstruction (Fig. 32.13). The inlet cannula should be located in the mid-RA providing unobstructed flow of blood into the circuit. In peripheral VA ECMO, although the tip of the return cannula is not visible using TOE, arterial cannulation can be confirmed by demonstration of the guidewire in the aorta. Echocardiography is then used to ensure there is no inappropriate unloading of one of the ventricles (progressive dilatation/failure to decompress). This may additionally be suggested by retrograde diastolic transmitral flow and/or retrograde systolic waves in pulmonary venous flow [18]. Where decompression is not achieved, venting is required either by a surgical or percutaneous approach.

The frequency of echocardiographic assessment in VA ECMO is debated; however, echocardiography should be performed when a complication is suspected (see Complications of extracorporeal support). Although this would usually be indicated by haemodynamic instability, on occasion a change in oxygenation should prompt echocardiographic evaluation. First, a paradoxical improvement in oxygenation may be due to impedence to mechanical flow (i.e. tamponade) rather than deterioration in respiratory function or the oxygenator. In this situation a comprehensive examination of the heart and circuit should be undertaken. Second,

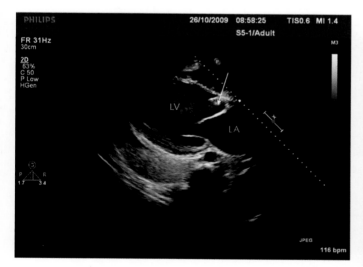

Fig. 32.9 Transthoracic echocardiogram (parasternal long-axis view) in systole of a patient requiring extracorporeal mechanical circulatory support for cardiogenic shock following implantation of a trans-catheter aortic valve (TAVI). Due to continuous delivery of flow to the ascending aorta, the TAVI has displaced inferiorly into the left ventricle (LV) resulting in severe AR. As equal pressures were present in the ascending aorta and LV, no colour flow was seen on colour Doppler. Consequently there was severe LV dilatation with progressive mitral annular dilatation and free MR during systole and diastole.

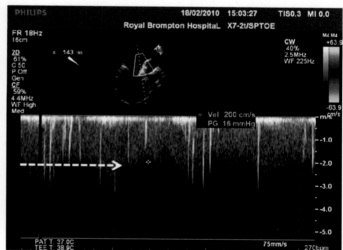

Fig. 32.10 Transoesophageal echocardiogram in a patient on veno-arterial extracorporeal membrane oxygenation for cardiac support post-aortic valve replacement. CW Doppler reveals continuous aortic regurgitation (broken arrow), with a low pressure difference between the ascending aorta and left ventricle (16 mmHg). In this patient the pressure in the ascending aorta was 65 mmHg indicating a high LV pressure in systole and diastole.

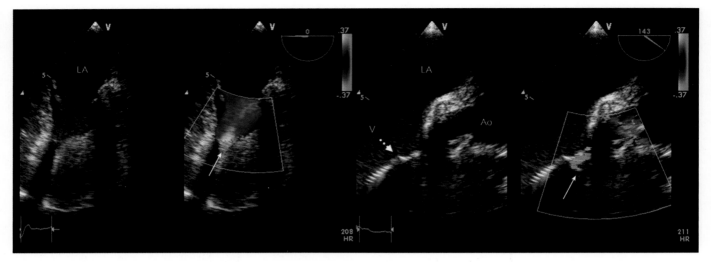

Fig. 32.11 Transoesophageal echocardiography (mid-oesophageal view) in a patient requiring insertion of an apical left ventricular vent due to persistent and worsening AR when on veno-arterial extracorporeal membrane oxygenation (VA ECMO) post-aortic valve replacement. In the image on the left, flow into the vent can be seen (arrowed). Monitoring the position of all cannulae during extracorporeal support is vital. In the image on the right taken 24 hours later, the vent (V, broken arrow) has migrated beneath the anterior mitral valve leaflet to the sub-aortic area. If not repositioned, this can result in worsening aortic regurgitation.

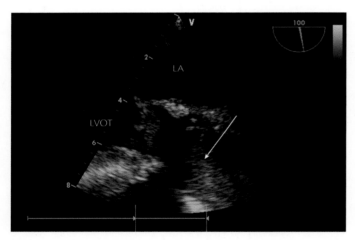

Fig. 32.12 Transoesophageal echocardiogram in a patient requiring veno-arterial extracorporeal membrane oxygenation 3 days after failure to wean from cardiopulmonary bypass for aortic valve replacement. Due to very severe left ventricular failure, no aortic valve opening was possible. Despite full anticoagulation there is extensive thrombus seen from the left ventricular outflow tract (LVOT) across the aortic valve replacement and extending to the ascending aorta (arrowed). The thrombus additionally occluded both coronary artery ostia. LA, left atrium.

in a patient requiring cardiorespiratory support, where there is persistent severe respiratory failure, as the heart begins to recover and eject this can result in the upper body being supplied by profoundly deoxygenated blood, whilst the lower body is hyperoxygenated (supplied by the ECMO circuit)—the Harlequin syndrome. If cardiac recovery is seen in this situation the echocardiographer should warn the attending team that their monitoring should be changed accordingly, and possibly consider changing to VV ECMO if cardiac function is adequate. In general, daily assessment should be considered if the patient has potential to be weaned [19, 20]. This would generally be suggested by haemodynamic

stability, persistent LV ejection with only minimal inotropic support, and adequate gas exchange. Echocardiographic parameters suggesting the patient is potentially weanable include an EF >35%, LVOT VTI >10 cm, absence of LV dilatation, and no tamponade [11]. Although there are no universally applied protocols for predicting successful weaning from VA ECMO, in general, this requires staged reduction in flows, monitored by clinical, haemodynamic, and echocardiographic variables. Various regimens exist including gradual reduction to 0.6 l/min/m² over a few minutes, or sequential reduction (66% 15 min, 22% 15 min). Failure should be determined in the context of each patient. Where a weaning trial is deemed successful, echocardiographic guidance of removal is indicated. If weaning is not feasible, and isolated cardiac support required, ventricular assist should be considered.

Ventricular assist devices

Ventricular assist devices (left/right/biventricular) are used according to existing guidelines and registries as longer term support for cardiac failure. Echocardiography plays a key role in the management of such patients [19, 20]. Some of the echocardiographic contraindications to VAD insertion are shown in ⊃ Table 32.3. With LVAD insertion a major echocardiographic challenge is predicting the tolerance of the RV to the increased preload [21]. This is important as RV dysfunction post-LVAD insertion is associated with increased mortality and morbidity [22]. Further, where significant RV dysfunction occurs, it limits function of the LVAD. A number of parameters have been proposed to predict adequate RV function, including RV transverse diameter <3.8 cm, FAC >40%, TAPSE >1.5 cm, and systolic strain/strain rate <16%/1.1 m/s; however, none taken alone is ideal. The strongest pre-implantation predictors of RV failure are pulmonary hypertension (PASP >50 mmHg) and severe RV systolic dysfunction [23]. As with all types of LVAD, AR may become continuous, and

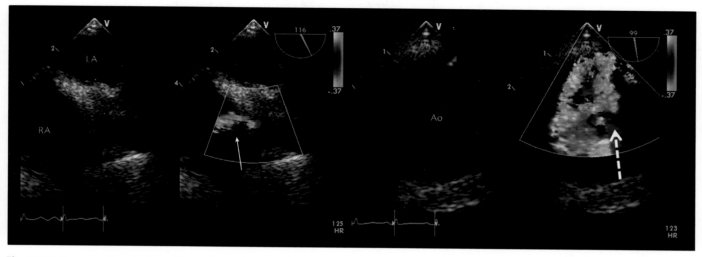

Fig. 32.13 Transoesophageal echocardiogram in a patient receiving veno-arterial extracorporeal membrane oxygenation. On the left (bicaval view) the inlet cannula is seen, with the inlet jet (arrowed) in mid-right atrium (RA). Note the inter-atrial septum is not impeding flow into the cannula. LA, left atrium. On the right (descending aorta, Ao) the return jet is seen (broken arrow) directed to the centre of the aortic lumen.

increase PCWP and PASP, further impairing RV function. When judged to be severe, AR may require surgical intervention at the time of VAD implantation.

Intra-operative TOE is used to assist in optimal placement of both inflow and outflow cannulae, ensuring they do not impact on any intra-cardiac structure and are orientated appropriately [19, 20]. Immediately after implantation, echocardiography is used to assist de-airing, and optimize LV filling whilst increasing pump speed to the required level of support. Here, using the mid-oesophageal 4-chamber view, the inter-ventricular septum should be in the midline. A rightward shift suggests too high a pump speed, and leftward too low. Finally, the aortic valve should be seen to open every few beats, although this may not be achievable in all patients. Various protocols have been suggested in order to achieve the goals of (a) adequate LV offloading whilst (b) maintaining intermittent aortic valve opening and (c) avoiding RV dysfunction. One such protocol is an echo ramped speed study. Here the RPM are decreased until one or more of the following are seen; the aortic valve opens with each beat, the LV becomes more dilated, and/or MR worsens (minimal speed). In order to determine the maximal speed the RPM are increased from the set speed until there is septal shift and/or development of ventricular dysrhythmias. The ideal state is that which allows tolerance of normal alterations in volume status, and is generally approximately 400 ml/min below the maximal speed. PW Doppler of VAD and mitral inflow confirms appropriately low velocities (⊃ Fig. 32.14).

Longer term assessment of LVAD using echocardiography has five main components:

◆ LV unloading: for continuous flow devices measure LVESD and LVEDD, for pulsatile devices (becoming obsolete) the largest LVEDD (at the end of diastole, just after MV closure) and smallest LVESD [20].

◆ RV function and pulmonary hypertension: requires a comprehensive right heart examination [19–23].

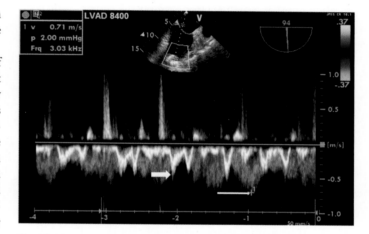

Fig. 32.14 Transoesophageal echocardiogram in a patient with a left ventricular assist device showing PW Doppler of inflow into the cannula (thin arrow), and simultaneously showing transmitral flow (thick arrow). In the miniaturized 2D image at the top of the figure, the inflow cannula at the apex of the left ventricle can be seen.
Image courtesy of Spectrum Health, Grand Rapids, USA.

◆ Cardiac output: right-sided CO should be estimated in parallel with degree of AV opening assessed by M-mode (normal/intermittent/complete closure) [24–26].

◆ Valvular function: demonstration of minimal TR, no worsening of AR, no aortic thrombus (⊃ Fig. 32.10) and ideally intermittent AV opening [19, 20].

◆ Ventricular recovery: there are no uniformly accepted criteria or protocols for predicting successful weaning from LVAD, although a number exist. The decision for explantation is based on clinical stability, echocardiography (with or without dobutamine stress), and measurement of invasive haemodynamics [27, 28]. Here, application of strain/strain rate imaging is a potentially exciting avenue for future research [29].

Echocardiographic detected complications of extracorporeal support

Echocardiography is key in detecting complications resulting from extracorporeal support. The most frequent include:

- Cannula displacement.
- Worsening regurgitation.
- Tamponade.
- Thrombus (from clotted aortic valve), or clotted pulmonary valve.
- Inadvertent overload/excessive offloading of one/both ventricles.

Cannula displacement

This may be major or minor, and result in significant disruption to circuit flow by obstruction to the inlet/outlet, or compression/obstruction of other structures (for example the suprahepatic vein; ⊃ Figs 32.15). The echocardiographer should know the anticipated position of the cannulae, and compare sequential studies.

Worsening valvular regurgitation

In VV ECMO, worsening TR is common, but difficult to assess due to hugely increased non-pulsatile forward flow. In patients undergoing VA ECMO, AR is important, in particular where there is no AV opening (⊃ Figs 32.7–32.9). Where inappropriate offloading is suspected (worsening LV dilatation, high LV diastolic pressure, and/or LA pressure) venting should be considered (⊃ Figs 32.10 and 32.11).

Tamponade

Tamponade (compromise of cardiac output and/or the circuit filling/emptying) due to a pericardial collection is common, particularly early after institution of therapy. Echocardiographic diagnosis is challenging, in particular in the presence of non-pulsatile flow and small/no tidal volume ventilation plus severe ventricular impairment (possibly with no ejection). Further, a large collection, even causing significant compression of a cardiac chamber, may have no clinical relevance until weaning from extracorporeal support is attempted (⊃ Fig. 32.16). If tamponade is clinically suspected, however, and a collection is demonstrated that is impeding filling/emptying, evacuation should be considered.

Thrombus

Despite full anticoagulation, thrombus may be detected using echocardiography, which may be related to the cannulae, cardiac chambers, or across the ventriculo-arterial valves (⊃ Figs 32.12, 32.17, and 32.18). Where VAD or VA ECMO are used following aortic valve replacement, valve thrombosis has been reported, in particular where the heart is not ejecting. Pulmonary artery thrombosis has also been described in VA ECMO in the absence of right heart ejection. Thrombus related to the cannulae is not uncommon, but when small, are usually not clinically important. Large thrombi and/or the presence of an inter-atrial communication, or thrombi in the systemic circulation, may require intervention. The situation with long-term LVAD differs in that the consequences of thrombosis of an indwelling device may be catastrophic. Direct evidence may be found where thrombus is seen related to the cannula inlet. Indirect evidence may be provided by insensitivity of echo parameters to change with altering pump speed, and/or when new AV opening is seen.

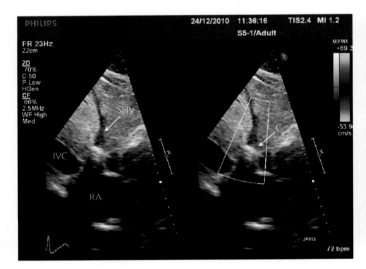

Fig. 32.15 Transthoracic echocardiogram, modified subcostal view. Cannula displacement in a patient on veno-venous extracorporeal membrane oxygenation where the cannula (C) has become displaced from the superior vena cava and migrated into the suprahepatic vein (SHV). Due to the small diameter of this vessel (<10 mm) it has become collapsed around the cannula with high velocity aliasing flows (arrowed).

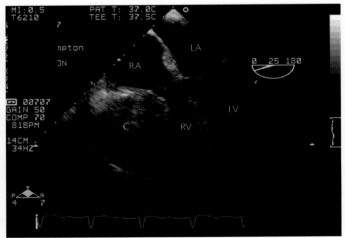

Fig. 32.16 Transoesophageal echocardiogram, modified mid-oesophageal 4-chamber view. An incidental finding of a pericardial collection (C) in a patient receiving peripheral extracorporeal cardiac support following repeat cardiotomy for coronary artery disease. The collection is localised and compressing the right ventricle (RV) but there was no compromise to haemodynamics or the extracorporeal support. LA, left atrium; RA, right atrium; LV, left ventricle; RV, right ventricle.

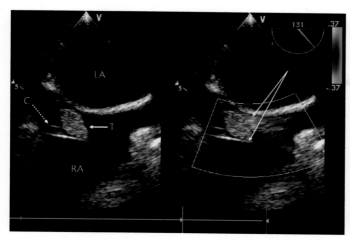

Fig. 32.17 Transoesophageal echocardiogram bicaval view in a patient with haemodynamic and circuit instability on extracorporeal membrane oxygenation (ECMO). The inlet cannula (C) is seen in the right atrium (RA) (broken arrow). Associated with the tip of the cannula is a thrombus (T, solid arrow). This is obstructing inlet flow, as shown on colour Doppler on the right (double-headed arrow).

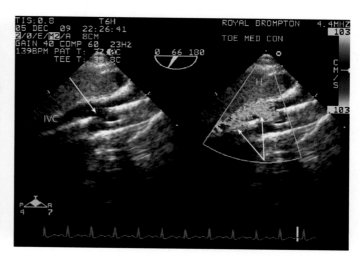

Fig. 32.19 Transthoracic echocardiogram, modified trans hepatic view, focusing on the inferior inlet section of a dual lumen cannula in a patient on veno-venous extracorporeal membrane oxygenation with juddering circuit lines. The cannula is seen in the inferior vena cava (IVC) with one of the inlet orifices arrowed. Colour Doppler reveals high velocity aliasing flow (double headed arrow) both into the cannula, and around it from the collapsed distal IVC. This indicates the patient either needs volume resuscitation or a reduction in RPM of the circuit. H, liver; RPM, revolutions per minute.

Excessive/inadequate offloading of one or both ventricles

Where excessive offloading is attempted, cardiac tissue may be seen prolapsing towards the cannula, resulting in partial obstruction and high Doppler velocities (◌ Fig. 32.19). This is usually associated with juddering of the cannulae and swings in flows. Inadequate offloading of one or both ventricles may be due to inadequate circulatory assist or inappropriate discharge. In these circumstances comprehensive echocardiographic examination, performed in the context of the degree of mechanical and inotropic circulatory support is mandated.

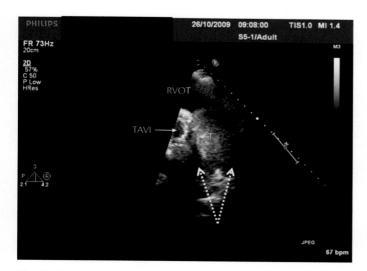

Fig. 32.18 Transthoracic echocardiogram, modified short-axis aortic valve view, focusing on the right ventricular outflow tract (RVOT), pulmonary valve, main pulmonary artery, and pulmonary artery bifurcation (double-headed arrow). This image is from a patient 5 days after initiation of veno-arterial extracorporeal membrane oxygenation for severe biventricular failure following trans-catheter aortic valve implantation (TAVI). There had been no right heart ejection, and despite full anticoagulation, the patient thrombosed (T) his main pulmonary artery extending beyond the pulmonary artery bifurcation.

Conclusion

Echocardiography is of unique importance for this patient population, where CMR is contraindicated, and cardiac CT has limited applications. As the role of extracorporeal support expands, this will require echocardiographers to become familiar with the normal and abnormal features of the hearts and circuits of these highly complex patients, as well as the pathophysiology of critical illness. The main challenges remain predicting the response of the heart to the load imposed by extracorporeal support, and the optimal time for weaning.

References

1. Stoney WS. Historical perspectives in cardiology evolution of cardiopulmonary bypass. *Circulation* 2009; 119: 2844–53.
2. McMurray JJV, Adamopoulos S, Anker SD, et al. ESC Guidelines for the diagnosis and treatment of acute and chronic heart failure 2012. The Task Force for the Diagnosis and Treatment of Acute and Chronic Heart Failure 2012 of the European Society of Cardiology. *European Heart Journal* 2012; 33: 1787–847.
3. Peura JL, Colvin-Adams M, Francis GS, et al. Recommendations for the use of mechanical circulatory support: device strategies and

patient selection: a scientific statement from the American Heart Association. *Circulation* 2012; 126: 3648–3667.

4. Park PK, Napolitano LM, Bartlett RH Extracorporeal membrane oxygenation in adult acute respiratory distress syndrome. *Crit Care Clin* 2011; 27: 627–46.

5. Beckmann A, Benk C, Beyersdorf F, et al. Position article for the use of extracorporeal life support in adult patients. *Eur J Cardiothorac Surg* 2011; 40: 676–80.

6. Dalton HJ. Extracorporeal life support: moving at the speed of light. *Respir Care* 2011; 56: 1445–56.

7. Terragni P, Maiolo G, Ranieri VM. Role and potentials of low-flow CO(2) removal system in mechanical ventilation. *Curr Opin Crit Care* 2012 Feb; 18 (1): 93–8.

8. Noah MA, Peek GJ, Finney SJ, et al. Referral to an extracorporeal membrane oxygenation center and mortality among patients with severe 2009 influenza A(H1N1). *JAMA* 2011; 306 (15): 1659–68.

9. ELSO Registry. http://www.elsonet.org/

10. Vignon P, AitHssain A, Brancois B, et al. Echocardiographic assessment of pulmonary artery occlusion pressure in ventilated patients: a transoesophageal study. *Crit Care* 2008; 12 (1): R18. doi: 10.1186/cc6792. Epub 2008 Feb 19.

11. Platts DG, Sedgwick JF, Burstow DJ, Mullany DV, Fraser JF. The role of echocardiography in the management of patients supported by extracorporeal membrane oxygenation. *J Am Soc Echocardiogr* 2012; 25: 131–41.

12. Cullen S, Shore D, Redington A. Characterization of right ventricular diastolic performance after complete repair of Tetralogy of Fallot. Restrictive physiology predicts slow postoperative recovery. *Circulation* 1995; 91 (6): 1782–9.

13. Javidfar J, Wang D, Zwischenberger J, et al. Insertion of bicaval dual lumen extracorporeal membrane oxygenation catheter with image guidance. *ASAIO J* 2011; 57: 203–5.

14. Dixon SR, Henriques JP, Mauri L, et al. A prospective feasibility trial investigating the use of the Impella. *JACC Cardiovasc Interv* 2009; 2: 91–6.

15. Boening A, Friedrich C, Caliebe D, Cremer J. Efficacy of intra-cardiac right ventricular microaxial pump support during beating heart surgery. *Interact CardioVasc Thorac Surg* 2004; 3 (3): 495–98.

16. Koenig PR, Ralston MA, Kimball TR, Meyer RA, Daniels SR, Schwartz DC. Balloon atrial septostomy for left ventricular decompression in patients receiving extracorporeal membrane oxygenation for myocardial failure. *J Pediatr* 1993; 122: S95–9.

17. O'Connor TA, Downing GJ, Ewing LL, Gowdamarajan R. Echocardiographically guided balloon atrial septostomy during extracorporeal membrane oxygenation (ECMO). *Pediatr Cardiol* 1993; 14: 167–8.

18. Vargas F, Gruson D, Valentine R et al. Transesophageal Pulsed Doppler echocardiography of pulmonary venous flow to assess left ventricular filling pressure in ventilated patients with acute respiratory distress syndrome. *J Crit Care* 1999; 19: 197–79.

19. Ammar K, Umland MM, Kramer C, et al. The ABCs of left ventricular assist device echocardiography: a systematic approach. *Eur Heart J Cardiovasc Imaging* 2012; 13:885–99.

20. Estep JD, Stainback RF, Little SH, Torre G, Zoghbi WA. The role of echocardiography and other imaging modalities in patients with left ventricular assist devices. State of the art paper. *J Am Coll Cardiol Img* 2010; 3 (10): 1049–64. doi: 10.1016/j.jcmg.2010.07.012

21. Fitzpatrick JR, Frederick JR, Hsu VM, et al. Risk score derived from pre-operative data analysis predicts the need for biventricular mechanical circulatory support. *J Heart Lung Transplant.* 2008; 27 (12): 1286–92. doi: 10.1016/j.healun.2008.09.006

22. Miller LW, Pagani FD, Russell SD. HeartMate II Clinical investigators use of a continuous-flow device in patients awaiting heart transplantation. *N Engl J Med* 2007; 357: 885–96.

23. Matthews JC, Koelling TM, Pagani FD, Aaronson KD. The right ventricular failure risk score: a pre-operative tool for assessing the risk of right ventricular failure in left ventricular assist device candidates. *J Am Coll Cardiol* 2008; 51 (22): 2163–72.

24. Lam KM, Ennis S, O'Driscoll G, Solis JM, Macgillivray T, Picard MH. Observations from non-invasive measures of right heart hemodynamics in left ventricular assist device patients. *J Am Soc Echocardiogr* 2009; 22: 1055–62.

25. Stainback RF, Croitoru M, Hernandez A, Myers TJ, Wadia Y, Frazier OH. Echocardiographic evaluation of the Jarvik 2000 axial-flow LVAD. *Tex Heart Inst J* 2005; 32: 263–70.

26. Myers TJ, Frazier OH, Mesina HS, Radovancevic B, Gregoric ID. Hemodynamics and patient safety during pump-off studies of an axial-flow left ventricular assist device. *J Heart Lung Transplant* 2006; 25: 379–83.

27. Dandel M, Weng Y, Siniawski H. Prediction of cardiac stability after weaning from left ventricular assist devices in patients with idiopathic dilated cardiomyopathy. *Circulation* 2008; 118 (Suppl 14): S94–105.

28. George RS, Yacoub MH, Tasca G. Hemodynamic and echocardiographic responses to acute interruption of left ventricular assist device support: relevance to assessment of myocardial recovery. *J Heart Lung Transplant* 2007; 26: 967–73.

29. Dandel M, Lehmkuhl H, Knosalla C, Suramelashvili N, Hetzer R. Strain and strain rate imaging by echocardiography—basic concepts and clinical applicability. *Curr Cardiol Rev* 2009; 5 (2): 133–48.

SECTION VI

Cardiomyopathies

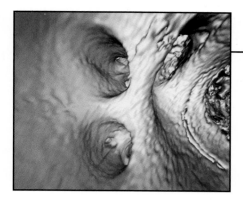

CHAPTER 33

Hypertrophic cardiomyopathy

Frank A. Flachskampf, Oliver Bruder, Ruxandra Beyer, and Petros Nihoyannopoulos

Contents

Introduction

Hypertrophic cardiomyopathy (HCM) is a genetically determined disease with familial and spontaneous occurrence. The disease is often asymptomatic. Symptoms typically develop in young adulthood or later. With advanced disease, the leading symptoms are dyspnoea, angina, and syncope. Because of the risk of syncope and of ventricular arrhythmias and sudden death, detection is important, even in the absence of symptoms in daily life.

On physical examination, findings may be entirely normal or a systolic murmur may be heard over the base of the heart at the left sternal border, which is not transmitted to the carotids. The ECG usually shows signs of left ventricular hypertrophy with strain or left bundle branch block.

The echocardiographic hallmark of HCM is an increase in wall thickness of the left ventricle, with a corresponding increase in left ventricular mass (⊃ Table 33.1). This increase is extremely variable, both in localization as in extent. In fact, localized thickening has been observed in all regions of the left ventricle with this disease, although the most frequent site is the septum. Besides an increase in wall thickness, classical echo signs of the disease include a particular echo texture ('granular sparkling') of the diseased myocardium, changes in mitral valve morphology with increased leaflet size, an anterior shift in papillary muscle position, signs of dynamic systolic left ventricular outflow tract obstruction, including narrowing of the left ventricular outflow tract, systolic anterior motion of the mitral valve, mid-systolic closure of the aortic valve, occurrence of a systolic outflow tract gradient or, less frequently, a systolic gradient at the mid-ventricular level, and mitral regurgitation. The latter signs indicate the presence of the obstructive form of the disease (hypertrophic obstructive cardiomyopathy). However, the degree of obstruction is often fluctuating, depending on sympathetic drive, load conditions, and other factors, and at least a low degree of obstruction is a very frequent finding, even if the full-blown picture of hypertrophic obstructive cardiomyopathy is not present.

Pathophysiology of hypertrophic cardiomyopathy

Hypertrophy

Degree and location of increased left ventricular wall thickness are very variable, ranging from the 'typical' sigmoid shape of the septum with 'asymmetric hypertrophy' (ratio of end-diastolic septal to posterior wall thicknesses >1:1.3) to apical hypertrophy or bizarre localized myocardial 'bumps' (⊃ Fig. 33.1). Hypertrophy usually is concentric

Table 33.1 Echocardiographic signs of HCM; note that none of these signs is absolutely specific for the diagnosis of HCM

◆ Left ventricular wall thickness increase and hypertrophy, especially, but not exclusively, with asymmetric septal hypertrophy (septal/posterior end-diastolic wall thickness >1.3) in the absence of other causes of hypertrophy; any left ventricular segment may be affected, and right ventricular hypertrophy also occurs.
◆ Decreased basal longitudinal myocardial velocities (e' <13.5 cm/s).
◆ Left ventricular systolic outflow tract obstruction or mid-ventricular obstruction
  • systolic anterior motion of the mitral valve with or without septal contact of leaflet tips
  • mid-systolic closure of aortic valve
  • presence of an increased systolic flow velocity (>2 m/s) in the left ventricular outflow tract, with a late systolic peak. In some instances the obstruction is mid-ventricular. Continuous-wave Doppler should be used to record maximal velocities, and pulsed-wave Doppler and colour flow imaging to identify the site of obstruction (left ventricular outflow tract, midventricular, or apical).
◆ Abnormalities of the mitral valve are frequent, including all degrees of mitral regurgitation (which may be dynamic), prolapse, leaflet thickening, and papillary muscle abnormalities.

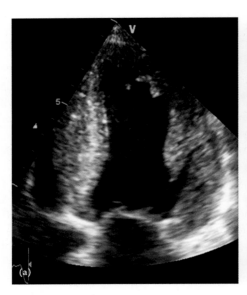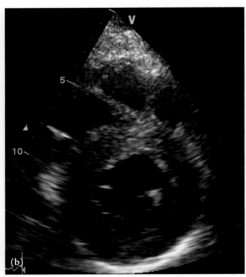

Fig. 33.1 (a) End-diastolic apical 4-chamber view of patient with hypertrophic cardiomyopathy. The maximal septal thickness is 31 mm, and the lateral wall is also massively thickened. Note bright echo texture of septal myocardium. (b) Diastolic parasternal short-axis view of left ventricle of same patient.

(without increase in cavity diameter), although eccentric hypertrophy with impaired left ventricular ejection fraction has been described in end-stage HCM. A pronounced, localized increase in wall thickness is suggestive of HCM, except for the basal septal bulge often found in long-standing hypertension. In any case, differentiation from long-standing severe hypertensive heart disease is difficult based on wall thickness or mass alone, except that very large increases in wall thickness and mass (e.g. end-diastolic thicknesses in excess of 20 mm) are indicative of cardiomyopathy. An overlap form of 'hypertensive hypertrophic cardiomyopathiy of the elderly' has been described [1]. Thus, in a patient with extensive wall hypertrophy and a history of substantial hypertension, additional HCM cannot be excluded. Similarly, aortic stenosis or infiltrative cardiomyopathy (e.g. cardiac amyloidosis) can produce left ventricular hypertrophy difficult to distinguish from HCM. Recently, reduced peak systolic longitudinal deformation (strain) averaged over all left ventricular walls was reported to distinguish hypertensive from cardiomyopathic hypertrophy, with values for deformation (strain) <10.6% (in absolute value, neglecting the negative sign) predicting HCM with a sensitivity of 85% and specificity of 100%. A ratio of end-diastolic septal to posterior wall thickness >1.3 combined with evaluation of systolic strain yielded a predictive accuracy of 96% [2].

Apical HCM is more frequently seen in Asia, especially in Japan, than in Western countries. In this subset of HCM, there is systolic apical cavity obliteration (⊃ Fig. 33.2), and giant negative T waves are seen in the precordial ECG leads. Left ventricular contrast echocardiography may aid in the delineation of apical hypertrophy. Apical aneurysms, which occur in only approximately 2% of patients with HCM [3, 4], are mostly associated with apical or midventricular hypertrophy, and seem to affect prognosis negatively. These aneurysms, which usually are small, may escape two-dimensional echo detection because of either suboptimal apical image quality (which may be improved by echo contrast) or foreshortening of the left ventricular apex. If this form of HCM is suspected, CMR may be helpful. Paradoxical diastolic flow directed towards the mitral valve may be present and detectable by Doppler.

The basic functional disorder in HCM occurs during diastole with slowed relaxation, impaired filling and decreased compliance of the ventricles. Far from being uniform, myocardial dysfunction is regional and irregular depending upon the extent and distribution of the underlying myofibrillar lesions. Early studies using M-mode echocardiography showed that the rates of filling and relaxation of the left ventricle were abnormal in patients with hypertrophic cardiomyopathy. However, pulsed-wave Doppler

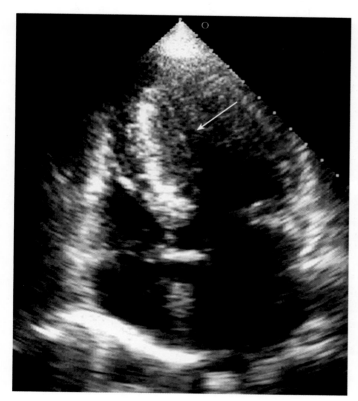

Fig. 33.2 Apical 4-chamber view of apical HCM with left ventricular cavity obliteration in systole (right, arrow).

echocardiographic recordings of transmitral flow are easier to obtain and provide a good overall estimate of diastolic filling abnormalities of the left ventricle [5]. In HCM patients, the period during which the heart is isovolumic (isovolumic relaxation time) is often prolonged, left ventricular filling is slow, and the proportion of filling volume resulting from atrial systole may be increased. As long as left atrial pressures are still normal, impaired ventricular relaxation results in prolonged isovolumic relaxation time, slower early ventricular filling (E wave), and a compensatory exaggerated atrial systolic filling (A wave), with a reduced E/A ratio [5]. In more severe cases, with increased mean diastolic left atrial pressure (>15 mmHg), rapid filling is increased with a consequent reduction of the atrial contribution, giving the wrong impression of 'normalization' of left ventricular filling (pseudonormalization). Such 'normalization' of the diastolic filling pattern in HCM can also happen in the presence of significant mitral regurgitation. More advanced still, with decreased compliance and high left ventricular filling pressures, there is accelerated and shortened rapid early filling and normal or reduced late filling similar to patients with restrictive cardiomyopathy. It is, therefore, understandable that in a non-homogeneous HCM population where patients exhibit different degrees of functional disability, they will be presenting with a spectrum of mitral and pulmonary venous inflow waveforms. Colour Doppler flow imaging can distinguish the high pre-systolic inflow velocity (A wave) from the lower velocity of the early diastolic filling flow (E wave) by the increased brightness of the red-orange colour occurring in late diastole, which also often

aliases. Since patients with HCM usually have small left ventricular cavity dimensions, the higher velocity in late diastole may be seen into the left ventricular cavity and even on occasion reaching the cardiac apex.

The texture of myopathic walls, especially the septum, has been described as 'granular sparkling', highlighting the increased brightness and strong speckle pattern of the myocardium (⊃ Figs 33.1 and 33.2). A stringent definition of this descriptive term, however, does not exist and the finding is rather unspecific, also occurring in severe hypertrophy of other aetiologies.

Obstruction

Basal septal hypertrophy per se leads to a narrowing of the outflow tract during systole (⊃ Figs 33.3 and 33.4). In addition, in the full-blown picture of obstructive HCM, the attachment of the papillary muscles is shifted anteriorly, thus contributing to the narrowing of the left ventricular outflow tract. HCM also frequently affects the mitral valve, with enlargement especially of the anterior leaflet [6]. This leaflet partakes in the obstructive mechanism, moving—together with the whole mitral apparatus—anteriorly into the left ventricular outflow tract and towards the septum in systole, a phenomenon termed systolic anterior motion (SAM; ⊃ Figs 33.3 and 33.6). The extent of the SAM is variable between patients and also in a given patient according to sympathetic drive, load conditions, and medication. The ultimate mechanism of this characteristic sign of obstruction is still debated, but elegant work from Robert A. Levine's group in Boston makes it likely that the mechanism is slack in the chordal tethering of the enlarged anterior mitral leaflet, at least partly due to the malposition of the papillary muscles, which allows leaflet tissue to be dragged into the outflow tract by the blood propelled towards the aortic valve [7, 8]. An alternative mechanism that has been proposed is a Venturi force sucking the mitral leaflet towards the septum by the increased flow velocity in the outflow tract [9]. The latter mechanism sees the systolic anterior motion as consequence, not cause, of left ventricular outflow tract obstruction, while the former explanation implies a causal contribution of SAM to obstruction.

Although left ventricular obstruction in HCM is most frequent at the outflow tract level (⊃ Figs 33.7–33.9), mid-ventricular obstruction at the papillary muscle level is not uncommon and can be detected and distinguished from classical obstructive HCM by registering systolic flow turbulence at the mid-ventricular (papillary) muscle level rather than at the outflow tract level by colour and spectral Doppler.

Changes in mitral valve morphology and function

As mentioned before, analyses of autopsy material have shown that mitral leaflet sizes are increased in patients with obstructive HCM, and that papillary muscle position, insertion, and morphology are often abnormal, with anterior and medial displacement and hypertrophy. These changes are related to SAM, obstruction, and the occurrence of mitral regurgitation, which is present to some degree in nearly all obstructive HCM patients and may be severe.

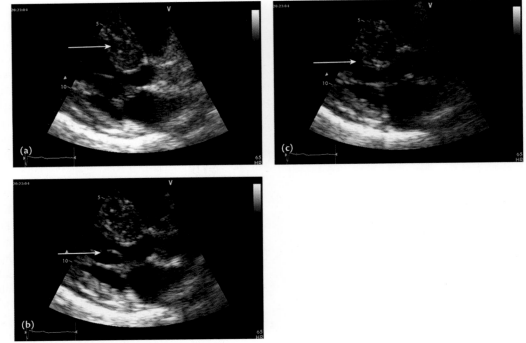

Fig. 33.3 Typical example of hypertrophic obstructive cardiomyopathy. Parasternal long-axis view (zoom). (a) End-diastolic frame, showing thickened septum (20 mm; arrow). Note that the posterior wall is less thickened (12 mm). (b) Early systole. The tip of the anterior mitral leaflet (arrow) approaches the septum. (c) Mid-systole: septal contact of the anterior leaflet (arrow). Note the narrowed outflow tract.

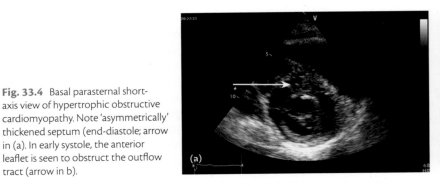

Fig. 33.4 Basal parasternal short-axis view of hypertrophic obstructive cardiomyopathy. Note 'asymmetrically' thickened septum (end-diastole; arrow in (a). In early systole, the anterior leaflet is seen to obstruct the outflow tract (arrow in b).

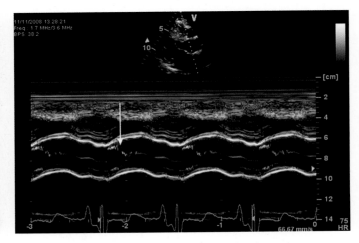

Fig. 33.5 M-mode of mitral valve in hypertrophic obstructive cardiomyopathy. Note typical systolic anterior motion pattern (arrow) with mid-systolic contact with the massively thickened septum.

Fig. 33.6 M-mode of the aortic valve in hypertrophic obstructive cardiomyopathy. Note mid-systolic partial closure of the aortic valve due to increasing obstruction (arrow).

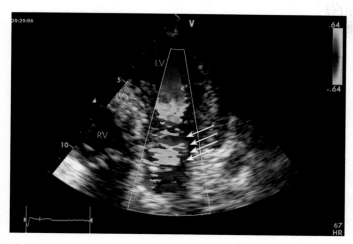

Fig. 33.7 Apical 5-chamber view in hypertrophic obstructive cardiomyopathy. Colour Doppler mapping in systole shows flow acceleration and turbulence in the left ventricular outflow tract (arrows). IVS, ventricular septum; LV, left ventricle; RV, right ventricle.

Myocardial velocity and deformation

In spite of usually preserved left ventricular ejection fraction (which mainly represents radial systolic inward motion), the longitudinal systolic and early diastolic velocities of the left ventricular myocardium are decreased, which is best detected at the mitral annulus level (➲ Fig. 33.10). In a study of 36 individuals who were genotyped and positive for a familial HCM form and 36 controls, a decrease of early diastolic tissue velocity e' (averaged from basal septal, lateral, anterior and posterior walls) below 13.5 cm/s had a sensitivity of 75% and a specificity of 86% to detect individuals genetically positive for HCM, although half of the 36 genetically positive individuals were asymptomatic and without hypertrophy on echo (➲ Fig. 33.11). Similar data were reported from another group [10, 11]. Myocardial longitudinal deformation (strain) is decreased at the site of hypertrophy; in a recent publication, mid-septal maximal strain was −1.3 ± 8.2% in HCM (including some patients with reversed midseptal strain, i.e. systolic elongation), versus 17.6 ± 5.0% in controls, with an inverse correlation between midseptal wall thickness and strain [12] (➲ Fig. 33.11), and averaged peak systolic longitudinal strain <10.6% has been used to distinguish HCM from hypertensive hypertrophy [2]. In the hypertrophic cardiomyopathy associated with Friedreich's ataxia, a neurodegenerative disease, significantly lower systolic and particularly early diastolic strain rates were noted in homozygously

affected patients than in age-matched controls [13]. Note, however, that such decreases in tissue velocities and deformation indices also occur in infiltrative cardiomyopathies (see Chapter 34) and hypertrophic remodelling of other aetiologies. In obstructive HCM, there may be a very short mid-systolic deceleration of longitudinal tissue velocity detectable, corresponding to mid-systolic aortic closure.

Diagnosis

The most recent pertinent recommendations of the European Society of Cardiology and of the American cardiac societies stipulate that 'The clinical diagnosis of HCM is established most easily and reliably with two-dimensional echocardiography by demonstrating left ventricular hypertrophy (LVH) (typically asymmetric in distribution, and showing virtually any diffuse or segmental pattern of left ventricular (LV) wall thickening). Left ventricular wall thickening is associated with a nondilated and hyperdynamic chamber (often with systolic cavity obliteration) in the absence of another cardiac or systemic disease (e.g. hypertension or aortic stenosis) capable of producing the magnitude of hypertrophy evident, and independent of whether or not LV outflow obstruction is present' [14–16].

A mild increase in wall thickness of the left ventricle is a very frequent echocardiographic finding and mostly due to hypertension. Exercise also leads to modest increases in wall thickness, and a study in 947 word-class athletes found an end-diastolic wall thickness >12 mm in only 1.7% of them, with a maximum of 16 mm [17]. Thus, substantial increases in wall thickness in the absence of hypertension are always suspicious of HCM. However, no unambiguous cut-off of septal thickness exists for the diagnosis of HCM. The pattern of 'asymmetric septal hypertrophy' is particularly typical of obstructive HCM, but balanced concentric hypertrophy may also occur and localized increases in wall thickness, e.g. in circumscribed regions of the left ventricular free wall, have been described as well. A particular form of HCM has been described predominantly in Asian patients, but also in others, where hypertrophy is confined to the left ventricular apex. Typically, these patients have deep negative symmetric T waves in their precordial ECG leads.

Obstruction can be suspected in the presence of 'turbulent' intraventricular flow on colour Doppler, which also precisely identifies

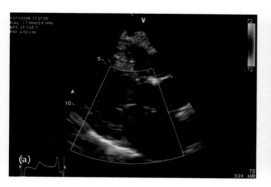
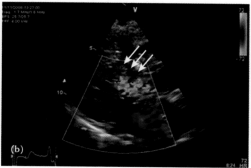

Fig. 33.8 Parasternal long-axis view in hypertrophic obstructive cardiomyopathy. (a) End-diastolic frame for orientation. (b) Colour Doppler mapping in systole shows flow acceleration and turbulence in the left ventricular outflow tract, well proximal of the aortic valve (arrows).

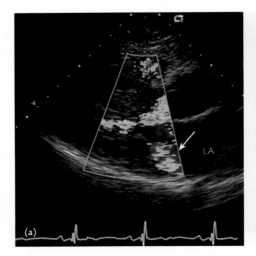
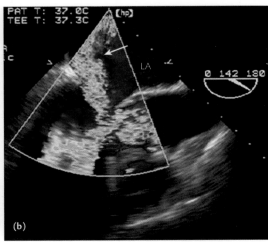

Fig. 33.9 Hypertrophic obstructive cardiomyopathy with severe mitral regurgitation (arrow): (a) parasternal long-axis view, b) transoesophageal long-axis view. Note also systolic high-velocity flow (turbulence) in the left ventricular outflow tract.

the location of maximal flow acceleration and thus, obstruction (⊃ Figs 33.7–33.9). This is especially important if interventional therapy is contemplated. The findings can be corroborated by carefully moving the sample volume of the pulsed-wave Doppler in an apical long-axis or five-chamber view along the septum from the left ventricular cavity towards the outflow tract from an apical window, identifying the location of obstruction where the peak systolic flow velocity starts to abruptly increase and aliasing occurs. Peak outflow tract velocities should be acquired by continuous-wave Doppler and typically show a late systolic maximum, giving the spectral curve a 'dagger shape' (⊃ Fig. 33.12). Peak velocities vary with the degree of obstruction, but can exceed 5 m/s. It is common practice to report the peak velocities or gradients and not mean gradients in this disease. The normal upper limit of left ventricular outflow tract velocities is not well defined, but is generally assumed to be 1.5 m/s; on the other hand, a peak subaortic flow velocity of >2.7 m/s or a gradient of >30 mmHg are currently recommended by guidelines to diagnose the obstructive form of HCM [14, 15]. Further, if a peak gradient >30 mmHg is present at rest, this is termed 'basal obstruction'; if not, HCM is

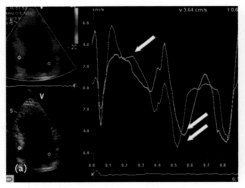
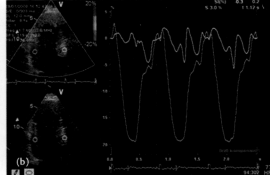

Fig. 33.10 Deformation imaging in HCM. (a) Longitudinal tissue velocities of basal septum (yellow) and lateral wall (green). Systolic (single arrow) and early diastolic velocities (double arrows) are severely depressed (<6 cm/s). (b) Longitudinal strain from hypertrophied septum (green) and lateral of wall of normal thickness (yellow). Note severely depressed longitudinal peak strain in the septum (<5%).

Fig. 33.11 Tissue Doppler parameters in the detection of subclinical hypertrophic cardiomyopathy. Longitudinal tissue velocities in normals, genetically affected patients *without* phenotypically manifest hypertrophy (M + /LVH−), and genetically affected patients *with* echocardiographic hypertrophy (M + /LVH +). (a) Shows peak systolic longitudinal velocities (Sa); (b) early diastolic velocities (Ea), measured at the lateral mitral annulus region. The differences are statistically significant.
Reproduced, with permission, from Nagueh SF, Bachinski LL, Meyer D, et al. Tissue Doppler imaging consistently detects myocardial abnormalities in patients with hypertrophic cardiomyopathy and provides a novel means for an early diagnosis before and independently of hypertrophy. *Circulation* 2001; 104: 128–30.

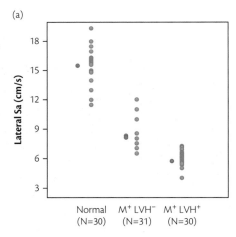
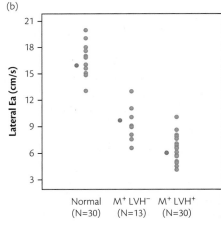

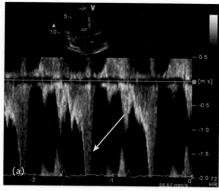

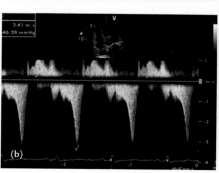

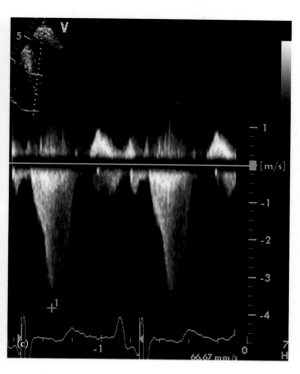

Fig. 33.12 (a) Pulsed Doppler recording of systolic flow in the left ventricle in a patient with hypertrophic obstructive cardiomyopathy. Note that sample volume is about 25 mm distant from the aortic valve, well within the left ventricle. Systolic flow velocities towards the outflow tract (arrow) are clearly elevated (>2 m/s) and there is aliasing. (b) Continuous-wave Doppler recording of outflow tract velocities in same patient. Note late-peaking elevated velocities (peak gradient, 46 mmHg). (c) Continuous-wave Doppler recording of outflow tract velocities from another patient with hypertrophic obstructive cardiomyopathy and a peak gradient of 60 mmHg.

'non-obstructive', and if only a provokable gradient >30 mmHg (by exercise, nitrates, or Valsalva) exists, this is called labile obstruction. The reported gradient is exclusively the peak gradient. If borderline velocities are detected, measurement after physical exercise or after administering sublingual nitroglycerine (one to two puffs) may be considered. Shape and timing distinguishes the continuous-wave signal of outflow tract obstruction from the signal of concomitant mitral regurgitation, which may be similar in peak velocity, but starts earlier and finishes later than the obstruction signal, and has a symmetric shape. Often one can see both spectra superimposed. If in doubt, mitral regurgitation should be recorded by pulsed Doppler at the mitral annulus level and the timing compared to the signal in question.

Morphologic signs of obstruction are:

◆ SAM, which can vary from a barely perceptible buckling to clear contact between the anterior mitral leaflet and the septum during systole. A systolic anterior motion confined to the chordae (chordal SAM) is a more unspecific finding not diagnostic of obstructive HCM. Even leaflet SAM, however, can occur in a number of other situations than obstructive HCM, namely during dobutamine stress in otherwise normal ventricles with excellent function, in states of volume depletion or external compression of the left ventricle (e.g. by a large right ventricle), and after surgical mitral valve repair with a ring.

◆ Mid-systolic (incomplete) closure of the aortic valve, best seen by M-mode (⊃ Fig. 33.6), due to the mid-systolic peak in obstruction.

Additional confirmation of HCM may be sought from tissue Doppler and deformation imaging (⊃ Fig. 33.10). Both show markedly decreased velocities and deformation parameters in the presence of HCM, in spite of preserved ejection fraction, and—based on published studies in small numbers of patients—may be able to detect HCM before hypertrophy becomes apparent or in genetically, but not phenotypically affected individuals. Special attention should be paid to a decrease in e' velocity when screening relatives of patients with HCM. However, these changes are not specific and also found in other cardiomyopathies or hypertrophy of other origins.

Current guidelines for HCM [15] recommend initial detailed evaluation of patients suspected of HCM by echo and, if the diagnosis is confirmed, a repeat echo if new symptoms occur. Echo (in particular transoesophageal echo) is also recommended for intraprocedural guidance during surgical or interventional treatment (class I recommendations). Class IIa recommendations are made for 1–2 yearly follow-up echo exams in symptomatic but stable patients, and of exercise echo to quantify dynamic outflow tract obstruction in patients without gradient at rest. For screening purposes, serial echo exams are felt to be reasonable for asymptomatic first-degree relatives of patients with proven HCM if they are not genetically tested. Suggested echo intervals are 5 years for adults and 12–18 months for children and adolescents. In the risk stratification for sudden cardiac death, and thus the evaluation for implantation of an implantable cardioverter/defibrillator, massive hypertrophy (ventricular wall thickness >30 mm) is an established risk factor with a class IIa recommendation for device implantation in the US. Other factors with less clear prognostic role are the presence of obstruction and of apical aneurysms. Exercise stress echo may be useful to document provokable obstruction or significant mitral regurgitation, both of which may be absent at rest, especially if symptoms suggest exercise dependency [15].

Pitfalls

An erroneous diagnosis of presence or absence of HCM can occur due to the following mistakes [18]:

◆ Left ventricular hypertrophy due to hypertension (often with a basal septal bulge), aortic stenosis, infiltrative cardiomyopathy, or heavy exercise. Left ventricular non-compaction may mimic HCM. This is a cardiomyopathy characterized by a two-layered left ventricular wall structure with a heavily trabecularized inner layer (the non-compacted layer) showing prominent inter-trabecular spaces and a thickness at least twice as large as the compacted outer layer [19].

◆ Over-reliance on M-mode measurements of septal and posterior wall thickness. M-mode measurements frequently are oblique to the true short axis of the left ventricle. Attention to this problem, measurements from 2D images or from anatomic M-mode help to avoid this problem.

◆ Apical hypertrophy may go undetected due to near-field artefact and a transducer position anterior and superior to the LV anatomic apex. Insufficient delineation of the lateral wall may also obscure localized hypertrophy. In cases of doubt, left heart contrast injection may be helpful.

◆ In conditions of volume depletion, during dobutamine stress, in acute anterior myocardial infarction, or with Takotsubo cardiomyopathy, unspecific systolic ventricular gradients may occur. These do not indicate the presence of cardiomyopathy.

◆ In hypertrophied ventricles, isolated mid-ventricular obstruction may occur without other typical signs of hypertrophic cardiomyopathy.

◆ Subaortic membranes create left ventricular outflow tract gradients and may be difficult to visualize by transthoracic echocardiography.

When recording left ventricular (outflow tract) gradients by continuous-wave Doppler, care must be taken not to confound them with mitral regurgitation signals. Mitral regurgitation starts earlier (immediately after the end of the transmitral A wave) and ends later (at the onset of the transmitral E wave). If in doubt, the timing of the systolic high velocity signal on continuous-wave

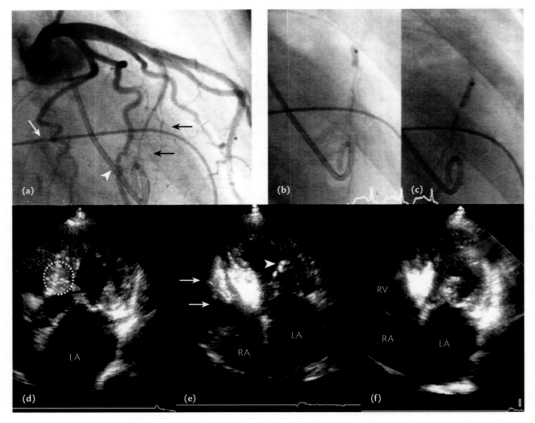

Fig. 33.13 Interventional and echocardiographic sequence of a (super-selective) septal ablation procedure for symptomatic HOCM. Angio sequence: first major septal perforator artery with two sub-branches (black arrows) as the presumed target vessel (a, white arrow: lead of the temporary pacemaker, white arrowhead: pigtail catheter in the left ventricle), balloon within the proximal part of the septal perforator, (b) distal vessel bed with two sub-branches contrasted angiographically, (c) balloon advanced super-selectively into the left/basal sub-branch. Corresponding echo sequence: subaortic septum as target region in typical SAM-associated, subaortic obstruction (d, dotted line), (e) test injection of the echo contrast agent in balloon position of (b) highlighting the basal half of the septum plus a right ventricular papillary muscle (white arrows), (f) after super-selective balloon position of (c), correct opacification of the target region is achieved. RA, right atrium; RV, right ventricle; LA, left atrium.

Reproduced from Faber L, Seggewiss H, Welge D, et al. Echo-guided percutaneous septal ablation for symptomatic hypertrophic obstructive cardiomyopathy: 7 years of experience. *European Journal of Echocardiography* (2004) 5 (5): 347–55, by permission of Oxford University Press.

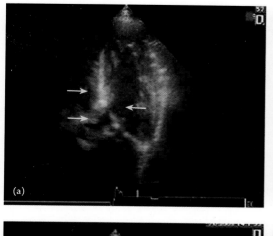

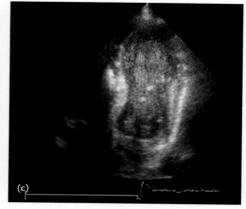

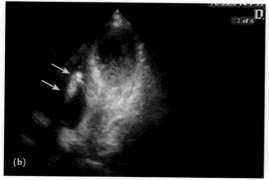

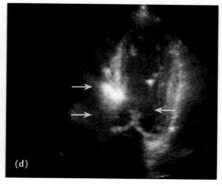

Fig. 33.14 Variety of structures at risk for alcohol-induced necrosis as detected by intra-procedural echocardiography. (a) Baseline 4-chamber view in a patient who had myectomy 5 years ago and underwent septal ablation because of class III symptoms and significant SAM-associated (arrow) recurrent obstruction. Target region marked by arrowheads. Test injection into the first presumed target vessel produces opacification of a right papillary muscle (b, arrows), test injection into a second septal perforator leads to LV cavity contrast (c) without any opacification within the target region, injection into the third target vessel correctly highlights the target region (d, arrowheads).

Reproduced from Faber L, Seggewiss H, Welge D, et al. Echo-guided percutaneous septal ablation for symptomatic hypertrophic obstructive cardiomyopathy: 7 years of experience. *European Journal of Echocardiography* (2004) 5 (5): 347–55, by permission of Oxford University Press.

Doppler assumed to be due to ventricular obstruction should be compared to the timing of pulsed-wave recordings of mitral regurgitation and outflow tract velocities. Finally, subaortic membranes in the left ventricular outflow tract may create high, turbulent outflow tract velocities, which can be confounded with obstructive HCM. The gradient created by a subaortic membrane has a mid-systolic, not late-systolic peak, and the membrane can be directly visualized by close attention to the outflow tract, best by transoesophageal echo.

Imaging in guiding the interventional treatment of hypertrophic obstructive cardiomyopathy

While medical therapy with beta-blockade and calcium antagonists is the first therapeutic step in symptomatic individuals, percutaneous septal alcohol ablation or surgical septal myectomy/myotomy are performed in patients with persisting severe symptoms. Echo is used in a few centres performing percutaneous alcohol ablation to define the perfusion territory of the targeted septal branch of the left anterior descending artery [20, 21] (⊃ Figs 33.13 and 33.14). For this purpose, echo contrast is injected during coronary angiography into the respective septal branch through the lumen of an over-the-wire balloon catheter after guidewire removal. The balloon is inflated to prevent spillover of contrast into the left anterior descending artery. Impressive variability in the perfusion territory of such branches has been reported. The delineation of the perfusion territory serves to:

- identify if the corresponding septal area is adjacent to the region of flow acceleration, and
- identify other structures perfused by the septal branch, e.g. right ventricular myocardial regions, papillary muscles, and other areas, which would be jeopardized by the planned alcohol ablation.

In the largest reported series of 337 patients who had intracoronary echo contrast application before intended septal ablation [21], in 18 (6%) patients the procedure was aborted because atypical perfusion territories were found at risk (right and left papillary muscles, right ventricular free wall) by the septal contrast injection.

During surgical myectomy/myotomy, intra-operative echo can guide the surgeon as to the necessary extent of removal of septal myocardium, while avoiding creation of a ventricular septal defect. Sometimes after myectomy small fistulas can be seen from coronary branches, which have been cut and now drain into the left ventricle (⊃ Fig. 33.15).

Role of cardiovascular magnetic resonance imaging in hypertrophic cardiomyopathy

Echocardiography is the first-line method for the diagnosis of hypertrophic cardiomyopathy. However, if image quality is limited with echocardiography, cardiovascular magnetic resonance

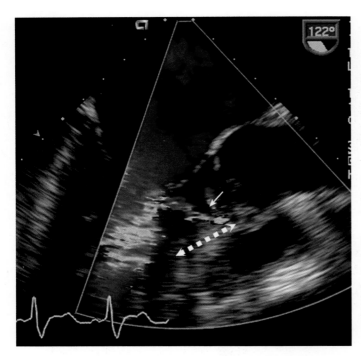

Fig. 33.15 Coronary fistulae (solid arrow) with diastolic flow into the left ventricle after surgical myectomy/myotomy in a patient with hypertrophic obstructive cardiomyopathy. The dotted double arrow delineates the approximate extent of the myectomy. Transoesophageal long-axis view.

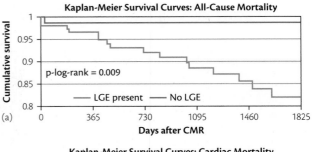

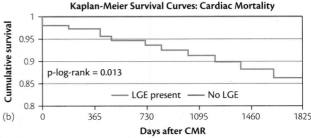

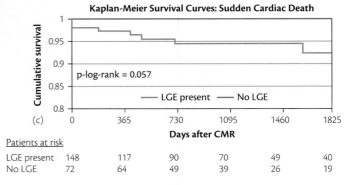

Patients at risk					
LGE present	148	117	90	70	49	40
No LGE	72	64	49	39	26	19

Fig. 33.16 Kaplan–Meier survival curves with regard to all-cause mortality (a), cardiac mortality (b), and sudden cardiac death (c). Note that in the group without any scar not a single patient suffered cardiac death (b) or sudden cardiac death (c) during the first five years of follow-up.

Reprinted from the *Journal of the American College of Cardiology*, 56:11, Bruder O et al, Myocardial scar visualized by cardiovascular magnetic resonance imaging predicts major adverse events in patients with hypertrophic cardiomyopathy, 875–87, Copyright 2010 with permission from Elsevier.

(CMR) cine imaging accurately visualizes the distribution and degree of left ventricular hypertrophy in all myocardial segments due to the complete short-axis coverage of the left ventricle and readily identifies patients with atypical or apical variants of hypertrophic cardiomyopathy [22].

In addition to anatomy and function, CMR late gadolinium enhancement offers a unique tool for high-resolution fibrosis or scar imaging [29]. The characteristic HCM pattern of late gadolinium enhancement distribution is intramural and within segments of hypertrophy, mainly the inter-ventricular septum, and the regions where the right ventricle inserts into the left ventricle [23, 24]. The presence of late gadolinium enhancement in patients with hypertrophic cardiomyopathy is related to progressive disease with left ventricular dysfunction [22] and the occurrence and frequency of ventricular tachyarrhythmias on ambulatory Holter ECG (25).

The annual mortality rate ranges from 1% to 2% in an unselected population (26). In particular, hypertrophic cardiomyopathy is the most common cause of sudden cardiac death in young people [33]. Unfortunately, recommended clinical factors for risk stratification in hypertrophic cardiomyopathy are limited by a very low positive predictive value [28, 29]. However, myocardial scars as displayed by late gadolinium enhancement are the likely substrate for potentially lethal ventricular tachyarrhythmias. Two recent studies simultaneously reported the prognostic impact of late gadolinium enhancement in asymptomatic or mildly symptomatic patients with HCM undergoing CMR [30, 31]. Bruder et al. [30] demonstrated in 220 patients, with a mean follow-up time of 3 years, that the presence of late gadolinium enhancement was the

best independent predictor of all-cause mortality, cardiac mortality, and sudden cardiac death (⊃ Fig. 33.16). Importantly, no patient without late gadolinium enhancement died during follow-up, whereas some patients without clinical risk factors but extensive late gadolinium enhancement suffered sudden cardiac death or aborted cardiac death (⊃ Fig. 33.17).

Obviously, future clinical trials that randomize patients to implantable cardioverter/defibrillator therapy depending on the presence or extent of late gadolinium enhancement, and the results of the EuroCMR registry [32] are needed to redefine current indications for implantable cardioverter/defibrillator placement in hypertrophic cardiomyopathy. At present, whenever in selected patients SCD risk stratification remains inconclusive after clinical risk assessment by conventional risk factors, late gadolinium enhancement can be used as a risk modifier to guide clinical decision-making with regard to implantable cardioverter/defibrillator implantation [15].

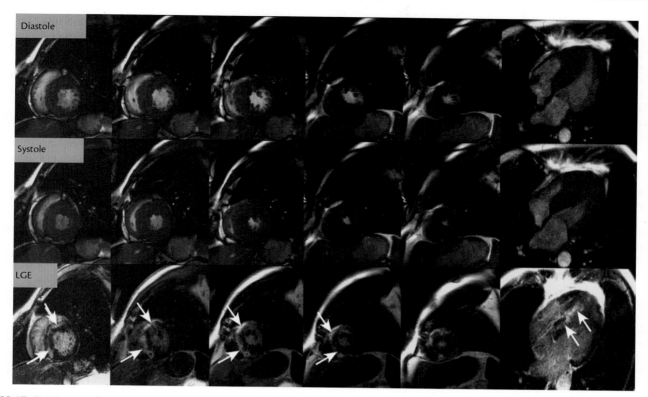

Fig. 33.17 CMR images of a 64 years old white male without any clinical risk factors. However, LGE revealed substantial myocardial scarring (white arrows). The patient suffered sudden cardiac death during follow-up, underscoring that myocardial scarring may be a better predictor of cardiac mortality than conventional risk factors.

Reprinted from the *Journal of the American College of Cardiology*, 56:11, Bruder O et al, Myocardial scar visualized by cardiovascular magnetic resonance imaging predicts major adverse events in patients with hypertrophic cardiomyopathy, 875–87, Copyright 2010 with permission from Elsevier.

References

1. Topol EJ, Traill TA, Fortuin NJ. Hypertensive hypertrophic cardiomyopathy of the elderly. *N Engl J Med* 1985; 312: 277–83.

2. Kato TS, Noda A, Izawa H, et al. Discrimination of nonobstructive hypertrophic cardiomyopathy from hypertensive left ventricular hypertrophy on the basis of strain rate imaging by tissue Doppler ultrasonography. *Circulation* 2004; 110: 3808–14.

3. Matsubara K, Nakamura T, Kuribayashi T, Azuma A, Nakagawa M. Sustained cavity obliteration and apical aneurysm formation in apical hypertrophic cardiomyopathy. *J Am Coll Cardiol* 2003; 42: 288–95; Erratum in: *J Am Coll Cardiol* 2003; 42: 1338.

4. Maron MS, Finley JJ, Bos JM, et al. Prevalence, clinical significance, and natural history of left ventricular apical aneurysms in hypertrophic cardiomyopathy. *Circulation* 2008; 118: 1541–9.

5. Nihoyannopoulos P, Karatasakis G, Frenneaux M, McKenna WJ, Oakley CM. Diastolic function in hypertrophic cardiomyopathy; relation to exercise capacity. *J Am Coll Cardiol* 1992; 19: 536–40.

6. Klues HG, Maron BJ, Dollar AL, Roberts WC. Diversity of structural mitral valve alterations in hypertrophic cardiomyopathy. *Circulation* 1992; 85: 1651–60.

7. Jiang L, Levine RA, King ME, Weyman AE. An integrated mechanism for systolic anterior motion of the mitral valve in hypertrophic cardiomyopathy based on echocardiographic observations. *Am Heart J* 1987; 113: 633–44.

8. Levine RA, Vlahakes GJ, Lefebvre X, et al. Papillary muscle displacement causes systolic anterior motion of the mitral valve. Experimental validation and insights into the mechanism of subaortic obstruction. *Circulation* 1995; 91: 1189–95.

9. Maron BJ, Bonow RO, Cannon RO, III, et al. Hypertrophic cardiomyopathy: Interrelations of clinical manifestations, pathophysiology and therapy. *N Engl J Med* 1987; 316: 780–9 and 844–52.

10. Nagueh SF, Bachinski LL, Meyer D, et al. Tissue Doppler imaging consistently detects myocardial abnormalities in patients with hypertrophic cardiomyopathy and provides a novel means for an early diagnosis before and independently of hypertrophy. *Circulation* 2001; 104: 128–30.

11. Ho CY, Sweitzer NK, McDonough B, et al. Assessment of diastolic function with Doppler tissue imaging to predict genotype in preclinical hypertrophic cardiomyopathy. *Circulation* 2002; 105: 2992–7.

12. Yang H, Sun JP, Lever HM, et al. Use of strain imaging in detecting segmental dysfunction in patients with hypertrophic cardiomyopathy. *J Am Soc Echocardiogr* 2003; 16: 233–9.

13. Dutka DP, Donnelly JE, Palka P, Lange A, Nunez DJ, Nihoyannopoulos P. Echocardiographic characterization of cardiomyopathy in Friedreich's ataxia with tissue Doppler echocardiographically derived myocardial velocity gradients. *Circulation* 2000; 102: 1276–82.

14. Maron BJ, McKenna WJ, Danielson GK, et al.; American College of Cardiology Foundation Task Force on Clinical Expert Consensus Documents; European Society of Cardiology Committee for Practice Guidelines. American College of Cardiology/European Society of Cardiology Clinical Expert Consensus Document on Hypertrophic

Cardiomyopathy. A report of the American College of Cardiology Foundation Task Force on Clinical Expert Consensus Documents and the European Society of Cardiology Committee for Practice Guidelines. *Eur Heart J* 2003; 24: 1965–91.

15. Gersh BJ, Maron BJ, Bonow RO, et al. American College of Cardiology Foundation/American Heart Association Task Force on Practice Guidelines. 2011 ACCF/AHA Guideline for the Diagnosis and Treatment of Hypertrophic Cardiomyopathy: a report of the American College of Cardiology Foundation/American Heart Association Task Force on Practice Guidelines. Developed in collaboration with the American Association for Thoracic Surgery, American Society of Echocardiography, American Society of Nuclear Cardiology, Heart Failure Society of America, Heart Rhythm Society, Society for Cardiovascular Angiography and Interventions, and Society of Thoracic Surgeons. *J Am Coll Cardiol* 2011; 58: e 212–60.

16. Nagueh SF, Bierig SM, Budoff MJ, et al. American Society of Echocardiography; American Society of Nuclear Cardiology; Society for Cardiovascular Magnetic Resonance; Society of Cardiovascular Computed Tomography. American Society of Echocardiography clinical recommendations for multimodality cardiovascular imaging of patients with hypertrophic cardiomyopathy: Endorsed by the American Society of Nuclear Cardiology, Society for Cardiovascular Magnetic Resonance, and Society of Cardiovascular Computed Tomography. *J Am Soc Echocardiogr* 2011; 24: 473–98.

17. Spirito P, Pelliccia A, Proschan MA, et al. Morphology of the 'athlete's heart' assessed by echocardiography in 947 elite athletes representing 27 sports. *Am J Cardiol* 1994; 74: 802–6.

18. Prasad K, Atherton J, Smith GC, McKenna WJ, Frenneaux MP, Nihoyannopoulos P. Echocardiographic pitfalls in the diagnosis of hypertrophic cardiomyopathy. *Heart* 1999; 82, Suppl 3: III8–15.

19. Oechslin E, Jenni R. Isolated left ventricular non-compaction: increasing recognition of this distinct, yet 'unclassified' cardiomyopathy. *Eur J Echocardiogr* 2002; 3: 250–1.

20. Faber L, Seggewiss H, Gleichmann U. Percutaneous transluminal septal myocardial ablation in hypertrophic obstructive cardiomyopathy: results with respect to intraprocedural myocardial contrast echocardiography. *Circulation* 1998; 22: 2415–21.

21. Faber L, Seggewiss H, Welge D, et al. Echo-guided percutaneous septal ablation for symptomatic hypertrophic obstructive cardiomyopathy: 7 years of experience. *Eur J Echocardiogr* 2004; 5: 347–55.

22. Rickers C, Wilke NM, Jerosch-Herold M, et al. Utility of cardiac magnetic resonance imaging in the diagnosis of hypertrophic cardiomyopathy. *Circulation* 2005; 112(6): 855–61.

23. Moon JC, Reed E, Sheppard MN, et al. The histologic basis of late gadolinium enhancement cardiovascular magnetic resonance in hypertrophic cardiomyopathy. *J Am Coll Cardiol* 2004; 43(12): 2260–4.

24. Moon JC, McKenna WJ, McCrohon JA, Elliott PM, Smith GC, Pennell DJ. Toward clinical risk assessment in hypertrophic cardiomyopathy with gadolinium cardiovascular magnetic resonance. *J Am Coll Cardiol* 2003 May 7; 41(9): 1561–7.

25. Adabag AS, Maron BJ, Appelbaum E, et al. Occurrence and frequency of arrhythmias in hypertrophic cardiomyopathy in relation to delayed enhancement on cardiovascular magnetic resonance. *J Am Coll Cardiol* 2008; 51(14): 1369–74.

26. Maron BJ, Olivotto I, Spirito P, et al. Epidemiology of hypertrophic cardiomyopathy-related death: revisited in a large non-referral-based patient population. *Circulation* 2000; 102(8): 858–64.

27. Maron BJ. Hypertrophic cardiomyopathy. *Lancet* 1997; 350(9071): 127–33.

28. Elliott PM, Poloniecki J, Dickie S, et al. Sudden death in hypertrophic cardiomyopathy: identification of high risk patients. *J Am Coll Cardiol* 2000; 36: 2212–8.

29. Spirito P, Seidman CE, McKenna WJ, Maron BJ. The management of hypertrophic cardiomyopathy. *N Engl J Med* 1997; 336: 775–85.

30. Bruder O, Wagner A, Jensen CJ, et al. Myocardial scar visualized by cardiovascular magnetic resonance imaging predicts major adverse events in patients with hypertrophic cardiomyopathy. *J Am Coll Cardiol* 2010; 56(11): 875–87.

31. O'Hanlon R, Grasso A, Roughton M, et al. Prognostic significance of myocardial fibrosis in hypertrophic cardiomyopathy. *J Am Coll Cardiol* 2010; 56(11): 867–74.

32. Bruder O, Schneider S, Nothnagel D, et al. EuroCMR (European Cardiovascular Magnetic Resonance) registry: results of the German pilot phase. *J Am Coll Cardiol* 2009; 54(15): 1457–66.

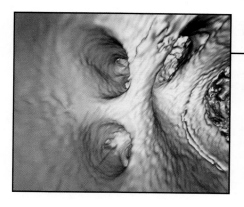

CHAPTER 34

Infiltrative cardiomyopathy

Joseph B. Selvanayagam, Majo Joseph,
Theodoros Karamitsos, and Stefan Neubauer

Contents

Amyloidosis

Amyloidosis is a clinical disorder caused by extracellular deposition of insoluble abnormal fibrils, derived from aggregation of misfolded, normally soluble, protein [1, 2]. About twenty different unrelated proteins are known to form amyloid fibrils *in vivo*, which share a pathognomonic ultrastructure. Systemic amyloidosis, in which amyloid deposits are present in the viscera, blood vessel walls, and connective tissues, is usually fatal and is the cause of about one per thousand deaths in developed countries. There are also various localized forms of amyloidosis in which the deposits are confined to specific foci or to a particular organ or tissue. 'Cardiac amyloidosis' describes involvement of the heart by amyloid deposition, whether as part of systemic amyloidosis (as is most commonly the case) or as a localized phenomenon.

Amyloid subtype classification

Systemic AA amyloidosis, formerly known as secondary amyloidosis, rarely involves the heart. Systemic AL amyloidosis, previously known as primary amyloidosis, is the most commonly diagnosed form of clinical amyloid disease in developed countries. AL fibrils are derived from monoclonal immunoglobulin light chains and consist of the whole or part of the variable (VL) domain. The heart is affected pathologically in up to 90% of AL patients, in 50% of whom diastolic heart failure with physical signs of right heart failure is a presenting feature. Conversely, less than 5% of patients with AL amyloidosis involving the heart have clinically isolated cardiac disease. Death in more than half of these patients is due to either heart failure or arrhythmia.

Rapezzi et al. conducted a longitudinal study on 233 patients with cardiac amyloidosis in two large tertiary Italian centres [3]. They found significant differences in pathophysiology and courses in the three types of amyloidosis that affect the heart. AL cardiomyopathy seems to be associated with only slightly increased wall thickness, but shows the highest frequency of haemodynamic derangement and low QRS voltage on ECG, and its clinical course is aggressive. The transthyretin (TTR) related cardiomyopathies, especially senile systemic amyloidosis (SSA), are associated with notably increased left ventricular (LV) wall thickness but less frequently with haemodynamic alterations. Their clinical course is less aggressive than in the AL type patients, despite the patients' average higher age and greater morphological abnormalities.

It has been postulated that the circulating free light chains in AL amyloid have direct toxic effects on the myocardium and the TTR related amyloid is predominantly an infiltrative cardiomyopathy.

Echocardiography

Echocardiography can show several features that are suggestive of cardiac amyloidosis (➲ Fig. 34.1), though the classical features are commonly only present in the later stages

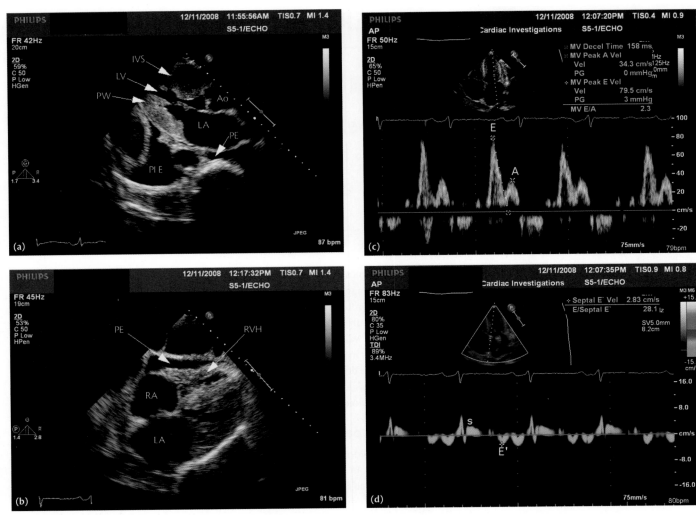

Fig. 34.1 TwoD echocardiogram (parasternal long-axis view) showing marked concentric left ventricular hypertrophy (IVS, inter-ventricular septum; PW, posterior wall) and a non-dilated left ventricular cavity (LV). There is also left atrial enlargement (LA) and a small pericardial (PE) and larger pleural effusion (PE) (a). TwoD echo (sub-costal view) highlighting markedly increased right ventricular thickness (RVH, right ventricular hypertrophy). There is also bi-atrial enlargement (RA, right atrium; LA, left atrium), and the presence of a small pericardial effusion (PE) (b). Spectral Doppler of mitral inflow of the same patient with advanced amyloid heart disease. There is a restrictive pattern with marked shortening of DT (deceleration time) and diminution of atrial contribution with E/A ratio >2 (c). Tissue Doppler velocity (apical window) of the medial mitral annulus in the same patient showing marked decrease in E' (early diastolic wave). The E/E' ratio was calculated at 28, which corresponds to significant elevation in left-sided filling pressures. There is also a striking decrease in the systolic positive wave (s) illustrating a significant decrease in longitudinal contractile function (d).

of disease and there is a wide spectrum of echocardiographic findings. It cannot confirm diagnosis in isolation and the images should be interpreted in the context of the clinical picture and other investigations. AA amyloid very rarely affects the heart and the common types that do, i.e. AL and variant/wild-type TTR types, cannot be distinguished by echo. Although extremely rare, hereditary apolipoprotein A-I amyloidosis can involve the heart, again producing similar echocardiographic abnormalities.

The commonest echocardiographic feature is increased thickness of the left ventricular (LV) wall, particularly in the absence of hypertension. This is often referred to incorrectly as 'hypertrophy' since the pathological process is infiltration, not myocyte hypertrophy. This feature has poor specificity for amyloidosis due to its occurrence in other conditions, e.g. hypertensive heart disease, hypertrophic cardiomyopathy and other infiltrative cardiac

diseases (glycogen storage diseases, sarcoidosis, haemochromatosis). The combination of increased LV mass in the absence of high ECG voltages may be more specific for infiltrative diseases of which amyloid is the commonest (Fig. 34.2). High sensitivity (72–79%) and specificity (91–100%) have been reported for this combination [4], though some study sizes are small and may be influenced by referral bias.

Increased echogenicity of the myocardium, particularly with a granular or 'sparkling' appearance, has been reported in several studies [5]. This can occur in other causes of left ventricular hypertrophy [6–8], however, and although high specificity rates are quoted (71–81%) [4], the populations studied were those referred with suspected amyloid, and this specificity may not be reflective of 'real-life' practice. Moreover, sensitivity tends to be low with this pattern seen in 26–36% of cardiac amyloid cases, apart from a

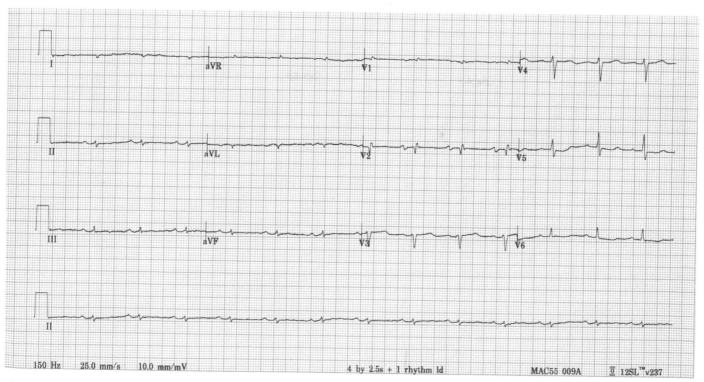

Fig. 34.2 Twelve lead ECG demonstrating small voltages in limb and chest leads (in same patient as Fig. 34.1). There is also poor R wave progression in the anterior leads (pseudoinfarct pattern). This appearance in combination with marked LV thickness on echocardiogram (see Fig. 34.1a) in the same patient is strongly suggestive of an infiltrative cardiomyopathy (cardiac amyloid).

single study suggesting a sensitivity of 87% [6]. It should be noted that this granular pattern only applies to standard echocardiographic imaging, without tissue harmonics being applied, as this increases myocardial echogenicity in general. Newer echocardiographic image processing techniques may also reduce the granular appearance. Thus, although increased echogenicity is common in amyloid, its usefulness as a discriminating factor is limited.

LV systolic function is usually normal until late stages of the disease process. Systolic function can in some cases be hyperdynamic (hence can be mistaken for hypertrophic or hypertensive cardiomyopathy) in initial stages but in advanced stages systolic function can be depressed without cavity dilation resulting in marked reduction in stroke volume and cardiac output.

Diastolic dysfunction, however, is the fundamental abnormality in cardiac amyloidosis and is abnormal prior to systolic dysfunction, which is often normal even with advanced symptoms. Early in the disease process, there may be an abnormal relaxation pattern with progression to a restrictive pattern in advanced and symptomatic disease (➲ Fig. 34.1c). Not only do diastolic parameters correlate with severity of symptoms but they are prognostic with a restrictive filling pattern (DT<150 msec; see ➲ Fig. 34.1c) associated with a mortality of 50% at one year. Atrial enlargement is a common finding in amyloid heart disease and reflects the abnormal diastolic function.

Tissue Doppler imaging can measure regional myocardial motion and velocity and can detect changes in systolic and diastolic function prior to more conventional measurements of cardiac dysfunction (➲ Fig. 34.1d). However, tissue Doppler velocity imaging suffers from the confounding effects of tethering and translation and hence newer techniques that assess regional longitudinal myocardial deformation, such as strain and strain rate, may be more sensitive. These tissue myocardial changes may be present prior to increased left ventricular wall thickness and symptoms, and hence may have a role in preclinical detection.

Other echocardiographic features are the result of diffuse infiltration with resultant increased wall thickness of the right ventricle, cardiac valves, and inter-atrial septum (➲ Fig. 34.1). Though cardiac valves may be focally or diffusely thickened, significant dysfunction is not common. Inter-atrial septal thickening, along with speckling, is a distinctive sign of amyloid with high specificity. Right ventricular abnormalities are common and may manifest as systolic or more commonly diastolic dysfunction. RV dilatation, if present, may reflect a more advanced disease process and is associated with a more adverse prognosis. Atrial involvement with demonstrable dysfunction using strain echocardiography has also been observed and may be contributory to cardiac symptoms in primary amyloidosis. Small to moderate sized pericardial effusion due to pericardial involvement is also common, particularly in end-stage disease. A high frequency of intra-cardiac thrombosis has been noted in patients with cardiac amyloidosis, especially those with the AL type, despite the presence of sinus rhythm and preserved ejection fraction [9].

Despite the number of echocardiographic features found in amyloid heart disease, none, taken individually, are diagnostic and they can be seen in other cardiac diseases. The diagnosis is still based on the combination of various echocardiographic findings with the integration of clinical findings and (where available) further imaging with CMR. However, marked myocardial hypertrophy along with valvular thickening, abnormality of diastolic function (particularly restrictive physiology), and presence of pericardial effusion in combination with characteristic ECG findings makes amyloid disease an important diagnostic consideration.

Cardiovascular magnetic resonance imaging (CMR)

A strength of CMR using late gadolinium enhancement (LGE) technique is the ability to 'phenotype' various forms of cardiomyopathy with high spatial resolution and reproducibility. Maceira et al. [10] studied 29 patients with systemic amyloidosis and 16 hypertensive controls using gadolinium-enhanced CMR. Amyloidosis was associated with qualitative global and sub-endocardial gadolinium enhancement of the myocardium. Sub-endocardial longitudinal relaxation time (T1) in amyloid patients was shorter than in controls, and was correlated with markers of increased myocardial amyloid load, such as left ventricular (LV) mass, wall thickness, inter-atrial septal thickness, and diastolic function. Global sub-endocardial late gadolinium enhancement was found in approximately two-thirds of patients. Based on pathological correlates in a patient from this study, the CMR hyper-enhancement probably represents interstitial expansion from amyloid infiltration.

Perugini et al. [11] studied an Italian population of patients with histologically proven systemic amyloidosis and echocardiographic diagnosis of cardiac involvement. Gadolinium enhancement by CMR was detected in 16 of 21 (76%) patients. In contrast to the study of Maceira et al., where the pattern of late enhancement was global and sub-endocardial, Perugini et al. reported a much more variable pattern of late enhancement, that could be localized or diffuse, and sub-endocardial or transmural. Transmural extension of hyper-enhancement (i.e. how much of the LV wall thickness was enhanced) within each patient significantly correlated with left ventricular (LV) end systolic volume. The number of enhanced segments correlated with LV end diastolic volume, end systolic volume, and left atrial size. An especially unique feature of LGE appearances in this population is the blood pool appearing atypically dark. This reflects the similar myocardial and blood T1 values due to high myocardial uptake and fast blood pool washout of the contrast agent. Although yet to be proved, imaging with a highly reproducible and quantifiable technique, such as CMR, may help to estimate the prevalence of cardiac involvement in systemic amyloidosis when cardiac morphological changes are not apparent by echocardiography.

Syed et al. performed LGE CMR in 120 patients referred to a tertiary centre with confirmed amyloidosis; 97% of the histologically confirmed cardiac amyloidosis (35/120) had abnormal LGE and 91% had increased LV wall thickness on echocardiography [12]. The pattern of LGE was global (transmural and sub-endocardial)

in 83%. Of the patients without cardiac histology and a normal echocardiogram, 30% had LGE (patchy focal or global), and the LGE presence was strongly associated with clinical, morphological, functional, and biochemical markers of prognosis. The absence of endomyocardial biopsy data in patients with a normal echocardiogram, however, is a weakness of the study and leaves the findings in this study subset as speculative rather than confirmatory.

A novel, quantitative, CMR technique, which may assist further the identification of sub-clinical early cardiac involvement in amyloidosis, is T1-mapping. Each tissue type exhibits a characteristic normal range of T1 values. T1-maps provide pixel-wise estimates of the T1 relaxation times of the underlying tissues and allow the visual differentiation of tissues using colour scales [13]. Recently, Karamitsos et al. showed that non-contrast T1 mapping has high diagnostic accuracy for detecting cardiac AL amyloidosis [14]. They recruited 53 patients with biopsy-proven, systemic AL amyloidosis and grouped them into three categories by echocardiographic wall thickness measures, diastolic functional assessment, and biomarkers: no cardiac involvement (26% of the cohort), possible involvement (21%), and definite involvement (53%). Comparison cohorts of healthy controls and patients with aortic stenosis matched by left ventricular mass to the amyloid patients with cardiac involvement were also recruited. Non-contrast T1 values were highest among patients with definite cardiac amyloidosis (mean 1,140±61 ms) as compared to either healthy controls (958±20 ms) or those with aortic stenosis (979±51 ms). There was a stepwise increase in T1 values as the probability for cardiac involvement increased. The authors concluded that non-contrast T1-mapping may be more sensitive than late gadolinium enhancement CMR for detecting cardiac amyloid, given that all amyloid patients with non-specific patchy enhancement had increased T1 values. Further studies are needed to investigate this intriguing hypothesis. Measurements of native T1 values can be combined with T1-maps post-gadolinium contrast to measure myocardial extracellular volume. Expansion of the myocardial extracellular volume represents a nonspecific increase in free water in myocytes and occurs in a variety of pathologies, including focal and diffuse fibrosis or myocardial oedema [15]. However, the massive elevation of myocardial extracellular volume evidenced in patients with cardiac amyloidosis, has not been seen in other diseases [16]. Therefore, T1-mapping with and without gadolinium contrast appears to be a useful addition in the imager's armamentarium for differentiating cardiomyopathies and holds out promise for increasing sensitivity in detecting early amyloid infiltration. Improved non-invasive surveillance may also potentially aid in the evaluation of new chemotherapeutic agents.

⊃ Figure 34.3 illustrates the typical CMR features of amyloid heart disease.

Nuclear imaging

Nuclear imaging of cardiac amyloidosis is predominantly accomplished with bone-seeking radiotracers, with variable results in

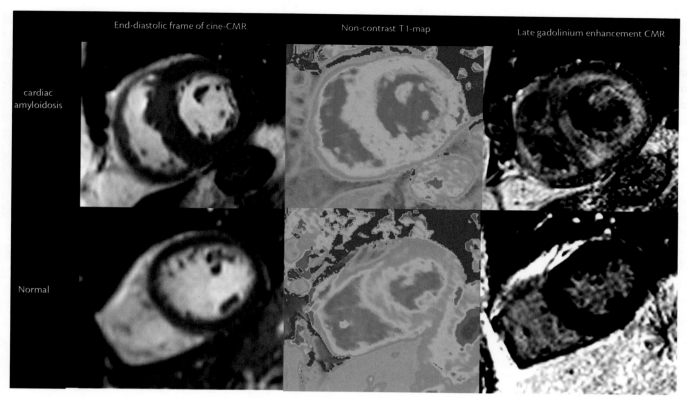

Fig. 34.3 Cardiac magnetic resonance (CMR) end-diastolic frame from short-axis cine (left panel), ShMOLLI non-contrast T1 map (middle panel), and late gadolinium enhancement (LGE) images (right panel) in a cardiac amyloid patient and a normal healthy individual. In the cine frame, note the marked left and right ventricular hypertrophy in the amyloid patient compared to the normal. In the non-contrast T1 map, note the markedly elevated myocardial T1 time in the cardiac amyloid patient (1,140 ms, giving a reddish appearance in the myocardium) compared to the normal control (965 ms, myocardium appears green). In the LGE image, note the extensive enhancement of the left and right ventricular walls associated with an abnormally dark blood-pool in the amyloid patient. In contrast, there is complete nulling of myocardial signal (myocardium is black) in the LGE image of the normal volunteer and blood pool is grey.

terms of diagnostic performance. Radiolabelled serum amyloid P component (SAP) distributes between the circulating and the amyloid bound SAP pools in proportion to their size and can then be imaged and quantified [17]. This safe non-invasive method provides unique information on the diagnosis, distribution, and extent of amyloid deposits throughout the body, and serial scans monitor progress and response to therapy. Serial SAP scans have unequivocally demonstrated that amyloid deposits of all types regress in a proportion of patients when the supply of the respective amyloid fibril precursor protein is sufficiently reduced. For cardiac amyloidosis, more promising nuclear method may be labelling derivatives of thioflavin-T. In a recent study, promising results were obtained using specific amyloid ligand C-11-PIB and PET imaging, but further studies and larger populations are required.

Sarcoidosis

Sarcoidosis is a systemic disorder of unknown aetiology involving granulomatous infiltration of various organs including the heart. The pathophysiology is thought to be related to an excessive cell-mediated immune response to an unknown antigen with accumulation of mononuclear inflammatory cells, mostly CD4 +

lymphocytes [18]. The resultant inflammatory response produces tissue injury and fibrosis, which may be focal or diffuse.

There is a striking variance in prevalence, with the disease more common in blacks and Scandinavians [19]. Cardiac involvement occurs in up to 30–40% in post-mortem studies [20, 21] and is associated with poorer prognosis, particularly if patients exhibit cardiac symptoms [22]. Clinically, cardiac involvement occurs in 5% and its presentation may include rhythm disturbance (particularly heart block), cardiac failure, cor pulmonale, and even sudden death [23]. However, diagnosis of cardiac involvement is difficult due to the numerous different manifestations of the disease process and the lack of sensitivity or specificity of various cardiac imaging tests. The Japanese Ministry of Health and Welfare guidelines for diagnosis of cardiac sarcoid, which incorporates the use of ECG, cardiac imaging, and histopathology is the most well-known and currently presides as the reference standard. More recently, Mehta et al., found that including advanced cardiac imaging with PET scanning or CMR increased sensitivity above the previously established criteria [24].

Echocardiography

Sarcoid involvement of the heart is a great masquerader and may present with a variety of echocardiographic abnormalities, including wall motion abnormalities (particularly regional thinning and aneurysms) [25], systolic and diastolic dysfunction, pulmonary hypertension, and pericardial effusions. Case reports have sarcoidosis mimicking coronary artery disease, Takotsubo cardiomyopathy, right ventricular cardiomyopathy [6], hypertrophic cardiomyopathy, and valvular dysfunction. However, in most cases of systemic sarcoidosis, there are no distinctive morphological or functional abnormalities of the heart. Tissue Doppler [26] and ultrasonic tissue characterization by myocardial integrated backscatter [27] have demonstrated abnormalities in the absence of other 2D-echocardiographic features and hence may have the ability to diagnose early cardiac involvement. ➲ Figure 34.4 shows an echocardiographic example of a patient with cardiac sarcoidosis.

Nuclear imaging

Thallium-201 scintigraphy in sarcoidosis can be distinctive with a pattern of reverse redistribution in which a resting perfusion defect improves with stress imaging. This can be helpful in differentiating sarcoid heart disease from an ischaemic cause [28]. However, these findings are non-specific, particularly in the absence of cardiac symptoms, and hence are of limited value as a screening test. Gallium-67 scintigraphy has also been used to diagnose cardiac sarcoid as it accumulates in the presence of active inflammation. Hence the absence of uptake may not exclude sarcoid involvement but suggests lack of active disease and has been shown to predict response to corticosteroid therapy [29]. More recently, a study by Ishimaru et al. using (18)F-fluoro-2-deoxyglucose positron emission tomography ((18)F-FDG PET)) demonstrated focal myocardial uptake in cardiac sarcoidosis [30].

Cardiovascular magnetic resonance imaging

The superior spatial resolution of CMR is particularly useful in identifying even small areas of myocardial oedema and fibrosis leading to post-inflammatory scarring that is typically seen in cardiac sarcoidosis. Both global and regional contractile dysfunction has been described, although, similar to cardiac amyloidosis, the late gadolinium enhancement (LGE) technique has been most widely evaluated in clinical studies using CMR. In the largest study to-date, Smedma and colleagues evaluated the utility of LGE in 58 patients with biopsy proven pulmonary sarcoidosis, 25% of whom also had symptoms suggestive of cardiac involvement [31]. All patients underwent clinical assessment, 12-lead electrocardiography (ECG), ambulatory ECG monitoring, transthoracic echocardiography, 201thallium single-photon emission computed tomography (SPECT), and CMR (cine and LGE). The modified Japanese Ministry of Health criteria was used as the gold-standard. CMR revealed LGE, mostly involving the epicardium of basal and lateral segments in 73% of patients diagnosed with cardiac involvement by the Japanese criteria. In about half of these patients, scintigraphy was normal; while patchy LGE was present underlining the differences in spatial resolution. This study is limited in that only a minority of patients had correlation between LGE-CMR results and endomyocardial biopsy. Other studies have confirmed the

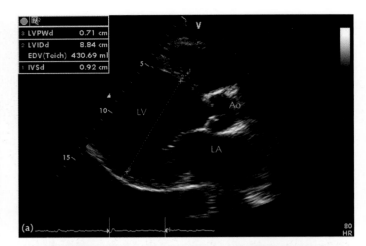

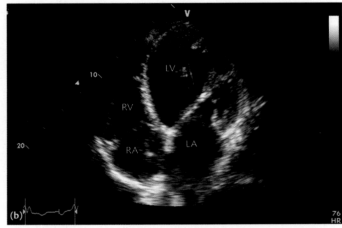

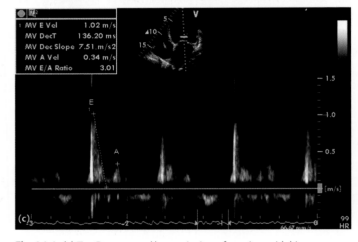

Fig. 34.4 (a) TwoD parasternal long-axis view of a patient with biopsy proven cardiac sarcoidosis. The appearance is typical of a dilated cardiomyopathy with globally reduced contraction. The end-diastolic dimension (LVEDd) is increased and there is normal thickness of the posterior wall (LVPWd) and the interventricular septum (IVSd). LV, left ventricle; Ao, aorta; LA, left atrium (b) TwoD echocardiogram of an apical 4-chamber showing a LV that is significantly dilated and spherical in shape. This patient had endomyocardial biopsy proven sarcoidosis, but the appearance is indistinguishable from a typical dilated cardiomyopathy. RV, right ventricle; RA, right atrium. Pulse Wave Doppler of mitral valve (MV) inflow in a patient with dilated cardiomyopathy due to sarcoidosis showing a restrictive filling pattern with a E (early diastolic filling) to A (late filling due to atrial contraction) ratio of greater than 2 and a short deceleration time (DT) (c).

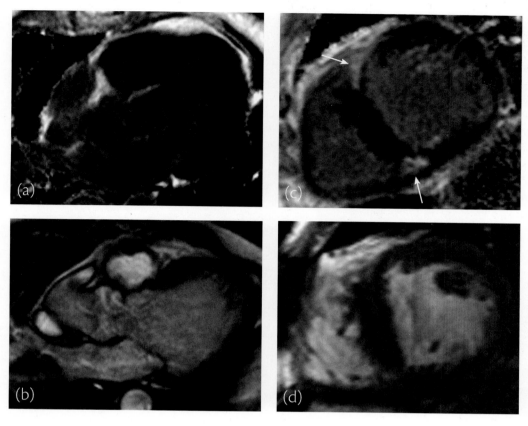

Fig. 34.5 CMR delayed enhancement. Left ventricular outflow tract view (a) and short-axis view and cine (c), left ventricular outflow tract view (b) and short-axis view (d) images from a patient with cardiac sarcoidosis. Images show typical CMR features: septal wall thinning, increased overall LV mass, and patchy late gadolinium hyper-enhancement (white arrows).

predilection of LGE for the basal-lateral segments, although sub-endocardial or transmural hyper-enhancement has been also observed, mimicking the ischaemic pattern. More recently, Patel and colleagues prospectively studied 81 patients with biopsy proven extra-cardiac sarcoidosis for a parallel and masked comparison of cardiac involvement between LGE CMR and standard clinical evaluation, with the use of consensus criteria based on JMHW guidelines [32].

Obstructive coronary disease was excluded by X-ray angiography in the LGE-CMR positive patients. They found that LGE CMR identified myocardial abnormalities in significantly more patients than a standard clinical evaluation based on JMHW guidelines (26% vs. 12%). LGE-CMR positive patients had a higher rate of adverse events, including cardiac death, during a 21-month follow-up, compared to LGE-CMR negative patients. Myocardial damage detected by LGE CMR appears to be associated with future adverse events including cardiac death, but there were few events in this small cohort and, therefore, a large-scale study is required. The long-term prognostic implications of LGE in cardiac sarcoidosis are not yet available.

Apart from LGE, both functional and anatomical ('white blood' and 'black blood') CMR sequences can help in detecting cardiac sarcoid by demonstrating some of its characteristic features—septal thinning, LV/RV dilatation and systolic dysfunction, pericardial effusion (see ⊃ Fig. 34.5) [33, 34]. T2-weighted sequences may also help in identifying myocardial oedema [35]. CMR also identifies pulmonary features of sarcoid, such as enlarged hilar lymph nodes and lung fibrosis.

Anderson–Fabry disease

Fabry's disease is an X-linked condition with systemic and cardiac manifestations. It is an enzyme deficiency of ∝-galactosidase [36], which results in accumulation of glycosphingoplipids in lysosomes of various cells and organs including the heart. Cardiac involvement is frequent [37] and results in myocyte vacuolation, hypertrophy, and regional fibrosis [38, 39]. This can result in heart failure and conduction abnormalities and is an important cause of death in these patients [40]. Currently, the diagnosis is based on one or more of biochemical testing, genetic mapping, and endomyocardial biopsy. However, imaging of the myocardium has been explored as a non-invasive way of early screening and diagnosing patients. Correct diagnosis is of vital importance as, unlike many other forms of infiltrative cardiomyopathy, the condition is potentially reversible with treatment by enzyme replacement therapy [41]. Fabry's cardiomyopathy is not as rare as initially thought and can be difficult to distinguish from other forms of infiltrative or hypertrophic cardiomyopathies. A recent study discovered that 6% of male patients diagnosed with hypertrophic cardiomyopathy in fact had Fabry's disease on biochemical and genetic testing [42]. Another study found that Fabry's disease was present in 10% of patients referred to their cardiac unit with unexplained hypertrophy [7].

Echocardiography

The principal echocardiographic finding is concentric LVH with often initially preserved systolic function and without cavity

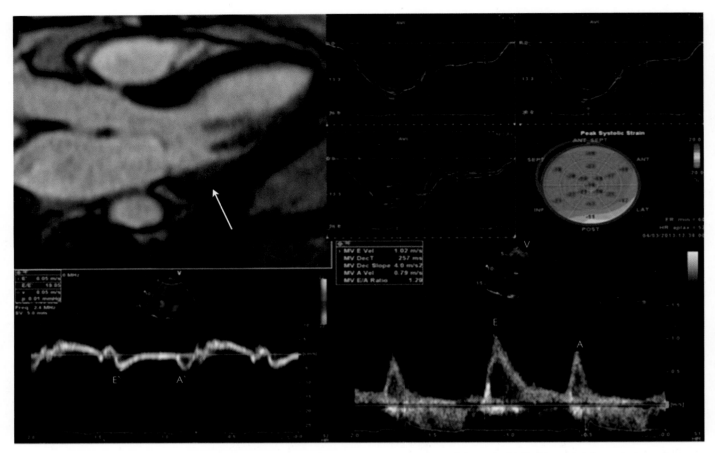

Fig. 34.6 LGE cardiovascular magnetic resonance and echocardiographic images in an FD patient. Top left panel: LGE-CMR image in left ventricular outflow tract view showing late gadolinium enhancement involving the basal inferolateral left ventricular (LV) wall (arrow), a site classical for FD. Top right panel: LV segments represented by a coloured bulls-eye chart (apex in the middle and base of the heart being the outer ring,) demonstrating reduced strain (<−18) in the basal inferolateral wall, corresponding to the area of LGE positivity. Bottom right panel: Spectral Doppler of LV inflow (velocity/time) demonstrating passive E wave (ventricular suction) and active A wave (atrial contraction) during ventricular diastole. Bottom left panel: Tissue (myocardial) velocity representing ventricular relaxation during passive filling (e') and atrial contraction (A). The e' is markedly depressed representing abnormal relaxation and the combined profile with the spectral Doppler is suggestive of moderate diastolic dysfunction (grade 3).

dilatation. The main functional abnormality, like in other infiltrative cardiomyopathies, is abnormal diastology, though restrictive physiology is also possible, but not as common. Cardiac valves may be thickened, but severe valve dysfunction is rare. There is also increased incidence of aortic root dilatation [43].

Recent studies using tissue Doppler imaging have shown a reduction in both relaxation and contraction tissue Doppler velocities in patients (see ⮑ Fig. 34.6). These findings are detectable before the onset of LVH and other morphological changes [44]. Strain and strain rate imaging reflect regional myocardial function and contractility, respectively. They are also reduced early in the disease process and can be reversed with treatment [41]. Strain imaging has the advantage over tissue Doppler velocity in that it can detect regional heterogeneity in myocardial function, which is characteristic of Fabry's with strain abnormalities being most pronounced in the inferolateral wall [8]. Interestingly, this is also the area where LGE-CMR abnormalities are most pronounced.

More recently, Pieroni and colleagues [45] have described the so-called binary sign, which is an abnormal appearance of the left ventricular endocardial border thought to be related to glycosphingolipid compartmentalization. They found this to be both a specific and sensitive marker for Fabry's disease. However, other authors have disputed this finding and suggested this binary appearance is non-specific and affected by instrumental settings [46].

As with other infiltrative and storage cardiomyopathies, the progression and spectrum of disease are not static. In the initial stages, standard morphological and functional changes may not be apparent and hence these newer tissue imaging techniques could provide earlier diagnosis with prompt consideration for enzyme replacement. Regardless, the higher than expected incidence of Fabry's should alert the imaging clinician to this diagnosis in anyone with unexplained left ventricular hypertrophy.

Cardiovascular magnetic resonance

Systematic reporting of CMR features in this disease (see ⮑ Fig. 34.7) is sparse. Moon et al. have reported LGE patterns in a unique distribution involving the basal inferolateral wall,

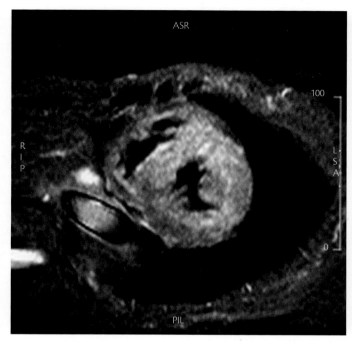
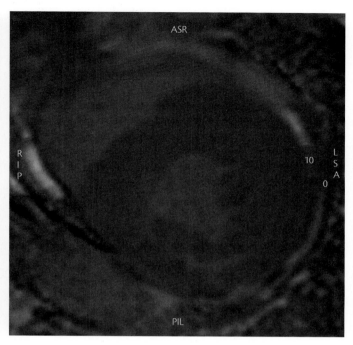

Fig. 34.7 CMR tissue characterization in a patient with Fabry's disease and cardiac involvement (LV Mass index 138g/m² (NR: 35–64)). Short-axis diastolic steady-state free-precession cine, showing normal LV dimension and increased mass (a). T2 STIR short-axis showing homogenous signal indicating absence of oedema and short-axis PSIR late enhancement (b). Showing infero-lateral uptake in a non-ischaemic distribution pattern (c).

sparing the endocardium, in 50% of affected patients [47]. LGE in this respect probably represents interstial expansion secondary to replacement fibrosis, although why this region of the myocardium is favoured is unclear. Nevertheless, the finding of substantial areas of myocardial fibrosis by CMR LGE may in future have important implications for the treatment of Fabry's disease, as enzyme replacement therapy may be less effective in patients with extensive areas of myocardial scarring.

Prolongation of myocardial T2 relaxation time has also been shown in studies of patients with genotype positive Fabry's disease, probably related to the marked deposition of glycolipid in the myocardium [48]. This has been suggested by some as a useful marker of this disease. However, there is a wide overlap in myocardial T2 values of Fabry's disease patients when compared with patients with LVH from other causes, such that T2 times *alone* are unlikely to be useful in clinching the diagnosis [48].

As with cardiac amyloidosis, non-contrast myocardial T1-mapping has the potential to become a useful, quantitative measure in Anderson–Fabry disease. In a recent study that included 44 patients with genetically proven Fabry disease, Sado and colleagues showed that septal T1 relaxation times were significantly lower in patients with Fabry disease (882±47 ms) compared to healthy volunteers (968±32ms, $P<0.001$) [49]. Furthermore, in patients with other causes of left ventricular hypertrophy, T1 times were generally elevated (1018±74 ms). The exact mechanism of T1 lowering in Fabry disease has not been fully elucidated but the accumulation of glycosphingolipids in myocytes is a postulated contributing mechanism. On segmental analysis, the inferolateral segment, which commonly shows midwall fibrosis on late gadolinium CMR, there was pseudo-normalization or

elevation of T1 times, correlating with the presence or absence of late gadolinium enhancement. Therefore, non-contrast T1 septal assessment is a simple and useful add-on to clinical CMR, providing a new parameter that appears to be useful in the the detection of early cardiac involvement in Fabry disease, with potential for therapy monitoring but further studies are needed to assess this.

Other infiltrative cardiomyopathies

In glycogen storage diseases (GSD), deficiencies in enzymes responsible for metabolizing muscle glycogen not only cause systemic diseases, but can involve the myocardium. Many types have been described, most of which can involve the heart, although in a number of cases (e.g. GSD Type 2a-Pompe's disease) the disease is invariably fatal in early infancy, and is unlikely to be encountered by the adult cardiologist. Danon disease (GSD Type 2b), characterized by an X-linked dominant inheritance pattern, can present in childhood and early adulthood. Among males, the key features are cardiomyopathy, skeletal myopathy, and intellectual disability ranging from mild learning problems to mental retardation. In a recent seminal study, Arad et al. showed that cardiac disease can be the initial and predominant manifestation of defects in human glycogen metabolism [50]. It was found that specific glycogen metabolism mutations, LAMP2 and PRKAG2, cause multi-system glycogen-storage disease and can also present as primary cardiomyopathy, mimicking hypertrophic or infiltrative cardiomyopathy.

Haemochromatosis can also be considered an infiltrative cardiomyopathy as it is a deposition disease in which iron is deposited intra-cellularly, causing cell damage with associated cardiac dysfunction. Echocardiography demonstrates features of dilated cardiomyopathy, including left ventricular dilatation and global systolic dysfunction. Cardiac involvement is progressive and in the later stages can manifest restrictive physiology that clinically can mimic constrictive disease. Non-invasive determination of the cardiac iron load is possible using CMR by measuring myocardial relaxation time T2*.

Myocardial T2* correlates well with cardiac iron concentration measured from biopsy specimens and T2* values <20 ms are associated with heart failure in patients with ß-thalassaemia major.

Summary

The evaluation and management of patients with infiltrative cardiomyopathy remains clinically challenging. Cardiac involvement in amyloidosis and sarcoidosis is associated with a more adverse prognosis and hence early identification is warranted.

Echocardiography, though able to detect gross morphological and functional abnormalities, lacks specificity and sufficient sensitivity. Newer methods using tissue imaging may prove to have a role in the future by their ability to define focal abnormalities and detect subclinical disease. Nuclear imaging is helpful in differentiating sarcoid from other cardiac diseases when symptoms are present, as well as predicting response to treatment. More recently, cardiac MRI has shown promise for all types of infiltrative cardiomyopathy, in not only identifying typical morphological and functional changes, but also in assessing disease activity. T1-mapping techniques, with or without the use of gadolinium contrast, hold promise of allowing early identification of cardiac involvement in infiltrative diseases and have the potential to be used for treatment monitoring. However, no imaging technique stands alone, and even the 'gold-standard' of endomyocardial biopsy may often not be conclusive, given the focal nature of cardiac infiltration in some cases. The integration of clinical assessment, tissue biopsy, and cardiac imaging will still need to form the basis of any future diagnostic framework.

References

1. Merlini G, Westermark P. The systemic amyloidoses: clearer understanding of the molecular mechanisms offers hope for more effective therapies. *J Intern Med* 2004; 255(2): 159–78.
2. Selkoe DJ. Folding proteins in fatal ways. *Nature* 2003; 426(6968): 900–4.
3. Rapezzi C, et al. Systemic cardiac amyloidoses: disease profiles and clinical courses of the 3 main types. *Circulation* 2009; 120(13): 1203–12.
4. Rahman JE, et al. Noninvasive diagnosis of biopsy-proven cardiac amyloidosis. *J Am Coll Cardiol* 2004; 43(3): 410–5.
5. Selvanayagam JB, et al. Evaluation and management of the cardiac amyloidosis. *J Am Coll Cardiol* 2007; 50(22): 2101–10.
6. Yared K, et al. Cardiac sarcoidosis imitating arrhythmogenic right ventricular dysplasia. *Circulation* 2008 118(7): e113–5.
7. Nakao S, et al. An atypical variant of Fabry's disease in men with left ventricular hypertrophy. *N Engl J Med* 1995; 333(5): 288–93.
8. Weidemann F, et al. The variation of morphological and functional cardiac manifestation in Fabry disease: potential implications for the time course of the disease. *Eur Heart J* 2005; 26(12): 1221–7.
9. Feng D, et al. Intracardiac thrombosis and embolism in patients with cardiac amyloidosis. *Circulation* 2007; 116(21): 2420–6.
10. Maceira AM, et al. Cardiovascular magnetic resonance in cardiac amyloidosis. *Circulation* 2005; 111(2): 186–93.
11. Perugini E, et al. Noninvasive etiologic diagnosis of cardiac amyloidosis using 99mTc-3,3-diphosphono-1,2-propanodicarboxylic acid scintigraphy. *J Am Coll Cardiol* 2005; 46(6): 1076–84.
12. Syed IS, et al. Role of cardiac magnetic resonance imaging in the detection of cardiac amyloidosis. *JACC Cardiovasc Imaging* 2010; 3(2): 155–64.
13. Piechnik SK, et al. Normal variation of magnetic resonance T1 relaxation times in the human population at 1.5 T using ShMOLLI. *J Cardiovasc Magn Reson* 2013; 15: 13.
14. Karamitsos TD, et al. Noncontrast t1 mapping for the diagnosis of cardiac amyloidosis. *JACC Cardiovasc Imaging* 2013; 6(4): 488–97.
15. Sado DM, et al. Cardiovascular magnetic resonance measurement of myocardial extracellular volume in health and disease. *Heart* 2012; 98(19): 1436–41.
16. Banypersad SM, et al. Quantification of myocardial extracellular volume fraction in systemic AL amyloidosis: an equilibrium contrast cardiovascular magnetic resonance study. *Circ Cardiovasc Imaging* 2013; 6(1): 34–9.
17. Hawkins PN. Serum amyloid P component scintigraphy for diagnosis and monitoring amyloidosis. *Curr Opin Nephrol Hyperten*s 2002; 11(6): 649–55.
18. Ionize MC, Rybicki BA, Teirstein AS. Sarcoidosis. *N Engl J Med* 2007; 357(21): 2153–65.
19. Dubrey SW, Bell A, Mittal TK. Sarcoid heart disease. *Postgrad Med J* 2007; 83(984): 618–23.
20. Silverman KJ, Hutchins GM, Bulkley BH. Cardiac sarcoid: a clinicopathologic study of 84 unselected patients with systemic sarcoidosis. *Circulation* 1978; 58(6): 1204–11.
21. Thomsen TK, Eriksson T. Myocardial sarcoidosis in forensic medicine. *Am J Forensic Med Pathol* 1999; 20(1): 52–6.
22. Roberts WC, McAllister Jr HA, Ferrans VJ. Sarcoidosis of the heart. A clinicopathologic study of 35 necropsy patients (group 1)and review of 78 previously described necropsy patients (group 11). *Am J Med* 1977; 63(1): 86–108.
23. Licka M, et al. Troponin T concentrations 72 hours after myocardial infarction as a serological estimate of infarct size. *Heart* 2002; 87(6): 520–4.
24. Mehta D, et al. Cardiac involvement in patients with sarcoidosis: diagnostic and prognostic value of outpatient testing. *Chest* 2008; 133(6): 1426–35.
25. Burstow DJ, et al. Two-dimensional echocardiographic findings in systemic sarcoidosis. *Am J Cardiol* 1989; 63(7): 478–82.
26. Fahy GJ, et al. Doppler echocardiographic detection of left ventricular diastolic dysfunction in patients with pulmonary sarcoidosis. *Chest* 1996; 109(1): 62–6.

27. Hyodo E, et al. Early detection of cardiac involvement in patients with sarcoidosis by a non-invasive method with ultrasonic tissue characterisation. *Heart* 2004; 90(11): 1275–80.

28. Fields CL, et al. Thallium-201 scintigraphy in the diagnosis and management of myocardial sarcoidosis. *South Med J* 1990; 83(3): 339–42.

29. Okayama K, et al. Diagnostic and prognostic value of myocardial scintigraphy with thallium-201 and gallium-67 in cardiac sarcoidosis. *Chest* 1995; 107(2): 330–4.

30. Ishimaru S, et al. Focal uptake on 18F-fluoro-2-deoxyglucose positron emission tomography images indicates cardiac involvement of sarcoidosis. *Eur Heart J* 2005; 26(15): 1538–43.

31. Smedema JP, et al. Evaluation of the accuracy of gadolinium-enhanced cardiovascular magnetic resonance in the diagnosis of cardiac sarcoidosis. *J Am Coll Cardiol* 2005; 45(10): 1683–90.

32. Patel MR, et al. Detection of myocardial damage in patients with sarcoidosis. *Circulation* 2009; 120(20): 1969–77.

33. Doughan AR, Williams BR, Cardiac sarcoidosis. *Heart* 2006; 92(2): 282–8.

34. Serra JJ, et al. Images in cardiovascular medicine. Cardiac sarcoidosis evaluated by delayed-enhanced magnetic resonance imaging. *Circulation* 2003; 107(20): e 188–9.

35. Vignaux O, et al. Clinical significance of myocardial magnetic resonance abnormalities in patients with sarcoidosis: a 1-year follow-up study. *Chest* 2002; 122(6): 1895–901.

36. Brady RO, et al. Enzymatic defect in Fabry's disease. Ceramidetrihexosidase deficiency. *N Engl J Med* 1967; 276(21): 1163–7.

37. Kampmann C, et al. Cardiac manifestations of Anderson-Fabry disease in heterozygous females. *J Am Coll Cardiol* 2002; 40(9): 1668–74.

38. Chimenti C, et al. Prevalence of Fabry disease in female patients with late-onset hypertrophic cardiomyopathy. *Circulation* 2004; 110(9): 1047–53.

39. Funabashi N, et al. Images in cardiovascular medicine. Myocardial fibrosis in Fabry disease demonstrated by multislice computed tomography: comparison with biopsy findings. *Circulation* 2003; 107(19): 2519–20.

40. MacDermot KD, Holmes A, and Miners AH, Natural history of Fabry disease in affected males and obligate carrier females. *J Inherit Metab Dis* 2001; 24 Suppl 2: 13–4; discussion 11–2.

41. Weidemann F, et al. Improvement of cardiac function during enzyme replacement therapy in patients with Fabry disease: a prospective strain rate imaging study. *Circulation* 2003; 108(11): 1299–301.

42. Sachdev B, et al. Prevalence of Anderson-Fabry disease in male patients with late onset hypertrophic cardiomyopathy. *Circulation* 2002; 105(12): 1407–11.

43. Linhart A, et al. New insights in cardiac structural changes in patients with Fabry's disease. *Am Heart J* 2000; 139(6): 1101–8.

44. Pieroni M, et al. Early detection of Fabry cardiomyopathy by tissue Doppler imaging. *Circulation* 2003; 107(15): 1978–84.

45. Pieroni M, et al. Fabry's disease cardiomyopathy: echocardiographic detection of endomyocardial glycosphingolipid compartmentalization. *J Am Coll Cardiol* 2006; 47(8): 1663–71.

46. Kounas S, et al. The binary endocardial appearance is a poor discriminator of Anderson-Fabry disease from familial hypertrophic cardiomyopathy. *J Am Coll Cardiol* 2008; 51(21): 2058–61.

47. Moon JCC, et al. Gadolinium enhanced cardiovascular magnetic resonance in Anderson-Fabry disease: Evidence for a disease specific abnormality of the myocardial interstitium. *Eur Heart J* 2003; 24(23): 2151–55.

48. Imbriaco M, et al. MRI characterization of myocardial tissue in patients with Fabry's disease. *AJR Am J Roentgenol* 2007; 188(3): 850–3.

49. Sado DM, et al. The identification and assessment of Anderson Fabry Disease by cardiovascular magnetic resonance non-contrast myocardial T1 mapping. *Circ Cardiovasc Imaging* 2013.

50. Arad M, et al. Glycogen storage diseases presenting as hypertrophic cardiomyopathy. *N Engl J Med* 2005; 352(4): 362–72.

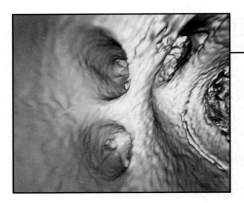

CHAPTER 35

Dilated cardiomyopathy

Tjeerd Germans, Massimo Lombardi, Danilo Neglia, Petros Nihoyannopoulos, and Albert C. van Rossum

Contents

Introduction

Definition of dilated cardiomyopathy

According to a recent statement of the European Society of Cardiology, dilated cardiomyopathy (DCM) is defined by the presence of left ventricular (LV) dilatation and systolic dysfunction in the absence of coronary artery disease (CAD) sufficient to cause global systolic impairment, or abnormal loading conditions (hypertension, valvular heart disease, and congenital heart disease). Right ventricular dilation and dysfunction may also be present but are not necessary for the diagnosis (⊃ Table 35.1) [1, 2].

First, the use non-invasive imaging techniques to exclude CAD and primary valvular pathology as causes of DCM will be briefly discussed. Then, the diagnostic and prognostic capabilities of echocardiography, nuclear techniques including single-photon emission computed tomography (SPECT) and positron emission tomography (PET), and cardiovascular magnetic resonance imaging (CMR) will be described in various causes of familial and non-familial DCM, such as idiopathic DCM, chronic myocarditis, sarcoidosis, Chagas' disease, various forms of vasculitis, cardiotoxins and cardiomyopathy associated with pregnancy and parturition. Also, unclassified forms of cardiomyopathies, such as isolated LV non-compaction, and Takotsubo cardiomyopathy will be addressed. All these cardiomyopathies are characterized by dilatation of the LV cavity and impairment of LV myocardial function and therefore further classification heavily depends on information provided by the different imaging modalities. Optimal diagnostic and prognostic information is obtained by integrating the specific characteristics unique to each of these modalities.

Differentiating DCM from CAD in LV dysfunction

Determining whether newly recognized LV dysfunction is due to CAD or to DCM, is a critical early step in the risk stratification and management of patients with a dilated left ventricle with systolic dysfunction. Generally, the diagnosis can be anticipated on a clinical ground, with CAD patients tending to be older than 40, while DCM patients usually present at a younger age. The final diagnosis is, however, conclusively achieved

Table 35.1 Definition of dilated cardiomyopathy

DCM is diagnosed when dimensions or volumes exceed 2 SD above the mean + 5% and LV ejection fraction is <45%

Indexed normal LV end-diastolic values presented as 95% confidence interval; 2 SD + 5% above mean.*

		Females	**Males**
Echocardiography	LVED dimension	2.4–3.2; 3.3 cm.m^{-2}	2.2–3.1; 3.2 cm.m^{-2}
	LVED volume	35–75; 78 ml.m^{-2}	35–75; 78 ml.m^{-2}
CMR†	LVED volume	50–93; 97 ml.m^{-2}	64–99; 103 ml.m^{-2}

*Indexed to body surface area.
†Reference values are presented for age group 40-49 years.
CMR, cardiovascular magnetic resonance imaging steady-state free precession cine imaging; DCM, dilated cardiomyopathy; ED, end diastolic; LV, left ventricular; SD, standard deviations.

by demonstration of the presence or absence of a significant stenosis in the main branches of coronary arteries at invasive coronary angiography.

The non-invasive work-up of patients with heart failure symptoms will start with echocardiography, since this is the most practical and widely available imaging modality. Once LV dilatation and impaired function have been assessed in the absence of abnormal loading conditions, such as in valvular and congenital heart disease, DCM must be differentiated from CAD. Typically, patients with CAD often have a dilated LV with regional wall motion abnormalities, sometimes with thin and echogenic myocardium due to old myocardial infarction. DCM patients present with a more diffuse dilatation, often with relatively preserved myocardial wall thickness.

The right ventricle is not often involved in CAD, unless there is proximal right coronary artery occlusion, while it is frequently affected in DCM. Nonetheless, multi-vessel coronary artery disease with extensive scarring from previous myocardial infarcts in multiple territories may mimic DCM, and additional testing to exclude significant CAD will be required. Then, CMR is of great value as a second-line imaging tool, since it is capable of demonstrating or excluding with high accuracy the presence of CAD-related infarct scarring using late gadolinium enhancement (LGE) imaging, and providing information on pathologic myocardial tissue composition. At the expense of radiation burden, nuclear techniques may also be applied to exclude CAD-related myocardial perfusion and metabolic defects. Finally, non-invasive evaluation of coronary morphology by multi-slice computed tomography (MSCT) has a very high negative predictive value for CAD, and may be employed to exclude CAD [3].

Differentiating DCM from primary valvular disease in LV dysfunction

LV dilatation will lead to mitral annular enlargement, which will cause the mitral leaflets not to appose properly and consequently lead to functional mitral regurgitation. This can be visualized with colour Doppler and quantified when necessary. While in some occasions the causal link between mitral regurgitation and a dilated left ventricle may be difficult to establish, the association of a globally hypokinetic LV with mitral regurgitation in the presence of otherwise structurally normal mitral leaflets, directs toward primary myocardial disease. One should note that secondary mitral regurgitation in DCM is not often severe and when this happens, it is more difficult to rule out mitral regurgitation as the prime culprit of LV dysfunction.

Aetiology of DCM

The DCM phenotype can be caused by (1) primary familial/genetic myocardial defects resulting in reduced force generation and/or transmission, (2) myocardial inflammation and cell damage (mainly due to infective, immunologic or toxic mechanisms), or (3) a complex interplay of unclear familial, immune-mediated, toxic, or infectious mechanisms that ultimately result in non-specific abnormalities of myocardial function, perfusion, and metabolism and subsequent DCM. This form of DCM is referred to as idiopathic DCM.

It is estimated that 20–50% of patients with DCM have evidence of familial disease [4]. Familial DCM is diagnosed when two or more closely related affected individuals are present in a single family and should also be suspected when there is a family history of premature cardiac death, conduction system disease, and/or skeletal myopathy [1, 4]. Autosomal dominant patterns of inheritance are predominantly caused by mutations in genes encoding for cytoskeletal, sarcomeric protein/Z-band, nuclear membrane, and intercalated disc proteins. X-linked diseases associated with DCM often involve skeletal muscular dystrophies (e.g. Becker and Duchenne). A matrilinear inheritance pattern and involvement of different organs suggest mitochondrial disease. Also, inherited metabolic disorders such as haemochromatosis or familial autoimmune disease may cause a DCM phenotype [5].

The electrocardiogram is often abnormal and may show conduction abnormalities (e.g. in Lamin A/C mutations, Lyme disease, Chagas' disease), extremely low QRS amplitude (phospholamban mutation), or bundle branch block [5].

Importantly, clinicians should be aware that disease penetrance may be variable and when family history is negative, first-degree relatives of newly diagnosed DCM patients should always be encouraged to undergo cardiological screening with ECG and echocardiography/CMR. Large series have shown that screening first-degree family members of patients with idiopathic DCM with echocardiography and ECG reveals familial disease in 20–35% [4]. Three to five-yearly follow-up is recommended since early diagnosis of DCM is crucial to institute early management.

Idiopathic DCM

Echocardiography in DCM

Two-dimensional (2D) echocardiography

Two-dimensional (2D) echocardiography is the cornerstone for the diagnosis of LV dysfunction, with or without ventricular dilation (➲ Figs 35.1 and 35.2). While ventricular dysfunction may be diffuse, which will distinguish it from regional myocardial dysfunction as a result of myocardial infarction, it is not always easy to rule out

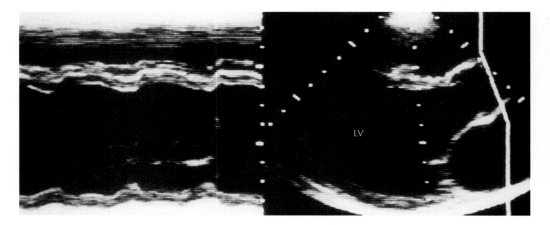

Fig. 35.1 M-mode echocardiogram (left) and 2D parasternal long-axis (right) from a patient with DCM and heart failure. The left ventricle is severely dilated with global hypokinesia and an EF estimated at 30%.

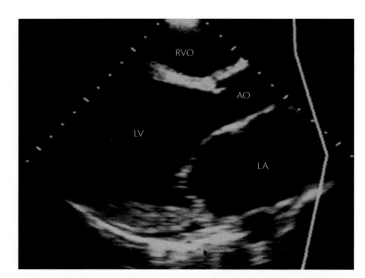

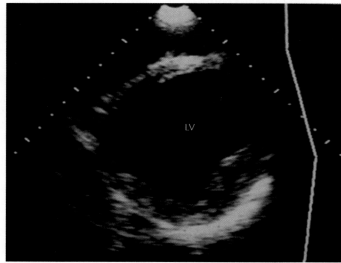

Fig. 35.2 Parasternal long-axis (top) and short-axis (bottom) from a patient with DCM. Note the marked dilatation of the left ventricle.

ischaemic LV dysfunction. This is why, ultimately, once ventricular dysfunction has been identified by echocardiography, it is imperative to rule out coronary artery disease by performing additional invasive or non-invasive testing. However, LV dimensions may remain normal and the only abnormality may be diffuse LV dysfunction

(📹 Video 35.1). This may well represent a milder form or an earlier stage of cardiomyopathy, or result from a recent myocarditic event. Regular follow-up with repeated echocardiographic examinations is warranted in this group of mild DCM patients to demonstrate changes of ventricular dimensions over time since prognosis of this phenotype is comparable to patients with DCM [1].

Quantification of LV geometry

Quantification of LV geometry is obviously important for patient follow-up and echocardiography is ideally suited for regular assessment. LV dimensions are usually sufficient, but assessing LV volumes may offer a better way to assess DCM severity and progression. Importantly, therapeutic options in idiopathic DCM, such as institution of ACE-inhibitors or selecting candidates for cardiac resynchronization therapy (CRT), need precise measures of ejection fraction (EF). To this end 2D-echocardiography provides the first line assessment of LV volumes and dyssynchrony. The recommended method to measure EF is the modified Simpson's method from two apical planes, including the four-chamber and two-chamber views. If the endocardial border cannot be delineated sufficiently with standard 2D-echocardiography, the use of ultrasound contrast agents or real-time three-dimensional echocardiography is recommended (➲ Figs 35.3 and 35.4) in order to accurately calculate LV volumes and EF [6, 7]. See 📹 Video 35.2.

Real-time three-dimensional imaging

Real-time three-dimensional imaging of the left ventricle has now been made available by the vast majority of ultrasound vendors. This allows a more accurate and reproducible measurement of LV volumes in a semi-automated fashion, thus importantly shortening the time to quantify LV function and dimensions. It has been demonstrated that LV volumes are more accurately measured with three-dimensional echocardiography and match those obtained by CMR with less test–retest variability and better inter-observer reproducibility than 2D-echocardiography [8]. These observations appear to be independent of LV morphology, with an accuracy comparable to CMR and exceeding that of nuclear techniques [9].

Intra-ventricular thrombus formation

Intra-ventricular thrombus formation is a considerable risk in ventricular dilatation due to diffuse hypokinesia and low

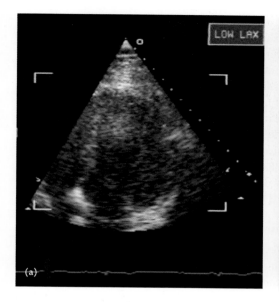
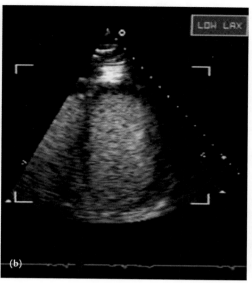

Fig. 35.3 (a) Apical projections from a patient with poor apical imaging with no endocardial border delineation. (b) The same patient after 0.3 ml of Sonovue injection. The entire endocardial border is now clearly visualized.

intra-ventricular velocities. These thrombi are believed to constitute a major risk of systemic embolization. Echocardiography can readily identify the presence of an intra-ventricular thrombus and lead to prompt anticoagulant treatment. Thrombi are usually attached at the apex (➲ Fig. 35.5) and may be laminar or protruding with a narrow point of attachment on the endocardial surface.

Nuclear imaging in DCM

Abnormalities in the myocardial energy production process, which can be recognized in the DCM heart not specifically linked to specific aetiologies, are implicated in the development of progressive cardiac failure. This pathogenesis is common to other cardiovascular disorders and could be linked to inappropriate perfusion due to coronary endothelial and microvascular abnormalities, abnormal mitochondrial function or metabolic derangement. These mechanisms, together with alterations in myocardial innervation, may contribute to the progressive myocardial damage and could represent reversible targets of treatment.

Myocardial perfusion imaging

Myocardial perfusion imaging has a high accuracy for excluding CAD in patients with LV dysfunction; thus in the absence of rest or

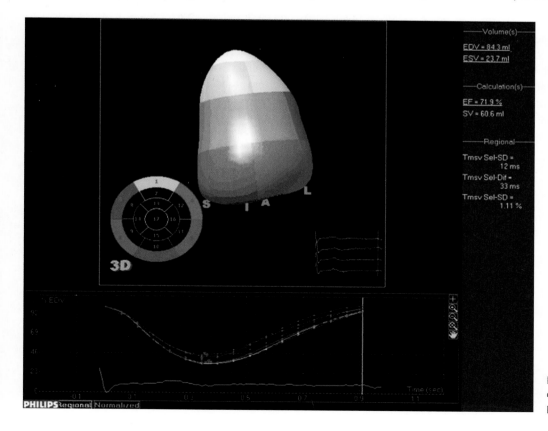

Fig. 35.4 Real-time three-dimensional echocardiography from a person with a normal heart.

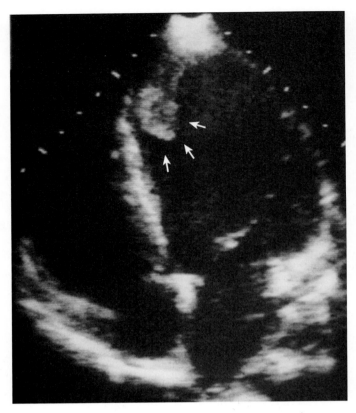

Fig. 35.5 Apical 4-chamber view from a patient with DCM. Note the presence of an apical thrombus. The patient was not receiving anticoagulation.

Using $^{15}O\text{-}H_2O$ or $^{13}N\text{-}NH_3$ as flow tracers in rest-stress protocols, quantitative evaluation of MBF in patients with DCM often demonstrates a diffuse impairment of myocardial perfusion and MBF reserve. This is interpreted as a result of coronary microvascular dysfunction, abnormal myocardial contractility, and wall stress, but is independent of myocardial fibrosis. A global and severe reduction in MBF reserve may occur even in the earlier stages of DCM. It is a distinctive marker of the severity of the disease and of an increased risk of progressive myocardial dysfunction, heart failure, and sudden death (⊃ Fig. 35.6) [11]. It must be kept in mind that a similar pattern of globally depressed myocardial perfusion may also occur in multi-vessel CAD, which still needs to be ruled out.

Myocardial metabolic imaging

Myocardial metabolic imaging for the assessment of myocardial metabolism using $^{18}F\text{-}FDG$ in patients with LV dysfunction is the most frequent clinical application of cardiac PET. It can be combined either with a $^{13}N\text{-}NH_3$ PET or a SPECT perfusion study. It allows identification of different characteristics of the dysfunctional myocardium based on the relationship between glucose metabolism and perfusion at rest. Residual metabolic activity is an indicator of myocardial viability and thus of potential reversibility of myocardial dysfunction. Increased regional FDG uptake relative to myocardial perfusion (perfusion/metabolism mismatch) indicates viability, while regional reduction of FDG uptake in proportion to perfusion (perfusion/metabolism match) indicates irreversibly damaged myocardium. It was generally believed that the demonstration of a regional 'match' or 'mismatch' pattern in patients with newly discovered LV dysfunction could help to identify a CAD aetiology. Actually, regionally matched perfusion and metabolic defects, indicating myocardial scar as well as regional flow metabolic 'mismatch' indicating ischaemia, can be frequently found in patients with idiopathic DCM (⊃ Fig. 35.7) [12]. However, data on the potential prognostic meaning of these findings in idiopathic DCM are still sparse.

The additional purpose of metabolic imaging in DCM is to assess abnormalities of intermediate myocardial metabolism that may further impair and/or be a consequence of reduced

stress-induced perfusion defects on SPECT or PET images, the likelihood of significant CAD as a cause of LV dysfunction is extremely low [10]. Conversely, the specificity is suboptimal mainly due to the frequent occurrence of regional perfusion abnormalities in a significant number of patients with LV dysfunction without detectable CAD (⊞ Video 35.3). PET has the specific advantage of precisely measuring the absolute myocardial blood flow (MBF, $ml.min^{-1}.g^{-1}$) at rest and during pharmacologic stress (i.v. dipyridamole or adenosine), and hence to measure regional and global MBF reserve.

Fig. 35.6 In patients with DCM and without overt heart failure, the extent of myocardial blood flow impairment at rest and during stress, measured by PET, predicts cardiac death and/or worsening of heart failure at follow-up [11].

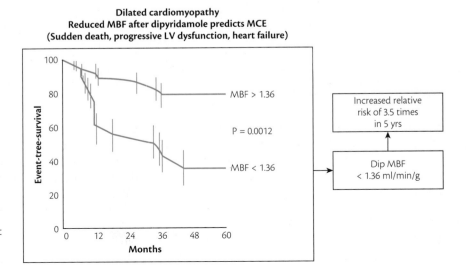

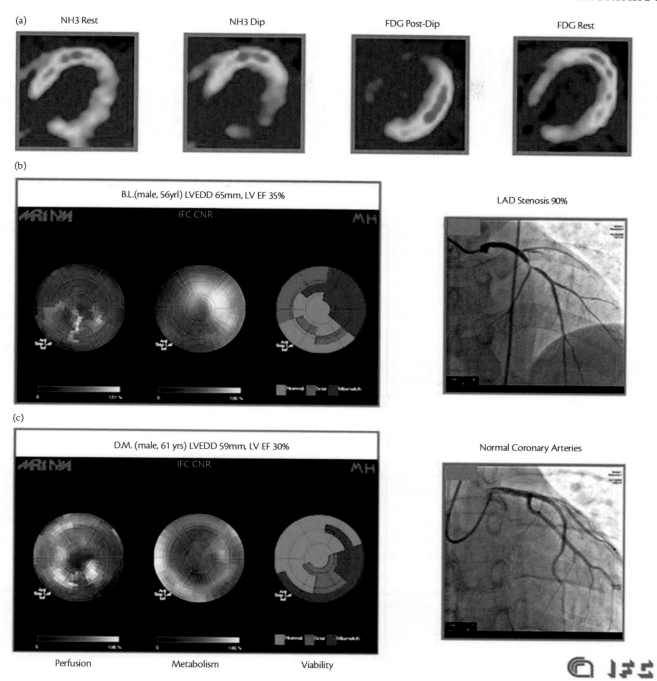

Fig. 35.7 (a) Four PET images obtained in a patient with DCM by ^{13}N-NH$_3$ and ^{18}F-FDG PET at rest and during dipyridamole stress showing a regional 'mismatch' pattern suggesting myocardial ischaemia. (b) Bull's-eye plots derived from ^{13}N-NH$_3$ and ^{18}F-FDG PET studies of a patient with DCM, showing regional flow-metabolism 'match' and 'mismatch'. (c) Bull's-eye plots of comparable PET studies obtained in a patient with CAD with poor LV function, demonstrating a typical flow-metabolism 'match' (green for normal and red for scar segments) and 'mismatch' (blue for viable segments).

contractile performance of the myocardium. Myocardial free fatty acid (FFA) metabolism is decreased and glucose metabolism increased in patients with idiopathic DCM proportionally to the severity of LV dysfunction. This compensatory metabolic shift towards the more efficient fuel glucose, as well as the effects of metabolic treatment, can be documented by PET imaging using ^{11}C-glucose, ^{11}C-palmitate and ^{11}C-acetate [13, 14]. In idiopathic DCM, myocardial metabolism, as well as myocardial perfusion, may not only globally, but also regionally improve after chronic treatment with beta blockers. Myocardial metabolic efficiency can be assessed by combining the PET measurement of oxidative metabolic rate (washout constant (k) from ^{11}C-acetate myocardial time–activity curve) and independent measurements of stroke work. Using this approach in patients with idiopathic DCM, oxidative metabolism and metabolic efficiency were shown to be reduced in proportion to the reduction of LV function and of the integrity of presynaptic innervations as assessed using ^{11}C-hydroxyephedrine PET imaging [15].

Sympathetic nerve imaging

Sympathetic nerve imaging can be performed with 123-iodine metaiodobenzylguanidine (^{123}I MIBG) SPECT. ^{123}I MIBG is an imaging tracer that shares similar myocardial uptake, storage, and release characteristics as endogenous norepinephrine in sympathetic nerve endings. Cardiac sympathetic denervation documented by this approach in patients with LV dysfunction is associated with arrhythmias. Performing ^{123}I MIBG SPECT imaging in candidates for implantation of a cardioverter-defibrillator (ICD), the documentation of a large MIBG defect is an independent predictor for appropriate therapy or cardiac death [16].

Nuclear imaging of LV function and dyssynchrony

Nuclear imaging of LV function and dyssynchrony is performed using gated acquisitions of perfusion and metabolic imaging studies or by equilibrium radionuclide ventriculography (ERNV). The addition of gating to myocardial perfusion scintigraphy or FDG PET studies has been demonstrated to be of great clinical value in CAD and DCM [17]. For patients with DCM, ECG-gated blood pool SPECT correlates well with CMR for the assessment of biventricular parameters, although RV indices should be cautiously interpreted [18]. Patients with DCM frequently present with left bundle branch block (LBBB), causing dyssynchronous activation of the left ventricle (early septal contraction against a relaxed LV free wall), which may further deteriorate cardiac function. CRT re-coordinates ventricular activation and may translate into improvement of cardiac function, symptoms, and prognosis. SPECT and PET imaging in patients with DCM and LBBB are helpful to recognize the efficacy of CRT. The septal-to-lateral perfusion ratio may be reduced in DCM with LBBB, when evaluated with ^{99m}Tc-sestamibi and SPECT or with ^{15}O-H$_2$O and PET, normalizing after CRT [19]. However, septal perfusion has also been demonstrated to be normal, when evaluated with ^{13}N-NH$_3$ and PET, without changes after CRT. Independently from regional distribution at rest, absolute measurement of MBF by PET demonstrates that an increase in hyperaemic MBF and MBF reserve after CRT is associated with improvement in LV wall stress and contractile function [19]. The effects of CRT on regional myocardial metabolism may be even more evident. In fact, LBBB is frequently associated with a reduced uptake of FDG in the septal wall which normalizes after CRT, expressing a more homogeneous myocardial oxygen consumption and improved metabolic efficiency [20]. There is preliminary evidence that a 'reverse mismatch' pattern in the septum, i.e. preserved perfusion with reduced FDG uptake, in patients with DCM and LBBB may predict a favourable prognosis after CRT.

The efficacy of pharmacological treatment

The efficacy of pharmacological treatment in patients with DCM can also to some extent be predicted by nuclear imaging. The favourable effect of carvedilol, a beta blocker, and trimetazidine on myocardial perfusion and metabolism have been assessed by nuclear medicine technologies [21]. However, the demonstration of the role of PET or SPECT specific patterns of myocardial perfusion and metabolism to predict response to treatment and outcome in DCM requires further extensive confirmative clinical research.

Hybrid imaging

Hybrid imaging with SPECT/CT or PET/CT scanners may expand the role of nuclear imaging in the evaluation of patients with DCM in the near future. Thus, in addition to the functional assessments obtained with SPECT and/or PET (i.e. myocardial perfusion, metabolism, and innervation), the new hybrid SPECT-PET/CT technology allows non-invasive anatomic exclusion of underlying coronary atherosclerosis in the same session (⊃ Fig. 35.8) [3]. Moreover, the analysis of the ventriculographic phase of CT could add a detailed evaluation of regional and global ventricular function. Independently from the availability of hybrid scanners, however, SPECT or PET may be combined with multi-detector CT

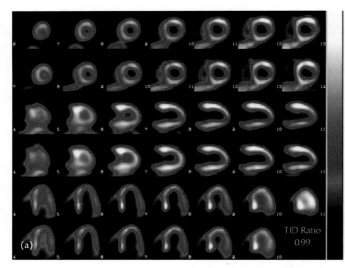
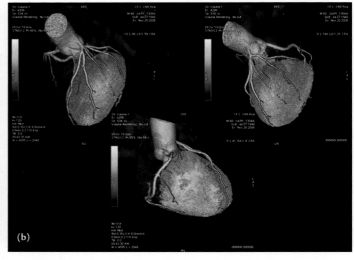

Fig. 35.8 (a) A perfusion ^{13}N-NH$_3$ PET study at rest (row of upper images) and during dipyridamole stress (row of lower images), performed in a patient with recent onset LBBB and LV EF 38% to exclude CAD as a cause of LV dysfunction. A non-reversible perfusion defect involving the middle-apical portions of the lateral wall is evident both at rest and during stress.(b) CT angiography performed soon after the PET study shows angiographically normal coronary arteries allowing the diagnosis of DCM.

in a new conceptual framework to provide a unique non-invasive work-up to exclude CAD, predicting risk, addressing treatment, and testing its efficacy. Contemporary rapid SPECT cameras and hybrid PET-CT techniques, coupled with the availability of new F-18 fluorine-labelled PET perfusion tracer and new quantitative methods and software for image processing, will most probably expand the use of nuclear cardiology in the clinical characterization of early stages of the development of DCM [22]. In addition, this approach might help to study the relationships between non-obstructive atherothrombosis, microvascular disease and progressive myocardial dysfunction and to evaluate new medical treatments targeted to alter or reverse the progression of heart failure. Prospective outcome studies are warranted to assess the value of this new approach in the evaluation of patients with DCM also taking into account cost-benefit and radiation exposure issues.

Cardiac magnetic resonance imaging in DCM

The value of CMR in the diagnosis of DCM relies on detailed determination of LV function using fast cine techniques (steady-state free-precession; SSFP), and the assessment of myocardial texture based on the application of techniques that accentuate differences in relaxation properties of the myocardium. The second may help to differentiate normal myocardium from pathologic processes associated with oedema, fibrosis, haemorrhage, iron, and protein fibril deposition using T1- and T2-weighted imaging, LGE imaging, T2-star imaging, and combinations of these techniques, respectively. Generally, the detailed functional measurement is useful to confirm a previous abnormal finding on echocardiography, whereas the assessment of pathological myocardial texture is unique to CMR and may provide a key to the aetiology of an idiopathic DCM.

Quantification of LV geometry

Quantification of LV geometry with CMR is generally performed using SSFP cine imaging [2]. The superior quality of images obtained by this technique facilitate the detection of regional abnormalities allowing an easier differentiation between ischaemic and non-ischaemic LV impairment. Nonetheless, this task may remain difficult in advanced ischaemic disease when extreme LV remodelling with subsequent LV dilation has developed.

Late gadolinium enhancement imaging (LGE)

Late gadolinium enhancement imaging (LGE) may be decisive based on the pattern of hyper-enhancement representing necrosis and fibrosis. Hyper-enhancement in ischaemic cardiomyopathy characteristically spreads from the sub-endocardium up to the epicardium and is confined to the perfusion territories of the coronary arteries. The prevalence of a sub-endocardial enhancement pattern in ischaemic cardiomyopathy is between 81 and 100%. In idiopathic DCM, hyper-enhancement was either absent (59–88% of cases) or appeared as a midwall rim of hyper-enhancement not related to specific coronary artery perfusion territories (9–28% of the cases) (⊃ Fig. 35.9). A minority of patients without obstructive CAD, however, may demonstrate the typical ischaemic sub-endocardial enhancement pattern. It has been postulated that this may result from missed infarcts due to transient occlusion and recanalization of the infarct-related vessel or vasospasm. Interestingly, the midwall enhancement pattern was shown to be present in patients with biopsy proven active and borderline myocarditis. This finding points to an aetiology of sustained myocarditis in at least a number of dilated cardiomyopathies so far classified as being 'idiopathic'.

Recently, midwall enhancement was shown to be an independent predictor of adverse outcome in terms of combined endpoints for all-cause mortality and hospitalization for heart failure, sudden cardiac death, inducible ventricular arrhythmias, and appropriate ICD therapy in patients with DCM [23–25]. Moreover, the predictive value of midwall hyper-enhancement remained significant after correction for LV volumes and EF. Thus, LGE may play an important role in selection of candidates for ICD implantation. Future studies will need to corroborate these expectations.

DCM and myocarditis

Myocarditis is strongly suspected when a previously healthy patient suddenly develops congestive cardiac failure, often after a

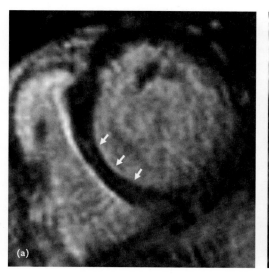 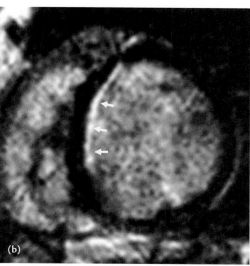

Fig. 35.9 Short-axis late gadolinium enhancement images of two patients with heart failure, dilated LV and poor EF. (a) A patient with DCM; a small rim of subtle intra-septal midwall hyper-enhancement that is observed in one-third of patients with DCM, indicating replacement fibrosis. (b) A patient with coronary artery disease; a bright sub-endocardial pattern of hyper-enhancement, typical of ischaemic origin due to coronary artery disease.

period of flu-like illness. Following standardization of the histo-pathological diagnosis of myocarditis by the Dallas criteria [26], evidence of myocarditis in dilated cardiomyopathy varies between 18 and 55%. The therapeutic implications, however, are limited, as the mere presence of inflammatory infiltrates does not necessarily signify active myocarditis.

Myocarditis due to viral infection, is a more frequent finding in DCM than is clinically obvious and can be identified as a cause of disease in almost 10% of cases using endomyocardial biopsy [27]. Inflammatory DCM is defined by the presence of chronic inflammatory cells in association with LV dilatation and reduced EF; histology and/or immunocytochemistry are therefore necessary for the diagnosis. Myocarditis increases the risk of sudden cardiac death in young adults during sports, and accounts for approximately 10% of sudden cardiac death cases in macroscopically normal hearts. The diagnosis may be difficult to establish and is generally based on a diversity of clinical signs supported by electrocardiographic and laboratory abnormalities. Endomyocardial biopsy still is considered the gold-standard for diagnosis, but this method has limited sensitivity inherent to the focal nature of myocarditis.

Echocardiography in myocarditis

Myocarditis is suspected when a patient is acutely ill and echocardiography demonstrates a non-dilated LV with global hypokinesia. Often, however, there is only regional ventricular dysfunction involving the septum or even the right ventricle, which may be more difficult to detect. When this regional ventricular dysfunction is present, it is difficult to rule out acute coronary syndrome. The patient's age and clinical presentation, however, often allow correct diagnosis. After the acute phase, the clinical course may be highly variable, ranging from complete recovery of LV function to the development of overt DCM. Therefore, serial follow-up with echocardiographic examinations is warranted to timely initiate therapy, when indicated.

Nuclear techniques in myocarditis

SPECT imaging, coupled with imaging agents of chronic inflammation or labelled antibodies may be used in myocarditis and inflammatory DCM [28]. [67]Gallium citrate scintigraphy has been tested in DCM patients showing that 87% of patients with histologically proven myocarditis had a positive [67]Gallium scan, while histology was positive only in 1.8% in the negative scintigraphic group. Indium-111 radiolabelled antimyosin antibodies have been shown to detect myocardial necrosis in human myocarditis. Using planar and SPECT cardiac imaging, the sensitivity of antimyosin imaging for the detection of histologically proven myocarditis is very high (91–100%) with a high negative predictive value (93–100%). By contrast, the specificity and positive predictive value of this approach are below 50%. However, a positive antimyosin scan can predict more accurately than myocardial biopsy a subsequent improvement in EF in acute onset DCM patients. Limitations to this technique include its current limited availability, radiation exposure, and 48-hour delays in obtaining imaging after injection to prevent interference of blood pool signal.

Cardiovascular magnetic resonance imaging in myocarditis

Several CMR techniques are used in non-invasive detection of myocarditis, including T2-weighted oedema imaging, T1-weighted spin-echo early gadolinium enhancement imaging and LGE imaging [29, 30]. When these techniques were compared in patients with clinically suspected acute myocarditis, T2-weighted imaging demonstrated the highest sensitivity (84%) and LGE imaging the highest specificity (100%). The best diagnostic accuracy, however, was obtained when any two of the three techniques were positive in the same patient (85%). Recommendations on the use of CMR for myocarditis were summarized in an expert consensus document [31].

The pattern of hyper-enhancement in the acute phase of myocarditis typically has multiple foci within the lateral wall of the LV, originating primarily from the epicardium (⊃ Fig. 35.10) (🖳 Video 35.4). When biopsies were taken from the regions with hyper-enhancement, histopathologic analysis revealed active myocarditis, which was less consistently observed when the biopsy specimens could not be retrieved from the hyper-enhanced regions. This suggests that CMR-guided biopsy may lead to a higher yield of positive findings than routine right ventricular biopsy in patients with acute myocarditis. In patients with idiopathic DCM, however, such a correlation has not been shown.

Differences in sensitivity of CMR techniques presumably are related to temporal changes of the inflammatory and healing process. Histologically, oedema and islets of necrosis are dispersed throughout the myocardium in the acute and subacute phase of inflammation and ongoing healing of the myocardium [30]. Depending on the time window after onset of inflammation, oedema-sensitive T2-weighted signal or necrosis and fibrosis sensitive LGE signal may both concur or one of the two may prevail [29]. After healing, LVEF and dimensions often restore, and the areas of hyper-enhancement almost completely resolve. Similar to the shrinkage of myocardial infarct size in the chronic phase, shrinkage of the islets of fibrotic areas to sizes smaller than the dimensions of a voxel has been suggested as an underlying mechanism of the resolution of hyper-enhancement. However, in some patients in whom LV dysfunction and dilation persists, a small remnant midwall rim of subtle hyper-enhancement may be observed that was shown to be associated with biopsy proven active and borderline myocarditis according to the Dallas criteria. This midwall rim is more often found in patients with idiopathic DCM and may reflect patchy areas of replacement fibrosis after sustained myocarditis. Importantly, the presence of hyper-enhancement in patients with biopsy proven viral myocarditis has shown to be a strong prognostic marker for all cause and cardiac mortality (hazard ratio 8.4 and 12.8, respectively), superior to LVEF [32].

DCM in cardiac sarcoidosis

Sarcoidosis is a systemic immunological disorder characterized by multiple non-caseating granulomas. Cardiac involvement

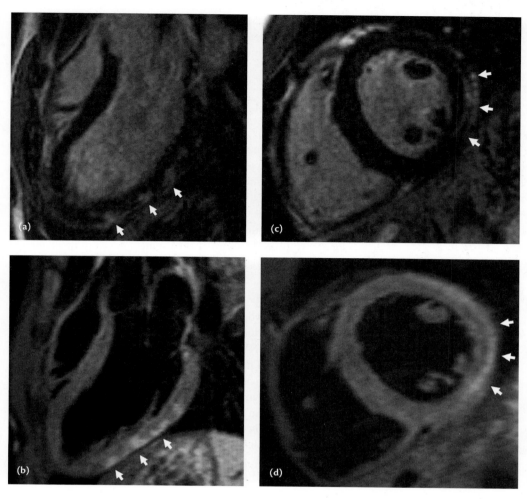

Fig. 35.10 A patient presenting with clinical signs of acute myocarditis. (a) Late gadolinium enhancement (LGE) image of a three-chamber view demonstrating a slightly dilated LV and focal, sub-epicardial enhancement of the inferolateral wall, indicating fibrosis or oedema, see arrowheads. (b) The same three-chamber view showing that the hyper-enhanced myocardial areas on the LGE image also have a high signal intensity on a T2-weighted image indicating oedema as a result of active inflammation. (c) LGE short-axis view of the same patient with typical epicardial hyper-enhancement. (d) T2-weighted short-axis image of the same patient with high signal intensity indicating oedema.

occurs in 20–60% of patients [33]. Most (80%) patients with cardiac sarcoidosis have conduction disturbance or arrhythmia and/or impaired LV function (31%) [34]. In patients who die in the active phase of myocardial sarcoidosis, granulomas may either be distributed evenly throughout the myocardium or occur as a localized mass, commonly in the basal portion of the ventricular septum. The frequency of sudden cardiac death reflects the high risk that the conduction system will be affected in both the focal and diffuse forms.

Echocardiography in sarcoidosis

Echocardiographic abnormalities indicating cardiac involvement in sarcoidosis include regional wall motion abnormalities, often not confined to perfusion territories of coronary arteries, ventricular aneurysms, pericardial effusion, LV systolic or diastolic dysfunction, valvular abnormalities, and abnormal wall thickness (either thinning or thickening). The most typical forms are those with proximal septal thinning and akinesia, while the distal septum and apex are contracting normally (◑ Fig. 35.11). In a small study population of 22 patients, ultrasonic tissue characterization with integrated backscatter showed a significant improvement in sensitivity over 2D-echocardiography [35]. Further studies will be necessary to confirm the usefulness of this technique. Other

techniques such as strain imaging have not been formally investigated but show reduced regional strain values.

Nuclear imaging in sarcoidosis

Myocardial SPECT with ^{99m}Tc-sestamibi has been used to detect myocardial involvement. Perfusion defects are more common in the right ventricle than in the left ventricle and correlate with atrioventricular block, heart failure, and ventricular tachycardia of right ventricular origin. These defects are frequently reversible, which makes it unlikely that they represent granulomatosis or fibrosis. ^{67}Gallium scintigraphy has been used in sarcoidosis as a marker of the activity and extent of the disease and for predicting the efficacy of corticosteroids, but it has been largely replaced by serial other tests. Heterogeneous myocardial FDG uptake at PET imaging may be a useful diagnostic marker of disease activity [36].

Cardiovascular magnetic resonance imaging in sarcoidosis

The non-caseating granulomas within the myocardium implicate an increase of extracellular space, so hyper-enhancement on LGE CMR is likely to occur. Hyper-enhancement was reported to be present in 19 of 58 patients (33%) with biopsy-proven pulmonary

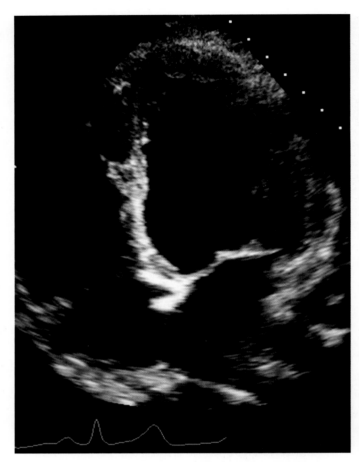

Fig. 35.11 A patient with sarcoidosis who presented with recurrent VT. Echocardiography showed proximal septal thinning and akinesia. It also showed very echogenic myocardium, likely suggestive of scar. The distal septum and apex were contracting normal.

sarcoidosis and in all patients with cardiac involvement according to guideline criteria [33]. Hyper-enhanced areas are focal, epicardial, or confluent transmural, and predominantly located in the basal and lateral LV segments (➲ Fig. 35.12), thereby showing similarity to LGE in myocarditis. Interestingly, the areas of hyper-enhancement were also present in patients with no LV dilation,

indicating that CMR may help prevent the development of heart failure by early detection of cardiac involvement, which accounts for up to 85% of mortality in this patient group.

DCM and Chagas' disease

Chagas' disease is an inflammatory infectious disease caused by the parasite *Trypanosoma cruzi* and is endemic in South America. The clinical course of the disease can be subdivided into three stages: an acute stage with fever and headache, an indeterminate phase in which patients are asymptomatic, and a chronic phase in which the heart is the most frequently affected organ, resulting in heart failure and the onset of potentially life-threatening ventricular arrhythmias. This cardiac involvement develops in 30–40% of patients, sometimes decades after the initial infection.

Nuclear imaging in Chagas' disease

Chagas' cardiomyopathy has several distinctive features in comparison with DCM due to viral myocarditis. Radionuclide functional imaging with ERNV and perfusion imaging by SPECT may detect LV regional wall motion abnormalities and perfusion defects in the absence of epicardial CAD, while right ventricular dysfunction is common in asymptomatic patients with no other clinical signs of heart failure. An association between regional defects in sympathetic denervation detected by ^{123}I-MIBG, and perfusion defects detected by ^{201}Tl scintigraphy have also been shown [37].

Cardiovascular magnetic resonance imaging in Chagas' disease

Localized aneurysm formation can be detected using SSFP cine imaging with predilection sites at the apex and basal inferolateral wall, which are difficult to evaluate with echocardiography (See 📺 Video 35.5). Using LGE imaging, areas of predominantly sub-endocardial hyper-enhancement can be observed within these regions in 20% of seropositive patients within the indeterminate phase of the disease, 85% with clinical Chagas' cardiomyopathy, and 100% with Chagas' cardiomyopathy and ventricular tachycardia (➲ Fig. 35.13)

Fig. 35.12 Late gadolinium enhancement (LGE) in patient with cardiac sarcoidosis. (a) LGE two-chamber view image showing multiple focal areas of hyper-enhancement observed in the epicardium and midwall, which partially become confluent and transmural. (b) LGE four-chamber view image of the same patient demonstrating the extent of scarring also present in the lateral wall and septum.

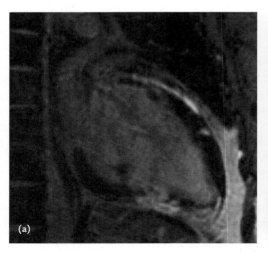
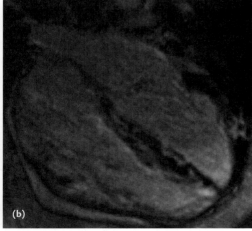

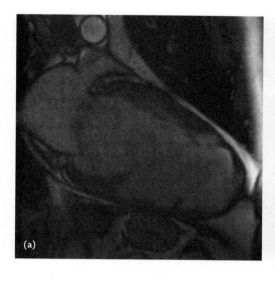
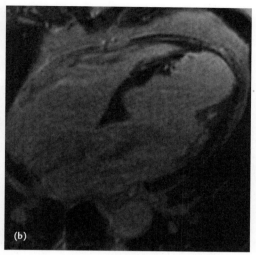

Fig. 35.13 Chronic stage of Chagas' disease with cardiac involvement. (a) SSFP two-chamber view cine image. The aneurysms at the apex and inferior wall result from recurrent episodes of inflammatory disease. (b) Late gadolinium enhancement four-chamber view image. Within the apical aneurysm a sub-endocardial rim of hyper-enhancement due to fibrosis is visible.

[38]. The hyper-enhancement pattern is indistinguishable from the ischaemic pattern, and predilection sites are thought to be terminal portions of the microcirculation, which are most vulnerable to become ischaemic in recurrent episodes of inflammatory disease and subsequent vasodilatation. Also, LGE imaging allows visualization of thrombus formation that may develop within the aneurysms.

DCM in vasculitis

Inflammatory states of the blood vessels may also affect the coronary arteries and the myocardium, leading to impaired LV function and heart failure.

Churg–Strauss syndrome

Churg–Strauss syndrome is a rare systemic small-vessel vasculitis with eosinophilic myocardial infiltration and subsequent cardiomyopathy. Subclinical cardiac involvement of disease can be diagnosed using LGE imaging, which may show areas of hyper-enhancement. These areas of hyper-enhancement may reflect either active inflammation that may require therapy, or fibrosis. To discriminate between both disease states, T2-weighted imaging can be used to visualize oedema indicating acute inflammation. Alternatively, ^{18}F-FDG PET also allows detection of increased FDG uptake that ensues from active inflammation in hyper-enhanced areas [39]. Using PET, the regional pattern of enhanced ^{18}F-FDG uptake and reduced ^{13}N-NH$_3$ uptake (the pattern of flow-metabolism mismatch) may be reversible after anti-inflammatory treatment and predicts improvement of cardiac function (◖ Fig. 35.14).

Takayasu arteritis

Myocardial damage and dilatation may ensue from large and small coronary vessels involvement. ^{99m}Tc-sestamibi and ^{18}F-FDG SPECT may reveal evidence of myocardial ischaemic damage.

Kawasaki disease

In children, cardiovascular manifestations can be prominent in the acute phase and are the leading cause of long-term morbidity and mortality. During this phase, the pericardium, myocardium, endocardium, valves, and coronary arteries all may be involved. Nuclear stress perfusion imaging for reversible ischaemia is indicated to assess the existence and functional consequences of coronary artery abnormalities in children with Kawasaki disease and coronary aneurysms. Myocarditis has been demonstrated in autopsy and myocardial biopsy studies to be a common feature of early Kawasaki disease. Myocardial inflammation has been documented in 50–70% of patients using ^{67}Ga citrate SPECT scans and ^{99m}Tc-labelled white blood cell scans.

With CMR, ectatic, but not aneurysmatic, coronary arteries in combination with an ischaemic pattern of hyper-enhancement have also been described [40].

DCM in neuromuscular disorders

In addition to conduction disorders, cardiac muscle involvement leading to progressive DCM is common in neuromuscular disorders and occurs in up to 90% and 70% of patients with Duchenne and Becker muscular dystrophy, respectively.

Echocardiography in neuromuscular disorders

In patients with Duchenne muscular dystrophy, and presumably other familial forms of DCM, tissue Doppler imaging (TDI) can be employed to detect early LV dysfunction, prior to any clinical manifestation of heart failure [41]. This may have therapeutic implications while early treatment might prevent LV remodelling. TDI may be used to detect regional or global myocardial dysfunction, particularly in patients with normal LV dimensions. Early ventricular dysfunction affects predominantly the longitudinal function of the left ventricle, which can better be assessed from apical projections. TDI is ideally suited to assess the LV longitudinal function by measuring mitral annular velocities, as well as myocardial velocity gradients or LV strain and strain rate. In addition, radial strain rate of the LV posterior wall at peak systole and early diastole may be reduced, while conventional echocardiography may be normal [42].

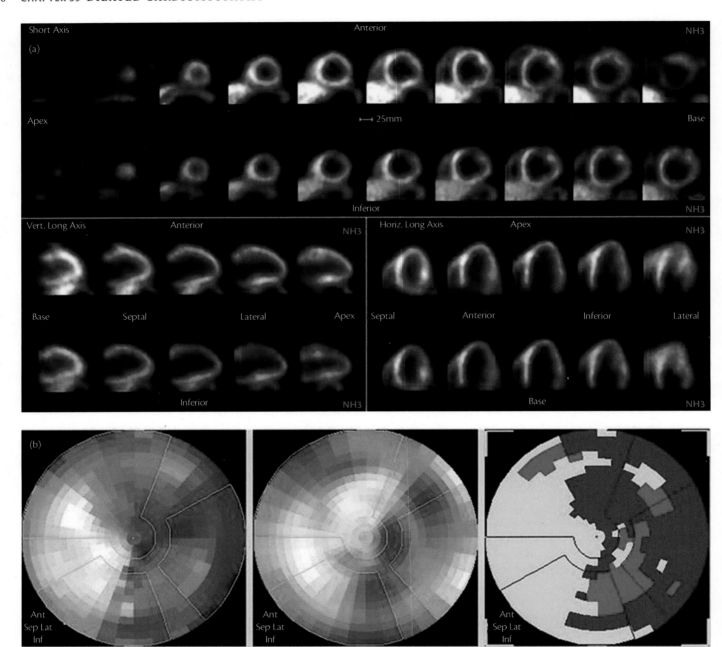

Fig. 35.14 (a) A perfusion ^{13}N-NH$_3$ PET study performed at rest (upper row of images) and during dipyridamole stress (lower row of images) in a patient with an active phase of Churg–Strauss disease. A perfusion defect involving the basal portion of the lateral wall is evident in both conditions, while a stress induced perfusion defect is present in the middle and apical portions of the anterior wall of the LV. (b) The resting ^{13}N-NH$_3$ perfusion images are compared with ^{18}F-FDG metabolic images. The tracer is injected after oral glucose loading on another day in a typical viability study. Extensive 'mismatch' pattern (blue segments) indicating ischaemia is evident in the anterolateral wall of the LV with some 'match' areas (red segments) indicating myocardial necrosis.

Doppler-based strain imaging has found only limited access into clinical practice due to several limitations, including angle dependency, a low signal-to-noise ratio, limited spatial resolution, and potential interactions by cardiac translational motion and tethering.

Tracking of acoustic markers (speckles) from frame-to-frame on the basis of 2D-echocardiography can now accurately determine regional and global LV function. This novel technique overcomes most of the limitations of conventional Doppler-based strain imaging (➲ Fig. 35.15). In addition, new measures of quantifying LV function have been widely accepted, such as LV rotation and torsion [21]. This type of new quantification tools are exciting and may well prove to be more accurate in predicting outcomes than the more traditional EF.

Cardiovascular magnetic resonance imaging in neuromuscular disorders

In paediatric patients with Duchenne muscular dystrophy, occult regional cardiac dysfunction with reduced

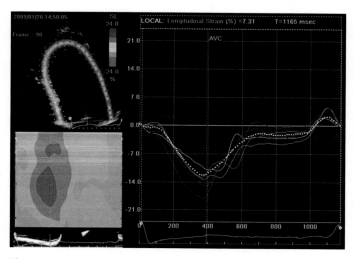

Fig. 35.15 Apical four-chamber view from a patient with DCM. Using speckle tracking, it is possible to quantify the longitudinal strain in every segment and express it as global longitudinal strain (dotted line). In this case, strain is markedly reduced.

circumferential strain was detected in patients with normal LV volumes and EF, using CMR tissue tagging [43]. In a study involving 74 patients (range of 8–26 years), 32% was found to have hyper-enhancement involving the posterobasal subepicardial region of the LV with a possible transmural and inferior or left lateral spreading [44]. In patients with Becker muscular dystrophy, hyper-enhancement has been demonstrated in 11 of 15 patients (73%, range 11–56 years), with a similar regional extension (➲ Fig. 35.16). CMR revealed abnormal findings including wall motion abnormalities, reduced LVEF, and LGE in 80% of patients, compared to 53% by echocardiography [45]. In both studies hyper-enhancement was associated with higher age and adverse LV remodelling with decreased EF, but serial studies are needed to clarify whether hyper-enhancement precedes LV dysfunction and may serve as an early marker for initiation of heart failure management.

DCM and cardiotoxic agents

Echocardiography and cardiotoxic drugs

A variety of substances can affect the heart leading to DCM. Perhaps the commonest toxin is alcohol. Macrocytosis is a useful indicator of chronically high alcohol consumption, even in the absence of abnormal liver function. A raised gamma-glutamyltransferase may be an indicator of only recent rather than long-term alcohol intake, whereas raised levels of other liver enzymes may be due to chronic alcohol hepatitis.

There is an individual susceptibility to the adverse effects of alcohol on the myocardium, which may well be genetically predisposed. The heart is typically markedly dilated with global ventricular dysfunction and it may show dramatic improvement after a patient has stopped excessive alcohol consumption. Therefore, evaluation of LV dimensions and function is recommended 6 months after alcohol abstinence.

Anthracyclines are widely used for treatment of malignancies and have a dose-related cardiac toxicity. The estimated risk of developing cardiomyopathy after anthracycline therapy has been reported to be 4.5% at 10 years and increases to 9.8% at 20 years after therapy among patients with cumulative doses of 300 mg/m^2 [46]. In addition, mediastinal irradiation, young age at exposure, female sex, and genetic susceptibility are known risk factors for the development of anthracycline cardiotoxicity. The prevalence of overt anthracycline-induced clinical heart failure is estimated between 0% and 16% [47].

Nuclear imaging and cardiotoxic drugs

ERNV provides initial and longitudinal quantitative assessment of LV function. EF should be measured in all patients before receiving doxorubicin; those with pre-existing heart disease and/or LV dysfunction are at greater risk of congestive heart failure. Continued use of doxorubicin after LV dysfunction has developed, causes progressive chamber dilatation and deterioration in systolic function.

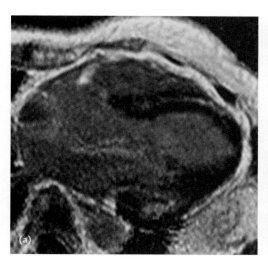

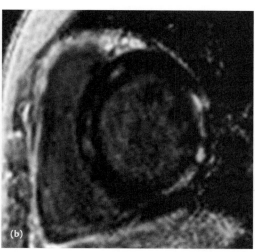

Fig. 35.16 Late gadolinium enhancement (LGE) imaging in a patient with Becker's muscular dystrophy. (a) LGE three-chamber view. (b) LGE short-axis view. Hyper-enhancement is predominantly apparent in the basal lateral wall and to a lesser degree in the interventricular septum.

Cardiovascular magnetic resonance imaging and cardiotoxic drugs

In long-term survivors of childhood cancer, focal myocardial hyper-enhancement is rare. In contrast, myocardial fibrosis is ubiquitous in post-mortem pathologic examinations of patients treated with anthracyclines. Indeed, reduction of both left and right ventricular function in this patient group has recently been demonstrated without hyper-enhancement on LGE imaging [48]. Although LGE imaging is well suited to qualitatively assess replacement fibrosis, it lacks the sensitivity to quantify diffuse fibrosis, due to its reliance on regional differences in gadolinium concentrations to generate image contrast [49]. With a more recently developed technique referred to as post-contrast T1-mapping, the gadolinium contrast tissue concentration can be quantified as an extracellular volume fraction [50]. An increased extracellular volume fraction indicates the presence of diffuse fibrosis. In long-term cancer survivors treated with anthracyclines, increased extracellular volume fractions were found in patients with both reduced and preserved LVEF. The increased extracellular volume fraction was related to diastolic dysfunction, underscoring that myocardium is diffusely affected in this disease [50].

DCM associated with pregnancy and parturition

Peripartum cardiomyopathy is an idiopathic cardiomyopathy presenting with heart failure secondary to LV systolic dysfunction towards the end of pregnancy or in the months following delivery, when no other cause of heart failure is found. The majority of patients who are diagnosed during pregnancy develop heart failure in the third trimester. Because of the low incidence, limited data is available on the aetiology of disease. Several mechanisms have been suggested, such as an abnormal maternal immunologic response and oxidative stress-mediated cleavage of the nursing hormone prolactin resulting in myocardial hypoxaemia and apoptosis [51]. Also, predisposing factors such as multiparity, race, hypertension, and genetic predisposition have been identified [52].

Peripartum cardiomyopathy can evolve in three ways of approximately equal thirds: one-third of patients completely recover in up to a year post-delivery and in one-third of patients cardiac function gradually deteriorates and evolves into overt DCM with poor LVEF requiring cardiac transplantation. Persisting cardiomegaly at 6 months is usually associated with high mortality and the women may be candidates for cardiac transplantation. Therefore, strict follow-up is mandatory.

Echocardiography in peripartum cardiomyopathy

The echocardiographic findings are usually those of a non-dilated left ventricle with global hypokinesia (increased end systolic dimensions), similar to myocarditis. Occasionally, the differential diagnosis with viral myocarditis is difficult and should rely mainly on clinical grounds. LV thrombus needs to be excluded, as this will carry a high risk for embolization and requires anticoagulation therapy. When LV dysfunction is discovered in the context of arrhythmias and congestive cardiac failure during the third trimester or immediately post-delivery, the diagnosis is straightforward.

Cardiovascular magnetic resonance imaging in peripartum cardiomyopathy

Although CMR is probably safe during pregnancy, it should only be used when acoustic windows do not allow sufficient image quality with echocardiography. CMR studies performed after delivery demonstrated a DCM with midwall hyper-enhancement [53], but the prognostic value of the absence of hyper-enhancement in patients with peripartum cardiomyopathy seems limited [54].

Isolated left ventricular non-compaction

As genetic evidence emerges, there is no consensus on whether left ventricular non-compaction is a separate cardiomyopathy, or merely a congenital or acquired morphological trait shared by many phenotypically distinct cardiomyopathies [1].

It is macroscopically characterized by an extensive layer of non-compacted myocardium aligning a compact layer of myocardium and is typically located in the apical and lateral regions of the left ventricle. Patients with isolated LV non-compaction often suffer from heart failure as first symptom of disease, but are also prone to thromboembolic events, since the hyper-trabecularization is believed to be a risk factor for cardiac thrombus formation. Isolated LV non-compaction may be present in neonates and children, but also in young adults. It is rarely diagnosed for the first time in middle or advanced ages.

Echocardiography in non-compaction cardiomyopathy

The diagnosis is made by echocardiography in the vast majority of patients by the combination of the clinical presentation of breathlessness or palpitations and the echocardiographic appearance of a coarsely trabeculated left ventricle, often localized towards the apex and presenting with sub-endocardial recesses. Jenni et al. proposed the following criteria: (1) no coexisting abnormalities, (2) a two-layered myocardial structure with a thin compacted epicardial band and a thick non-compacted endocardial layer of trabecular meshwork with deep endomyocardial spaces with a non-compacted/compacted ratio of 2.0 in end-systole, (3) non-compaction predominantly in the mid-lateral, mid-inferior, and apical segments, (4) colour Doppler evidence of deep-perfused inter-trabecular recesses [55]. This is best visualized in the apical four-chamber and parasternal short-axis views. Because of the limitations of 2D-echocardiography to visualise the cardiac apex, the use of transvenous contrast agents will improve the visualization of apical recesses. With the dissemination of transthoracic three-dimensional echocardiography the cardiac apex can also be better identified and the myocardial recesses better visualized.

Nuclear imaging in non-compaction cardiomyopathy

PET with ^{13}N-NH$_3$ has been shown to demonstrate restricted myocardial perfusion and decreased flow reserve in these myocardial areas in children. The myocardial perfusion defects may contribute to myocardial damage and possibly to cause arrhythmias and pump failure.

Cardiovascular magnetic resonance imaging in non-compaction cardiomyopathy

With the advent of high-resolution imaging techniques such as CMR, abnormal trabeculation is more easily recognized,

requiring stricter criteria for diagnosis of non-compaction than the previously defined echocardiographic criteria of a non-compacted to compacted layer ratio >2 in end-systole. Based on a comparison between CMR images of patients with several forms of cardiomyopathy and hypertrophy, and a limited number of patients with previously demonstrated non-compaction cardiomyopathy, a non-compacted to compacted ratio >2.3 in end-diastole has been proposed, yielding a sensitivity of 86% and specificity of 99% [56] (⊃ Fig. 35.17) (See 🎥 Videos 35.6 and 35.7). However, in our experience, measuring non-compacted to compacted ratios >2.3 are also frequently found in a low pre-test likelihood population with other cardiomyopathies, such as ischaemic DCM and HCM and even in healthy volunteers. Therefore, in general population, higher cut-off may be warranted. Also, crypt formation has been described in genetically proven carriers of hypertrophic cardiomyopathy without overt hypertrophy [57] (⊃ Fig. 35.18) (🎥 Videos 35.8 and 35.9). Although by CMR clearly distinct from the typical hyper-trabecularization pattern

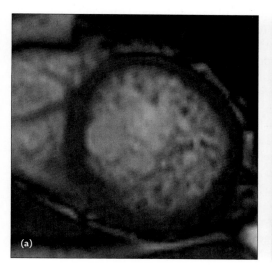

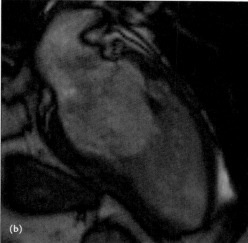

Fig. 35.17 A patient with isolated left ventricular non-compaction cardiomyopathy demonstrating a meshwork of trabeculae predominantly in the apex. The end-diastolic non-compacted to compacted ratio exceeds 2.3. (a) SSFP cine short-axis view. (b) SSFP cine two-chamber view.

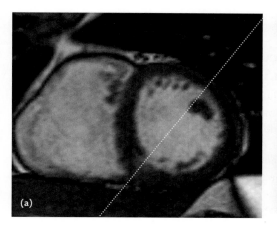

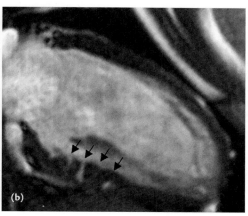

Fig. 35.18 Myocardial crypts in the inferoseptal wall as observed in genetically proven carrier of a hypertrophic cardiomyopathy mutation without overt hypertrophy. The appearance is clearly distinct from hypertrabecularization in non-compaction cardiomyopathy (see Fig. 35.17). (a) SSFP end-diastolic cine short-axis view with a dashed line through a bright, blood containing triangle in the inferoseptum indicating the transsection of modified two-chamber view to best visualize the crypts. (b) In the SSFP cine end-diastolic modified two-chamber view, the crypts are clearly visible in the inferoseptum, see arrow heads.

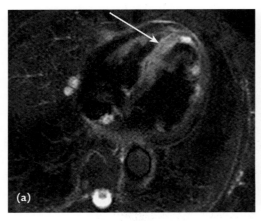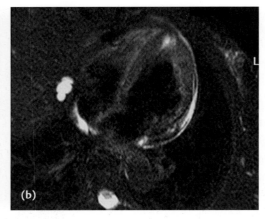

Fig. 35.19 MRI case of Tako Tsubo. (a) T2 image obtained during the acute phase. A clear enhancement of the signal due to the presence of myocardial oedema at the level of the inter-ventricular septum is evident (arrow). (b) At the same level, the T2 image obtained 3 months later, no signal abnormality could be observed. With kind persmission of Dr Lorenzo Montu, Humanitas, Milan, Italy.

of non-compaction cardiomyopathy, prominent crypts may have been misdiagnosed by echocardiography as non-compaction cardiomyopathy in the past. Therefore, further refinement of the criteria to diagnose LV non-compaction cardiomyopathy with CMR is necessary. Of note, no specific hyper-enhancement pattern has been reported so far in this particular patient group.

Takotsubo cardiomyopathy

Takotsubo cardiomyopathy was first described in 1990 as a unique clinical entity among acute coronary syndromes characterized by sudden onset of chest symptoms, electrocardiographic changes consistent with myocardial ischaemia, transient LV dysfunction (apical or mid-segment, or both) without significant coronary stenosis on angiography [58]. This rare clinical variant is unique and has a favourable prognosis compared with other causes of acute coronary syndromes, despite the similarity in presentation. To date, the precise aetiologic basis of this syndrome is not clear. Takotsubo cardiomyopathy has been linked to an excess sympathetic nervous activity, which is proposed as a central mechanism in the pathogenesis of transient left-ventricular apical dysfunction (apical ballooning syndrome). Acute multi-vessel coronary vasospasm (epicardial or microvascular), abnormalities in coronary endothelial function, and catecholamine-mediated cardiotoxicity have also been suggested.

Echocardiography in Takotsubo cardiomyopathy

Echocardiography is typical of an extensive acute left coronary artery syndrome with extensive apical akinesia or even dyskinesia (➲ Fig. 35.19). The diagnosis, however, is based on the natural history of the disease, which is based on the restoration of the ventricular function within 2–4 weeks [58, 59].

Nuclear imaging in Takotsubo cardiomyopathy

SPECT imaging can be used to evaluate myocardial damage and the pathogenesis of the syndrome. Using myocardial ^{123}I-MIBG and ^{99m}Tc-sestamibi to assess myocardial perfusion in patients with LV angiographically proven Takotsubo cardiomyopathy has demonstrated a decreased heart-to-mediastinum ratio of ^{123}I-MIBG at early (20 minutes) and delayed (4 hours) image acquisition, with an increased cardiac washout rate indicating a functional alteration in presynaptic sympathetic neurotransmission [60]. The neuronal tracer was evidently reduced in the akinetic apex and the perfusion tracer showed a modest defect. It has also been documented that the severity of the apical perfusion defects, assessed by measurements of the TIMI myocardial perfusion grade at angiography, correlates with the extent of acute myocardial injury suggesting a catecholamine-mediated endothelial/microvascular dysfunction as a pathogenic mechanism in this disease. SPECT and PET perfusion-metabolic studies in these patients have shown a sort of 'reverse mismatch' pattern (FDG defect in excess of perfusion defect) at the apex suggesting that the myocardial damage caused by sympathetic overload may involve abnormalities of both perfusion and glucose metabolism with a scintigraphic 'fingerprint' of reversibility [61].

Cardiovascular magnetic resonance imaging in Takotsubo cardiomyopathy

Using CMR, Takotsubo cardiomyopathy is characterized by wall motion abnormalities and increased T2-weighted signal indicating oedema without signs of hyper-enhancement (➲ Fig. 35.20) [62]. It is worth noting that the pattern of oedema during the acute phase is different from the other non-ischaemic acute syndromes. Thus, CMR is particularly useful to confirm a suspected diagnosis of Takotsubo cardiomyopathy, since it can differentiate from other ACS mimicking syndromes with normal coronary arteries such as myocarditis and infarction due to coronary embolisation.

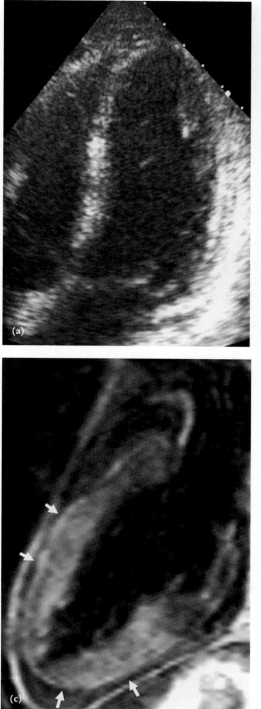

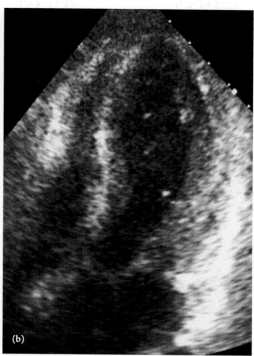

Fig. 35.20 A patient with Takotsubo cardiomyopathy. (a) 2D-echocardiography end-diastolic four-chamber view showing normal LV dimensions. (b) 2D-echocardiography end-systolic four-chamber view showing apical ballooning. (c). CMR T2-weighted two-chamber view of the left ventricle. Note the higher signal intensity of the mid and apical segments indicating myocardial oedema (arrows), not confined to the boundaries of a perfusion territory of an epical coronary artery suggesting an acute inflammatory process.

References

1. Elliott P, Andersson B, Arbustini E, et al. Classification of the cardiomyopathies: a position statement from the European Society Of Cardiology Working Group on Myocardial and Pericardial Diseases. *Eur Heart J* 2008; 29(2): 270–6.

2. Maceira AM, Prasad SK, Khan M, Pennell DJ. Normalized left ventricular systolic and diastolic function by steady state free precession cardiovascular magnetic resonance. *J Cardiovasc Magn Reson* 2006; 8(3): 417–26.

3. Andreini D, Pontone G, Bartorelli AL, et al. Sixty-four-slice multidetector computed tomography: an accurate imaging modality for the evaluation of coronary arteries in dilated cardiomyopathy of unknown etiology. *Circ Cardiovasc Imaging* 2009; 2(3): 199–205.

4. Hershberger RE, Siegfried JD. Update 2011: clinical and genetic issues in familial dilated cardiomyopathy. *J Am Coll Cardiol* 2011; 57(16): 1641–9.

5. Rapezzi C, Arbustini E, Caforio AL, et al. Diagnostic work-up in cardiomyopathies: bridging the gap between clinical phenotypes and final diagnosis. A position statement from the ESC Working Group on Myocardial and Pericardial Diseases. *Eur Heart J* 2013:34(19); 1448–58.

6. Mor-Avi V, Jenkins C, Kuhl HP, et al. Real-time 3-dimensional echocardiographic quantification of left ventricular volumes: multicenter study for validation with magnetic resonance imaging and investigation of sources of error. *JACC Cardiovasc Imaging* 2008; 1(4): 413–23.

7. Senior R, Becher H, Monaghan M, et al. Contrast echocardiography: evidence-based recommendations by European Association of Echocardiography. *Eur J Echocardiogr* 2009; 10(2): 194–212.

8. Hare JL, Jenkins C, Nakatani S, Ogawa A, Yu CM, Marwick TH. Feasibility and clinical decision-making with 3D echocardiography in routine practice. *Heart* 2008; 94(4): 440–5.

9. Chan J, Jenkins C, Khafagi F, Du L, Marwick TH. What is the optimal clinical technique for measurement of left ventricular volume after myocardial infarction? A comparative study of 3-dimensional echocardiography, single photon emission computed tomography, and cardiac magnetic resonance imaging. *J Am Soc Echocardiogr* 2006; 19(2): 192–201.

10. Klocke FJ, Baird MG, Lorell BH, et al. ACC/AHA/ASNC guidelines for the clinical use of cardiac radionuclide imaging—executive summary: a report of the American College of Cardiology/American Heart Association Task Force on Practice Guidelines (ACC/AHA/ASNC Committee to Revise the 1995 Guidelines for the Clinical Use of Cardiac Radionuclide Imaging). *J Am Coll Cardiol* 2003; 42(7): 1318–33.

11. Neglia D, Michelassi C, Trivieri MG, et al. Prognostic role of myocardial blood flow impairment in idiopathic left ventricular dysfunction. *Circulation* 2002; 105(2): 186–93.

12. van den Heuvel AF, van Veldhuisen DJ, van der Wall EE, et al. Regional myocardial blood flow reserve impairment and metabolic changes suggesting myocardial ischaemia in patients with idiopathic dilated cardiomyopathy. *J Am Coll Cardiol* 2000; 35(1): 19–28.

13. Davila-Roman VG, Vedala G, Herrero P, et al. Altered myocardial fatty acid and glucose metabolism in idiopathic dilated cardiomyopathy. *J Am Coll Cardiol* 2002; 40(2): 271–7.

14. Tuunanen H, Engblom E, Naum A, et al. Trimetazidine, a metabolic modulator, has cardiac and extracardiac benefits in idiopathic dilated cardiomyopathy. *Circulation* 2008; 118(12): 1250–8.

15. Bengel FM, Permanetter B, Ungerer M, Nekolla SG, Schwaiger M. Alterations of the sympathetic nervous system and metabolic performance of the cardiomyopathic heart. *Eur J Nucl Med Mol Imaging* 2002; 29(2): 198–202.

16. Boogers MJ, Borleffs CJ, Henneman MM, et al. Cardiac sympathetic denervation assessed with 123-iodine metaiodobenzylguanidine imaging predicts ventricular arrhythmias in implantable cardioverter-defibrillator patients. *J Am Coll Cardiol* 2010; 55(24): 2769–77.

17. Hesse B, Lindhardt TB, Acampa W, et al. EANM/ESC guidelines for radionuclide imaging of cardiac function. *Eur J Nucl Med Mol Imaging* 2008; 35(4): 851–85.

18. Xie BQ, Tian YQ, Zhang J, et al. Evaluation of left and right ventricular ejection fraction and volumes from gated blood-pool SPECT in patients with dilated cardiomyopathy: comparison with cardiac MRI. *J Nucl Med* 2012; 53(4): 584–91.

19. Knaapen P, van Campen LM, de Cock CC, et al. Effects of cardiac resynchronization therapy on myocardial perfusion reserve. *Circulation* 2004; 110(6): 646–51.

20. Lindner O, Sorensen J, Vogt J, et al. Cardiac efficiency and oxygen consumption measured with 11C-acetate PET after long-term cardiac resynchronization therapy. *J Nucl Med* 2006; 47(3): 378–83.

21. Naya M, Tsukamoto T, Morita K, et al. Myocardial beta-adrenergic receptor density assessed by 11C-CGP12177 PET predicts improvement of cardiac function after carvedilol treatment in patients with idiopathic dilated cardiomyopathy. *J Nucl Med* 2009; 50(2): 220–5.

22. Dilsizian V, Taillefer R. Journey in evolution of nuclear cardiology: will there be another quantum leap with the F-18-labeled myocardial perfusion tracers? *JACC Cardiovasc Imaging* 2012; 5(12): 1269–84.

23. Gulati A, Jabbour A, Ismail TF, et al. Association of fibrosis with mortality and sudden cardiac death in patients with nonischaemic dilated cardiomyopathy. *JAMA* 2013; 309(9): 896–908.

24. Wu KC, Weiss RG, Thiemann DR, et al. Late gadolinium enhancement by cardiovascular magnetic resonance heralds an adverse prognosis in nonischaemic cardiomyopathy. *J Am Coll Cardiol* 2008; 51(25): 2414–21.

25. Nazarian S, Bluemke DA, Lardo AC, et al. Magnetic resonance assessment of the substrate for inducible ventricular tachycardia in nonischaemic cardiomyopathy. *Circulation* 2005; 112(18): 2821–5.

26. Aretz HT, Billingham ME, Edwards WD, et al. Myocarditis. A histopathologic definition and classification. *Am J Cardiovasc Pathol* 1987; 1(1): 3–14.

27. Felker GM, Thompson RE, Hare JM, et al. Underlying causes and long-term survival in patients with initially unexplained cardiomyopathy. *N Engl J Med* 2000; 342(15): 1077–84.

28. Skouri HN, Dec GW, Friedrich MG, Cooper LT. Noninvasive imaging in myocarditis. *J Am Coll Cardiol* 2006; 48(10): 2085–93.

29. Abdel-Aty H, Boye P, Zagrosek A, et al. Diagnostic performance of cardiovascular magnetic resonance in patients with suspected acute myocarditis: comparison of different approaches. *J Am Coll Cardiol* 2005; 45(11): 1815–22.

30. Mahrholdt H, Goedecke C, Wagner A, et al. Cardiovascular magnetic resonance assessment of human myocarditis: a comparison to histology and molecular pathology. *Circulation* 2004; 109(10): 1250–8.

31. Friedrich MG, Sechtem U, Schulz-Menger J, et al. Cardiovascular magnetic resonance in myocarditis: A JACC White Paper. *J Am Coll Cardiol* 2009 Apr 28; 53(17): 1475–87.

32. Grun S, Schumm J, Greulich S, et al. Long-term follow-up of biopsy-proven viral myocarditis: predictors of mortality and incomplete recovery. *J Am Coll Cardiol* 2012; 59(18): 1604–15.

33. Smedema JP, Snoep G, van Kroonenburgh MP, et al. Evaluation of the accuracy of gadolinium-enhanced cardiovascular magnetic resonance in the diagnosis of cardiac sarcoidosis. *J Am Coll Cardiol* 2005; 45(10): 1683–90.

34. Valantine H, McKenna WJ, Nihoyannopoulos P, et al. Sarcoidosis: a pattern of clinical and morphological presentation. *Br Heart J* 1987; 57(3): 256–63.

35. Hyodo E, Hozumi T, Takemoto Y, et al. Early detection of cardiac involvement in patients with sarcoidosis by a non-invasive method with ultrasonic tissue characterisation. *Heart* 2004; 90(11): 1275–80.

36. Tahara N, Tahara A, Nitta Y, et al. Heterogeneous myocardial FDG uptake and the disease activity in cardiac sarcoidosis. *JACC Cardiovasc Imaging* 2010; 3(12): 1219–28.

37. Miranda CH, Figueiredo AB, Maciel BC, Marin-Neto JA, Simoes MV. Sustained ventricular tachycardia is associated with regional myocardial sympathetic denervation assessed with 123I-metaiodobenzylguanidine in chronic Chagas cardiomyopathy. *J Nucl Med* 2011; 52(4): 504–10.

38. Rochitte CE, Oliveira PF, Andrade JM, et al. Myocardial delayed enhancement by magnetic resonance imaging in patients with Chagas' disease: a marker of disease severity. *J Am Coll Cardiol* 2005; 46(8): 1553–8.

39. Marmursztejn J, Guillevin L, Trebossen R, et al. Churg–Strauss syndrome cardiac involvement evaluated by cardiac magnetic resonance imaging and positron-emission tomography: a prospective study on 20 patients. *Rheumatology (Oxford)* 2013; 52(4): 642–50.

40. Mavrogeni S, Bratis K, Karanasios E, et al. CMR evaluation of cardiac involvement during the convalescence of Kawasaki disease. *JACC Cardiovasc Imaging* 2011; 4(10): 1140–1.

41. Giatrakos N, Kinali M, Stephens D, Dawson D, Muntoni F, Nihoyannopoulos P. Cardiac tissue velocities and strain rate in the early detection of myocardial dysfunction of asymptomatic boys with Duchenne's muscular dystrophy: relationship to clinical outcome. *Heart* 2006; 92(6): 840–2.

42. Dutka DP, Donnelly JE, Palka P, Lange A, Nunez DJ, Nihoyannopoulos P. Echocardiographic characterization of cardiomyopathy in Friedreich's ataxia with tissue Doppler echocardiographically derived myocardial velocity gradients. *Circulation* 2000; 102(11): 1276–82.

43. Ashford MW, Jr, Liu W, Lin SJ, et al. Occult cardiac contractile dysfunction in dystrophin-deficient children revealed by cardiac magnetic resonance strain imaging. *Circulation* 2005; 112(16): 2462–7.

44. Puchalski MD, Williams RV, Askovich B, et al. Late gadolinium enhancement: precursor to cardiomyopathy in Duchenne muscular dystrophy? *Int J Cardiovasc Imaging* 2009; 25(1): 57–63.

45. Yilmaz A, Gdynia HJ, Baccouche H, et al. Cardiac involvement in patients with Becker muscular dystrophy: new diagnostic and pathophysiological insights by a CMR approach. *J Cardiovasc Magn Reson* 2008; 10: 50.

46. van Dalen EC, van der Pal HJ, Kok WE, Caron HN, Kremer LC. Clinical heart failure in a cohort of children treated with anthracyclines: a long-term follow-up study. *Eur J Cancer* 2006; 42(18): 3191–8.

47. Kremer LC, van Dalen EC, Offringa M, Voute PA. Frequency and risk factors of anthracycline-induced clinical heart failure in children: a systematic review. *Ann Oncol* 2002; 13(4): 503–12.

48. Ylanen K, Poutanen T, Savikurki-Heikkila P, Rinta-Kiikka I, Eerola A, Vettenranta K. Cardiac magnetic resonance imaging in the evaluation of the late effects of anthracyclines among long-term survivors of childhood cancer. *J Am Coll Cardiol* 2013; 61(14): 1539–47.

49. Mewton N, Liu CY, Croisille P, Bluemke D, Lima JA. Assessment of myocardial fibrosis with cardiovascular magnetic resonance. *J Am Coll Cardiol* 2011; 57(8): 891–903.

50. Neilan TG, Coelho-Filho OR, Shah RV, et al. Myocardial extracellular volume by cardiac magnetic resonance imaging in patients treated with anthracycline-based chemotherapy. *Am J Cardiol* 2013; 111(5): 717–22.

51. Sliwa K, Blauwet L, Tibazarwa K, et al. Evaluation of bromocriptine in the treatment of acute severe peripartum cardiomyopathy: a proof-of-concept pilot study. *Circulation* 2010; 121(13): 1465–73.

52. Elkayam U. Clinical characteristics of peripartum cardiomyopathy in the United States: diagnosis, prognosis, and management. *J Am Coll Cardiol* 2011; 58(7): 659–70.

53. Barone-Rochette G, Rodiere M, Lantuejoul S. Value of cardiac MRI in peripartum cardiomyopathy. *Arch Cardiovasc Dis* 2011; 104(4): 263–4.

54. Mouquet F, Lions C, de Groote P, Bouabdallaoui N, et al. Characterisation of peripartum cardiomyopathy by cardiac magnetic resonance imaging. *Eur Radiol* 2008; 18(12): 2765–9.

55. Thavendiranathan P, Dahiya A, Phelan D, Desai MY, Tang WH. Isolated left ventricular non-compaction controversies in diagnostic criteria, adverse outcomes and management. *Heart* 2013; 99(10): 681–9.

56. Petersen SE, Selvanayagam JB, Wiesmann F, et al. Left ventricular non-compaction: insights from cardiovascular magnetic resonance imaging. *J Am Coll Cardiol* 2005; 46(1): 101–5.

57. Germans T, Wilde AA, Dijkmans PA, et al. Structural abnormalities of the inferoseptal left ventricular wall detected by cardiac magnetic resonance imaging in carriers of hypertrophic cardiomyopathy mutations. *J Am Coll Cardiol* 2006; 48(12): 2518–23.

58. Tsuchihashi K, Ueshima K, Uchida T, et al. Transient left ventricular apical ballooning without coronary artery stenosis: a novel heart syndrome mimicking acute myocardial infarction. Angina Pectoris-Myocardial Infarction Investigations in Japan. *J Am Coll Cardiol* 2001; 38(1): 11–8.

59. Bybee KA, Kara T, Prasad A, et al. Systematic review: transient left ventricular apical ballooning: a syndrome that mimics ST-segment elevation myocardial infarction. *Ann Intern Med* 2004; 141(11): 858–65.

60. Burgdorf C, von HK, Schunkert H, Kurowski V. Regional alterations in myocardial sympathetic innervation in patients with transient left-ventricular apical ballooning (Tako-Tsubo cardiomyopathy). *J Nucl Cardiol* 2008; 15(1): 65–72.

61. Cimarelli S, Sauer F, Morel O, Ohlmann P, Constantinesco A, Imperiale A. Transient left ventricular dysfunction syndrome: pathophysiological bases through nuclear medicine imaging. *Int J Cardiol* 2010; 144(2): 212–8.

62. Eitel I, Behrendt F, Schindler K, et al. Differential diagnosis of suspected apical ballooning syndrome using contrast-enhanced magnetic resonance imaging. *Eur Heart J* 2008; 29(21): 2651–9.

⊃ For additional multimedia materials please visit the online version of the book (http://www.esciacc.oxfordmedicine.com)

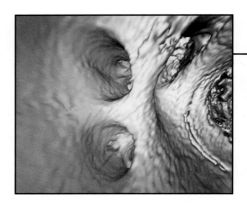

CHAPTER 36

Other genetic and acquired cardiomyopathies

Petros Nihoyannopoulos, Perry Elliott, and Gaby Captur

Contents

Arrhythmogenic right ventricular cardiomyopathy/dysplasia (ARVC/D)

Introduction and definitions

The right ventricle may be the seat of ventricular tachycardia of left bundle branch block pattern [1]. Recent interest has centred on its pathophysiology because early reports suggested that an apparent absence of gross organic heart disease indicated a more favourable prognosis [2]. The term 'arrhythmogenic right ventricular cardiomyopathy' was first proposed in 1977 by Fontaine et al. [3] when he reported right ventricular tachycardia associated with right-sided structural disorders.

Although ARVC/D is a cardiomyopathy affecting primarily the right ventricle (RV) [4], the left ventricle (LV) is also affected in many patients. It is a heterogeneous group of conditions characterized by right ventricular dysfunction and dilatation from very subtle abnormalities located at the RV to a most extensive RV and LV dysfunction.

Men are more frequently affected than women and it is usually discovered between the second and fourth decade of life. The most common presentation is arrhythmia, specifically ventricular tachycardia originating from the RV with the characteristic LBBB morphology. ARVC/D is also an important cause of sudden death in individuals <30 years of age and has been found in up to 20% of sudden deaths in young people [4].

In most patients ARVC/D is a genetic trait disease with variable penetrance and incomplete expression. The first gene mutations were identified in a recessive, syndromic variant of ARVC known as Naxos disease caused by a two-base pair deletion in the gene encoding plakoglobin [5, 6], a component of cell-to-cell junctions. This discovery led to the identification of disease-causing mutations in other genes encoding desmosomal proteins in the more common autosomal dominant forms of ARVC [7]. Latterly, very similar clinical phenotypes have been identified in patients with mutations in non-desmosomal genes, including titin [8], desmin [9], and lamin [10].

ARVC is characterized by replacement of myocardial tissue in the right ventricular wall by adipose tissue and fibrosis that starts on the right ventricular sub-epicardium and progresses to the endocardium with replacement of myocytes and thinning of the wall (⊃ Fig. 36.1).

The regions of the RV most frequently involved are the RV inflow area, the apex, and the infundibulum. These three areas form the 'triangle of dysplasia' (⊃ Fig. 36.2). When the LV is also involved, the fibro-fatty replacement can affect both the septum and left ventricular free wall.

Criteria for diagnosis of ARVC/D

A definite diagnosis of ARVC/D requires the histological finding of transmural fibro-fatty replacement of RV myocardium. However, in the living patient histological diagnosis is

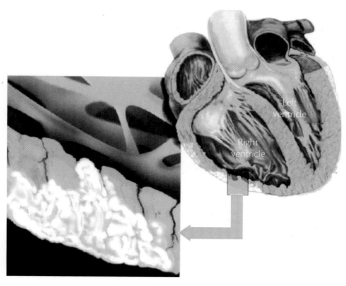

Fig. 36.1 Diagrammatic representation of the histology in arrhythmogenic right ventricular cardiomyopathy.

difficult as small amounts of adipose tissue are also present in the epicardial layer, as well as within the RV myocardium in normal subjects and increases with the advancing age.

The non-specific nature of most clinical findings and the absence of a single diagnostic test make the diagnosis of ARVC extremely challenging. In 1994 an International Task Force guideline proposed standardized diagnostic criteria based upon the identification of structural, morphological, ECG, and arrhythmic features and the evaluation of families [11]. Specific features were classified as major and minor according to their perceived specificity but many were subjective and not supported by good evidence. For this reason, the criteria were updated in 2010 (see ➲ Table 36.1) using the same basic scheme, but adding three new diagnostic criteria [12]:

◆ **Definite:** two major, or one major and two minor or four minor criteria from different diagnostic categories.

◆ **Borderline diagnosis:** one major and one minor or three minor criteria from different diagnostic categories.

◆ **Possible diagnosis:** one major or two minor criteria from different diagnostic categories.

Global or regional right ventricular dysfunction

The right ventricle is difficult to image using echocardiography because of its proximity to the anterior chest wall and its complex shape and orientation. Cardiovascular magnetic resonance overcomes some of these difficulties by providing three-dimensional visualization of the heart and other thoracic structures. It also provides a method for detecting fat and fibrosis using tissue characterization, but as the RV wall is very thin, partial volume effects can affect the image and differentiation between pericardial fat, and fatty infiltration of the RV can be difficult.

While the 1994 criteria relied on mostly qualitative assessment of the RV size and function, the new criteria provide precise cut-offs for RV dimensions and exclude regional wall motion abnormalities because of their low specificity.

A major change is the recognition of LV involvement, which is frequent with disease progression and a poor prognostic marker. When LV involvement predominates, terminology becomes very confusing and the differentiation from dilated cardiomyopathy somewhat arbitrary. On the other hand, the presence of late gadolinium enhancement and, less commonly, myocardial fat in the left ventricle in the absence of overt left ventricular dysfunction, may help to identify affected individuals.

Echocardiography

Echocardiography in expert hands can identify subtle RV abnormalities in the form of RV free wall thinning (➲ Fig. 36.3) or RV apical aneurysms (➲ Fig. 36.4) by careful and systematic evaluation of the RV [13–15]. Echocardiography is probably the diagnostic test of choice but this needs to be performed comprehensively by experts following standardized protocols for the detailed imaging of the right ventricle [16]. As ARVC/D affects primarily the RV, it is important to perform all right ventricular views, which include the RV inflow and outflow views. The typical presentation will be that of a young patient with ventricular arrhythmias of right ventricular origin. This patient will be first referred for an echocardiographic examination, which will have to be conducted in an expert department to look for subtle RV abnormalities. The earliest abnormalities that can be detected may be focal areas of myocardial dysfunction, which may involve the RV inflow, apex, and/or the RV outflow tract. Those three locations constitute the 'triangle of dysplasia'. These

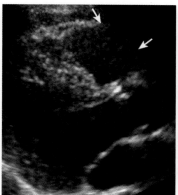

RV Outflow

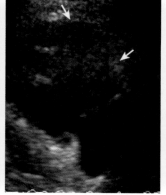

RV inflow

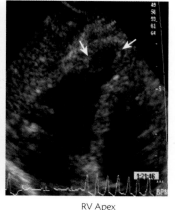

RV Apex

Fig. 36.2 Echocardiographic views from a patient with ARVC/D illustrating the 'triangle of dysplasia'. On the left panel, the outflow track seen from parasternal long-axis view (arrows) and demonstrate a subtle thinning of the free wall. In the middle panel, the RV inflow track view shows the localized akinetic region in the free wall (arrows). On the right panel, apical 4-chamber projection demonstrating an apical aneurysm on the RV (arrows).

Table 36.1 2010 Task Force criteria for the diagnosis of ARVC

I Global and/or regional dysfunction and structural alterations
MAJOR
By 2D echo: Regional RV akinesia, dyskinesia, or aneurysm and one of the following (end-diastole):
—PLAX RVOT ≥ 32 mm (corrected for body size [PLAX/BSA] ≥19 mm/m²)
—PSAX RVOT ≥36 mm (corrected for body size [PSAX/BSA] ≥21 mm/m²)
—or fractional area change ≤33%
By MRI: Regional RV akinesia or dyskinesia or dyssynchronous RV contraction and one of the following:
—Ratio of RV end-diastolic volume to BSA ≥110 ml/m² (male) or ≥100 ml/m² (female)
—or RV ejection fraction ≤40%
By RV angiography: Regional RV akinesia, dyskinesia, or aneurysm
MINOR
By 2D echo: Regional RV akinesia or dyskinesia and 1 of the following (end-diastole):
—PLAX RVOT ≥29 to <32 mm (corrected for body size [PLAX/BSA] ≥16 to <19 mm/m²)
—PSAX RVOT ≥32 to <36 mm (corrected for body size [PSAX/BSA] ≥18 to <21 mm/m²)
—or fractional area change > 33% to ≤40%
By MRI: Regional RV akinesia or dyskinesia or dyssynchronous RV contraction and one of the following:
—Ratio of RV end-diastolic volume to BSA ≥100 to <110 ml/m² (male) or ≥90 to <100 ml/m² (female)
—or RV ejection fraction > 40% to ≤45%
II Tissue characterization of walls
MAJOR
Residual myocytes <60% by morphometric analysis (or <50% if estimated), with fibrous replacement of the RV free wall myocardium in ≥1 sample, with or without fatty replacement of tissue on endomyocardial biopsy
MINOR
Residual myocytes 60% to 75% by morphometric analysis (or 50% to 65% if estimated), with fibrous replacement of the RV free wall myocardium in ≥1 sample, with or without fatty replacement of tissue on endomyocardial biopsy
III Repolarization abnormalities
MAJOR
Inverted T-waves in right precordial leads (V1, V2, and V3) or beyond in individuals >14 years of age (in the absence of complete right bundle-branch block QRS ≥120 ms)
MINOR
Inverted T-waves in leads V1 and V2 in individuals >14 years of age (in the absence of complete right bundle-branch block) or in V4, V5, or V6
Inverted T-waves in leads V1, V2, V3, and V4 in individuals >14 years of age in the presence of complete right bundle-branch block
IV Depolarization/conduction abnormalities
MAJOR
Epsilon wave (reproducible low-amplitude signals between end of QRS complex to onset of the T wave) in the right precordial leads (V1 to V3)
MINOR
Late potentials by SAECG in ≥1 of 3 parameters in the absence of a QRS duration of ≥110 ms on the standard ECG: filtered QRS duration (fQRS) ≥114 ms; duration of terminal QRS <40 µV (low-amplitude signal duration) ≥38 ms; root-mean-square voltage of terminal 40 ms ≤20 µV
Terminal activation duration of QRS ≥55 ms measured from the nadir of the S wave to the end of the QRS, including R′, in V1, V2, or V3, in the absence of complete right bundle-branch block
V Arrhythmias
MAJOR
Non-sustained or sustained ventricular tachycardia of left bundle-branch morphology with superior axis (negative or indeterminate QRS in leads II, III, and aVF and positive in lead aVL)
MINOR
Non-sustained or sustained ventricular tachycardia of RV outflow configuration, left bundle-branch block morphology with inferior axis (positive QRS in leads II, III, and aVF and negative in lead aVL) or of unknown axis
> 500 ventricular extrasystoles per 24 hours (Holter)

VI Family history

MAJOR

ARVC/D confirmed in a first-degree relative who meets current Task Force criteria
ARVC/D confirmed pathologically at autopsy or surgery in a first-degree relative
Identification of a pathogenic mutation categorized as associated or probably associated with ARVC/D in the patient under evaluation

MINOR

History of ARVC/D in a first-degree relative in whom it is not possible or practical to determine whether the family member meets current Task Force criteria
RVC/D confirmed pathologically or by current Task Force criteria in second-degree relative

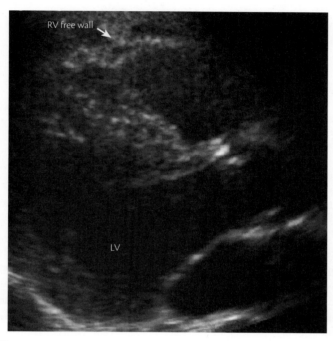

Fig. 36.3 Parasternal long-axis projection from a patient with ventricular tachycardia demonstrating a non-dilated RV outflow but a localized RV free wall thinning (arrow) and absent contraction, suggestive of ARVC/D.

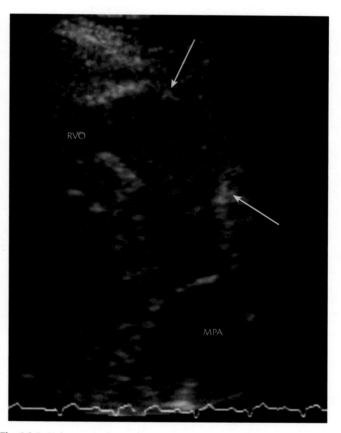

Fig. 36.5 Right ventricular outflow track view demonstrating a clear aneurysm below the pulmonary valve (arrows) taking the form of a 'mushroom'.

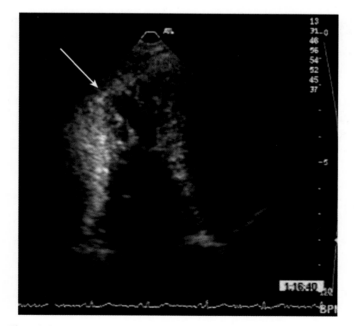

Fig. 36.4 Same patient as in Fig. 36.3. Apical 4-chamber demonstrating the discrete aneurysm at the apex (arrow).

areas, however, may easily be missed if particular attention has not been made. The more obvious and pathognomonic abnormalities are those of localized aneurysmal regions of the triangle of dysplasia in the form of systolic bulges (➲ Fig. 36.5). As long as the RV inflow and outflow tract projections are carefully recorded, missing those regional dyskinetic regions will be difficult. In a more advanced stage of ARVC/D, extended areas of RV free wall may become thin and akinetic, which, together with RV dilatation, will form the 'typical' pattern of ARVC/D (➲ Figs 36.6 and 36.7). Ultimately, the whole of the RV will be thinned, dilated, and hypokinetic. The diagnosis here is difficult to miss and is straightforward with any imaging modality. Lastly, in the most severe and advanced cases, the LV will also become involved and could mimic that of non-specific dilated cardiomyopathy. Global RV dysfunction is most common in patients with cardiac arrest, although this is not necessarily true in patients with first presentation. ➲ Figures 36.5 and 36.6 are from

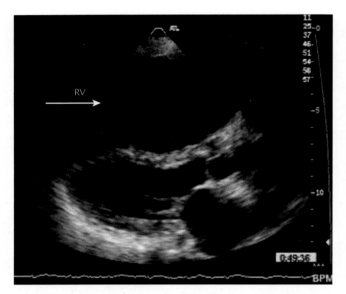

Fig. 36.6 Parasternal long-axis view from a patient with advanced ARVC/D demonstrating a dilated RV (arrow) with marked global hypokinesia. Notice that the LV size is normal.

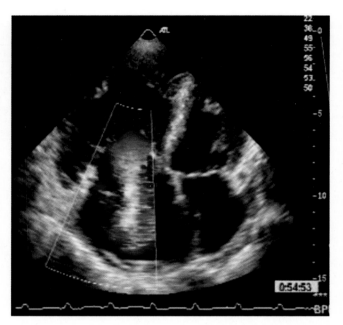

Fig. 36.8 Apical 4-chamber projection with colour Doppler demonstrating the presence of almost free tricuspid regurgitation secondary to the marked dilatation of the tricuspid annulus. Notice the low velocity flow as seen by the deep blue colour of the velocity jet.

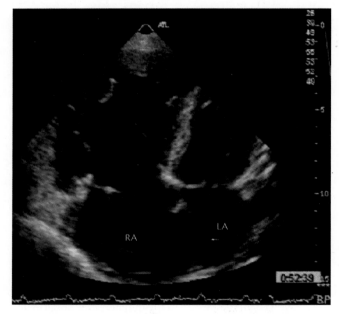

Fig. 36.7 Apical 4-chamber view from the same patient as in Fig. 36.6 demonstrating the markedly dilated RV. This patient can be compared with patient in Fig. 36.4 where the aneurysm was very discrete.

a 55-year-old lady with ARVC/D. The marked dilatation of the RV will lead to functional tricuspid regurgitation (⊃ Fig. 36.8). The differential diagnosis here with pulmonary hypertension is straightforward by directing the continuous wave Doppler beam along the tricuspid regurgitant jet in order to estimate the RV systolic pressures. 🎥 Video 36.1 shows a discrete RV apical aneurysm while the patient developed her usual arrhythmia (movie).

Cardiac magnetic resonance

In recent years, MRI scanners and imaging protocols have rapidly been developed [9]. At present, imaging is generally performed

on 1.5 Tesla systems, using dedicated cardiac phased-array coils with multiple elements and ECG triggering, although 3T scanners offering better spatial resolution rapidly develop. CMR evaluation of ARVC/D was initially focused on the detection of fat tissue infiltration at the level of RV free wall. First reports in the early nineties [17, 18] included T1-weighted spin echo images showing bright signal intensity corresponding to RV free wall fatty infiltration. After a period of initial enthusiasm that almost gave CMR the same value as histology for the detection of fat replacement, both in formalin-fixed hearts and *in vivo* [19, 20], the role of CMR in the detection of fat was redefined. Since fat infiltration has been described in normal hearts and given that CMR tissue characterization (fat infiltration) is often difficult, the clinical and diagnostic utility at present is limited [21, 22] (⊃ Table 36.2).

CMR abnormalities described in patients with ARVC/D (⊃ Table 36.3) can be divided into two groups: functional anomalies and morphological changes, both of them most commonly found in the 'triangle of dysplasia'.

Table 36.2 CMR advantages for the evaluation of ARVC/D

Non-invasive
Absence of ionizing radiation
Non-iodinated contrast agents
High spatial and temporal resolution
Multiple planes
High contrast between blood pool and myocardium
No acoustic window problems
High reproducibility on RV volume and function parameters
Tissue characterization

ARVC/D, arrhythmogenic right ventricular dysplasia.

Table 36.3 CMR findings on ARVC/D

	Task Force criteria		
	Major	**Minor**	**None**
Functional abnormalities			
Severe RV dilatation	+		
RV severe systolic dysfunction without LV involvement	+		
Localized RV aneurysm (akinetic, dyskinetic areas with diastolic bulging)	+		
Severe segmental dilatation of RV	+		
Mild global RV dilatation		+	
Mild RV ejection fraction reduction		+	
Mild segmental dilatation RV		+	
Regional RV hypokinesia		+	
Morphological abnormalities			
RV free wall thinning			+
RV moderator band or trabeculae hypertrophy			+
RVOT enlargement			+
RV fat infiltration			+
Delayed enhancement (intra-myocardial fibrosis)			+

CMR, cardiac magnetic resonance; ARV/CD, arrythmogenic right ventricular dysplasia; RV, right ventricle; LV, left ventricle; RVOT, right ventricular outflow tract.

Functional evaluation

As with echocardiography, among functional abnormalities described by CMR in ARVC/D, dilatation and RV systolic dysfunction are most commonly found in patients who meet Task Force criteria. Other abnormalities include regional wall motion abnormalities (hypokinesia or akinesia) and focal aneurysm with persistent diastolic bulging (⊃ Table 36.1). CMR allows the evaluation of RV volumes and global and regional function. ECG-gated breath-hold gradient echo sequences (steady-state free-precession) achieve an excellent contrast between blood and myocardium with good delineation of RV endocardial borders. Image planes include classical long-axis cardiac views, as well as RV outflow tract (RVOT), short-axis and axial images from the level of the RVOT to the diaphragm (📹 Video 36.2). RV volume and systolic function are calculated from serial short-axis cine loops tracing end-diastolic and end-systolic areas. Suppression of premature ventricular beats with antiarrhythmic therapy is recommended to avoid blurring and age, height, and weight should be recorded in all cases. RV volumes and ejection fraction (EF) should be matched according to age, sex, and body surface area. Ventricular dilatation is defined when end-diastolic volume (EDV) is 117% above predicted [23]. Wall motion abnormalities are subjectively assessed in order to detect localized aneurysm defined as akinetic or dyskinetic regions of the RV wall showing diastolic bulging (📹 Videos 36.3 and 36.4). Since normal variations of RV regional function are frequently seen on healthy subjects (📹 Video 36.5), especially on axial planes and near moderator band insertion [24], the significance of their presence should be interpreted with caution. For this reason, performance and interpretation of ARVC/D suspected CMR should be limited to high-volume centres, with experts in CMR who are familiar with the disease, in order to avoid false-positive ARVC/D diagnosis.

Morphological evaluation

Morphological abnormalities include focal wall thinning (⊃ Fig. 36.9), moderator band or trabeculae hypertrophy, RVOT enlargement, and intra-myocardial fibro-fatty infiltration. Although a first approach to wall thickness and RVOT diameter can be done using previously described ECG-gated fast gradient echo sequences, a better spatial resolution is achieved by the use of black blood spin echo sequence. Current black blood sequences use a breath-hold fast spin echo with a dual magnetization preparation pulse (double inversion-recovery), which provides end-diastolic T1-weighted images for detailed morphological analysis (⊃ Fig. 36.10). Fat infiltration is also evaluated with this sequence;

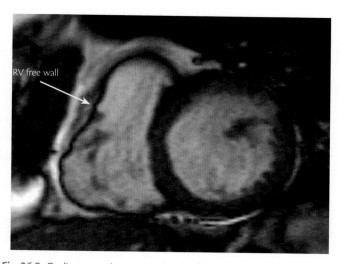

Fig. 36.9 Cardiac magnetic resonance imaging from a patient with ARVC/D. Note the clarity of the thinned RV free wall (arrow) and the dilation of the RV cavity.

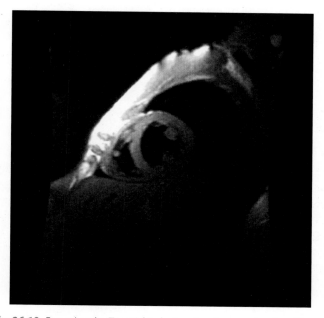

Fig. 36.10 Fast spin echo T1-weighted spin echo of a normal patient. Note anatomical detail of right ventricular wall.

since signal intensity of fat on T1-weighted images is high (bright), much higher than normal myocardium, the presence of a bright focal or diffuse area within the right or left ventricular myocardium is suggestive of fat infiltration. However, high signal intensity on T1-weighted images is not specific of fat; proximity to surface coil, motion-related artefacts, and other technical issues may cause projection of high signal intensity onto the myocardium causing the false diagnosis of fatty infiltration. Along with T1-weighted images, a fat suppressed sequence should always be performed. The presence of a bright signal spot within the myocardium on T1-weighted images that darkens or disappears on fat-suppressed images is diagnostic of fatty infiltration (➲ Fig. 36.11). High spatial resolution on spin echo images is mandatory [25]. Even though fat detection with CMR is not a Task Force criterion for the diagnosis of ARVC/D, most CMR protocols include T1-weighted and T2-weighted STIR (fat suppression) images on axial and short-axis planes. Importantly, planning of both sequences should be the same, so the very same

image can be seen without and with fat suppression. This approach has proved to increase inter-observer agreement and confidence in diagnosis and evaluation of intra-myocardial fatty infiltration in patients suspected of having ARVC/D [26]. Fat RV infiltration detected with cine CMR has also been described in patients without any other ARVC/D abnormalities [27] and its presence should be evaluated with caution (➲ Fig. 36.12).

Delayed enhancement

In recent years, delayed enhancement imaging in the CMR evaluation of patients with ARVC/D for detecting fibrosis has gained acceptance. Studies have shown that delayed-enhancement can be detected in biopsy-proven ARVC/D patients in areas with wall thinning and regional dysfunction [28, 29]. Fibro-fatty infiltration is more common in ARVC/D patients than fatty infiltration alone. Detection of fibrotic tissue using delayed enhancement may be more important than the detection of fat replacement alone

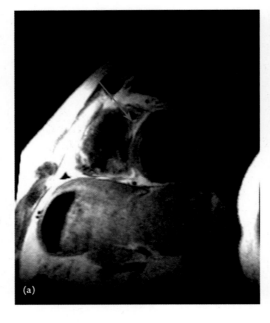
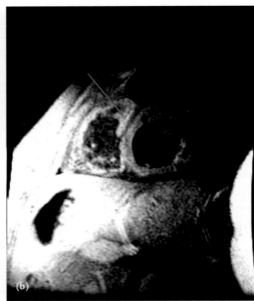

Fig. 36.11 (a) Fat spin echo T1-weighted image showing high signal intensity suggestive of fat infiltration in the septum (arrow). (b) Same image as (a) with fat suppression. Septal high signal intensity has disappeared, confirming the diagnosis of fat infiltration in this patient diagnosed with arrhythmogenic right ventricular dysplasia.

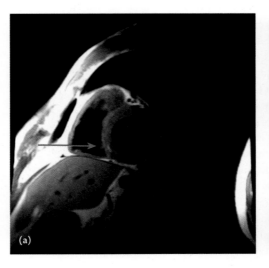
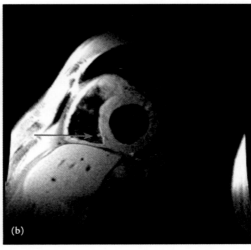

Fig. 36.12 (a) T1-weighted image of a patient with unexplained syncope. Linear high signal intensity is noted in the inferior septum (arrow) that disappears on fat suppressed images (b) corresponding to fat infiltration. No other abnormalities were noted.

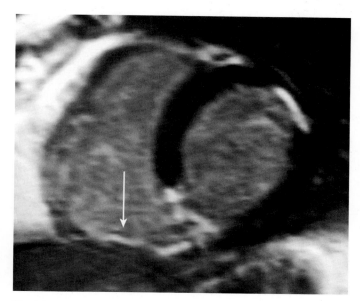

Fig. 36.13 Delayed gadolinium enhancement from a patient with ARVC/D. Short-axis projection demonstrating the scar in the inferior-basal portion of the RV but also extending into the LV. Image obtained with permission from [9].

(⊃ Figs 36.13 and 36.14). However, prognostic implications and its clinical utility for diagnosis and prognostic purposes are not defined yet. At present, inclusion on CMR protocols (⊃ Table 36.4), which are already long and technically demanding, is a question of debate. Further studies are needed in order to address these issues and to establish the feasibility of delayed enhancement detection within the thin RV wall.

CMR limitations

Despite the excellent image quality and reproducibility, CMR has some disadvantages: the data acquisition and analysis requires expertise and is rather time-consuming, without clear validated and standardized protocols. Some patient groups, such as claustrophobic or patients with pacemakers, cannot undergo CMR.

The lack of widespread availability of CMR scanners, however, may constitute the most significant limitation of this technique. In ARVC/D, localized RV aneurysms may be detected with CMR but they can also be missed when the plane of section is outside a localized aneurysm.

Other imaging techniques

Recently, multi-detector computed tomography (MDCT) was used in the evaluation of patients suspected of having ARVC/D. Also, patients with a pacemaker and cardioverter-defibrillators can be studied using CT, which at present cannot be imaged with CMR. Increased RV trabeculation and RV intra-myocardial fat and scalloping were associated with ARVC/D RV volumes. Also RV inlet dimensions and RV outflow tract surface areas are increased in patients with ARVC/D. Further studies are warranted to ensure the accuracy of CT in the detection of ARVC/D [30]. Also multi-detector CT can be used to detect fibro-fatty infiltrations. However, with increasing experience, it became apparent that the differentiation of myocardial fibro-fatty infiltration from the fatty tissue normally present in the pericardium is inaccurate, unless of course the infiltration is extensive. Furthermore, myocardial fat can be present not only in ARVC/D, but is often related to aging, prior myocardial infarction, and chronic ischaemia [31]. The separation between myocardial infiltration versus normal pericardial fat is almost impossible in the presence of thinned RV free wall.

The recent development of radionuclide blood-pool SPECT imaging allows also regional assessment of the left and right ventricular function. In one prospective study it was found that detecting localized dysfunction by gated SPECT was accurate in the detection of ARVC (sensitivity 100%, specificity 81%) [32] but obviously more studies are needed to assess the value of this technique in this setting.

An interesting alternative for detecting right ventricular involvement in ARVC/D is using imaging of cardiac neural innervation. In two earlier studies this method was found to be a very sensitive marker of ARVC/D [33, 34] but no large prospective trials have been published.

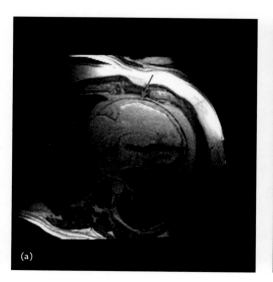

(a)

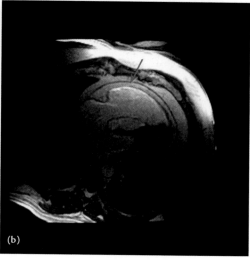

(b)

Fig. 36.14 Double inversion-recovery sequence after gadolinium injection showing diffuse right ventricular wall enhancement (arrows) indicative of myocardial fibrosis (a, b).

Table 36.4 Basic CMR study protocol for ARVC/D

1. Localizers (real time, 3 plane ...)			
2. 4-chamber, 2-chamber, LVOT and RVOT	Gradient echo sequence (SSFP)	7 mm/3 mm 8 mm/2 mm	Functional assessment (global and regional)
3. Sequential short-axis slices from base to apex	Gradient echo sequence (SSFP)	7 mm/3 mm 6 mm/4 mm	Ventricular volumes, mass, EF. Global and regional RV function
4. Axial sequential cine images from RVOT to the diaphragm	Gradient echo sequence (SSFP)	7 mm/3 mm 6 mm/4 mm	Regional RV functional evaluation (RVOT)
5. Black blood T1 images, sequential short-axis view	T1-weighted double inversion-recovery fast spin echo	6 mm/4 mm FOV 26–28	Fat infiltration (intra-myocardial high signal intensity)
6. Black blood T1 fat-suppressed images, short-axis	T1-weighted double inversion-recovery fast spin echo with fat suppression	Same planning as T1-weighted images, same parameters	Fat infiltration (suppression of intra-myocardial high signal intensity)
7. Same sequences (5 and 6) on axial plane from RVOT to the diaphragm			
8. Delayed enhancement (optional)	Inversion recovery prepared breath-hold cine gradient-echo images	6–7 mm/4–3 mm 8 mm/2 mm	Intra-myocardial fibrosis (fibro-fatty infiltration)

CMR, cardiac magnetic resonance; ARVC/D, arrythmogenic right ventricular dysplasia; RV, right ventricle; LV, left ventricle; RVOT, right ventricular outflow tract; SSFP, steady-state free-precession; FOV, field of view.

Histological demonstration of fibro-fatty replacement of myocardium

The second major criterion for the diagnosis of ARVC/D is the histological demonstration of fibro-fatty replacement of myocardium on endomyocardial biopsy. The problem, however, with endomyocardial biopsy is that it is difficult to perform in patients with thin walls, risking the danger of perforating the myocardium and biopsy of the pericardium instead leading to misleading diagnosis. Furthermore, in its earlier stages of the disease progression the fibro-fatty replacement has a patchy distribution, thus making myocardial biopsy even less helpful (➲ Figs 36.15 and 36.16).

Repolarization and depolarization/conduction abnormalities

The electrocardiogram is central to the diagnosis of ARVC. One of the key features of ARVC is the presence of T-wave inversion in right precordial leads in absence of complete right bundle branch block (RBBB), which is considered specific enough to be a major abnormality. T-wave inversion in V1–V2 (in individuals beyond 14 years of age and in the absence of complete RBBB) is considered a minor abnormality. LV involvement is reflected in the repolarization criteria, which include the presence of T-wave inversion in lateral leads V4, V5, or V6 (typically seen in cases of LV involvement) as minor criterion. Epsilon waves are small-amplitude

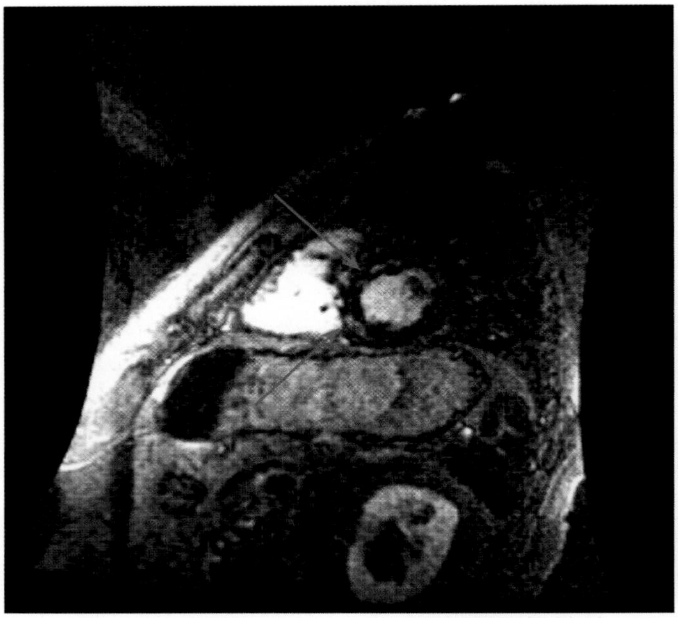

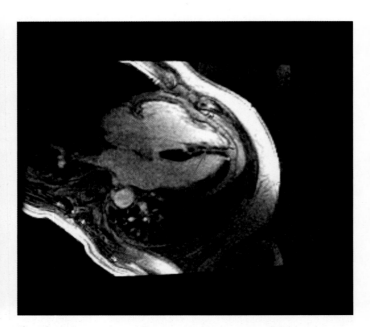

Fig. 36.15 Diffuse intra-myocardial septal delayed enhancement in a patient with arrhythmogenic right ventricular dysfunction, short-axis view (arrows).

Fig. 36.16 Same patient as Fig. 36.10. Septal intra-myocardial delayed enhancement, 4-chamber view.

electrical potentials that occur at the end of the QRS complex and at the beginning of the ST segment detected in the right precordial leads. They are thought to represent areas of delayed activation in the right ventricle as a consequence of fibrous and/or fibro-fatty replacement of RV myocardium and are considered a major criterion. Late potentials detected by signal-averaged ECG are considered a minor criterion in the new diagnostic algorithm.

Ventricular arrhythmias are common in patients with ARVC and are often the initial presentation of the disease. Sustained and non-sustained ventricular tachycardia and ventricular ectopics typically have a left bundle branch block morphology (LBBB) reflecting their RV origin. When LV involvement is present, ventricular arrhythmias with a right bundle branch block morphology may be observed. The right ventricular outflow tract is also the site of origin for idiopathic RV outflow tract ventricular tachycardia, which is usually a benign condition occurring in patients with structurally normal hearts. The new ARVC criteria take this into account by considering VT with left bundle branch block morphology and an inferior axis, as a minor criterion, but VT with LBBB configuration and a superior axis a major criterion. The presence of more than 500 ventricular ectopics in a 24-hour tape is a minor criterion.

Family history

The final and perhaps the most significant major diagnostic criterion is the presence of familial disease confirmed at necropsy or surgery (hard evidence). The new ARVC criteria acknowledge unequivocal disease in a first-degree relative or a history of ARVC confirmed pathologically at autopsy or surgery a major criterion A premature young (<35 years of age) sudden cardiac death due to suspected ARVC is a minor criterion. The new ARVC criteria include the presence of a pathogenic mutation associated, or probably associated, with ARVC in an individual with clinical suspicion of the disease, but it is important to adhere to conventional rules for assignment of pathogenicity to genetic variants as variation in desmosomal genes is relatively common in normal individuals.

Because of the genetic character of ARVC/D, it is important to screen all members of the family once the diagnosis has been made. This can be performed non-invasively by routine ECG and echocardiography.

Conclusions

Arrhythmogenic RV cardiomyopathy has been recognized as an important cause of sudden death in association with exercise and athletic participation. Physicians should consider this condition in young subjects who die suddenly or in people with unexplained cardiac arrhythmias. Diagnosis relies predominantly on imaging using echocardiography and CMR, which are complementary as long as they are performed by experts. Management involves the suppression of malignant arrhythmias with anti-arrhythmic medication but is increasingly directed toward placement of automatic implantable defibrillators as the most effective treatment to prevent sudden cardiac death.

Left ventricular non-compaction
Introduction

The term non-compaction is used to describe the appearance of excessive trabeculations and deep recesses within the left and sometimes right ventricular myocardium that result from abnormal intra-uterine cardiac development and persistence of the foetal myocardial meshwork [35, 36]. Typically, there is an increase in the relative thickness of the trabeculated layer of the ventricular wall compared to the compact layer (Fig. 36.17). In some patients, non-compaction is associated with left ventricular (LV) dilatation and systolic dysfunction.

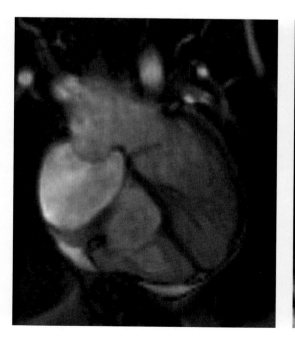
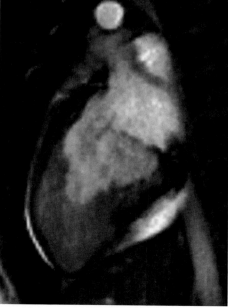

Fig. 36.17 Apical 4-chamber view (left) and parasternal short-axis view (right) from a patient with left ventricular non-compaction. Note the deep trabeculations in the distal part of the ventricle also seen in the short-axis view below the papillary muscle level.

Aetiology

Left ventricular non-compaction occurs in association with numerous congenital heart defects including atrioseptal and ventriculoseptal defects, congenital aortic stenosis and aortic coarctation [37–41]. Isolated LV non-compaction (NC) is a rare disorder with prevalence rates ranging from 0.05 to 0.24% of the general population [42, 43]. Familial disease occurs in 18% to 50% of adults with isolated LVNC, mostly with an autosomal dominant mode of inheritance [44–46]. Numerous mutations in genes encoding cardiac sarcomere proteins have been reported, including ß-myosin heavy chain (MYH7) cardiac troponin T (TNNT2), and alpha-cardiac actin (ACTC1), as well as calcium-handling genes and other cardiomyopathy genes such as lamin A/C, LDB3, and Taffazin. Many of the genetic mutations that cause LVNC also cause hypertrophic, dilated, and restrictive cardiomyopathies [47] and disease expression varies even within families. Prominent trabeculations are also reported in the right ventricle in some patients with arrhythmogenic right ventricular cardiomyopathy [48]. The implication of these findings is that LVNC is often a non-specific manifestation of an underlying familial myocardial disorder.

Some reports have suggested that isolated ventricular non-compaction may appear during adult life in patients with muscular dystrophy [49], or as a transient phenomenon during myocarditis [50] but it may be more appropriate to label such cases as 'hypertrabeculation' rather than non-compaction, accepting that it may be impossible to distinguish the two entities using imaging alone.

Clinical presentation

Presentation with heart failure, arrhythmias, and systemic thromboembolism occurs at all ages and, in general, complications mirror the severity of LV dilatation and systolic dysfunction [47, 51].

Several studies have suggested that patients with LVNC have poor left ventricular function and a high incidence of ventricular arrhythmias and systemic emboli, but recent reports suggest a much lower incidence of death, stroke, or sustained ventricular arrhythmia, probably reflecting the identification of pre-clinical or mild cases [52].

Diagnostic criteria

LVNC is a clinical diagnosis based on the appearance of prominent and excessive trabeculae on echocardiography or cardiac magnetic resonance imaging (⊃ Fig. 36.18) but there is no single diagnostic standard. Several criteria are in current use but all share an emphasis on prominent trabeculation at the left ventricular apex [53–65]. All were established from retrospective analyses of small populations of patients presenting with left ventricular dysfunction and there are few data on trabecular patterns in normal individuals.

The most widely used echo criteria are those described by Jenni et al., which require a 2:1 ratio of non-compacted to compacted myocardium and colour Doppler evidence of deep perfused inter-trabecular recesses. Strictly applying imaging criteria leads to over-diagnosis of LVNC, particularly in those with systolic heart failure and in people of Afro-Caribbean origin [66]. Therefore, careful evaluation of symptoms, family history, and left ventricular function must accompany imaging investigations.

Treatment

There is no specific clinical management for LVNC. Heart failure is treated with standard pharmacotherapy. Anticoagulation with warfarin is recommended in the presence of LV dilatation and systolic dysfunction (EF<40%). Arrhythmias should be managed using anti-arrhythmic agents or implantable defibrillators according to guidelines (⊃ Table 36.5).

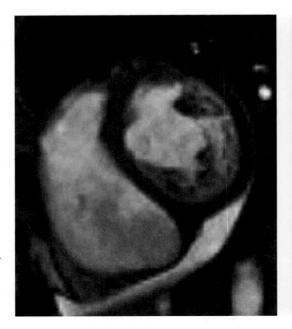 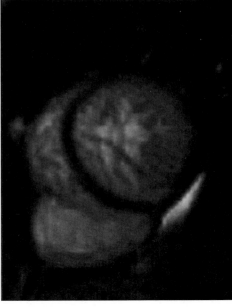

Fig. 36.18 Cardiac MRI from another patient with left ventricular non-compaction demonstrating again the deep trabeculations predominantly in the distal lateral wall.

Table 36.5 Summary of echocardiographic, CMR and CT diagnostic criteria for LVNC

Modality	Year	Author	Measurement	Phase	Plane	Reproducibility Intra-O	Reproducibility Inter-O	Pathoanatomical Correlation
Echo	1990	Chin [53]	2-layered structure of the myocardium (epicardial compacted, endocardial non-compacted layer). Determination of the X-to-Y ratio (≤0.5) X—Distance between the epicardial surface & through inter-trabecular recess Y—Distance between epicardial surface & peak of trabeculation	ED	PLAX for basal & mid X/Y SC & A4C for apical X/Y	✗	✓*	✓†
	2000	Jenni [64]	Thickened myocardium with a 2-layered structure consisting of a thin compacted epicardial layer (C) & a thicker, non-compacted endocardial layer (N) or trabecular meshwork with deep endomyocardial spaces; N/C ratio >2.0 Predominant location of the pathology: mid-lateral, mid-inferior, apex Colour Doppler evidence of deep inter-trabecular recesses filled with blood from the LV cavity Absence of coexisting cardiac abnormalities (in the presence of isolated LVNC)	ES	PSAX for N/C measurements A4C to assess colour Doppler	✗	✓ [37]	✓‡
	2002	Ströllberger [66]	>3 trabeculations protruding from the LV wall, apical to the papillary muscles, visible in one image plane at ED Trabeculations form the non-compacted part of a 2-layered myocardial structure, best visible at ES Trabeculations with the same echogenicity as the myocardium & synchronous movement with ventricular contractions Perfusion of the inter-trabecular spaces from the LV cavity N/C ratio >2.0 at ED (this criterion was introduced later)	ED ES	PSAX A4C & modified views	✗	✓ [55]	✓ [57]
	2008	Belanger [48]	No evidence of congenital heart disease, hypertrophic or infiltrative cardiomyopathy, or documented coronary artery disease Evidence of prominent trabeculations in the apex in any view without the traditional requirement for a ratio of non-compacted (NC) to compacted (C) wall thickness >2 Concentration of the NC area in the apex Blood flow through the area of NC Maximal linear NC/C ratio measured in the A4C view Also digital planimetry of the area of non-compaction	ES ES	A4C A4C	✗	✗	✗

Classification

Classification	NC/C Ratio	LVNC Area by Planimetry
None	0	0
Mild	>0 and <1	≥0 cm² and <2.5 cm²
Moderate	≥1 and <2	≥2.5 cm² and <2.5 cm²
Severe	2+	≥5.0 cm²

(Continued)

Modality	Year	Author	Measurement	Phase	Plane	Reproducibility		Pathoanatomical Correlation
						Intra-O	Inter-O	
	2012	Gebhard [59]	Maximal systolic thicknesses of 'non-compacta' & 'compacta' measured in standard short-axis views at the apical or midventricular level, in the segment with most prominent recesses/trabeculation LVNC if maximal systolic 'compacta' thickness <8 mm	ES	SAX	X	X	X
CMR	2005	Petersen [60]	Non-compaction assessed by qualitative analysis of all segments (excluding segment 17), a distinct two-layered appearance In each of the three diastolic long-axis views, the segment with the most pronounced trabeculations is chosen for measurement of the thickness of NC/C ratio perpendicular to the wall. Only the maximal ratio is considered: LVNC if NC/C >2.3	ED	HLA VLA LVOT	X	✓~	X
	2010	Jacquier [61]	Compacted LV mass: endocardial border drawn to include papillary muscle and exclude LV trabeculation Global LV mass: endocardial border drawn to include papillary muscles and trabeculation Trabeculated mass therefore = global LV mass—compacted LV mass LVNC if trabeculated LV mass >20%	ED	SAX	✓§	✓	X
	2012	Grothoff [62]	Calculation of: Total LV myocardial mass index (LV-MMI) Compacted (LV-MMIcompacted) Non-compacted (LV- MMInon-compacted) Percentage LV-MMnon-compacted LVNC if Total LV-MMInon-compacted > 15 g/m2 or percentage LV- MMnon-compacted >25% In addition to: Demonstrating trabeculation in basal segments and a ratio of NC/C ≥3: 1	ED	SAX	✓	✓	X
CT	2012	Melendez-Ramirez [63]	NC/C ratio in all segments except segment 17 LVNC if NC/C ratio >2.2 at ED involving ≥2 segments.	ED	SAX: base, mid, apical 2C 4C 3C	✓	✓	X

Courtesy of Dr Gaby Captur, UCL.

*Inter-observer variation for X/Y ratios significant at the LV apex (**P**<0.001).

†Necropsy (**n** = 3) comparison of endomyocardial patterns visually to echo without formal quantification.

‡Echo and pathoanatomical correlation in 9 patients.

~A separate group [30] investigated reproducibility for these criteria reporting <10% variability (statistical methods and significance levels not provided).

§Intra-observer data previously published by another group [31].

Echo, transthoracic echocardiography; CMR, cardiovascular magnetic resonance; CT, computerized tomography; Intra-O, intra-observer reproducibility; Inter-O, inter-observer reproducibility; ED, end-diastole; PLAX, parasternal long axis; SC, subcostal; A4C, apical 4-chamber; PSAX, parasternal short axis; LV, left ventricular; HLA, horizontal long axis; VLA, vertical long axis; LVOT, left ventricular outflow tract view; SAX, short axis; ✓, data published; X, no data published; LVNC, left ventricular non-compaction.

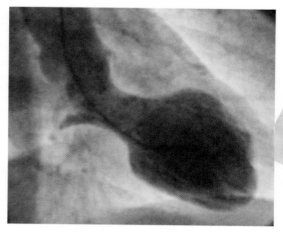
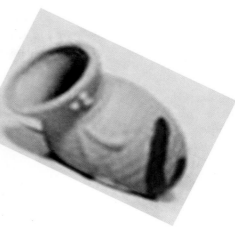

Fig. 36.19 Left ventriculography from a 65-year-old female who presented as a primary angioplasty call showing a typical apical ballooning with dynamic proximal ventricular contraction. This patient had unobstructed coronaries. On the right, a picture of a Japanese fishing pot with a narrow neck and wide base that is used to trap octopus.

Takotsubo cardiomyopathy (stress cardiomyopathies)

Introduction and definitions

Takotsubo cardiomyopathy (TC) is a syndrome of transient left ventricular apical dysfunction occurring with excess catecholamine during periods of stress, most prevalent amongst postmenopausal women. The original description arises from the mechanism of closure of the Japanese octopus trap in the early 1990s [67]. The pathophysiology is complex and unclear and involves catecholamine-mediated myocardial stunning. Patients with TC have exaggerated sympathetic activation with plasma catecholamine levels several times those of age- and sex-matched patients with extensive myocardial infarction. It has important implications because its clinical presentation mimics that of an acute coronary syndrome.

Diagnosis

The diagnosis is often made following an emergency admission simulating an acute coronary syndrome with electrocardiographic changes in the form of acute ST segment elevation or depression, a dilated cardiac apex (apical ballooning) during ventriculography (⬥ Fig. 36.19) but unobstructed coronary arteries [68, 69]. Usually, levels of creatine kinase-MB and troponin T are mildly elevated, out of proportion to the extensive myocardial dysfunction. Echocardiography typically demonstrates a large apical aneurysm with hypercontraction of the basal segment. However, the final diagnosis lies in the reversibility of the apical ballooning over a relatively short period between 1–3 weeks.

The syndrome of transient apical ballooning and stress cardiomyopathy has been well documented in the last two decades. However, the onset mechanism that ultimately results in reversible myocardial dysfunction with inflammatory infiltrate on biopsy, as opposed to myocardial necrosis with an acute infarct, remains unclear.

Several mechanisms have been proposed, such as multi-vessel epicardial spasm with regional myocardial stunning [67] and

catecholamine-excess toxicity mediated by intracellular Ca^{2+} overload [70]. Neurogenic pathways enhancing catecholamine toxicity particularly in post-menopausal women lacking oestrogen have recently been suggested [71]. Acute microvascular dysfunction represents the common endpoint with visible perfusion defects, which improved with adenosine infusion and resolved spontaneously at 4 weeks [72].

Enhanced sympathetic activity appears to play a very important role in the pathophysiology of TC [73]. Triggering factors, such as intense emotional stress, are frequently seen in patients with this syndrome and excessive levels of catecholamines have been found in patients with TC (⬥ Table 36.6).

Although some cases of basal ballooning have been reported, it is the cardiac apex that is typically involved [74]. The reason for this is unclear but several hypotheses have been put forward that make the apex more sensitive to catecholamine surge: (1) the apex does not have a 3-layered myocardial configuration that makes it structurally vulnerable, (2) it has a limited elasticity reserve, (3) it can easily become ischaemic as a consequence of its relatively limited coronary circulation, and (4) it is more responsive to adrenergic stimulation.

Table 36.6 Basic findings in patients with Takotsubo cardiomyopathy

- A preponderant occurrence of the syndrome in elderly or postmenopausal females
- Onset consequent to acute emotional stress or an acute medical condition
- ST-segment elevation or depression, or T-wave changes
- A prolonged QT interval
- A mild increase in cardiac enzymes
- Typical akinesis of the apical and distal anterior wall together with hypercontraction of the basal wall
- The occasional presence of transient intracavitary pressure gradients in some patients
- A need for acute haemodynamic support in some cases
- Complete resolution of the apical wall motion abnormality and the depressed LVSF.

Echocardiography

Echocardiography is the imaging modality of choice. It shows a large apical aneurysm with full-thickness myocardium (⊃ Fig. 36.20). The basal portion of the left ventricle is often contracting vigorously and it may be accompanied by a high outflow track gradient, systolic anterior motion of the mitral valve, and mitral regurgitation. Patients are usually very ill with severe heart failure at the start but subsequently they recover. Often within days, the left ventricular function improves with resolution of the apical aneurysm (⊃ Fig. 36.21). Complications may include the formation of an apical thrombus (⊃ Fig. 36.22), and the presence of pericardial effusion. Contrast echocardiography will delineate the left ventricular apex better and may show some apical hypoperfusion (⊃ Fig. 36.23).

Cardiac magnetic resonance

Typically, CMR will show the same pattern of apical dyskinesia (⊃ Fig. 36.24), although in the acute phase when the patient is very ill it may be difficult for the patient to go into the magnet. Perhaps the most useful information that CMR will provide is the absence of myocardial scar, which is typically found in myocardial infarction [75].

Conclusions

TC should be considered in the differential diagnosis of acute myocardial infarction given that it is the underlying cause for patients labelled with acute coronary syndrome in >1%.

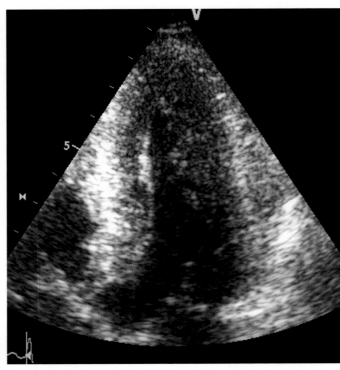

Fig. 36.21 Same patient as in Fig. 36.20 8 days later. Note the complete recovery of left ventricular function.

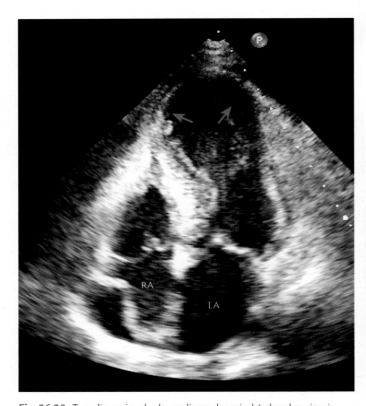

Fig. 36.20 Two-dimensional echocardiography apical 4-chamber view in end-systole from a patient with Takotsubo cardiomyopathy. There is typical apical aneurysm (arrows) with dynamic basal septal contraction. Note the small pericardial effusion at the back of the right atrium. LA, left atrium; RA, right atrium.

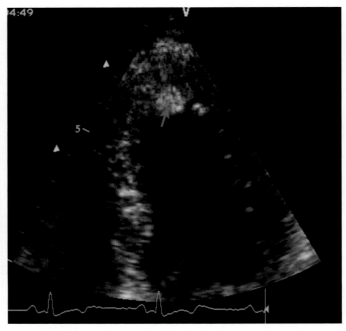

Fig. 36.22 Apical 4-chamber view from a patient with Takotsubo cardiomyopathy and an apical thrombus (arrow).

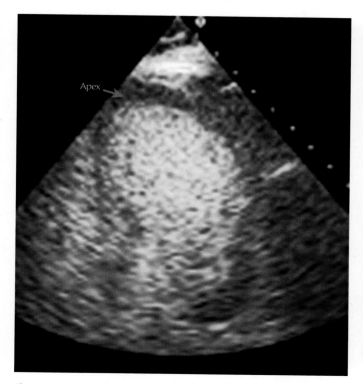

Fig. 36.23 Myocardial contrast echocardiography showing apical hypoperfusion reduced opacification of the apex (arrow).

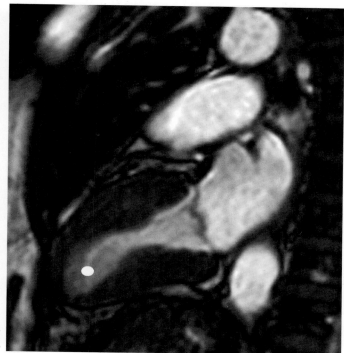

Fig. 36.24 Cardiac magnetic resonance imaging demonstrating apical ballooning.

The diagnosis is often made in the cardiac catheterization laboratory after the patient presents with an acute coronary syndrome and unobstructed coronary arteries have been found.

Echocardiography quickly shows an extensive apical aneurysm (ballooning) with dynamic basal contraction.

TC is an acute and transient form of stress-induced heart failure, although occasionally there is no recollection of a preceding stressful event.

Management of TC is supportive with inotropic agents and intra-aortic balloon pumps, whilst heparin prevents LV thrombus formation.

References

1. Foale RA, Nihoyannopoulos P, Ribeiro P, et al. Right ventricular abnormalities in ventricular tachycardia of right ventricular origin: relation to electrophysiological abnormalities. *Heart* 1986; 56: 45–54.
2. Pietras RJ, Mautner R, Denes P, et al. Chronic recurrent right and left ventricular tachycardia: comparison of clinical, haemodynamic and angiographic findings. *Am J Cardiol* 1977; 40: 32–7.
3. Fontaine G, Frank R, Vedel J, Grosgogeat Y, Cabrol C, Facquet J. Stimulation studies and epicardial mapping in ventricular tachycardia: study of mechanisms and selection for surgery. In: Kulbertus HE, editor. *Reentrant Arrhythmias*. Lancaster, PA: MTP Publishing, 1977: 334–50.
4. Corrado D, Basso C, Thiene G. Arrhythmogenic right ventricular cardiomyopathy: diagnosis, prognosis, and treatment. *Heart* 2000; 83: 588–95.
5. McKoy G, Protonotarios N, Crosby A, et al. Identification of a deletion in plakoglobin in arrhythmogenic right ventricular cardiomyopathy with palmoplantar keratoderma and woolly hair (Naxos disease). *Lancet* 2000; 355: 2119–24.
6. Norgett EE, Hatsell SJ, Carvajal-Huerta L, et al. Recessive mutation in desmoplakin disrupts desmoplakin-intermediate filament interactions and causes dilated cardiomyopathy, woolly hair and keratoderma. *Hum Mol Genet* 2000; 9: 2761–6.
7. Rampazzo A, Nava A, Malacrida S, et al. Mutation in human desmoplakin domain binding to plakoglobin causes a dominant form of arrhythmogenic right ventricular cardiomyopathy. *Am J Hum Genet* 2002; 71: 1200–6.
8. Taylor M, Graw S, Sinagra G, et al. Genetic variation in titin in arrhythmogenic right ventricular cardiomyopathy-overlap syndromes. *Circulation* 2011; 124: 876–85.
9. Gerull B, Heuser A, Wichter T, et al. Mutations in the desmosomal protein plakophilin-2 are common in arrhythmogenic right ventricular cardiomyopathy. *Nat Genet* 2004; 36: 1162–4.
10. Quarta G, Syrris P, Ashworth M, et al. Mutations in the Lamin A/C gene mimic arrhythmogenic right ventricular cardiomyopathy. *Eur Heart J* [Epub ahead of print].
11. McKenna WJ, Thiene G, Nava A, et al. Diagnosis of arrhythmogenic right ventricular dysplasia/cardiomyopathy: task force of the working group myocardial and pericardial disease of the European Society of Cardiology and the Scientific Council on Cardiomyopathies of the

International Society and Federation of Cardiology. *Br Heart J* 1994; 71: 215–8.

12. Marcus FI, McKenna WJ, Sherrill D, et al. Diagnosis of arrhythmogenic right ventricular cardiomyopathy/dysplasia: proposed modification of the task force criteria. *Circulation* 2010; 121: 1533–41.

13. Ho SY, Nihoyannopoulos P. Anatomy, echocardiography, and normal right ventricular dimensions. *Heart* 2006; 92: i2–13.

14. Bleeker GB, Steendijk P, Holman ER, et al. Acquired right ventricular dysfunction. *Heart* 2006; 92: i14–18.

15. Foale RA, Nihoyannopoulos P., McKenna WJ, et al. The echocardiographic measurements of the normal adult right ventricle. *Br Heart J* 1986; 56: 33–44.

16. G B Bleeker, P Steendijk, E R Holman, et al. Assessing right ventricular function: the role of echocardiography and complementary technologies. *Heart* 2006; 92: i19–26.

17. Blake LM, Scheinman MM, Higgins CB. MR feature of arrhythmogenic right ventricular dysplasia. *AJR* 1994; 162: 809–12.

18. Aufferman W, Wichter T, Breihardt G, Joachimsen K, Peters PE. Arrhythmogenic right ventricular disease: MR imaging vs angiography. *AJR* 1993; 161: 549–55.

19. Basso C, Thiene G, Corrado D, et al. Arrhythmogenic right ventricular cardiomyopathy. Dysplasia, dystrophy, or myocarditis? *Circulation* 1996; 94: 983–91.

20. Menghetti L, Basso C, Nava A, et al. Spin-echo nuclear magnetic resonance for tissue characterisation in arrhythmogenic right ventricular cardiomyopathy. *Heart* 1996; 76: 467–70.

21. MR imaging of arrhythmogenic right ventricular cardiomyopathy: morphologic findings and interobserver reliability. *Cardiology* 2003; 99: 153–62.

22. Tandri H, Calkins H, Marcus FI. Controversial role of magnetic resonance imaging in the diagnosis of arrhythmogenic right ventricular dysplasia. *Am J Cardiol* 2003; 92: 649.

23. Sen-Chowdhry S, Prasad SK, Syrris P, et al. Cardiovascular magnetic resonance in arrhythmogenic right ventricular cardiomyopathy revisited comparison with task force criteria and genotype. *J Am Coll Cardiol* 2006; 48: 2132–40.

24. Sievers B, Addo M, Franken F, Trappe HJ. Right ventricular wall motion abnormalities found in healthy subjects by cardiovascular magnetic resonance imaging and characterized with a new segmental model. *J Cardiovasc Mag Resonance* 2004; 6: 601–8.

25. Castillo E, Tandri H, Rodriguez ER, et al. Arrhythmogenic right ventricular dysplasia: ex vivo and in vivo fat detection with black-blood MR imaging radiology 2004; 232: 38–48.

26. Abbara S, Migrino RQ, Sosnovik DE, et al. Value of fat suppression in the MRI evaluation of suspected arrhythmogenic right ventricular dysplasia. *AJR* 2004; 182: 587–91.

27. Macedo R, Prakasa K, Tichnell C, et al. Marked lipomatous infiltration of the right ventricle: MRI findings in relation to arrhythmogenic right ventricular dysplasia. *AJR* 2007; 188: W423–7.

28. Tandri H, Saranathan M, Rodríguez ER, et al. Noninvasive detection of myocardial fibrosis in arrhythmogenic right ventricular cardiomyopathy using delayed-enhancement magnetic resonance imaging. *J Am Coll Cardiol* 2005; 45: 98–103.

29. Hunold P, Wieneke H, Bruder O, et al. Late enhancement: a new feature in MRI of arrhythmogenic right ventricular cardiomyopathy? *Journal of Cardiovascular Magnetic Resonance* 2005; 7: 649–55.

30. Bomma C, Dalal D, Tandri H, et al. Evolving role of multidetector computed tomography in evaluation of arrhythmogenic right ventricular dysplasia/cardiomyopathy. *Am J Cardiol* 2007; 100: 99–105.

31. Mariano-Goulart D, Déchaux L, Rouzet F, et al. Diagnosis of diffuse and localized arrhythmogenic right ventricular dysplasia by gated blood-pool SPECT. *J Nucl Med* 2007; 48: 1416–23.

32. Jacobi AH, Gohari A, Zalta B, Stein MW, Haramati LB. Ventricular myocardial fat: CT findings and clinical correlates. *J Thorac Imaging* 2007; 22: 130–5.

33. Takahashi N, Ishida Y, Maeno M, et al. Noninvasive identification of left ventricular involvements in arrhythmogenic right ventricular dysplasia: comparison of 123I-MIBG, 201TlCl, magnetic resonance imaging and ultrafast computed tomography. *Ann Nucl Med* 1997 Aug; 11: 233–41.

34. Lerch H, Bartenstein P, Wichter T, et al. Sympathetic innervation of the left ventricle is impaired in arrhythmogenic right ventricular disease. *Eur J Nucl Med* 1993; 20: 207–12.

35. Elliott P, Andersson B, Arbustini E, et al. Classification of the cardiomyopathies: a position statement from the European Society of Cardiology Working Group on Myocardial and Pericardial Diseases. *Eur Heart J* 2008; 29: 270–6.

36. Jenni R, Oechslin E, Schneider J, Attenhofer Jost C, Kaufman PA. Echocardiographic and pathoanatomical characteristics of isolated left ventricular non-compaction: a step towards classification as a distinct cardiomyopathy. *Heart* 2001; 86: 666–71.

37. Nugent AW, Daubeney PE, Chondros P et al.; National Australian Childhood Cardiomyopathy Study. The epidemiology of childhood cardiomyopathy in Australia. *N Engl J Med* 2003; 348: 1639–46.

38. Stollberger C, Finsterer J. Left ventricular hypertrabeculation/noncompaction. *J Am Soc Echocardiogr* 2004; 17: 91–100.

39. Bellet S, Gouley BA. Congenital heart disease with multiple cardiac abnormalities: report of a case showing aortic atresia, fibrous scar in myocardium and embryonal sinusoidal remains. *Am J Med Sci* 1932; 183: 458–65.

40. Lauer RM, Fink HP, Petry EL, et al. Angiographic demonstration of intramyocardial sinusoids in pulmonary-valve atresia with intact ventricular septum and hypoplastic right ventricle. *N Engl J Med* 1964; 271: 68–72.

41. Dusek J, Ostadal B, Duskova M. Postnatal persistence of spongy myocardium with embryonic blood supply. *Arch Pathol* 1975; 99: 312–7.

42. Ritter M, Oechslin E, Sütsch G, Attenhofer C, Schneider J, Jenni R. Isolated non-compaction of the myocardium in adults. *Mayo Clin Proc* 1997; 72: 26–31.

43. Pignatelli RH, McMahon CJ, Dreyer WJ, et al. Clinical characterization of left ventricular non-compaction in children: a relatively common form of cardiomyopathy. *Circulation* 2003; 108: 2672–8.

44. Sasse-Klaassen S, Gerull B, Oechslin E, Jenni R, Thierfelder L. Isolated non-compaction of the left ventricular myocardium in the adult is an autosomal dominant disorder in the majority of patients. *Am J Med Genet A* 2003; 119: 162–7.

45. Klaassen S, Probst S, Oechslin E, et al. Mutations in sarcomere protein genes in left ventricular non-compaction. *Circulation* 2008; 117: 2893–2901.

46. Hoedemaekers YM, Caliskan K, Michels M, et al. The importance of genetic counseling, DNA diagnostics, and cardiologic family screening in left ventricular non-compaction cardiomyopathy. *Circ Cardiovasc Genet* 2010; 3: 232–9.

47. Probst S, Oechslin E, Schuler P, et al. Sarcomere gene mutations in isolated left ventricular non-compaction cardiomyopathy do not predict clinical phenotype. *Circ Cardiovasc Genet* 2011; 4(4): 367–74.

48. Wlodarska EK, Wozniak O, Konka M, Piotrowska-Kownacka D, Walczak E, Hoffman P. Isolated ventricular non-compaction mimicking arrhythmogenic right ventricular cardiomyopathy—a study of nine patients. *Int J Cardiol* 2010; 145(1): 107–11.

49. Finsterer J, Stöllberger C, Gaismayer K, Janssen B. Acquired non-compaction in Duchenne muscular dystrophy. *Int J Cardiol* 2006; 106(3): 420–1

50. Pfammatter JP, Paul TH, Flik J, Drescher J, Kallfelz HC. Fieberassoziierte Moykarditis bei einem 14 jährigen Jungen. *Z Kardiol* 1995; 84: 947–50.

51. Oechslin EN, Attenhofer Jost CH, Rojas JR, Kaufmann PA, Jenni R. Long-term follow-up of 34 adults with isolated left ventricular non-compaction: a distinct cardiomyopathy with poor prognosis. *J Am Coll Cardiol* 2000; 36: 493–500.

52. Murphy RT, Thaman R, Blanes JG, et al. Natural history and familial characteristics of isolated left ventricular non-compaction. *Eur Heart J* 2005; 26(2): 187–92.

53. Chin TK, Perloff JK, Williams RG, Jue K, Mohrmann R. Isolated non-compaction of left ventricular myocardium. A study of eight cases. *Circ* 1990; 82: 507–13.

54. Oechslin E, Jenni R. Left ventricular non-compaction revisited: a distinct phenotype with genetic heterogeneity? *Eur Heart J* 2011; 32: 1446–56.

55. Saleeb SF, Margossian R, Spencer CT, et al. Reproducibility of echocardiographic diagnosis of left ventricular non-compaction. *J Am Soc Echocardiogr* 2012; 25: 194–202.

56. Stöllberger C, Finsterer J, Blazek G. Left ventricular hypertrabeculation/non-compaction and association with additional cardiac abnormalities and neuromuscular disorders. *Am J Cardiol* 2002; 90: 899–902.

57. Finsterer J, Stöllberger C, Feichtinger H: Histological appearance of left ventricular hypertrabeculation/non-compaction. *Cardiology* 2002; 98: 162–4.

58. Belanger AR, Miller MA, Donthireddi UR, Najovits AJ, Goldman ME. New classification scheme of left ventricular non-compaction and correlation with ventricular performance. *Am J Cardiol* 2008; 102: 92–96.

59. Gebhard C, Stähli BE, Greutmann M, Biaggi P, Jenni R, Tanner FC. Reduced left ventricular compacta thickness: a novel echocardiographic criterion for non-compaction cardiomyopathy. *J Am Soc Echocardiogr* 2012; 25: 1050–57.

60. Petersen SE, Selvanayagam JB, Wiesmann F, et al. Left ventricular non-compaction: insights from cardiovascular magnetic resonance imaging. *J Am Coll Cardiol* 2005; 46: 101–5.

61. Jacquier A, Thuny F, Jop B, et al. Measurement of trabeculated left ventricular mass using cardiac magnetic resonance imaging in the diagnosis of left ventricular non-compaction. *Eur Heart J* 2010; 31: 1098–104.

62. Grothoff M, Pachowsky M, Hoffmann J, et al. Value of cardiovascular MR in diagnosing left ventricular non-compaction cardiomyopathy and in discriminating between other cardiomyopathies. *Eur Radiol* 2012; 22: 2699–709.

63. Melendez-Ramirez G, Castillo-Castellon F, Espinola-Zavaleta N, Meave A, Kimura-Hayama ET. Left ventricular non-compaction: A proposal of new diagnostic criteria by multidetector computed tomography. *J Cardiovasc Comput Tomogr* 2012; 6: 346–54.

64. Dellegrottaglie S, Pedrotti P, Roghi A, Pedretti S, Chiariello M, Perrone-Filardi P. Regional and global ventricular systolic function in isolated ventricular non-compaction. Pathophysiological insights from magnetic resonance imaging. *Int J Cardiol* 2012; 26; 158: 394–99.

65. Fernández-Golfín C, Pachón M, Corros C, et al. Left ventricular trabeculae: quantification in different cardiac diseases and impact on left ventricular morphological and functional parameters assessed with cardiac magnetic resonance. *J Cardiovasc Med (Hagerstown)* 2009; 10: 827–33.

66. Kohli SK, Pantazis AA, Shah JS, et al. Diagnosis of left-ventricular non-compaction in patients with left-ventricular systolic dysfunction: time for a reappraisal of diagnostic criteria? *Eur Heart J* 2008; 29(1): 89–95. Epub 2007 Nov 9.

67. Dote, K, Satoh, H, Tateishi, H, et al. Myocardial stunning due to simultaneous multivessel coronary spasm: a review of 5 cases. *Journal of Cardiology* 1991; 21: 203–14.

68. Kurisu S, Sato H, Kawagoe T, et al. Tako-tsubo-like left ventricular dysfunction with ST-segment elevation: a novel cardiac syndrome mimicking acute myocardial infarction. *Am Heart J* 2002; 143: 448–55.

69. Abe Y, Kondo M, Matsuoka R, Araki M, Dohyama K, Tanio H. Assessment of clinical features in transient left ventricular apical ballooning. *J Am Coll Cardiol* 2003; 41: 737–42.

70. Frustaci A, Loperfido F, Gentiloni N, et al. Catecholamine-induced cardiomyopathy in multiple endocrine neoplasia. A histologic, ultrastructural, and biochemical study. *Chest* 1991; 99; 382–5.

71. Akashi Y, Goldstein D, Barbaro G, et al. Takotsubo cardiomyopathy: a new form of acute, reversible heart failure. *Circulation* 2008, 118: 2754–62.

72. Galiuto L, Ranieri De Caterina A, Porfidia A, et al. Reversible coronary microvascular dysfunction: a common pathogenetic mechanism in apical ballooning or tako-tsubo syndrome. *Eur Heart J* 2010; 31: 1319–27.

73. Wittstein IS, Thiemann DR, Lima JA, et al. Neurohumoral features of myocardial stunning due to sudden emotional stress. *N Engl J Med* 2005; 352: 539–48.

74. Virani SS, Khan AN, Mendoza CE, Ferreira AC, de Marchena E. Takotsubo cardiomyopathy, or broken-heart syndrome. *Tex Heart Inst J* 2007; 34 (1): 76–9.

75. Eitel I, Behrendt F, Schindler K, et al. Differential diagnosis of suspected apical ballooning syndrome using contrast-enhanced magnetic resonance imaging. *Eur Heart J* 2008; 29: 2651–9.

⊃ **For additional multimedia materials, please visit the online version of the book (⌂ http://www.esciacc.oxfordmedicine.com)**

SECTION VII

Peri-myocardial disease

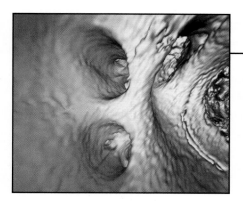

CHAPTER 37

Pericardial effusion and cardiac tamponade

Paul Leeson and Harald Becher

Contents

Background to pericardial effusions and cardiac tamponade

Pericardial space

A pericardial effusion is an accumulation of fluid within the pericardial space created by the serous pericardium. The serous pericardium consists of two membranes: one lines the inside of the fibrous pericardium and the other extends over the outer surface of the heart (visceral pericardium). The serous membranes are continuous with each other and therefore form a deflated sac. This provides a potential space for fluid to accumulate and as the amount of fluid increases there is an associated increase in intra-pericardial pressure [1].

The vascular connections to the heart pass through the pericardium via two irregular holes. One hole accommodates the great vessels—aorta and pulmonary artery—and the other the venous connections—pulmonary veins and vena cavae. At each point the serous pericardium has to wrap around the blood vessels and therefore two pockets (or sinuses) are created; the transverse sinus between aorta and pulmonary artery, and the oblique sinus between the pulmonary veins on the back of the left atrium [2]. These are of particular importance in pericardial effusions because collections can localize in the sinuses. These localized collections may cause clinical symptoms because of restricted flow in the associated blood vessels, such as pulmonary vein flow when fluid localizes in the oblique sinus.

Causes of pericardial effusions

Normally within the pericardial space there is a small amount of pericardial fluid, around ten to fifteen millilitres. This fluid is a transudate produced by the visceral pericardium and ensures the two layers of serous membrane move freely over each other to allow unrestricted motion of the cardiac chambers during systole and diastole. Diagnosis of a pericardial effusion implies the presence of an abnormal increase in fluid within the pericardial space [3].

Pericardial fluid accumulates for similar reasons to fluid accumulation in any other body space and typically is either a transudate or exudate. The most common cause of effusion is in response to pericardial inflammation, as in pericarditis or post-cardiac surgery. If infective then the effusion may be purulent. Effusions also occur in response to malignant processes, both those in direct proximity to the heart, such as pericardial or cardiac, and also those more distant, such as breast or lung [4]. Metabolic changes, such as hypothyroidism or uraemia, can also lead to fluid collection and rarely effusions occur due to abnormalities in lymphatic drainage, described as a chylous effusion. Haemopericardium occurs after coronary surgery and if there is any other pathological or iatrogenic cardiac or coronary rupture that allows blood to be released into the pericardial space.

The characteristics or location of an effusion, as well as the presence of intra-pericardial structures may help determine the underlying diagnosis. Fibrin strands or loculated effusions are often seen in response to inflammation, whereas haematoma is very suggestive of a haemopericardium. Irregular or invasive masses may suggest tumour, cyst, or fungal infection.

Size of pericardial effusions

Pericardial effusions vary significantly in size and haemodynamic effect. These two factors are not directly related and haemodynamic effects are more closely related to the speed of fluid accumulation. In conditions such as malignancy, where fluid has accumulated over several months, the pericardium has had time to adapt and accommodates larger volumes before haemodynamic problems occur [4]. In sudden fluid accumulation, which can occur following iatrogenic cardiac or coronary puncture, only a small amount of fluid is required to limit cardiac function.

Global effusions are usually graded as mild, moderate, or large based on their depth, which is the distance between pericardial and cardiac surface [5]. This depth is sometimes used to approximate to volume. Less than 0.5 cm usually equates to around 50 to 100ml of fluid, whereas a depth of 0.5 to 1 cm is considered a mild effusion and is associated with volumes of around 100 to 250 ml. A moderate effusion is usually 1 to 2 cm, or 250 to 500 ml, and a large effusion tends to be over 2 cm deep and is associated with over 500 ml of fluid. These approximations do not hold for localized or loculated effusion. (Table 37.1).

Cardiac tamponade

Pericardial effusions have haemodynamic consequences when they restrict normal cardiac function [2, 4]. The presence of cardiac tamponade specifically refers to diagnosis of the severe haemodynamic compromise that leads to clinical symptoms and signs. This diagnosis is based on tachycardia (>100 bpm), hypotension (<100 mmHg systolic), pulsus paradoxus (>10 mmHg drop in blood pressure on inspiration), and a raised JVP with prominent x descent [5].

For clinical symptoms to emerge the effusion must be sufficient to increase intra-pericardial pressure to levels greater than intra-cardiac pressure. The first visible signs of haemodynamic impact therefore occur in chambers at lower pressure and at points within the cardiac cycle when pressure is at a minimum. After a general reduction in chamber size, the right atrium starts to appear to collapse in atrial systole. As intra-pericardial pressure increases further this is followed by parts of the right ventricle starting to collapse at the end of ventricular systole. The combination of rapid atrial collapse in atrial systole, followed by rapid ventricular collapse at the end of ventricular systole, creates the appearance of a swinging right atrium and ventricle [6]. Cardiac efficiency is impaired as a result and blood flow through the heart becomes limited, eventually leading to symptoms.

Table 37.1 Estimates of fluid volume based on depth of effusion

Depth of effusion (cm)	Estimate of volume (ml)
<0.5	50–100
0.5–1	100–250
1–2	250–500
>2	>500

Table 37.2 Imaging features of tamponade

Imaging features of tamponade
Pericardial effusion
Right atrial collapse in atrial diastole
Right ventricular collapse from end-systole into diastole
Respiratory variation of Doppler at mitral valve of >15% (typically >40% in tamponade)
Respiratory variation of Doppler at tricuspid valve of >25%
Respiratory variation of Doppler in left and right ventricular outflow of >10%
Septal fluttering—early diastolic notching on M-mode
Dilatation of inferior vena cava and hepatic veins

Intra-cardiac pressure is also affected by respiration, which is normally associated with a swing of 5 mmH_2O in intra-thoracic pressure. During inspiration there is an increase in blood flow into the lungs, which increases flow into the right heart and reduces flow into the left heart. Expiration forces blood out of the lungs into the left heart and reduces flow into the right heart. These changes in flow can normally be identified by a small variation in blood pressure with respiration. As intra-pericardial pressure begins to approach intra-cardiac pressure and influence blood flow into the right heart the drop in blood pressure with inspiration becomes more exaggerated and is described as *pulsus paradoxus* when it exceeds 10 mmHg [5, 6] (Table 37.2).

Imaging pericardial effusions

Overview

Pericardial imaging is usually based on a staged, multi-modality approach [7, 8]. The combination of echocardiography, cardiac CT, and cardiac MR provide sufficient spatial resolution to visualize the pericardium, a wide field of view to look for associated pathology within the chest, a high temporal resolution to provide detailed information on myocardial function (and acute changes in function), and a means to differentiate tissue characteristics, such as calcium, blood, tumour, and fibrosis. However, echocardiography is usually the main modality used in management of pericardial effusions, with cardiac CT and cardiac MR reserved for patients in whom there is a need to investigate possible underlying diagnoses, such as malignancy, or there is concern about very localized effusions. Alternatively, assessment of effusions by cardiac MR and cardiac CT may be carried out as part of image acquisition for broader cardiac pathology or effusions may be noted incidentally. The key roles of cardiovascular imaging when there is a pericardial effusion are to identify the size and location of the effusion, likely cause, haemodynamic effects and the best approaches to remove the effusion (pericardiocentesis).

Chest X-ray

The chest X-ray remains the standard first-line investigation in patients with chest pain or shortness of breath. The pre-dominant symptom of a pericardial effusion is shortness of breath

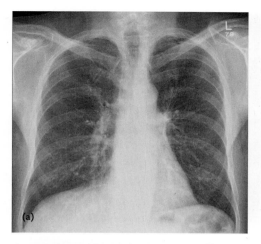
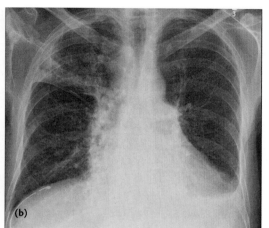
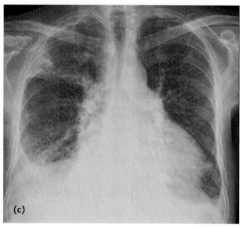

Fig. 37.1 Series of chest X-rays (a–c) of the same patient taken over six months. Note the gradual change in shape of the cardiac silhouette into a globular heart as a pericardial effusion develops. In the final image (c) a thin lower attenuation band can be noted around the lateral border of the heart consistent with the fluid layer within the pericardium.
Images courtesy of Radiology Department, John Radcliffe Hospital, Oxford.

and, therefore, very frequently, the chest X-ray is the first image acquired before the diagnosis is made. The strengths of the chest X-ray are: its wide availability; wide field of view to pick up alternative or related pathology, such as chest infection; ability to provide an outline of cardiovascular structures against the lung; and ability to pick up calcification [9]. The pericardium itself is not normally visible on the chest X-ray, except when it becomes calcified and in the majority of patients the most useful information is obtained from changes in the shape of the cardiac silhouette (⊃ Fig. 37.1). *Pericardial effusions* classically cause a large, globular heart [10]. Such a finding should prompt further imaging with echocardiography. Other information may be gathered from the chest X-ray about possible underlying or alternative pathologies such as chest infections, tuberculosis or malignancy.

Echocardiography

Advantages and disadvantages of echocardiography

Identification of a pericardial effusion was one of the first uses of echocardiography and echocardiography remains the imaging modality of choice for initial investigation of pericardial effusion [11]. This is because it is readily available at the bedside, in the clinic, and, increasingly, in the community. Echocardiography

has the spatial and temporal resolution to provide information on quantity and position of fluid accumulation within the pericardial space combined with related changes in haemodynamics [5]. Information on cardiac size, function, and mass can be collected at the same time. In combination with transoesophageal imaging, the whole of the pericardial space can be viewed, including the sinuses [6, 11]. Presence of thrombus or fibrin can also be noted from changes in echo characteristics and masses associated with the pericardium can be identified. Echocardiography may be limited by body habitus and is not able to differentiate accurately fluid types or assess pericardial thickness. The modality also lacks the field of view to assess related pathology in the lungs. However, echocardiography is particularly useful in the emergency setting when there is concern about acute haemodynamic compromise due to pericardial fluid accumulation, for which it can also be used to aid pericardial drainage.

Appearances on echocardiography

Part of the pericardium and pericardial space can be seen in all standard echocardiography views (⊃ Fig. 37.2 and 📹 Videos 37.1-37.4). However, the best transthoracic views to see a pericardial effusion are usually the parasternal long and short axes, apical four-chamber and subcostal views. During transoesophageal echocardiography, the most useful additional views are the four-chamber view (mid-oesophageal 0° view) as it allows assessment of

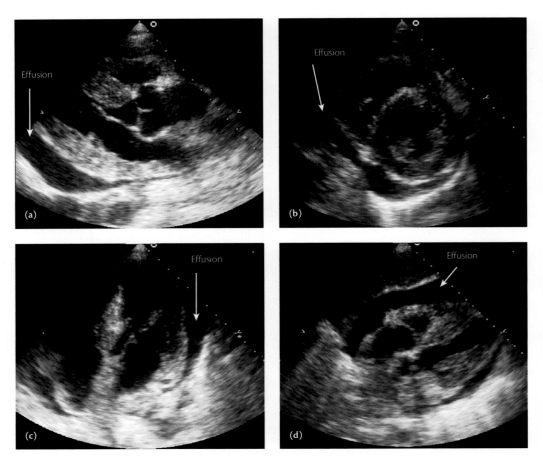

Fig. 37.2 Four standard echocardiography views. A pericardial effusion can be noted in each view. Images courtesy of Radiology Department, John Radcliffe Hospital, Oxford.

localized collections around the pulmonary veins and right heart, and the aortic valve views (mid-oesophageal short-axis 50° and long-axis 135° views) to assess the transverse sinus [5]. Transgastric short-axis views can also be used to assess depth of effusions.

The pericardial surfaces may be apparent as a thin, slightly brighter line around the heart (⊃ Fig. 37.3 and ▣ Video 35.5). The acoustic properties of the pericardium are close to those of surrounding tissues and therefore it is difficult to see, which makes measures inaccurate. Gross changes in thickness or calcifications (which are seen as echo-lucent areas with associated shadowing) may be seen. The normal pericardial space is a thin

black line around the heart and there should only be a few millimetres of fluid, which is usually only evident during systole [12]. A pericardial effusion will be seen as an abnormal increase in size of this echo-lucent space. Pleural fluid has a similar appearance and it is important to differentiate this from a pericardial collection. This can usually be achieved because the pericardium is visible (⊃ Fig. 37.3) or from the position of the collection relative to the aorta [13]. As the pericardium lies between the aorta and heart, pericardial fluid will track along the inferolateral surface of the heart, whereas pleural fluid will abut the aorta (⊃ Fig. 37.3). Echocardiography will be able to assess the size, location, possible

Fig. 37.3 2D-echocardiography example of a pleural and pericardial collection. Note the bright white pericardium and how the pericardial fluid passes between aorta and heart, whereas the pleural fluid lies outside the aorta. Images courtesy of Radiology Department, John Radcliffe Hospital, Oxford.

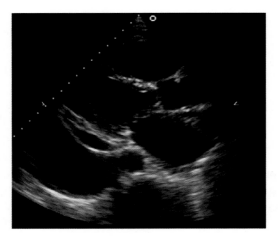

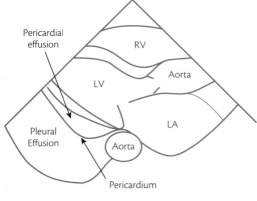

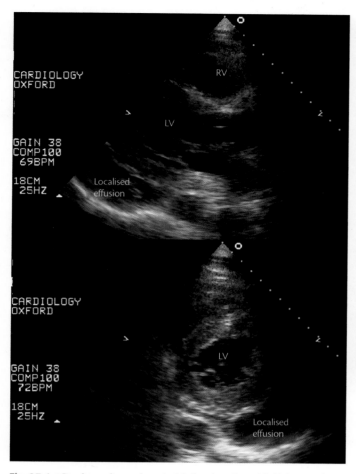

Fig. 37.4 2D-echocardiography apical 4-chamber view with fibrin strands evident within the effusion along the lateral wall of the left ventricle.
Images courtesy of Radiology Department, John Radcliffe Hospital, Oxford.

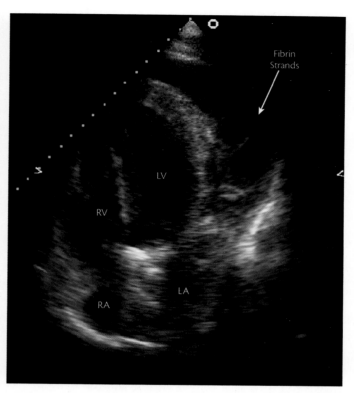

Fig. 37.5 2D-echocardiography parasternal long-axis and parasternal short-axis views of a pericardial effusion localized against the inferolateral wall of the left ventricle.
Images courtesy of Radiology Department, John Radcliffe Hospital, Oxford.

underlying diagnosis, and haemodynamic effects of an effusion. Furthermore, it will be able to determine whether the effusion is global, localized or loculated (⊃ Fig. 37.4 and ▣ Video 37.6).

Echocardiography can approximate volume of fluid based on depth with more accurate volume measures obtainable from planimetry of pericardial and cardiac borders in apical views or from 3D-echocardiography. Pericardial fluids (serous, blood, or pus) are all seen as black echo-lucent areas and it is difficult to differentiate between fluid type with echocardiography. Strands (fibrin) can easily be seen (⊃ Fig. 37.5 and ▣ Video 37.7) and haematoma may be evident, although it has similar echocardiographic density to myocardium. Transoeosphageal echocardiography may be particularly useful for assessment of possible localized effusions in patients with haemodynamic problems after cardiac surgery (⊃ Fig. 37.6 and ▣ Video 37.8) and, in this setting, transgastric views can be used to assess the size of the effusion.

Cardiac tamponade and echocardiography

Echocardiography is of great importance for assessment of cardiac tamponade. A key feature that can be identified with echocardiography is the 2D evaluation of the abnormal collapse of the right atrium and ventricle (⊃ Fig. 37.7 and ▣ Video 37.9). The first part

of the heart to be affected is the right atrium at end-diastole. As pressure increases further the right ventricle starts to be affected and collapses at end-systole [5]. Clinical haemodynamics usually intervene before intra-pericardial pressure is sufficient to influence the left ventricle and atrium.

Cardiac tamponade is associated with *pulsus paradoxus*, which is the abnormal exaggeration of the variation in systolic blood pressure with respiration. This occurs due to changes in blood flow through the heart and therefore Doppler is ideally suited to identify these variations in blood flow [6]. To demonstrate the respiratory variation, Doppler inflow across one of the valves can be measured and change in E-wave recorded (⊃ Fig. 37.8). Respiration can be tracked using a physio trace or annotated on the recording. Normally, peak flow across the mitral valve varies by <15% and <25% at the tricuspid valve (⊃ Fig. 37.9). Greater than this supports tamponade but clinical signs are usually associated with >40% variation at the mitral valve. Exaggerated flow changes through the heart during respiration can also be demonstrated in the left and right ventricle outflow tracts (increased flow in inspiration on the right and in expiration on the left) with variation of greater than 10%. Increases in filling pressures may also be evident with dilatation of the inferior vena cava and hepatic veins. Septal motion may be abnormal with fluttering of the septum as left and right ventricles fill during diastole, probably due to waves of competitive filling of the two ventricles. This is reported as early diastolic notching on M-mode. The septum may also 'bounce' towards the left ventricle on inspiration because of the reduced left ventricular filling.

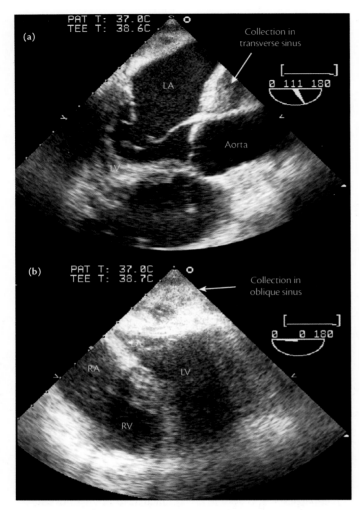

Fig. 37.6 Transoesophageal echocardiography views of localized collections. (a) A 0° four-chamber view with a localized, haematoma filled collection behind the left atrium consistent with an oblique sinus collection. (b) A 135° long-axis view of the aortic valve. As well as the oblique sinus collection, fluid and haematoma is also present in the transverse sinus between aorta and left atrium. Images courtesy of Radiology Department, John Radcliffe Hospital, Oxford.

Cardiac CT

Advantages and disadvantages of cardiac CT

Cardiac CT provides a modality when more detailed imaging of pericardial pathology is required and may be particularly useful to assess loculated or localized effusions not well visualized on echocardiography [14, 15]. Furthermore, CT may be indicated to investigate underlying causes, such as malignancy. Effusions may be identified on CT as an incidental finding during chest CT imaging for investigation of symptoms, such as shortness of breath. Strengths of cardiac CT are its ability to identify easily calcification, including microcalcifications, provide soft tissue contrast with tissue characterization—including fluid assessment based on attenuation—and a wide field of view to identify associated chest pathology. Multi-detector CT has enabled motion-free imaging of the pericardium to improve resolution, multi-planar reformation, and options to assess associated changes in cardiac function [16]. Without gating, motion artefacts can make measurements difficult, including complicating differentiation of thickened pericardium from fluid. The major limitations of cardiac CT are the requirement for ionising radiation and use of iodinated contrast agents.

Appearances on cardiac CT

The normal pericardial surfaces are seen as a thin grey line of soft-tissue density usually well delineated between the pericardial and epicardial fat layers [3, 16]. Therefore the pericardium is most evident on the anterior surface of the heart in front of the right ventricle and right atrium where the fat is more prominent and there is an area of ventral mediastinal fat. Pericardial fluid usually has attenuation characteristics of water and is seen as a thin line between the pericardial surfaces and the heart (⊃ Fig. 37.10). Attenuation characteristics may allow differentiation of the contents of an effusion. The more common transudate effusions have the attenuation of water, whereas those with higher protein content such as haemopericardium, purulent exudates, malignancy or chylous effusions have high attenuation

Fig. 37.7 2D-echocardiography apical four chamber view of a large global pericardial effusion. The image is stopped in end-diastole and end-systole to demonstrate right atrial and right ventricular collapse, respectively. This observation is supportive of cardiac tamponade.
Images courtesy of Radiology Department, John Radcliffe Hospital, Oxford.

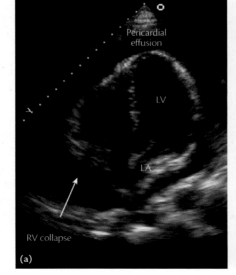

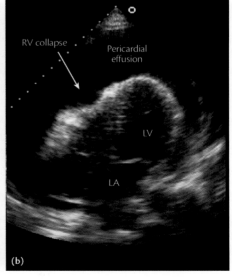

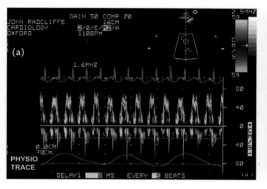

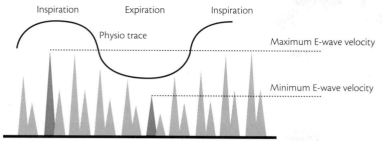

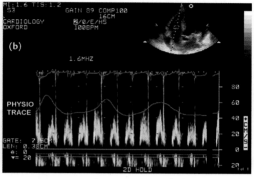

Fig. 37.8 Demonstrates pulse wave Doppler echocardiography of mitral valve inflow during cardiac tamponade with variation in E-wave velocity on inspiration and expiration.
Reproduced from Leeson, Augustine, Mitchell & Becher, *Echocardiography*, 2edn, 2012 with permission from Oxford University Press.

Fig. 37.9 Doppler recordings of normal (minimal) respiratory variation in tricuspid inflow and an exaggerated variation in inflow in a patient with a pericardial effusion.
Images courtesy of Radiology Department, John Radcliffe Hospital, Oxford.

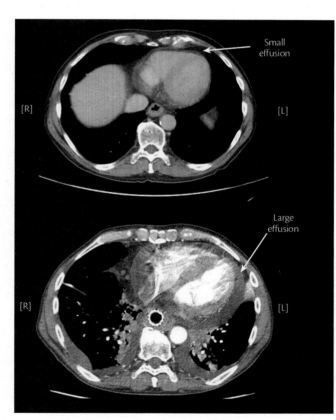

Fig. 37.10 Two standard transverse CT slices demonstrate a small and a large effusion. Note the attenuation characteristics of the effusion.
Images courtesy of Radiology Department, John Radcliffe Hospital, Oxford.

[3, 15]. The attenuation of haemopericardium varies with age, with a gradual reduction over time and the emergence of mixed areas due to the presence of thrombus. Inflammatory effusions may be associated with contrast uptake by the pericardium [16]. A limitation of cardiac

CT is the differentiation of a small effusion from pericardial thickening or when the effusion is the same attenuation as pericardium because of volume averaging. Because the whole heart is seen in every acquisition loculated or localized effusions and those around the anterior heart can be imaged within a standard protocol [14]. Another feature of cardiac CT is the wide field of view, which can be used to assess for related pathology in the lungs and also more clearly define the extent of masses associated with the pericardium. Cardiac CT is therefore particularly useful for more detailed assessment of pericardial pathology associated with the effusion, in particular, pericardial thickness (⊃ Fig. 37.11), calcification, and size, extent and functional effects of pericardial masses (⊃ Fig. 37.12).

Cardiac tamponade and cardiac CT

Cardiac tamponade should have been identified clinically and on echocardiography. However, multi-detector CT allows visualization of the cardiac cycle and may identify chamber collapse or changes in cardiac chamber size. If these findings are noted to be present during CT examination then urgent referral for treatment is warranted.

Cardiac MR

Advantages and disadvantages of cardiac MR

Cardiac MR provides a modality for more detailed assessment of pericardial effusions [17]. Cardiac MR can be useful to diagnose localized effusions around the right atrium, aorto-pericardial reflection and posterior to the left ventricle [18]. Effusions may also be evaluated by cardiac MR as part of other cardiac pathology being imaged or noted incidentally. Strengths of cardiac MR are its ability to provide unrestricted planes of view, differentiation

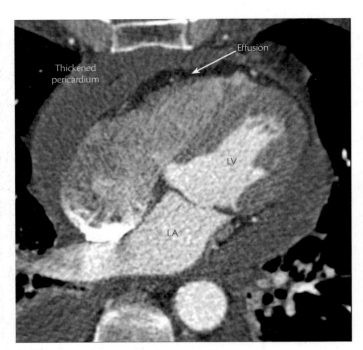

Fig. 37.11 Cardiac CT appearances of a patient with a grossly thickened pericardium and small effusion.
Images courtesy of Dr Ed Nicol, Royal Brompton Hospital, London.

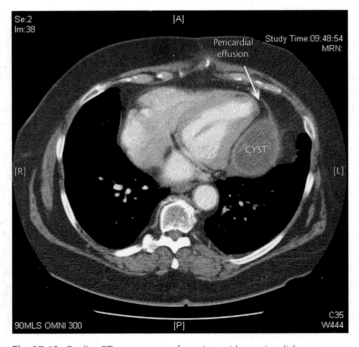

Fig. 37.12 Cardiac CT appearances of a patient with a pericardial cyst associated with an effusion.
Images courtesy of Radiology Department, John Radcliffe Hospital, Oxford.

of tissue, and fluid characteristics based on T1 and T2 characteristics and provision of functional cardiac imaging [19, 20]. Assessment of the myocardium, alongside the pericardium, and the use of gadolinium contrast can provide important information on cardiomyopathic processes that may complicate a pericardial effusion [21, 22]. Cardiac MR has a wide field of view to study related chest pathology or define extent of pericardial masses, and avoids ionizing radiation.

Appearances on cardiac MR

The normal pericardium is visible as a thin dark line on most cardiac MR sequences. It is dark on both T1 and T2 weighted sequences because it is fibrous, with a low water content [22]. Fat has different magnetic resonance characteristics and therefore the pericardial and epicardial fat help delineate the pericardium [23]. Transudates will have low-signal on T1 and high-signal on T2 with complex exudative effusions exhibiting greater signal intensity on T1 (⊃ Fig. 37.13 and ▣ Video 37.10). SSFP-cine imaging is associated with greater signal intensity in the presence of a greater T2/T1 ratio and therefore transudates tend to have high intensity (Fig. 37.13). On inversion recovery gadolinium late enhancement imaging effusions appear strikingly black (⊃ Fig. 37.14). The wide field of view means cardiac MR provides detailed assessment of loculated effusions, particularly around the aortic-pericardial reflection and at the left ventricular apex [18]. In sequences with high-signal from the pericardial fluid it is important to differentiate the effusion from the epicardial and pericardial fat. The presence of inflammatory or protein-rich material within the effusion also creates patchy changes in signal intensity (⊃ Fig. 37.15 and ▣ Video 37.11). The wide field of view allows detailed assessment of size and extent of pericardial masses and tissue characteristics can be used to aid diagnosis [24, 25].

Cardiac tamponade and cardiac MR

Cine images of cardiac function and free-breathing sequences allow identification of haemodynamic changes, such as reduced chamber size or collapse associated with pericardial fluid. In cardiac tamponade there could also be dilatation of the inferior vena cava and free breathing sequences may demonstrate abnormal septal motion. The classic right heart signs of ventricular and atrial collapse if present should prompt referral for treatment [26] (⊃ Fig. 37.16).

Other modalities

The pericardium is not seen during angiography and because of the 'windowing' used the cardiac silhouette is also not as clear as on chest radiography. Therefore changes in size of the cardiac silhouette that may be present in pericardial effusions are more subtle. In iatrogenic pericardial effusion following intervention on a coronary artery the pericardial space may become evident due to accumulation of contrast around the heart. During pericardiocentesis, contrast can be purposefully injected to identify the pericardial space and fluoroscopy can be used to guide needle position.

Pericardial effusions are not seen on nuclear perfusion imaging. FDG-PET is not indicated for investigation of pericardial disease but as FDG-PET measures metabolic activity, changes in uptake within the pericardium can occur [27] in pericardial tumours or in chronic inflammatory pericarditis. It is usually difficult to distinguish uptake from that seen in the myocardium. However, this may be simplified if a pericardial effusion is present and separates the peri- and myocardium [28].

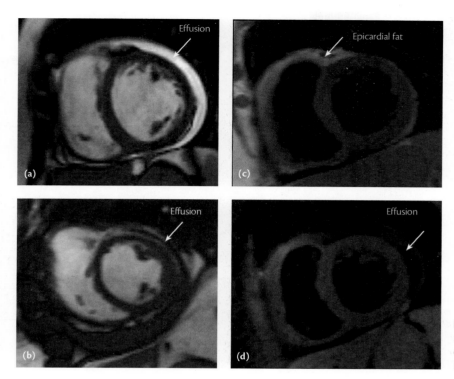

Fig. 37.13 Four short-axis cardiovascular magnetic resonance views demonstrate the appearances of an effusion on (a and b) SSFP-imaging and T1 turbo spin echo image without (c) and with (d) fat saturation.

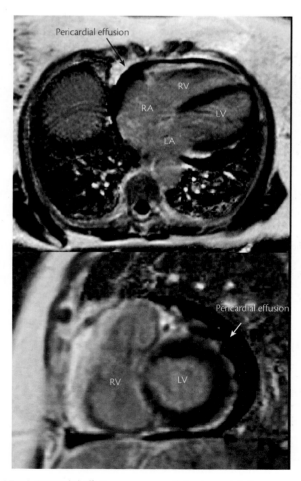

Fig. 37.14 Pericardial effusion appearances following gadolinium on a cardiovascular magnetic resonance inversion recovery sequence.
Images courtsey of Oxford Centre for Clinical Magnetic Resonance Research.

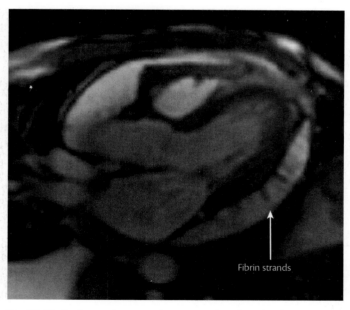

Fig. 37.15 Cardiovascular magnetic resonance SSFP four-chamber (horizontal long-axis) view demonstrates the high intensity effusion and strands of low intensity along the lateral wall consistent with fibrin strands.
Images courtsey of Oxford Centre for Clinical Magnetic Resonance Research.

Pericardiocentesis

Overview

Pericardiocentesis is used to drain pericardial effusions for diagnostic purposes or to treat cardiac tamponade. The aims of pericardiocentesis are to enter the pericardial space with a needle and insert a drain via a Seldinger technique. Imaging can help

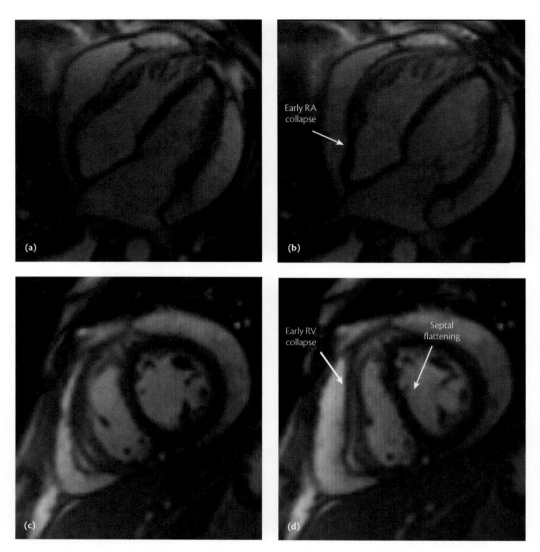

Fig. 37.16 Cardiovascular magnetic resonance SSFP views of a large global effusion with evidence of mild right atrial collapse in end-diastole and right ventricular collapse in late systole. Images courtesy of Oxford Centre for Clinical Magnetic Resonance Research.

by guiding the insertion of the needle, confirming position of the needle or drain within the pericardial space, and monitoring removal of fluid.

Chest X-ray and angiography

Fluoroscopy can aid pericardial drainage because the needle is clearly seen on screening. The needle can be followed according to the landmarks of the ribs and spines to a position where the pericardial space should be present.

Echocardiography

Echocardiography is the modality of choice for imaging-guided pericardiocentesis. Pericardiocentesis is usually done from subcostal or apical positions and echocardiography allows pre-procedural evaluation of location and depth of fluid in these positions [5]. In particular, for an apical approach, the operator can search for the position where the effusion is closest to the chest wall and reaches its largest width. During the procedure the angle of the echo probe used to achieve images can be used as

a guide to the angle to be used for the needle. Imaging can then be maintained from the alternative position (apical or subcostal) and the needle can sometimes be seen advancing into pericardial space. If it is not clear whether the needle is in the pericardial space then injection of a small amount of agitated saline contrast down the needle should be seen filling the pericardial space (➲ Fig. 37.17).

Conclusions

The pericardium has a key function to maintain cardiac efficiency and function by allowing free movement of the heart. Impairment of this normal function due to the accumulation of a pericardial effusion can lead to a range of symptoms from mild discomfort to haemodynamic collapse. Presentation with pericardial effusion can present a diagnostic conundrum because of the similarities between symptoms and other pathologies; for example, chest pain of pericardial or cardiac origin, breathlessness of chest disease, heart failure, or cardiomyopathies. Multi-modality cardiovascular

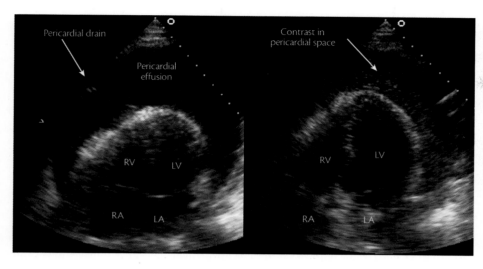

Fig. 37.17 2D-echocardiography apical 4-chamber echocardiography views acquired during pericardiocentesis. In (a) a part of the pericardial drain is just visible and in (b) agitated saline contrast has been injected down the pericardiocentesis needle to confirm position of the needle within the pericardial space.
Images courtesy of Radiology Department, John Radcliffe Hospital, Oxford.

imaging is an essential and incredibly powerful tool to aid diagnosis. Echocardiography provides the modality of choice for immediate, simple assessment of pericardial effusions and evaluation of possible cardiac tamponade. Furthermore, echocardiography can guide intervention and provide follow up assessments. Cardiac CT and MR provide means for detailed investigation of localized effusions and also of wider pathology that may be related to the presence of a pericardial effusion.

References

1. Stephen WM. Imaging pericardial disease. *Radiol Clin North Am* 1989; 27: 1113.
2. Breen JF. Imaging of the pericardium. *J Thorac Imaging* 2001; 16 (1): 47–54.
3. Kim JS, Kim HH Yoon Y. Imaging of pericardial diseases. *Clin Radiol* 2007; 62 (7): 626–31.
4. Camm A, Luscher T, Serruys PW. *ESC Textbook of Cardiovascular Medicine.* 2006, Oxford: Blackwell Publishing.
5. Leeson P, Mitchell A, Becher H. *Echocardiography*, 2nd edn. 2012, Oxford: Oxford University Press.
6. Merce, J, et al. Correlation between clinical and Doppler echocardiographic findings in patients with moderate and large pericardial effusion: implications for the diagnosis of cardiac tamponade. *Am Heart J* 1999; 138 (4 Pt 1): 759–64.
7. Yared, K, et al. Multimodality imaging of pericardial diseases. *JACC Cardiovasc Imaging* 2010; 3 (6): 650–60.
8. Schairer JR, et al. A systematic approach to evaluation of pericardial effusion and cardiac tamponade. *Cardiol Rev* 2011; 19 (5): 233–8.
9. Weinreb JC, et al. ACR clinical statement on noninvasive cardiac imaging. *J Am Coll Radiol* 2005. 2 (6): 471–7.
10. Carsky EW, Azimi F, Mauceri R. Epicardial fat sign in the diagnosis of pericardial effusion. *JAMA* 1980; 244 (24): 2762–4.
11. Feigenbaum H. Echocardiographic examination of the left ventricle. *Circulation* 1975; 51 (1): 1–7.
12. Feigenbaum H, Armstrong WF, Ryan T. *Feigenbaum's Echocardiography*, 6th edn. 2004, Philadelphia: Lippincott Williams and Wilkins.
13. Otto CM. *Textbook of Clinical Echocardiography*, 3rd edn. 2004, Philadelphia: Saunders.
14. Levy-Ravetch M, et al. CT of the pericardial recesses. *AJR* 1985; 144: 707–14.
15. Lopez Costa I, Bhalla S. Computed tomography and magnetic resonance imaging of the pericardium. *Semin Roentgenol* 2008; 43 (3): 234–45.
16. Wang ZJ, et al. CT and MR imaging of pericardial disease. *Radiographics* 2003; 23 Spec No: S167–80.
17. Jeudy J, White CS. Cardiac magnetic resonance imaging: techniques and principles. *Semin Roentgenol* 2008; 43 (3): 173–82.
18. Mulvagh SL, et al. Usefulness of nuclear magnetic resonance imaging for evaluation of pericardial effusions, and comparison with two-dimensional echocardiography. *Am J Cardiol* 1989; 64 (16): 1002–9.
19. Lardo AC, et al. *Cardiovascular Magnetic Resonance: Established and Emerging Applications.* 2003, London: Taylor and Francis.
20. Misselt AJ, et al. MR imaging of the pericardium. *Magn Reson Imaging Clin N Am* 2008; 16 (2): 185–99, vii.
21. Leeson CP, et al. Atrial pathology in cardiac amyloidosis: evidence from ECG and cardiovascular magnetic resonance. *Eur Heart Journal* 2006; 27: 1670.
22. Smith WH, et al. Magnetic resonance evaluation of the pericardium. *Br J Radiol* 2001; 74 (880): 384–92.
23. Maksimovic R, et al. Magnetic resonance imaging in pericardial diseases. Indications and diagnostic value. *Herz* 2006; 31 (7): 708–14.
24. Sechtem U, Tscholakoff D, Higgins CB. MRI of the abnormal pericardium. *AJR Am J Roentgenol* 1986; 147 (2): 245–52.
25. Sechtem U, Tscholakoff D, Higgins CB. MRI of the normal pericardium. *AJR Am J Roentgenol* 1986; 147 (2): 239–44.
26. Olson MC, et al. Computed tomography and magnetic resonance imaging of the pericardium. *Radiographics* 1989; 9 (4): 633–49.
27. Strobel K, Schuler R, Genoni M. Visualization of pericarditis with fluoro-deoxy-glucose-positron emission tomography/computed tomography. *Eur Heart J* 2008; 29 (9): 1212.
28. Leeson P. *Cardiovascular Imaging.* 2011, Oxford: Oxford University Press.

➲ **For additional multimedia materials please visit the online version of the book** (⬆ http://www.esciacc.oxfordmedicine.com)

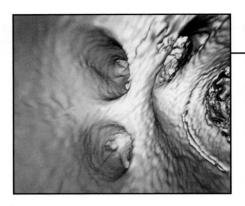

CHAPTER 38

Constrictive pericarditis

Jérôme Garot and Frank Rademakers

Contents

Introduction

Constrictive pericarditis (CP) and restrictive cardiomyopathy (RCMP) have some similarities in presentation but their pathophysiology and therapeutic approach are quite different [1]. It is imperative that the correct diagnosis be made before installing a therapy, which, if applied for the wrong diagnosis, could be deleterious. In some patients, various components of fluid accumulation, constriction, and abnormalities in myocardial compliance and function can coexist, making the diagnostic process difficult [2]. To better understand the contribution of various imaging modalities, the pathophysiology and the clinical presentations will be reviewed. Since some transitions exist, tamponade will also be covered [3]. Most diagnostic signs on imaging are direct illustrations and consequences of the underlying pathophysiology.

Pathophysiology of the pericardium

The normal human pericardium is a relatively stiff sac, enveloping the heart and returning on itself at the origins of the vessels; it is attached to the adventitia of the arteries and to the sternum, vertebral column, and diaphragm [4]. The pressure in the pericardium is between 0 and 3 mmHg and slightly less than right atrial pressure (RAP). As such, it counteracts the distension pressure of the cardiac cavities and mostly so for the thin-walled, low pressure right heart, where the structure of the wall itself resists volume and shape changes less and where the relaxation process in the myocardium contributes less to overall filling than in the left heart (suction pump). The driving force for the expansion of a heart cavity is the active relaxation generating a negative force during the brief, early diastolic suction period and the difference between the intra-cavitary and pericardial pressure during the passive dilation or filling period and during active atrial contraction.

When fluid accumulates in the pericardium, the pressure in the pericardium increases, the transmural diastolic distending pressures of the atria drop to zero (tamponade sets in), and the increased atrial pressures equalize. As the effect of a decreased distension pressure is more pronounced in the right heart, a compression of the right atrium and ventricle occurs at the time of lowest intra-cavitary pressure, i.e. early diastole, impeding early filling, and consequently limiting total filling volume and ultimately stroke volume; with increasing pericardial volume and pressure, the atrium remains collapsed throughout diastole. Left ventricular (LV) filling and output become compromised by the decreased right-heart output and the increased left–right interaction. The increase in pericardial pressure depends on the speed of fluid accumulation, since the pressure–volume relation of the pericardium is relatively flat in the first part, but becomes exponential thereafter. With slow accumulation, the pericardium can grow and adapt to accommodate large amounts of fluid with only a small increase in pressure. Every acute intervention that increases the venous return to the heart increases total heart volume and, as such, intra-pericardial total volume and pressure; if this occurs on the steep portion of the pericardial

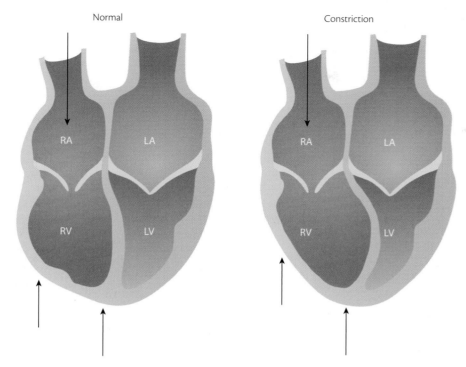

Fig. 38.1 Ventricular interdependence in normal conditions during inspiration with increased filling of the right heart and in pericardial constraint leading to a shift of the inter-ventricular septum toward the left.

P–V relation, it will ensue in an upward shift of the LV diastolic P–V relation. On the other hand, a significant hypovolaemia with overall small heart cavities can mask the haemodynamic effects and clinical signs of tamponade.

Since the left and right heart occupy the pericardial sac together, a ventricular interdependence or coupling exists, i.e. the more space one side of the heart occupies, less is available for the other side, leading to increased diastolic pressures in the contralateral part (⊃ Fig. 38.1). This interdependence is present in normal circumstances during breathing and is exaggerated by

fluid accumulation in the pericardium or by pericardial stiffening. The depth and speed of respiration also significantly determine the size of the effect on cardiac haemodynamics and should be recorded during imaging. During inspiration, pressure in the thorax and the pericardium drops, and flow toward (inferior vena cava; IVC) and from the right heart increases (with an increased total right heart volume and pressure), while the reverse occurs on the left side (when exaggerated this causes pulsus paradoxus); during expiration, the opposite changes take place (⊃ Fig. 38.2). While cardiac tamponade counteracts distension pressures throughout

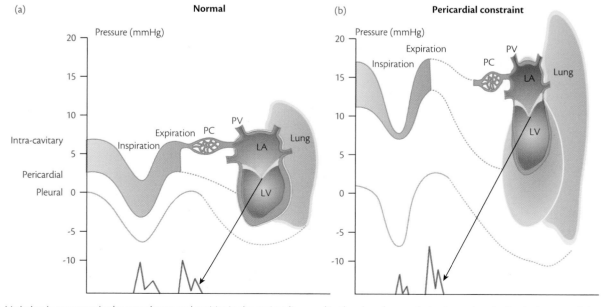

Fig. 38.2 Variation in pressures in the vasculature and cavities in the pericardium and in the pleural space during in- and expiration in the normal situation (a) and in conditions of pericardial constraint (b); in (a), the gradients remain the same with a constant transmural filling pressure and inflow over the mitral valve as a consequence; in (b), the gradients vary with a decrease during inspiration and a subsequent variation in the mitral inflow pattern.

the entire filling period, the restraint in CP is nearly absent during early filling when overall cardiac volume is lowest, but rapidly increases thereafter, giving rise to the characteristic square root sign on LV pressure traces. Another characteristic of CP is the belated transmission of changes in intra-thoracic pressures to the intra-pericardial structures, creating the exaggerated acute changes in filling gradients at the onset of the inspiratory and expiratory motions. During inspiration, the increased venous return is not coupled to the characteristic drop in RA pressure and systemic venous pressure may actually increase, i.e. Kussmaul's sign in the superior caval vein (SVC) (➲ Fig. 38.3). In patients with CP, the pulmonary wedge pressure is influenced by the inspiratory fall in thoracic pressure, while the LV pressure is shielded from respiratory pressure variations by the stiff pericardium. Thus, inspiration lowers the pulmonary wedge pressure and, presumably, left atrial pressure (LAP), but not LV diastolic pressure, thereby decreasing the pressure gradient for ventricular filling accounting for the decline in filling efficiency. Reciprocal changes occur in the volume of right ventricular filling (➲ Fig. 38.4). These reciprocal changes are mediated by the ventricular septum, not by increased systemic venous return. When the pressure gradient

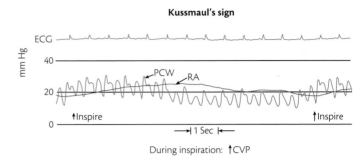

Kussmaul's sign

During inspiration: ↑CVP

Fig. 38.3 Kussmaul's sign with a paradoxical increase of right atrial pressure during early inspiration due to the belated transmission of decreased intra-thoracic pressure to the intra-pericardial structures. *RA*, right atrium; *CVP*, central venous pressure; *PCW*, pulmonary capillary wedge pressure.

between the left and right heart shifts, the inter-atrial and inter-ventricular septum can move; in normal conditions, the pressures on the left are higher than on the right, leading to the characteristic shape of the septa; with CP, a sudden shift of the prevailing pressure gradient between left and right ventricle during early diastole causes a septal bouncing motion that is characteristic

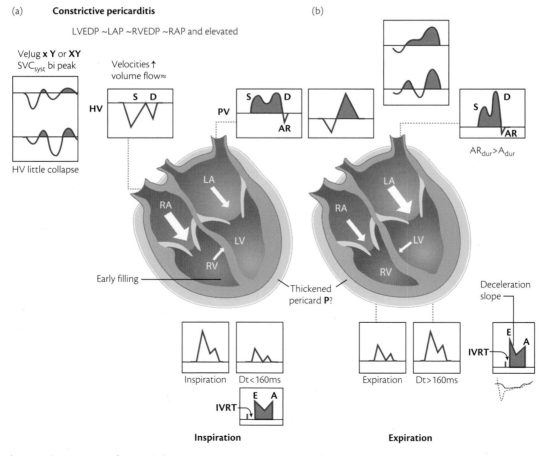

Fig. 38.4 Haemodynamic characteristics of pericardial constriction. Various pressures and flow patterns are illustrated during inspiration (a) and expiration (b). *RA*, right atrium; *LA*, left atrium; *RV*, right ventricle; *LV*, left ventricle; *LVEDP*, left ventricular end-diastolic pressure; *LAP*, left atrial pressure; *RVEDP*, right ventricular end-diastolic pressure; *RAP*, right atrial pressure; *SVC*, superior vena cava; *HV*, hepatic vein; *VeJug*, jugular vein; *PV*, pulmonary vein; *diast*, diastole; *P*, pressure; *s*, systolic; *d*, diastolic; *AR*, atrial reversal; *dur*, duration; *E*, early filling velocity; *A*, atrial contraction velocity; *Dt*, deceleration slope of early filling velocity; *IVRT*, isovolumic relaxation time.

Table 38.1 Common and distinct pathophysiologic features in CP and RCMP

Pathophysiologic features	CP	RCMP
Non-dilated ventricles	+	+
Ventricular filling limited to early diastole	+	+
High venous pressures (dilated IVC with reduced respiratory collapse)	+	+
Ventricular dip-and-plateau	+	+
Large atria	–	+
Pronounced respiratory filling changes (increased interdependence)	+	–
No or less respiratory variation in left-sided flows	–	+
Immediate haemodynamic variation on 1st beat after onset of respiratory variation	+	–
Hepatic vein flow reversal on atrial contraction	+	–
– more pronounced in expiration	–	+
– more pronounced in inspiration	+	–
Prolonged IVRT variable with respiration	–	+
Low myocardial early diastolic velocities (e')		

for this condition. Since respiratory interdependence in CP decreases at higher absolute LA pressures and with the severity of constriction, examining a patient in the upright position (decrease of filling pressures) can unmask interdependence. In comparison to CP, tamponade exhibits a more marked pulsus paradoxus and a fall in RAP with onset of inspiration (no Kussmaul's sign) because the intra-thoracic pressure changes are readily transmitted to the intra-cardiac cavities. CP must also be differentiated from RCMP, where the compliance problem resides within the myocardium (⊃ Table 38.1) (⊃ Fig. 38.5) [5].

Clinical findings

History

CP is the end result of a number of diseases that cause pericardial inflammation (⊃ Table 38.2). Tuberculous pericarditis traditionally accounted for most cases, but post-viral pericarditis, cardiac surgery, thoracic radiotherapy, and idiopathic diseases are now the most common causes [6]. Morphologically, there is

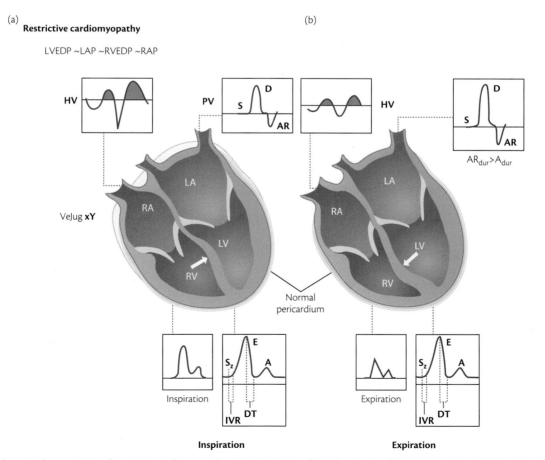

Fig. 38.5 Haemodynamic characteristics of restrictive cardiomyopathy during inspiration (a) and expiration (b). *RA*, right atrium; *LA*, left atrium; *RV*, right ventricle; *LV*, left ventricle; *LVEDP*, left ventricular end-diastolic pressure; *LAP*, left atrial pressure; *RVEDP*, right ventricular end-diastolic pressure; *RAP*, right atrial pressure; *SVC*, superior vena cava; *HV*, hepatic vein; *VeJug*, jugular vein; *PV*, pulmonary vein; *diast*, diastole; *P*, pressure; *s*, systolic; *d*, diastolic; *AR*, atrial reversal; *dur*, duration; *E*, early filling velocity; *A*, atrial contraction velocity; *Dt*, deceleration slope of early filling velocity; *IVRT*, isovolumic relaxation time.

Table 38.2 Aetiologies of pericarditis

Aetiologies
Idiopathic
Infectious (viral, tuberculous, bacterial or fungal)
Radiotherapy
Neoplasm
Autoimmune (systemic lupus erythematosus, rheumatoid arthritis, systemic sclerosis or ankylosing spondylitis)
Uraemia
Cardiac injury (surgery or trauma)
Myocardial infarction (acute or chronic (Dressler's syndrome))

thickening and fibrosis of the visceral and parietal pericardium, often with adhesions to the adjacent myocardium. About 50% of patients show some pericardial calcification [7]. A prior history of pericarditis (e.g. tuberculosis, infectious disease, connective tissue disease such as rheumatoid arthritis, malignancy), trauma, or cardiac surgery makes the diagnosis of CP more likely. A history of an infiltrative disease that may involve the heart muscle (e.g. amyloidosis, haemochromatosis, or sarcoidosis) or a therapy that can cause myocardial apoptosis and fibrous replacement (chemotherapy) favours the diagnosis of RCMP. Prior mantle radiation or cardiac surgery can result in both pericardial restriction and/or RCMP.

Physical examination

The clinical presentation of CP and RCMP may be strikingly similar. Patients may complain of dyspnoea, fatigue, peripheral oedema, weakness, and exercise intolerance. Physical examination is notable for jugular venous distention, pedal oedema, and in severe cases hepatomegaly, ascites, and anasarca. Using only a systemic venous pressure tracing or observing the venous neck pulse, it is not possible to distinguish between CP, RCMP, and tricuspid regurgitation with an enlarged compliant right atrium, right heart failure (e.g. due to right ventricular infarction or pulmonary hypertension), or circulatory overload with systemic congestion.

The contour of the jugular venous pulse in all these conditions is dominated by a deep, steep Y descent. The abrupt cessation of early diastolic filling may be manifested in either CP or RCMP by an early diastolic sound, which is called a pericardial knock in patients with CP.

Kussmaul's sign

The presence of Kussmaul's sign (◐ Fig. 38.3) is often sought in patients with suspected CP. Kussmaul's sign represents the lack of the expected inspiratory decline in jugular venous pressure due to a decrease in effective operative compliance of the right ventricle. In severe cases, the pressure actually increases with inspiration. In most cases of CP studied during quiet respiration, Kussmaul's sign takes a '*forme fruste*'; respiratory variation of the mean central venous pressure is absent rather than reversed. Importantly, Kussmaul's sign is also observed in right heart failure or systemic venous congestion of any cause, and in severe tricuspid regurgitation. Doppler flow measured in the superior vena cava or the jugular vein is the imaging correlate of this clinical sign. In contrast, the venous pulse in cardiac tamponade (with a continuous counteraction of filling) has a truly abnormal waveform characterized by the attenuation of the Y descent, or its replacement by an upwardly sloping segment. Kussmaul's sign is usually absent in tamponade.

Non-invasive imaging

Imaging modalities

Chest X-ray

Calcification of the pericardium (excepting scattered plaques) strongly suggests CP (◐ Fig. 38.6). However, the absence of calcification is compatible with either diagnosis, since pericardial stiffening can occur without calcification. Mild cardiomegaly on chest X-ray is common in both conditions, but more prominent in RCMP. It is due to atrial rather than ventricular enlargement.

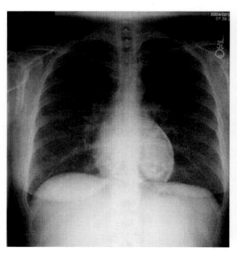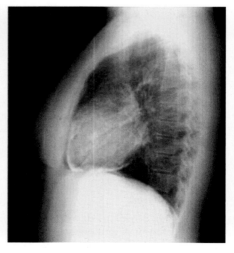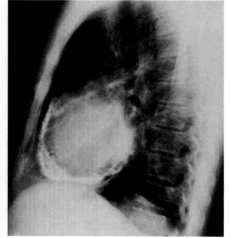

Fig. 38.6 Pericardial calcifications on chest X-ray.

Echocardiography

Echocardiography is the first-line investigation for assessing pericardial disease. It is a quick and simple test, widely and readily available. However, this examination is limited in its ability to assess the pericardium because of limited acoustic window, limited field of view, and its inability to image the entire pericardium and surrounding structures. The parietal pericardium produces one of the most strongly reflective echo-producing areas of the heart. Pericardial thickness exceeding 3–5 mm is highly suggestive of CP (⮌ Fig. 38.7). Transoesophageal echocardiography (TOE) can be useful to establish pericardial thickening [8]. However, constriction can also be caused by a thin tight peel of visceral pericardium. Thus, a normal appearing parietal pericardium does not rule out CP [9]. Patients who have had radiation therapy or open heart surgery may have areas of thickened pericardium that do not cause haemodynamic compromise.

CP exhibits the following features that are supportive of the diagnosis, but not necessarily diagnostic:

♦ Pericardial thickening and adhesion: lack of 'sliding'; heart motion transmitted to other organs ('tugging').

♦ Septal bounce—abrupt transient rightward movement.

♦ Plethoric IVC and unresponsive to respiration; dilated hepatic veins.

♦ Left and right ventricular size decreased; heart tubular in shape.

♦ Mild biatrial enlargement.

Septal bounce is the 2D counterpart of the M-mode septal notch and is often the first and best clue that constriction is present. Haemodynamic variations during respiration are easily obtained by echocardiography. The registration of the respiratory trace is important. In CP, haemodynamic alterations occur very quickly during the first beat after onset of in- or expiration.

It should be differentiated from less specific changes occurring after 2 or 3 beats that may be seen in COPD, or due to exaggerated respiratory motion. In comparison to CP, RCMP findings on 2D-echocardiography include absence of pericardial adhesion and thickening, normal or increased LV mass, increased myocardial reflectance, moderate to severe biatrial enlargement, frequent AV valve regurgitation, pulmonary hypertension, and AV valve excursion unaffected by respiration on M-mode.

An echo free space between pericardial layers is the hallmark of a pericardial effusion. Not all pericardial spaces represent effusion. Pericardial fat is the most common source of non-effusive pericardial space. Fat is absent above the right atrium in the 4-chamber view and just posterior to the base of the LV; low intensity echoes within the space are often present, and the motion of the pericardium is normal.

Pericardial tamponade has certain features on 2D-echocardiography: moderate or large effusion, right atrial expiratory collapse, RV expiratory compression collapse, plethoric IVC with diminished respiratory response, left atrial compression, small chamber volumes (especially the RV), and reciprocal size changes with respiration between RV and LV, and mitral and tricuspid valves. Many of the RV findings may be absent in a patient with significant pulmonary artery hypertension.

By its ability to view cardiac structures from any desired angulation, 3D transthoracic and TOE have shown promise and potential advantages over 2D in certain clinical situations. In particular, it offers incremental value in assessing the anatomy of the pericardium including echo densities within the effusion, fibrinous bands, and loculated effusions. It may be advantageous in post-cardiac surgery follow up of haemopericardium, quantification of the effusion, evaluation of pericardial masses, differentiating pericardial effusion from ascites and pleural effusion, and for the assessment of the extent of the disease in CP [10].

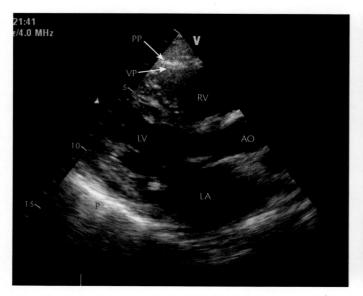

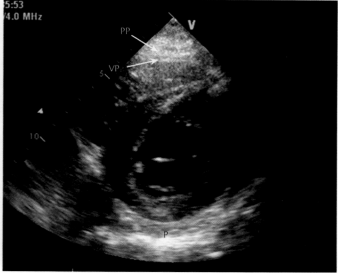

Fig. 38.7 2D echocardiogram with the bright echo signals at the anterior and posterior surface of the heart representing the calcified pericardial structures. *RV*, right ventricle; *LV*, left ventricle; *AO*, aorta; *P*, posterior pericardium; *PP*, parietal pericardium; *VP*, ventricular pericardium.

Doppler echocardiography

CP and RCMP have a number of Doppler characteristics in common. Most notable is a restrictive mitral inflow or ventricular filling pattern with striking E dominance and a short deceleration time, indicating early rapid filling in both entities. Colour M mode Doppler shows an excessively rapid transit of blood flow from the mitral and tricuspid (⊃ Fig. 38.8) orifice to the apex in CP, whereas the transit is much slower than normal in RCMP.

It is mainly the changes with respiration that can help in establishing the correct diagnosis between CP and RCMP [11, 12]. These include respiratory changes in the mitral E velocity (early diastolic LV filling increases with expiration) and reciprocal changes in right-sided Doppler flows (⊃ Fig. 38.9) [13]. The respiratory variations in ventricular filling velocity in RCMP are usually minimal (less than 10%), whereas patients with CP may have alterations as large as 30–40%, and almost always at least 15% with clinically significant constriction. However, the ventricular filling velocity is highly influenced by preload; thus, when LAP is greatly elevated, respiratory variation in this parameter may not be seen in CP. Reducing preload by head-up tilting may reveal the abnormality in such cases. The highly variable RR'-intervals make the diagnosis of respiratory variations in CP difficult when atrial fibrillation is present. Respiratory variation in mitral E velocity, like pulsus paradoxus, can also be present in patients with chronic obstructive pulmonary disease. These patients have a marked increase in inspiratory SVC systolic flow velocity on pulsed-wave

Doppler (⊃ Fig. 38.10), which is not seen to that extent in those with CP (⊃ Fig. 38.11). There are both false-positive and false-negative results when examining the respiratory variation of the mitral flow velocity to differentiate CP from RCMP. Measurement of other parameters may be helpful:

◆ In CP, there is a reversal of forward hepatic venous flow during expiration (⊃ Fig. 38.11), since the RV becomes less compliant as the LV fills more.

◆ Atrial and ventricular diastolic compliance are determined by the pericardium in CP. Blood can transfer easily from atrium to ventricle because no change in total cardiac volume occurs. By contrast, the ventricles of patients with RCMP are much stiffer than the atria. The atria typically enlarge considerably, and ultimately fail. Thus, late ventricular filling velocity is reduced, and diastolic flow reversal occurs; in comparison, flow reversal in CP occurs either in systole or in both systole and diastole [13].

Tissue doppler imaging

Pulsed-wave tissue Doppler imaging may help to distinguish between CP and RCMP by measuring the myocardial velocity gradient or strain [14]. Doppler myocardial velocities (⊃ Fig. 38.12), as measured from the LV posterior wall on the apical views in early diastole and during ventricular ejection, are significantly lower in patients with RCMP compared to those with CP and to normal controls [15]. The early diastolic Doppler tissue velocity at the mitral

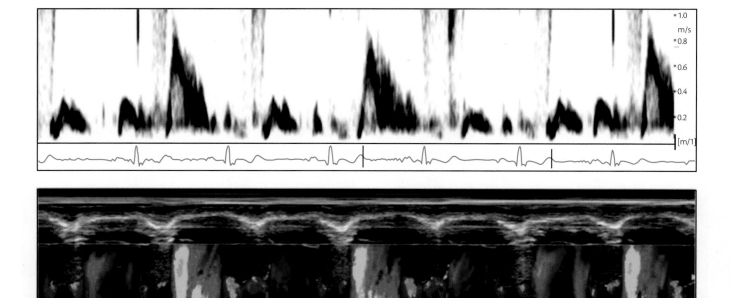

Fig. 38.8 Tricuspid Doppler flow and colour M-mode of the RV in a patient with CP. Flow in the RV is very fast and limited to early diastole; notice the large variation with respiration.

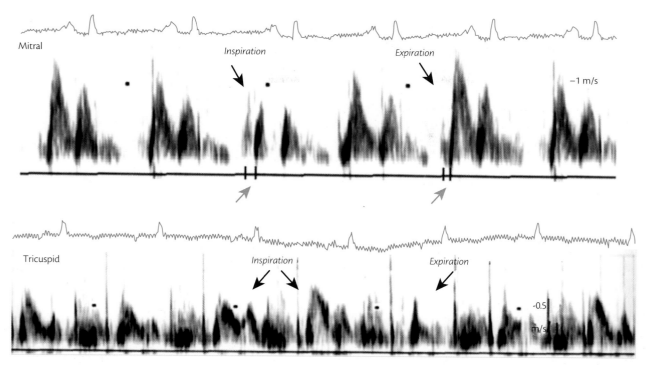

Fig. 38.9 The variation in mitral and tricuspid inflow with respiration in a patient with CP. Not only peak velocities but also deceleration varies considerably: mitral DT 120–70–160– 125 ms, tricuspid DT 140–180–100–140 ms.

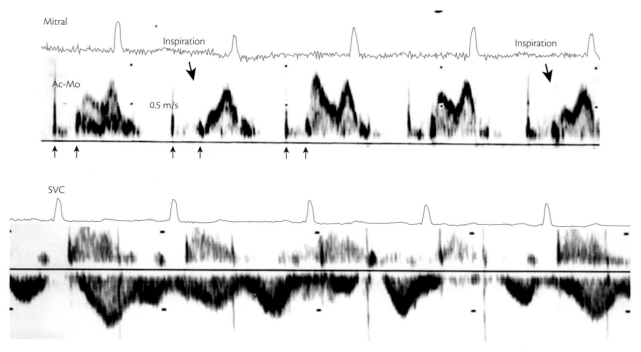

Fig. 38.10 A case of left ventricular hypertrophy and pulmonary obstructive disease: similar to CP, a significant variation exists in mitral inflow velocities with respiration; in contrast to CP, the flow in the superior vena cava also varies significantly with respiration.

annulus (e′) can be helpful in diagnosis [16]. The transmitral e′ is decreased in RCMP due to an intrinsic decrease in myocardial contraction and relaxation, while the transmitral e′ is increased in CP because the longitudinal movement of the myocardium is enhanced in compensation of the limited radial motion [17, 18].

A high e′ velocity (>12 cm/s) usually indicates CP, while a low e′ velocity (<8 cm/s) usually indicates restrictive myocardial disease. However, a large number of patients fall in between these numbers, and diagnosis remains unclear. In those patients, the time difference between mitral inflow and e′ can be helpful [19].

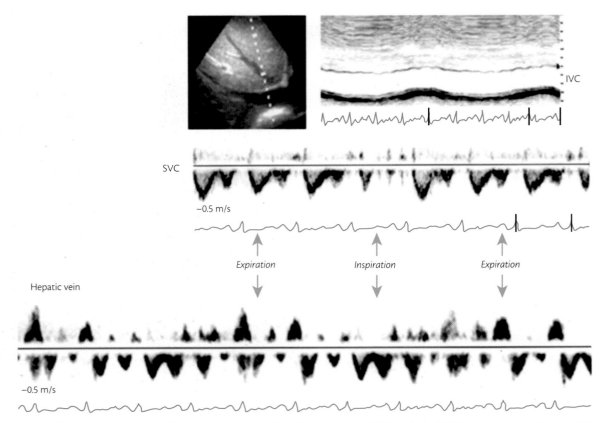

SVC

−0.5 m/s

Hepatic vein

−0.5 m/s

IVC

Expiration   *Inspiration*   *Expiration*

Fig. 38.11 Patient with CP shows the absence of respiratory variation of the inferior vena cava (IVC), the lack of significant variation of flow velocities of the superior vena cava (SVC), and the significant variation in the hepatic vein with flow reversal during expiration.

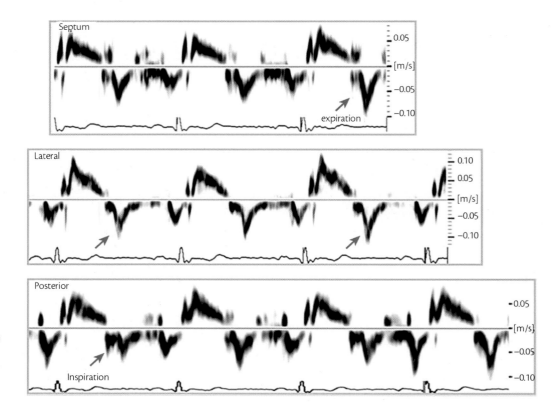

Fig. 38.12 Tissue Doppler traces in a patient with CP showing normal systolic velocities; diastolic velocities are in the non-diagnostic range and vary with respiration.

Speckle tracking echocardiography (STE)

By its ability to demonstrate distinct patterns of LV mechanics in CP and RCMP, STE may be a helpful adjunctive tool to echocardiography. Indeed, the deformation of the LV is constrained in the circumferential direction in CP, whereas it is more altered in the longitudinal direction in RCMP [20].

Cardiac CT

Cross-sectional imaging techniques (CT and CMR) are now widely accepted as the imaging modalities of choice for a comprehensive and accurate assessment of the pericardium. CT and CMR can provide 3D images of the heart and pericardium in any anatomical plane as well as structural and functional information. They are less operator-dependent than echocardiography and provide greater soft-tissue contrast. Unlike echo, they offer the capability of imaging the surrounding structures of the heart and the entire pericardium.

CT scanning of the heart gated to the cardiac cycle is extremely useful in the diagnosis of CP [21]. The pericardium is identified as a higher attenuation linear structure between the low density epicardial and mediastinal fat. The thickness of the pericardium is readily measured, with the upper limit of normal being 2 mm (⊃ Fig. 38.13). Enhancement of thickened pericardium can also be determined, which is useful in cases of suspected pericarditis or tumour infiltration. CT is particularly sensitive for identifying pericardial calcification that is often associated with CP (⊃ Fig. 38.14). The density of pericardial effusion can be

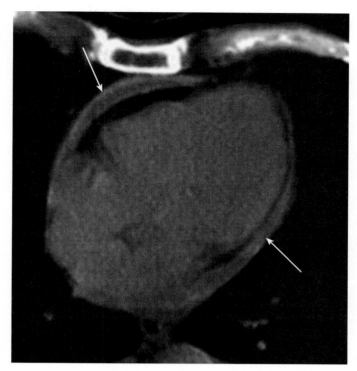

Fig. 38.13 CT scan in a patient with CP and severely thickened pericardium (8 mm, arrows).

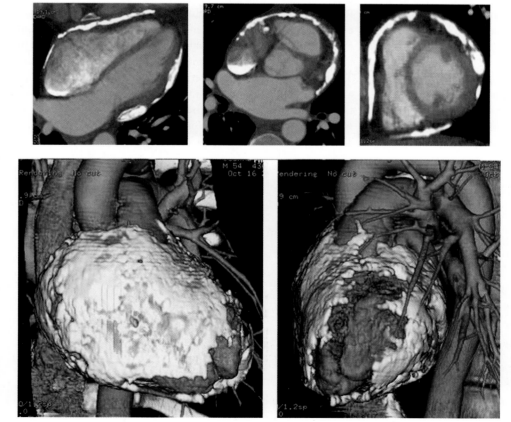

Fig. 38.14 CT scan in a patient with CP and severe pericardial calcifications (upper panel). 3D volume rendered images showing extensive calcifications (lower panel). Courtesy of Dr Erik Bouvier, ICPS, Massy.

determined, with a simple effusion having uniform low attenuation (with a Hounsfield unit of 0), whereas complex effusions, e.g. those resulting from blood or infection, are of increased density. CT has a short acquisition time of a few seconds. A normal appearance or non-visualization of the pericardium does not rule out the diagnosis of CP.

Other findings include dilatation of the inferior vena cava, deformed ventricular contours, and angulation of the ventricular septum. Ventricular functional parameters can be acquired with retrospective ECG-gated acquisitions, but are associated with an increased radiation dose. Failure of the immediately adjacent pulmonary structures to pulsate during the cardiac cycle, in the presence of a regionally or globally thickened pericardium, is suggestive of constrictive physiology.

CMR

The standard CMR protocol for investigating pericardial disease involves sequences to assess pericardial structure, ventricular function, flow, and tissue characterization.

Breath-hold ECG-gated fast spin echo segmented black blood T1-weighted images can accurately determine the thickness of the pericardium [22]. The use of a small field of view is recommended. Scanning in two perpendicular planes through the heart with no or a minimal gap between slices guarantees optimal depiction of the entire pericardium. These images are often of higher quality when a saturation band is applied to the anterior chest wall [23]. This reduces signal from the soft tissues in the chest wall and more clearly distinguishes the anterior pericardium from the RV free wall. The pericardium is composed of fibrous tissue and has a low MRI signal intensity (⊃ Fig. 38.15) [24]. It is therefore easily seen when adjacent to high signal fat. Typical morphologic features of CP include increased pericardial thickening (normal thickness is ≤2 mm, a pericardium ≥4 mm is highly suggestive of CP) (⊃ Fig. 38.16 and 38.17) and dilatation of the inferior vena cava (⊃ Fig. 38.18). In some studies, pericardial thickening on CMR of >4 mm differentiates CP from RCMP with a sensitivity and specificity of 88% and 100%, respectively [25]. Thickening may be patchy and consequently

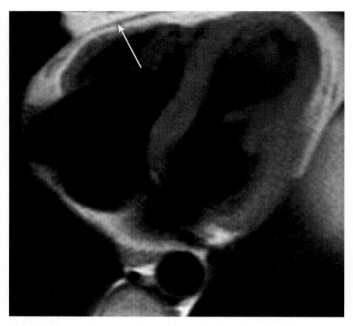

Fig. 38.15 Appearance of normal pericardium over the right ventricle on a CMR image. Arrow points to normal thickness pericardium.

imaging of the entire pericardium is needed. Pericardial thickening alone, in the absence of fitting physiology, should not lead to the diagnosis of CP. Morphological features that indirectly suggest a constrictive physiology may be present. Evidence of high ventricular filling pressures, such as dilatation of the vena cava, hepatic veins, coronary sinus, and atria, are seen in both CP and RCMP. Ascites and pleural effusions are common, reflecting elevated RAP. Spin-echo sequences are useful in the assessment of the contents of a pericardial effusion. A simple effusion is of low signal on T1-weighted images and uniform high signal on T2- and STIR (short tau inversion recovery) images. Complex and septated effusions can be identified by CMR more accurately than with CT. The signal of these complex effusions is variable, with haemorrhagic effusions often showing increased signal on T1- imaging.

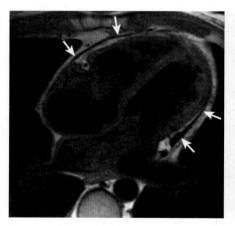
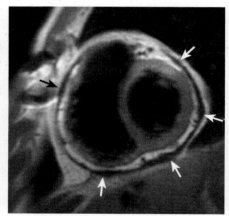
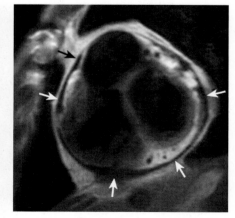

Fig. 38.16 Some typical features of CP on CMR: thickening of the pericardium (low signal intensity, arrows). Tissue with high intensity signal around pericardium is pericardial fat.

Cine MR diastole   Cine MR systole   T1 Spin echo

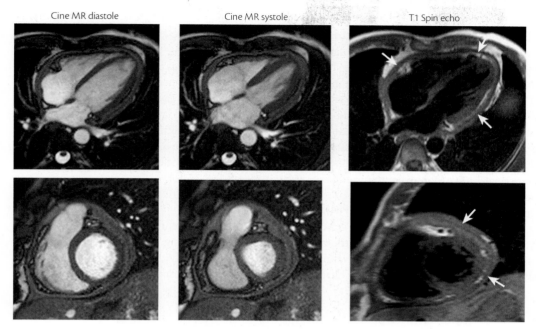

Fig. 38.17 Typical features of CP on cine CMR and black-blood *T1*-weighted spin echo CMR with thickened pericardium (arrows).

Steady-state free-precession gradient echo cine sequences allow for functional imaging that is crucial for the diagnosis of CP. More specific to CP is the distortion of the ventricular chambers leading to a tubular shape, particularly around the AV groove (⊃ Fig. 38.19). Real-time sequences provide rapidly acquired, relatively low-resolution cine images, which can be performed during free breathing, so that the effects of respiration on cardiac function can be determined. During inspiration, a negative intra-thoracic pressure causes increased systemic venous return to the RV, leading to a paradoxical displacement

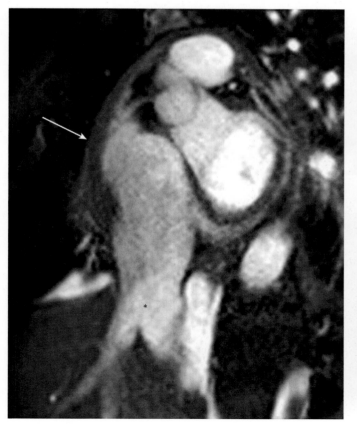

Fig. 38.18 Dilatation of the inferior vena cava (asterisk) and hepatic veins in a patient with CP and thickened pericardium (arrow).

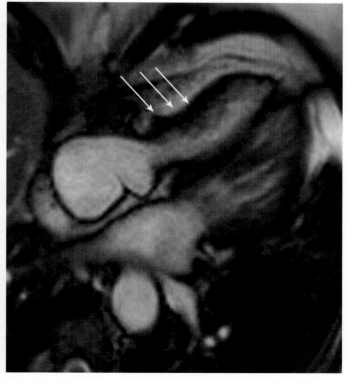

Fig. 38.19 Image extracted from a SSFP cine sequence in a patient with CP, showing a narrowed, tubular shaped right ventricle, particularly around the atrio-ventricular groove (arrows).

of the septum towards the LV (septal bounce) (➲ Fig. 38.20) [26].Conversely, during expiration, pulmonary venous return will be increased and LV filling will be preferred, allowing normalization of inter-ventricular septal position. In some studies, this finding differentiates CP from RCMP with a sensitivity of 81%, specificity of 100%, and a positive predictive value of 100% [27]. More recently, other functional parameters directly driven from the exaggerated ventricular interdependence have been proposed [28]. Pericardial mobility can also be assessed with high spatial and temporal resolution, and is appealing to differentiate normal from rigid pericardium. Moreover, the restricted expansion of the myocardium during cardiac filling abutting against the stiff pericardium can be well appreciated. These issues may be important in diagnosing patients with minimally or non-thickened CP. Pericardial thickness should not be measured on cine CMR images. Mainly because of motion artefact, the limits of spatial resolution and chemical-shift

artefact that may occur at the pericardial fat–fluid interface, the pericardium can appear thicker on cine imaging than on black-blood spin-echo images.

In CP, the pericardium is seen as a rigid, non-compliant structure with adhesions between the pericardial layers and the adjacent myocardium. CMR tagging may be helpful by showing those adhesions between the epicardial layers of the myocardium and the fibrotic pericardium [29], resulting in the lack of myocardial slippage well characterized by the lack of deformation of the tag lines at the interface between myocardium and pericardium during the cardiac cycle (➲ Fig. 38.21).

Phase-contrast flow imaging
Velocity-encoded CMR allows accurate assessment of flow across the atrioventricular valves. Owing to high atrial pressure, the ventricles fill very rapidly in early diastole upon opening of the mitral and tricuspid valves. If present, CP then causes an abrupt

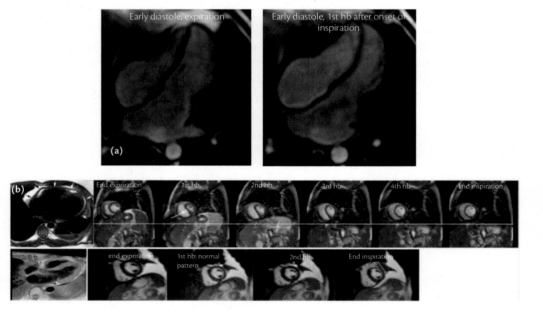

Fig. 38.20 (a) Real-time cine MR images in the 4-chamber view during early diastole in a patient with CP. Note the marked septal bounce occurring on the first heart beat (hb) after the onset of inspiration. (b) Variation in septal shape with respiration as measured with real-time CMR in a patient with CP (top) and a patient with RCMP (bottom). Notice the immediate septal bounce with the onset of inspiration in CP, which disappears by end inspiration; no such shape change occurs in RCMP.

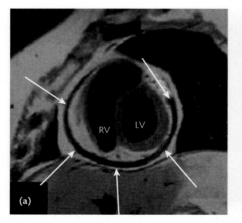
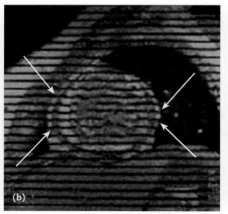
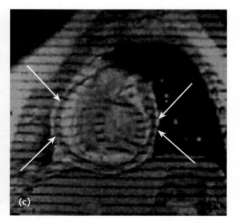

Fig. 38.21 CMR study of a patient with CP. (a) The thickened pericardium (arrows); (b) and (c) are tagged images; arrows point to uninterrupted tag lines at the level of the pericardium, showing the adhesion of the epi- and pericardial structures.

T1-weighted spin echo   LGE-CMR

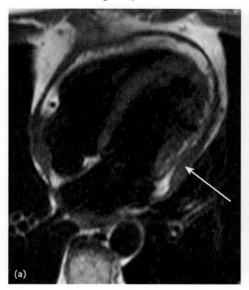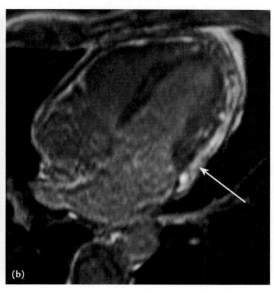

Fig. 38.22 *T1*-weighted black-blood CMR in a patient with active tuberculous disease, pericardial thickening (a, arrow) and fitting physiology of CP. Notice the enhancement of the pericardium on contrast-enhanced CMR (b, arrow), indicative of ongoing pericardial inflammatory process.

cessation of ventricular filling. This is manifest on phase-contrast imaging as a dominant E wave in early diastole and a very small or absent A wave in late diastole.

Late gadolinium enhanced (LGE) CMR

LGE CMR can be used to depict late enhancement of the pericardium that is indicative of ongoing focal or diffuse inflammatory processes (➲ Fig. 38.22). Along with biological inflammatory markers, this parameter has recently been proposed for the prediction of the reversibility of sub-acute CP after anti-inflammatory medical therapy [30].

In difficult cases, particularly when there are multiple potential aetiologies for heart failure, invasive cardiac catheterization may be required for diagnosis. Elevation and equalization of diastolic filling pressures occur in patients with CP. The dip-and-plateau configuration of diastolic ventricular pressures (the square root sign) corresponds to a rapid early filling, aided by augmented suction followed by a hampered further filling caused by rapidly increasing pressures. These haemodynamic alterations may also occur in other cardiac disorders, but their presence is mandatory

for the diagnosis of CP. Diastolic equalization may not be present in patients with constriction and a low volume state. In these patients, the cardiac output will be low. Therefore, the presence of normal cardiac output with normal filling pressures precludes the presence of haemodynamically significant CP.

Clinical syndromes

There are several presentations of CP that do not have the typical features [31].

Effusive CP

The pericardial cavity is typically obliterated in patients with CP. Thus, even the normal amount of pericardial fluid is absent. However, pericardial effusion may be present in some cases (➲ Fig. 38.23). In this setting, the scarred pericardium not only constricts the cardiac volume, but can also put pericardial fluid under increased pressure, leading to signs suggestive of cardiac tamponade. This combination is called effusive CP [32]. The diagnosis of effusive CP often becomes apparent during

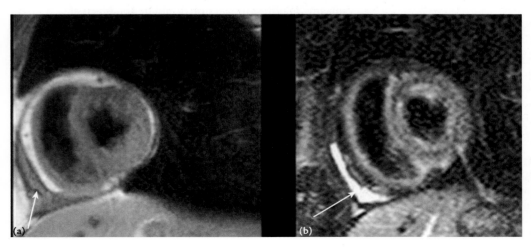

Fig. 38.23 Effusive CP. Arrow points to low signal thickened pericardium on black blood *T1*-weighted spin echo image (a). Arrow points to high signal pericardial effusion on short tau inversion-recovery black blood *T2*-weighted spin echo image (b).

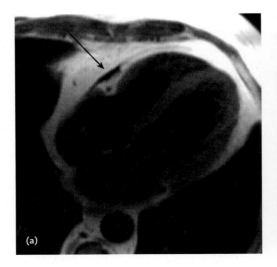
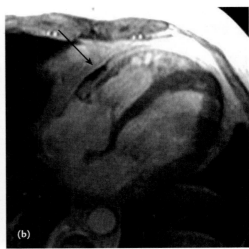

Fig. 38.24 Focal pericardial thickening (arrows) in a patient with clinical features of right-sided constriction (*T1*-weighted spin echo (a), cine CMR (b)).

pericardiocentesis in patients initially considered to have uncomplicated cardiac tamponade [32]. Indeed, unexpected persistence of the v wave of RAP is a clue to the possibility of effusive CP. After pericardiocentesis, despite lowering of the pericardial pressure to near zero, persistence of elevated RAP suggests effusive CP, defined by the failure of the RAP to fall by 50% or to a level below 10 mmHg. Some clinical clues suggest that a patient with manifestations of CP may actually have effusive CP:

♦ Pulsus paradoxus is often present; this finding is uncommon in classical CP because the inspiratory decline in intra-thoracic pressure is not transmitted to the right heart chambers.

♦ A pericardial knock is absent.

♦ The Y descent is less marked than expected.

♦ Kussmaul's sign is frequently absent.

CP without pericardial thickening

Up to 18% of patients with surgically proven CP have no evidence of significant pericardial thickening (≤2 mm) [9]. The most common causes of constriction in this group are cardiac surgery, irradiation, previous infarction, and idiopathic causes. Showing the typical haemodynamic features of constriction is, therefore, important. Also, the lack of myocardial slippage on CMR tagging may be very helpful (⊃ Fig. 38.21) [29].

Regional CP

A regional fluid accumulation, pericardial adhesion, or a combination (effusive constrictive) can be very difficult to diagnose with

haemodynamic features limited to the underlying cavity, rather than the entire heart and often occurring over the RV (tubular-shaped). CMR is generally the best way to identify localized thickening (⊃ Fig. 38.24) and adhesion (tagging).

Transient CP

Some patients with acute CP appear to resolve on follow-up echocardiography and clinical assessment. In one series, 17% of patients showed resolution over 2–3 months [33]. Although most patients with acute pericarditis proceed to complete resolution, some of them may have transient constrictive physiology, whereas others develop chronic CP. In acute presentations, it may therefore be worth pursuing a period of medical therapy before proceeding to surgery.

Conclusion

The diagnosis of CP generally requires both the demonstration of an appropriate physiology and evidence of pericardial thickening. Differential diagnosis in pericardial disease remains difficult and challenging to the clinician. When a discrepancy exists between clinical findings and haemodynamic evaluation with imaging, multiple modalities should be combined and, if a very low or very high atrial pressure is suspected, an intervention to increase or lower this pressure can be required to unmask characteristic findings during respiration and with respect to ventricular interdependence.

References

1. Maisch B, Seferovic PM, Ristic AD, et al. Guidelines on the diagnosis and management of pericardial diseases executive summary; The Task Force on the diagnosis and management of pericardial diseases of the European Society of Cardiology. *Eur Heart J* 2004; 25: 587–610.
2. Hancock EW. Differential diagnosis of restrictive cardiomyopathy and constrictive pericarditis. *Heart* 2001; 86: 343–9.
3. Goldstein JA. Cardiac tamponade, constrictive pericarditis, and restrictive cardiomyopathy. *Curr Probl Cardiol* 2004; 29: 503–67.
4. Shabetai R. *The Pericardium*. Norwell, MA: Kluwer; 2003: 227.
5. Lavine SJ. Genesis of the restrictive filling pattern: pericardial constraint or myocardial restraint. *J Am Soc Echocardiogr* 2004; 17: 152–60.

6. Ling L, Oh J, Schaff H, et al. Constrictive pericarditis in the modern era: evolving clinical spectrum and impact on outcome after pericardiectomy. *Circulation* 1999; 100: 1380–6.

7. O'Leary SM, Williams PL, Williams MP, et al. Imaging the pericardium: appearances on ECG-gated 64-detector row cardiac computed tomography. *Br J Radiol* 2010; 83: 194–205.

8. Ling LH, Oh JK, Tei C, et al. Pericardial thickness measured with transesophageal echocardiography: feasibility and potential clinical usefulness. *J Am Coll Cardiol* 1997; 29: 1317–23.

9. Talreja DR, Edwards WD, Danielson GK, et al. Constrictive pericarditis in 26 patients with histologically normal pericardial thickness. *Circulation* 2003; 108: 1852–7.

10. Scohy TV, Maat AP, McGhie J, ten Cate FJ, Bogers AJ. Three-dimensional transesophageal echocardiography: diagnosing the extent of pericarditis constrictiva and intraoperative surgical support. *J Card Surg* 2009; 24: 305–8.

11. Hatle LK, Appleton CP, Popp RL. Differentiation of constrictive pericarditis and restrictive cardiomyopathy by Doppler echocardiography. *Circulation* 1989; 79: 357–70.

12. Hurrell DG, Nishimura RA, Higano ST, et al. Value of dynamic respiratory changes in left and right ventricular pressures for the diagnosis of constrictive pericarditis. *Circulation* 1996; 93: 2007–13.

13. Oh JK, Hatle LK, Seward JB, et al. Diagnostic role of Doppler echocardiography in constrictive pericarditis. *J Am Coll Cardiol* 1994; 23: 154–62.

14. McCall R, Stoodley PW, Richards DA, Thomas L. Restrictive cardiomyopathy vs. constrictive pericarditis: making the distinction using tissue Doppler imaging. *Eur J Echocardiogr* 2008; 9: 591–4.

15. Palka P, Lange A, Donnelly JE, Nihoyannopoulos P. Differentiation between restrictive cardiomyopathy and constrictive pericarditis by early diastolic doppler myocardial velocity gradient at the posterior wall. *Circulation* 2000; 102: 655–62.

16. Ha JW, Oh JK, Ling LH, et al. Annulus paradoxus: transmitral flow velocity to mitral annular velocity ratio is inversely proportional to pulmonary capillary wedge pressure in patients with constrictive pericarditis. *Circulation* 2001; 104: 976–8.

17. Ha JW, Ommen SR, Tajik AJ, et al. Differentiation of constrictive pericarditis from restrictive cardiomyopathy using mitral annular velocity by tissue Doppler echocardiography. *Am J Cardiol* 2004; 94: 316–9.

18. Garcia MJ, Rodriguez L, Ares M, Griffin BP, Thomas JD, Klein AL. Differentiation of constrictive pericarditis from restrictive cardiomyopathy: assessment of left ventricular diastolic velocities in longitudinal axis by Doppler tissue imaging. *J Am Coll Cardiol* 1996; 27: 108–14.

19. Choi EY, Ha JW, Kim JM, et al. Incremental value of combining systolic mitral annular velocity and time difference between mitral inflow and diastolic mitral annular velocity to early diastolic annular velocity for differentiating constrictive pericarditis from restrictive cardiomyopathy. *J Am Soc Echocardiogr* 2007; 20: 738–43.

20. Sengupta PP, Krishnamoorthy VK, Abhayaratna WP, et al. Disparate patterns of left ventricular mechanics differentiate constrictive pericarditis from restrictive cardiomyopathy. *JACC Cardiovasc Imaging* 2008; 1: 29–38.

21. Isner JM, Carter BL, Bankoff MS, et al. Differentiation of constrictive pericarditis from restrictive cardiomyopathy by computed tomographic imaging. *Am Heart J* 1983; 105: 1019–25.

22. Misselt AJ, Harris SR, Glockner J, Feng D, Syed IS, Araoz PA. MR imaging of the pericardium. *Magn Reson Imaging Clin N Am* 2008; 16: 185–99.

23. Bogaert J, Francone M. Cardiovascular magnetic resonance in pericardial disease. *J Cardiovasc Magn Reson* 2009; 11: 14.

24. Sechtem U, Tscholakoff D, Higgins CB. MRI of the normal pericardium. *AJR Am J Roentgenol* 1986; 147: 239–44.

25. Masui T, Finck S, Higgins CB. Constrictive pericarditis and restrictive cardiomyopathy: evaluation with MR imaging. *Radiology* 1992; 182: 369–73.

26. Francone M, Dymarkowski S, Kalantzi M, et al. Assessment of ventricular coupling with real-time cine MRI and its value to differentiate constrictive pericarditis from restrictive cardiomyopathy. *Eur Radiol* 2006; 16: 944–51.

27. Giori B, Mollett NRA, Dymarkowski S, Rademakers FA, Bogaert J. Assessment of ventricular septal motion in patients clinically suspected of constrictive pericarditis, using magnetic resonance imaging. *Radiology* 2003; 228: 417–24.

28. Anavekar NS, Wong BF, Foley TA, et al. Index of biventricular interdependence calculated using cardiac MRI: a proof of concept study in patients with and without constrictive pericarditis. *Int J Cardiovasc Imaging* 2013; 29: 363–9.

29. Kojima S, Yamada N, Goto Y. Diagnosis of constrictive pericarditis by tagged cine magnetic resonance imaging. *N Engl J Med* 1999; 341: 373–4.

30. Feng D, Glockner J, Kim K, et al. Cardiac magnetic resonance imaging pericardial late gadolinium enhancement and elevated inflammatory markers can predict the reversibility of constrictive pericarditis after antiinflammatory medical therapy: a pilot study. *Circulation* 2011; 124: 1830–7.

31. Sagrista-Sauleda J. Pericardial constriction: uncommon patterns. *Heart* 2004; 90: 257–8.

32. Sagrista-Sauleda J, Angel J, Sanchez A, Permanyer-Miralda G, Soler-Soler J. Effusive-constrictive pericarditis. *N Engl J Med* 2004; 350: 469–75.

33. Haley JH, Tajik AJ, Danielson GK, Schaff HV, Mulvagh SL, Oh JK. Transient constrictive pericarditis: causes and natural history. *J Am Coll Cardiol* 2004; 43: 271–5.

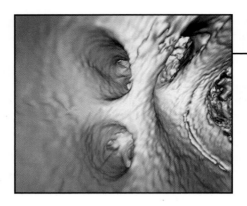

CHAPTER 39

Myocarditis

Heiko Mahrholdt, Ali Yilmaz,
and Udo Sechtem

Contents

Introduction

The symptoms and signs of myocarditis are non-specific. Thus, myocarditis is a differential diagnosis in many patients with heart complaints. As myocarditis may accompany common viral infections of the upper respiratory and gastrointestinal tracts, and mild ECG changes are not uncommon in such patients, the diagnosis needs to be considered in large patient cohorts. Establishing the correct diagnosis is of importance as the disease may lead to sudden cardiac death or dilated cardiomyopathy.

As clinical tools such as history taking, physical examination, blood tests, the ECG, and the chest X-ray are not sufficient to ascertain the diagnosis of myocarditis [1], additional information from cardiac imaging techniques, or endomyocardial biopsy, are necessary to confirm or exclude the disease. In daily clinical routine, however, the use of biopsy is limited to severely ill patients with reduced left ventricular function due to its invasiveness and potential complications. Thus, this chapter reviews how non-invasive cardiac imaging techniques can be used in clinical practice to diagnose myocarditis.

Imaging modalities other than cardiac magnetic resonance imaging

Echocardiography

Echocardiography still represents the first-choice imaging modality in patients with a clinical suspicion of myocarditis, since it offers the acquisition of comprehensive anatomic and functional data very quickly at the bedside of the patient. Especially in haemodynamically unstable patients in whom their clinical state precludes the application of other, potentially more accurate imaging modalities, such as cardiac magnetic resonance imaging, echocardiography is the most helpful imaging tool.

In the last years, new developments have broadened the armamentarium of echocardiographic methods: apart from traditional M-mode and 2-dimensional echocardiography, new techniques such as tissue Doppler, strain-rate imaging, or contrast-enhanced echocardiography have become available for evaluation of patients with clinical symptoms suggestive of myocarditis. Recently, longitudinal and circumferential strain parameters (measured by 2-dimensional speckle tracking echocardiography) were shown to be not only of diagnostic, but also prognostic value in young patients with suspected acute myocarditis [2, 3]: deterioration of LV function and overall event-free survival were significantly related to these measurements (◔ Fig. 39.1). However, the additional value of these new echocardiographic imaging techniques compared to established non-invasive imaging modalities such as CMR in patients with myocarditis is yet unknown and echocardiographic data in larger patient groups are not available. Using M-mode and 2-dimensional

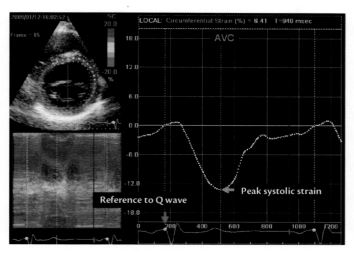

Fig. 39.1 Circumferential strain–time plot. Peak strain was measured on strain-time curve (white dots) with electrocardiographic reference. The strain zero reference was set at the Q-wave (red arrow). Aortic valve closure (AVC) was set at the vertical green dashed line using M-mode timing measurements. With permission from Khoo et al. [3].

echocardiography in patients with histologically proven myocarditis, a multitude of different echocardiographic patterns comprising dilated, hypertrophic, restrictive, or even ischaemic cardiomyopathy can be detected, but these echocardiographic features are non-specific in comparison to biopsy results [4].

However, echocardiography may help to differentiate between fulminant and non-fulminant acute myocarditis. While fulminant myocarditis is characterized by a rapid onset of illness with severe haemodynamic compromise, non-fulminant acute myocarditis is believed to have a less distinct presentation with less severe haemodynamic compromise but with a greater likelihood to progress to dilated cardiomyopathy. Using echocardiography, normal left ventricular diastolic diameters, combined with an increased thickness of the inter-ventricular septum (⊃ Fig. 39.2) and/or an impaired right ventricular systolic function at initial presentation, are more suggestive of fulminant myocarditis [5]. Those patients who initially suffer from fulminant myocarditis with severe impairment of cardiac function are more likely to recover quickly, while those patients presenting with non-fulminant myocarditis are more prone to develop progressive cardiac dysfunction.

Myocardial scintigraphy

Two scintigraphic methods, gallium-67 scintigraphy and indium-111 radiolabelled antimyosin imaging (⊃ Fig. 39.3) have been used in the past for diagnosis and evaluation of prognosis in patients with clinical suspicion of myocarditis. These techniques have a high sensitivity [6, 7] but data are only available from patients with severely impaired left ventricular (LV) function (indicating severe forms of myocarditis), and the gold-standard against which the sensitivity of the techniques was evaluated was

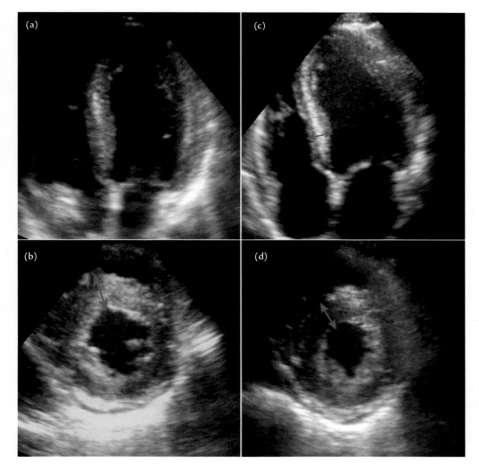

Fig. 39.2 2D-echocardiographic images of a patient presenting with fulminant myocarditis: An increased thickness of the inter-ventricular septum is seen at acute onset in the long- (a) and short-axis (b) views. Five days after presentation the thickness of the septum has already decreased (c and d).

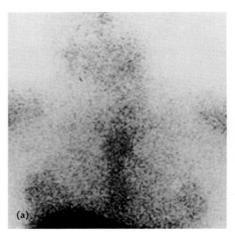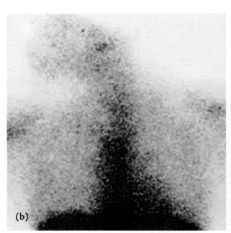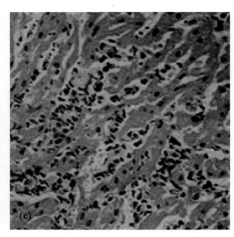

Fig. 39.3 Antimyosin scan of a healthy patient with normal findings (a). Significant myocardial antimyosin uptake in a patient with myocarditis (b) with the corresponding right ventricular endomyocardial biopsy (c) demonstrating lymphomononuclear cell infiltrate diagnostic of myocarditis.
Reprinted by permission of the Society of Nuclear Medicine from Martin et al., *J Nucl Med* 2004; 45: 429-37, ⊃ Fig. 39.1.

endomyocardial biopsy without immune histology, which itself suffers from a low sensitivity [8]. Gallium-67 is a non-specific marker of inflammation. Gallium imaging should be performed 72 h after the injection of the tracer to avoid false-positive results from remaining gallium circulating in the blood. In clinical practice, owing to this disadvantage, gallium scintigraphy is rarely used today.

The disease process of myocarditis is histologically characterized by myocardial inflammation with accumulation of immune cells leading to myocardial damage with necrosis of cardiomyocytes. Since necrotic cardiomyocytes lose the integrity of their cell membranes, intracellular proteins such as myosin are exposed to the extracellular space. Indium-111 labelled antimyosin is able to localize and visualize those myocardial areas. In practice, antimyosin antibodies are coupled with indium-111 and administered intravenously. Scintigraphic imaging (single photon emission computed tomography, SPECT) is performed 48 h after intravenous administration of the radionuclide. Qualitative or (semi-) quantitative analysis of the scans is then performed. The semiquantitative calculation of the heart-to-lung ratio may be used to objectively assess the extent of antimyosin-coupled indium-111 labelled radionuclide accumulation in the myocardium. Although a cut-off heart-to-lung ratio <1.6 has been suggested to be normal, such a cut-off value needs to be established individually in each centre by studying a healthy control group.

The strength of scintigraphy in the work-up of myocarditis is based on many studies suggesting that a positive biopsy result (indicative of myocarditis) is almost always associated with a positive scintigraphic result, while a negative scintigraphic result is excluding a biopsy-based diagnosis of myocarditis with a high degree of reliability. However, the specificity (31–44%), and the positive predictive value (28–33%) of indium-111 scintigraphy are quite low [8]. In consideration of this limited specificity, the radiation burden and the practical difficulties of myocardial scintigraphy, the use of scintigraphic techniques has declined over the past years.

Multi-detector computed tomography

The diagnostic capacity of multi-detector-computed tomography (MDCT) has tremendously increased with recent technological advancements. MDCT-based coronary angiography is becoming increasingly popular for non-invasive evaluation of coronary artery disease comprising the assessment of coronary diameters, plaque calcification, and vessel wall pathology. Hence, MDCT coronary angiography is increasingly used in low- and intermediate-risk patients presenting with chest pain suggestive of coronary artery disease. As myocarditis may be a differential diagnosis in these patients, tissue information from MDCT images would be helpful to not only rule out coronary disease, but to also establish the diagnosis of myocarditis.

Preliminary investigations suggest that contrast-enhanced MDCT may be helpful for myocardial tissue characterization. Such delayed enhancement (DE)-MDCT images are acquired 5–10 min after contrast injection with a lower tube current and voltage compared to MDCT coronary angiography in order to reduce radiation dose and perhaps also increase signal-to-noise [9].

The combination of MDCT coronary angiography and DE-MDCT can be used to differentiate ischaemic from non-ischaemic cardiomyopathy (⊃ Fig. 39.4): ischaemic myocardial damage is characterized by sub-endocardial or transmural delayed enhancement, while non-ischaemic forms are characterized by epicardial or intramural patterns of DE [10]. Preliminary data suggest that diagnostic agreement of MDCT with contrast-enhanced cardiovascular magnetic resonance (CMR) is excellent [10]. In acute myocarditis, DE-MDCT is also able to detect patterns of damage in the epicardial portion of the left ventricular myocardium similar to contrast-enhanced CMR [11].

A combined procedure of MDCT coronary angiography and DE-MDCT could become attractive for the diagnosis of acute myocarditis in the emergency department, since it allows the acquisition of comprehensive data in a single study within 15 min. However, the clinical use of such a combined procedure is limited

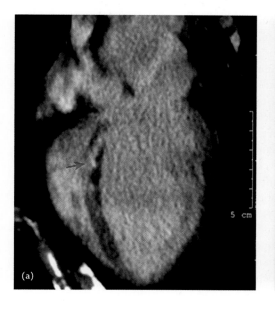

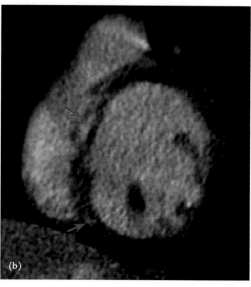

Fig. 39.4 Delayed-enhancement (DE) multi-detector-computed tomography in patient with myocarditis demonstrating intramural DE in the septal wall in a long- (a) and short-axis (b) view.
Kindly provided by le Polain de Waroux et al., *Eur Heart J* 2008; 29: 2544–51.

due to the radiation burden (up to 20 mSv with ~30% from DE-MDCT) with a risk of radiation-induced cancer [12], especially in young patients who present with myocarditis. The lower image quality as compared to LGE-CMR may also result in a lower sensitivity of detecting small areas of myocardial damage.

Hybrid imaging techniques

Emerging hybrid PET/CT and PET/MRI techniques may have considerable potential for future cardiovascular inflammation imaging because they combine PET, a highly sensitive and quantitative modality to detect even low grade inflammation, with CT or MRI that enable non-invasive assessment of cardiovascular anatomy with excellent spatial resolution. PET performed with, for example, fluorine-18-fluorodeoxyglucose (FDG) has the unique ability to depict metabolically active regions. Use of FDG PET/CT is well established for the diagnosis and management of malignancies; however, it is also well suited for assessing infectious and inflammatory processes of the myocardium [13]. For example, high FDG uptake was demonstrated in the area of myocardial infarction (MI) on day 5 after MI, largely reflecting myocardial inflammation

caused by accumulated macrophages (➲ Fig. 39.5). Unfortunately, larger studies evaluating the diagnostic value of PET/CT or MRI in patients with acute myocarditis are still missing. Moreover, FDG-based PET assessment of myocardial disease can be challenging because FDG may also accumulate in normal myocardium and techniques to prevent this are required. Novel PET tracers that specifically target monocytes/macrophages are being tested in preclinical studies and could overcome these limitations in the future.

Cardiovascular magnetic resonance (CMR) imaging

Due to its non-invasiveness, the lack of radiation exposure, its image quality, which helps assessing and quantifying cardiac function, and its high tissue contrast, which can be modified using various pulse sequences, CMR has become an important technique for evaluating patients with suspected myocarditis. In many institutions CMR is now routinely applied clinically in such patients and many reports confirmed the feasibility and diagnostic accuracy of CMR protocols.

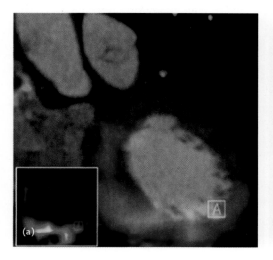

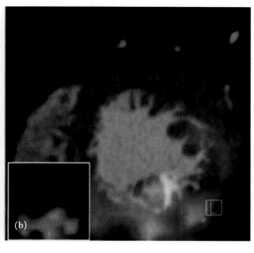

Fig. 39.5 FDG PET/CT in a patient 5 days after right coronary artery occlusion showed increased PET signal in the injured/inflamed inferior left ventricular wall.
With permission from Lee et al. [8].

Anatomic and functional abnormalities

For just depicting anatomic and functional abnormalities in patients with suspected myocarditis, CMR has few advantages as compared to echocardiography. It is mainly in patients with a suboptimal ultrasound window, in those in whom a 3-dimensional visualization of the ventricles is needed to detect subtle abnormalities of regional anatomy and function, and in those in whom details of the right ventricle are of interest, that CMR should be employed for this purpose only.

Similar to echocardiography, CMR detects an increase in myocardial mass in patients with fulminant myocarditis, and is able to document normalization of mass with disappearance of myocardial oedema. CMR is more sensitive than echocardiography in depicting small and often localized pericardial effusions, which may be found adjacent to the myocardial region mostly affected by myocardial inflammation [14]. The presence of pericardial effusion in a patient suspected to have myocarditis supports on-going active inflammation.

Tissue characterization

The following three tissue features potentially associated with myocardial inflammation may be visualized by CMR:

1. Hyperaemia seems to be the cause of an increased signal on T1-weighted spin-echo images following gadolinium administration (elevated global relative enhancement (gRE)).

2. Tissue oedema, which may result in an elevated T2 signal.

3. Myocardial necrosis or scarring, as indicated by the presence of late gadolinium enhancement (LGE).

Hyperaemia CMR (early myocardial gadolinium enhancement ratio)

The myocardium in patients with the clinical manifestations of acute myocarditis shows hyper-enhancement relative to skeletal muscle on T1-weighted contrast-enhanced images in the early wash-out period (➲ Fig. 39.6) [15]. Scanning is started immediately following the first pass of contrast media, such as gadolinium diethylenetriamine pentaacetic acid (Gd-DTPA), using a standard fast spin-echo pulse sequence with sufficient T1-weighting, and is completed at 5 min after the injection [16].

The mechanism of signal increase related to tissue hyperaemia in the myocardium remains unclear. Tissue hyperaemia may lead to faster distribution of contrast medium into the interstitial space. However, it is also conceivable that the increased T1 signal is caused by the same mechanism of tissue destruction, which explains the late gadolinium enhancement effect. Whatever the exact cause, an increased T1 signal can be observed during the first minutes after injection of the contrast agent. It is usually difficult to visually appreciate the diffuse rise in signal intensity on these images and thus quantification of signal changes is necessary. As spin-echo imaging often yields low contrast between inflamed and normal myocardium, and suffers from image artefacts, it turned out to be advantageous to relate the signal increase in the myocardium to that observed in neighbouring skeletal muscle [15]. Thus, relative enhancement depends on the assumption that skeletal muscle is normal, which may be erroneous if the inflammation also involves skeletal muscles. Although early gadolinium enhancement ratio suffers from several artefacts, several studies confirm the diagnostic usefulness of this parameter (➲ Table 39.1). Nevertheless, this pulse sequence is only used in a few centres around the world.

Oedema imaging by CMR

Acutely inflamed tissue shows an increase in water content due to oedema formation. Isolated oedema usually indicates reversible myocardial injury. However, oedema also accompanies necrosis, as shown in myocardial infarction. Once myocarditis has healed, oedema should disappear.

T2-weighted CMR [16] today is usually performed by short inversion time recovery (STIR) pulse sequences. These pulse sequences are sensitive to the long T2 of water protons to generate images with a higher signal intensity of oedematous myocardial tissue as compared to non-inflamed muscle tissue in the vicinity. Depending on the distribution of oedema within the left ventricular myocardium, there may be visible regional signal differences within an image. Regions with a signal intensity of more than 2 standard deviations above the mean of normal appearing myocardial tissue within the same slice are regarded as indicative of

Fig. 39.6 T1-weighted cross-sectional views at the mid-ventricular level of a patient with myocarditis. The left panel displays a view obtained before gadopentate dimeglumine (Gd-DTPA). The right panel depicts the same view after the administration of 0.1 mmol/kg Gd-DTPA. Note diffuse signal enhancement in the left ventricle.
Reproduced from Friedrich MG, Contrast media–enhanced magnetic resonance imaging visualizes myocardial changes in the course of viral myocarditis. *Circulation*, 97:18, 1802–1809, Copyright 1998, with permission from Wolters Kluwer.

Pre contrast

Post contrast

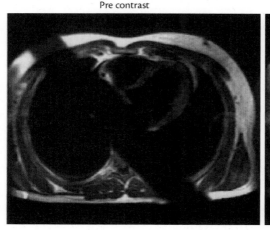
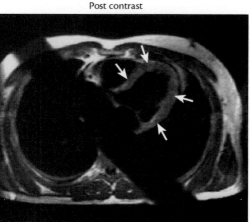

Table 39.1 Sensitivity and specificity of global relative enhancement (T1 spin-echo) in myocarditis

SENSITIVITY	n	Sensitivity	SPECIFICITY	n	Specificity
Friedrich et al. [8]	19	84%°	Friedrich et al. [1]	34	90%°
Abdel-Aty et al. [14]	25	80%°	Abdel-Aty et al. [6]	23	74%°
Laissy et al. [*]	20	85%°			
Laissy et al. [**]	24	100%°	Laissy et al. [**]	7	100%°
Gutberlet et al. [15]	48	63%°°	Gutberlet et al. [15]	35	86%°°
Total	**136**	**79%**		**99**	**86%**

* Laissy JP, Messin B, Varenne O, et al. MRI of acute myocarditis: a comprehensive approach based on various imaging sequences. *Chest* 2002; 122(5): 1638–48.
** Laissy JP, Hyafil F, Feldman LJ, et al. Differentiating acute myocardial infarction from myocarditis: diagnostic value of early- and delayed-perfusion cardiac MR imaging. *Radiology* 2005; 237(1): 75–82.
° Sensitivity and specificity to detect inflammation as defined by clinical picture.
°° Sensitivity and specificity to detect inflammation as defined by immunohistochemistry.

regional oedema. One has to be careful not to look at too-small regions as signal inhomogeneity on T2 images in normals may be considerable. However, the often diffuse nature, especially in less aggressive inflammation, makes quantitative analysis of the signal of the entire slice of myocardium superior to visual analysis. Signal intensity of the myocardium is normalized to that of nearby skeletal muscle and ratios of 1.9 or higher are regarded as indicative of oedema. However, this cut-off ratio is based on small-sized studies and every centre is advised to establish its own cut-off value.

An obvious drawback of this type of analysis is the dependence on absence of inflammation in the skeletal muscle, which is not uncommon in systemic viral illness. Another shortcoming of T2-weighted CMR is that in patients with arrhythmias or motion artefacts from breathing, image quality may not allow reliable visualization or quantification of oedema. Moreover, in studies looking at the diagnostic value of T2 oedema imaging it is usually not specifically mentioned how the diagnosis was made (visually or by quantification or by both methods). The results of several studies are shown in ⊃ Table 39.2.

Necrosis and fibrosis imaging by CMR (late gadolinium enhancement)

The more severe forms of myocarditis may result in tissue necrosis, which is often focal in nature just as the disease itself. New contrast enhanced CMR techniques employing inversion pulses to null the signal of normal myocardium were initially developed for infarct imaging (⊃ Fig. 39.7). However, they also show necrotic or fibrotic myocardium in patients with myocarditis as bright areas and provide high contrast between diseased and normal myocardium. Imaging is performed at about 5–10 min after contrast injection (late gadolinium enhancement; LGE). The mechanism by which contrast enhancement can be explained is as follows: when serious membrane damage has occurred in early necrosis, gadolinium molecules enter the intracellular space. This results in an increased volume of distribution for the contrast agent within a voxel of tissue with an associated increase in signal intensity. In the chronic stage of myocarditis, areas of scar are histologically characterized by abundant loose connective tissue with a few fibrocytes. Again, voxels within such areas of myocardium exhibit a higher concentration of contrast medium as compared to normal myocardial tissue. In contrast to necrotic or fibrotic tissue, densely packed myocytes forming most of the normal myocardium are not accessible to gadolinium compounds. Hence, the volume of distribution and the concentration of the contrast agent within a voxel remain low.

When such inversion recovery gradient echo-techniques are used in patients with clinically suspected myocarditis (history of respiratory or gastrointestinal symptoms with 8 weeks of

Table 39.2 Sensitivity and specificity of T2-weighted imaging in myocarditis

SENSITIVITY	n	Sensitivity	SPECIFICITY	n	Specificity
Rieker et al. [*]	11	100%°			
Abdel-Aty et al. [6]	25	84%°	Abdel-Aty et al. [1]	23	74%°
Laissy et al. [**]	20	62%°			
Laissy et al. [***]	24	61%°			
Gutberlet et al. [15]	48	67%°°	Gutberlet et al. [15]	35	69%°°
Total	**128**	**71%**		**58**	**71%**

*Rieker O, Mohrs O, Oberholzer K, Kreitner KF, Thelen M. [Cardiac MRI in suspected myocarditis]. Rofo Fortschr Geb Rontgenstr Neuen Bildgeb Verfahr 2002; 174(12): 1530–6.
**Laissy JP, Messin B, Varenne O, et al. MRI of acute myocarditis: a comprehensive approach based on various imaging sequences. *Chest* 2002; 122(5): 1638–48.
***Laissy JP, Hyafil F, Feldman LJ, et al. Differentiating acute myocardial infarction from myocarditis: diagnostic value of early- and delayed-perfusion cardiac MR imaging. *Radiology* 2005; 237(1): 75–82.
°Sensitivity and specificity to detect inflammation as defined by clinical picture.
°°Sensitivity and specificity to detect inflammation as defined by immunohistochemistry.

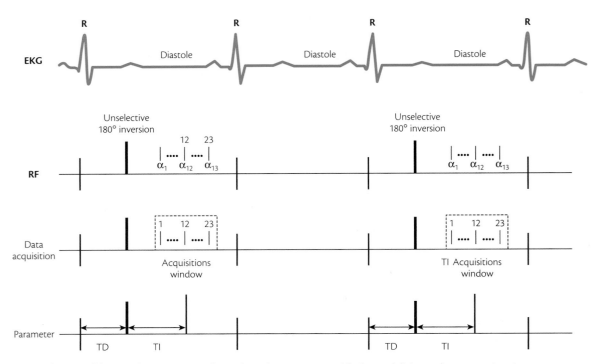

Fig. 39.7 Schematic diagram of the inversion recovery gradient echo pulse sequence used for late gadolinium enhancement imaging.
Reprinted with permission from Simonetti et al. *Radiology* 218: 215–23, 2001.

admission in combination with fatigue/malaise, chest pain, dyspnoea, or tachycardia plus ECG changes such as conduction block, ST abnormalities, supraventricular tachyarrhythmia, or ventricular tachycardia) LGE is found in up to 90% of the patients [17]. The regions of LGE have a patchy distribution throughout the left ventricle. They are frequently located in the lateral free wall (⊃ Fig. 39.8), and originate from the epicardial quartile of that wall. Another frequently seen pattern is the mid-wall stria pattern in the basal inter-ventricular septum in patients with chronic myocarditis (⊃ Fig. 39.9) [18]. LGE-CMR also has a good sensitivity in

patients with a more chronic form of myocarditis by clinical criteria [10]. However, in this series of biopsy confirmed patients with chronic myocarditis, borderline myocarditis—the less severe form of the disease by the DALLAS criteria—was less often associated with LGE than active myocarditis by the DALLAS criteria [10].

If scarring occurs in acute myocarditis it will usually remain visible on LGE images when the acute inflammation has long subsided. However, chronic scar following acute myocarditis is often significantly smaller than in the acute stage due to scar shrinking. When the initial areas of scarring are just large enough to be

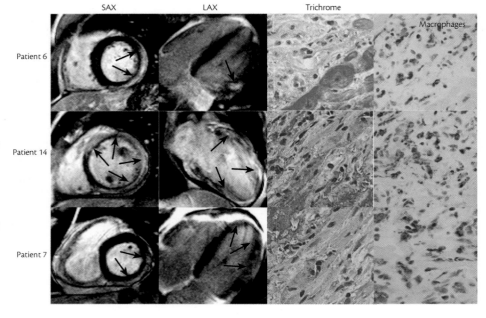

Fig. 39.8 Late gadolinium enhanced (LGE) CMR images and histopathology of typical patients in whom biopsies were obtained from the area of contrast enhancement. The panels show cases of active myocarditis with myocyte damage as well as infiltration of macrophages. Note that contrast enhancement is often located in the sub-epicardial region of the posterolateral wall.
Reproduced from Mahrholdt H, et al. Cardiovascular magnetic resonance assessment of human myocarditis: a comparison to histology and molecular pathology. *Circulation*, 109:10, 2004, 1250–8, with permission from Wolters Kluwer.

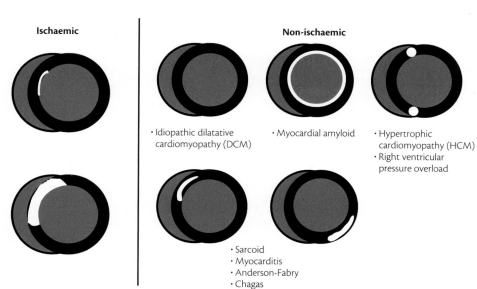

Ischaemic

Non-ischaemic

· Idiopathic dilatative
cardiomyopathy (DCM)

· Myocardial amyloid

· Hypertrophic
cardiomyopathy (HCM)
· Right ventricular
pressure overload

· Sarcoid
· Myocarditis
· Anderson-Fabry
· Chagas
· Other infiltrative disorders

Fig. 39.9 Late gadolinium enhancement patterns that one may encounter in clinical practice. If hyper-enhancement is present, the endocardium should be involved in patients with ischaemic disease. Isolated mid-wall or epicardial hyper-enhancement strongly suggests a 'non-ischaemic' aetiology.
Reproduced from Mahrholdt H, et al. Delayed enhancement cardiovascular magnetic resonance assessment of non-ischaemic cardiomyopathies. *European Heart Journal*, 26:15, 2005, 1461–74, by permission of Oxford University Press.

visible, scar shrinking may lead to disappearance of LGE in some patients (⊃ Fig. 39.10).

LGE-CMR is the most widely used approach in the diagnosis of myocarditis and this is reflected in the literature. ⊃ Table 39.3 shows the results of published studies including the average weighted sensitivity and specificity.

Which CMR pulse sequences should be used?

A disadvantage of the LGE-CMR technique is the inability to demonstrate diffuse myocardial changes as encountered in diffuse acute myocarditis with diffuse oedema formation. In addition, localized oedema without accompanying myocyte death will not

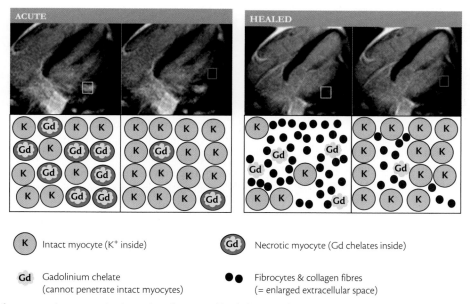

ACUTE

HEALED

K Intact myocyte (K⁺ inside)

Gd Necrotic myocyte (Gd chelates inside)

Gd Gadolinium chelate
(cannot penetrate intact myocytes)

●● Fibrocytes & collagen fibres
(= enlarged extracellular space)

Fig. 39.10 Mechanism of contrast enhancement in the setting of acute and healed myocarditis. Upper images show LGE images using inversion recovery gradient echo images. Bottom images show a schematic view of contrast enhancement. Just as in infarcts, acute necrosis in the setting of myocarditis is characterized by ruptured sarcolemmal membranes and surrounding interstitial oedema, allowing the contrast agent to accumulate in the interstitium, as well as to diffuse into the intracellular space. Thus, the general mechanism of hyper-enhancement in myocarditis is the same as in infarction. During healing some amount of interstitial oedema persists and necrotic myocytes are slowly replaced by fibrous tissue, comparable to small chronic infarcts. Thus, hyper-enhancement will remain present during this phase of the disease. However, when healing is completed, oedema has resolved while scars shrink and remodel over time. Consequently, voxels may now contain so many previously bordering surviving myocytes that hyper-enhancement in these voxels may not be visible any longer, resulting in the area of hyper-enhancement to decrease significantly. This effect is likely magnified by the patchy distribution of scars in myocarditis and the fact that interstitial oedema mainly occurs in areas of myocardial necrosis. Thus, all areas of visible hyper-enhancement may disappear in some cases after healing, just leaving minimal diffuse signal enhancement.

Table 39.3 Sensitivity and specificity of LGE-CMR in myocarditis

SENSITIVITY	n	Sensitivity	SPECIFICITY	n	Specificity
Rieker et al. [*]	11	45%°	Rieker et al. [*]	10	100%°
Mahrholdt et al. [10]	32	88%°°	Roiditi et al. [**]	8	100%°
Abdel-Aty et al. [14]	25	44%°	Abdel-Aty et al. [6]	23	100%°
Hunold et al. [*****]	6	100%			
Laissy et al. [******]	24	79%°	Laissy et al. [***]	31	97%°
Ingkanisorn et al. [****]	21	100%°			
DeCobelli et al. [12]	23	84%°°			
Gutberlet et al. [15]	48	27%°°	Gutberlet et al. [15]	35	80%°°
Mahrholdt et al. [11]	87	95%°°			
Yilmaz et al. [#]	71	46%°°			
Total	**348**	**68%**		**107**	**93%**

* Rieker O, Mohrs O, Oberholzer K, Kreitner KF, Thelen M. [Cardiac MRI in suspected myocarditis]. Rofo Fortschr Geb Rontgenstr Neuen Bildgeb Verfahr 2002; 174(12): 1530–6.
** Roditi GH, Hartnell GG, Cohen MC. MRI changes in myocarditis--evaluation with spin echo, cine MR angiography and contrast enhanced spin echo imaging. Clin Radiol 2000; 55: 752–58.
*** Laissy JP, Hyafil F, Feldman LJ, et al. Differentiating acute myocardial infarction from myocarditis: diagnostic value of early- and delayed-perfusion cardiac MR imaging. Radiology 2005; 237(1): 75–82.
**** Ingkanisorn WP, Paterson I, Calvo KR, et al. Cardiac magnetic resonance appearance of myocarditis caused by high dose IL-2: similarities to community-acquired myocarditis. J Cardiovasc Magn Res 2006; 8: 353–60.
***** Hunold P, Schlosser T, Vogt FM, et al. Myocardial late enhancement in contrast-enhanced cardiac MRI: distinction between infarction scar and non-infarction-related disease. AJR Am J Roentgenol 2005; 184: 1420–6.
****** Laissy JP, Messin B, Varenne O, et al. MRI of acute myocarditis: a comprehensive approach based on various imaging sequences. Chest 2002; 122(5): 1638–48.
# Yilmaz A, Mahrholdt H, Athanasiadis A, et al. Coronary vasospasm as the underlying cause for chest pain in patients with PVB19 myocarditis. Heart 2008; 94: 1456–63.

result in enough increase in extracellular space to cause LGE [19]. Thus, the sensitivity of LGE to detect milder forms of myocarditis may be suboptimal.

CMR imaging optimized at detecting hyperaemia or oedema may be more sensitive for identifying patients with acute myocarditis. A study comparing early gadolinium enhancement, oedema imaging, and late gadolinium enhancement, using the appropriate pulse sequences in patients with cardiac symptoms suggestive of myocarditis, made the following observations [20]:

1. T1-weighted early gadolinium enhancement (using a turbo spin echo sequence) yields a significantly higher global myocardial relative enhancement in patients compared to volunteers. A cut-off value of 4.0 has a sensitivity of 80% and a specificity of 73% to identify myocarditis.

2. T2-weighted oedema imaging (using a triple inversion recovery pulse sequence) shows significantly higher global myocardial signal intensity in patients than in volunteers, although there is overlap. A cut-off value of 1.9 has a sensitivity of 84% and a specificity of 74% to identify the disease.

3. Necrosis LGE imaging (using an inversion recovery gradient echo pulse sequence) has a lower sensitivity of only 44% but the specificity is high (100%).

4. The best diagnostic performance was obtained when myocarditis was diagnosed in patients in whom any two of the criteria obtained by the three techniques were positive [20].

One needs to remember, however, that in this series the gold-standard for identifying myocarditis was the clinical presentation of the patient and endomyocardial biopsy was not performed. In addition, gRE imaging does not work equally well in all centres.

When performing the same CMR protocol consisting of a T1-weighted gRE, a T2-weighted oedema, and a LGE pulse sequence in patients with clinically suspected *chronic* myocarditis, increased myocardial gRE (obtained from the T1 images) and increased oedema ratio (obtained from the T2 images) are common findings, whereas LGE is less often detected than reported for acute myocarditis [21]. This suggests that clinically active inflammation is usually associated with T2 signal elevation, as well as an increase in gRE ratio, irrespective of whether the onset of clinical symptoms has been recent or whether the clinical presentation is a more chronic one. One may also conclude that scar in chronic myocarditis may have shrunk to an extent that LGE-CMR has reduced sensitivity (➲ Fig. 39.10). Also, in chronic myocarditis, the approach of diagnosing myocarditis by CMR, when two out of the three pulse sequences performed resulted in pathologic results, yielded the best accuracy [21].

Follow-up of patients with myocarditis by CMR

Clinical improvement of myocarditis patients is paralleled by normalization of gRE and oedema ratio in many patients [22]. Serial assessment of the relative T2 signal, gRE ratio, and LGE at initial presentation and after 18 months in 36 patients diagnosed with acute myocarditis by clinical criteria showed a decrease of the mean T2 signal ratio from 2.4 to 1.9, a decrease of the gRE signal ratio from 7.6 to 4.4, and a decrease of the amount of LGE from 38% to 22% of left ventricular mass. These findings are in line with previous publications describing the individual time courses of each of those CMR parameters [23, 24] in myocarditis patients. Hence, the CMR approach combining a contrast enhanced T1-weighted pulse sequence, a T2-weighted sequence, plus an LGE pulse sequence may be capable of differentiating reversible and healing (elevated T1 gRE ratio and T2 oedema ratio, which normalizes over time) myocarditis and irreversible myocardial damage with or without on-going inflammation (persistent LGE with or without accompanying elevations of T1 gRE ratio and T2 oedema ratio) non-invasively.

In patients with on-going cardiac symptoms, the clinical question is often whether the acute inflammatory process has healed. If none or just one of T2 or gRE ratios is elevated, this constellation may have a very high negative predictive value for excluding on-going active myocarditis in living patients [22].

However, data on the value of CMR in identifying healed from on-going active myocarditis are far from being conclusive. The largest study examining patients with clinically suspected chronic myocarditis by CMR and endomyocardial biopsy [21] found absence of T2 elevation in 33%, and no elevated gRE ratio in 37% of those shown to have inflammation by histology. Hence, there will be several patients with persisting inflammation who will have elevation of only one of these two CMR parameters.

Another important clinical question is risk stratification of patients with myocarditis and suspected myocarditis with regard to mortality and major adverse cardiac events. Grün et al. [25] recently evaluated the long-term mortality in patients with viral myocarditis, to establish the prognostic value of various clinical, functional, and CMR parameters. They concluded that among their population with a wide range of clinical symptoms biopsy

proven viral myocarditis was associated with a long-term mortality of up to 19.2% in 4.7 years, and that the presence of LGE was the best independent predictor of all-cause and of cardiac mortality. Importantly, no patient without LGE suffered cardiac or sudden cardiac death during follow-up despite biopsy proven myocarditis (➲ Fig. 39.11). In a population of patients with clinically suspected myocarditis (consecutive all comers) a normal CMR (defined as LV-EF ≥ 60% and LV-EDV≤ 180ml and no LGE) has a very low risk for death or other adverse cardiac events [26].

CMR or endomyocardial biopsy?

Biopsies obtained from the area of LGE show acute or borderline myocarditis [17] in a higher percentage than reported from biopsies taken randomly (usually from the right ventricle) in some reports. These findings may be explained by the fact that more LGE may be associated with more intense inflammation permitting the operator to direct the bioptome towards the area of maximum injury. Myocarditis was found less consistently in patients in whom the biopsy could not be obtained from the region of contrast enhancement [17]. However, the data on CMR guided biopsy remain controversial. Yilmaz et al. reported that a preferential biopsy in regions showing late gadolinium enhancement on cardiovascular magnetic resonance did not increase the number of positive diagnoses of myocarditis [27]. Irrespective of the precise location of biopsy taking the available data show: (1) biventricular biopsies have a higher diagnostic yield compared to selective biopsies and (2) that left ventricular biopsies give a higher diagnostic yield compared to right ventricular biopsies, while having a lower risk for minor complications.

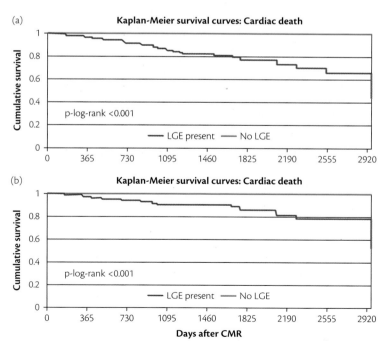

Fig. 39.11 Kaplan–Meier survival curves with regard to cardiac mortality (a) and sudden cardiac death (b) of patients with biopsy proven myocarditis. Note that no patient without the presence of LGE suffered an event.

Reprinted from Grun S, et al, Long-term follow-up of biopsy-proven viral myocarditis: predictors of mortality and incomplete recovery. *Journal of the American College of Cardiology*, 58:18 1604–1615, Copyright 2012, with permission from Elsevier

When managing patients with inflammatory heart disease today, it should be kept in mind that endomyocardial biopsy remains the only technique that can directly assess the presence and intensity of myocardial inflammation *in vivo*. Therefore, it is the technique of choice if clinically indicated to differentiate between active and healed myocarditis. Endomyocardial biopsy also provides information on the underlying cause of inflammation, such as viral or bacterial infection of the myocardium, or myocardial autoimmune processes, on the presence of giant cells, or Churg-Strauss syndrome [28]. This information cannot be obtained by CMR imaging but is essential for patient management decisions. The importance of endomyocardial biopsy is reflected in the current guidelines [28] recommending it in basically all patients developing non-ischaemic heart failure, as well as for several other non-ischaemic conditions.

Clinical recommendations

The optimal CMR approach for diagnosing myocarditis may depend on the clinical presentation of the patient. The patient with less impressive symptoms may be more likely to have pathologic hyperaemia and oedema imaging with normal LGE. Recent expert consensus suggests that CMR should be performed in patients who are symptomatic, have clinical evidence suggesting myocarditis, and in whom CMR will likely affect clinical management

[16]. A positive diagnosis of myocarditis may result in a recommendation to refrain from exercise, beta blockade may be instituted in patients with arrhythmias, and clinical follow-up may be scheduled. Some patients may require additional follow-up by echocardiography or CMR. In patients with occupations associated with strenuous exercise, the indication to perform CMR should even be broader, as the consequences of having the disease are more severe. In these patients clinical symptoms may be absent, and the mere presence of an abnormal ECG should trigger a request of performing CMR (⊃ Table 39.4).

In most centres only two sets of images (T2 oedema and LGE) are acquired (⊃ Table 39.5), whereas myocardial global relative enhancement is not measured due to the fact that T1-weighted spin-echo images are often of poor quality. When all three sets of images are acquired, myocarditis is defined to be present when at least two of the three sets of images show pathologic results [16]. Other centres feel that LGE is the most stable pulse sequence with the fewest number of artefacts, and they rely on the result of this set of images alone. This approach may result in some underdiagnosis of myocarditis but has a good specificity. These different approaches at different centres reflect the fact that there are still not enough data available at the moment, especially in patients who also had endomyocardial biopsy, to give final recommendations on CMR in patients with suspected myocarditis.

Table 39.4 Indications for CMR in myocarditis

Suspected myocarditis based on various combinations of clinical symptoms such as fatigue, palpitations, arrhythmias, unexplained dyspnoea, unexplained chest pain in the absence of coronary artery disease or any other structural heart disease, and/or abnormal resting ECG.
Clinical presentation with acute coronary syndrome in the absence of coronary artery disease or culprit lesion.
Clinical presentation with successful resuscitation after sudden cardiac death in the absence of coronary artery disease or any structural heart disease.
Clinical presentation with new onset of heart failure in the absence of coronary artery disease or any structural heart disease.
CMR guidance of endomyocardial biopsy to increase sensitivity.
Follow-up of known myocarditis.
Follow-up of known myocarditis after antiviral or immunosuppressive treatment.

Table 39.5 CMR protocol for work-up of myocarditis

Requirements
Patient should be able to hold his/her breath for 15–20 seconds.
Limited diagnostic performance with frequent extrasystoles (>10/min), atrial fibrillation.
Step 1: LV structure and function module
1. Scout imaging—axial, coronal, sagittal.
2. Axial (8–10 mm) set of steady-state free precession (SSFP) or half Fourier single shot turbo spin echo images through the chest.
3. Scout to line up short-axis images—this can either be a single shot image or a cine acquisition.
a) 2-chamber long-axis (also called the vertical long-axis) prescribed off an axial view showing the apex and mitral valve, bisecting the mitral valve and apex.
b) Horizontal long-axis prescribed off of the 2-chamber long-axis bisecting the apex and centre of the mitral valve.
4. Steady-state free-precession (SSFP) short-axis cine images, from the mitral valve plane through the apex prescribed from the previously acquired horizontal long-axis image.
a) Slice thickness 6–8 mm, with 2 mm inter-slice gaps.
b) Temporal resolution <45 msec between phases.
c) Parallel imaging used as available, speed up factor 2×.

5. SSFP long-axis cine images.

    a) 4-chamber long-axis, prescribed off a basal short-axis image, bisecting the inter-ventricular septum.

    b) 2-chamber long-axis, prescribed off of a basal short-axis image, bisecting the anterior and inferior walls.

    c) 3-chamber long-axis, prescribed off of the most basal short-axis including the plane of the LVOT, bisecting the LVOT and the posterolateral wall.

6. Analysis.

    a) All short-axis images are evaluated with computer-aided analysis packages for planimetry of endocardial and epicardial borders at end-diastole and end-systole.

    b) The inclusion or exclusion of papillary muscles in the LV mass should be the same as that used in normal reference ranges used for comparison.

    c) Care must be used at the 1 or 2 most basal slices. Due to systolic movement of the base towards the apex, the end-systolic phase will include only left atrium. However, this slice at end-diastole will include some of the LV mass and volume.

Step 2: T2-weighted black blood imaging module

1. Breath-hold, segmented fast spin-echo imaging with dark blood preparation (double inversion recovery).

2. Perform imaging prior to contrast administration.

3. Selected slices based on cine imaging findings (e.g. 2- and 4-chamber long-axis and 3 representative short-axis slices).

4. Adjust readout to mid-diastole.

5. Slice thickness 8 mm slice thickness of dark blood prep should be greater than the base-apex motion of the mitral annulus.

6. Analysis.

    a) Visual analysis of all T2-weighted images for focal signal enhancement matching morphological abnormalities, wall motion abnormalities and/or regions of late gadolinium enhancement. Caution: sub-endocardial slow flow artefact!

    b) Quantitative analysis comparing average signal intensity (SI) with the average signal intensity of skeletal muscle. Depending on the individual scanner (at least 20 healthy volunteers must be scanned and evaluated before starting to evaluate patients), the normal ratio $SI_{myocardium}/SI_{skeletal\ muscle}$ is reported to be <1.8-2.0 [14].

Step 3: Late gadolinium enhancement

1. Need at least 10-min wait after contrast administration (0.15–0.2 mmol/kg). Note: the delay may be shorter than 10 min if lower doses are used as blood pool signal falls below that of late enhanced myocardium.

2. 2D segmented inversion recovery GRE imaging during diastolic stand-still.

3. Same views as for cine imaging (short- and long-axis views).

4. Slice thickness, same as for cine imaging.

5. In-plane resolution, ~1.4–1.8 mm.

6. Acquisition duration per R-R interval below 200 msec but should be less in the setting of tachycardia.

7. Inversion time set to null normal myocardium. Alternative is to use fixed TI with a phase-sensitive sequence.

8. Read-out is usually every other heartbeat but can be modified to every heartbeat in the setting of bradycardia, and every third heartbeat in the setting of tachycardia or arrhythmia.

9. Optional: single-shot imaging (SSFP readout) performed as backup for patients with irregular heartbeat, difficulty breath holding.

10. Analysis—examine the 'pattern' of enhancement as certain non-ischaemic myocardial diseases have predilection for scarring in various myocardial regions (Fig. 39.9).

References

1. Magnani JW, Dec GW. Myocarditis: current trends in diagnosis and treatment. *Circulation* 2006; 113: 876–90.

2. Hsiao JF, Koshino Y, Bonnichsen CR, et al. Speckle tracking echocardiography in acute myocarditis. *Int J Cardiovasc Imaging* 2013; 29(2): 275–84.

3. Khoo NS, Smallhorn JF, Atallah J, Kaneko S, Mackie AS, Paterson I. Altered left ventricular tissue velocities, deformation and twist in children and young adults with acute myocarditis and normal ejection fraction. *J Am Soc Echocardiogr* 2012; 25(3): 294–303.

4. Pinamonti B, Alberti E, Cigalotto A, et al. Echocardiographic findings in myocarditis. *Am J Cardiol* 1988; 62: 285–91.

5. Felker GM, Boehmer JP, Hruban RH, et al. Echocardiographic findings in fulminant and acute myocarditis. *J Am Coll Cardiol* 2000; 36: 227–32.

6. Narula J, Khaw BA, Dec GW, et al. Diagnostic accuracy of antimyosin scintigraphy in suspected myocarditis. *J Nucl Cardiol* 1996; 3: 371–81.

7. O'Connell JB, Henkin RE, Robinson JA, Subramanian R, Scanlon PJ, Gunnar RM. Gallium-67 imaging in patients with dilated cardiomyopathy and biopsy-proven myocarditis. *Circulation* 1984; 70: 58–62.

8. Lee WW, Marinelli B, van der Laan AM, et al. PET/MRI of inflammation in myocardial infarction. *J Am Coll Cardiol.* 2012; 10; 59(2): 153–63.

9. le Polain de Waroux JB, Pouleur AC, Goffinet C, Pasquet A, Vanoverschelde JL, Gerber BL. Combined coronary and late-enhanced multidetector-computed tomography for delineation of the etiology of left ventricular dysfunction: comparison with coronary angiography and contrast-enhanced cardiac magnetic resonance imaging. *Eur Heart J* 2008; 29: 2544–551.

10. DeCobelli CF, Pieroni M, Esposito A, et al. Delayed gadolinium-enhanced cardiac magnetic resonance in patients with chronic myocarditis presenting with heart failure or recurrent arrhythmias. *J Am Coll Cardiol* 2006; 47: 1649–54.

11. Redheuil AB, Azarine A, Garrigoux P, Mousseaux E. Images in cardiovascular medicine. Correspondence between delayed enhancement patterns in multislice computed tomography and magnetic resonance imaging in a case of acute myocarditis. *Circulation* 2006; 114: e571–L e572.

12. Einstein AJ, Henzlova MJ, Rajagopalan S. Estimating risk of cancer associated with radiation exposure from 64-slice computed tomography coronary angiograph. *JAMA* 2007; 298(3): 317–23.

13. James OG, Christensen JD, Wong TZ, Borges-Neto S, Koweek LM. Utility of FDG PET/CT in inflammatory cardiovascular disease. *Radiographic* 2011; 31(5): 1271–86.

14. Ong P, Athansiadis A, Hill S, et al. Usefulness of pericardial effusion as new diagnostic criterion for noninvasive detection of myocarditis. *Am J Cardiol* 2011; 108(3): 445–52.

15. Friedrich MG, Strohm O, Schulz-Menger J, Marciniak H, Luft FC, Dietz R. Contrast media-enhanced resonance imaging visualizes myocardial changes in the course of viral myocarditis. *Circulation* 1998; 97: 1802–9.

16. Friedrich MG, Sechtem U, Schulz-Menger J, et al. Cardiovascular magnetic resonance in myocarditis. *J Am Coll Cardiol* (in press), 2009.

17. Mahrholdt H, Goedecke C, Wagner A, et al. Cardiovascular magnetic resonance assessment of human myocarditis: a comparison to histology and molecular pathology. *Circulation* 2004; 109: 1250–8.

18. Mahrholdt H, Wagner A, Deluigi C, et al. Presentation, patterns of myocardial damage and clinical course of viral myocarditis. *Circulation* 2006; 114: 1581–90.

19. Li G, Xiang B, Dai G, et al. Tissue edema does not change gadolinium-diethylenetriamine pentaacetic acid (Gd-DTPA)-enhanced T1 relaxation times of viable myocardium. *J Magn Reson Imaging* 2005; 21: 744–51.

20. Abdel-Aty H, Boyé P, Zagrosek A, et al. The sensitivity and specificity of contrast-enhanced and T2-weighted cardiovascular magnetic resonance to detect acute myocarditis. *J Am Coll Cardiol* 2005; 45: 1815–22.

21. Gutberlet M, Spors B, Thoma T, et al. Suspected chronic myocarditis at cardiac MR: diagnostic accuracy and association with immunohistologically detected inflammation and viral persistence. *Radiology* 2008; 246: 401–9.

22. Zagrosek A, Abdel-Aty A, Boyé P, et al. Cardiovascular magnetic resonance monitors reversible and irreversible myocardial injuries in myocarditis: insights from a comprehensive approach. *J Am Coll Cardiol Imag* 2009 (in press).

23. Zagrosek A, Wassmuth R, Abdel-Aty H, Rudolph A, Dietz R, Schulz-Menger J. Relation between myocardial edema and myocardial mass during the acute and convalescent phase of myocarditis—a CMR study. *J Cardiovasc Magn Reson* 2008; 10: 19.

24. Wagner A, Schulz-Menger J, Dietz R, Friedrich MG. Long-term follow-up of patients paragraph sign with acute myocarditis by magnetic paragraph sign resonance imaging. *Magma* 2003; 16: 17–20.

25. Grün S, Schumm J, Greulich S, et al. Long-term follow-up of biopsy-proven viral myocarditis: predictors of mortality and incomplete recovery. *J Am Coll Cardiol* 2012; 59(18): 1604–15.

26. Schumm J, Greulich S, Grün S, et al. Risk stratification by CMR in patients with suspected myocarditis.

27. Yilmaz A, Kindermann I, Kindermann M, et al. Comparative evaluation of left and right ventricular endomyocardial biopsy: differences in complication rate and diagnostic performance. *Circulation* 2010; 122(9): 900–9.

28. Cooper LT, Baughman KL, Feldman AM, et al. The role of endomyocardial biopsy in the management of cardiovascular disease: a scientific statement from the American Heart Association, the American College of Cardiology, and the European Society of Cardiology. Endorsed by the Heart Failure Society of America and the Heart Failure Association of the European Society of Cardiology. *Eur Heart J* 2007; 28: 3076–93.

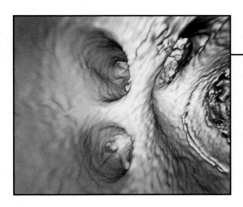

CHAPTER 40

Cardiac masses and tumours

Peter Buser, Thomas Buck, and Björn Plicht

Contents

Introduction

Cardiac tumours represent a rare but important cause of morbidity and mortality in clinical cardiology and are often challenging in diagnostic cardiac imaging. There is a broad spectrum of differential diagnosis for cardiac masses (⊃ Table 40.1). This chapter is mainly focused on the diagnosis of primary and secondary cardiac tumours and intra-cardiac thrombi. Primary cardiac tumours are rare with a prevalence between 0.001 and 0.3% [1]. Based on autopsy studies, secondary cardiac tumours, including metastases from distant malignomas or local invasion from neoplasms in the chest, are at least 20 times more common [2]. Three-quarters of the primary cardiac tumours are benign, and nearly half of those are myxomas, the rest being lipomas, papillary fibroelastomas, haemangioma, and rhabdomyomas. Of the malignant primary cardiac tumours, 95% are sarcomas, and the more common types are angiosarcomas (37%), undifferentiated sarcomas (24%),

Table 40.1 Differential diagnosis of cardiac masses

Primary Cardiac Tumours	
Benign	Myxoma
	Lipoma
	Papillary fibroelastoma
	Rhabdomyoma
	Fibroma
Malignant	Angiosarcoma
	Malignant fibrous histiocytoma
	Leiomyosarcoma
	Rhabdomyosarcoma
	Osteosarcoma
	Liposarcoma
	Primary cardiac lymphoma
Secondary Cardiac Tumours, Metastases	
Thrombus	
Vegetation	
Abscess	
Anatomic Variants (Crista Terminalis, etc.)	
Focal Myocardial Hypertrophy	
Lipomatous Hypertrophy of Inter-atrial Septum	
Cysts (Bronchogenic, Pericardial)	

Table 40.2 MR characteristics of primary cardiac tumours. Typical signal intensities on T1- (T1-TSE) and T2- (T2-TSE) weighted images, bright blood gradient echo (GE) cine sequences, and uptake of contrast media

	T1-TSE	T2-TSE	GE	Contrast
Primary Benign Cardiac Tumours				
Myxoma	↔	↑	↓	+
Lipoma	↑	↑	↑	−
Fibroelastoma	↔	↑	↔	+
Haemangioma	↔	↑	↔	+
Rhabdomyoma	↔/↑	↔/↑	↔	as myocardium
Fibroma	↔/↑	↔/↓	↔	−
Primary Malignant Cardiac Tumours				
Angiosarcoma	inh	inh	inh	+
Leiomyosarcoma	var	var	var	+
Osteosarcoma	inh	inh	inh	+
Liposarcoma				
Lymphoma	↔	↔	↔	inh
Thrombus				
Fresh thrombus				
Older thrombus				

Tumour signal intensity relative to signal intensity of myocardium: hyperintense, ↑; hypointense, ↓; isointense, ↔; inh, inhomogeneous signal intensity within the tumour; var, variable signal intensity with same histology.

malignant fibrous histiocytomas (11–24%), leiomyosarcomas (8%), and osteosarcomas (3–9%) [3].

The treatment for different types of cardiac masses differs greatly. Diagnostic imaging of cardiac tumours provides important clinical decision-making information, such as origin, size, extension, morphology, and mobility of the tumour, involvement of cardiac chambers, valves, myocardium and pericardium, invasiveness, vascularization, and tissue characterization. Echocardiography is usually the first imaging modality providing high sensitivity in detecting cardiac masses, particularly by transoesophageal approach, and detailed analysis of mass characteristics by the use of different imaging modalities, including 3D imaging, tissue Doppler imaging, and contrast imaging. A large number of cardiac tumours, in fact, are detected incidentally during routine echocardiographic examinations. Cardiac magnetic resonance (CMR) also offers distinct advantages in diagnosing cardiac masses and tumours including 3D and multi-planar views, a large field of view, excellent contrast resolution, adequate temporal and high spatial resolution, and the unique potential to characterize specific tissues based on their signal intensity with different imaging sequences and during contrast enhancement. In patients with contraindications for CMR, cardiac CT is an alternative, although irradiation exposure has to be taken in to account.

Primary cardiac tumours

Primary benign cardiac tumours

Myxoma

Myxomas comprise approximately 50% of primary benign cardiac tumours. They typically arise from the inter-atrial septum or the fossa ovalis, although they can arise from any endocardial area. Of myxomas, 75% are located within the left atrium, 20% in the right atrium, and rarely in the ventricles [4]. Myxomas typically manifest as intra-cardiac masses attached to the endocardium by a narrow pedicle, although broad-based and immobile masses have been reported. Myxomas may be lobular and smooth or may have villous extensions. They frequently have organized thrombi on the surface. Internally, myxomas are heterogeneous and frequently contain cysts, necrosis, haemorrhage, and calcifications [5]. Most cardiac myxomas are sporadic, but occasionally they occur multiple and familial, and may include the LAMB (lentigines, atrial myxoma, mucocutaneous myxomas, and blue naevi) and the NAME (naevi, atrial myxoma, myxoid neurofibromas, and ephelides) syndromes, which are listed under the nomenclature of the Carney complex and are associated with the germline mutation PRKAR1A [6]. Patients with cardiac myxomas often present with signs and symptoms of cerebral or systemic embolism, haemodynamic obstruction, or signs of systemic disease such as fatigue, arthralgias, weight loss, high sedimentation rate, and anaemia due to IL-6 and TNF production.

In echocardiographic imaging, myxomas are usually isodense to the myocardium. Transoesophageal echocardiography has a higher sensitivity in detecting myxomas compared to transthoracic echocardiography, especially in case of small myxomas, and should be performed in any case with suspicion for intra-cardiac tumour or source of embolism. Differentiation between myxoma and thrombus can be difficult. Compared to thrombi, myxomas usually are single masses, and they are typically located at the inter-atrial septum near the aortic root (⮪ Fig. 40.1, 📹 Videos 40.1a, b, and d). Morphology, mobility, and attachment to endocardium

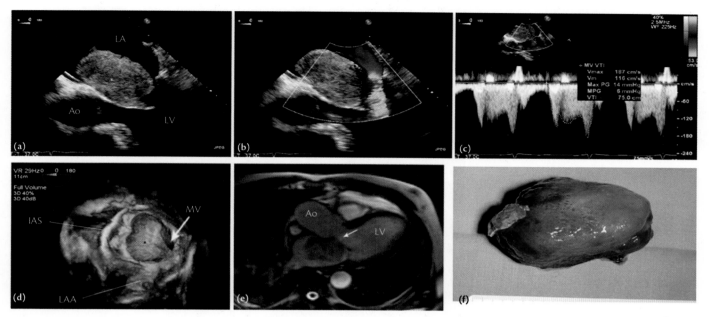

Fig. 40.1 Large left atrial myxoma (6.5 × 3.4 cm) with typical origin at the basal inter-atrial septum in a 60-year-old male patient with history of two recent cerebral embolic strokes. (a–c) Transoesophageal echocardiographic imaging shows the myxoma (*asterisk) as a highly mobile mass of heterogeneous texture and isodensity relative to the myocardium. Large myxomas can occlude the mitral valve during diastolic filling with flow obstruction demonstrated by colour Doppler (b), causing functional mitral stenosis with mean PG of 6 mmHg measured by continuous wave Doppler in this case (c). Real-time 3D echocardiographic imaging (d) reveals the true extension of the myxoma (*asterisk) in relation to the left atrium and mitral valve. In cardiac MR the myxoma (arrow) appears as a hypointense mass with heterogeneous texture (e). Photographic representation of the resected myxoma shows a glassy-elastic tumour with a vascularized, myxoid matrix in histology proving myxoma (f). LA, left atrium; Ao, aorta; LV, left ventricle; IAS, inter-atrial septum; LAA, left atrial appendage; M, mitral valve.

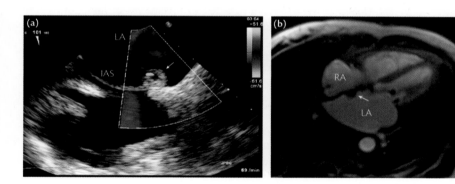

Fig. 40.2 Small left atrial myxoma (1.2 × 1.1 cm) with typical origin at the fossa ovalis in a 62-year-old female patient with moderate-to-severe mitral stenosis. In the severely dilated left atrium with spontaneous echo contrast, the mass (arrow) was initially diagnosed as a thrombus. But evidence of flow by transoesophageal colour Doppler echocardiography (a) within the mass indicating vascularization of the tumour proven to be a myxoma by histology. Cardiac MR representation (b) of the myxoma in the same patient (arrow). LA, left atrium; IAS, inter-atrial septum; RA, right atrium.

do not provide reliable discrimination between myxomas and thrombi. The presence of a tumour in the pulmonary veins, renal veins, or vena cava extension has been described as a useful aid in the differentiation of a malignant neoplasm from myxoma because myxomas with venous involvement have not been reported [7]. Although usually presenting as a homogeneous, gelatinous mass, myxoma can present an inhomogeneous echo due to intra-tumoural haemorrhage, necrosis, or calcification. Sometimes cystic formations can be displayed. Detection of flow within the myxoma by colour Doppler with a sufficiently reduced pulse repetition frequency indicates vascularization and makes thrombus less likely (⊃ Fig. 40.2, 📹 Video 40.2). However, colour Doppler is not sensitive in detecting vascularization in every myxoma. In large left atrial myxomas occluding the mitral valve during diastolic filling, functional mitral stenosis can be detected by colour Doppler and continuous wave Doppler measurement of elevated pressure gradient (⊃ Fig. 40.1, 📹 Videos 40.1a, b, c, d).

On CMR examination, cardiac myxomas are usually isointense to the myocardium on T1-weighted images and hyperintense on T2-weighted images. Less commonly, they can appear heterogeneous on both T1-weighted and T2-weighted images due to the presence of haemorrhage, necrosis, and calcification (⊃ Fig. 40.3, 📹 Video 40.3). With cine CMR low signal intensity, mobile masses are revealed, and the origin, size, mobility, extension into the different cardiac chambers, and haemodynamic obstruction can be depicted. After intravenous injection of contrast, media myxomas usually show a heterogeneous contrast enhancement to some degree.

With cardiac CT, myxomas usually have heterogeneous low attenuation reflecting gross pathologic features. Calcifications can be found frequently.

Papillary fibroelastoma

Papillary fibroelastomas are the second most common benign primary cardiac tumour after myxoma and represent 10% of all

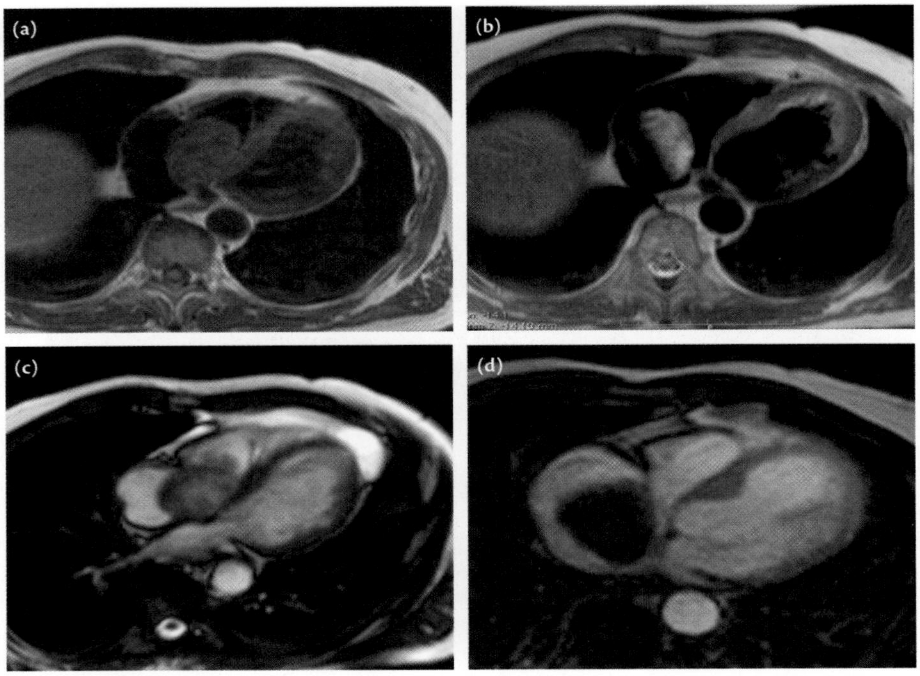

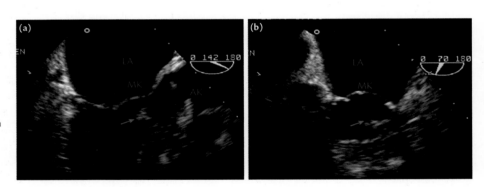

Fig. 40.3 Typical tissue signal intensities of a right atrial myxoma with different CMR sequences. (a) T1-weighted image with isointense signal of the myxoma relative to myocardium. (b) T2-weighted image shows heterogeneous signal intensity with hyperintense parts of the myxoma relative to myocardium. (c) Cine TRUFI image shows heterogeneous signal intensity of the myxoma. (d) Contrast enhanced image early after contrast administration shows enhancement of the normal myocardium, but no enhancement of the myxoma.

Fig. 40.4 Transoesophageal echocardiographic representation of a histologically proven papillary fibroelastoma (arrow) as an incidental finding in a 56-year-old male with origin from the endocardium at the anterolateral wall of the left ventricular outflow tract shown in long-axis (a) and short-axis (b) view of the aortic outflow tract. LA, left atrium; MV, mitral valve; AK, aortic valve.

primary cardiac tumours [3, 5]. On histology, a collection of non-vascular fronds of dense connective tissue lined by endothelium are found [3]. The reported prevalence varies considerably, because papillary fibroelastomas are usually asymptomatic and may therefore be underrepresented in patient series. When symptoms occur, they are usually related to embolization from thrombi on the tumour surface, but embolization of parts of the fibroelastoma is not unlikely. Of fibroelastomas, 90% occur on valve surfaces, and they are slightly more common on the aortic (29%) and the mitral valves (25%) than on the pulmonary (13%) and tricuspid valves (17%). However, this may be influenced by the increased prevalence of symptoms associated with the left-sided valves. Of fibroelastomas, 16% arise from non-valvular surfaces [3]. Fibroelastomas are usually small (<1 cm) tumours, although they have been reported as large as 5 cm.

In echocardiographic imaging, papillary fibroelastomas typically present as small, mobile masses. They have a characteristic stippled edge with a shimmer or vibration at the tumour–blood interface [8]. Finger-like projections can produce the impression of a sea anemone. Most likely they are attached to the endocardium either on the aortic or left ventricular side of the aortic

valve or neighbouring endocardium (➲ Fig. 40.4, 🎥 Videos 40.4a and b). Due to their small size, fibroelastomas are rarely detected by transthoracic echocardiography. Even in transoesophageal echocardiography, fibroelastomas are usually incidental findings. Fibroelastomas often appear alike infectious vegetations or Lambl's excrescences, which makes differentiation difficult.

On CMR examination, papillary fibroelastomas are often hard to depict due to their small size, adherence to valvular and, therefore, rapidly moving structures. They are mostly detected on cine CMR as small tumours with low signal intensity attached to moving valves. In sporadic case reports, fibroelastomas have been shown to have intermediate signal intensity on T1-weighted images and intermediate to low signal intensity on T2-weighted images [9, 10, 11]. On delayed enhancement images after administration of Gd-DTPA, a hyperintense signal intensity caused by the fibroelastic tissue has been reported [9].

With cardiac CT, papillary fibroelastomas can be found occasionally. With ECG-gated contrast enhanced 64-slice spiral CT, a well-defined, pedunculated, mobile, spherical structure with a density of 64 ± 21 Hounsfield units has been described [10].

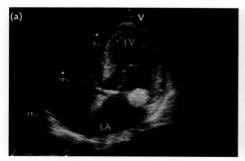 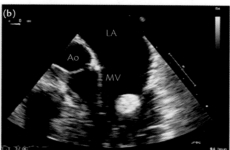 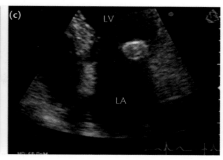

Fig. 40.5 Three examples of cardiac masses with similar echocardiographic appearance located at the posterior mitral leaflet or mitral ring. Because masses were considered benign, histology is unknown. (a) A 60-year-old patient with chronic dialysis with transthoracic echocardiography showing shadowing of the echolucent, immobile mass at the posterior mitral ring being most evident of severe mitral ring calcification. (b) A 37-year-old otherwise healthy female patient with the incidental echocardiographic finding of a hyperintense, highly mobile mass on the posterior mitral leaflet without shadowing. All criteria summarized make the mass most likely to be a haemangioma or fibroma. (c) Transthoracic echocardiographic detection of a mobile mass at the posterior mitral ring with a hyperdense outer region and a more isodense centre region and discrete echo shadowing as an incidental finding in a 56-year-old otherwise healthy patient. Differential diagnosis includes mitral ring calcification as well as lipoma, haemangioma, or fibroma. LV, left ventricle; LA, left atrium; MV, mitral valve; Ao, aorta.

Lipoma and lipomatous hypertrophy of the inter-atrial septum

Primary cardiac lipomas are benign neoplasms composed of mature adipose tissue and are histologically similar to extra-cardiac soft-tissue lipomas [3]. In autopsy studies they constitute 8–12% of primary cardiac tumours. This, however, may not represent the true prevalence, since small lipomas may remain undiagnosed in asymptomatic patients, and, on the other hand, lipomatous hypertrophy of the inter-atrial septum has been included in reports of cardiac lipomas. Lipomatous hypertrophy of the inter-atrial septum is defined as 'any deposit of fat in the atrial septum which exceeds 2 cm in transverse dimension' [3], is caused by an increase in the number of adipocytes, spares the fossa ovalis, is associated with advanced age and obesity, and does not represent a true cardiac neoplasy. Lipomas are encapsulated, homogeneous fatty tumours. They may arise from the epicardium, from the endocardium, or from the inter-atrial septum [12, 13, 14]. They grow as broad-based, pedunculated masses into any of the cardiac chambers and may reach giant sizes and weigh up to 4,800 g [15]. Many patients are asymptomatic, and the tumour is found incidentally because of chest X-ray abnormalities or heart murmur. Symptoms include shortness of breath, signs of haemodynamic obstruction, or arrhythmias.

In echocardiographic imaging, the finding of cardiac tumours suspicious of being primary cardiac lipomas is extremely rare. Because those tumours are commonly considered benign they are not surgically resected and, therefore, definite histological evidence of a lipoma is lacking (⊃ Fig. 40.5, 🎦 Videos 40.5a–c). In echocardiography, lipomas usually appear as sharply circumscribed, hypodense masses broadly attached on the adjacent wall. There is no shadowing, no necrosis, or intra-tumoural haemorrhage as a discriminating criterion to sclerotic masses. In contrast, lipomatous hypertrophy of the inter-atrial septum is a more frequent finding in transthoracic and transoesophageal echocardiography, without further diagnostic or therapeutic consequences, however. Characteristic thickening of the inter-atrial septum of more than 2 cm spares the fossa ovalis. In rare cases, vena cava

inflow obstruction can occur. A tangential imaging by a multi-plane probe is important to distinguish between true septal hypertrophy or malprojection mimicking hypertrophy.

On CMR examination, the diagnosis of a lipoma can be made with a high degree of certainty. On T1-weighted images, lipomas have a homogeneous increased signal intensity that is comparable to the signal intensity of subcutaneous fat. Necrosis, haemorrhages, or calcifications are not found. On T2-weighted images, they appear with intermediate signal intensity. By application of a fat saturation, preparation pulse with T1-weighted sequences signal intensity is decreased parallel to subcutaneous fat. Cardiac lipomas do not enhance with administration of contrast media (⊃ Fig. 40.6).

On cardiac CT, lipomas appear as homogeneous, low-attenuation masses with approximately –50 Hounsfield units.

Haemangioma

Haemangiomas are benign vascular tumours that represent less than 2% of all cardiac tumours and 5–10% of benign cardiac tumours. They are classified according to the size of their vascular channels into capillary, cavernous, or venous haemangiomas [16]. They can occur in any cardiac location and arise from the epicardium, endocardium, myocardium, and pericardium. Cardiac haemangiomas are often clinically insignificant, exist unrecognized, and are mostly diagnosed incidentally. Symptoms depend on the location within the heart and the extent of the tumour. Conduction disturbances, AV-block, arrhythmias, pericardial effusion, and angina have been reported [17].

Echocardiographic finding of cardiac tumours suspicious of being haemangiomas is extremely rare, and, similar to lipomas, histological evidence usually is lacking. They vary in size between less than 1 cm and more than 8 cm and are pediculated, non-calcified but hyperdense, and most often attached to the left or right ventricular wall but can occur in any cardiac cavity [18].

On CMR examination, cardiac haemangiomas show intermediate signal intensity on T1-weighted images, which is comparable to myocardium. On T2-weighted images, high signal intensity is typically observed. Cardiac haemangiomas enhance intensely and

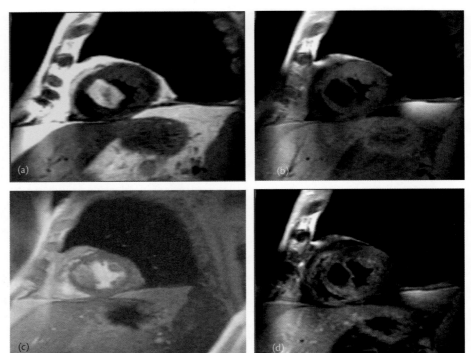

Fig. 40.6 Typical tissue signal intensities with different CMR sequences of a lipoma located within the inter-ventricular septum. (a) T1-weighted image shows hyperintense signal of the lipoma which is similar to subcutaneous fat; (b) T1-weighted image with preparation pulse for fat saturation shows hypointense signal of the lipoma relative to myocardium. Similar signal loss of subcutaneous fat; (c) cine TRUFI image shows isointense signal of the lipoma relative to myocardium; (d) T1-weighted image with preparation pulse for fat saturation after contrast administration shows no contrast enhancement of the lipoma.

very rapidly after administration of contrast media indicating a high vascularity. However, early enhancement after gadolinium administration can be inhomogeneous because of interspersed calcifications and fibrous septations within the tumour [19].

On unenhanced cardiac CT haemangiomas are shown as well-delineated mass heterogeneous to low density. They intensely enhance after intravenous contrast administration [19].

Rhabdomyoma

Rhabdomyomas are the most common primary cardiac tumour in children. They are myocardial hamartomas, and up to 50% occur in association with tuberous sclerosis [20]. Most frequently, rhabdomyomas are located in the myocardium of both ventricles and multiplicity is common. The size of the tumours may vary from miliary nodules measuring less than 1 mm up to masses of 10-cm diameter, and they tend to disappear spontaneously, although occasionally surgical resection is necessary.

Echocardiography may be diagnostic of an intra-cardiac mass by demonstrating the presence of an intra-cavitary, echodense structure. Rhabdomyomas will more frequently be lobulated in shape and ventricular in origin [21]. When occurring intramurally, a circumscribed ventricular wall thickening of the left and/or right ventricle can be detected. Multifocal lesions are common.

On CMR examination, rhabdomyomas show a homogeneous isointense signal on T1-weighted images compared to the surrounding myocardium. On T2-weighted images, hyperintense signal is observed within the mass, which is different from the surrounding myocardium. Perfusion imaging shows complete opacification of the full thickness of the mass with almost immediate opacification of the central portion. Early gadolinium uptake is more intense compared to the surrounding myocardium, and

abnormal late gadolinium enhancement may be observed across the entire thickness of the mass [22].

Fibroma

Cardiac fibroma is a congenital neoplasm and is the second most common cardiac tumour in children. It is the paediatric cardiac tumour most commonly resected. However, 15% of cardiac fibromas occur in adolescents and adults. There is an increased risk of cardiac fibromas in patients with Gorlin syndrome, which is characterized by multiple naevoid basal cell carcinomas of the skin, jaw cysts, and bifid ribs. Less than 14% of these patients have cardiac fibromas (20). The morphological features of cardiac fibromas are characteristically solitary, circumscribed, firm, grey–white, and often centrally calcified. The cellularity of the lesion decreases as fibrosis and the patient's age increase. Common clinical manifestations in patients with cardiac fibromas are heart failure, arrhythmias, and sudden death. Cardiac fibromas are usually located within the myocardium of the ventricles and the inter-ventricular septum and the lateral wall of the left ventricle are most commonly involved. The size of the tumours is rather large and varies between 2 and 5 cm.

In the echocardiographic evaluation, cardiac fibromas appear as non-contractile solid masses often attached to the left ventricular septum and well demarcated from the surrounding myocardium by multiple calcifications.

On CMR examination, cardiac fibromas may manifest as a discrete mural mass or focal myocardial thickening. These lesions appear isointense to hyperintense relative to myocardium on T1-weighted images and hypointense with T2-weighted images, findings which are characteristic for fibrous tissue. After intravenous administration of gadolinium, contrast media cardiac fibromas do not show enhancement during first-pass perfusion, suggesting a low vascularity. However, 10 min after contrast administration, intense late gadolinium enhancement was observed reflecting an increased extracellular volume of distribution within the ventricular myocardium [23].

Primary malignant cardiac tumours

The majority of primary malignant cardiac tumours are sarcomas. Primary cardiac sarcomas by definition are confined to the heart or pericardium at the time of diagnosis. The most common types are angiosarcoma (37%), unclassified or undifferentiated sarcoma (24%), malignant fibrous histiocytoma (11–24%), leiomyosarcoma (8%), and osteosarcoma (3–9%) [3]. Primary cardiac sarcomas most commonly metastasize to the lungs but also to the lymph nodes, bone, liver, brain, bowel, spleen, adrenal glands, pleura, diaphragm, kidneys, thyroid, and skin [24].

Cardiac sarcomas that typically affect the left atrium are malignant fibrous histiocytoma, osteosarcoma, and leiomyosarcoma. Patients present with symptoms of mitral valve obstruction such as dyspnoea and heart failure.

Approximately 80% of cardiac angiosarcomas occur in the right atrium and involve the pericardium. Therefore, symptoms of right-sided heart inflow obstruction or cardiac tamponade are common.

Angiosarcoma

Echocardiographic imaging helps to differentiate between benign myxomas and malignant infiltrative growing angiosarcomas by evidence of infiltration of the cardiac wall. With the evidence of haemorrhagic pericardial effusion, a malignant tumour should be considered. Angiosarcomas appear as an inhomogeneous mass with hypodense necrotic and haemorrhagic zones, usually located in the right atrium. A possible infiltration of the pericardium, the tricuspid valve, and the vena cava can be displayed.

On CMR examination, angiosarcomas are depicted as large, heterogeneous, invasive right atrial masses frequently with extensive pericardial involvement and haemorrhagic pericardial effusion. Pericardial and extra-cardiac invasion, valvular destruction, tumour necrosis, and metastases are frequently seen. Cardiac angiosarcomas have a marked heterogeneity of signal intensity on T1-weighted and T2-weighted images. Hyperintense foci in T1-weighted images may correspond to intra-tumoural haemorrhage, whereas hyperintense foci on T2-weighted images may represent cystic or necrotic parts of the tumour [25]. Vascular structures within the tumour may appear hyperintense on cine sequences, which has been described as 'cauliflower' in appearance [16]. Cardiac angiosarcomas typically show diffuse and intense contrast enhancement that has been described as 'sunray' appearance [26].

Other sarcomas

Undifferentiated sarcoma, malignant fibrous histiocytoma, leiomyosarcoma, rhabdomyosarcoma, osteosarcoma, fibrosarcoma, and liposarcoma are rare primary malignant cardiac tumours. However, approximately 10% of surgically resected cardiac tumours are primary sarcomas.

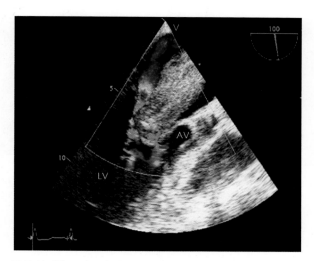

Fig. 40.7 Undifferentiated primary cardiac sarcoma (*asterisk) in a 67-year-old female patient with the history of progressive dyspnoea due to functional mitral stenosis caused by diastolic occlusion of mitral inflow by the large sarcoma shown by colour Doppler. Note the similar appearance of the sarcoma in transoesophageal echocardiographic imaging compared to the myxoma in Fig. 40.1 except of the sarcoma's origin from the left atrial roof. LV, left ventricle; AV, aortic valve.

For the echocardiographic evaluation of the other cardiac sarcomas, the same rules may be applied as for angiosarcomas, except they are not characteristically located within the right atrium but elsewhere in the heart predominantly within the left atrium. They typically originate from the roof of the left atrium as a criterion of discrimination from myxomas (⬇ Fig. 40.7, 📹 Video 40.7), as well as infiltration of the surrounding cardiac wall or pericardial structures (⬇ Fig. 40.8, 📹 Video 40.8). They appear as large, mobile, and inhomogeneous masses with zones of necrosis and haemorrhage and are indistinguishable from angiosarcoma. Only osteosarcomas can be differentiated by typically showing calcification.

On CMR examination, cardiac sarcomas are typically shown as large, heterogeneous, broad-based masses that frequently occupy most of the affected cardiac chamber or multiple chambers (📹 Video 40.9). Pericardial and extra-cardiac invasion, tumour necrosis, and metastases are all characteristic features of malignant lesions. Cardiac sarcomas enhance heterogeneously with non-enhancing areas corresponding to necrosis.

Cardiac CT is very helpful in the evaluation of cardiac osteosarcoma because it typically shows calcifications [3].

Primary cardiac lymphoma

Primary cardiac lymphoma involves only the heart or pericardium at the time of diagnosis with no evidence of extra-cardiac lymphoma [3]. Although 16–28% of patients with disseminated lymphoma have cardiac involvement, primary cardiac lymphoma is very rare. It is seen mostly in immunocompromised patients, particularly in association with the acquired immunodeficiency syndrome.

In the echocardiographic evaluation, an immobile, sometimes polypoid mass appears, predominantly in the right atrium. It is commonly combined with a pericardial effusion. Infiltration of the cardiac structures can occur (⬇ Fig. 40.10, 📹 Video 40.10).

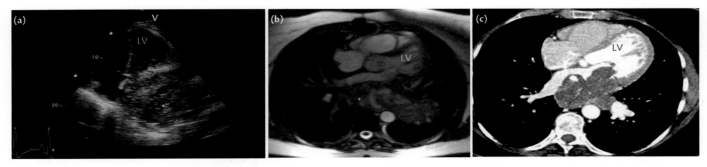

Fig. 40.8 Large rhabdomyosarcoma (*asterisk) first detected by transthoracic echocardiography (a) in an 83-year-old female patient with signs of progressive dyspnoea. The tumour that fills out the entire dilated left atrium in echocardiography appears of heterogeneous texture with hypodense zones of necrosis and hyperdense sclerotic spots. Cardiac MR (b) revealed a large rhabdomyosarcoma (7.0 = 13.1 cm) with cystic areas and strong contrast agent uptake in border regions, as well as with extensive infiltration of the left lung and less infiltration of the right lung, but no metastases. Cardiac CT 1 mo after cardiac MR (c) reveals rapid progression of tumour size now being 9.1 × 14.3 cm with progressive building of a wall around the left lung hilus and compression of the oesophagus. LV, left ventricle.

Fig. 40.9 Cine TRUFI demonstrating a large leiomyosarcoma with invasion of large parts of the right atrial wall and free wall of the right ventricle, destruction of the anterior leaflet of the tricuspid valve and pericardial and pleural effusion. Isointense signal of the leiomyosarcoma relative to myocardium.

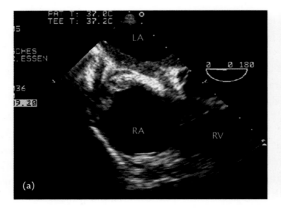
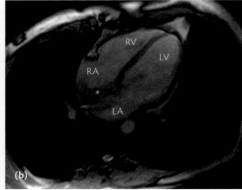

Fig. 40.10 Primary cardiac lymphoma in a 25-year-old male patient with acute myeloid leukaemia. Transoesophageal echocardiographic imaging shows massive growth of a heterogeneous tumour mass (*asterisk) within the inter-atrial septum with infiltration of the right atrial roof. Cardiac MR reveals tumour manifestation beginning in the right atrial roof or superior vena cava entrance, which is walled in by the tumour, and tumour growth up to pulmonary artery descending aorta, into the posterior right atrial wall and the inter-atrial septum and caudal up to the inferior vena cava and coronary sinus. The tumour (*asterisk) is clearly hyperintense on the T2-weighted image and enhances markedly after contrast administration, but no myocardial late enhancement was found. LA, left atrium; RA, right atrium; RV, right ventricle; LV, left ventricle.

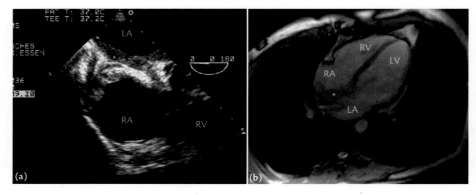

On CMR examination, poorly marginated and heterogeneous lesions are observed, which are isointense to slightly hypointense on T1-weighted images and isointense on T2-weighted images relative to myocardium. Contrast administration produces a heterogeneous pattern of enhancement [20].

With cardiac CT, primary cardiac lymphomas are hypoattenuating or isoattenuating relative to myocardium and demonstrate heterogeneous enhancement after intravenous contrast administration [27].

Secondary cardiac tumours, metastases

Tumours within the chest can cause displacement and compression of the heart or infiltrate the heart and pericardium directly. High-resolution imaging of such tumours and proof of infiltration is important because such tumours are usually non-resectable. Cardiac metastases can arise from almost any malignant tumour,

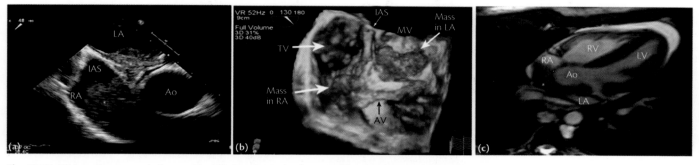

Fig. 40.11 High-malignant, cerebellar non-Hodgkin lymphoma in a 19-year-old male patient with secondary cardiac lymphoma manifestation in both atria. Transoesophageal echocardiographic imaging shows growth of lymphoma masses (*asterisks) of heterogeneous texture on both sides of the inter-atrial septum (IAS) (a). Real-time 3D echocardiography (b) provides greater information on the location and extent of lymphoma manifestation. Cardiac MR (c) shows lymphoma growth isointense to the myocardium into left and right atrium (*asterisk), as well as subtotal occlusion of vena cava superior causing thrombus formation into right vena subclavia, left vena brachiocephalica, and right vena jugularis. LA, left atrium; RA, right atrium; Ao, aorta; RV, right ventricle; TV, tricuspid valve; MV, mitral valve; LV, left ventricle.

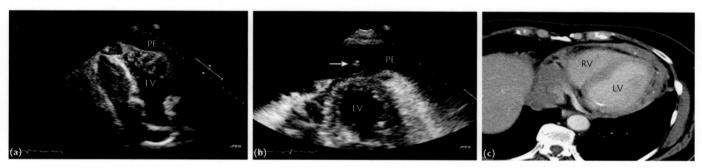

Fig. 40.12 Secondary cardiac manifestation of a low-malignant non-Hodgkin lymphoma in a 77-year-old female patient. Transthoracic echocardiography shows massive intra-pericardial lymphoma growth with compression of the right heart chambers as well as infiltrative growth into right ventricular apex (*asterisk) (a). At the time of echocardiographic examination, cardiac lymphoma manifestation was unknown, and diagnosis of haemodynamic important pericardial effusion (PE) was priority. Surprisingly, echo-guided pericardiocentesis (b) with the needle tip safely placed in the echo-free pericardial space (arrow) did not allow fluid aspiration. Cardiac CT (c) revealed the diagnosis of circular intra-pericardial lymphoma growth (*asterisks) as the explanation of the punctio sicca. PE, pericardial effusion; LV, left ventricle; RV, right ventricle.

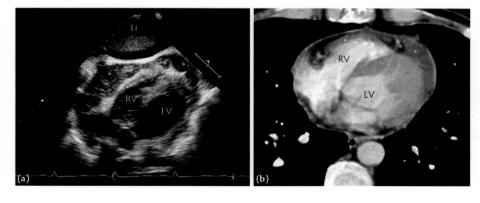

Fig. 40.13 Secondary cardiac manifestation of thymus carcinoma in a 52-year-old male patient with infiltrative pericardial and myocardial growth. Transthoracic echocardiographic image from a subcostal view (a) shows the tumour (*asterisks) hypodense relative to the myocardium and with heterogeneous appearance. Cardiac CT shows the tumour reaching from above the aortic arch to the heart apex with displacement of the entire heart and marked intra-pericardial growth (*asterisks) and compression of right heart chambers. Li, liver; RV, right ventricle; LV, left ventricle.

and melanomas have been reported to have the highest frequency of seeding into the heart at autopsy.

Secondary cardiac lymphoma show similar echocardiographic characteristics as primary cardiac lymphomas (⊃ Figs 40.11 and 40.12, 🎥 Videos 40.11a, b, and 40.12a, b). Common echocardiographic findings associated with cardiac metastases are malignant pericardial effusion sometimes with enclosed tumour masses with partially bizarre surface structures. The infiltrated cardiac walls appear with a hyperdense thickening (⊃ Figs 40.13 and 40.14, 🎥 Videos 40.13 and 40.14). Wall motion abnormalities in these regions are common. Application of echo contrast agents can reveal the tumour perfusion and helps

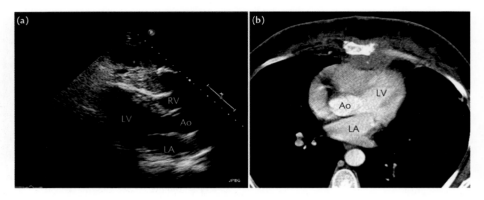

Fig. 40.14 Sternal metastasis of breast carcinoma in a 47-year-old female patient with marked displacement of the heart and compression of right heart chambers. Transthoracic echocardiographic imaging in a parasternal view (a) shows an isodense tumour mass of heterogeneous appearance (*asterisk) with infiltrative growth into right heart pericardium. Cardiac CT with contrast application (b) shows the large sternal metastasis (8.2 × 6.4 cm) (*asterisk) with infiltrative growth into the mediastinum and pericardium. LV, left ventricle; R, right ventricle; LA, left atrium; Ao, aorta.

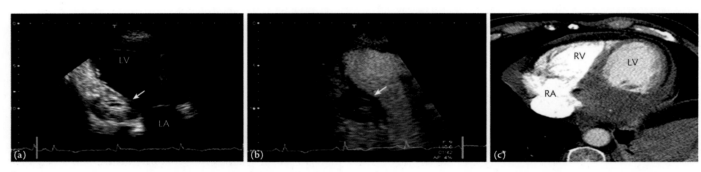

Fig. 40.15 Cardiac metastasis of urothel carcinoma in a 70-year-old male patient. In transthoracic echocardiography the metastasis located in the basal inferior wall of the left ventricle (arrow) appears with a typical pattern of a hypodense outer region that is clearly demarcated from myocardial tissue and a hyperdense central region (a), which enhances markedly after myocardial contrast application (b) indicating central perfusion of the metastasis. Cardiac CT (c) shows the metastasis (*asterisk) as a homogeneous mass, which is isointense relative to the myocardium. LV, left ventricle; LA, left atrium; RV, right ventricle; RA, right atrium.

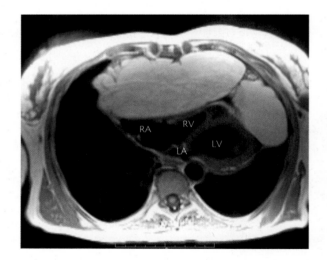

Fig. 40.16 T1-weighted image of metastases in the chest of a cystadeno-carcinoma. Huge fluid-containing cysts with septations are shown to compress and dislocate the cardiac chambers without signs of tumour invasion. The patient suffered from severe dyspnoea.

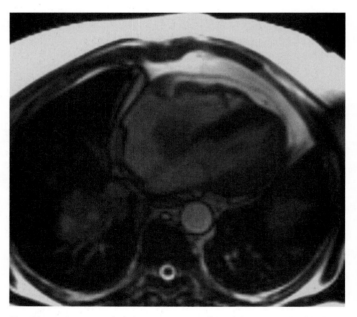

Fig. 40.17 Cine CMR showing a metastasis of a melanoma attached to the right sided interatrial septum. A large and several smaller metastases in both lungs are also demonstrated.

discrimination of the metastasis from the surrounding tissue (➲ Fig. 40.15, 🎥 Videos 40.15a, b).

On CMR examination, the extension of tumours within the chest (➲ Fig. 40.16, 🎥 Video 40.16), their relation to cardiac structures, signs of invasion (🎥 Video 40.17), evidence of haemorrhagic, and serous pericardial effusion can be demonstrated very effectively due to the large field of view and the high contrast resolution. This information is necessary to assess potential

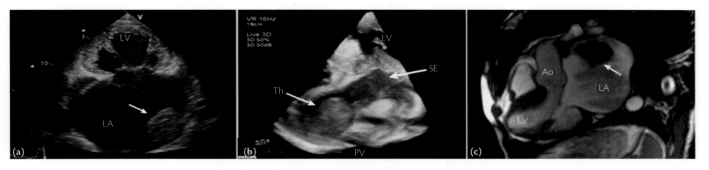

Fig. 40.18 Left atrial thrombus in a monstrous dilated left atrium (10.0 × 10.5 cm) in a 46-year-old male patient with long-standing hypertrophic restrictive cardiomyopathy. Transthoracic echocardiographic imaging (a) shows the isodense appearance of the large immobile thrombus (4 × 5 cm) (arrow) broadly attached to left atrial wall. Note the marked spontaneous echo contrast (SE) passing from the left atrium through the mitral valve. Real-time 3D-echocardiography reveals the true shape and size of the thrombus (Th) (b) and its exact location relative to pulmonary vein (PV) entrance. Cardiac MR (c) shows the thrombus (arrow) with hypointense appearance and no contrast uptake after contrast application. LV, left ventricle; LA, left atrium; Ao, aorta.

resectability of the tumour (📼 Video 40.18). Cardiac CT, with its excellent spatial resolution, may provide comparable information as CMR; however, CMR has been shown to be even more effective in demonstrating invasion of the pericardium and myocardium [28].

Thrombus

Thrombi represent the most frequently found intra-cardiac masses. Mitral valve disease and atrial fibrillation are the predominant risk factors for thrombus formation within the left atrium, especially within the left atrial appendage. Thrombi within the left ventricle are typically found in areas of severe wall motion abnormalities such as akinetic, dyskinetic, or aneurysmal myocardial segments after myocardial infarction. Severe impairment of global left ventricular function may also increase the risk for thrombus formation within the left ventricular cavity. Thrombus morphology correlates with the risk for systemic embolization: mobile or exophytically growing thrombi carry a risk of 50% for systemic embolism, whereas this risk is 10% for immobile, mural thrombi. Right-sided thrombi are found less frequently and may represent transitory thrombi in patients with deep vein thrombosis and pulmonary embolism. However, in patients with rather rare systemic diseases such as Behçet disease, Löffler's endocarditis, Churg–Strauss syndrome, and coagulopathies, thrombi can be found in all cardiac chambers.

Echocardiographic appearance of intra-cardiac thrombi is heterogeneous. Because thrombi can mimic any other cardiac mass, echocardiography cannot reliably differentiate between thrombi and tumours (➲ Figs 40.18, 40.19, 40.20, 40.21, 40.22, 📼 Videos 40.19a, b, 40.20a–d, 40.21, 40.22, 40.23a–c). Thrombi show a different echodensity, depending on age and degree of thrombus organization (➲ Fig. 40.19). Even vascularization can be found in some cases. Sometimes a layering phenomenon can be found, indicating appositional thrombus growth. Confounding risk factors for thrombus formation, such as wall motion abnormalities

(➲ Fig. 40.20, 📼 Video 40.21), atrial dilatation (➲ Fig. 40.18, 📼 Video 40.19), and slow flow with spontaneous echo contrast (➲ Fig. 40.18, 📼 Video 40.19), allow differentiation to cardiac tumours. Reduced velocities within the left atrial appendage due to atrial fibrillation can be detected by pulsed wave Doppler and can predict the risk for thrombus formation (➲ Fig. 40.22, 📼 Video 40.23).

On CMR examination, the appearance of thrombus is dependent on the composition and physico-chemical properties of its components. Paramagnetic haemoglobin degradation products, such as intracellular methemoglobin, haemosiderin, and ferromagnetic ferritin, accumulate with ageing of the thrombus. On T1-and T2-weighted images these haemoglobin degradation products are hypointense. Detection and characterization of thrombi with dark-blood prepared T1-and T2-weighted images is, however, suboptimal, because slow blood flow around thrombi may produce slow flow artefacts and thereby impede the detection of thrombi. With cine sequences, however, fresh thrombus may show hyperintense signal intensity (➲ Fig. 40.23) and subacute and old thrombi low signal intensity (➲ Fig. 40.24). Thrombi generally do not enhance after administration of contrast media; however, chronic organized thrombi may occasionally show patchy peripheral contrast uptake [29]. Delayed contrast CMR has been shown to be highly helpful in detecting intra-cardiac thrombi, which have very low signal intensity (black) with this technique. On the other hand, adjacent infarcted myocardium shows very high signal intensity (white). During first pass of the contrast media through the cardiac chambers, left ventricular cavity is strongly enhanced with abnormal intra-ventricular structures appearing dark in comparison [30]. Contrast enhanced inversion recovery CMR allows visualization of small thrombi (<1 cm), although some may be missed due to flow turbulence in proximity to dysfunctional myocardial wall segments or lack of contrast between a mural thrombus and the adjacent myocardium. In this case, a combination of cine CMR sequences and contrast enhanced inversion recovery CMR sequences may overcome that problem [31].

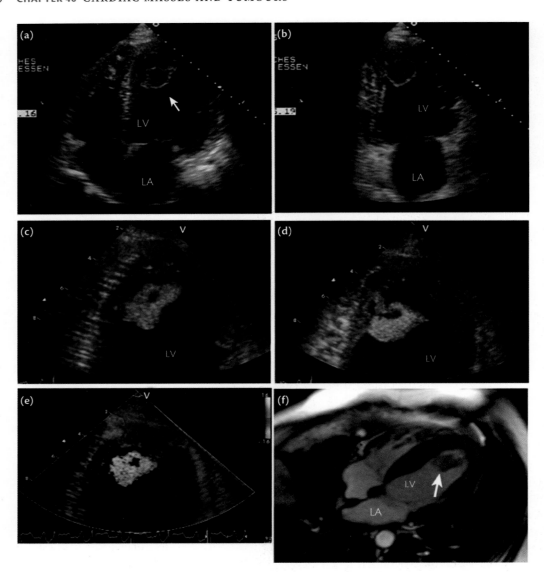

Fig. 40.19 Apical left ventricular thrombus in a 32-year-old male patient with thrombophilia due to factor X mutation. Transthoracic echocardiographic imaging in apical 4-chamber (a) and 2-chamber view (b) shows typical appearance of a fresh thrombus (arrow) with hyperdense outer border and hypodense centre. The jelly-like thrombus is highly mobile and deformable and only partly attached to the infero-apical wall. In 10 days follow-up under intensive anticoagulation the thrombus became markedly more organized and stiffer (c, d). Colour-coded tissue Doppler imaging (TDI) provides still image documentation of incoherent thrombus motion relative to cardiac tissue (e). In cardiac MR (f) the jelly-like thrombus (arrow) appears to be only attached by thin threadlike structures to the apical wall. LV, left ventricle; LA, left atrium.

Fig. 40.20 Large thrombus formation in an apical left ventricular aneurysm in a 54-year-old male patient after apical myocardial infarction. Transthoracic echocardiographic imaging (a) shows a large immobile thrombus (*asterisk) with heterogeneous appearance with hypodense areas and hyperdense sclerotic spots. Cardiac MR (b) shows the thrombus (*asterisk) with hypointense appearance and no contrast uptake after contrast application. AV, aortic valve; LV, left ventricle; LA, left atrium.

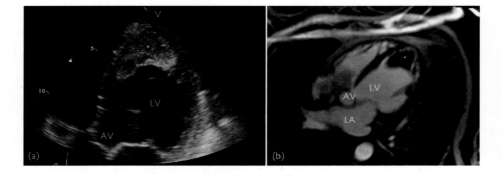

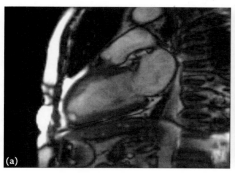
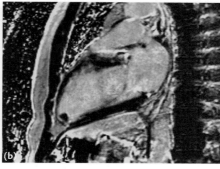

Fig. 40.21 Multiple right atrial thrombi in a 60-year-old male patient with history of cerebral transient ischaemia attacks. Transoesophageal echocardiographic imaging (a) shows multiple mobile hypodense thrombi attached to the right-sided inter-atrial septum and right atrial walls. In cardiac MR (b) 2 days later only one thrombus (arrow) was detectable, shown hypointense in TrueFISP-Sequences. LA, left atrium; RA, right atrium.

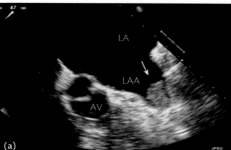
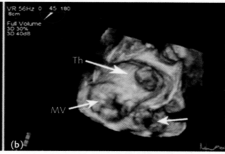
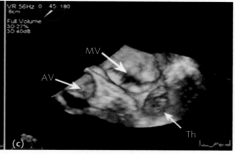

Fig. 40.22 Cardiac thrombus in the left atrial appendage in a 74-year-old male patient with moderate–severe mitral stenosis and dilated left atrium. Transoesophageal echocardiographic imaging in 2D mode (a) shows a 1.0 × 1.9 cm large isodense, slightly mobile thrombus (arrow) in the left atrial appendage (LAA). Real-time 3D imaging provides improved orientation by showing neighbouring cardiac structures in an *en face* view from left atrium to mitral valve (MV) (b) as well as exact dimension of the thrombus (Th) within the appendage (c). LA, left atrium, AV, aortic valve.

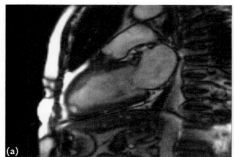
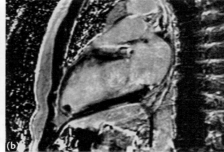

Fig. 40.23 Fresh thrombus in the left ventricular apex assessed with CMR. (a) A single image frame from a cine CMR loop in a left ventricular long-axis 2-chamber view shows the thinned wall of the left ventricular apex after myocardial infarction containing a thrombus depicted as a bright spherical mass surrounded by a dark rim. (b) With late gadolinium enhancement the infarcted area of the left ventricular apex is depicted hyperintense (white, scar) and the thrombus black without any uptake of contrast media.

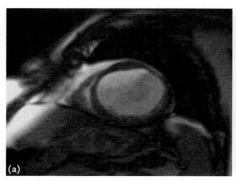
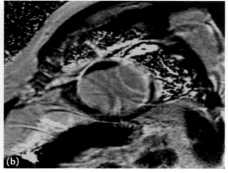

Fig. 40.24 Chronic mural thrombus in a patient with chronic anteroseptal myocardial infarction and heart failure as assessed by CMR. (a) A single image frame from a cine CMR loop in a left ventricular short-axis view shows the thinned anteroseptal wall with chronic myocardial infarction and a hypointense mural mass (thrombus) in the infarct zone. (b) With late gadolinium enhancement the infarct area (white, scar) is depicted transmurally in the anteroseptal segments and sub-endocardially (non transmural) in the lateral segment. In the anteroseptal segments the mural thrombus is depicted hypointense (black) inside the white myocardial scar without any uptake of contrast media.

References

1. Butany J, Nair V, Naseemuddin A, Nair GM, Catton C, Yau T. Cardiac tumours: diagnosis and management. *Lancet Oncol* 2005; 6: 219–28.

2. Lam KY, Dickens P, Chan AC. Tumours of the heart. A 20-year experience with a review of 12,485 consecutive autopsies. *Arch Pathol Lab Med* 1993; 117: 1027–31.

3. Burke A, Virmany R. Tumours of the heart and great vessels. In: *Atlas of Tumour Pathology*, 3rd series, fasc 16. Washington, DC: Armed Forces Institute of Pathology; 1996.

4. Araoz PA, Mulvagh SL, Tazelaar HD, Julsrud PR, Breen JF. CT and MR imaging of benign primary cardiac neoplasm with echocardiographic correlation. *Radiographics* 2000; 20: 1303–19.

5. Tazelaar HD, Locke TJ, McGregor CG. Pathology of surgically excised primary cardiac tumours. *Mayo Clin Proc* 1992; 67: 957–65.

6. Stergiopoulos SG, Stratakis CK. Human tumours associated with Carney complex and germline PRKAR1A mutations: a protein kinase A disease. *FEBS Lett* 2003; 546: 59–64.

7. Edwards LC, III, Louie EK. Transthoracic and transoesophageal echocardiography for evaluation of cardiac tumours, thrombi, and valvular vegetations. *Am J Cardiac Imaging* 1994; 8: 45–48.

8. Klarich KW, Enriquez-Sarano M, Gura GM, Edwards WD, Tajik AJ, Seward JB. Papillary fibroelastoma: echocardiographic characteristics for diagnosis and pathologic correlation. *JACC* 1997; 30: 784–90.

9. Kelle S, Chiribiri A, Meyer R, Fleck E, Nagel E. Papillary fibroelastoma of the tricuspid valve seen on magnetic resonance imaging. *Circulation* 2008; 117: e190–91.

10. Lembcke A, Meyer R, Kivelitz D, Thiele H, Barho C, Albes JM, Hotz H. Papillary fibroelastoma of the aortic valve. Appearance in 64-slice spiral CT, magentic resonance imaging and echocardiography. *Circulation* 2007; 115: e3–6.

11. Kondruweit M, Schmid M, Strecker T. Papillary fibroelastoma of the mitral valve: appearance in 64-slice spiral CT, magnetic resonance imaging and echocardiography. *Eur Heart J* 2008; 29: 831.

12. Grande AM, Minizioni G, Perderzolli C, et al. Cardiac lipomas. Description of 3 cases. *J Cardiovasc Surg* 1998; 39: 813–5.

13. Vanderheyden M, De Sutter J, Wellens F, Andries E. Left atrial lipoma: case report and review of the literature. *Acta Cardiol* 1998; 53: 31–32.

14. Mousseaux E, Idy-Peretti I, Bittoun J, et al. MR tissue characterization of a right atrial mass: diagnosis of a lipoma. *J Comput Assist Tomogr* 1992; 16: 148–51.

15. Lang-Lazdunski L, Oroudji M, Pansard Y, Vissuzaine C, Hvass U. Successful resection of giant intrapericardial lipoma. *Ann Thorac Surg* 1994; 58: 238–40.

16. Krombach GA, Saeed M, Higgins CB. Cardiac masses. In: Higgins CB, de Roos A (eds). *Cardiovascular MRI and MRA*. Philadelphia, PA: Lippincott Williams & Wilkins; 2003. 136–44.

17. Kober G, Magedanz A, Mohrs O, Nowak B, Scherer D, Bug R, Voigtländer T. Non-invasive diagnosis of a pedunculated left ventricular haemangioma. *Clin Res Cardiol* 2007; 96: 227–31.

18. Kojima S, Sumiyoshi M, Suwa S, et al. Cardiac haemangioma: a report of two cases and review of the literature. *Heart Vessels* 2003; 18: 153–6.

19. Oshima H, Hara M, Kono T, Shibamoto Y, Mishima A, Akita S. Cardiac haemangioma of the left atrial appendage: CT and MR findings. *J Thorac Imag* 2003; 18: 204–6.

20. Grebenc ML, Rosado de Christenson ML, Burke AP, Green CE, Galvin JR. Primary cardiac and pericardial neoplasms: Radiologic-pathologic correlation. *Radiographics* 2000; 20: 1073–1103.

21. Fischer DR, Beerman LB, Prak SC, Bahnson HAT, Fricker FJ, Mathews RA. Diagnosis of intra-cardiac rhabdomyoma by two-dimensional echocardiography. *Am J Cardiol* 1984; 53: 978–9.

22. Wage R, Kafka H, Prasad S. Cardiac rhabdomyoma in an adult with previous presumptive diagnosis of septal hypertrophy. *Circulation* 2008; 117: e469–70.

23. Yan AT, Coffey DM, Li Y, et al. Myocardial fibroma in Gorlin Syndrome by cardiac magnetic resonance imaging. *Circulation* 2006; 114: e376–9.

24. Burke AP, Cowan D, Virmani R. Primary sarcomas of the heart. *Cancer* 1992; 69: 387–95.

25. Frank H. Cardiac and paracardiac masses. In: Manning W, Pennell D (eds). *Cardiovascular Magnetic Resonance*. New York: Churchill Livingstone; 2002. 342–454.

26. Kaminaga T, Takeshita T, Kimura I. Role of magnetic resonance imaging for the evaluation of tumours in cardiac region. *Eur Radiol* 2003; 13: L1–10.

27. Ceresoli Gl, Ferreri AJ, Bucci E, Ripa C, Ponzoni M, Villa E. Primary cardiac lymphoma in immunocompetent patients. *Cancer* 1997; 80: 1497–506.

28. Mader MT, Poulton TB, White RD. Malignant tumours of the heart and great vessels: MR imaging appearance. *Radiographics* 1997; 17: 145–53.

29. Paydarfar D, Krieger D, Dib N, et al. In vivo magnetic resonance imaging and surgical histopathology of intra-cardiac masses: distinct features of subacute thrombi. *Cardiology* 2001; 95: 40–47.

30. Attili AK, Espinosa L, Gebker R. AJR teaching file: Left ventricular mass in a patient with ischemic heart disease. *AJR* 2007; 188: S31–34.

31. Barkhausen J, Hunold P, Eggebrecht H, et al. Detection and characterization of intra-cardiac thrombi on MR imaging. *AJR* 2002; 179: 1539–44.

⊃ **For additional multimedia materials please visit the online version of the book (⌐ http://www.esciacc.oxfordmedicine.com)**

SECTION VIII

Adult congenital heart disease

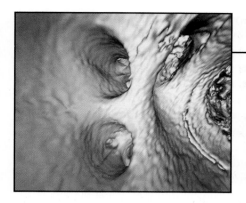

CHAPTER 41

The role of echocardiography in adult congenital heart disease

Luc Mertens and Mark K. Friedberg

Contents

Introduction

Congenital malformations of the heart affect at least 1% of newborn infants. Without intervention, the prognosis for more complex forms is poor. Over the last few decades advances in paediatric cardiology and cardiac surgery have significantly improved patient management, and the majority of patients now survive into adulthood [1, 2]. This has led to new challenges as increasing numbers of adult patients with congenital heart disease transition into the care of adult cardiac services. Caring for these patients requires expert knowledge and a new subspecialty of adult congenital heart disease (CHD) has emerged. This patient population also has specific imaging requirements due to variability in morphology and haemodynamics.

Overview of the main non-invasive imaging modalities

The different non-invasive modalities are, to a large extent, complementary. More than one modality is likely to be needed to address all the relevant clinical questions, particularly in the more complex cases.

Chest X-ray

Chest X-ray (postero-anterior ± lateral) provides an inclusive overview of the heart, mediastinum, pulmonary vessels, lung fields, and thoracic skeleton. It remains a valuable and inexpensive modality, with only a low dose of ionizing radiation, for the serial comparison of heart size, pulmonary vascularity, and peripheral lung fields in adults with CHD.

Transthoracic echocardiography (TTE)

Transthoracic echocardiography (TTE) is generally the first-line cardiovascular imaging modality because of its convenience, availability, real-time acquisition, relatively modest cost, and safety. Its usefulness is, however, operator-dependent, particularly in adults with CHD. Limited echocardiographic acoustic windows and the suboptimal penetration of ultrasound represent important limitations in adults after cardiovascular surgery.

Transoesophageal echocardiography (TOE)

Transoesophageal echocardiography (TOE) has the advantage of clear access to more posterior parts of the heart, particularly for 3D visualizations of valves and the atrial septum.

A disadvantage, however, is its invasive nature, generally requiring sedation or anaesthesia, making it less acceptable than cardiac magnetic resonance (CMR) for serial investigation. The field of view provided by TOE also is relatively narrow, with limited access to extra-cardiac structures, and the alignment of the Doppler beam with unusually oriented flow jets can be challenging. Perioperative TOE is for assessing the immediate post-surgical.

Cardiovascular magnetic resonance (CMR)

Cardiovascular magnetic resonance (CMR) is not restricted by body size or poor acoustic windows and is versatile, offering a repertoire of velocity mapping and tissue contrast options, without any ionizing radiation. CMR is widely regarded as the gold-standard for measurements of right as well as left ventricular volumes, although analysis takes time and requires rigorously consistent methods of acquisition and measurement that may be hard to maintain in practice. It also provides flow quantification and tissue characterization, which can be important in adults with CHD.

Multi-slice computed tomography (MSCT)

Multi-slice computed tomography (MSCT) also offers robust spatial localization, plus excellent spatial resolution in much shorter investigation times than CMR. It is well suited for imaging the epicardial coronary arteries and aorto-pulmonary collateral arteries, and for the investigation of parenchymal lung disease, if present. ECG-gated cine MSCT allows measurements of biventricular size and function, albeit at a lower temporal resolution than CMR, and subject to adequate opacification of the intra-ventricular blood volumes. In patients with a pacemaker or ICD, CT provides an alternative to CMR. The main drawback of MSCT is exposure to a substantial dose of ionizing radiation and the need of contrast media. Other drawbacks compared with CMR include less versatile tissue contrast and an inferior ability to evaluate cardiovascular physiology.

Describing abnormal cardiovascular connections

For the description of anatomy a common methodology can be used by all imaging techniques. This is called the segmental approach [3]. The heart is viewed as consisting of certain segments (the systemic and pulmonary veins, the atria, the ventricles and the great vessels), which are defined by unique morphological characteristics. The segments need to be identified and the connections between the segments are to be described. These are the veno-atrial connections, the atrioventricular connections, and the ventriculo-arterial connections.

Segmental analysis begins by defining the cardiac position and atrial arrangement (situs). The cardiac position may be levocardia, dextrocardia, or mesocardia. The atrial situs is 'usual' (situs solitus, i.e. a right atrium (RA) on the right and a left atrium (LA) on the left), or 'inverted' (situs inversus) or there can be bilateral duplication of one type of atrium known as right or left atrial 'isomerism'. Isomerism is generally associated with accompanying

malformations. Atrio-ventricular (AV) and ventriculo-arterial connections are described as concordant (e.g. RA to right ventricle (RV), or left ventricle (LV) to aorta), discordant (e.g. LA to RV), double inlet (e.g. double inlet left ventricle), or single inlet (left AV-valve atresia). This requires identification of the ventricular chambers as morphological left or right ventricles, which is based on unique morphological characteristics for each ventricle. A RV typically has more coarse apical trabeculations, has a tricuspid valve at the inlet, has a moderator band, and the inlet and outlet are separated by an infundibulum. Afterwards the great vessels are identified and the ventriculo-arterial connections are described. These connections can be concordant (normal), discordant (transposition of the great arteries), double outlet (double outlet RV), or single outlet (pulmonary atresia, common arterial trunk). Finally, communications between the left and right side need to be described (ventricular septal defect, VSD; atrial septal defect, ASD; patent ductus arteriosus, PDA).

The role of echocardiography in different congenital defects

Atrial septal defects (ASD)

ASDs are common also in the adult population. When diagnosing patients with ASDs, the following questions should be addressed.

Type and location of the ASD

- Secundum ASD (70%). The defect is localized centrally in the intra-atrial septum (Fig. 41.1; Videos 41.1a,b). There can be multiple defects and the defect can be fenestrated.

- Primum ASD (11%). Belongs to the spectrum of atrioventricular septal defects (Fig. 41.2; Videos 41.2a,b). This is always associated with an abnormal left atrioventricular valve ('cleft' AV-valve).

- Sinus venosus ASD (SVC 5.3–10%, IVC 2%). This defect is located outside the limbus of the fossa ovalis, on the right septal surface adjacent to the drainage site of the superior (or inferior) vena cava (Fig. 41.3; Video 41.3). This is commonly associated with partially anomalous venous return of the right upper pulmonary vein.

- Coronary sinus ASD. This defect is in the wall which separates the coronary sinus from the left atrium (LA). It may be fenestrated or completely absent. An enlarged coronary sinus with a drop out between the LA and the coronary sinus is seen. Best view is a posteriorly tilted 4-chamber view (Fig. 41.4).

Haemodynamic effects

The atrial left-to-right (L→R) shunt can cause right heart dilatation and can be associated with pulmonary hypertension. Signs of a haemodynamically significant ASD are:

- RA and RV dilatation.
- Abnormal 'paradoxical' septal motion.
- Elevated RV pressure (rare).

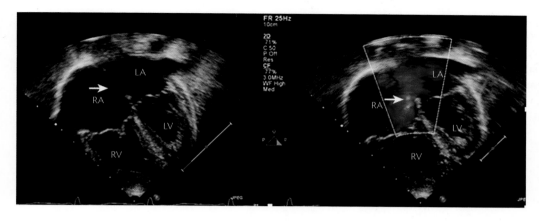

Fig. 41.1 Large secundum ASD. There is a large central defect with secondary right atrial and right ventricular dilatation. The arrow points to the secundum ASD. The colour Doppler image on the right shows the left to right shunt through the ASD (arrow). RA, right atrium; RV, right ventricle; LA, left atrium; LV, left ventricle.

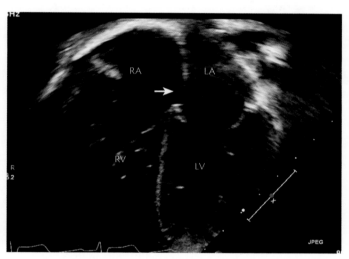

Fig. 41.2 Large primum defect. The defect is located low in the atrial septum just above the atrioventricular junction (arrow). The left and right AV-valve are inserted at the same level and this is associated with abnormal left AV-valve anatomy ('cleft' mitral valve). The right atrium and right ventricle are dilated. RA, right atrium; RV, right ventricle; LA, left atrium; LV, left ventricle.

◆ The right to left (L→R) shunt can be quantified using the continuity equation (RV outflow tract VTI×RV outflow tract area/LVOT VTI×LVOT area) and a Qp/Qs > 2/1 is generally considered to be haemodynamically significant.

Associated anomalies

A full segmental analysis needs to be performed as nearly any congenital anomaly can be associated with an atrial septal defect [4]. Important to exclude before interventional closure of secundum defects are pulmonary venous anomalies and interrupted inferior vena cava (IVC).

Mostly ASDs can be diagnosed using TTE. However, if right heart dilatation is found without identifying an ASD, additional imaging including TOE or CMR can be indicated to diagnose a sinus venosus defect or anomalous pulmonary venous connections.

Imaging is important during interventional closure of secundum ASDs. Currently interventional closure is monitored either by TOE or by intra-cardiac echocardiography (ICE) [5]. Before device closure adequacy of the ASD rims need to be defined.

Three-dimensional echocardiography (3DE) allows an *en face* view of the defects with a more accurate assessment of its size, morphology, as well as morphology of surrounding structures [6, 7].

Imaging post-surgery or intervention

Post-surgery or intervention, echocardiographic follow-up should focus on the following aspects:

◆ Residual atrial shunt through the patch/device.

◆ Position of the patch or device relative to other cardiac structures.

◆ Complications related to device implantation like erosion of the aorta or atrial roof, thrombosis, infectious endocarditis, and device embolization.

◆ Residual RA and RV dilatation.

◆ Presence of pulmonary hypertension (PHT).

◆ AV-valve regurgitation (especially after ASD primum correction).

Role of other imaging techniques

Generally ASDs can be imaged fully using transthoracic echocardiography and in case of poor echocardiographic windows, TOE is a very useful additional diagnostic technique. In case there is still uncertainty regarding the location (especially sinus venosus defects can be difficult to image by echocardiography in adults), or associated congenital abnormalities (particularly pulmonary vein abnormalities), CMR can be performed. Apart from the detailed anatomical imaging, CMR also allows a more accurate quantification of the systemic and pulmonary blood flow and calculation of Qp/Qs, which can be helpful for therapeutic decision-making.

Ventricular septal defects (VSD)

In the newborn period, ventricular septal defects are one of the most common structural abnormalities diagnosed due to the high prevalence of small muscular VSDs in this population. As most of the small muscular defects close spontaneously and since large defects are treated surgically or percutaneously during childhood, VSDs are less common in the adult population.

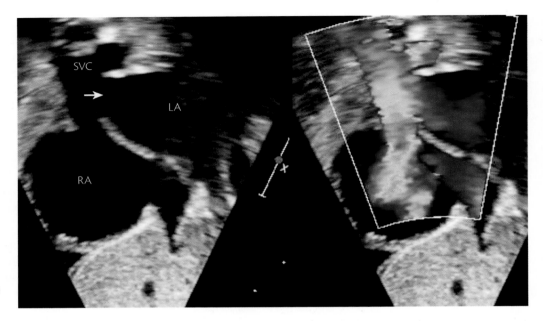

Fig. 41.3 Sinus venosus defect. Subcostal view on the atrial septum (sagittal plane) A defect is noted in the superior part of the atrial septum (arrow). Typically there is overriding of the superior vena cava over the defect. There is a left to right shunt caused by the defect as shown on the colour image.

The type and location of the VSD

♦ Perimembranous VSDs (60%) are localized in the membranous part of the septum and are characterized by fibrous continuity between the leaflets of the atrioventricular and arterial valve (⊃ Fig. 41.5; Videos 41.4a,b,c). These defects may have inlet, trabecular, or outlet extensions. Anterior deviation of the outlet part of the septum can cause RV outflow tract obstruction (tetralogy of Fallot). Posterior deviation can cause LV outflow tract obstruction and can be associated with aortic arch anomalies (coarctation, interrupted aortic arch)

♦ Muscular VSD (20%) defects are localized in the muscular septum. The muscular VSDs can be divided into the inlet, trabecular or outlet types. There may occasionally be multiple defects.

♦ Doubly committed VSDs (5%) are localized just below the aortic and pulmonary valve and are characterized by fibrous continuity between the aortic and pulmonary valve.

Assessment of defect size and haemodynamic significance

♦ Size of the VSD should be measured in at least two dimensions. A VSD is small (<5 mm), moderate (5–10 mm), or large (>10 mm). 3DE by allowing an *en face* visualization of the defects allows an accurate assessment of its size and morphology [8].

♦ The L → R shunt can cause LA and LV dilatation. LA size, volume and LV dimensions should be measured. There can be associated secondary mitral insufficiency due to LV dilatation. Associated structural abnormalities of the mitral valve are possible and should always be excluded.

♦ A VSD can be unrestrictive (with no significant pressure difference between both ventricles) or restrictive due to small size or tissue partially covering the VSD.

♦ A VSD can be associated with PHT. RV pressures should be assessed based on calculating the VSD pressure Doppler gradient or tricuspid regurgitant jet. Obstructive PHT can develop and result in R → L shunting across the VSD (Eisenmenger's syndrome).

♦ The shunt can be calculated and a Qp/Qs >1.5–2.0/1 is considered as haemodynamically significant.

Associated anomalies

Any congenital heart defect can be associated with a VSD. A full segmental analysis is therefore crucial. Commonly associated lesions are:

♦ Prolapse of the right coronary leaflet with progressive AR.

♦ Development of double chambered RV due to the presence of hypertrophic RV muscle bands.

♦ Development of LV outflow tract obstruction due to the development of a fibromuscular ridge or sub-aortic membrane, or due to the presence of posterior malignment of the outlet septum.

♦ Anterior malaligment of the outlet septum can cause right ventricular outflow tract obstruction and aortic override (tetralogy of Fallot).

Imaging post-surgery or interventions

Most large VSDs will have been surgically closed during childhood. Percutaneous device closure of certain perimembranous and muscular VSDs is possible. Post-surgical or device closure of a VSD, the following needs to be assessed:

♦ Residual VSDs due to patch leaks or additional VSDs.

♦ The development of sub-aortic stenosis (membrane or fibromuscular ridge).

♦ The development of right ventricular muscle bundles causing right ventricular outflow tract obstruction.

♦ Aortic insufficiency.

♦ Tricuspid insufficiency (after perimembranous VSD closure), pulmonary insufficiency (after surgical closure of doubly committed VSD).

♦ Residual PHT.

Role of other imaging techniques

Most VSDs can be imaged using TTE. Rarely TOE or other imaging modalities may be indicated. CMR can help quantifying the Qp/QS. In case there is uncertainty regarding the pulmonary vascular resistance or the presence of obstructive PHT, cardiac catheterization may be indicated.

Atrioventricular septal defects (AVSD)

Most AVSDs are diagnosed in adulthood and will have been treated surgically in childhood. In adulthood, unoperated AVSDs with large ventricular components are associated with obstructive pulmonary hypertension (Eisenmenger syndrome). Isolated septum primum septum defects or intermediate AVSDs can be diagnosed in adulthood.

Types of AVSDs and morphologic description

The essential morphological feature of an AVSD is the presence of a common atrioventricular (AV) junction with a common AV-valve at the entrance of both ventricles [9, 10]. When imaging, the following features are important:

◆ Variable shunting across the AVSD. Different relationships between the bridging leaflets and the atrial and ventricular septal components determine different levels of shunting. In a complete defect, shunting is present at the level of the atrial septum (primum defect) and the inlet ventricular septum (➲ Fig. 41.6a; 📹 Video 41.7a). If the bridging leaflets attach to the crest on the inter-ventricular septum, they can close the VSD, and shunting can be present only at atrial level (primum defect). If the bridging leaflets are attached to the underside of the atrial septum, shunting can only be present at the ventricular level (inlet VSD). The bridging leaflets can close all septal defects resulting in a common AV-junction with no atrial or ventricular communication (➲ Fig. 41.4).

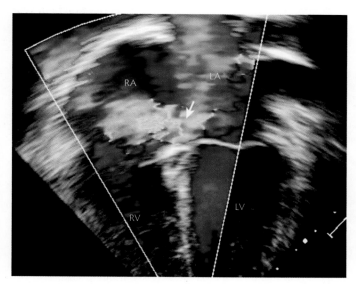

Fig. 41.4 Coronary sinus ASD. This is a posteriorly directed apical 4-chamber view. In this view a defect is shown in the area where the coronary sinus drains into the right atrium (arrow) with a left to right shunt from the left atrium (LA) through the coronary sinus into the right atrium (RA).

◆ The common AV valve at the entrance of the ventricles is abnormal and is made up of five leaflets (➲ Fig. 41.6b; 📹 Video 41.7b). It differs from a normal mitral and tricuspid valve. There is a variable degree of functional AV-valve abnormalities associated with this lesion. This mainly left or right AV-valve regurgitation with valve stenosis being more uncommon. Three-dimensional echocardiography can be helpful in defining the AV-valve morphology and determining the mechanisms of AV-valve regurgitation.

◆ The left ventricular outflow tract (LVOT) is elongated in the parasternal long axis. This is due to the presence of a single AV junction and unwedging of the aorta. LVOT obstruction can be present.

◆ Most defects have balanced ventricular chambers with dilatation of the RV mainly related to the atrial shunt. Unbalanced AVSD with RV or LV dominance can be present however.

Haemodynamic assessment

◆ Variable degrees of atrial and/or ventricular shunting can be present. These shunts can result in atrial as well as ventricular dilatation.

◆ PHT can be present mainly related to the presence of an unrestrictive VSD or, more rarely, related to the primum ASD.

◆ AV valve regurgitation severity needs to be assessed and the mechanism needs to be described

◆ If uncorrected, AVSD with large VSD components will give rise to obstructive PHT and Eisenmenger's syndrome

Associated lesions

Any associated congenital heart defect can be present and a full segmental analysis is essential. Commonly associated lesions are:

◆ Additional secundum ASD and additional muscular VSDs.

◆ Associated PDA which can be difficult to detect in case of PHT.

◆ Anterior deviation of the outlet septum can result in RV outflow tract obstruction (AVSD + tetralogy of Fallot).

◆ LVOT obstruction can be present and this can be associated with aortic coarctation or interrupted aortic arch.

◆ AVSD can be associated with more complex situs anomalies (isomerism).

Post-surgical imaging

Surgical repair typically consists of closing the atrial and ventricular communications and involves variable interventions on the atrioventricular valve dependent on a variable degree of atrioventricular valve regurgitation. Typically the 'cleft' in the left AV-valve is closed surgically. Residual lesions include:

◆ Residual atrial and/or ventricular shunts.

◆ Left and right AV-valve regurgitation or stenosis. Left AV-valve regurgitation is common and often is due to the presence of a residual 'cleft'. Other mechanisms related to AV-valve dysplasia may be present. The description of the severity and associated AV-valve stenosis is important. Three-dimensional

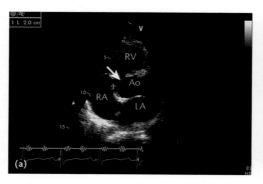
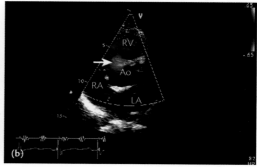

Fig. 41.5 (a) Perimembranous VSD as shown on a parasternal short-axis view (arrow). The size is measured from this view. Typically the VSD is adjacent to the septal leaflet of the tricuspid valve. There is fibrous continuity between the aortic and tricuspid valve. (b) Perimembranous VSD. Colour flow demonstrates left to right shunting during systole (arrow).

echocardiography can be helpful in determining the mechanisms contributing to residual AV-valve regurgitation.

- LVOT obstruction can be present often related to the development of sub-aortic obstruction.
- PHT can be present post-operatively.

Role of other imaging techniques

Generally echocardiography should be able to describe the anatomical and haemodynamic features of patients with AVSD pre and post-operatively. In case of poor echocardiographic windows, TOE can be helpful. In adults aortic arch imaging and imaging of a PDA can be challenging and CMR or MSCT might be needed if clinically indicated. For patients with suspicion of elevated pulmonary vascular resistance, cardiac catheterisation may be required to determine pulmonary vascular resistance.

Patent ductus arteriosus

A PDA is not an uncommon lesion in adulthood. The L→R shunt causes left LV volume overload. If large it may cause progressive obstructive PHT and the Eisenmenger syndrome.

Morphology of the PDA

In a left aortic arch, the duct is usually located between the descending aorta and the left pulmonary artery. If the arch is right-sided, the duct can be present between the descending aorta and the right pulmonary artery, but other locations like between the

left subclavian artery and the left pulmonary artery are possible. This variability in location of the duct makes the echocardiographic diagnosis sometimes difficult. Colour flow Doppler can be helpful in identifying the duct location (➲ Fig. 41.7a).

Haemodynamic consequences of a PDA

For the haemodynamic assessment of a PDA, the size of the duct, the presence of restriction to pressure, the direction of shunting, and the pressure and volume loading caused by the PDA need to be assessed (➲ Fig. 41.7b). The shunt size and direction can be assessed by 2D-echocardiography, colour Doppler, pulsed Doppler, and continuous wave Doppler. If the pulmonary vascular resistance (PVR) is normal, the flow is left to right (L→R) and continuous. Flow velocity is high in a restrictive PDA. The peak and mean gradient between the aorta and pulmonary artery can be measured. With increasing PVR, flow becomes bidirectional with R→L flow in systole and L→R shunting in diastole. With progressive pulmonary vascular disease, the shunt can be exclusively R→L. The L→R shunt will cause an increase in pulmonary blood flow and can result in LA and LV dilatation caused by LV volume loading. In case the duct is unrestrictive, PHT will be present causing pressure loading to the RV.

Associated anomalies

In the adult population, an isolated PDA is the most common presentation, but associated congenital anomalies need always be

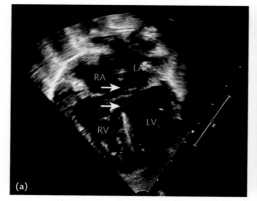
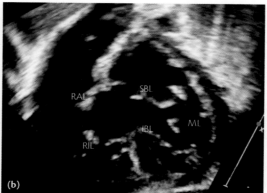

Fig. 41.6 (a) Complete atrioventricular septal defect. There is a single AV-valve at the entrance of both ventricles. There is a large atrial primum component (upper arrow) and a large inlet ventricular septum defect (lower arrow). There is a single AV-valve at the entrance of both ventricles. (b) Subcostal 'en face' view on the AV-valve. There is a single AV-valve at the inlet of both ventricles. This valve has 5 leaflets: superior bridging leaflet (SBL), mural leaflet (ML), inferior bridging leaflet (IBL), right anterior leaflet (RAL), right inferior leaflet (RIL).

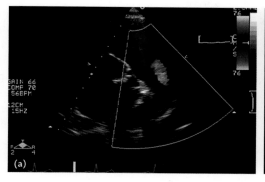
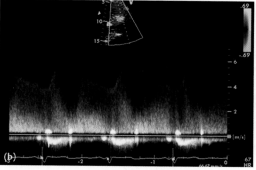

Fig. 41.7 (a) Patent ductus arteriosus. Colour flow doppler demonstrating aortic to pulmonary flow in the short-axis view. The red colour represents the diastolic flow though the arterial duct. (b) Patent ductus arteriosus. There is continuous left to right shunting from the aorta to the pulmonary artery through the duct. The high velocity across the duct excludes the presence of significant pulmonary hypertension.

excluded. As for any congenital defect, a full segmental analysis is required.

Imaging post-surgery or intervention

A PDA can be closed surgically or interventionally by placement of a coil or a duct occluder [11]. After PDA closure the following should be evaluated:

- Residual shunting through the duct.
- Residual PHT.
- Residual LV dilatation and mitral regurgitation.
- Obstruction on the left pulmonary artery after coil/device placement.

Role of other imaging techniques

A PDA can usually be diagnosed using TTE. Rarely CMR or MSCT might be required especially if the origin of the duct is unusual. In case of PHT, a cardiac catheterization may be required to assess the PVR and its responsiveness to pulmonary vasodilators may be helpful in therapeutic decision-making.

Coarctation of the aorta

In classic coarctation there is a narrowing of the aorta located distal to the origin of the left subclavian artery in proximity to the level of insertion of the arterial duct [12]. The morphology of the narrowing is variable but typically is discrete with variable degrees of hypoplasia of the isthmus and the transverse aortic arch. The more extreme form is interruption of the aortic arch, which obviously is extremely rare to be diagnosed in adulthood. The diagnosis should be clinical with arterial hypertension associated with poor or absent femoral pulses and an arm-leg blood pressure gradient. Typically large collaterals develop providing blood supply to the lower part of the body.

Imaging the morphology of coarctation of the aorta

In adults, imaging coarctation of the aorta using echocardiography can be challenging due to the limited echocardiographic penetration and often limited visualization of the descending aorta. The best screening method for diagnosing coarctation of

the aorta is scanning the abdominal aorta in a subcostal long-axis view (➲ Fig. 41.8). If there is a decreased systolic flow with diastolic run-off, this is suggestive for the presence of a narrowing on the thoracic aorta. To further identify the location of the narrowing, the suprasternal view should be used but this gives very often only very limited windows in adult patients (➲ Fig. 41.9; ⏺ Video 41.8). Colour flow Doppler can be helpful. If the distal aorta cannot be viewed in the presence of an abnormal abdominal flow pattern and clinical suspicion, additional imaging by CMR and MSCT may be required.

Haemodynamic significance

To determine the haemodynamic significance of the coarctation, the blood pressure gradient between a limb proximal and distal to the narrowing has to be measured. Continuous wave Doppler can be used to interrogate the gradient across the narrowed segment. The coarctation is significant if high velocities and anterograde diastolic flow is seen (diastolic runoff due to continued pressure

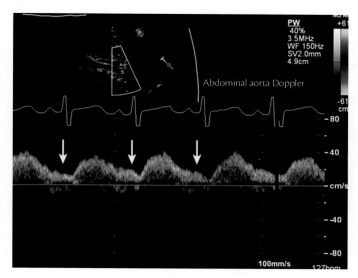

Fig. 41.8 Coarctation of the aorta. Abdominal aortic flow in aortic coarctation. Typically there is a continuous flow pattern in the abdominal aorta with diastolic forward flow (arrows) instead of the normal pulsatile pattern.

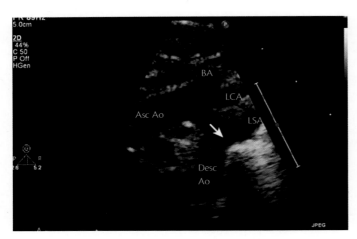

Fig. 41.9 Coarctation of the aorta. The coarctation with an obvious posterior shelf is located just distal to the origin of the left subclavian artery. There is a localized narrowing in the juxtaductal region with a prominent posterior shelf. BA, brachiocephalic artery; LCA, left carotid artery; LSA, left subclavian artery; Asc Ao, ascending aorta; Desc Ao, descending aorta.

gradient in diastole) (⊃ Fig. 41.10). The CW Doppler gradient may be misleading due to different factors: (1) the presence of a PDA or the development of arterial collaterals may reduce the gradient across the coarctation; (2) the simplified Bernoulli equation is less accurate for long segment lesion or segments with multiple stenosis; (3) often multiple obstructive lesions in series are present (like hypoplasia of the transverse arch) that lead to an increased peak velocity proximal to the descending aortic narrowing. The expanded Bernoulli equation should be used if the proximal velocity exceeds 1 m/s:

Peak gradient = $4v^2$max-coarctation – $4v^2$max-pre coarctation.

The arterial hypertension associated with coarctation, can cause secondary left ventricular hypertrophy (LVH) with increased LV wall thickness and mass. Secondary LV systolic and diastolic dysfunction can be present.

Associated lesions

Coarctation can be associated with multiple other cardiac defects. The most common ones include:

♦ Bicuspid aortic valve with variable degree of aortic valve stenosis insufficiency.

♦ Sub-aortic stenosis due to a small outflow tract or sub-aortic membrane can be present.

♦ Mitral valve anomalies like a parachute-type mitral valve with mitral valve stenosis.

♦ Supravalvar mitral stenosis related to the presence of a supramitral membrane.

♦ Ventricular septal defects.

Imaging post-surgery or intervention

After surgery or interventional treatment (balloon dilatation and/or stent implantation), follow-up imaging should focus on diagnosing residual arch narrowing (aortic arch hypoplasia), residual

narrowing at the coarctation site, detection of aneurysm formation, and studying the secondary effects on LV mass and systolic and diastolic function. Especially the detection of aneurysm formation can be challenging by echocardiography in adults and additional imaging using CMR or MSCT might be required. In case of stent implantation MSCT is the modality of choice. Early development of coronary artery disease and ischaemic heart disease is possible and might also require additional imaging.

Role for additional imaging techniques

In adults with coarctation of the aorta, there is an important role for CMR and MSCT in the pre-operative and post-operative assessment due to the limited visualization of the area of the coarctation area and the aortic arch using echocardiography.

Right ventricular outflow tract obstruction (RVOTO)

The two most common lesions causing RVOTO are pulmonary valve stenosis and subvalvular pulmonary stenosis caused by RV muscle bundles.

Morphology of RVOTO

The most common form of RVOTO is caused by pulmonary valve (PV) stenosis. The valve can be tricuspid, bicuspid, or unicuspid with variable degree of dysplasia of the leaflets (⊃ Fig. 41.11; ≞ Video 41.9). There can be tethering of the valve leaflets in the supravalvular area causing additional supra valve narrowing, which can influence the success of balloon dilatation of the pulmonary valve. Subvalvular stenosis is caused by hypertrophy of RV muscle bundles causing dynamic obstruction in the RVOT. Muscle bundles dividing the RV into a proximal and distal chamber characterize double-chamber RV. Double-chamber RV is differentiated from infundibular narrowing in that the obstruction is located lower within the body of the RV. A concomitant perimembranous VSD may be identified (⊃ Fig. 41.12; ≞ Video 41.10).

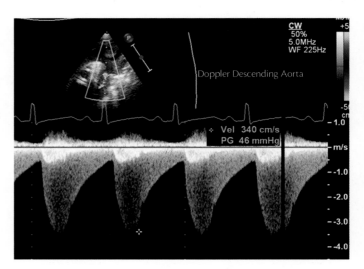

Fig. 41.10 Coarctation of the aorta. Continuous wave Doppler through the coarctation region. The typical 'saw-tooth' pattern is identified with the typical diastolic run-off.

Haemodynamic assessment

RVOT obstruction can generally be well diagnosed using TTE. The valve morphology can be assessed and before intervention the annulus size can be measured. If the gradient is muscular, it often has a dynamic component, which is characterized by a high peak late in systole. Continuous wave Doppler can be used to grade the severity of the obstruction. Generally RVOT obstruction is considered severe if the Doppler peak gradient measures >80 mmHg. Different factors can influence the gradient however: an atrial L→R shunt can lead to increased velocities and gradient overestimation. Conversely, RV dysfunction, severe tricuspid regurgitation, atrial R→L shunting, high pulmonary artery pressures due to a large PDA all result in a lower Doppler velocity across the stenosis and can cause underestimation of the severity. There can be secondary RV hypertrophy (RVH) indirectly reflecting the degree of obstruction but RVH is very difficult to quantify echocardiographically.

Associated lesions

Multiple associated lesions can be present. The most common ones are:

◆ Atrial septal defects.
◆ Ventricular septal defects.

Imaging post-surgery or intervention

Generally echocardiography can be used for post-interventional follow-up. After balloon dilatation or surgical valvotomy, residual pulmonary valve stenosis can be present and Doppler can measure the gradient. Pulmonary regurgitation can be present and the severity can be evaluated by colour Doppler and continuous wave Doppler. If severe, this can result in progressive RV dilatation and dysfunction as after tetralogy of Fallot repair. After muscle bundle resection, residual muscular obstruction can be present.

Role of other imaging techniques

In the majority of patients the diagnosis of RVOT obstruction can be made using echocardiography. In case of very poor transthoracic images, TOE can be helpful defining the level of obstruction (valvar, subvalvar, supravalvar). CMR can be used in the post-intervention assessment particulary in patients with severe pulmonary regurgitation (PR) causing RV dilatation. CMR allows quantifying the pulmonary regurgitant fraction and regurgitant volume as well as the RV volumes and ejection fraction.

Left ventricular outflow tract obstruction

Congenital abnormalities of the left ventricular outflow tract can be present in the adult population. This includes congenital aortic stenosis, subvalvar aortic stenosis, and supravalvar stenosis. The evaluation of congenital valve abnormalities does not differ from acquired aortic valve disease and the reader is referred to the chapters on aortic valve disease in this book.

Morphology of sub-aortic and supravalvar stenosis

Sub-aortic stenosis

Sub-aortic stenosis is a narrowing in the LVOT below the aortic valve (➲ Fig. 41.13). Three subtypes can be identified: a membranous form, a fibromuscular ridge, and a fibromuscular tunnel. Colour flow Doppler detects turbulence, while pulse wave Doppler helps to localize the origin of acceleration. M-mode and 2D imaging may demonstrate early systolic closure of the aortic valve or fluttering of the aortic valve leaflets. Continuous wave Doppler should be used to assess the peak and mean gradients across the lesion. Diagnosis can be made by TTE and only rarely additional imaging modalities are required. Defining the exact location of the narrowing, describing the mechanism and the relationship to the aortic valve is the information required for surgical treatment. 3DE can visualize the LVOT *en face* and it allows assessment of the morphology of the obstruction, its severity as well as relationships with aortic valve and aortic valve anatomy.

Supravalvular stenosis

Supravalvular stenosis is a rarer form of LVOT obstruction. The stenosis is typically localized at the level of the sinotubular junction. It can be membranous, hourglass-shaped and be associated with hypoplasia of the ascending aorta and also the more distal aortic arch. The coronary arteries may be involved in the supravalvular narrowing, which puts these patients at risk for ischaemia, especially

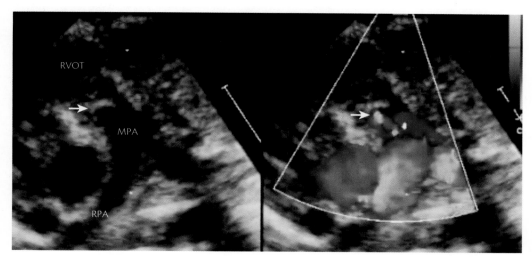

Fig. 41.11 Critical valvular pulmonary stenosis. The pulmonary valve is thickened (arrow left panel) and there is limited opening of the valve leaflets with minimal antegrade flow (arrow right panel).

when arterial pressure decreases (general anaesthesia). In patients with elastin gene mutations associated pulmonary branch stenosis is not uncommon. Supravalvular stenosis can be secondary to surgery such as after the arterial switch procedure.

Haemodynamic assessment

The haemodynamic assessment of an LVOT obstruction includes measurement of the peak and mean gradients by Doppler techniques. The gradient is best measured from the apical outflow tract views. For subvalvar stenosis a peak gradient >50 mmHg is considered haemodynamically significant. Subvalvar stenosis can cause damage to the aortic valve resulting in associated aortic regurgitation. For supravalvar stenosis the gradient is best measured from suprasternal windows. The secondary effect on the LV needs to be assessed including the occurrence of LVH and LV systolic and diastolic dysfunction.

Associated lesions

In adult congenital patients, sub-aortic stenosis is typically seen in patients after VSD closure, after repair of double outlet RV and in patients with AVSD. It can also be present as an isolated lesion.

Supravalvar stenosis is typically present in patients with elastin gene mutations and patients with Williams' syndrome. It is associated in these patients with supravalvar pulmonary stenosis and pulmonary artery branch stenosis, hypoplasia of the aortic arch, arterial hypertension and coronary artery narrowing. Supravalvar stenosis can be present after sugery involving the ascending aorta like after an arterial switch operation or a Ross operation.

Post-operative evaluation

After surgical intervention, residual outflow tract obstruction and aortic valve function need to be evaluated. Recurrence of subvalvar stenosis is common and requires serial follow-up. Aortic valve function needs to be monitored, especially for the presence of progressive aortic regurgitation.

Role of other imaging techniques

Generally subvalvar and supravalvular stenosis can be diagnosed using TTE. For subvalvar stenosis TOE can be helpful in those cases where the LVOT cannot be visualized well. TOE can help to determine the mechanism of the obstruction better. In patients with supravalvular stenosis in the context of elastin gene abnormalities the coronary arteries can be involved in the disease process. As the origins of the coronary arteries can be extremely difficult to image using TTE, additional imaging techniques may be required. These include TOE, CMR, MSCT or angiography. These imaging modalities also allow a better assessment of the entire aortic arch and the pulmonary artery branches.

Ebstein's anomaly

Ebstein's anomaly is a relatively rare congenital abnormality that sometimes can be diagnosed in adulthood.

Morphology

Ebstein's anomaly of the tricuspid valve is defined by apical displacement of the septal and postero-inferior leaflets of the tricuspid valve [14] (➲ Fig. 41.14; 📹 Video 41.11). Typically the tricuspid valve orifice is rotated superiorly towards the RV outflow tract. The antero-superior leaflet is large and redundant (sail-like). The displacement can be very significant and results in significant atrialization of the basal part of the RV reducing the stroke volume. This is associated with variable degrees of tricuspid stenosis and regurgitation (➲ Fig. 41.15; 📹 Video 41.12). The severity of Ebstein malformation is largely determined by the degree of apical displacement and the severity of the tricuspid valve regurgitation (TR). Significant atrialization of the RV cavity results in a reduction of stroke volume and together with the TR this reduces RV output.

Haemodynamic assessment

In the haemodynamic assessment the evaluation of tricuspid valve regurgitation and tricuspid valve stenosis is important. Colour Doppler echocardiography can be extremely helpful to determine the degree of tricuspid regurgitation. Tricuspid stenosis is uncommon and the evaluation requires alignment with the tricuspid inflow, which can be challenging. The severity of the stenosis can be underestimated by a gradient measurement due to the presence of a PFO/ASD.

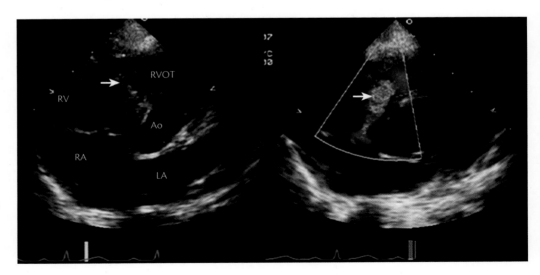

Fig. 41.12 Double-chambered right ventricle. A hypertrophied muscle band is noted with flow acceleration (arrows) in the RV cavity between the RV inflow and outflow. This patient also had a spontaneously closed perimembranous ventricular septal defect.

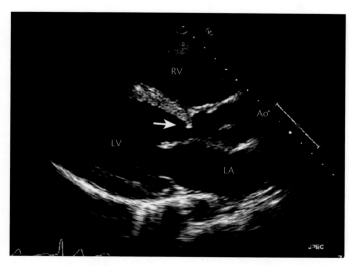

Fig. 41.13 Subaortic stenosis. There is a fibromuscular ridge (arrow) in the left ventricular ouflow tract below the insertion of the aortic valve.

Associated lesions

An ASD or PFO is often present and can result in R → L shunting causing desaturation and is associated with a risk for paradoxical emboli. There can be associated pulmonary valve stenosis. Other common associated lesions include LV non-compaction cardiomyopathy and VSDs.

Post-operative evaluation

Surgery consists of either a valvuloplasty of the TV or a TV replacement in case the valve is not deemed repairable. The recently introduced cone technique provides an anatomical repair of the valve. Post-operative evaluation involves assessment of tricuspid valve function (degree of regurgitation or stenosis), assessment of RV size and function and also LV functional assessment.

Role of other imaging techniques

Generally, Ebstein malformation can be diagnosed well by TTE. In adults with poor echocardiographic windows TOE can be a useful additional imaging technique for assessing tricuspid valve function and to identify the presence of a PFO/ASD. For certain patients CMR can be useful to determine RV volumes and function or to quantify the severity of tricuspid regurgitation. For patients needing surgical repair or replacement of the tricuspid valve, tricuspid valve function can generally be followed using TTE and no additional imaging techniques are required.

Congenital mitral valve anomalies

In adults, acquired mitral valve disease is much more common than congenital abnormalities of the valve. The evaluation of mitral valve stenosis and insufficiency is discussed in another chapter in this book. The same techniques apply to patients with congenital valve abnormalities but the mechanisms for valve dysfunction are different.

Morphology of congenital mitral valve abnormalities

Different types of mitral valve anomalies can be distinguished.

Parachute mitral valve

This defect is characterized by an abnormality of the subvalvar apparatus with the support provided to the anterior and posterior leaflets by a single papillary muscle (most commonly the posteromedial papillary muscle). Typically this results in decreased mobility of the leaflets with the presence of mitral stenosis. It can be associated with other left ventricular abnormalities such as subaortic stenosis, aortic valve disease and coarctation of the aorta.

Double-orifice mitral valve

This is a left AV valve with two orifices each having their own attachments. The first type is associated with an AVSD. The second type is a mitral valve with two orifices each having their own chordal attachments and papillary muscles. The orifices can be stenotic or regurgitant. A short-axis view generally is diagnostic although the orifices might be in different planes.

Isolated cleft in the mitral valve

In an AVSD the zone of apposition between the superior and the mural leaflets is sometimes called a 'cleft'. An isolated cleft in the anterior mitral leaflet not associated with an AVSD is a rare lesion that can cause progressive mitral regurgitation (➲ Fig. 41.16). While in an AVSD the cleft is oriented towards the inter-ventricular septum, in an isolated cleft, the cleft is oriented towards the LVOT.

The morphology of the mitral valve anomaly can generally be well described using 2DE. 3DE with an *en face* view of the mitral valve from the ventricular perspective will allow a better definition of the valve anomaly and the subvalvar apparatus.

Haemodynamic assessment

The different anatomic abnormalities can be associated with variable degrees of mitral valve stenosis and insufficiency. The evaluation is identical to acquired mitral valve disease but prior to valve surgery, the surgeon should be aware of the exact mechanism causing valve dysfunction.

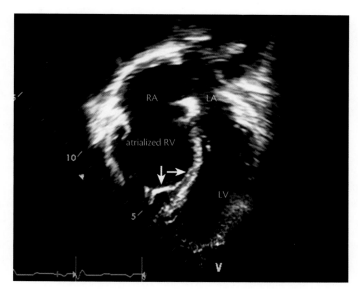

Fig. 41.14 Ebstein's anomaly. The apical 4-chamber view shows the apical displacement of the tricuspid septal leaflet (arrows) and the normally inserted anterior leaflet. There is a large atrialized portion of the RV.

Associated lesions

Mitral valve anomalies can be isolated but can be associated with other types of LV congenital abnormalities. This includes LVOT obstruction, aortic valve disease and coarctation of the aorta. Other congenital defects associated include double outlet RV (parachute mitral valve).

Post-operative assessment

Post-operative evaluation includes mitral valve function and left ventricular function.

Role of other imaging techniques

Generally, TTE provides sufficient imaging but in case of poor windows, TOE may be required. There is a limited role for other imaging techniques as CMR and MSCT do not image the leaflets well.

Tetralogy of Fallot and tetralogy of Fallot with pulmonary atresia

Tetralogy of Fallot is the most common cyanotic lesion, which is rare to diagnose in adulthood as most of the patients will have been diagnosed and treated during childhood. Most patients in the adult congenital clinic are postoperative patients.

Morphologic description

Tetralogy of Fallot (TOF) is defined as the combination of a large outlet VSD with overriding of the aorta associated with various degrees of RV outflow tract obstruction and secondary RV hypertrophy. The key anatomical feature of tetralogy of Fallot is anterocephalad deviation of the outlet septum causing various degrees of muscular/infundibular RV outflow tract obstruction (⊃ Fig. 41.17; ▦ Videos 41.13a,b,c). This is associated with variable degrees of pulmonary valve obstruction and hypoplasia of pulmonary artery branches. Tetralogy of Fallot

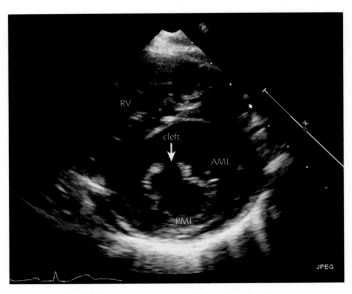

Fig. 41.16 Isolated cleft in the anterior leaflet of the mitral valve. Short-axis view at the level of the valve leaflets. AML, anterior mitral valve leaflet; PML, posterior mitral leaflet. Typically the cleft is anteriorly oriented.

with pulmonary atresia can be considered as an extreme form where no connection is present between the RV and the pulmonary circulation. The pulmonary perfusion can be duct-dependent to central pulmonary arteries or be dependent on aorto-pulmonary collaterals [15].

The pre-operative assessment of an uncorrected patient with TOF includes the following:

◆ Define the size and localization of the VSD + degree of aortic override (⊃ Fig. 41.18): perimembranous to outlet (92%), doubly committed (5%), inlet VSD or AVSD (2%). If aorta overrides the VSD by more than 50%, this is called a double outlet RV.

◆ Define the mechanism + severity of RV outflow tract obstruction: infundibular, valvular and/ or supravalvular (⊃ Fig. 41.19).

◆ Define whether the pulmonary arteries (PA) are present and confluent. Measure the size of the proximal and distal PAs and look for PA branch stenosis. Exclude the presence of aorta-pulmonary collaterals.

◆ Identify coronary artery abnormalities especially any coronary artery crossing the RV outflow tract. This can be an abnormal left anterior descending (LAD) from the right coronary artery (RCA), an accessory LAD from the RCA, or a prominent conal branch from RCA. Typically the origins of the coronary arteries are clockwise rotated. Before any intervention on the right outflow tract the relationship of the outflow tract including stenting and pulmonary valve implantation, the relationship of the coronaries to the outflow tract and proximal pulmonary artery branches needs to be determined.

◆ Determine aortic arch anomalies: TOF can be associated with a right aortic arch and other arch anomalies. The presence of aorto-pulmonary collaterals needs to be determined.

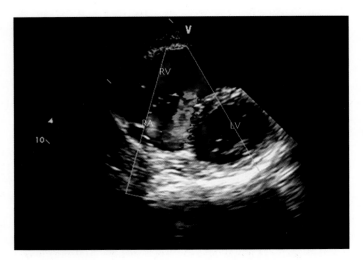

Fig. 41.15 Tricuspid regurgitation associated with Ebstein's disease. This is viewed from a short-axis view as typically in Ebstein's malformation the tricuspid valve opens in the direction of the right ventricular outflow tract. The regurgitant jet generally is best viewed from this view. The arrow indicates the tricuspid regurgitant jet at valve level.

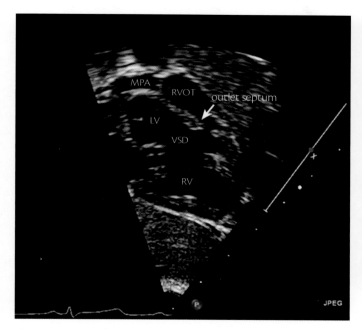

Fig. 41.17 Tetralogy of Fallot. Subcostal view demonstrating the anterior deviation of the outlet septum causing subvalvar obstruction. The arrow indicates the anterocephalad deviation of the outlet septum, causing right ventricular outflow tract obstruction. LV, left ventricle; RV, right ventricle; VSD, ventricular septal defect; RVOT, right ventricular outflow tract; MPA, main pulmonary artery.

Pre-operative haemodynamic assessment

The pre-operative haemodynamic assessment mainly includes the determination of the severity of the RVOT obstruction and identifying the different levels of obstruction (infundibular, valvar, supravalvar). Different Doppler techniques need to be combined. The direction of shunting across the VSD needs to be determined.

Associated anomalies

TOF can be associated with other lesions and, like for any congenital defect, a full segmental evaluation is required:

- Associated abnormalities like ASDs, left superior vena cava draining to the coronary sinus, additional VSDs, abnormal pulmonary venous return.
- AVSD can be associated if the VSD extends to the inlet part of the septum.
- Aortic arch anomalies: right aortic arch, double aortic arch.
- Aortic root dilatation and progressive aortic regurgitation.

Post-operative imaging

Surgical repair of tetralogy of Fallot includes closure of the VSD and surgical relief of RV outflow tract obstruction using different techniques. If the pulmonary valve annulus is too small, a transannular patch is required to relieve the RVOT obstruction, resulting in severe pulmonary regurgitation (PR). This can cause progressive RV dilatation and dysfunction.

Post-operative evaluation includes the assessment of:

- Residual RV outflow tract obstruction.
- Pulmonary regurgitation.

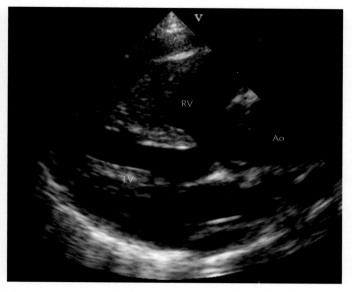

Fig. 41.18 Tetralogy of Fallot. Parasternal long-axis view demonstrating the ventricular septal defect extending to the outlet part of the septum and the overriding of the aorta over the defect (in this case around 50% override).

- Residual VSD.
- RV size and function.
- Pulmonary artery branch stenosis.
- Aortic root dilatation and aortic insufficiency.
- LV function.

The most common residual lesion is pulmonary regurgitation resulting in RV dilatation and dysfunction (⊃ Fig. 41.20; 📷 Videos 41.14a,b). Timely replacement of the pulmonary valve can prevent irreversible damage to the RV but timing of the valve replacement is still controversial and seems largely dependent on RV volume. Different imaging techniques can be used for the assessment of RV function in these patients [16–18].

Role of different imaging techniques

For the pre-operative assessment, in children generally echocardiography can provide all the necessary information. Only in case of pulmonary atresia with complex pulmonary perfusion through major aorto-pulmonary collaterals, additional imaging may be required to delineate the pulmonary blood supply. CMR and MST both provide excellent images of the pulmonary circulation but angiography remains the clinical gold standard in the pre-operative assessment of this lesion, especially if pressure measurements are required.

For the post-operative assessment, echocardiography remains the first-line imaging technique. It allows assessment of the presence of a residual VSD, residual RV outflow tract obstruction, the severity of pulmonary regurgitation, tricuspid valve regurgitation, aortic root dilatation, and aortic regurgitation. In adults the pulmonary branches can be difficult to visualize, especially more distally. In patients with significant pulmonary regurgitation, RV dimensions and RV functional parameters can be obtained for serial assessment. We propose using tricuspid annular systolic plane annular excursion (TAPSE), fractional area change, and pulsed tissue Doppler. 3DE can be used to measure RV volumes and ejection fraction if the windows allow for a good volumetric data acquisition. Strain imaging is an emergent technique that can be used to assess RV longitudinal function but has not found its way yet into the routine clinical practice. Apart from assessing RV function, the assessment of LV function is very important for this patient population as progressive LV dysfunction carries a poor prognosis for this patient population.

Especially in the post-operative evaluation, there is an important role for the use of CMR mainly for quantifying RV volumes and ejection fraction, pulmonary regurgitant fraction and volumes and for better delineating the pulmonary branch anatomy. Timing of pulmonary valve replacement may be influenced by measurement of RV volumes with a cut-off value between 170–190 ml/m^2. In patients with contraindications to CMR, MSCT can be an alternative for measurement of RV size and function.

Transposition of the great arteries

Transposition of the great arteries (TGA) obviously is a neonatal diagnosis as it causes significant cyanosis, which is not compatible with life if not treated. There is a growing population of adult patients who underwent surgical treatment for TGA in the first years of life.

Morphology of TGA and associated anomalies

In TGA the aorta arises from the morphological RV and the pulmonary artery from the morphological LV resulting in ventriculo-arterial discordance [19]. In this section we will discuss ventriculo-arterial discordance with atrio-ventricular concordance. Most commonly in this condition the aorta is positioned rightward and anterior relative to the position of the pulmonary artery.

Commonly associated lesions are:

◆ VSD in up to 50% of all patients. The VSD is most commonly located in the perimembranous area but can be located anywhere of the septum. In case of inlet extension, straddling of the tricuspid valve may occur.

◆ LVOT obstruction: subpulmonary and pulmonary stenosis, which can preclude an arterial switch procedure.

◆ Coarctation of the aorta can be associated.

◆ Variable coronary artery anatomy. This is important when performing an arterial switch operation, which involves a coronary artery transfer. The usual, is the left coronary artery (left anterior descending originating from the right facing sinus and the right coronary artery from the left sinus). The most common coronary variant is the circumflex originating from the RCA (18%). A single coronary artery or an intramural course of a coronary artery can make an arterial switch procedure more challenging.

The pre-operative anatomy can generally be accurately diagnosed by TTE. Additional imaging is nowadays rarely required. The treatment for TGA has undergone an historical evolution as the atrial switch procedure (Senning or Mustard operation) was performed until the mid-1980s to early 1990s, to be replaced by the arterial

switch operation afterwards [20]. For TGA with VSD and LVOT obstruction, the Rastelli operation is performed although this was recently replaced by the Nikaidoh procedure in selected cases.

Post-operative imaging

The post-operative imaging differs according to which type of surgery the patient underwent. For all patients, TTE is the first-line imaging technique. For specific indications, other imaging techniques may be used.

Evaluation after the atrial switch procedure (Senning or Mustard)

The principle of both surgeries is the same: the systemic venous return is rerouted to the left ventricle and the pulmonary circulation and the pulmonary venous return is redirected to the right ventricle and aorta. This redirects the systemic venous blood to the pulmonary circulation and the pulmonary venous blood to the systemic circulation. In a Mustard operation an intra-atrial tunnel is constructed using artificial patch material, while in a Senning operation the intra-atrial rerouting is performed using native atrial tissue. The diagnostic imaging performed for both procedures is similar and requires [21]:

◆ Identifying the venous pathways to rule out tunnel obstruction or baffle leaks (⊃ Fig. 41.21). Pathway obstruction is the most common problem, especially after Mustard procedure. The superior vena cava and inferior vena cava pathways, as well as the pulmonary venous pathways, need to be imaged. This requires multiple imaging windows and views, which sometimes can be difficult to image in adults. 3DE can be helpful in visualizing the pathways and their spatial relationships. TOE and CMR can be needed in case TTE cannot define the pathways well. Contrast echocardiography with injection of agitated saline through a peripheral intravenous cannula can be helpful to detect pathway obstruction and baffle leaks.

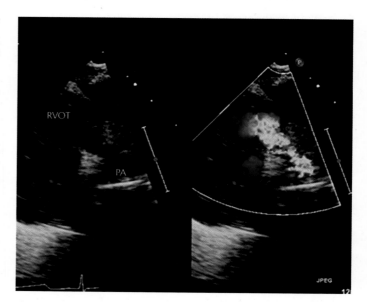

Fig. 41.19 Tetralogy of Fallot. Parasternal long-axis view tilted towards the right ventricular outflow tract. There is flow acceleration from below the valve, at the valve level due to the small pulmonary valve that domes and also tethers at the supravalvular level.

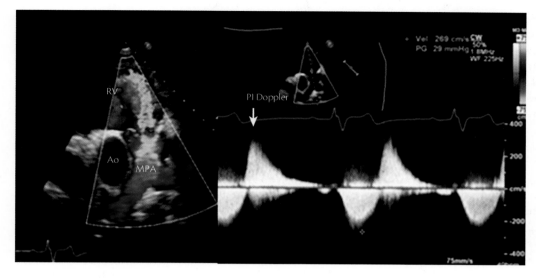

Fig. 41.20 Tetralogy of Fallot. Postoperative image. Severe pulmonary regurgitation after tetralogy of Fallot repair. The left panel shows a diastolic frame with a wide regurgitant jet at valve level and backflow originating from distally into the pulmonary branches (red colour in the branches). The Doppler (arrow) shows the short deceleration time typical for severe pulmonary regurgitation with flow only in early and mid diastole.

◆ Assessment of systemic RV function and tricuspid regurgitation. Progressive tricuspid regurgitation and systemic RV dysfunction are common problems after the atrial switch procedure (⮊ Fig. 41.22). Quantification of systemic RV function by echocardiography remains challenging. For RV functional assessment we suggest using a combination of different methods for serial follow-up. These include TAPSE, fractional area change and tissue Doppler echocardiography. Strain imaging is emerging but its clinical use for this indication still remains to be proven. Also 3DE could be used but generally the image acquisition is challenging with limited image resolution. Progressive tricuspid regurgitation after the atrial switch generally is a sign of RV dysfunction and failure, in patients after the switch procedure. For RV functional assessment, CMR remains the clinical reference technique.

Evaluation after the arterial switch procedure

The adult population of patients who underwent the arterial switch procedure is quickly growing as the atrial switch procedure has become obsolete in paediatric cardiac surgery. After the arterial switch procedure, the following problems may occur:

◆ Progressive neo-aortic root dilatation associated with neo-aortic valve regurgitation.

◆ In a switch procedure the pulmonary trunk is put in front of the ascending aorta with the right pulmonary artery to the right and the left pulmonary artery to the left of the ascending aorta. Pulmonary branch stenosis can be caused by stretching the proximal pulmonary artery branches. Imaging the RV outflow tract and pulmonary arteries is required and can be difficult in post-operative patients after the switch procedure (⮊ Fig. 41.23). Peak velocities ≤2 m/s (predicted maximum instantaneous gradient ≤16 mm Hg) across the distal main pulmonary artery and branch pulmonary arteries are within normal limits after arterial switch procedure. TOE generally does not help to visualize the anteriorly located pulmonary arteries and MSCT of CMR might be the only non-invasive alternative.

◆ Coronary artery stenosis can develop after the coronary transfer and has been reported to cause coronary artery stenosis in 10–15% of all patients. Coronary stenosis, and especially kinking, can result in myocardial ischaemia. Monitoring of global and regional myocardial performance is important. Dobutamine stress echocardiography can be used to identify perfusion problems. Direct visualization of the coronaries is possible using cardiac CMR and MSCT. Coronary angiography should be considered in patients in whom coronary stenosis or occlusion is highly suspected.

◆ Ventricular size and function: evaluation of LV size and function is required in every patient after the arterial switch procedure. In patients with PA branch stenosis, assessment of RV function is also important.

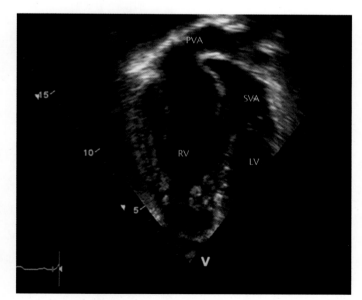

Fig. 41.21 Apical 4-chamber view of patient after the Senning operation. The pulmonary venous atrium (PVA) is directing the pulmonary venous blood to the right ventricle. The systemic venous blood is directed through the systemic venous atrium (SVA) to the left ventricle. The RV becomes the systemic ventricle after this operation.

Evaluation after the Rastelli procedure

In patients who underwent the Rastelli procedure, the VSD has been closed creating a tunnel between the LV and the aorta and the RV is connected with a conduit to the pulmonary arteries. Imaging the patients after the Rastelli procedure involves:

◆ Evaluation of the RV-to-pulmonary artery conduit and branch pulmonary arteries by 2DE, colour, and spectral Doppler using several approaches.

◆ Evaluation of the LV-to-aortic valve pathway for obstruction and aortic regurgitation.

◆ Evaluation of LV function as LV dysfunction is a potential late complication after the Rastelli operation.

◆ Exclude the presence of residual VSDs.

Congenitally corrected transposition of the great arteries

Congenitally corrected transposition of the great arteries (ccTGA), is defined as atrio-ventricular discordance associated with ventriculo-arterial discordance. This results in 'physiological correction' as the oxygenated pulmonary venous blood enters the LA, which connects through the tricuspid valve to the morphological RV into the aorta [21]. Systemic venous deoxygenated blood enters the RA, which connects, to the morphologic LV through the mitral valve into the pulmonary circulation. This can be associated with situs anomalies, VSDs, tricuspid valve anomalies. In 20% of cases there is dextrocardia [22]. Any imaging technique should describe the full anatomy, as well the functional impact (systemic RV function and tricuspid regurgitation).

Generally this can be done using TTE, but in adults TOE or CMR might be required.

Morphology of ccTGA

TTE is the first-line technique to diagnose ccTGA (⊃ Figs 41.24–41.26; ≛Videos 41.15, 41.16). In usual atrial situs arrangement, the tricuspid valve and the RV are located on the left and the mitral valve and LV are positioned on the right. This can be easily detected on the apical 4-chamber view due to the more apical insertion of the tricuspid valve relative to the mitral valve. As the tricuspid valve is often abnormal in this condition with some Ebstein-like features, the apical displacement of the TV is more obvious. The presence of the moderator band and the more heavily trabeculated RV on left also provides an imaging sign for ccTGA. Typically for this condition, the ventricles and the inter-ventricular septum are oriented in a more vertical plane than usual, which requires vertical rotation of the probe in the parasternal views. In the short-axis view of the great arteries, the aorta is positioned anterior to the left of the pulmonary artery.

Commonly associated anomalies

◆ VSD (~60–70%). Commonly perimembranous but other locations are possible.

◆ LV outflow tract and pulmonary stenosis (~40–70%). Commonly subvalvular (aneurysmal valve tissue, chords, discrete fibrous obstruction) and valvar.

◆ Tricuspid valve abnormalities (~83–90%).Variable pathology (increased apical displacement of septal leaflet (Ebstein's like), thickened/malformed leaflets, straddling). Tricuspid regurgitation is common and can be progressive.

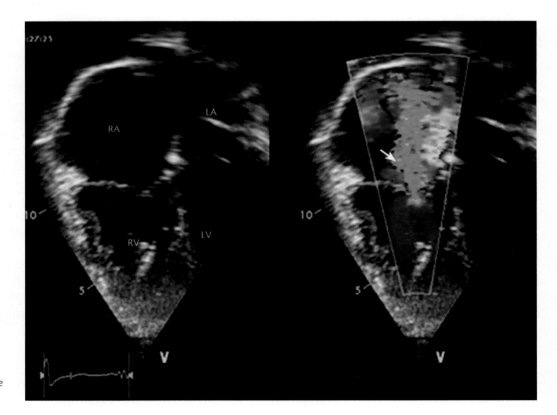

Fig. 41.22 Severe tricuspid regurgitation after the Senning operation. The RV is dilated and hypertrophied. Notice the broad jet of regurgitation at the tricuspid valve level (arrow).

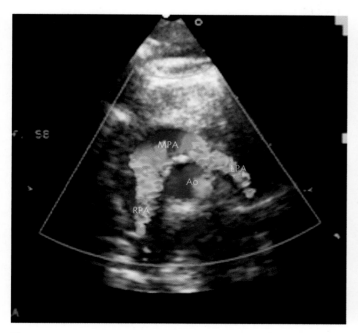

Fig. 41.23 The arterial switch operation. Position of the pulmonary arteries after the arterial switch procedure. Due to the commonly used Lecompte manoeuvre the pulmonary artery bifurcation is located anterior to the aorta. MPA, main pulmonary artery, LPA, left pulmonary artery; RPA, right pulmonary artery.

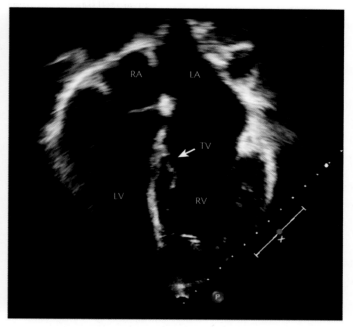

Fig. 41.24 ccTGA. Apical 4-chamber view in a patient with congenitally corrected transposition of the great arteries (atrio-ventricular and ventricular arterial discordance). The left atrium (LA) connects through the more apically displaced tricuspid valve to the morphologic right ventricle (RV), situated on the left. The right atrium (RA) connects through the mitral valve to the morphologic left ventricle (LV) situated on the right.

◆ Mitral valve abnormalities (~50%). Cleft mitral valve is possible and if a VSD is present straddling through the VSD.

◆ ASD (43%).

◆ Other associated lesions: aortic stenosis, aortic coarctation, left atrial isomerism, coronary artery variants, complete heart block.

Haemodynamic assessment

In any patient with ccTGA, haemodynamic assessment is focused on the systemic RV function and the severity of tricuspid regurgitation (TR). Progressive TR is common in this condition related to the frequent anatomical abnormalities of the TV and this is generally not well-tolerated by the systemic RV and can result in progressive RV dilatation and dysfunction. Severe TR should be treated surgically before irreversible RV dysfunction develops. LVOT obstruction (subpulmonary obstruction) can be present and requires assessment of the gradient together with a description of the mechanism causing the obstruction.

Pre- and post-operative assessment

Most of the assessment can be performed by TTE or by TOE in case of poor imaging windows. Assessment of patients with ccTGA should focus on:

◆ Tricuspid valve regurgitation for possible repair or replacement.

◆ Evaluation of RV function.

◆ Assess feasibility of biventricular repair (double switch-type procedure) or need for pulmonary artery banding (LV retraining).

◆ After pulmonary artery banding assess LV function, hypertrophy, and tricuspid regurgitation.

◆ After atrial switch and Rastelli procedures assess leak or obstruction across tunnels and conduits.

◆ Assess for worsening ventricular function and atrioventricular valve regurgitation.

Role for other imaging techniques

CMR can be used in case of poor echocardiographic windows and for quantification of RV volumes and ejection fraction. CMR is also used for evaluating the effect of pulmonary artery banding and LV retraining on LV hypertrophy and LV function. CMR allows quantifying systemic and pulmonary blood flows. There is a role for MSCT in these patients as complete heart block is very common in this population and pacemakers are frequently needed. In patients with pacemakers who develop systolic dysfunction, the possibility of RV dyssynchrony as a contributing factor to the development of systolic dysfunction should be considered. Strain imaging to study timing of myocardial events can be helpful in understanding the mechanisms.

The functionally univentricular heart

This is a wide anatomic spectrum of patients in which one of the chambers is too small to sustain either the pulmonary or systemic circulation [23, 24]. The dominant ventricle can be an RV or an LV. A second smaller ventricle is invariably present. Sometimes two adequately sized ventricles are present, but anatomy prevents septation (such as straddling of the atrioventricular valves). The segmental approach needs to be used to describe the morphology. This can generally be done using TTE although in adults poor echocardiographic windows may require additional imaging techniques. Most adult patients with univentricular hearts will have been palliated by the Fontan operation. The principle is that the dominant ventricular chamber is used for the systemic circulation while the systemic venous blood is directed to the pulmonary arteries, bypassing the heart [25]. Since its introduction, the Fontan operation has undergone many modifications. Currently the total cavo-pulmonary connection with the lateral tunnel or the use of an extra-cardiac conduit is the most commonly used. A fenestration is often placed between the systemic venous pathway and the pulmonary venous atrium. The fenestration allows a R→L shunt that decompresses the systemic venous pathway and maintains adequate cardiac output. In case of favourable haemodynamics, the fenestration can be device-closed. As different types of Fontan connections exist, the echocardiogrpher must be aware of which type of surgical connection was performed. Being aware of the surgical history is key to interpretation of the images.

Before looking at the Fontan connection it is important to know the underlying morphology of the heart. This includes a description of the atrial situs (solitus, inversus, isomerism), the AV-connections (double inlet, single inlet with left/right absent connection), common inlet (unbalanced AVSD) (see ⊃ Figs 41.27–41.30). It is important to determine ventricular morphology of the dominant ventricle (left/right). A small

superior and rightward subarterial outlet chamber is typically a morphologic RV. A small inferior-posterior rudimentary chamber is typically a morphologic LV. The outflow tract to the aorta should be visualized and should be unobstructive. AV-valve function should be assessed, as well as ventricular function.

Imaging a patient after the Fontan operation should include the following.

Visualizing the Fontan connections

The patency of the connections and absence of obstruction and thrombi should be assessed. This involves:

◆ Evaluation of the superior cavo-pulmonary anastomosis (⊃ Fig. 41.31), as well as the entire IVC to pulmonary artery connection.

◆ Flow measurements in the superior and IVC should be obtained and the effect of respiration on the flows should be studied. In general there is low-velocity flow with increase in flow velocities with inspiration.

◆ Evaluation of the patency and size of the fenestration. The mean gradient across the fenestration provides an estimate of the transpulmonary pressure gradient.

◆ In case of an intra-cardiac-type of connection, baffle leaks should be excluded.

◆ Flow to both pulmonary arteries should be assessed using colour and spectral pulsed Doppler.

Visualization of the entire conduit might be extremely difficult and a TOE or CMR are excellent non-invasive alternatives.

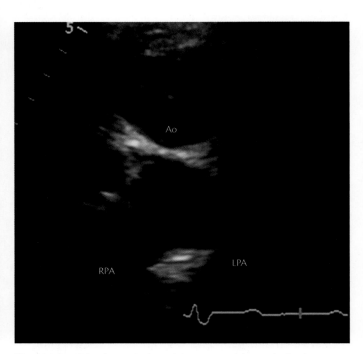

Fig. 41.25 ccTGA long-axis view. Parasternal long-axis view in a patient with congenitally corrected transposition of the great arteries. The left atrium (LA) connects to the anteriorly located right ventricle (RV), which connects to the anteriorly located aorta (Ao). The pulmonary artery (PA) is positioned posteriorly to the aorta.

Fig. 41.26 ccTGA short-axis view. High parasternal short-axis view in a patient with congenitally corrected transposition of the great arteries. The aorta (Ao) is seen anterior and slightly leftward of the pulmonary artery, which is posterior and branches into the left (LPA) and right (RPA) pulmonary arteries.

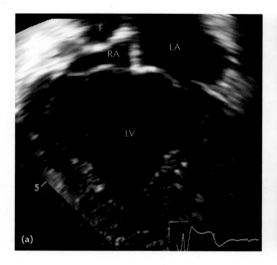

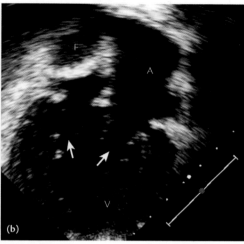

Fig. 41.27 (a and b) Double inlet left ventricle. Apical view of double inlet left ventricle. (a) In this systolic frame, two separate AV valves connect the left atrium (LA) and right atrium (RA) to a single ventricle of left ventricular morphology (LV). The Fontan (F) connection is seen posteriorly. (b) Diastolic frame from an apical 4-chamber view in a patient with double inlet left ventricle. The right atrium and left atrium (A) connect via separate atrioventricular valves (arrows) to the dominant left ventricle (V). The Fontan circuit (F) is seen behind the right atrial cavity.

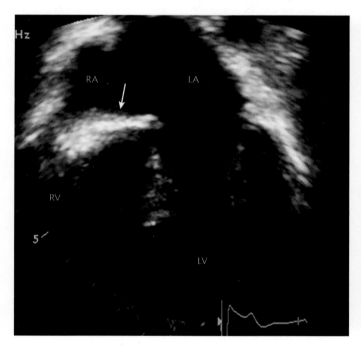

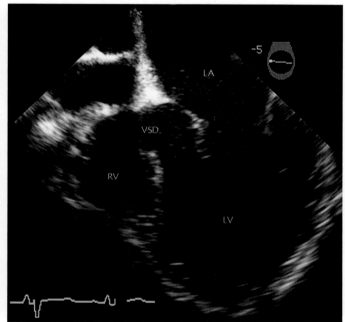

Fig. 41.28 Tricuspid atresia. Apical 4-chamber view in patient with absent right atrioventricular connection (tricuspid atresia). The absent right atrioventricular connection is seen echocardiographically as an echogenic border between the right atrium and small right ventricle (arrow). The atrial communication between the right (RA) and left atria (LA) is widely patent. The mitral valve and left ventricle (LV) dominate the image. The right ventricle (RV) is barely seen in this image.

Fig. 41.29 Tricuspid atresia. 4-chamber view obtained at transoesophageal echocardiography in patient with absent right atrioventricular connection (tricuspid atresia). The left atrium (LA) connects through the mitral valve to the left ventricle (LV). No atrioventricular valve is discernible on the right and the absent connection is seen echocardiographically as an echogenic border between the right atrium and small right ventricle (RV). The posterior aspect of ventricular septal defect (VSD) is seen and is non-restrictive.

Visualizing the pulmonary veins

Pulmonary venous obstruction should be excluded. All four pulmonary veins should therefore be identified after the Fontan operation and pulmonary venous flow should be evaluated using colour and spectral pulsed Doppler techniques. If pulmonary vein problems are suspected, additional imaging techniques like MSCT, CMR, and cardiac catheterization are required.

AV-valve function

Low atrial pressure is a condition for optimal Fontan function. AV-valve stenosis and more commonly AV valve regurgitation should be evaluated.

Ventricular function assessment

Ventricular function assessment is an important part of postoperative Fontan evaluation but due to the lack of quantitative techniques it is largely a subjective qualitative approach. Also the evaluation of diastolic function is extremely difficult due to abnormal AV-valve anatomy and abnormal pulmonary venous flow.

Detection of aortic-to-pulmonary collateral flow

An estimated 80% of patients undergoing Fontan-type operations already have, or subsequently develop, systemic arterial-to-pulmonary arterial collaterals as a consequence of preoperative, or continued, hypoxaemia. Competitive flow from these aorto-pulmonary vessels can increase right-sided pressures, thereby reducing systemic venous flow to the pulmonary arteries. These collaterals can be detected by TTE using suprasternal aortic views but MSCT, CMR and angiography are more sensitive non-invasive techniques for detecting collateral flow.

Eisenmenger's syndrome

Eisenmenger's syndrome is characterized by irreversible pulmonary vascular disease as a result of a systemic-to-pulmonary communication (e.g. ASD, non-restrictive VSD, non-restrictive PDA, AVSD, aorto-pulmonary window, surgical systemic-to-pulmonary shunt). An initial L → R shunt reverses direction following an increase in pulmonary vascular resistance and arterial pressures [26]. The R → L shunt causes systemic desaturation, which is progressive with the increase in pulmonary vascular resistance. Due to the presence of a shunt the RV will never reach suprasystemic pressures and becomes less dysfunctional compared with patients with primary pulmonary hypertension.

Follow-up of these patients involves defining the underlying structural defect causing the increased pulmonary pressures, the direction of shunting across the defect, the presence of associated lesions, and RV and LV function. As for the other congenital lesions, TTE is the first-line diagnostic technique. Usually, TTE generally can:

- Identify RV hypertrophy, flattening and bowing of the interventricular septum in systole. ('D' sign, see ⊃ Fig. 41.32). Diastolic flattening occurs with disease progression.

- Pulmonary artery systolic and diastolic pressures (septal configuration), peak gradient from RV to RA from tricuspid regurgitation jet using modified Bernoulli equation (RV systolic pressure mmHg=tricuspid regurgitation peak velocity^2 (m/s)×4+estimated RA pressure). This pressure will be equal to pulmonary systolic pressure if no gradient exists across the RV outflow tract.

- Mean pulmonary artery pressure estimated from peak early diastolic pulmonary regurgitation velocity and the diastolic pulmonary artery pressure estimated from the end-diastolic pulmonary regurgitation velocity.

- Qualitative and quantitative assessment of RV function. With disease progression, RV enlargement and dysfunction may occur.

- LV function (prognostic factor).

- Worsening tricuspid regurgitation (increasing afterload, annular dilatation, and RV dysfunction) and RA enlargement.

- Underlying structural defect, coexisting structural abnormalities, surgical shunts.

- Obstruction or aneurysm in main pulmonary artery and proximal branches

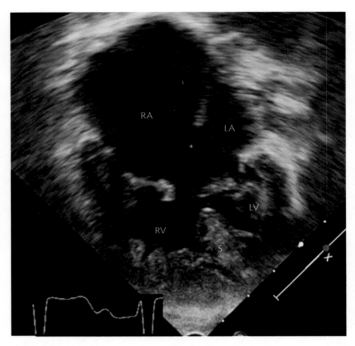

Fig. 41.30 Unbalanced AVSD. Apical 4-chamber view in a patient with unbalanced atrioventricular septal defect. The right atrium (RA) is considerably larger than the left atrium (LA). The large primum atrial septal defect is denoted with an asterisk. The common atrioventricular valve opens preferentially to the right ventricle (RV) which is dominant. The left ventricle (LV) is small. The ventricular septal defect is seen as the space between the inter-ventricular septum (S) and the atrioventricular valve.

- Colour flow Doppler helps define the anatomical defect and direction of shunting. Increased R → L shunting during supine bicycle ergometry, although the shunt may be small and difficult to demonstrate due to a low gradient. Contrast echo can enhance visualization of the shunt.

Role of TOE

- Can be performed relatively safely and is usually well tolerated (even when baseline oxygen saturation levels are < 80%).

- May be useful for detecting ASDs/PDA and for imaging posterior structures (pulmonary veins).

- Should be performed in lung transplant candidates (detect unsuspected intra-cardiac defects/shunts, proximal pulmonary artery thrombus).

Role of CMR

- Not routinely required but may be useful in selected cases for anatomical definition and to estimate magnitude of R → L shunt.

Special topics in adult congenital imaging

Echocardiography in the pregnant woman with congenital heart disease

Pregnancy is associated with increased blood volume, which results in increased cardiac chamber sizes. There is an increase in cardiac output to the increased circulatory volume in combination with the reduction in systemic vascular resistance due to the presence of the low resistance placental circulation. Physiologic pulmonary and tricuspid regurgitation and trivial mitral regurgitation are common. In patients with CHD this increased blood volume and the higher circulatory demand can cause problems. Careful monitoring of the circulatory adaptation using imaging may be required [27]. High-risk patients include patients with significant aortic stenosis (mean gradient >30–40 mmHg, valve area <0.7 cm² before pregnancy), significant aortic coarctation, significant mitral stenosis (valve area <2 cm²), reduced systemic ventricular function (EF <40%), mechanical prosthetic valve, Marfan's syndrome (especially when ascending aorta diameter >44 mm), and cyanotic heart disease. Pregnancy is contraindicated in Eisenmenger physiology and significant PHT. In every woman with CHD, a foetal echocardiogram has to be performed to rule out CHD in the foetus. A screening foetal echocardiography in a specialized centre should be performed at around 17–19 weeks. TOE can be performed if TTE windows are not sufficient. CMR is also safe during pregnancy and can be used for specific indications (RV function, aortic root dilatation).

Tissue Doppler, strain and strain rate in congenital heart disease

Quantification of ventricular function in patients with congenital heart disease can be very challenging using echocardiography. For the assessment of RV function, as well as single ventricular function, most of the time subjective visual assessment of ventricular function (eyeballing) is used. Alternative more quantitative methods should be used for follow-up and early detection of ventricular dysfunction. Tissue Doppler quantifies myocardial velocities and either pulsed or colour Doppler can be used. The introduction of speckle-tracking echocardiography made strain imaging more easily applicable in clinical practice. Strain measures myocardial deformation, while strain rate measures the speed of myocardial deformation. Both reflect myocardial function but are influenced by loading conditions.

Although still considered emerging techniques for clinical use, the research data on the clinical applicability and utility of both tissue Doppler and strain techniques are accumulating [28–31].

* Tissue Doppler velocities are considered useful for:
  * Diastolic function assessment.
  * Evaluation of dyssynchrony.
* Strain and strain rate imaging are promising techniques:
  * Evaluation of global and regional systolic RV function.
  * Evaluation of global and regional LV function.
  * Evaluation of dyssynchrony.

Three-dimensional echocardiography in congenital heart disease

3DE is useful for anatomical definition and for functional assessment, facilitating spatial recognition of intra-cardiac anatomy, thereby enhancing diagnostic confidence. 3DE is an emerging application. Full-volume data acquisition in a single cardiac cycle and 3D myocardial strain are now being applied. TOE 3DE facilitates peri-operative assessment.

Functional assessment

* 3DE measurements compare well with CMR for measurement of LV volumes, ejection fraction and mass.
* RV volumes and EF also compare reasonably with CMR measurements [32]. There is a systemic underestimation of RV volumes by around 25%. There is a growing role of 3DE in the assessment and management of RV volumes in patients after tetralogy of Fallot repair atrial switch procedures, and congenitally corrected transposition of the great vessels.

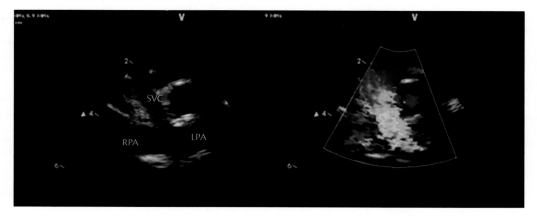

Fig. 41.31 Bidirectional cavopulmonary anastomosis (bidirectional Glenn shunt). Suprasternal view. The superior vena cava (SVC) is connected end-to-side to the right pulmonary artery (RPA). The functionally proximal left pulmonary artery can be visualized. With colour Doppler the flow through the connection and the proximal pulmonary arteries can be imaged.

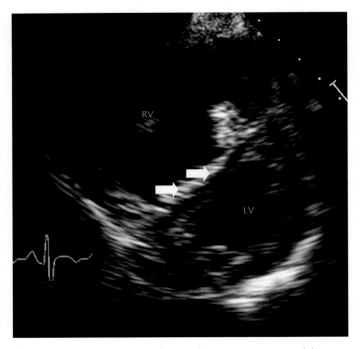

Fig. 41.32 Septal flattening in pulmonary hypertension. Parasternal short-axis view. The inter-ventricular septum is flat in systole due to the elevated pulmonary pressures. Due to the flattening, the LV has the configuration of a capital 'D'.

Assessment of AV valve regurgitation

◆ Allows visualization of the entire regurgitant jet.

◆ Orthogonal planes placed through the jet yield true vena contracta jet area.

◆ Ability to overlay colour Doppler on transparent grey-scale image and transient suppression of the colour image facilitates understanding of regurgitant mechanism.

Acknowledgement

We would like to acknowledge the contributions of Dr Edgar Tay and Dr Michael Gatzoulis to the first edition of this chapter.

References

1. Hoffman JI, Kaplan S. The incidence of congenital heart disease. *J Am Coll Cardiol* 2002; 39(12): 1890–900.

2. Hoffman JI, Kaplan S, Liberthson RR. Prevalence of congenital heart disease. *Am Heart J* 2004; 147(3): 425–39.

3. Anderson RH, Ho SY. Sequential segmental analysis: description and characterization for the millenium. *Cardiol Young.* 1997: 98–116.

4. Ferreira Martins JD, Anderson RH. The anatomy of interatrial communications—what does the interventionist need to know? *Cardiol Young* 2000; 10(5): 464–73.

5. Bartel T, Konorza T, Arjumand J, et al. Intra-cardiac echocardiography is superior to conventional monitoring for guiding device closure of interatrial communications. *Circulation* 2003; 107(6): 795–7.

6. Handke M, Heinrichs G, Moser U, et al. Transesophageal real-time three-dimensional echocardiography methods and initial in vitro and human in vivo studies. *J Am Coll Cardiol* 2006; 48(10): 2070–6.

7. van den Bosch AE, Ten Harkel DJ, McGhie JS, et al. Characterization of atrial septal defect assessed by real-time 3-dimensional echocardiography. *J Am Soc Echocardiogr* 2006; 19(6): 815–21.

8. Zipes DP, Camm AJ, Borggrefe M, et al. ACC/AHA/ESC 2006 guidelines for management of patients with ventricular arrhythmias and the prevention of sudden cardiac death—executive summary: A report of the American College of Cardiology/American Heart Association Task Force and the European Society of Cardiology Committee for Practice Guidelines (Writing Committee to Develop Guidelines for Management of Patients with Ventricular Arrhythmias and the Prevention of Sudden Cardiac Death) Developed in collaboration with the European Heart Rhythm Association and the Heart Rhythm Society. *Eur Heart J* 2006; 27(17): 2099–140. Epub 2006/08/23.

9. Smallhorn JF, Tommasini G, Anderson RH, Macartney FJ. Assessment of atrioventricular septal defects by two dimensional echocardiography. *Br Heart J* 1982; 47(2): 109–21.

10. Smallhorn JF. Cross-sectional echocardiographic assessment of atrioventricular septal defect: basic morphology and preoperative risk factors. *Echocardiography* 2001; 18(5): 415–32.

11. Giroud JM, Jacobs JP. Evolution of strategies for management of the patent arterial duct. *Cardiol Young* 2007; 17 Suppl 2: 68–74.

12. Matsui H, Adachi I, Uemura H, Gardiner H, Ho SY. Anatomy of coarctation, hypoplastic and interrupted aortic arch: relevance to interventional/surgical treatment. *Expert Review of Cardiovascular Therapy* 2007; 5(5): 871–80.

13. Knauth Meadows A, Ordovas K, Higgins CB, Reddy GP. Magnetic resonance imaging in the adult with congenital heart disease. *Semin Roentgenol* 2008; 43(3): 246–58.

14. Paranon S, Acar P. Ebstein's anomaly of the tricuspid valve: from fetus to adult: congenital heart disease. *Heart* 2008; 94(2): 237–43.

15. Bashore TM. Adult congenital heart disease: right ventricular outflow tract lesions. *Circulation* 2007; 115(14): 1933–47.

16. Redington AN. Determinants and assessment of pulmonary regurgitation in tetralogy of Fallot: practice and pitfalls. *Cardiol Clin* 2006; 24(4): 631–9, vii.

17. Mertens LL, Friedberg MK. Imaging the right ventricle—current state of the art. Nature reviews *Cardiology* 2010; 7(10): 551–63. Epub 2010/08/11.

18. Valsangiacomo Buechel ER, Mertens LL. Imaging the right heart: the use of integrated multimodality imaging. *Eur Heart J* 2012; 33(8): 949–60.

19. Anderson RH, Weinberg PM. The clinical anatomy of transposition. *Cardiol Young* 2005; 15 Suppl 1: 76–87.

20. Pretre R, Tamisier D, Bonhoeffer P, Mauriat P, Pouard P, Sidi D, et al. Results of the arterial switch operation in neonates with transposed great arteries. *Lancet* 2001; 357(9271): 1826–30.

21. Warnes CA. Transposition of the great arteries. *Circulation* 2006; 114(24): 2699–709.

22. Graham TJ, Bernard Y, Mellen B, et al. Long-term outcome in congenitally corrected transposition of the great arteries: a multi-institutional study. *J Am Coll Cardiol* 2000; 36: 255–61.

23. Cook AC, Anderson RH. The functionally univentricular circulation: anatomic substrates as related to function. *Cardiol Young* 2005; 15 Suppl 3: 7–16.

24. Anderson RH, Cook AC. Morphology of the functionally univentricular heart. *Cardiol Young* 2004; 14 Suppl 1: 3–12.

25. Gewillig M. The Fontan circulation. *Heart* 2005; 91(6): 839–46.

26. Vongpatanasin W, Brickner M, Hillis L, Lange R. The Eisenmenger syndrome in adults. *Ann Intern Med* 1998; 128: 745–55.

27. Siu SC, Colman JM. Heart disease and pregnancy. *Heart* 2001; 85(6): 710–5.

28. Mertens L, Ganame J, Eyskens B. What is new in pediatric cardiac imaging? *Eur J Pediatr* 2008; 167(1): 1–8.

29. Friedberg MK, Mertens L. Deformation imaging in selected congenital heart disease: is it evolving to clinical use? *J Am Soc Echocardiogr* 2012; 25(9): 919–31.

30. Friedberg MK, Mertens L. Tissue velocities, strain, and strain rate for echocardiographic assessment of ventricular function in congenital heart disease. *Eur J Echocardiogr* 2009; 10(5): 585–93.

31. Forsey J, Friedberg MK, Mertens L. Speckle tracking echocardiography in pediatric and congenital heart disease. *Echocardiography* 2013; 30(4): 447–59.

32. Niemann PS, Pinho L, Balbach T, et al. Anatomically oriented right ventricular volume measurements with dynamic three-dimensional echocardiography validated by 3-Tesla magnetic resonance imaging. *J Am Coll Cardiol* 2007; 50(17): 1668–76.

33. Zanchetta M, Onorato E, Rigatelli G, et al. Intra-cardiac echocardiography-guided transcatheter closure of secundum atrial septal defect: A new efficient device selection method. *J Am Coll Cardiol* 2003: 1677–82.

⊃ **For additional multimedia materials, please visit the online version of the book (⤵ http://www.oxfordmedicine.com)**

CHAPTER 42

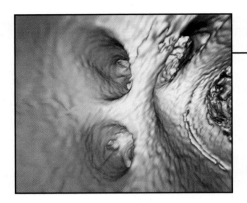

The roles of CMR and MSCT in adult congenital heart disease

Philip Kilner, Ed Nicol, and Michael Rubens

Contents

Introduction

The relatively unrestricted access provided by CMR and MSCT allows the assessment of clinically important regions that may lie beyond ultrasonic access. These include the pulmonary veins and the sinus venosus regions of the atrial septum, the right ventricular free wall and outflow tract, the pulmonary arteries, the whole aorta and the para-mediastinal regions which may be crossed by aorto-pulmonary collateral arteries [1, 2]. Both CMR and MSCT allow 3D contrast enhanced angiography and regional or global assessment of biventricular function with good blood–tissue differentiation. MSCT offers the better spatial resolution and does not require specific predetermination of imaging planes as there is a complete volume of data that can be rotated and cut to any desired plane. CMR offers the possibility of 'dynamic' angiography, visualizing the sequential opacification of successive vascular regions. Besides freedom from radiation, the key additional strengths of CMR lie in its high temporal resolution, measurements of flow volumes, and characterization of tissues, if needed.

Comprehensive CMR acquisition in ACHD

Except in straightforward cases where the questions to be answered are well defined, it is prudent in a baseline or pre-surgical CMR study to perform a comprehensive examination that will allow review of the structure and function of the myocardium, valves and vessels through all regions of the heart and mediastinum. A stack of multiple transaxial ± coronal cines is simple and relatively quick to acquire using a contemporary CMR system. Such cine stacks are easily reviewed using suitable image display software. Dynamic contrast enhanced angiography or non-contrast 3D steady-state free-precession (SSFP) imaging can also be valuable, although these do not, on their own, yield cyclic functional information. Cine images should also be aligned with each inflow and outflow valve, and with any shunt flow, so that interconnections can be established and described according to sequential segmental analysis (see previous chapter).

Measurements of right and left ventricular function

Both CMR and MSCT allow volumetric analysis of both ventricles without geometric assumptions, which is particularly important given the variability of RV shape in ACHD [3]. However, the myocardium of the RV is extensively trabeculated in most individuals, with only a relatively thin layer of compact myocardium in the free wall. This makes reproducible delineation of the RV blood–muscle boundary challenging. For CMR the most reproducible approach is probably to place a relatively smooth boundary line (contributing to a reconstructed 3D surface) between the trabeculated and compact layers of the RV free wall [4]. However, this boundary can be hard to define where trabeculations come together in systole. In MSCT a more rapid and robust semi-automated boundary detection based on attenuation (or signal) differences between the (opacified) blood and myocardium is routinely used (⊃ Fig. 42.1). It may become feasible to apply a similar method to CMR cines, which could potentially be more accurate, although not necessarily directly comparable with the simplified, manually placed boundary method.

Additional considerations affecting RV volume measurements are the movements of the atrio-ventricular junction, which can contribute a significant part of the RV stroke volume, and the difficulty of locating pulmonary annular level after infundibular resection or patching in repairs of tetralogy of Fallot. We recommend that an aneurysmal or akinetic RV outflow tract is included in the RV volume, up to the expected level of the pulmonary valve.

It needs to be emphasized that, for serial comparisons of RV function, consistent methods of delineation need to be used. Contour data for volumetric analysis should ideally be stored in a database and remain available for comparison at the time of follow-up.

Flow measurements by CMR

The measurement of volume flow in a large vessel is potentially an unrivalled strength of CMR. Through-plane velocity mapping of ascending aortic and main pulmonary artery flow (⊃ Fig. 42.2) allow calculations of left- and right-sided output and therefore of shunting, and of the amount of regurgitation of the outflow valves. For these derived values, however, the measurements of velocity need to have a high standard of accuracy. This is not easy to achieve on all CMR systems, and care may be needed to minimize or correct errors introduced by background phase offset errors, particularly when the vessel is dilated [5].

Jet velocities and calculations of pressure difference

Measurements of the velocities of post-stenotic jets or of relatively broad regurgitant jets are feasible by phase contrast CMR, as long as the velocity mapping slice is located to transect the jet immediately downstream of the orifice so that voxels lie completely within the coherent jet core. As with Doppler ultrasound, pressure differences may be estimated by applying the modified Bernoulli equation. However, the velocities of narrow jets through

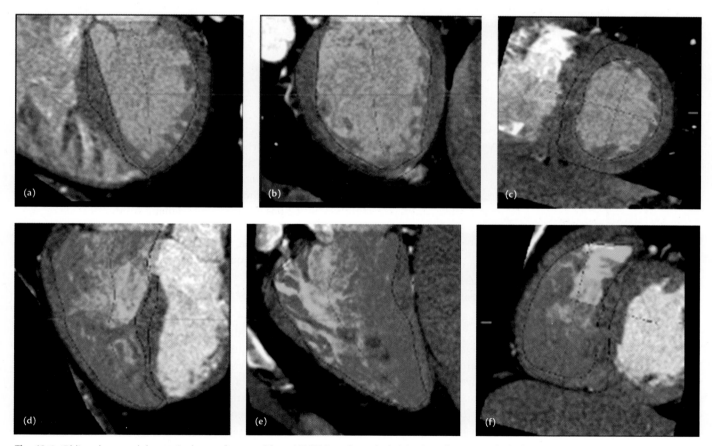

Fig. 42.1 Oblique long- and short-axis planes reformatted from MSCT data after a single injection of contrast, which also gave opacification of the coronary and pulmonary arteries. In the left ventricle (a–c) and right ventricle (d–f), the opacified blood regions identified for volume calculation are coloured pink.

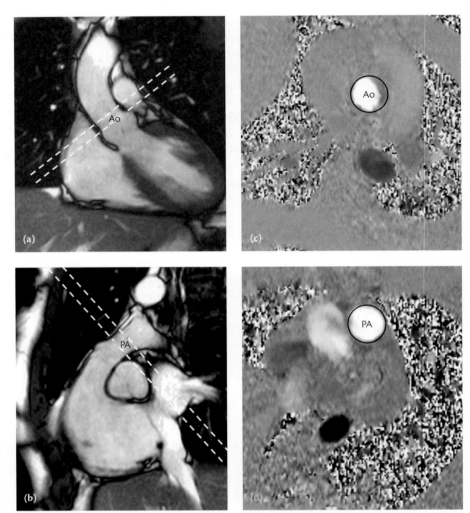

Fig. 42.2 CMR cine images (a and b) aligned with the ascending aorta (Ao) and main pulmonary artery (PA). Systolic frames of through-plane phase contrast velocity maps (c and d), located as indicated by the dotted lines, from which the volumes of aortic and pulmonary flow (and regurgitant volume, if present) can be derived.

mildly regurgitant tricuspid or pulmonary valves, which are used in echocardiography for estimations of RV or PA pressure, are unlikely to be accurately measured by CMR.

The roles of CMR or MSCT in specific diagnostic groups

Please note: Further anatomical and pathophysiological background can be found in the corresponding subsections of the preceding chapter on echocardiographic investigation.

Atrial septal defects (ASD)

While echocardiography is the first-line modality, CMR and MSCT (➲ Fig. 42.3a). can address unanswered questions about the location and size of unusual defects, biventricular size and function, and any associated anomalies, notably the possibility of anomalous pulmonary venous drainage [6]. With CMR the amount of shunting (Qp:Qs measurement) can also be assessed. A contiguous transaxial stack of cines and pulmonary venous angiography allow visualization of all pulmonary veins and any

sinus venosus defect. A contiguous atrial short-axis stack, parallel to ventricular short-axis planes, progressing from the A–V junction to the SVC, is suitable for visualization of an ASD, followed by through-plane velocity mapping of transecting flow through the defect. Both these views can be obtained by rotating and slicing the MSCT dataset to the required plane.

However, for the identification or exclusion of a small ASD or patent foramen ovale, CMR and MSCT are likely to be less effective than a (repeat) contrast echo study.

Ventricular septal defects (VSD)

VSDs can usually be visualized by echocardiography. They are easily identified by MSCT (➲ Fig. 42.3b). CMR can add Qp:Qs measurement, if required (➲ Fig. 42.1). The commonest way of identifying a small VSD by CMR is by the presence of a systolic jet on the RV side of the septum, seen in one of the ventricular short-axis cines that are acquired routinely for ventricular function measurement. The suspected jet should then be cross-cut with additional cine images. Mapping of velocities through a plane transecting the VSD jet can contribute to sizing of the defect.

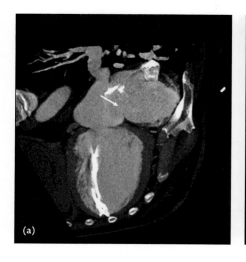

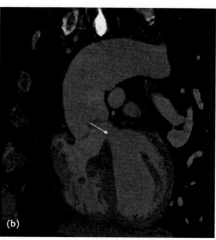

Fig. 42.3 Reformatted MSCT images showing an atrial septal defect (broad white arrow in a). Note the atrial and ventricular pacing leads that pass through the ASD and terminate in the left atrium and left ventricle, respectively. (b) A ventricular septal defect (thin white arrow) in a patient with tetralogy of Fallot.

Atrioventricular septal defect

CMR and MSCT can provide additional views of any (residual) defect or associated anomaly, and CMR can quantify any residual shunt or regurgitation of the left A-V valve.

Patent ductus arteriosus

Either CMR or MSCT can show the size of a duct and any associated abnormalities of anatomy or ventricular function. For screening, a routine contiguous coronal stack of steady-state free-precession (bright blood) images, one slice per heartbeat, is recommended as part of every ACHD CMR study. The jet through a small PDA can be identified in the distal pulmonary trunk in such images, and then interrogated further by cine imaging and velocity mapping, including Qp:Qs measurement. Note: when the shunt is from aorta to the distal PAs, the ascending aortic flow will be *more* than the MPA flow, whereas distal to the PDA, the actual pulmonary flow will be correspondingly greater than the systemic.

Coarctation of the aorta

CMR or MSCT contrast enhanced angiographies are helpful in the assessment of native coarctation diagnosed beyond childhood with a view to balloon dilatation and stenting or surgery. Either modality also allows visualization of recoarctation or aneurysm formation after repair. CMR can probably offer the more thorough assessment of any associated pathology such as stenosis or regurgitation of a bicuspid aortic valve, dilatation of the ascending aorta, or LV hypertrophy. The aortic arch with coarctation may not lie in a single plane, and when using cine imaging and velocity mapping, it is necessary to identify planes best orientated for the depiction and measurement of any jet flow through the coarctation. The presence of diastolic prolongation of forward flow, or a diastolic tail, is a useful sign of significant coarctation, which can be demonstrated by plotting a velocity–time curve of jet flow beyond the coarctation [7]. Following stent insertion for coarctation (➲ Fig. 42.4), MSCT may better visualize the stent position and possible intra-stent stenosis due to the signal drop out that may occur with CMR [8].

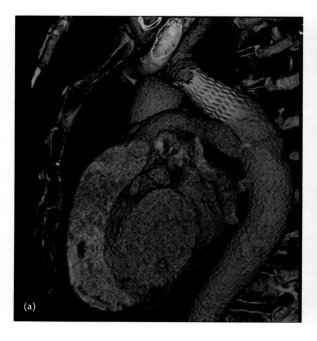

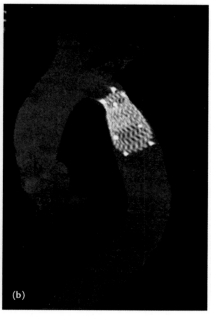

Fig. 42.4 Aortic coarctation with stent imaged by MSCT. Both volume rendered (a) and maximal intensity projections (b) show the position of the stent and allow its dimensions to be measured.

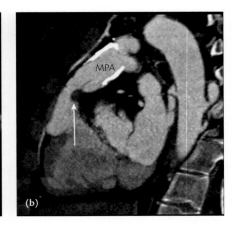

Fig. 42.5 The MSCT volume rendered image (a) shows a heavily calcified main pulmonary artery homograft conduit (MPA) and a corrugated tubular conduit (white arrowhead) to the right pulmonary arterial branches (RPA) after unifocalization surgery for pulmonary atresia with aorto-pulmonary collateral arteries. Panel (b) shows sub-pulmonary stenosis (white arrow) proximal to the calcified homograft.

Berry aneurysms of the circle of Willis or other cerebral vessels occur in up to 10% of patients with coarctation bearing the risk of rupture [9]. As rupture of a cerebral aneurysm is associated with high mortality, screening for cerebrovascular aneurysms by MRI may be wise, particularly, if symptoms develop.

Right ventricular outflow tract (RVOT) obstruction and double-chambered RV

The main contributions of CMR or MSCT lie in demonstrating the level(s) of RVOT obstruction, particularly in adults with poor acoustic windows. Stenosis may be present at more than one level of the RVOT, or in the pulmonary arteries (⊃ Fig. 42.5). Of note, a mild degree of pulmonary stenosis can result in marked post-stenotic dilatation, usually affecting the pulmonary trunk and LPA.

Sub-infundibular stenosis or double-chambered RV can be well demonstrated by CMR. The obstructing muscular bands or fibro-muscular ridge between the hypertrophied body of the RV and the non-hypertrophied and non-obstructive infundibulum, and the resulting systolic jet, should be well seen on at least one of the routine ventricular short-axis cines (⊃ Fig. 42.6, Video 42.1). Mapping of velocities through a plane transecting the jet, together with visualization of the degree of upstream RV hypertrophy and septal flattening, allows an assessment of severity. However, an associated VSD with its jet usually arising close to the tricuspid valve into the trabeculated, high pressure part of the RV may be hard to identify on CMR.

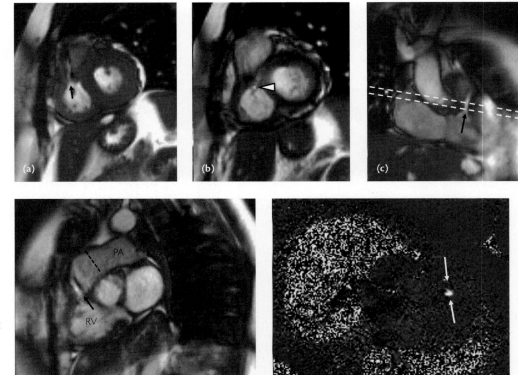

Fig. 42.6 Double-chambered right ventricle or sub-infundibular stenosis identified by CMR in a 53-year-old male. A routine short-axis SSFP cine (a) shows a systolic jet (arrowed) directed from the hypertrophied sinus of the RV into the non-hypertrophied infundibulum. A slightly more basal short-axis cine b) shows a systolic bright spot (arrowhead) indicative of flow through a small perimembranous VSD. The oblique coronal cine (c and Video 42.1) is aligned with the jet in panel a. The dotted lines indicate the slice location of through-plane jet velocity mapping (d), which recorded a peak systolic velocity of 3.8 m/s. An oblique sagittal RVOT cine (e) shows the RV jet in relation to the unobstructed infundibulum and pulmonary valve, whose level is marked by the dotted line. The patient went on to have surgical relief of the sub-infundibular stenosis and closure of the VSD by a right atrial approach, conserving the native pulmonary valve.

Left ventricular outflow tract obstruction (LVOTO) and aortic regurgitation

While echocardiography remains the first line of investigation, CMR cine imaging and jet velocity mapping can be valuable in assessing the level(s) and nature of obstruction, which may be present at more than one level. In the case of hypertrophic obstructive cardiomyopathy, late gadolinium imaging can contribute an assessment of myocardial fibrosis, which may be relevant to prediction of the risk of arrhythmia.

Assessment of aortic valve stenosis by MSCT has been found to show good correlation with transthoracic echocardiography [10] and transoesophageal echocardiography and there is no reason to believe that the same should not be true for other valves. Any calcification of valve structures can be seen, and cardiac gating also allows assessment of valve leaflet mobility and valve orifice dimensions through the cardiac cycle.

The amount of aortic regurgitation can be measured using CMR by mapping velocities through a plane transecting the ascending aorta. For reproducibility and longitudinal comparison, the plane is probably best located immediately above the sino-tubular junction. Although this approach is clinically valuable, the derived measurements of aortic regurgitation are highly susceptible to any background phase offset errors, which may need to be minimized or corrected [5]. Furthermore, upward diastolic movement of the aortic root relative to a fixed velocity mapping plane can result in significant underestimation of the regurgitant fraction if the root is mobile and dilated. In isolated aortic regurgitation, the excessive LV stroke volume relative to that of the RV can also quantify the regurgitation, as long as the volumes are accurately measured.

CMR assessment after Ross operation

The commonest post-operative complications are stenosis or regurgitation of the RV–PA homograft conduit. Stenosis may be due to shrinkage of the homograft tube or a suture line, or to stiffening of the valve leaflets. Any jet formation should be visualized by cine imaging and quantified by velocity mapping, and regurgitation measured by velocity mapping [11]. The autograft valve in aortic position should also be assessed for possible dilatation and regurgitation, particularly beyond the first decade after operation. Visualization of the re-implanted coronary arteries may be indicated using MSCT or CMR 3D SSFP acquisition. If there is a question of post-surgical LV ischaemia or infarction, perfusion imaging and/or late gadolinium enhancement may be considered.

Ebstein's anomaly and tricuspid regurgitation

CMR or MSCT allow thorough visualization of RA-RV anatomy, the ASD if present, tricuspid valve displacement and malfunction, the size and contractility of the functional part of the RV (➲ Fig. 42.7, 📹 Video 42.2). A stack of transaxial CMR cines,

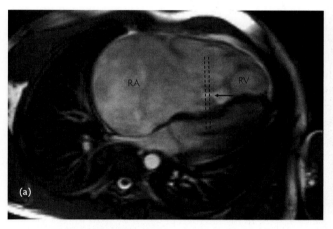
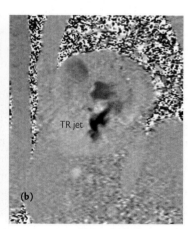
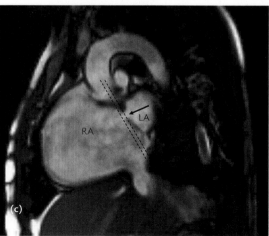
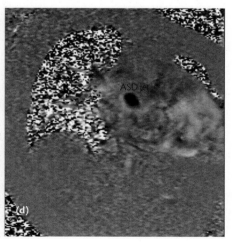

Fig. 42.7 Ebstein's anomaly imaged by CMR. Cine imaging in a 4-chamber plane (a) shows regurgitation (arrow) through the dysplastic tricuspid valve. The dotted lines indicate the plane through which velocities were mapped (b) to depict the cross-sectional size of tricuspid regurgitant jet (TR), assessed in this case as severe. An atrial short-axis cine in the same patient (c) shows bidirectional flow through an atrial septal defect (arrow). The dotted lines indicate the plane through which velocities were mapped (d) to depict the cross section of the ASD jet.

supplemented by 4-chamber and sagittal RVOT cines, is recommended. Transaxial cines may be used for volume measurements of the functional part of the Ebstein RV, which can be hard to delineate in short-axis slices. In spite of atrialization, higher RV volumes than normal may be found in the presence of severe tricuspid regurgitation. The severity of tricuspid regurgitation can be assessed using through-plane velocity mapping, the VENC typically set at 250 cm/s, to depict the cross-section of the regurgitant stream through a plane transecting the jet on the right atrial side of the orifice. A TR jet cross-section, reflecting the regurgitant defect, of 6×6 mm or more can be regarded as severe. An ASD, due in this setting to distension and gaping of a PFO, can be present in about 50% of adult Ebstein patients, and should be sought with an atrial short-axis cine stack. If present, the resting shunt can be measured by aortic and pulmonary velocity mapping. Cines may show diastolic compression of the LV by the dilated right heart, which can impair LV filling and so limit the cardiac output.

Congenital mitral valve dysfunction

While echocardiography remains the first line of investigation, CMR can contribute to the measurement of regurgitation and assessments of the structural cause and of any associated myocardial or other pathology. For identification of tethering, prolapse, or failure of coaptation, a contiguous stack of 5-mm thick cine images aligned perpendicular to the central part of the line of mitral coaptation is recommended [12]. Regurgitant or stenotic jets are visible on cine imaging, although appearances depend on the jet size and characteristics, and on the relative location and orientation of the imaging slice. Planimetry of an orifice, or rather of the cross-section of the jet immediately downstream of the orifice, is feasible in some but not all cases, depending on the structure of the jet and the relative thickness and location of the imaging slice. Jet velocity mapping can contribute to quantification of stenosis and the time course of jet flow. In the absence of another regurgitant or shunt lesion, mitral regurgitation can be quantified using ventricular stroke volume difference. However, a more widely applicable approach is to subtract the aortic outflow volume from the LV stroke volume.

Cor triatriatum sinister

Echocardiography is likely to be satisfactory, but a stack of contiguous CMR cines will show the intra-atrial membrane well if orientated orthogonal to it. Transaxial or 4-chamber orientations may be suitable. Transaxial cines can also show any anomalous pulmonary venous drainage. As in the case of an ASD, mapping of velocities through a plane orientated parallel and close to the membrane on its downstream side can delineate flow through the orifice(s).

Repaired tetralogy of Fallot

CMR has become the modality of choice for the assessment and follow up of adults with repaired tetralogy of Fallot (ToF). CMR measurements of RV and LV function, pulmonary regurgitation, right ventricular outflow tract obstruction, conduit or pulmonary artery stenoses, and possible residual shunting all contribute to decisions on management, notably the possibility of pulmonary valve replacement for pulmonary regurgitation (PR). Where CMR is unavailable or contraindicated MSCT can provide morphological assessment and ventricular function but not the flow or shunt data. The pathophysiology of PR differs from that of aortic regurgitation because of the situation of the sub-pulmonary right heart, connected in series with the more powerful left heart via the low-resistance pulmonary and high-resistance systemic vasculature. Free PR, with little or no effective valve function, is common after repair of ToF. It may be tolerated without symptoms for decades, and is typically associated with a regurgitant fraction of ~40% (➲ Fig. 42.8, 🎬 Video 42.3). However, RV dysfunction, arrhythmia, and premature death can result. Surgical pulmonary valve replacement is considered in such patients in most centres, but deciding when to operate remains controversial, particularly if the patient is asymptomatic, and bearing in mind that a homograft replacement may only function effectively for 15–20 years [13]. Once a conduit is in position, however, progressive stenosis or regurgitation may be treatable by percutaneous placement of a stented valve within the relatively rigid tube of the conduit [14, 15]. Studies by Therrien et al. [16] and Oosterhof et al. [17] compared CMR measurements of RV volumes before and after surgical pulmonary valve replacement, finding that patients with pre-operative indexed RV end-diastolic volumes above about 60 ml/m^2 and end-systolic volumes above about 82 ml/m^2 failed to recover to the normal RV volume range. Although this may be taken as a guide to RV volumes that should not be exceeded when waiting to replace a pulmonary valve, there are more factors to be considered. Even in the absence of an effective pulmonary valve, the amount of regurgitation depends on factors upstream and downstream. In occasional cases the regurgitant fraction can exceed 50%, which may be attributable to an unusually large and compliant RV, large and compliant pulmonary arteries whose elastic recoil contributes to the regurgitation, branch PA stenosis, or elevated peripheral resistance limiting the distal escape of flow, or combinations of these. However, branch pulmonary artery stenosis has been found to be associated with limited RV dilatation, perhaps due to development of a relatively restrictive RV [18]. Contrast enhanced 3D angiography may be used for the visualization of PA branch stenosis, and appropriately aligned cines can visualize jet formation and the reduced systolic expansion of PA branches distal to a stenosis that is obstructive enough to require relief, either percutaneously or at the time of surgery. Surgeons can resect any akinetic region of the RVOT that may have resulted from previous infundibular resection or patching, so regional as well as global RV function needs to be described. Tricuspid regurgitation needs to be identified and assessed, as does any residual VSD patch leak and consequent shunting. Global and regional LV function, and any aortic root dilatation or aortic regurgitation, also need assessment [19]. So, in summary, the evaluation of repaired ToF requires thorough assessment of the left and right heart, extending to the branch PAs. Each measurement should be interpreted in the context of circulatory factors upstream and downstream.

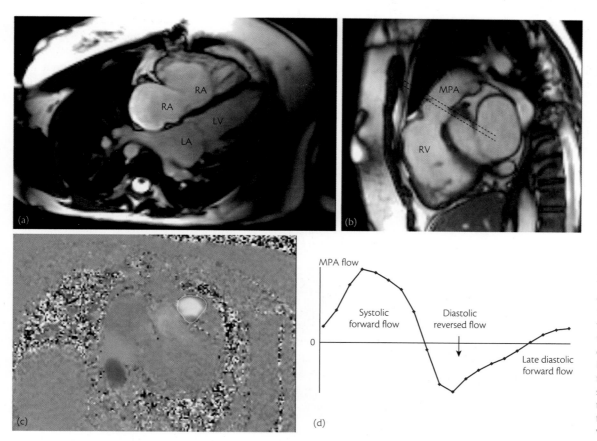

Fig. 42.8 Repaired tetralogy of Fallot imaged by CMR. The 4-chamber cine (a) shows evidence of mild tricuspid regurgitation. An oblique sagittal RVOT cine (b) shows evidence of pulmonary regurgitation, without effective valve function. The dotted lines indicate the slice through which pulmonary flow velocities were mapped (c, with the MPA outlined). (d) The pulmonary flow curve derived from the velocity data, from which a regurgitant fraction of 38% was calculated. Note the late diastolic forward flow occurring as atrial systole delivers flow forwards through the fully expanded right ventricle.

Common arterial trunk

CMR or MSCT can be useful in visualizing either the native pulmonary arterial branches, the conduit(s) following repair and can help to quantify biventricular function. CMR can additionally quantify any regurgitation of the truncal valve.

Transposition of the great arteries (TGA)

TGA treated by atrial switch operation (Mustard or Senning)

CMR or MSCT can assess the atrial pathways and systemic RV function [20]. With CMR experience, oblique cines and velocity maps can be aligned with respect to systemic and pulmonary venous atrial pathways (➲ Fig. 42.9, 📹 Video 42.4). Comprehensive coverage can, however, be achieved using a stack of contiguous transaxial or coronal cines or a 3-dimensional SSFP sequence. Baffle-leaks may not be easy to identify by CMR, the suture line being long and non-planar, but measurement of Qp:Qs may be helpful.

TGA treated by arterial switch operation

CMR or MSCT allow assessment of any RVOT or supravalvar pulmonary artery stenosis, branch PA stenosis, and function of both ventricles and the neo-aortic valve. MSCT or CMR can contribute to assessment of the patency of the re-implanted coronary arteries, and CMR perfusion imaging may be considered [21].

TGA treated by Rastelli operation

CMR or MSCT allow assessment of possible stenosis or incompetence of the RV-to-PA conduit, the LVOT, of biventricular function, and, with CMR, possible residual shunt.

Double-outlet RV

CMR or MSCT can be valuable, particularly after surgery if a conduit, PA branch stenosis, residual shunting, or ventricular dysfunction need assessment.

Congenitally corrected transposition of the great arteries

Either CMR or MSCT can demonstrate the abnormal anatomy and connections well, which can be helpful in adults with poor acoustic windows. A useful way of distinguishing which ventricle is morphologically the RV is to compare the two surfaces of the inter-ventricular septum. The LV surface is relatively smooth, with few trabeculations arising from it, in contrast to the RV side, which gives rise to the moderator band and multiple trabeculations in the apical region (➲ Fig. 42.10, 📹 Video 42.5).

The functionally univentricular heart

In patients with poor acoustic windows, any of the diagnostic issues listed in the preceding chapter can be addressed by CMR or MSCT, and also systemic or pulmonary venous anomalies, aortic

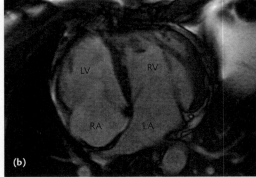

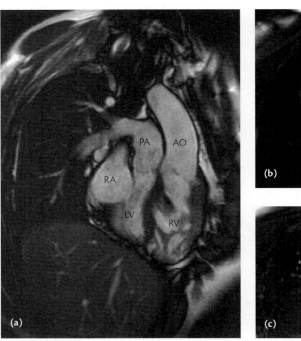

Fig. 42.9 Transposition of the great arteries after an atrial switch procedure (Mustard operation). An oblique sagittal cine (a) is aligned to show the discordant ventriculo-arterial connections. An oblique coronal cine (b) is aligned with the superior vena cava (SVC) and inferior vena cava (IVC) pathways, passing to the left of the surgically placed baffle, towards the sub-pulmonary left ventricle. An oblique long-axis cine (c) shows the pulmonary venous atrial compartment (PVAC), which carries blood from the pulmonary veins to the right ventricle. A mid short-axis cine (d) shows the expected hypertrophy of the systemic right ventricle.

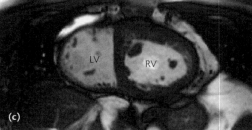

Fig. 42.10 Unoperated 'congenitally corrected' transposition of the great arteries imaged by CMR. Both the atrio-ventricular and the ventriculo-arterial connections are discordant (a and b). Note the expected apical displacement of the septal insertion of the tricuspid valve of the RV relative to that of the mitral valve of the LV. In the short-axis cine (c) note that, as in Fig. 42.9, the left ventricular cavity can be identified as the one on the smoother, less trabeculated side of the ventricular septum.

arch malformations, and branch PA stenoses. The global and regional function of the volume-loaded dominant ventricle can be assessed with either modality, with late gadolinium scar imaging by CMR if required.

The Fontan circulation

Fontan operations, performed in children in whom the abnormal cardiac anatomy precludes biventricular repair, results in a fundamental departure from normal circulatory dynamics. The systemic and pulmonary vascular beds are connected in series downstream of the single functional ventricle, so eliminating shunting at the cost of a critically elevated systemic venous pressure that is required to maintain flow through the lungs. Earlier procedures incorporated the right atrium between the caval veins and pulmonary arteries, whereas total cavo-pulmonary connection, connecting IVC flow to the PAs via a lateral tunnel or extra-cardiac conduit, has been favoured in recent years. CMR or MSCT allow assessment of the Fontan cavo-(atrio)-pulmonary connections, branch pulmonary arteries, pulmonary veins (which can be compressed by a dilated right atrium after an atrio-pulmonary connection), the atrio-ventricular valve(s), the ventricle(s), the ventricular outflow tract, and any residual leaks (with CMR) or collateral vessels. Comprehensive coverage using a stack of contiguous transaxial SSFP cines is recommended, this generally being suitable for the identification of any intra-atrial thrombus or suspected stenosis of the cavo-pulmonary connections. Velocity mapping can be used to assess flow through a suspected narrowing. In this setting, a peak jet velocity exceeding 1 m/s may represent significant stenosis. Should contrast injection for either MSCT or CMR angiography be considered, the connection of the SVC to the PAs and its relation to IVC flow should be borne in mind. Injection from a leg, or else non-contrast CMR 3D SSFP imaging, may be preferable. Evaluation of myocardial fibrosis by LGE may contribute to the assessment impaired ventricular function, if present.

Pulmonary arterial hypertension including Eisenmenger's syndrome

Although neither CMR nor MSCT can measure pulmonary arterial pressures, good visualization of any RV hypertrophy, ventricular septal flattening and any limitation of the systolic expansion of distended PAs means that the presence of pulmonary hypertension can be inferred and qualitatively assessed by CMR. CMR and MSCT also allow measurements of cardiac output, RV function, and hypertrophy, and CMR can be used, after gadolinium injection, for assessment of RV or septal fibrosis. In Eisenmenger's syndrome, either modality can give valuable information on the underlying malformation(s), and CMR allows shunt calculation at rest. Contrast PA angiography, particularly by MSCT, is used to identify any pulmonary arterial thrombus (⊃ Fig. 42.11) [22].

Coronary artery anomalies and acquired coronary disease

Contrast enhanced MSCT is superior to CMR for assessment of coronary artery patency and calcification, if present (⊃ Fig. 42.12) [23]. Both techniques are also able to determine global and regional myocardial function. The origin and proximal course of the coronary arteries can be visualized in most patients by CMR using cardiac gated 3D SSFP angiography, with fat suppression and without contrast agent and either diaphragm navigator or breathhold acquisition. However, the strength of CMR in this field lies in the complementary information that can be obtained on myocardial viability and perfusion [24].

Prospects for further development

Both CMR and MSCT continue to be developed and refined. There are particular needs for reliable and user-friendly postprocessing tools for the analysis of multidimensional image data. For example, rapid and reproducible segmentation and analysis of biventricular volumes from images of either modality would be a major step forward.

CMR is an inherently versatile modality. The repertoire of radio pulse and magnetic gradient sequences, and their uses with respect to tissue characteristics, movements, flows, and contrast agents, is being steadily extended and refined. 'Comprehensive' image acquisitions can potentially be less operator-dependent, delivering an inclusive dataset for subsequent review and measurement. However, prolonged acquisitions have to be gated or synchronized with respect to respiratory, as well as cardiac, cycles. Rapidly acquired 4-dimensional (time resolved 3-dimensional) CMR acquisitions have yet to achieve sufficient robustness and freedom from artefacts for clinical value. Comprehensive (3-dimensional, 3-directionally encoded and time resolved) velocity mapping has been implemented [25] and processed to give dynamic streamline or particle trace displays reconstructed from data acquired of many heart and respiratory cycles, but limitations include acquisition periods of 30 minutes or more, and the inability of this approach to accurately measure a wide range of velocities in the presence of jet flow.

Real-time CMR acquisition requires neither cardiac nor respiratory gating and has a place in the imaging of breathing related modifications of heart movement; for example, breathing-dependent

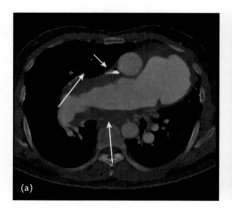
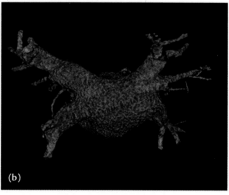

Fig. 42.11 Pulmonary arterial and pulmonary venous anatomy imaged by MSCT. (a) Demonstrates dilated main and right pulmonary arteries with both mural calcification (white arrow) and *in situ* thrombus (white arrowheads). The ratio of the diameters of the pulmonary arteries to the aorta is more than 1, an indicator of pulmonary hypertension. (b) Demonstrates normal pulmonary venous drainage into the left atrium.

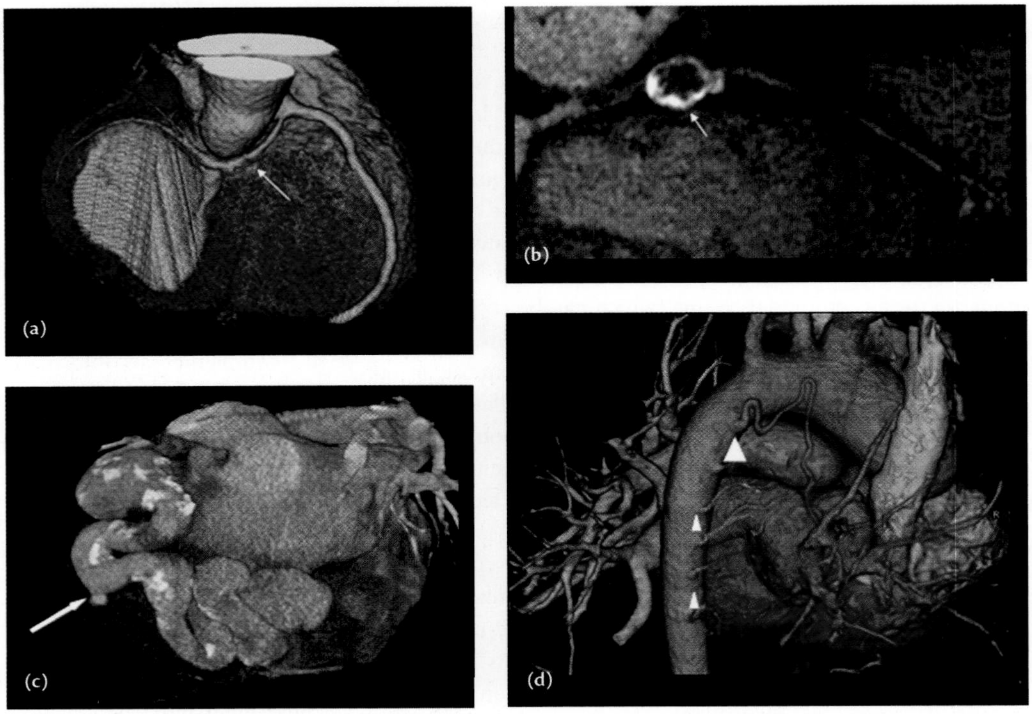

Fig. 42.12 Coronary anomalies imaged by MSCT include (a) aberrant coronary arteries, with the left circumflex artery (white arrow) arising from the right coronary artery, (b) coronary artery aneurysm in Kawasaki disease (note lack of contrast enhancement of aneurysm due to thrombus within it), and (c) a dilated and tortuous coronary arterio-venous fistula via a left circumflex artery (white arrow) that drains directly to the coronary sinus. Panel (d) shows aorto-pulmonary collateral arteries (arrow heads) arising from the descending aorta and supplying parts of the right lung.

deviation of the ventricular septum in constrictive pericarditis [26]. Real-time flow velocity acquisition may access novel information on haemodynamic pathophysiology, particularly in relation to respiratory movements and exercise. [27]

There is a major drive to reduce the ionizing radiation dose from MSCT with new and novel protocols and algorithms now standard on all new MSCT machines. Many of the newest generation of MSCT scanners have now complete cardiac coverage (256/320 detectors), allowing full angiography with no or minimal gantry movement and the possibility of contrast tracking allowing some flow data to be gained. This has led to a 50–90% reduction in ionizing radiation dose with the latest scanners delivering approximately 1 mSv for a CTA and less than 5 mSv for a combined CT coronary, pulmonary, and aortic angiogram.

One of the additional limitations of MSCT in patients with congenital heart disease has been the lack of tolerance to pharmacological rate control (usually β-blockers) and with the latest iteration of MSCT the temporal resolution has been reduced, albeit not to the current rate of CMR.

MSCT continues to develop rapidly and is likely to remain a significant modality in the assessment of adult congenital heart disease, particularly for the assessment of coronary artery pathology and pulmonary hypertension and if CMR is unable to be performed or unavailable locally.

References

1. Fratz S, John H, Annika S, et al. Routine clinical cardiovascular magnetic resonance in paediatric and adult congenital heart disease: patients, protocols, questions asked and contributions made. *J Cardiovasc Magn Reson* 2008; 10: 46.
2. Nicol ED, Gatzoulis M, Padley SP, Rubens M. Assessment of adult congenital heart disease with multi-detector computed tomography: beyond coronary lumenography. *Clin Radiol* 2007; 62(6): 518–27.
3. Blalock SE, Banka P, Geva T, Powell AJ, Zhou J, Prakash A. Interstudy variability in cardiac magnetic resonance imaging measurements of ventricular volume, mass, and ejection fraction in repaired tetralogy of Fallot: A prospective observational study. *J Magn Reson Imaging* 2013;38:829-35.
4. Winter MM, Bernink FJ, Groenink M, et al. Evaluating the systemic right ventricle by CMR: the importance of consistent and reproducible delineation of the cavity. *J Cardiovasc Magn Reson* 2008; 10(1): 40.
5. Gatehouse PD, Rolf MP, Graves MJ, et al. Flow measurement by cardiovascular magnetic resonance: a multi-centre multi-vendor study of background phase offset errors that can compromise the accuracy of derived regurgitant or shunt flow measurements. *J Cardiovasc Magn Reson* 2010; 12: 5.
6. Piaw CS, Kiam OT, Rapaee A, et al. Use of non-invasive phase contrast magnetic resonance imaging for estimation of atrial septal defect size and morphology: a comparison with transesophageal echo. *Cardiovasc Intervent Radiol* 2006; 29: 230–34.
7. Muzzarelli S, Meadows AK, Ordovas KG, et al. Prediction of hemodynamic severity of coarctation by magnetic resonance imaging. *Am J Cardiol* 2011; 108: 1335–40.
8. Budoff MJ, Shittu A, Roy S. Use of cardiovascular computed tomography in the diagnosis and management of coarctation of the aorta. *J Thorac Cardiovasc Surg* 2013;146:229-32.

9. Connolly HM, Huston J 3rd, Brown RD Jr, Warnes CA, Ammash NM, Tajik AJ. Intracranial aneurysms in patients with coarctation of the aorta: a prospective magnetic resonance angiographic study of 100 patients. *Mayo Clin Proc* 2003; 78: 1491–9.

10. Pouleur AC, le Polain de Waroux JB, Pasquet A, Vanoverschelde JL, Gerber BL. Aortic valve area assessment: multidetector CT compared with cine MR imaging and transthoracic and transesophageal echocardiography. *Radiology* 2007; 244: 745–54.

11. Crowe ME, Rocha CA, Wu E, Carr JC. Complications following the Ross procedure: cardiac MRI findings. *J Thorac Imaging* 2006; 21: 213–8.

12. Gabriel RS, Kerr AJ, Raffel OC, Stewart RA, Cowan BR, Occleshaw CJ. Mapping of mitral regurgitant defects by cardiovascular magnetic resonance in moderate or severe mitral regurgitation secondary to mitral valve prolapse. *J Cardiovasc Magn Reson* 2008; 10: 16.

13. Henkens IR, van Straten A, Schalij MJ, et al. Predicting outcome of pulmonary valve replacement in adult tetralogy of Fallot patients. *Ann Thorac Surg* 2007; 83: 907–11.

14. Lurz P, Coats L, Khambadkone S, et al. Percutaneous pulmonary valve implantation: impact of evolving technology and learning curve on clinical outcome. *Circulation* 2008; 117: 1964–72.

15. Quail MA, Frigiola A, Giardini A, et al. Impact of pulmonary valve replacement in tetralogy of Fallot with pulmonary regurgitation: a comparison of intervention and nonintervention. *Ann Thorac Surg* 2012; 94: 1619–26.

16. Therrien J, Provost Y, Merchant N, Williams W, Colman J, Webb G. Optimal timing for pulmonary valve replacement in adults after tetralogy of Fallot repair. *Am J Cardiol* 2005; 95(6): 779–82.

17. Oosterhof T, van Straten A, Vliegen HW, et al. Preoperative thresholds for pulmonary valve replacement in patients with corrected tetralogy of Fallot using cardiovascular magnetic resonance. *Circulation* 2007; 116: 545–51.

18. Maskatia SA, Spinner JA, Morris SA, Petit CJ, Krishnamurthy R, Nutting AC. Effect of branch pulmonary artery stenosis on right ventricular volume overload in patients with tetralogy of Fallot after initial surgical repair. *Am J Cardiol* 2013 2013; 111: 1355–60.

19. Geva T. Repaired tetralogy of Fallot: the roles of cardiovascular magnetic resonance in evaluating pathophysiology and for pulmonary valve replacement decision support. *J Cardiovasc Magn Reson* 2011; 13: 9.

20. Salehian O, Schwerzmann M, Merchant N, Webb GD, Siu SC, Therrien J. Assessment of systemic right ventricular function in patients with transposition of the great arteries using the myocardial performance index: comparison with cardiac magnetic resonance imaging. *Circulation* 2004; 110: 3229–233.

21. Taylor AM, Dymarkowski S, Hamaekers P, et al. MR coronary angiography and late-enhancement myocardial MR in children who underwent arterial switch surgery for transposition of great arteries. *Radiology* 2005; 234: 542–47.

22. Nicol ED, Kafka H, Stirrup J, et al. A single, comprehensive non-invasive cardiovascular assessment in pulmonary arterial hypertension: Combined computed tomography pulmonary and coronary angiography. *Int J Cardiol* 2009; 136: 278–88.

23. Nicol ED, Stirrup J, Roughton M, Padley SP, Rubens MB. 64-Channel cardiac computed tomography: intraobserver and interobserver variability (part 1): coronary angiography. *J Comput Assist Tomogr* 2009; 33: 161–8.

24. Wu HD, Kwong RY. Cardiac magnetic resonance imaging in patients with coronary disease. *Curr Treat Options Cardiovasc Med* 2008; 10(1): 83–92.

25. Markl M, Kilner PJ, Ebbers T. Comprehensive 4D velocity mapping of the heart and great vessels by cardiovascular magnetic resonance. *J Cardiovasc Magn Reson* 2011; 13: 7.

26. Francone M, Dymarkowski S, Kalantzi M, Rademakers FE, Bogaert J. Assessment of ventricular coupling with real-time cine MRI and its value to differentiate constrictive pericarditis from restrictive cardiomyopathy. *Eur Radiol* 2006; 16: 944–51.

27. Steeden JA, Jones A, Pandya B, Atkinson D, Taylor AM, Muthurangu V. High-resolution slice-selective Fourier velocity encoding in congenital heart disease using spiral SENSE with velocity unwrap. *Magn Reson Med* 2012; 67: 1538–46.

⊃ **For additional multimedia materials please visit the online version of the book (** http://www.esciacc.oxfordmedicine.com**)**

Aortic disease: aneurysm and dissection

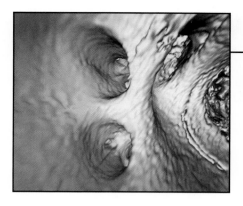

CHAPTER 43

Role of echocardiography

Covadonga Fernández-Golfín and José L. Zamorano

Contents

Introduction

Aortic diseases are an important source of morbidity and mortality. Usually (apart from acute aortic syndromes) aortic pathology gives no signs or symptoms and diagnosis and follow-up is performed by means of imaging techniques [1]. As a first-line diagnostic test in cardiovascular diseases, echocardiography plays an important role in the assessment of thoracic aorta diseases.

Normal anatomy and echocardiographic assessment of the normal aorta

The thoracic aorta is divided in the aortic root (aortic annulus, cusps, and the sinuses of Valsalva), the ascending aorta (from the sinotubular junction to the brachiocephalic artery origin), the aortic arch (from the brachiocephalic artery to the isthmus), and the descending thoracic aorta (from the isthmus to the diaphragm).

Thoracic aorta evaluation is part of the transthoracic echocardiographic (TTE) examination. Ascending aorta, mainly aortic root and proximal tubular segment, are clearly seen in most cases and TTE may be enough for diagnosis and follow-up. Evaluation of distal ascending aorta, arch and descending aorta is limited and further evaluation with other imaging techniques is warranted. All available image planes should be used to get the best assessment of normal thoracic aorta (see ⊃ Fig. 43.1 and ⊃ Fig. 43.2). Left and right parasternal long axes are essential for aortic root evaluation and measurements. Leading edge–leading edge measurement is performed in diastole, ideally in 2D images (M-mode tends to underestimate the measured values) at the level of aortic annulus, aortic sinuses, and sinotubular junction [2]. Measurements should be performed perpendicular to the

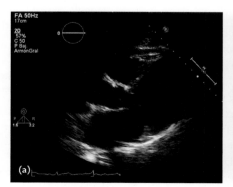
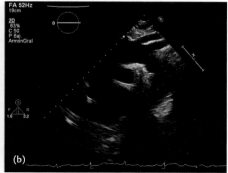

Fig. 43.1 TTE (a) parasternal long-axis view in diastole showing aortic root and proximal ascending aorta and (b) suprasternal view.

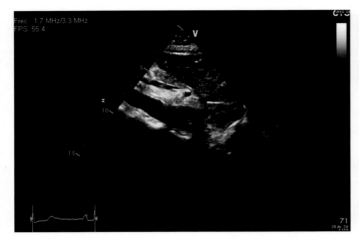

Fig. 43.2 Subcostal view showing longitudinal view of abdominal aorta.

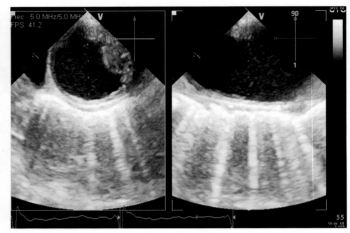

Fig. 43.4 Descending thoracic aorta, multi-plane acquisition with short-axis and long-axis aortic views. Prominent atherosclerotic plaque is seen.

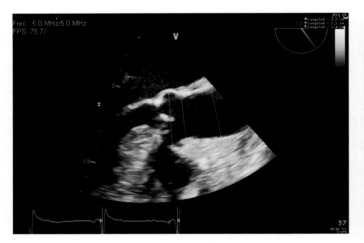

Fig. 43.3 TEE long-axis view showing aortic root anatomy and diameters

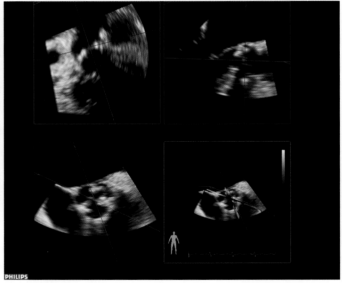

Fig. 43.5 3D aortic root multi-planar reconstruction for diameter and area measurements.

blood flow in specific anatomic landmarks. The widest diameters at the level of the Valsalva sinuses should be used for reporting aortic root diameters [1]. Suprasternal window should be performed in all cases to assess distal ascending aorta, arch and proximal descending aorta. If after a full comprehensive echocardiogram study, doubts remain, another image technique should be used.

Transoesophageal echocardiography (TEE) is superior to TTE for the evaluation of the thoracic aorta. TE probe's proximity to the oesophagus allows high-resolution images not only of the aortic root, but also from the thoracic descending aorta and aortic arch. Only a small portion of the distal ascending aorta is not evaluable with TEE due to the right bronchus and trachea interposition (blind spot). Aortic root assessment is performed in the 3-chambers' view at 120° (see ⊃ Fig. 43.3), with complementary images obtained in the short-axis view at 45°. Long- and short-axis views of the descending thoracic aorta are obtained after a 180° probe rotation with visualization of the descending aorta from the coeliac trunk to the aortic arch with the great vessels. New 3D ultrasound probes that allow simultaneous multi-plane assessment are useful in the evaluation of the aorta and aortic wall (see ⊃ Fig. 43.4). Acquisition of 3D images with posterior reformatting with different software, allows accurate measurements of aortic diameters perpendicular

to the blood flow and vessel overcoming some of the limitations of 2D echocardiography (see ⊃ Fig. 43.5) [3].

Normal echocardiographic diameters of the thoracic aorta strongly depend on age and body surface area [4]. Normal reference values for the different aortic segments are listed in ⊃ Table 43.1 [1].

Table 43.1 Normal thoracic aorta echocardiographic diameters

	Diameter	Indexed
Aortic annulus	20–31 mm	13 ± 1 mm/m^2
Sinuses of Valsalva	29–45 mm	19 ± 1 mm/m^2
Sinotubular junction	22–36 mm	15 ± 1 mm/m^2
Tubular ascending aorta	22–36 mm	15 ± 2 mm/m^2
Aortic arch	22–36 mm	
Descending aorta	20–30 mm	

From Evangelista A, et al. *European Journal of Echocardiography* 2010; 11: 645–8.

Role of echocardiography in aortic diseases: aneurysm and dissection

Aortic aneurysm

An aortic aneurysm (AA) is defined as a permanent and localized dilatation of an artery with a diameter at least 50% above its expected normal diameter. All vessel walls are present, but intima and media may be so thin that its non-invasive identification may be difficult [5]. They may be sacular or fusiforms.

Pseudoaneurysm is defined in cases where there is a disruption of the arterial wall with extravasation of blood contained by periarterial connective tissue. Arterial wall in the case of pseudoaneurysms lack the three-layer structure of the normal thoracic aorta [5].

In most cases AA is related to hypertension, atherosclerosis, aortic stenosis, or bicuspid aortic valve. Other aetiologies include Marfan syndrome and other connective tissue diseases. Medial degeneration with disruption and loss of elastic fibres and proteoglycans deposition characterize the histopathology of AA [5].

In many cases diagnosis is made as an incidental finding when the patient undergoes an imaging modality for other reasons (computed tomography, magnetic resonance, or echocardiography). In the remaining cases diagnosis is suspected based on an abnormal thorax X-ray or as part of a screening strategy in predisposing pathologies (bicuspid aortic valve or Marfan syndrome).

Echocardiographic diagnosis of AA depends on aneurysmal location. Aortic root and proximal ascending AA diagnosis is based on TTE (see ⊃ Fig. 43.6 and 📹 Video 43.1). AA is defined when aortic diameters exceed those expected for age and body surface area [5]. TTE allows AA diagnosis and possible associated cardiac abnormalities (bicuspid aortic valve). Rarely, alternative imaging techniques are needed for diagnosis or follow-up. On the contrary, when AA is located elsewhere along the thoracic aorta, alternative imaging techniques should be performed. Although TEE is able to evaluate most of the thoracic aorta, other imaging techniques like magnetic resonance or computed tomography are preferred since they allow a non-invasive comprehensive evaluation of the aorta without limitations of TEE (aortic tortuosity, semi-invasive). TEE should be used in combination with magnetic resonance or computed tomography in acute cases where aortic dissection or other complications are suspected.

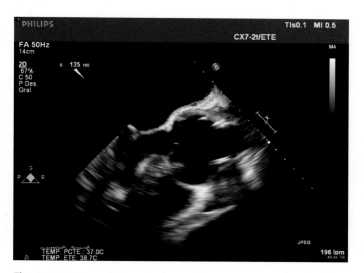

Fig. 43.7 TEE long-axis view showing aortic root aneurysm and proximal ascending aorta graft in a patient with previous Type A aortic dissection surgery.

Aortic root reconstruction or replacement is indicated in patients when the degree of dilatation of the aorta or aortic root reaches or exceeds 5.5 cm by echocardiography [6]. Patients with bicuspid aortic valves and dilatation of the aortic root or ascending aorta with a diameter greater than 4.0 cm should undergo serial evaluation. Aortic root reconstruction or replacement are indicated (IIb recommendation) in patients with bicuspid aortic valves if the diameter of the aortic root or ascending aorta is greater than 5.0 cm (see ⊃ Fig. 43.7 and 📹 Video 43.2) and risk factors (aortic coarctation, systemic hypertension, family history of aortic dissection, or >2mm/year increase in aortic diameter). In patients with Marfan syndrome, surgery is recommended when diameter is ≥5.0 cm. If risk factors are present (family history of aortic dissection and/or aortic size increase >2 mm/year, severe AR or mitral regurgitation, desire of pregnancy) surgery should be considered with diameters ≥4.5 cm [6].

In patients undergoing aortic valve replacement due to severe aortic regurgitation or aortic stenosis, lower thresholds (>4.5 cm) for concomitant aorta surgery may be considered depending on age, body surface area, aetiology of valvular disease, presence of a bicuspid aortic valve, and intra-operative shape and thickness of the ascending aorta [6].

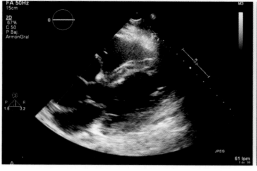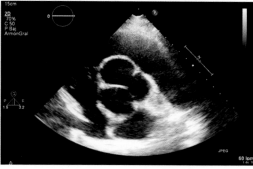

Fig. 43.6 TTE parasternal long- and short-axis views of a patient with an aortic root aneurysm after aortic dissection surgery (supracoronary graft).

Aortic dissection

Aortic dissection (ad) occurs when there is a disruption of the media and bleeding within and along the wall of the aorta occurs [5]. It is characterized by the formation of a false lumen in the tunica media of the aortic wall. Clinical presentation is in most cases in the form of acute onset chest pain with high mortality and morbidity. Depending on the anatomic characteristics, different types of aortic dissection can be differentiated, each with their own clinical, therapeutic and prognostic implications [7].

According to the Stanford classification of ad, there are two main types: type A and type B [8, 9]. An ad is type A if it includes the ascending aorta and type B if it does not involve the ascending aorta. The De Bakey classification subdivides the dissection process into: a type I dissection if it involves the entire aorta, a type II dissection if it involves the ascending aorta, and a type III dissection if it involves the descending aorta [9]. Intramural haematoma (IH) and aortic ulcers may be signs of evolving dissections or dissection subtypes. Bases on these findings, a new classification of the so-called aortic syndromes has been proposed [10]: class 1—classical ad with an intimal flap between true and false lumen; class 2—medial disruption with formation of intramural haematoma/haemorrhage; class 3—discrete/subtle dissection without haematoma, eccentric bulge at tear site; class 4—plaque rupture leading to aortic ulceration, penetrating aortic atherosclerotic ulcer with surrounding haematoma, usually subadventitial; class 5—iatrogenic and traumatic dissection. All types of aortic syndromes can also be classified into acute and chronic: chronic dissections are considered to be present if more than 14 days have elapsed since the acute event or if they are found occasionally.

A typical ad begins with the tearing of the aortic intima, which exposes the diseased underlying medial layer to the pulsating blood flow. The blood then penetrates this layer, dissecting it. This dissection can then extend distally for a variable distance, creating a false lumen. Shearing forces can then cause the tearing of the internal part of the dissected aorta wall, producing additional entry and exit zones. The most common locations for primary intimal tears are: in the ascending aorta 1–5 cm above the right sinus of Valsalva (65% of cases), in the proximal descending aorta under the left subclavian artery (20%), in the transverse aortic arch (10%), and in the distal thoracic-abdominal aorta (5%) (11).

Rapid and accurate diagnosis of ad and other forms of aortic syndromes, in many cases in critically ill patients are mandatory. Diagnosis accuracy of TEE, computed tomography and magnetic resonance are similar and decision depends on availability and experience of the staff present. In most centres, computed tomography is the first imaging technique, but during diagnosis work up, in the majority of cases especially if surgery is needed, another imaging modality (mainly TEE) is performed [1].

Echocardiographic diagnosis is based on the detection of an intimal flap that divides the aorta into the true and false lumen [1]. False lumen flow may be detected by colour flow but sometimes, in cases of thrombosis or retrograde dissection, colour flow is absent. TTE has been considered of limited value in the diagnosis of aortic dissection. However, recent technique development and use of contrast has increased its diagnostic accuracy, especially in cases of type A aortic dissection [12]. Due to its availability, rapid information, and capability of alternative and additional diagnosis, it is performed as the first-line imaging technique in the emergency department. Diagnosis is made when an intimal flap is seen (see ⊃ Fig. 43.8 and ▣ Video 44.3), usually at the level of the aortic root or ascending aorta. If no intimal flap is visible, other indirect signs that may accompany aortic dissection are: pericardial effusion, aortic regurgitation (⊃ Fig. 43.9), aortic dilatation, and segmental wall motion abnormalities. Even in the absence of a clear flap, the presence of these findings in the clinical context should raise suspicion of acute ad. However, its low negative predictive value does not allow ruling out the diagnosis and further studies are needed [1, 13].

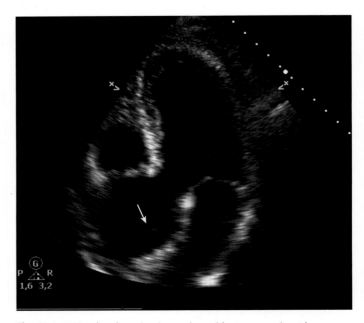

Fig. 43.8 TTE 5-chambers view in a patient with acute type A aortic dissection. An intimal flap (arrow) is seen on the aortic root.

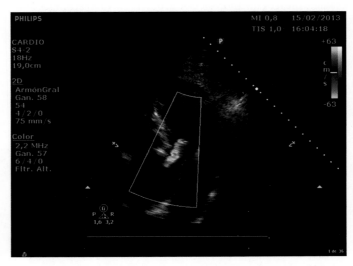

Fig. 43.9 Colour Doppler, TTE 5-chambers view of the same patient with type A acute aortic dissection. Significant central aortic regurgitation jet is seen.

TEE overcomes many of the limitations encountered with TTE. Several studies have demonstrated the accuracy of TEE in the diagnosis of aortic dissection with sensitivity of 86–100%, specificity 90–100%, and a negative predictive value of 86–100% [1]. The main diagnostic findings that TEE provides in a patient with an aortic dissection are: intimal dissection flaps (see ⊃ Fig. 43.10 and ▣ Video 43.4); M-mode ultrasound allows the detection and differentiation of intimal flaps in the aorta; enlargement of the aortic wall, dilation of the aortic root and enlarging of the posterior wall is possible; M-mode ultrasound has also been described as useful for differentiating between real flaps and artefacts [14].

◆ Identification of the true and false lumens (see ⊃ Table 43.2). The presence of flow does not absolutely distinguish the true lumen from the false lumen. The true lumen is characterized by: reduced size, greater pulsatility during systole, the presence of echocontrast is rare, clotting is also rare, and communication is from true lumen to false lumen during systole.

◆ Differentiation between communicating and non-communicating dissection: According to how the flow is visualized in the false lumen and to how tears are detected in the intimal flap, it is possible to differentiate between communicating and non-communicating dissections. When communication exists, the intimal flap shows wide movements during the cardiac cycle whereas movements are reduced in non-communicating dissections.

◆ Localizing entry and communication points.

◆ Pericardial effusion: the effusion of fluid in the pericardium and/or the pleural space is a sign of poor prognosis.

◆ Coronary artery ostium involvement (see ⊃ Fig. 43.11 and ▣ Video 43.5).

◆ Involvement of lateral branches of the aorta.

◆ Aortic valve involvement: TEE may evaluate the severity and mechanism of aortic regurgitation that complicates acute type A dissections. In case aortic valve is normal and aortic regurgitation is secondary to a repairable aortic lesion, the patient may undergo aortic valve repair but if there are non-repairable abnormalities, the patient should undergo valve replacement (see ⊃ Fig. 43.10).

◆ Thrombosis in the false lumen (see ⊃ Fig. 43.12 and ▣ Video 43.6).

Recently, case reports have illustrated the possible utility of 3D TEE echocardiography in ad (see ▣ Video 43.7). Moreover, it seems to be superior to 2D TEE echocardiography in the assessment of entry tear size in chronic dissection [15].

Other forms of acute aortic syndrome

IH has a distinctly different appearance on TEE: no intimal flap is visible and the aortic lumen has a normal shape. The aortic wall is thickened (>5 mm) with a typical circular or crescent shape (⊃ Fig. 43.11) that extends along the aorta without colour flow

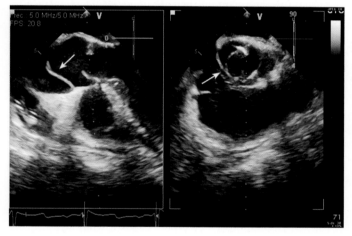

Fig. 43.10 TEE multi-plane image of the aortic valve and aortic root of a patient with type A acute aortic dissection. An intimal flap (solid arrow) is seen in the aortic root in patient with bicuspid aortic valve (dash arrow).

Table 43.2 Echocardiographic features of true and false lumen

	False lumen	True lumen
Size	Large	Small
Pulsation	No, systolic compression	Yes
Flow direction	Systolic antegrade flow reduced or absent, or retrograde flow	Systolic antegrade flow
Communication flow	From true to false lumen in systole	Absent
Spontaneous contrast	Frequent	Thick
Wall	Thin	No
Thrombosis	Yes	

Adapted from Evangelista A, et al. *European Journal of Echocardiography* 2010; 11: 645–8.

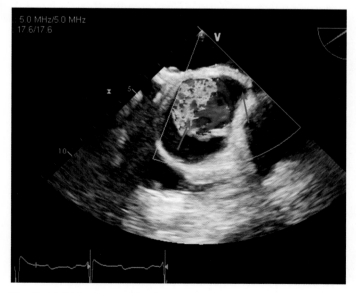

Fig. 43.11 TEE colour Doppler short-axis view. Systolic expansion with flow is seen in the true lumen (arrow). Left main coronary ostium is seen arising from the true lumen (dash arrow).

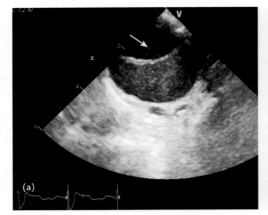 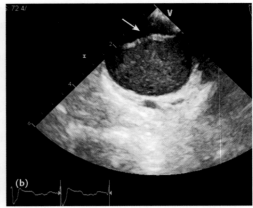

Fig. 43.12 Descending thoracic aorta with systolic expansion of the true lumen (arrow, a) and compression during diastole (arrow, b). Partial thrombosis of the false lumen is also seen.

[1, 5, 13]. Typically it shows a localized thickening of the aorta wall with echo-free central intramural spaces limited to one or two scanning planes. Multiple layers of aorta wall divided by the haemorrhage, an increased distance between the lumen and the oesophagus, and a periaortic area with no echo are seen on TEE. It is caused by, either a rupture of the aortic vasa vasorum, which provokes a bleeding that separates medial wall layers, or, less commonly, by a penetrating atheroscleroctic ulcer. Differential diagnosis with diffuse atherosclerosis or mural thrombus is sometimes difficult. The irregular surface of the protruding plaques or thrombus may give the clue for diagnosis along with the location of intimal calcification, if present (outside the thrombus or atherosclerotic plaque and in the most inner aortic border in the case of haematoma) [1].

IH can cause typical dissection in approximately 30% of patients [13] or heal spontaneously. In these patients, no false lumen is detected. One of the main characteristics of IH is its dynamic nature, with the possibility of its developing into a classic ad or an aortic rupture. Reabsorption may even occur (10% of cases). Nevertheless, recent studies confirm a poor prognosis with high in hospital mortality of this type of aortic syndrome [16].

Atherosclerotic lesions may cause erosion at the aortic surface. If this erosion invades the medial layer a penetrating aortic ulcer (PU) develops. In this type of lesion the internal elastic lamina always shows a rupture. Echocardiographic (TEE) diagnosis of PU ulcers is based on the image of crater-like outpouching of the aortic wall (➲ Fig. 43.12), generally associated with extensive aortic atheroma [1]. Some authors include the identification of blood flow in the interior and at the edges of the ulcer; IH may be associated. They are usually located in the descending thoracic aorta, and their clinical presentation is normally very similar to classic aortic dissection or IH. PU follows a very variable course and can lead to aortic dissection, aortic aneurysm, or even rupture. A common development is the progressive dilation of the aorta, but if ulceration continues to deepen it can cause a pseudoaneurysm or even aortic rupture. Computed tomography and magnetic resonance able to characterize the aortic wall with extended field of view are also available for diagnosis and follow-up [17, 18].

Pitfalls and limitations of the technique

In most cases, AA diagnosis is straightforward without pitfall or limitations. However, in the case of ad, artefacts in the aortic root are frequently seen. These false images are related to reverberation of the calcified aortic wall, pulmonary artery, or left atrial wall and appear as hyperechogenic lines in the aortic lumen. Location and movement are the best way to assure the diagnosis. Typically, false images in the aortic root appear located twice as far from the transducer as the posterior aortic wall, and their movement is parallel to the posterior aortic wall but with double displacement amplitude. Intra-luminal reverberations in ascending aorta are located at twice the distance from the right pulmonary artery posterior wall, as from the posterior aortic wall [1]. Extension of ad and great vessels involvement is best visualized with computed tomography or magnetic resonance.

The main limitation of TTE is poor acoustic window, especially in obese patients with pulmonary obstructive diseases and thorax deformities. Many patients are critically ill, which also limits image quality. Regarding TEE the main limitation is the operator's experience, which is crucial in the case of false images, differential diagnosis, and complete assessment of the pathology and complications. Correct imaging plane, avoiding angulations and foreshortening are also important issues, especially in AA diagnosis and follow-up. Care should be taken to avoid errors in the image acquisition and measurements.

Prognostic information provided by echo

Echocardiography plays an important role in prognosis stratification of AA. It allows not only diameter measurement, but also the rate of increase in diameter that in certain pathologies may be an indication for surgery.

In the acute phase of ad, echocardiographic parameters have prognosis significance. Pericardial effusion and periaortic haematoma are associated with worse outcome. In the subacute phase, the aortic diameter seems to be related to further aortic dilatation [1]. Absence of complete thrombosis of the false lumen is associated with worst outcome and different echocardiographic parameters assessing this feature have shown its prognostic significance: compression of the true lumen, partial false lumen thrombosis (opposed to false lumen thrombosis), communication between the true and false lumen, and presence of antegrade or retrograde flow in the false lumen [1]. In those cases where the false lumen is patent, entry tear proximal location and size after ad was associated with higher risk [19].

Follow-up

Patient follow-up depends on the type of aortic pathology and location. In the case of AA limited to the aortic root, TTE is the technique of choice, since reproducible measurements can be performed, it is non-invasive, and concomitant evaluation of cardiac structure can be performed. In cases of AA in the tubular ascending aorta or elsewhere, TTE is not appropriate and other imaging techniques must be chosen. Since TEE is semi-invasive with some limitations regarding visualization of distal ascending aorta, computed tomography or magnetic resonance are preferred [1, 5].

In the case of ad, the role of echocardiography is limited. Even though TEE can assess the structure of the dissection, surgical repair, healing of the dissection and obliteration of the false lumen, or blood flow dynamics in true and false lumina, computed tomography and magnetic resonance are superior in the follow-up [1].

Conclusions

Echocardiography plays an important role in the diagnosis and management of patients with aortic diseases. TTE is essential in the diagnosis and follow-up of aortic root aneurysm where TEE is seldom needed. When other parts of thoracic aorta are affected, or in cases of acute aortic syndromes, TEE is superior, being useful for diagnosis, surgery guidance, and follow-up. Alternative imaging modalities may complement information provided by echocardiography, especially if the distal ascending aorta, arch and descending aorta are affected.

References

1. Evangelista A, Flachskampf FA, Erbel R, et al. Echocardiography in aortic diseases: EAE recommendations for clinical practice. *Eur J Echocardiogr* 2010; 11: 645–58.

2. Lang R, Bierig M, Devereux R, et al. Recommendations for Chamber Quantification. A report from the American Society of Echocardiography's Nomenclature and Standards Committee, the Task Force on Chamber Quantification, and the European Association of Echocardiography. *Eur J Echocardiogr* 2006; 7: 79–108.

3. Joshi D, Bicer EI, Donmez C, et al. Incremental value of live/real time three-dimensional transoesophageal echocardiography over the two-dimensional technique in the assessment of aortic aneurysm and dissection. *Echocardiography* 2012; 29: 620–30.

4. Vasan RS, Larson MG, Levy D. Determinants of echocardiographic aortic root size. The Framingham heart study. *Circulation* 1995; 91: 734–40.

5. Hiratzka LF, Bakris GL, Beckman JA, et al. 2010 ACCF/AHA/AATS/ACR/ASA/SCA/SCAI/SIR/STS/SVM Guidelines for the diagnosis and management of patients with thoracic aortic disease. A Report of the American College of Cardiology Foundation/American Heart Association Task Force on Practice Guidelines, American Association for Thoracic Surgery, American College of Radiology, American Stroke Association, Society of Cardiovascular Anesthesiologists, Society for Cardiovascular Angiography and Interventions, Society of Interventional Radiology, Society of Thoracic Surgeons, and Society for Vascular Medicine. *J Am Coll Cardiol* 2010; 55: e27–129.

6. Vahanian A, Alfieri O, Andreotti F, et al. Joint Task Force on the Management of Valvular Heart Disease of the European Society of Cardiology (ESC); European Association for Cardio-Thoracic Surgery (EACTS). Guidelines on the management of valvular heart disease (version 2012). *Eur Heart J* 2012; 33: 2451–96.

7. Crawford ES, Svensson LG, Coselli JS, Safi HJ, Hess KR. Surgical treatment of aneurysm and/or dissection of the ascending aorta, transverse aortic arch, and ascending aorta and transverse aortic arch. Factors influencing survival in 717 patients. *J Thorac Cardiovasc Surg* 1989; 98: 659–74.

8. De Bakey ME, McCollum CH, Crawford ES, et al. Dissection and dissecting aneurysms of the aorta: twenty-year follow-up of five hundred and twenty-seven patients treated surgically. *Surgery* 1982; 92: 1118–34.

9. Svensson LG, Labib SB, Eisenhauer AC, Butterly JR. Intimal tear without haematoma. *Circulation* 1999; 99: 1331–6.

10. Roberts W. Aortic dissection: anatomy, consequences and causes. *Am Heart J* 1991; 101: 195–214.

11. Erbel R, Engberding R, Daniel W, et al. Echocardiography in diagnosis of aortic dissection. *Lancet* 1989; 1: 457.

12. Evangelista A, Avegliano G, Aguilar R, et al. Impact of contrast-enhanced echocardiography on the diagnostic algorithm of acute aortic dissection. *Eur Heart J* 2010; 31: 472–9.

13. Meredith EL, Masani ND. Echocardiography in the emergency assessment of acute aortic syndromes. *Eur J Echocardiogr* 2009; 10: i31–39.

14. Evangelista A, Garcia-del-Castillo H, Gonzalez-Alujas T, et al. Diagnosis of ascending aortic dissection by transoesophageal echocardiography: utility of M-mode in recognizing artifacts. *J Am Coll Cardiol* 1996; 27: 102.

15. Evangelista A, Aguilar R, Cuellar H, et al. Usefulness of real-time three-dimensional transoesophageal echocardiography in the assessment of chronic aortic dissection. *Eur J Echocardiogr* 201; 12: 272–77.

16. Harris KM, Braverman AC, Eagle KA, et al. Acute aortic intramural haematoma: an analysis from the International Registry of Acute Aortic Dissection. *Circulation* 2012; 126: S91–6.

17. Montgomery DH, Ververis JJ, McGorisc G, Frohwein S, Martin RP, Taylor WR. Natural history of severe atheromatous disease of the thoracic aorta: a transoesophageal echocardiography study. *J Am Coll Cardiol* 1996; 27: 95–101.

18. Atar S, Nagai T, Birnbaum Y, et al. Transoesophageal echocardiography Doppler findings in patients with penetrating atherosclerotic aortic ulcers. *Am J Cardiol* 1999; 83: 133–5.

19. Evangelista A, Salas A, Ribera A, et al. Long-term outcome of aortic dissection with patent false lumen predictive role of entry tear size and location. *Circulation* 2012; 125: 3133–41.

⊃ **For additional multimedia materials please visit the online version of the book (**⌀ **http://www.esciacc.oxfordmedicine.com)**

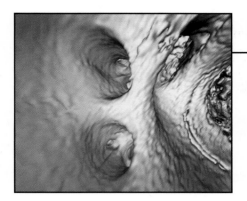

CHAPTER 44

Role of magnetic resonance imaging in aortic disease

Arturo Evangelista and Jérôme Garot

Contents

Introduction

MRI is increasingly becoming the first-line technique for evaluating diseases of the thoracic aorta [1,2]. MRI possesses the capability for multiplanar imaging. It may use a non-toxic contrast agent and does not involve ionising radiation. With recent advances in gradient hardware, much shorter repetition times are achievable, resulting in significant increase in acquisition speed.

Magnetic resonance imaging techniques

Black-blood sequences

To optimize the quality of MR aortic images, the acquisitions are performed with ECG gating and during repeated breath-holds. Blood circulating through the aorta is black on conventional spin-echo and turbo spin-echo sequences owing to the emptying signal produced by the transit time effect of moving blood in the short phase. These sequences provide great morphological information on the aortic wall and adjacent structures. T1- or T2-weighted images are useful for characterization of wall tissue. Spin-echo T1-weighted imaging provides the best pathoanatomic details of intramural haematoma, intimal flaps, or atheromas. T2-weighted images demonstrate oedema as high signal and can provide useful information regarding the activity of inflammatory aortic conditions. Post-contrast T1 imaging with fat suppression is useful in the diagnosis of some entities such as aortitis or mycotic aneurysms. ECG triggering is essential in minimizing motion and pulsatility artefact. A slice of 3–8 mm and echo time (TE) of 20–30 ms are standard, while repetition time (TR) is determined from the R–R' interval of the ECG. ECG-triggered, breath-hold turbo spin echo (TSE) has been the cornerstone of black-blood MRI for aortic disease. A double inversion-recovery technique is used to abolish the blood signal. The black-blood appearance is the result of nulling of the blood flowing into the slice by the first 180° inversion pulse at a specific inversion time (TI). Imaging occurs during mid to late diastole and the entire image is acquired over several heartbeats. Rapid black-blood spin-echo sequences such as HASTE or SS-FSE sequences (Half Fourier sampling, single-shot) permit correct morphological assessment of the aorta with very rapid acquisition times. Recently, a fast diffusion-prepared (DP) balanced SSFP-based magnetic resonance technique that allows for three-dimensional dark blood imaging has been described. Since this is a three-dimensional technique, the images offer improved slice resolution and more intuitive visualization of the thoracic aorta.

Cine-MR sequences

Cine-MR images are acquired using steady-state-free-precession (SSFP) sequences that provide excellent contrast between blood pool and surrounding tissue without the use of contrast agents. SSFP sequences (True FISP, Fiesta or Balanced FFE) permit high-contrast images with very short acquisition times since they have very low repetition times. They have become pivotal in providing vivid imaging of flowing blood. Due to high temporal resolution, images of multiple phases of the heart cycle can be obtained and blood flow visualized both during systole and diastole. Non-contrast SSFP imaging enables rapid exclusion of aortic dissection in the single shot mode and a more detailed evaluation in the cine mode, both visualizing dissected wall in any plane. The high signal-to-noise and contrast-to-noise renders SSFP particularly useful for patients incapable of breath-holding or in the setting of suspected aortic syndrome [3, 4]. SSFP sequences generate images of brilliant blood. The emptying signal determines turbulent flow in haemodynamically significant stenosis or valvular regurgitation that may be useful in the detection of aortic coarctation or valvular disease. When evaluating the aorta, which contains areas of turbulent high-velocity flow, the conventional gradient echo cine sequences can be helpful as they tend to be less prone to flow-related artefacts than SSFP.

Flow mapping

Accurate quantitative information on blood flow is obtained from modified gradient-echo sequences with parameter reconstruction from the phase rather than the amplitude of the MR signal. This is also known as flow mapping or phase contrast or velocity-encoded (VENC) cine MRI. VENC cine-MRI sequences provide great functional information owing to their capacity to quantify flow. Quantification of both flow velocity and volume permits physiopathological assessment of blood flow alterations in different aortic diseases. The information is processed using magnitude and phase images. Signal magnitude images display brilliant flowing blood and offer better anatomical assessment, while phase images show a map of flow velocities and direction. Using post-processing techniques, it is possible to obtain curves of flow vs. time, velocity vs. time, and peak velocity vs. time. Quantitative data on flow velocity and flow are estimated by multiplying the spatial mean velocity and cross-sectional area of the vessel. In this manner, the haemodynamic parameters can be quantified in different situations such as aortic coarctation or valvular disease, and also in the analysis of flow patterns in true and false lumina of aortic dissection. More recently, blood flow imaging with three-dimensional time-resolved phase-contrast cardiac magnetic resonance (four-dimensional flow) has been proposed as an innovative and visually appealing method for studying cardiovascular disease. The sequence allows for quantification of important secondary vascular parameters including wall shear stress (WSS) and oscillatory shear index (OSI) [5, 6].

Non-contrast-enhanced MR angiography

Because of the potential risk of contrast-induced nephrogenic systemic sclerosis in patients with severe renal failure, three-dimensional (3D) unenhanced MRA sequences have been proposed, such as the balanced steady-state free-precession (bSSFP) MR angiography, which enables high quality 3D datasets, including motion-free images of the aorta when combined with ECG gating and respiratory navigation [7, 8]. The whole dataset of the thoracic aorta can be acquired in only a few minutes with high signal-to-noise (SNR) and contrast-to-noise (CNR), with the pitfall of potential flow artefacts in the context of flow disturbance and high velocity jets.

Contrast-enhanced MR angiography (CE-MRA)

CE-MRA images are obtained by T1-weighted 3D-gradient echo sequences following endovenous contrast administration, through the shortening effect of T1 of gadolinium contrast. These sequences offer important anatomical information on both the aorta and main collateral vessels. This technique is suitable for the depiction of abnormalities such as penetrating atherosclerotic ulcer, dissection, coarctation, and aneurysm. The acquired images must be re-evaluated by post-process MIP and MPR reconstructions. By the application of ultra-rapid spoiled gradient-echo sequences in steady-state free-precession and the implantation of parallel acquisition techniques, multiphasic time-resolved 3D MRA images are obtained with high temporal and spatial resolution. These sequences are very useful in aortic dissection or shunts. In multiphasic time-resolved 3D MRA sequences, contrast injection is started at the same time as image acquisition, using the first set of images as a mask for posterior subtraction using post-processing techniques through MIP and MPR reconstructions.

If metallic devices related to the aorta are present (such as stents or adjacent embolization coils), the quality of MR images may be limited by off resonance artefacts that preclude optimal evaluation.

Normal aorta and common variants

The aorta is the largest and strongest artery in the body. The ascending thoracic aorta arises from the aortic valve annulus to the right of the midline and arches in a parasagittal plane to the left of the trachea to descend in the left paravertebral region, exiting the thorax via the diaphragmatic hiatus. In the human adult, normal diameter is considered to be within the limits of 40 mm in the aortic root, 37 mm in ascending aorta, and 28 mm in descending aorta. However, normal aortic dimensions should be normalized by body size and age. In a recent study [9] including 120 healthy volunteers, 10 of each gender in each decile from 20 to 80 years, aortic root measurement was assessed by MRI. Diastolic cusp-commissure dimensions showed evidence of an increase of 0.9 mm per decade in men and 0.7 mm per decade in women. The elastic properties of the aorta contribute crucially to its normal function. However, elasticity and distensibility of the aorta decline with age. The loss of elasticity and aortic compliance probably account for the increase in pulse pressure commonly seen in elderly persons and are accompanied by progressive dilatation of the aorta. This loss of elasticity is caused by structural changes, including an increase in collagen content and formation of intimal atherosclerosis.

The most common variant of normal aorta is the aberrant right subclavian artery arising distal to the left subclavian artery, coursing to the right and passing behind the oesophagus. This is only rarely associated with other anomalies and is usually of little significance. A right-sided aortic arch (aortic arch passing to the right of the trachea) is associated with two principal branching patterns: mirror-image branching, which is associated with a high rate of congenital cardiac anomaly, and right aortic arch with aberrant left subclavian artery, which has a low association with other abnormalities.

Diagnosis of thoracic aortic disease

Atherosclerosis

MRI is a non-invasive imaging modality that can visualize and characterize the composition of atherosclerotic plaques and differentiate tissue structure on the basis of proton magnetic properties with excellent soft tissue contrast. MRA sequences are highly useful for the detection of aortic atheroma, although they offer information on late repercussions of the plaque in the aortic lumen at an advanced stage of the disease. For accurate assessment of atheromatous plaques, structural alterations occurring in the aortic wall must be observed. Black-blood TSE sequences are very useful and promising in the identification and characterization of aortic plaque and for distinguishing its components *in vivo*. Being composed of cholesterol esters, the lipid nucleus has a short T2 and will appear as hypointense, while the fibrocellular components are hyperintense. Calcium deposits can be appreciated as hypointense regions within the plaque on T1-, proton density- and T2-weighted images. The fibrous cap and lipid core, organized thrombus and fresh thrombus or calcification and necrotic areas have been well characterized in studies performed both *in vitro* and *in vivo*. Fayad et al. [10] showed that MRI evaluation of the aorta compared well with transoesophageal echocardiography (TEE) for the assessment of aortic atherosclerotic plaque thickness, extent, and composition. Furthermore, high resolution non-invasive MRI demonstrates regression of aortic atherosclerotic lesions secondary to lipid lowering by simvastatin [11]. A very promising aspect is the capability of MRI to detect inflammatory activity of atheromatous plaque with the administration of contrast media. Inflammatory phenomena that determine the accumulation of macrophages can be demonstrated as hyper-uptake of gadolinium chelates in the plaque. This uptake is also produced with the use of other contrasts such as ultra-small superparamagnetic particles of iron oxides (USPIO) by macrophages of the atheromatous plaque [12, 13] (⊃ Fig. 44.1). Although commonly opposed as a limitation compared to TEE, MRI offers the possibility of assessing mobile atherosclerotic debris within the aortic lumen through the use of SSFP cine sequences.

Aortic aneurysms

Thoracic aortic aneurysmal disease usually occurs as a result of atherosclerotic or inherited conditions—Marfan's, Loeys–Dietz, Ehlers–Danlos, and Turner's syndromes. Aneurysms are often incidentally discovered on imaging, with the ascending aorta most commonly involved [14–18].

MRI is a robust tool for evaluation of aortic aneurysms. Three-dimensional contrast-enhanced MR angiography is highly accurate at depicting the location, extent, and precise diameter of an aneurysm and its relationship to the aortic branch vessels. It is recommended to combine MRA images with spin-echo in

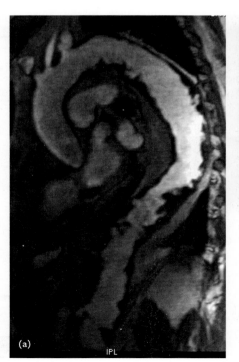
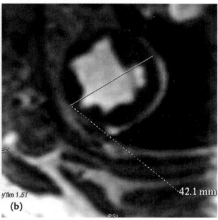

Fig. 44.1 Images extracted from a series of 3D MRA images of the thoracic aorta, in the parasagittal view (a) and in the transverse view (b), in a patient with severe and extensive atheroma of the aorta, 48 h after injection of USPIO. The uptake of USPIO by active macrophages of the atheromatous plaque leads to a signal void within the aortic wall.

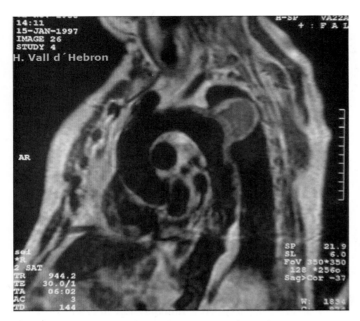

Fig. 44.2 T1-weighted black-blood image in sagittal view showing a thrombosed saccular aneurysm in proximal descending aorta.

black-blood images (Fig. 44.2), which are very useful for detecting alterations of the wall and adjacent structures. In mycotic aneurysm, T2-weighted and post-contrast T1-weighted images permit the identification of inflammatory changes in the aortic wall and adjacent fat, secondary to bacterial infection. Atherosclerotic lesions are visualized as areas of increased thickness with high signal intensity and irregular profiles. Periaortic haematoma and areas of high signal intensity within the thrombus may indicate instability of the aneurysm and are well depicted on spin-echo images. The information provided by MRA in aortic aneurysm is similar to that offered by current CT equipment. Both methods permit to accurately determine aortic diameters in sagittal plane. Post-processing techniques (MIP, MPR, and rendering volume) facilitate the visualization of the entire aorta and its principal branches, and are highly useful when planning treatment. The advantage of MRI over CT is that it is a non-ionizing technique that permits serial follow-up studies innocuously. For correct

monitoring, it is necessary to measure aortic diameter in the same location and same spatial plane. Diameters of the aortic annulus, the sinus of Valsalva, the sino-tubular junction and the ascending portion of the aorta should be measured in a standardized way. Absolute measurements are not a good predictor of the severity of abnormality, and measurements should be considered relative to age, gender and body surface area [15]. The sagittal plane allows for more reproducible measurements [19]. Contrast-enhanced 3D MRA can provide precise topographic information on the extent of an aneurysm and its relationship with the aortic branches [20] (Fig. 44.3 (Video 44.1)). The homogeneous enhancement of flowing blood within the lumen facilitates the delineation of thrombus. The capability of contrast MRA to visualize the Adamkiewicz artery represents an important advance in planning the surgical repair of a thoracic aneurysm, thereby avoiding postoperative neurological deficit secondary to spinal cord ischaemia. The newer non-contrast-enhanced SSFP MRA sequences have similar accuracy to CE-MRA [8]. As these sequences are quick and simple to perform, they have the potential to play a major role in the efficient follow-up of aneurysms. Combined information on aneurysm morphology and functional data provided by cine-MR sequences aids understanding of the physiopathology of aneurysmal dilatation. When the aneurysm affects the ascending aorta, it is recommended to conduct a functional study through the aortic valve using cine-MR and velocity-encoded sequences to rule out associated valvular disease. The aortic cusps should be assessed as bicuspid or tricuspid, which has a significant impact when tailoring therapeutic strategy (Fig. 44.4). The aortic root in the widest true short-axis image available has a trefoil shape, which favours the use of either three cusp-to-commissure or three cusp-to-adjacent cusp measurements [9]. Cusp-to-cusp measurements are easier to perform and may depict pathologic dilatation earlier since they are larger than cusp-to-commissure measurements [9]. They are also preferable for interimaging technique agreement since the right cusp-to-non-coronary cusp measurement in the parasternal long-axis window is standard in transthoracic echocardiography. Recently, MRI has been established as an accurate non-invasive tool for the assessment of aortic distensibility and pulse-wave velocity. These methods have been

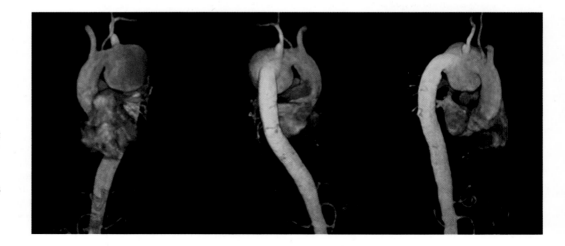

Fig. 44.3 Saccular atherosclerotic aneurysm. Volume rendering images from contrast-enhanced MR angiography shows a saccular aneurysm of the aortic arch and its relationships with the supra-aortic branches visualized in different projections.

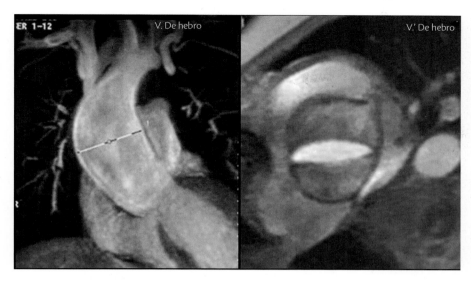

Fig. 44.4 Ascending aorta aneurysm (left) in a patient with bicuspid aortic valve (right) assessed by gradient echo MRI sequences.

used to assess aortic elasticity in patients with Marfan syndrome, bicuspid aortic valve, or aortic aneurysms [21–23]. They could be of clinical value for the identification of patients who are at high risk of aortic complications.

Acute aortic syndromes

Acute aortic syndromes carry high mortality and morbidity and early recognition of these conditions is vital to ensure prompt treatment [24]. Dissection, intramural haematoma (IMH), penetrating atherosclerotic ulcers (PAUs), and traumatic partial or total rupture are the primary pathologies in this group. They can share common imaging features, occur together or be *directly related*.

Aortic dissection

Aortic dissection is characterized by a laceration of the aortic intima and inner layer of the aortic media that allows blood to course through a false lumen in the outer third of the media. Diagnosis of aortic dissection is based on the demonstration of the intimal flap that separates the true from the false lumen (📹 Video 44.2). At the acute phase, MRI is often limited by poor availability, patient claustrophobia, and is hampered by a more time-consuming study. In suspected aortic dissection, the standard MRI examination should begin with black-blood sequences. In the axial plane, the intimal flap is detected as a straight linear image inside the aortic lumen. The true lumen can be differentiated from the false by the anatomical features and flow pattern: the true lumen shows a signal void, whereas the false lumen has higher signal intensity. A high signal intensity of pericardial effusion indicates bloody components and is considered to be a sign of impending rupture of the ascending aorta into the pericardial space. Similarly, the presence of pleural effusion is an indicator of impending aortic rupture (📹 Video 44.3). Detailed anatomical information of aortic dissection must indicate the extension of the dissection and the perfusion of branch vessels from the true or false channels. Therefore, a spin-echo sequence in the sagittal plane should be performed and, in stable patients, gradient-echo sequences or phase contrast images can help identify aortic regurgitation and entry or re-entry sites, as well as differentiate slow

flow from thrombus in the false lumen (➲ Fig. 44.5). Contrast CE-MRA has proved to be superior to black-blood sequences in the assessment of dissection extension and supraaortic trunk involvement. However, owing to the limitation of this technique to visualize the aortic wall and adjacent structures, the study protocol of aortic dissection should include black-blood sequences [25].

For planning surgery or endovascular repair, it is very useful to demonstrate the course of the flap, entry tear location, false lumen

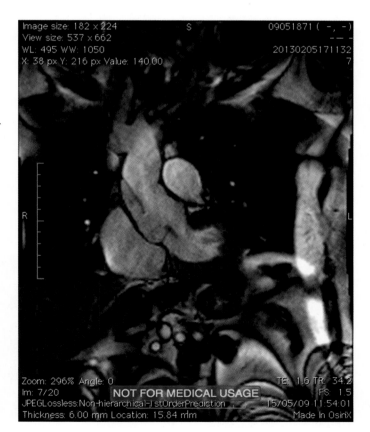

Fig. 44.5 SSFP cine mode showing the intimal flap (arrow) and mild aortic regurgitation in a patient with type A dissection.

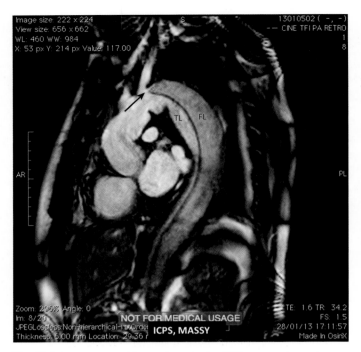

Fig. 44.6 Image extracted from a dynamic cine SSFP sequence in a patient with type B aortic dissection arising just after the take-off of the left subclavian. The arrow shows the entry tear. TL, true lumen; FL, false lumen.

thrombosis, aortic diameter, and main arterial trunk involvement by post-processed techniques with MPR reconstructions, MIP and volume rendering. It is mandatory to visualize the native images from CE-MRA since the flap may not be seen on volumetric reconstruction [26]. In type B dissection, it is important to acquire images with a wide field-of-view that includes the whole aorta from the arch to the aortic bifurcation. Time-resolved MRA provides additional functional information compared to conventional MRA, such as the dynamic assessment of blood flow in entry tears. In addition, the different evolution of contrast filling in both lumina of aortic dissection may be best depicted by applying rapid MRA sequences with maximum contrast at different phase. Subsecond CE-MRA can demonstrate sequential filling of the true and false lumen and may help identify the entry and exit points of the dissection (⊃ Fig. 44.6). In dissection of the ascending aorta,

it is mandatory to include cine-MRI sequences through the left ventricular outflow tract to rule out valvular regurgitation.

Intramural haematoma

Spontaneous acute IMH can be observed without any imaging features of intimal flap or penetrating atherosclerotic ulcer. Spontaneous IMH may be secondary to the rupture of the vasa vasorum, the capillary network of the adventitia and media [27, 28]. However, IMH may also be secondary to imperceptible microscopic intimal tears with limited wall dissection in which the false lumen is completely thrombosed. IMH is associated with hypertension and tends to occur preferentially in older patients and disproportionately in the descending aorta [29, 30]. A classic double-barrelled dissection in which the lumen is completely thrombosed at the time of initial imaging is very rare but indistinguishable from an IMH, and these conditions may have considerable overlap in natural history and require similar treatment [29, 30]. Although greater availability and rapidity favour the use of CT in acute diseases, MR plays a major role in the diagnosis of intramural haematoma. The greater contrast among tissues offered by MR often permits the depiction of small intramural haematomas, which may go unnoticed by CT [28]. The typical finding on MRI is the presence of wall thickening of the hyperintense aorta on T1-weighted black-blood sequences. In hyperacute phase, the haematoma shows an isotense signal in T1-weighted images and a hyperintense signal in T2-weighted images. From the first 24–72 hours, the change from oxyhaemoglobin to metahaemoglobin is responsible for a hyperintense signal in T1- and T2-weighted images (⊃ Fig. 44.7). Fat-suppression techniques are crucial to differentiate periaortic fat from intramural haematoma. Mural thrombi may present with semi-lumen morphology that mimics the morphology of IMH, rendering the differential diagnosis by CT or TEE difficult. This differentiation is easier by MR since mural thrombosis shows a hypo-or isointense signal in both T1-and T2-weighted sequences.

Penetrating atherosclerotic ulcer

PAU is defined as an atherosclerotic lesion that penetrates the elastic lamina, usually leading to haematoma within the media, but also potentially to true dissection or rupture. The diagnosis of

Fig. 44.7 Intramural haematoma diagnosed by MRI in ascending (a) and descending aorta (b). T1-weighted black-blood images show a thickening of the aortic wall with increased signal intensity (arrows).

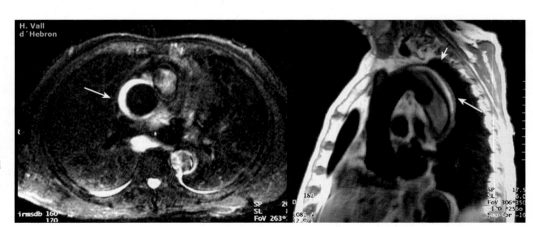

penetrating ulcer by MRI is based on the visualization of a crater-like ulcer located in the aortic wall. MRA is particularly suitable for depicting aortic ulcers along with the irregular aortic wall profile seen in diffuse atherosclerotic involvement. The aortic ulcer is easily recognized as a contrast-filled outpouching of variable extent with jagged edges (⊃ Fig. 44.8). Black-blood sequences may show disruption of the intima with extension of the ulcer to the thickened media that may be associated with intramural haematoma. It may be difficult to differentiate penetrating ulcer from the typical forms of dissection. The differential diagnosis should be established between arteriosclerotic ulcers that penetrate the middle layer and ulcer-like images that develop from a localised dissection of an intramural haematoma that appears as a pseudoaneurysm located in the area of the former intramural haematoma. Prognosis of these ulcer-like images is clearly more benign than that of symptomatic PAU.

Acute aortic syndrome in blunt trauma

Thoracic aortic injury is one of the leading causes of death in major blunt trauma and involves the partial or total transection of the aortic wall [31]. The aortic segment subjected to the greatest strain by rapid deceleration forces is located just beyond the isthmus. Aortic rupture occurs 90% of times at this site. Other less common sites are the distal ascending aorta or distal segments of the descending aorta. The lesion is transverse and involves all or part of the aortic circumference, penetrating the aortic layers to various degrees with the formation of a

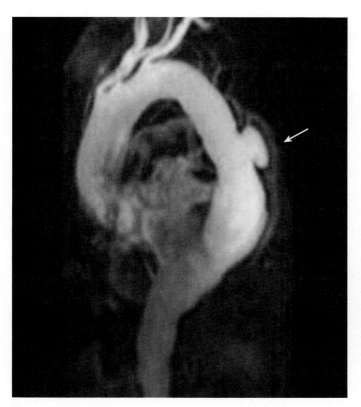

Fig. 44.8 Penetrating aortic ulcer in descending aorta showed by contrast-enhanced MR angiography.

false aneurysm. Intimal haemorrhage without any laceration has been described in pathological series but was not easily recognized before the advent of high-resolution imaging modalities. Periaortic haemorrhage occurs irrespective of the type of lesion. The closed bore design and long examination time have been considered to be the main limitations of MRI in acute aortic diseases and trauma patients. The development of fast MRI techniques has shortened the examination time to a few minutes and therefore MRI can be considered in critically-ill patients. The potential for MRI to detect the haemorrhagic components of a lesion by its high signal intensity is beneficial in trauma patients. On spin-echo images in the sagittal plane, the longitudinal view of the thoracic aorta makes it possible to distinguish a partial lesion from a lesion encompassing the entire aortic circumference. This discrimination is of prognostic significance since a circumferential lesion may be more likely to rupture. The presence of peri-adventitial haematoma and/or pleural and mediastinal haemorrhagic effusion may also be considered as a sign of instability. On the same sequence, the wide field-of-view of MRI provides a comprehensive evaluation of chest trauma such as lung contusion and oedema, pleural effusion and rib fractures. Furthermore, if delayed surgery is considered, MRI may be used to monitor thoracic and aortic lesions as it is non-invasive and repeatable [32]. MRA provides an excellent display of the aortic lesion and its relationship with supra-aortic vessels. However, it does not add any diagnostic value to spin-echo MRI, and it cannot supply information on parietal lesions and haemorrhagic lesions outside the aortic wall.

Aortitis

Inflammatory diseases of the aorta can be classified into two major subgroups: aortitis of non-specific or unknown aetiology (Takayasu's aortitis, Behçet disease, giant cell aortitis, Kawasaki disease, ankylosing spondylitis), and specific aortitis, in which the aortitis is the consequence of an inflammatory disease of known origin (e.g. syphilitic aortitis). Relevant ethnic differences have been observed in the epidemiological distribution of nonspecific aortitis—they are more common in Asian countries. Typical findings are marked irregular thickening of the aortic wall along with fibrous lesions that are the results of the inflammatory process of the media, which can lead to stenotic lesions (Takayasu's disease), aneurysms of the aorta and its major branches, or aortic insufficiency as a consequence of aortic root dilation. The high spatial and contrast resolution offered by newer MRI techniques permit the assessment of the aortic wall, and MRI is included as a routine test in the work-up of patients with vasculitis affecting large vessels, giant cell arteritis, and Takayasu's arteritis. Contrast spin-echo in black blood sequences is useful to identify the wall thickening in aortitis of various causes. In the initial stages of Takayasu's arteritis, short inversion-time inversion-recovery (STIR) and post-contrast T1-weighted sequences are particularly useful. Inflammatory changes in initial phases are reflected with contrast uptake and hyperintensity secondary to the wall oedema in STIR sequences (⊃ Fig. 44.9). Active inflammatory disease appears as variable thickening of the aortic wall and delayed

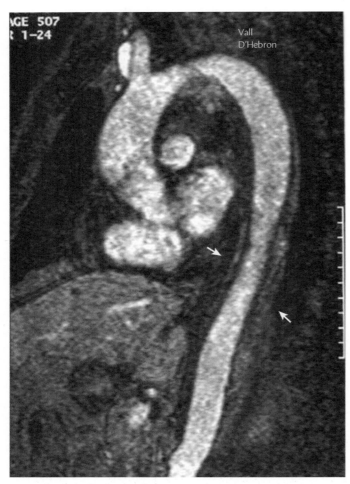

Fig. 44.9 Takayasu's arteritis. Sagittal STIR image shows a thickening of the aortic wall with increased signal (arrow) suggesting wall oedema.

contrast-enhancement after gadolinium administration can characterize the degree of inflammation in the aortic wall of patients with Takayasu's arteritis (33). In advanced stages of the disease, CE-MRA can determine the presence of stenosis in the aorta and its main branches secondary to chronic fibrous alterations. Recently, the capability of F-18 FDG hybrid PET camera combined with MRI to depict early stages of Takayasu's aortitis has been demonstrated [34]. Moreover, MRI can be useful in evaluating the response to medical treatment by depicting a decrease in arterial wall thickness.

Aortic coarctation

Coarctation of the aorta causes a more severe stenosis at the junction of the aortic arch and descending aorta and may be focal or more diffuse. Pseudocoarctation resembles a true coarctation but is caused by aortic kinking just distal to the origin of the left subclavian artery. It is usually not flow-limiting and therefore not associated with multiple collaterals. CE-MRA is the most useful technique for evaluating stenoses of the thoracic aorta. Temporally-resolved subsecond CE-MRA can depict aortic stenoses, but it is particularly useful in haemodynamically significant lesions such as coarctation, where it demonstrates gradual filling of chest wall collaterals (➲ Fig. 44.10). Phase contrast MRI can be used to measure velocity and flow, both proximal and distal to a stenosis, and helps assess the significance of a stenosis [35]. It may be very useful in monitoring disease progression over time. However, it is important to obtain measurements in similar anatomical locations to produce accurate and consistent results. MR is also well adapted for serial follow-up imaging after surgery of the aortic aorta with no radiation exposure.

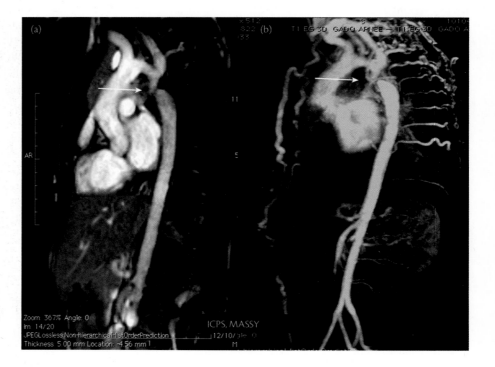

Fig. 44.10 Aortic coarctation. (a) Cine SSFP MR sequence showing the aortic coarctation (arrow). (b). Rapid dynamic subsecond CE-MRA in the same patient with aortic coarctation (arrow) showing extensive collaterals.

Pitfalls and limitations

The main limitations of MRI imaging include its low availability 24 hours per day, cost, patient claustrophobia, and the classical contraindications (pacemakers/defibrillators, metallic ocular implants, and cerebral vascular clips). MRI is not contraindicated in patients with mechanical prosthetic valves but the valve may induce a signal void artefact, which may preclude the study of the initial portion of the aorta. Big aortic stents make usually impossible the local study of the aorta. In acute aortic diseases, MRI is limited by lesser availability and is more time-consuming. For unstable patients, TEE or CT are better options. The use of gadolinium chelates is not possible in patients with severe renal insufficiency (clearance <30 ml/min), even in those on haemodialysis, since it carries the potential risk for the development of nephrogenic systemic fibrosis [36].

MRI in diagnostic strategies

Aortic atherosclerosis

TEE and MRI are powerful non-invasive tools for visualizing aortic atheromas. In patients with stroke or peripheral embolism, TEE is the technique of choice since it affords excellent assessment of the size and mobility of complicated plaques. MR imaging can non-invasively distinguish various components of the plaque such as fibrous cap, lipid core and thrombus, thereby assessing plaque stability [34]. Unlike TEE, MRI can visualize the entire thoracic aorta including the small section of ascending aorta, which is obscured by the tracheal air column. Furthermore, serial MRI can be used to monitor progression and regression of atheromatous plaques after lipid-lowering therapy. Cine MRI may also permit the assessment of complex plaque and aortic debris mobility with thrombus formation (➲ Fig. 44.11).

Aortic aneurysm

Aneurysms affecting the aortic root can be correctly assessed by TTE if the echocardiographic window is adequate. TEE will only be warranted when the acoustic window is poor or when the type of surgical treatment (repair or valve replacement) is being considered. In contrast, both TTE and TEE have limitations for adequate measurement of distal ascending aorta diameters, aortic arch and descending aorta. However, contrast-enhanced CT scanning and MRI very accurately detect the size of thoracic aortic aneurysms. Axial images often cut through the ascending aorta off-axis, resulting in a falsely large aortic diameter. Nevertheless, when the axial data are reconstructed into three-dimensional images (CT angiography), one can measure the tortuous aorta in true cross-section and obtain accurate measurement of aortic diameter. Such three-dimensional imaging should then always be used to follow patients with aortic aneurysms over time. MRI may be preferred for the follow-up of patients since it avoids the need for ionizing radiation [1, 2].

Acute aortic syndromes

For imaging suspected acute aortic syndromes, a primary consideration should be the accuracy and rapidity in the diagnosis. A meta-analysis [38] showed diagnostic accuracy to be practically the same (95–100%) for CT, TEE, and MRI. Most shortcomings are due to user-interpretation errors rather than the technique itself. However, the analysis of the International Registry of Aortic Dissection (IRAD) [39] showed that CT is the most frequently used imaging technique (61%), followed by echocardiography (33%). MRI does have potential limitations in this patient population. The scan times for MRI are significantly longer than for CT. Although cardiac rhythm, blood pressure, and oximetry can be monitored with MRI-appropriate equipment, caring for patients can be difficult in emergent or unstable clinical scenarios. Nevertheless, in stable patients with doubtful intramural haematoma diagnosed by CT, MRI is the technique of choice since the hyperintense signal in the aortic wall can facilitate a correct diagnosis. In addition, MRI is accurate for the study of aortic ulcers, particularly for intramural haemorrhage that complicates ulcers, and is indicated if kidney failure is present.

TEE, CT, and MRI are also very useful in the diagnosis of traumatic aortic lesions such as intimal dissection, medial laceration, pseudoaneurysm, or periaortic haemorrhage. Selection of the imaging test depends on the haemodynamic instability of the patient and the availability and experience of the centre. TEE offers

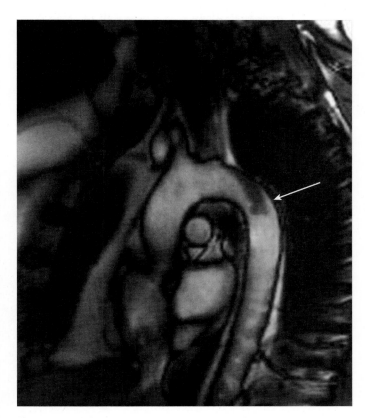

Fig. 44.11 Still frame extracted from SSFP cine MR showing extensive atherothrombotic debris (arrow) in a patient with aortic atheroma.

excellent information on aortic wall lesions, but both CT and MR have an advantage owing to their wider field-of-view.

MRI in prognosis and follow-up

Aortic aneurysm

The size of the aorta is the principal predictor of aortic rupture or dissection. In a large retrospective study gathering thoracic aortic aneurysms of different aetiologies, the risk of rupture or dissection was 6.9% per year and, including death, 15.6% per year for a size >60mm [15, 16]. The mean growth rate for all thoracic aneurysms was 1 mm/yr. The growth rate was significantly higher for aneurysms of the descending aorta, 1.9 mm/yr, than those of the ascending aorta, 0.7 mm/yr. In addition, dissected thoracic aneurysms grew significantly more rapidly (1.4 mm/yr) than non-dissected aneurysms (0.9 mm/yr). In a more recent study, Davies et al. [15] recommended elective operative repair before the patient enters the zone of moderate risk of an aortic size index greater than 2.75 cm/m².

MRI is the best technique in the follow-up of patients with inherited aortic disease. All patients with Marfan syndrome should have annual imaging of the ascending aorta (⊃ Fig. 44.12). TTE can be used for serial imaging follow-up of the dilated ascending aorta when correlation between the dimensions measured by TTE and CT/MRI have been documented. Repeat MRI is suggested at least every 3 years in patients with Marfan syndrome to reassess the aortic arch and descending aorta and reconfirm that TTE remains a reliable tool for measurement of the ascending aorta. Following elective aortic root replacement, CT/MRI are generally performed to establish a baseline aortic assessment for patients with Marfan syndrome [18–22] Annual TTE and MRI imaging of the aorta is generally recommended following aortic root replacement. The frequency of aortic imaging is individualized depending on patient characteristics, type of operation performed,

complications and duration of follow-up. Serial postoperative follow-up imaging should focus on progression of disease affecting the native aorta, and common postoperative complications including the development of pseudoaneurysm and coronary anastomotic aneurysms.

Aortic root aneurysms are present in the majority of Loeys–Dietz syndrome patients. Involvement of other aortic segments and smaller arteries in the form of aneurysms or marked tortuosity are characteristic in this population [40]. Although annual comprehensive arterial imaging protocol with MRI or MDCT has been recommended, the strategy for follow-up is not well-established and should be individualized from annually to every 2–3 years, depending on abnormalities present, family risk of complications, and the degree of evolution.

CT and MRI have better inter-observer variability than echocardiography for aortic diameter measurements. MRA permits us to define a plane in any arbitrary space orientation and easily find the plane orthogonal to the vessel walls (⊃ Fig. 44.13).

Acute aortic syndrome

Along with age, signs and/or symptoms of organ malperfusion, and clinical instability, fluid extravasation into the pericardium and periaortic haematoma have poor prognosis in acute phase. After discharge, variables related to greater aortic dilatation were entry tear size [42], maximum descending aorta diameter in subacute phase and the high-pressure pattern in false lumen [41, 43].

Survivors of initial aortic dissection repair still face considerable risk for future complications, including bleeding at the repair site, aortic graft infection, and pseudoaneurysm (▤ Video 44.4). Slight thickening around the graft caused by peri-graft fibrosis is a common finding. However, large or asymmetrical thickening around the tube-graft may represent localised haematoma caused by anastomotic leakage [41]. The higher incidence of bleeding has been reported at the site of re-implanted coronary arteries. Gadolinium-enhanced

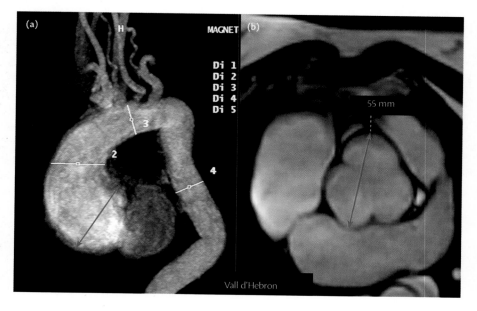

Fig. 44.12 MRI in Marfan patient. Left: parasagittal plane by MRA showing significant enlargement of the aortic root (arrow). Right: maximum diameter from right cusp-to-noncoronary cusp by non-contrast-enhanced SSFP (arrow).

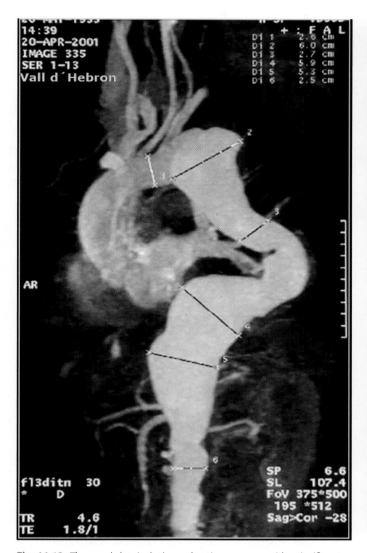

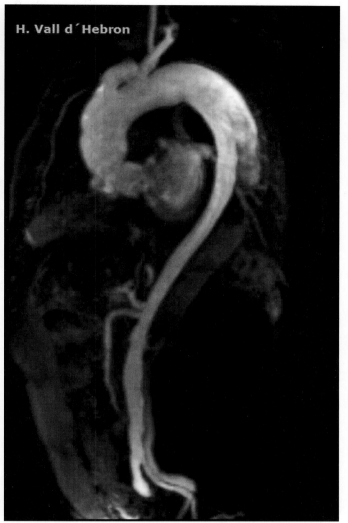

Fig. 44.13 Thoracoabdominal atherosclerotic aneurysms with a significant aorta tortuosity. By gradient-echo MR correct measurement of the aortic diameters perpendicular to the aortic walls can be performed.

Fig. 44.14 Type B aortic dissection. Time-resolved sagittal maximum-intensity-projection angiograms show time course of enhancement of both lumens.

MRI with standard spin-echo sequences can provide detailed information on suture detachment; the site of bleeding appears as high-signal intensity within the haematoma. Moreover, gadolinium-enhanced MRA is particularly effective in the depiction of the complex postoperative anatomy and in elucidating the prosthetic tube, distal and proximal anastomoses and residual distal dissection and, occasionally, dilated segments (📹 Video 44.5).

Because of these risks, patients commonly undergo post-operative monitoring. MRI offers many advantages for these patients, as aortic dimensions can be acquired with both precision and reproducibility, aspects that are critical for serial imaging, in which small changes in dimension may have significant clinical implications. Futhermore, the integrated study of anatomy and physiology on blood flow can provide very interesting data to clarify the mechanisms responsible for aortic dilatation. Time-resolved MRA can provide additional dynamic information on blood flow in entry tears (➲ Fig. 44.14).

Velocity-encoded cine-MR sequences have a promising role in the functional assessment of aortic dissection through the quantification of flow in both lumina and the possibility of establishing haemodynamic patterns of progressive dilatation risk (➲ Fig. 44.15). Increased false lumen pressure was another important factor implying false lumen enlargement. The high false lumen pressure was due, in the majority of cases, to a large entry tear without distal emptying flow or re-entry site of similar size. It is often difficult to identify the distal discharge communication; thus, indirect signs of high false lumen pressure such as true lumen compression, partial thrombosis of the false lumen [43] or the velocity pattern of false lumen flow by phase contrast sequences should be considered [44, 45].

The evolution of intramural haematoma may result in resorption, aneurysm formation or dissection [46]. Intramural haematoma may regress completely in 34% of patients, progress to aortic dissection in 12% and to aneurysm in 20% and evolve

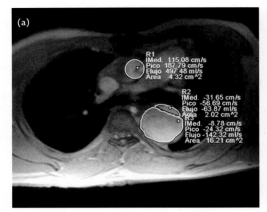

Fig. 44.15 Phase-contrast volumetric quantification of true and false lumen flows. (a) Cross-sectional area of both lumens. (b) Flow volume curves of the true lumen (red) and false lumen (green).

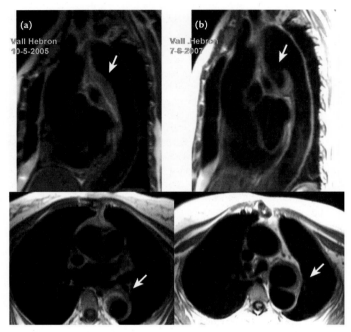

Fig. 44.16 Acute type B intramural haematoma (a) which evolved to localized dissection and pseudoaneurysm formations after a 2-year follow-up (b).

to pseudoaneurysm in 24% (⬧ Fig. 44.16). Given their wider field-of-view, MRI and CT are better than TEE for defining this dynamic evolution. MRI offers has the possibility of monitoring the evolution of intramural bleeding and depicting new asymptomatic intramural re-bleeding episodes.

The natural history of penetrating aortic ulcer is unknown. Like intramural haematoma, several evolution patterns have been described. Many patients with penetrating ulcer do not need immediate aortic repair but do require close follow-up with serial imaging studies, by CT or MRI, to document disease progression (⬧ Fig. 44.17). Although many authors have documented the propensity of aortic ulcers to develop progressive aneurysmal dilatation, the progression is usually slow. MRI may be helpful to show incidental and asymptomatic bleeding of aortic ulcers. Spontaneous, complete aortic rupture may occur. Some aortic ulcers are an incidental finding, similar to saccular aneurysms. In these cases, size and enlargement are the only predictors of complications.

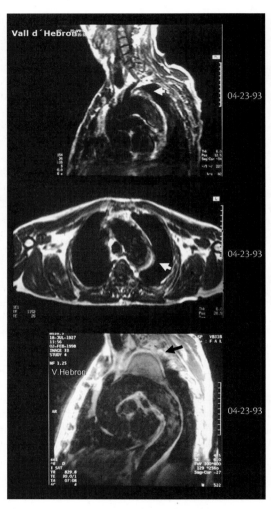

Fig. 44.17 Penetrating atherosclerotic ulcer with small intramural haemorrhage located in the upper part of the descending aorta. T1-weighted, in sagittal view reveals this ulceration (arrow). After 5 years of asymptomatic evolution, MRI shows a large saccular aneurysm formation (arrow) in the original site of the atherosclerotic ulcerated plaque.

Acknowledgements

The authors thank Dr Francesca Sanguineti (Hôpital Jacques Cartier, ICPS, Massy) for her contribution to the iconographic data.

References

1. François CJ, Carr JC. MRI of the thoracic aorta. *Cardiol Clin* 2007; 25: 171–84.

2. Russo V, Renzulli M, Buttazzi K, et al. Acquired diseases of the thoracic aorta: role of MRI and MRA. *Eur Radiol* 2006; 16: 852–65.

3. François CJ, Tuite D, Deshpande V, Jerecic R, Weale P, Carr JC. Unenhanced MR angiography of the thoracic aorta: initial clinical evaluation. *Am J Roentgenol* 2008; 190: 902–6.

4. Amano Y, Takahama K, Kumita S. Non-contrast-enhanced MR angiography of the thoracic aorta using cardiac and navigator-gated magnetization-prepared three-dimensional steady-state free precession. *J Magn Reson Imaging* 2008; 27: 504–9.

5. Hope MD, Hope TA, Crook SE, et al. 4D flow CMR in assessment of valve-related ascending aortic disease. *JACC Cardiovasc Imaging* 2011; 4: 781–7.

6. Frydrychowicz A, Stalder AF, Russe MF, et al. Three-dimensional analysis of segmental wall shear stress in the aorta by flow-sensitive four-dimensional-MRI. *J Magn Reson Imaging* 2009; 30: 77–84.

7. Miyazaki M, Lee VS. Nonenhanced MR angiography. *Radiology* 2008; 248: 20–43.

8. Krishnam MS, Tomasian A, Malik S, Desphande V, Laub G, Ruehm SG. Image quality and diagnostic accuracy of unenhanced SSFP MR angiography compared with conventional contrast-enhanced MR angiography for the assessment of thoracic aortic diseases. *Eur Radiol* 2010; 20: 1311–20.

9. Burman ED, Keegan J, Kilner PJ. Aortic root measurement by cardiovascular magnetic resonance. *Circulation Cardiovascular Imaging* 2008; 1: 104–13.

10. Fayad ZA, Nahar T, Fallon JT, et al. In vivo magnetic resonance evaluation of atherosclerotic plaques in the human thoracic aorta. *Circulation* 2000; 101: 2503–9.

11. Corti R, Fayad ZA, Fuster V, et al. Effects of lipid-lowering by simvastatin on human atherosclerotic lesions. A longitudinal study by high-resolution, noninvasive magnetic resonance imaging. *Circulation* 2001; 104: 249–52.

12. Briley-Saebo KC, Shaw PX, Mulder WJ, et al. Targeted molecular probes for imaging atherosclerotic lesions with magnetic resonance using antibodies that recognize oxidation-specific epitopes. *Circulation* 2008; 117: 3206–15.

13. Briley-Saebo KC, Mulder WJ, Mani V, et al. Magnetic resonance imaging of vulnerable atherosclerotic plaques: current imaging strategies and molecular imaging probes. *J Magn Reson Imaging* 2007; 26: 460–79.

14. Hiratzka LF, Bakris GL, Beckman JA, et al. ACCF/AHA/AATS/ACR/ASA/SCA/SCAI/SIR/STS/SVM guidelines for the diagnosis and management of patients with Thoracic Aortic Disease: a report of the American College of Cardiology Foundation/American Heart Association Task Force on Practice Guidelines, American Association for Thoracic Surgery, American College of Radiology, American Stroke Association, Society of Cardiovascular Anesthesiologists, Society for Cardiovascular Angiography and Interventions, Society of Interventional Radiology, Society of Thoracic Surgeons, and Society for Vascular Medicine. *Circulation* 2010; 121: e266–369.

15. Davies RR, Gallo A, Coady MA, et al. Novel measurement of relative aortic size predicts rupture of thoracic aortic aneurysms. *Ann Thorac Surg* 2006; 81: 169–77.

16. Elefteriades JA. Natural history of thoracic aortic aneurysms: indications for surgery, and surgical versus nonsurgical risks. *Ann Thorac Surg* 2002; 74: S1877–80.

17. Masuda Y, Takanashi K, Takasu J, Morooka N, Inagaki Y. Expansion rate of thoracic aortic aneurysms and influencing factors. *Chest* 1992; 102: 461–6.

18. Roman MJ, Rosen SE, Kramer-Fox R, Devereux RB. Prognostic significance of the pattern of aortic root dilation in the Marfan syndrome. *J Am Coll Cardiol* 1993; 22: 1470–76.

19. Kawamoto S, Bluemke DA, Traill TA, et al. Thoracoabdominal aorta in Marfan syndrome: MR Imaging findings of progression of vasculopathy after surgical repair. *Radiology* 1997; 203: 727–32.

20. Krinsky G. Gadolinium-enhanced three-dimensional magnetic resonance angiography of the thoracic aorta and arch vessels. A review. *Invest Radiol* 1998; 33: 587–605.

21. Nollen GJ, Groenink M, Tijssen JGP, et al. Aortic stiffness and diameter predict progressive aortic dilatation in patients with Marfan syndrome. *Eur Heart J* 2004; 25: 1146–52.

22. Groeninck M, de Roos A, Mudder BJ, et al. Changes in aortic distensibility and pulse wave velocity assessed with magnetic resonance imaging following beta-blocker therapy in the Marfan syndrome. *Am J Cardiol* 1998; 82: 203–8.

23. Grotenhuis HB, Ottenkamp J, Westenberg JM, et al. Reduced aortic elasticity and dilatation are associated with aortic regurgitation and left ventricular hypertrophy in nonstenotic bicuspid aortic valve patients. *J Am Coll Cardiol* 2007; 49: 1660–5.

24. Hagan PG, Nienaber CA, Isselbacher EM, et al. The International Registry of Acute Aortic Dissection (IRAD): new insights into an old disease. *JAMA* 2000; 283: 897–903.

25. Kunz RP, Oberholzer K, Kuroczynski W, et al. Assessment of chronic aortic dissection: contribution of different ECG-gated breath-hold MRI techniques. *Am J Roentgenol* 2004; 182: 1319–26.

26. Goldfarb JW, Holland AE, Heijstraten FM et al. Cardiac-synchronized gadolinium-enhanced MR angiography: preliminary experience for the evaluation of the thoracic aorta. *Magn Reson Imaging* 2006; 24: 241–8.

27. Nienaber CA, von Kodolitsch Y, Petersen B, et al. Intramural hemorrhage of the thoracic aorta: diagnostic and therapeutic implications. *Circulation* 1995; 92: 1465–72.

28. Nienaber CA, Sievers HH. Intramural haematoma in acute aortic syndrome: more than one variant of dissection? *Circulation* 2002; 106: 284–5.

29. Evangelista A, Domínguez R, Sebastià C, et al. Long-term follow-up of aortic intramural haematoma. Predictors of outcome. *Circulation* 2003; 108: 583–9.

30. Evangelista A, Mukherjee D, Mehta RH, et al. International Registry of Aortic Dissection (IRAD) Investigators. Acute intramural haematoma of the aorta: a mystery in evolution. *Circulation* 2005; 111: 1063–70.

31. Richens D, Kotidis K, Neale M, Oakley C, Fails A. Rupture of the aorta following road traffic accidents in the United Kingdom 1992–1999. The results of the co-operative crash injury study. *Eur J Cardiothorac Surg* 2003; 23: 143–8.

32. Fattori R, Celletti F, Descovich B, et al. Evolution of post-traumatic aneurysm in the subacute phase: magnetic resonance imaging follow-up as a support of the surgical timing. *Eur J Cardiothorac Surg* 1998; 13: 582–7.

33. Choe YH, Kim DK, Koh EM, et al. Takayasu arteritis: diagnosis with MR imaging and MR angiography in acute and chronic active stages. *J Magn Reson Imaging* 1999; 10: 751–7.

34. Meller J, Grabbe E, Becker W, et al. Value of F-18 FDG hybrid camera PET and MRI in early Takayasu aortitis. *Eur Radiol* 2003; 13: 400–5.

35. Mohiaddin RH, Kilner PJ, Rees, et al. Magnetic resonance volume flow and jet velocity mapping in aortic coarctation. *J Am Coll Cardiol* 1993; 22: 1515–21.

36. Shellock FG, Spinazzi A. MRI safety update 2008: part 1, MRI contrast agents and nephrogenic systemic fibrosis. *Am J Roentgenol* 2008; 191: 1129–39.

37. Shunk KA, Garot J, Atalar E, Lima JA. Transesophageal magnetic resonance imaging of the aortic arch and descending thoracic aorta in patients with aortic aterosclerosis. *J Am Coll Cardiol* 2001; 37: 2031–5.

38. Shiga T, Wajima Z, Apfel CC, et al. Diagnostic accuracy of transesophageal echocardiography, helical computed tomography, and magnetic resonance imaging for suspected thoracic aortic dissection. Systematic review and meta-analysis. *Arch Intern Med* 2006; 166: 1350–56.

39. Hagan PG, Nienaber CA, Isselbacher EM, et al. The international registry of acute aortic dissection (IRAD). *JAMA* 2000; 283: 897–903.

40. Loeys BL, Chen J, Neptune ER, Judge DP, et al. A syndrome of altered cardiovascular, craniofacial, neurocognitive and skeletal development caused by mutations in TGFBR1 or TG FB2. *Nat Genet Mar* 2005; 37 (3): 275–81.

41. Fattori R, Bacchi-Reggiani L, Bertaccini P, et al. Evolution of aortic dissection after surgical repair. *Am J Cardiol* 2000; 86: 868–72.

42. Evangelista A, Salas A, Cuellar H, Pineda V, et al. Long-term outcome of aortic dissection with patent false lumen-predictive role of entry tear size and location. *Circulation* 2012; 125: 3133–41.

43. Tsai TT, Evangelista A, Nienaber CA, et al. Partial thrombosis of the false lumen in patients with acute type B aortic dissection. *N Engl J Med* 2007; 357: 349–59.

44. Inoue T, Watanabe S, Sakurada H, et al. Evaluation of flow volume and flow patterns in the patent false lumen of chronic aortic dissection using velocity-encoded cine magnetic resonance imaging. *Jpn Circ J* 2000; 64: 760–4.

45. Strotzer M, Aebert H, Lehhart M, et al. Morphology and hemodynamics in dissection of the descending aorta. Assessment with MR imaging. *Acta Radiologica* 2000; 41: 594–600.

46. Evangelista A, Domínguez R, Sebastià C, et al. Long-term follow-up of aortic intramural haematoma. Predictors of outcome. *Circulation* 2003; 108: 583–9.

⊃ **For additional multimedia materials please visit the online version of the book** (⌂ http://www.esciacc.oxfordmedicine.com)

CHAPTER 45

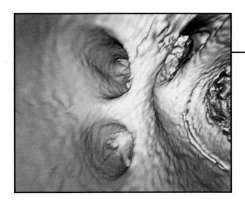

Role of multi-slice computed tomography (MSCT)

Raimund Erbel, Sofia Churzidse, Michael Horacek, Hagen Kälsch, Alexander Janosi, and Thomas Schlosser

Contents

Introduction

Multi-slice computed tomography (MSCT) is currently the most important technique for imaging the aorta allowing visualization of all aortic segments including the peripheral arteries. Using intravenous contrast the aortic wall and aortic dimensions can accurately be determined. Most important is the ability to image stent grafts and stent struts independent of the material used [1]. Currently MSCT with 16, 32, 64, 2 × 128, 320 or even 640 detector rows and fast tube rotation times. Thereby, high-resolution imaging is possible even in very sick patients without breath-hold. This is particularly important for emergency situations like the patient with polytrauma. It is not surprising, that MSCT is the most often used technique in patients with acute aortic syndrome studied in the international registry of aortic dissection [2].

The normal aorta

In children and young adults the aorta shows a strong association with body surface area [3]. At this age the results are derived from studies using echocardiography visualizing the ascending aorta [4]. In adults and the elderly, CT and MSCT data are available for the ascending and the descending thoracic aorta, as well as abdominal aorta (⊃ Table 45.1).

For the thoracic aorta, measurements of diameters are performed at the level of the pulmonary artery bifurcation (⊃ Fig. 45.1). Two aortic diameters perpendicular to each other are measured. For other questions, the diameters of the aortic ring, the aortic bulbus, the aortic arch, and other segments of the aorta can be selected.

Derived from EBCT (ultrafast CT, scan time 100 ms), the mean diameters of the ascending and descending aorta are 3.45 ± 0.4 cm/2.54 ± 0.3 cm for women and 3.71 ± 0.4/2.82 ± 0.3 cm for men (⊃ Table 45.1). These aortic diameters were measured based on non-contrast CTs, so that it is not possible to distinguish between the aortic wall and the aortic lumen. However, no general consensus has been presented on whether or not the aortic wall has to be included or excluded in CT measurements [10, 11].

The enlargement of the aorta over time means that the shape change of the aorta for those with a normal value is in the range of 0.2 cm/m^2 per year for the ascending aorta and 0.225 cm/m^2 per year for the descending aorta in women, and 0.2 cm/m^2 per year and 0.25 cm/m^2 per year for the ascending and descending aorta in men, respectively, taking into account in 90. percentile distribution (⊃ Fig. 45.2). This corresponds to an enlargement of the ascending aorta by 0.15 cm in 10 years in women and men, and of the

Table 45.1 Studies on mean aortic diameters measured by computed tomography

Author	Year	Sample size (*n*)	Age range (years)	Anatomic landmark of the Aorta	ATA diameter	DTA diameter
Aronberg et al. [5]	1984	102	21–61	Caudal to the aortic arch	3.5 cm	2.6 cm
Hager et al. [6]	2002	70	17–89	Caudal to the aortic arch 'at maximal size'	3.1 ± 0.4 cm	2.5 ± 0.4 cm
Kaplan et al. [7]	2008	214	24–87	Pulmonary artery level	3.4 ± 0.5 cm	n.a.
Lin et al. [8]	2008	103	51 ± 14	Pulmonary artery level	3.0 ± 0.3 cm	2.3 ± 0.2 cm
Mao et al. [9]	2008	1,442	55 ± 11	Pulmonary artery level	3.4/3.6 cm (females/ males)	n.a.
Wolak et al. [10]	2008	2,952	26–75	Pulmonary artery level	3.3 ± 0.4 cm	2.4 ± 0.3 cm
ACC-Guidelines [11]	2010			Pulmonary artery level	2.86 cm (females/males) (X-ray)	2.45-2.64/2.39-2.98 cm (females/males)
Kälsch et al. [4]	2013	4,129	45–75	Pulmonary artery level	3.45 ± 0.4/3.71 ± 0.4 cm (females/males)	2.54 ± 0.3/2.82 ± 0.3 cm (females/males)

(Kälsch et al. *Int J Cardiol* 2013; 163: 72–8)

ATA/DTA = ascending/descending thoracic aorta.

descending aorta we have seen the values are 0.16 cm and 0.17 cm in 10 years, respectively.

The aortic diameters increase over time. Gender- and age-dependent percentile distribution of diameters of the ascending and descending thoracic aorta showed within three decades from 45

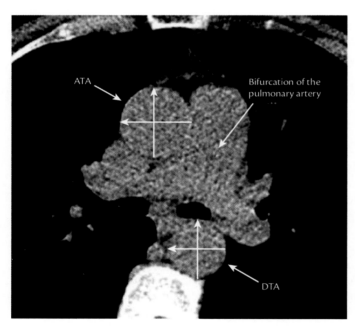

Fig. 45.1 Axial measurements of diameters of ascending thoracic aorta (ATA) and descending thoracic aorta (DTA) at the pulmonary artery bifurcation in non-contrast enhanced EBCT. Transaxial slice at the lower level of the pulmonary artery bifurcation from a computed tomography coronary artery calcium scan showing the method for deriving the ascending and descending thoracic aortic diameter. The white arrows represent outer wall ATA and DTA diameter measurements perpendicular to the axis of rotation of the aorta.

Reprinted from *International Journal of Cardiology*, 163:1, Hagen Kälsch et al, Body-surface adjusted aortic reference diameters for improved identification of patients with thoracic aortic aneurysms: Results from the population-based Heinz Nixdorf Recall study, 72–78, Copyright 2013 with permission from Elsevier.

years to 75 years an increase from 2.4 cm/m² to 2.7 cm/m² for females and 2.3 cm/m² to 2.5 cm/m² for males.

The aortic size increase is associated with age, height, weight, and body surface area, with no difference for men and women in univariable analysis. In multi-variable analysis age, systolic blood pressure, and body surface area were independently associated with the diameter increase of both the ascending and descending aorta.

For the abdominal aorta, most available studies have used ultrasound. Using CT, normal values were reported for eight aortic locations defined in ⊃ Fig. 45.3 and ⊃ Table 45.2 [13].

In addition to the aortic diameter, the increase in wall thickness has to be taken into account related to the aging process and development of atherosclerosis. Minimal intimal thickening and extensive intimal thickening are regarded as grade I and grade II aortic sclerosis [14].

Aortic aneurysms

The definition of aneurysm has not well been defined and is regarded as a discrete localized or generalized ectasia of the aorta. Usually a diameter of the ascending aorta ≥ 2.1 cm/m² is taken as a threshold [15]. This threshold is typically present for females, exceeding the 90. percentile of the aortic diameter between 45 and 70 years and for males beyond the age of 60 years (⊃ Fig. 45.1).

However, no correction for body surface area is performed when decision-making for surgery is discussed. Usually a threshold of 5.5 cm is regarded as indication for surgery [11]. This definition is derived from retrospective studies of patients developing aortic dissection or rupture. More prospective studies have to be performed in this field, before more details can be given.

Different to the normal aorta, aortic aneurysms are growing more rapidly at about 1 mm per year [16]. This is also seen in the percentile distribution of changes over time with higher

(a)

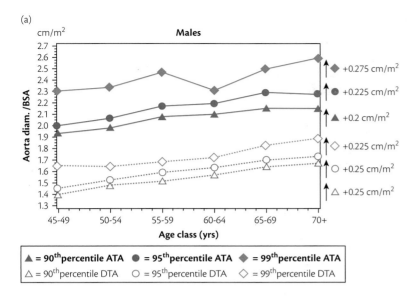

cm/m²

Males

Aorta diam. /BSA

2.7
2.6
2.5
2.4
2.3
2.2
2.1
2.0
1.9
1.8
1.7
1.6
1.5
1.4
1.3

↑ +0.275 cm/m²
↑ +0.225 cm/m²
↑ +0.2 cm/m²
↑ +0.225 cm/m²
↑ +0.25 cm/m²
↑ +0.25 cm/m²

45-49   50-54   55-59   60-64   65-69   70+

Age class (yrs)

▲ = 90ᵗʰpercentile ATA   ● = 95ᵗʰpercentile ATA   ◆ = 99ᵗʰpercentile ATA
△ = 90ᵗʰpercentile DTA   ○ = 95ᵗʰpercentile DTA   ◇ = 99ᵗʰpercentile DTA

(b)

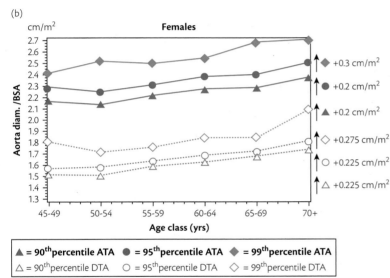

cm/m²

Females

Aorta diam. /BSA

2.7
2.6
2.5
2.4
2.3
2.2
2.1
2.0
1.9
1.8
1.7
1.6
1.5
1.4
1.3

↑ +0.3 cm/m²
↑ +0.2 cm/m²
↑ +0.2 cm/m²
↑ +0.275 cm/m²
↑ +0.225 cm/m²
↑ +0.225 cm/m²

45-49   50-54   55-59   60-64   65-69   70+

Age class (yrs)

▲ = 90ᵗʰpercentile ATA   ● = 95ᵗʰpercentile ATA   ◆ = 99ᵗʰpercentile ATA
△ = 90ᵗʰpercentile DTA   ○ = 95ᵗʰpercentile DTA   ◇ = 99ᵗʰpercentile DTA

Fig. 45.2 Association between aortic diameter (cm) of ascending thoracic aorta (ATA) and descending thoracic aorta (DTA) indexed for body surface area (BSA) in males (a) and females (b) with increasing age. The arrows demonstrate the constant increase of aortic diameters between the age of 45 and 75 years of both ATA and DTA for each percentile
Reprinted from *International Journal of Cardiology*, 163:1, Hagen Kälsch et al, Body-surface adjusted aortic reference diameters for improved identification of patients with thoracic aortic aneurysms: Results from the population-based Heinz Nixdorf Recall study, 72–78, Copyright 2013 with permission from Elsevier.

Table 45.2 Normal values of eight segments of the abdominal aorta

Anatomic segments	Men		Women	
	Mean	SD	Mean	SD
A (*n* = 62)	19.3	2.2	17.6	2.3
B (*n* = 70)	18.6	1.8	16.5	2.2
C (*n* = 64)	17.5	1.6	15.5	2.2
D (*n* = 41)	17.1	1.7	14.6	2.0
E1 (*n* = 77)	15,0	1.4	13.1	1.7
E2 (*n* = 70)	15.0	1.3	12.5	1.2
IL (*n* = 57)	9.8	1.3	8.0	0.9

(Reprinted from Fleischmann D et al., *J Vasc Surg* 2001; 33: 97–105, with permission from Elsevier) See Fig. 45.3.
A/B, above/below the common trunk, below the superior mesenteric artery; C/E1, above/below the renal arteries; E2, above the bifurcation; IL, iliac arteries.

diameter increase in the 99. percentile compared to the 90. percentile (➲ Fig. 45.2). The higher growth rate is related to the increase in wall stress (σ) taking into account the aortic radius (r), wall thickness (Th) and aortic pressure (P) according to the Law of LaPlace:

$$\text{wall stress } (\sigma) = Pxr/2Th$$

In order to estimate the growth rate, a mathematical equation has been developed [17]. Based on retrospective analyses Elefteriadis et al. could demonstrate, that the threshold for significant increase of risk for complications of aortic aneurysms was found for the ascending aorta at 6 cm and for the descending aorta at 6 or even more, 7 cm [18]. The aortic growth is silent, regular control of shape changes of the aorta are needed during follow-up in order to detect critical thresholds.

Abdominal aortic aneurysms

Abdominal aortic aneurysms (AAA) are associated with risk factors for atherothrombosis. Diabetes mellitus, is negatively associated with presence of AAA and progression [19, 20]. This observation of a protective role of diabetes against AAA development and progression was not supported by recent meta-analyses, which demonstrated that BMI and the waist–hip ratio are associated with the presence of AAA; waist–hip ratio being superior to BMI [21]. But no association was found between BMI and AAA growth.

Also, for total cholesterol a strong association with the presence of AAA was found (few results for randomized control trials) [22, 23]. Again, relationship to the AAA growth rate could not clearly be demonstrated [24–26]. In a meta-analysis it could be demonstrated that statin therapy is likely effective in prevention of growth of AAA (>55 mm), demonstrating an inhibitory effect on AAA growth.

The classification of AAA is most often done by CT. Three types with subdivision of type II in three parts are differentiated (➲ Fig. 45.4). The subdivision is dependent upon whether or not the renal arteries or the iliac arteries are involved. For treatment purposes the size of the healthy part of the aorta, as well as the diseased parts of iliac arteries, have to be measured. For endovascular

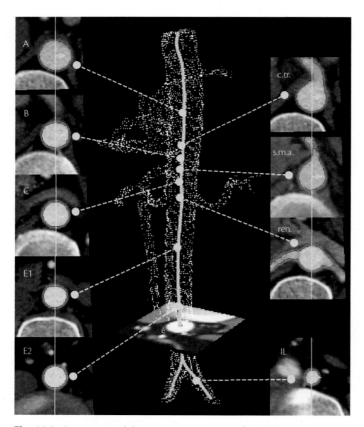

Fig. 45.3 Cross-sectional diameter measurements of the abdominal aorta in eight segments defined by the origin of peripheral arteries and the bifurcation. Reprinted from *Journal of Vascular Surgery*, 33:1, Fleischmann D, et al. Quantitative determination of age-related geometric changes in the normal abdominal aorta, 97–105, Copyright 2001, with permission from Elsevier.

grafting type I, IIa, and IIb are optimal indications, including about 50% of patients presenting with AAA (➲ Fig. 45.4) [27].

The progression of technologies enables digital segmentation and diameter, as well as volume measurements on CT angiography. It could be demonstrated that AAA volume measurements are more sensitive than diameter measurements to detect growth, while providing an equivalent and high reproducibility (➲ Fig. 45.5) [28].

MSCT-based angiography (CTA) produces better intra- and inter-observer correlations in measuring vessel length than digital subtraction angiography (DSA) and the potential to replace DSA as an imaging method before graft stent implantation [29]. This was confirmed by other authors for three-dimensional construction of complex anatomy [30–32].

Aortic sclerosis

Using MSCT the aortic wall can be imaged and signs of atherosclerotic plaque formation can be detected, which are subdivided into five grades by echocardiography and used for MSCT, too [14]:

Grade I	minimal intimal thickening
Grade II	extensive intimal thickening
Grade III	aortic atheroma
Grade IV	protruding atheroma
Grade V	mobile atheroma

Mural thrombus formation in aortic aneurysm is found in more than 85% of cases [34, 35]. Another problem may derive from diffuse enlargement of the descending aorta with smooth thrombus formation, as it may be present in chronic aortic dissection. Variable amounts of calcification is a sign of atherosclerosis. Even without using contrast, calcification of the aorta can be detected. It may also be present as a dystrophic sign in old thrombi of the aorta. The method for quantification is similar to the measurement of the coronary artery calcification using the Agatston-Score. In aortic aneurysm more severe calcifications are found than in dissection [36]. Calcification of the aorta has a similar sensitivity and predictive value for coronary and cardiovascular events as coronary artery calcification [37]. However, in comparison to coronary artery calcification, calcification of thoracic aorta does not yield any additional value when adjusted for risk factors.

The criteria for a differentiation of the aortic sclerosis from aortic dissection is shown in ➲ Table 45.3.

Penetrating ulceration of an atheroma resulting from plaque rupture of the internal elastic lumina can be accompanied by haemorrhage of the aortic wall (intramural haematoma). Typical intimal flaps and a false lumen are not seen. Particularly in elderly patients without aortic sclerosis, these findings are usually present in the abdominal part of the descending aorta and are called penetrating aortic ulcer (PAU), not rarely found in multiple locations. By MSCT the length, depth, and width of the PAU lumen can be

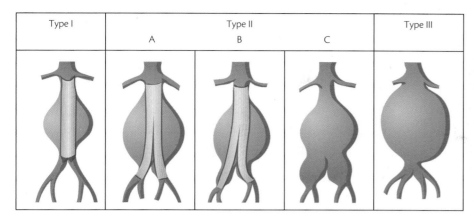

Fig. 45.4 Morphometric AAA definitions and possible graft configuration. Type I: proximal neck ≥15 mm and distal cuff ≥10 mm (tubular endograft), type IIA: proximal neck ≥15 mm and AAA down to aortic bifurcation (bifurcated endograft); type IIB: proximal neck ≥15 mm and aneurysmal involvement of the proximal CIAs (bifurcated endograft); type IIC: proximal neck ≥15 mm and AAA down to the iliac bifurcation (open surgery); and type III: proximal neck <15 mm and distal AAA expansion (open surgery). *Journal of Endovascular Surgery* 1997;4:39–44, Schumacher C, et al.

measured and signs of penetration with thinning of the aortic wall and haemorrhage of the surrounding tissue detected.

Inflammatory aortic diseases

The recognition of the important role of inflammation in acute aortic syndrome goes back to the early suggestion of R. Virchow, Berlin, who early supposed that inflammation plays an important role in atherosclerosis. The introduction of positron emission tomography in combination with MSCT allows an identification of patients with inflammation, which may play an important role in acute aortic syndrome but also in inflammatory diseases. Using the injection of (^{18}F) fluorodeoxyglucose, enhanced PET/CT of the body trunk is performed followed by a CT angiography of the entire aorta. In a first attempt, 33 patients with acute aortic syndrome were studied. PET-negative were 22 of 33 patients, but 11 (33%) were tracer positive (➲ Fig. 45.6). During follow-up of 224 ± 195 days, 32% of patients showed a progression of the acute aortic syndrome, when PET/CT was positive. PET/CT negative patients (55%) were stable or showed a regression of the disease. In comparison to the PET/CT results, elevated CRP and D-Dimer were not able to distinguish this high-risk patient population [38].

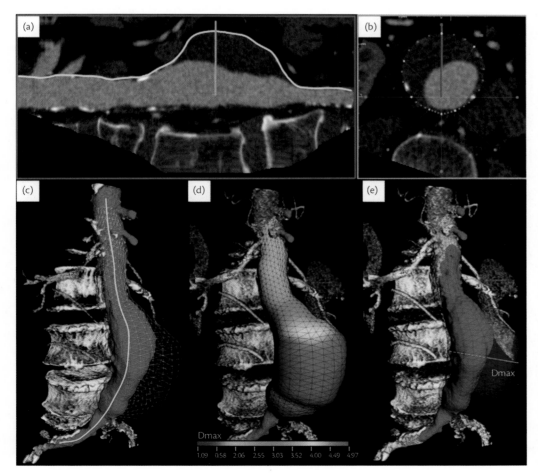

Fig. 45.5 AAA model in a 72-year-old man with a D-max of 6.97 cm. (a) Stretched longitudinal view of the path-based image. This path may be edited, if needed. The blue line represents the corresponding axial view. (b) Axial view shows AAA optimized path obtained by automated segmentation of aneurysm wall. The green lines represent the radial planes that can be edited in the orthogonal views. The red line represents the active stretched longitudinal view. (c) AAA surface model with optimized path (yellow line), lumen (red) and outer-wall mesh (green) of the AAA. (d) D-max values are colour-coded at each location: the smallest diameters are represented in blue and the largest in red. (e) The automatically calculated D-max is highlighted by the blue dashed line. Reprinted from *European Journal of Radiology*, 81:8, Kaufmann C, et al. Measurements and detection of abdominal aortic aneurysm growth: Accuracy and reproducibility of a segmentation software, 1688–94, Copyright 2012, with permission from Elsevier.

Table 45.3 Differential diagnosis of aortic sclerosis and aortic dissection

	Aortic sclerosis	Aortic dissection
Aortic diameter	↑↑	↑
Wall thickness	↑	Normal, except intramural haematoma and haemorrhage
Lumen surface	rough	smooth
Thrombus formation	lumen	False lumen
Floating thrombus	+	–
Intimal calcium displacement	+	+ +

Meanwhile further studies have been performed demonstrating the role of inflammation in aortic diseases. In patients with Takayasu-arteritis the role of [18F] FDG-PET could be shown [39, 40]. The rate of PET-positive findings in the aorta was higher in aortic syndrome than in the patients which could be studied in cancer, where the incidence was 7% (⊃ Fig. 45.7) [41].

In aortitis PET/CT can help to establish the diagnosis early before life-threatening sequelae of aortitis occur [42]. Similarly the formation of mycotic aneurysms of the aorta can be diagnosed using FDG PET/CT [43].

Meanwhile [18F] FDG PET (⊃ Fig. 45.7) has even been used to demonstrate the medication-associated attenuation of signs of inflammatory atherosclerotic plaque in patients with impaired glucose tolerance or diabetes. This could be demonstrated in a prospective randomized controlled study looking to the ascending aorta, as well as the carotid artery [44].

The PET/CT studies will get more attention in the future, when the 64 slice PET/CT systems are more widely used providing higher spatial and temporal resolution.

Aortic dissection

In aortic dissection, MSCT allows a differentiation of the true and false lumen according to a different contrast density and filling (⊃ Fig. 45.8). Contrast may be absent in the false lumen, when no communication between true and false lumen or intramural haematoma is present. Particularly in this situation, careful analysis of the true lumen often leads to the detection of small localized tears demonstrating a rupture point. When contrast fills the false lumen, the intimal flap can be visualized and often the entry and re-entry tear identified.

Whereas the exact localization of the entry tear is usually possible, due to a disrupture of the intimal flap, the re-entry is quite difficult to detect, particularly when it is located in peripheral arteries and not in the aorta itself. MSCT is able to visualize the exact location and extent of dissection. Malperfusion of peripheral arteries (⊃ Fig. 45.9) can be imaged but differentiation between static and dynamic obliteration is not always possible. But, most important, thrombus obliteration of false lumen (⊃ Fig. 45.10) is visible.

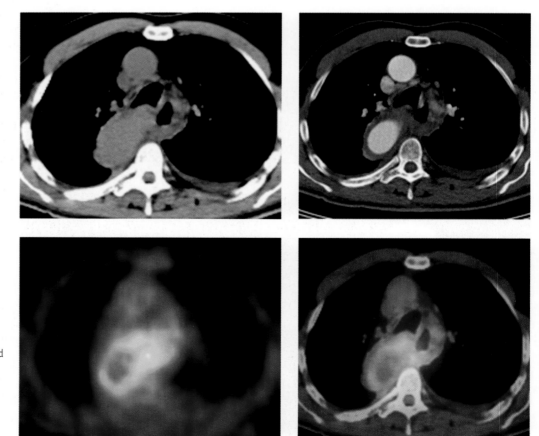

Fig. 45.6 CT and FDG-PET in a patient with acute aortic syndrome (intramural haematoma) who showed positive optic in the aortic arch and was treated successfully by graft stent implantation. Provided by Hilmar Kühl, Institute of Diagnostic and Therapeutic Radiology, University Clinic Essen, Germany.

Baseline

Post-treatment

Glimepiride

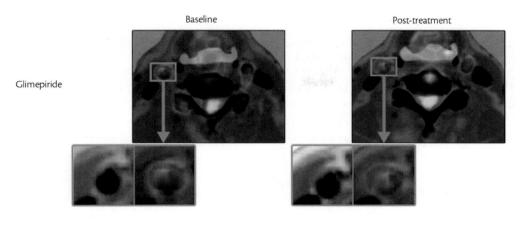

Baseline

Post-treatment

Pioglitazone

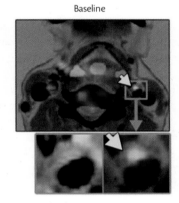

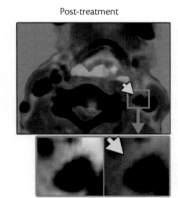

Fig. 45.7 Treatment effects on FDG uptake in atherosclerotic plaques. Treatment effects of pioglitazone and glimepiride on 18 F-flurodeoxyglucose (FDG) uptake in atherosclerotic plaques is presented with contrast images on the left and baseline and after 4-month treatment (right side) with pioglitazone (bottom) and glimepiride (top). Note reduction in FDG uptake in the atherosclerotic plaque. Reprinted from *JACC: Cardiovascular Imaging*, 4:10, Mizoguchi M, et al. Pioglitazone attenuates atherosclerotic plaque inflammation in patients with impaired glucose tolerance or diabetes: A prospective, randomized, comparator-controlled study using serial FDG PET/CT imaging study of carotid artery and ascending aorta, 1110-1118, Copyright 2011, with permission from Elsevier.

Particularly in the case of extensive motion of the intimal flap, exact decision-making is not possible. MSCT is not able to visualize or grade aortic regurgitation and define the exact mechanism, which may be valvular or dissection-related. Very important is, however, the ability of MSCT to demonstrate signs of emergency, including periaortic haematoma, mediastinal bleeding, pericardial effusion, and pleural effusion. Due to the measurement of the X-ray density Hounsfield units, acute and chronic haematoma can be differentiated based on differences in density, which is most important in the case of pleural effusion detected not rarely noted in

ascending but also descending aortic dissection. Thereby, MSCT is able to define ongoing aortic penetration or rupture.

A major role of MSCT is nowadays to assess the result of surgical or endovascular therapy: to define the presence of endoleaks after stent implantation and, if present, to differentiate the type of endoleak. Close follow-up of patients after stenting can best be done by MSCT.

It has to be taken into account that aortic dissection can occur even below the recommended criteria for surgery [45]. The cut-off value of 5.5 cm is now recommended as a good threshold for

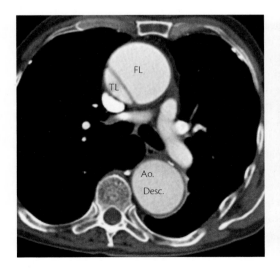

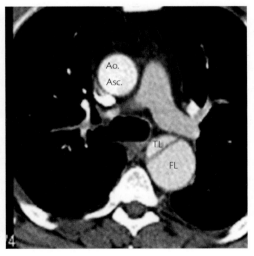

Fig. 45.8 Two examples of classical aortic dissection with a true and false lumen visualized in the ascending aorta (type A) aortic dissection (left side) limited to the ascending aorta (aortic dissection II). Aortic dissection type B (aortic dissection III) with clear separation of true and false lumen in the descending aorta but normal ascending aorta (Ao asc/desc = aorta ascendens/descendens).

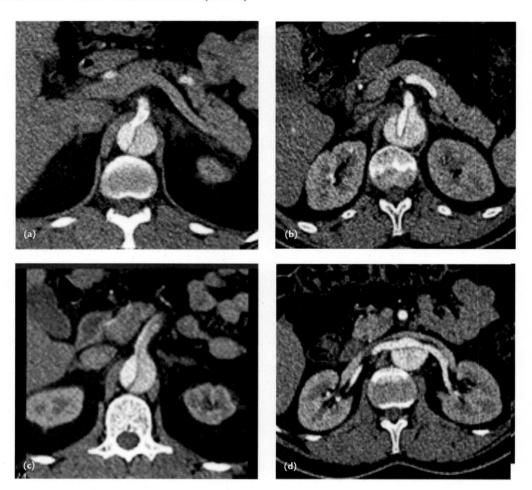

Fig. 45.9 Visualization of aortic dissection type B with involvement of peripheral arteries and malperfusion of the Truncus coeliacus. (a) Dissecting membrane obliterating the Truncus coeliacus. (b) Free arteria mesenterica superior. (c) Obliterated flow due to a dissection membrane of the arteria mesenterica inferior. (d) Both renal arteries have an origin in the true lumen.

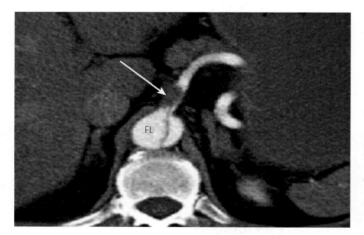

Fig. 45.10 Aortic dissection type B with thrombus in the false lumen occluding the Truncus coeliacus as sign of malperfusion which was responding after stenting and increasing flow in the true lumen and needed stenting of the Truncus coeliacus. FL, false lumen.

indication for surgery (15). But other authors have pointed out that only a small proportion of patients demonstrate dissection at small sizes and that the number of patients at risk increases dramatically, once the threshold of 6 cm is reached. In the Yale Aortic Center, patients were followed for a long period with an algorithm going for surgery by symptoms or aortic size ≥5.5 cm. With this algorithm no

aortic dissection and rupture occurred during close follow-up and optimal medical therapy. These data are supported by biomechanical testing showing that the enlargement of the aorta decreases the aortic wall distensibility, reaching a critical point at 6 cm [46]. At this point wall stress steeply increases and thus, the risk of rupture. At 6 cm the elastic properties of the aortic wall are exhausted [17].

Intramural haematoma

By MSCT a clear-cut differentiation can be given between the classical aortic dissection and the presence of intramural haematoma. Currently the latter is regarded as an initial step to classical dissection, which occurs after disruption of the intimal wall with antegrade or retrograde dissection of the wall disease creating a false and true lumen. Intramural haematoma do not show contrast within the thickened aortic wall, which is usually very smooth, crescent-shaped, has a relatively high density and localized to small parts of the aorta [47, 48]. This type of intramural haematoma (Type I) (◯ Fig. 45.11) has to be separate from secondary events with haemorrhage and haematoma formation in severe aortic sclerosis and PAU (Type II) [47].

Acute symptoms can occur related to the expansion of the adventitia and persist even for many days with changing intensity dependent on level of blood pressure.

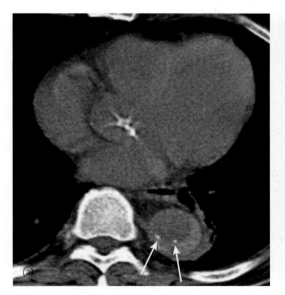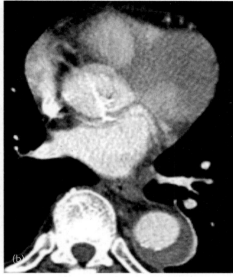

Fig. 45.11 Intramural haematoma demonstrating displacement of calcium spots in the non-contrast CT (left side). Crescent appearance of the intramural haematoma with wall thickening not involving the medial part of the aorta. The calcium spots are well visualized at the intima layer in the contrast enhanced CT (right side).

Discrete aneurysms

Using CT, even large aneurysms can incidentally be found. In case of acute aortic syndrome, MSCTs have to be analysed very carefully in order to detect any sign of intimal disruption and pseudoaneurysm formation, which can initially be very discrete, but progress very rapidly [49].

Penetrating aortic ulcer

Computed MSCT provides the best technology in order to analyse the structure of the atheroma with plaque ulceration in detail. In addition to the size (length, depth, and width), MSCT detects the presence of intramural haematoma and calcification, as well as the surrounding injury of tissue. Important is to check the whole aorta, because PAUs (⮕ Fig. 45.12) are most often

found in multiple aortic segments. Close follow-up is necessary in order to detect progression of the PAU, which can successfully be stented.

The surrounding tissue has to be taken into account in order to visualize, if contained chronic rupture is present leading from PAU to pseudoaneurysm and rupture [50]. Massive aneurysms can be found producing further symptoms related to compression or infiltration of tissue, bones, or nerves. Such contained rupture can even cause vertebral erosion leading to symptoms like back pain, even for years [51]. Contained rupture sizes are often called sealed, spontaneous healed, or leaking aneurysms [51, 52].

But such sealed aneurysms can also occur without any significant change in blood values because of restrictive blood loss. These patients are often clinically stable. Most often these contained ruptures are located posteriorly, producing smooth erosion that can be differentiated to erosion due to bacterial infections.

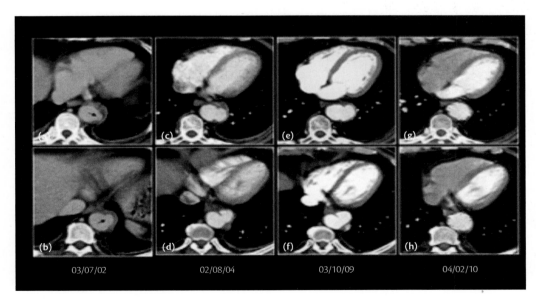

03/07/02   02/08/04   03/10/09   04/02/10

Fig. 45.12 Contrast-enhanced CT scans showing a penetrating aortic ulcer (PAU) of the distal descending thoracic aorta (a and b). Acute aortic syndrome (c to f) with rapid progression of the penetrating aortic ulcer during short follow-up. (g and h) Four months after successful graft stent implantation resolution of the ulcer (aortic remodelling).
Reprinted from *American Heart Journal*, 151:2, Eggerbrecht H, et al. Endovascular stent-graft treatment of penetrating aortic ulcer: Results over a median follow-up of 27 months, 530–6, Copyright 2006, with permission from Elsevier.

Blunt chest—iatrogenic thoracic injury

The use of aortic MSCT in blunt chest trauma has specific protocols in combination with TEE, especially in unstable and intubated patients, as reported recently [53, 54]. The protocol consists of an unenhanced phase, an arterial contrast-enhanced phase from the thoracic inlet to the symphysis pubis, and a delayed phase. Generate oblique reconstructions, resembled the images obtained in conventional angiography, as well as sagittal, coronal, and multi-planar reconstruction (MPR) are required [54]. The use of 100 ml intravenous iodinated contrast at 4 ml/s is suggested to get a maximal arterial enhancement, acquisition of axial images at 0.75 mm collimation, and reviewing images at a section thickness of 1.5 mm [55].

In less aggressive protocols, axial images are acquired at 1.5 mm collimation during a portal venous phase, after injection of 80 ml of iodinated contrast at 2 ml/s in order to minimize a contrast and radiation exposure compared to a three-phase vascular MDCT. When non-standardized, non-specific arterial MDC protocols are performed, up to 10% of less severe aortic injuries are missed [56].

In patients with traumatic thoracic injury, the Society of Vascular Surgery has published clinical practice guidelines [57]. The guidelines classified traumatic injury in four grades (⊃ Fig. 45.13), including intimal tears as grade I, intramural haematoma as grade II, pseudoaneurysms with transection of the aortic wall as grade III, and rupture as grade IV. For imaging purposes CT is used in order to classify the extent of the traumatic injury [58], in grade I aortic injury is limited to the intima and therefore careful watching is indicated, but surgery in the other types II, III and IV (Fig. 45.13).

This decision was based on the evidence that most type I injuries heal spontaneously [58]. But close follow-up is necessary, in order to detect late aortic/related complications, which on the other side may justify endovascular repair on body of low risk patients with small tears [53].

Iatrogenic aortic dissection

The development of surgical and interventional techniques have also led to iatrogenic aortic dissection like those after surgery with cardioplegia cannula insertion of the ascending aorta, during Bentall operation [59–63]. But also, iatrogenic aortic dissection after percutaneous coronary interventions, even in the situation of acute myocardial infarction, have been reported [64, 65]. In comparison, interventional procedures had a better outcome than surgical procedures as the course of iatrogenic aortic dissection type A [66]. The decision of surgical or non-surgical therapy remains challenging because the 10 years' survival with surgical treatment was reported to be 68% and not significantly different from spontaneous healing [67]. Similar results are reported by the IRAD register [68].

MSCT and, in some cases, in combination with transoesophageal echocardiography are the most important techniques [69].

Risk factors for retrograde iatrogenic aortic dissection seem to be diabetes mellitus and hypertension [68]. Less often, classical intimal flaps or patent false lumen are visualized, suggesting that iatrogenic aortic dissection often occurs in the form of intramural haematoma and has a more focal structure [69].

MSCT is the technique that usually is performed in order to detect iatrogenic dissection after surgery (>90%). The false lumen is usually found at the ascending but also in the descending aorta. Histological examinations demonstrated cystic medial necrosis in 22.2% and aortitis in 2.8%, while the remaining had other aortic findings [66]. The prognosis of these patients is poor, as after 10 years the survival rate is about 30%.

The large database of IRAD included 34 (5%) of 723 patients with iatrogenic aortic dissection (76%) type A and 24% type B aortic dissection. Most of the type A dissections were related to cardiac surgical procedures, whereas 88% of the type B iatrogenic aortic dissection were related to cardiac interventional

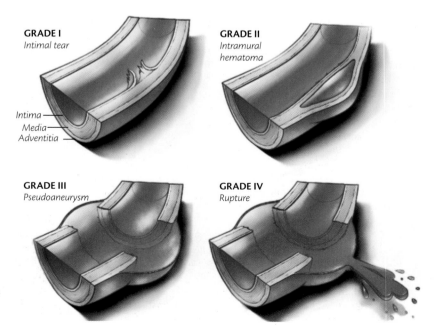

Fig. 45.13 MDCT base classification of traumatic aortic injury according to clinical practice guidelines of Society of Vascular Surgery.
Reprinted from *Journal of Vascular Surgery*, 53:1, Lee AW, et al. Endovascular repair of traumatic thoracic aortic injury: Clinical practice guidelines of the Society for Vascular Surgery, 187–92, Copyright 2011, with permission from Elsevier.

procedures [68]. In the IRAD register intimal flaps as well as open false lumen were less likely than in spontaneous aortic dissection [68].

Iatrogenic dissection related to PCI is not only restricted to the right coronary artery, but can also occur during PTCA of the left coronary artery, as recently reported in an emergency situation where MSCT revealed the extended dissection from the arch to the abdominal aorta [65]. The overall incidence in the emergency setting of myocardial infarction is higher than in elective cases [65].

The resolution of iatrogenic aortic dissection is best illustrated by MSCT. A potential risk factor has been the use of large ≥8 F Amplatz catheters, particularly in the right coronary artery [70]. Due to the stable situation, patients can be followed 4 days after the PCI. In a recent case report a significant reduction in the diameter of the false lumen could be demonstrated with complete resolution after 4 weeks. Instead of going to immediate surgery, the stenting of the ostium of the coronary artery may be enough to control the dissection [71]. Even rapid progression of the dissection with involvement of side branches leading to malperfusion or developement of myocardial infarction

or tamponade has been observed mandating immediate surgical intervention [70].

Limitations of MSCT

The highest resolution is received when ECG triggering is used and slice thickness is below 2 mm. As this protocol is more time-consuming, MSCT studies are done without ECG triggering and with slice thicknesses of 2 mm or more. In critical emergency situations, motion artefacts suggesting increased wall thickness and acute dissection may be present artificially. In contrast, in non triggered CT data sets, small aortic dissections and PAU may be missed due to motion artefacts.

The ECG triggering for CT is important not only to avoid artefacts, but also due to pulsation of the aorta, which may vary between 7.5% to 27.5% during one cardiac cycle (12, 72, 73).

Due to the elongation of the aorta during aging and particularly in patients with hypertension the assessment of diameters in axial images is difficult and can only be reliable, when three dimensional construction are done and cross-sections received orthogonal to the aortic long axis.

References

1. Eggebrecht H, Nienaber CA, Neuhäuser M, et al. Endovascular stent-graft placement in aortic dissection: a meta-analysis. *Eur Heart J* 2006; 27: 489–98.

2. Moore AG, Eagle KA, Bruckman D, et al. Choice of computed tomography, transesophageal echocardiography, magnetic resonance imaging, and aortography in acute aortic dissection: International Registry of Acute Aortic Dissection (IRAD). *Am J Cardiol* 2002; 89: 1235–8.

3. Roman MJ, Devereux RB, Kramer-Fox R, O'Loughlin J. Two-dimensional echocardiographic aortic root dimensions in normal children and adults. *Am J Cardiol* 1989; 64: 507–12.

4. Kälsch H, Lehmann N, Möhlenkamp S, et al. Body-surface adjusted aortic reference diameters for improved identification of patients with thoracic aortic aneurysms: results from the population-based Heinz Nixdorf Recall study. *Int J Cardiol* 2013; 163: 72–8.

5. Aronberg DJ, Glazer HS, Madsen K, Sagel SS. Normal thoracic aortic diameters by computed tomography. *J Comput Assist Tomogr* 1984; 8: 247–50.

6. Hager A, Kaemmerer H, Rapp-Bernhardt U, et al. Diameters of the thoracic aorta throughout life as measured with helical computed tomography. *J Thorac Cardiovasc Surg* 2002; 123: 1060–6.

7. Kaplan S, Aronow WS, Lai H, et al. Prevalence of an increased ascending and descending thoracic aorta diameter diagnosed by multi-slice cardiac computed tomography in men versus women and in persons aged 23 to 50 years, 51 to 65 years, 66 to 80 years, and 81 to 88 years. *Am J Cardiol* 2007; 100: 1598–9.

8. Lin FY, Devereux RB, Roman MJ, et al. Assessment of the thoracic aorta by multidetector computed tomography: age- and sex-specific reference values in adults without evident cardiovascular disease. *J Cardiovasc Comput Tomogr* 2008; 2: 298–308.

9. Mao SS, Ahmadi N, Shah B, et al. Normal thoracic aorta diameter on cardiac computed tomography in healthy asymptomatic adults: impact of age and gender. *Acad Radio* 2008; 15: 827–34.

10. Wolak A, Gransar H, Thomson LE, et al. Aortic size assessment by non-contrast cardiac computed tomography: normal limits by age, gender, and body surface area. *JACC Cardiovasc Imaging* 2008; 1: 200–9.

11. Hiratzka LF, Bakris GL, Beckman JA, et al.; American College of Cardiology Foundation/American Heart Association Task Force on Practice Guidelines; American Association for Thoracic Surgery; American College of Radiology; American Stroke Association; Society of Cardiovascular Anesthesiologists; Society for Cardiovascular Angiography and Interventions; Society of Interventional Radiology; Society of Thoracic Surgeons; Society for Vascular Medicine. 2010 ACCF/AHA/AATS/ACR/ASA/SCA/SCAI/SIR/STS/SVM Guidelines for the diagnosis and management of patients with thoracic aortic disease. A Report of the American College of Cardiology Foundation/American Heart Association Task Force on Practice Guidelines, American Association for Thoracic Surgery, American College of Radiology, American Stroke Association, Society of Cardiovascular Anesthesiologists, Society for Cardiovascular Angiography and Interventions, Society of Interventional Radiology, Society of Thoracic Surgeons, and Society for Vascular Medicine. *J Am Coll Cardiol* 2010; 55: e27–129.

12. Elefteriades JA, Farkas EA. Thoracic aortic aneurysm clinically pertinent controversies and uncertainties. *J Am Coll Cardiol* 2010; 55: 841–57.

13. Fleischmann D, Hastie TJ, Dannegger FC, et al. Quantitative determination of age-related geometric changes in the normal abdominal aorta. *J Vasc Surg* 2001; 33: 97–105.

14. Ribakove GH, Katz ES, Galloway AC, et al. Surgical implications of transesophageal echocardiography to grade the atheromatous aortic arch. *Ann Thorac Surg* 1992; 53: 758–61.

15. Erbel R, Aboyans V, Boileau C, et al. 2014 ESC Guidelines on the diagnosis and treatment of aortic diseases: Document covering acute and chronic aortic diseases of the thoracic and abdominal aorta of the adult. The Task Force for the Diagnosis and Treatment of Aortic Diseases of the European Society of Cardiology (ESC). *Eur Heart J* 2014;35:2873–926.

16. Coady MA, Rizzo JA, Hammond GL, Kopf GS, Elefteriades JA. Surgical intervention criteria for thoracic aortic aneurysms: a study of growth rates and complications. *Ann Thorac Surg* 1999; 67: 1922–6.

17. Rizzo JA, Coady MA, Elefteriades JA. Procedures for estimating growth rates in thoracic aortic aneurysms. *J Clin Epidemiol* 1998; 51: 747–54.

18. Coady MA, Rizzo JA, Hammond GL, et al. What is the appropriate size criterion for resection of thoracic aortic aneurysms? *J Thorac Cardiovasc Surg* 1997; 113: 476–91.

19. Reaven GM, Lithell H, Landsberg L. Hypertension and associated metabolic abnormalities—the role of insulin resistance and the sympathoadrenal system. *N Engl J Med* 1996; 334: 374–81.

20. Lederle FA, Johnson GR, Wilson SE, et al. Prevalence and associations of abdominal aortic aneurysm detected through screening. Aneurysm Detection and Management (ADAM) Veterans Affairs Cooperative Study Group. *Ann Intern Med* 1997; 126: 441–9.

21. Cronin O, Walker PJ, Golledge J. The association of obesity with abdominal aortic aneurysm presence and growth. *Atherosclerosis* 2013; 226: 321–7.

22. The UK Small Aneurysm Participants. Trial mortality results for randomised controlled trial of early elective aortic aneurysm. *Lancet* 1998; 352: 1649–55.

23. Brewster DC, Cronenwett JL, Hallett JW Jr, Johnston KW, Krupski WC, Matsumura JS; Joint Council of the American Association for Vascular Surgery and Society for Vascular Surgery. Guidelines for the treatment of abdominal aortic aneurysms. Report of a subcommittee of the Joint Council of the American Association for Vascular Surgery and Society for Vascular Surgery. *J Vasc Surg* 2003; 37: 1106–17.

24. Katz DA, Littenberg B, Cronenwett JL. Management of small abdominal aortic aneurysms. Early surgery vs watchful waiting. *JAMA* 1992; 268: 2678–86.

25. Nevitt MP, Ballard DJ, Hallett JW Jr. Prognosis of abdominal aortic aneurysms. A population-based study. *N Engl J Med* 1989; 321: 1009–14.

26. Brady AR, Thompson SG, Fowkes FG, Greenhalgh RM, Powell JT; UK Small Aneurysm Trial Participants. Abdominal aortic aneurysm expansion: risk factors and time intervals for surveillance. *Circulation* 2004; 110: 16–21.

27. Schumacher H, Eckstein HH, Kallinowski F, Allenberg JR. Morphometry and classification in abdominal aortic aneurysms: patient selection for endovascular and open surgery. *J Endovasc Surg* 1997; 4: 39–44.

28. Kauffmann C, Tang A, Therasse E, et al. Measurements and detection of abdominal aortic aneurysm growth: Accuracy and reproducibility of a segmentation software. *Eur J Radiol* 2012; 81: 1688–94.

29. Diehm N, Herrmann P, Dinkel HP. Multidetector CT angiography versus digital subtraction angiography for aortoiliac length measurements prior to endovascular AAA repair. *J Endovasc Ther* 2004; 11: 527–34.

30. Prinssen M, Verhoeven EL, Verhagen HJ, Blankensteijn JD. Decision-making in follow-up after endovascular aneurysm repair based on diameter and volume measurements: a blinded comparison. *Eur J Vasc Endovasc Surg* 2003; 26: 184–7.

31. Bley TA, Chase PJ, Reeder SB, et al. Endovascular abdominal aortic aneurysm repair: nonenhanced volumetric CT for follow-up. *Radiology* 2009; 253: 253–62.

32. van Keulen JW, van Prehn J, Prokop M, Moll FL, van Herwaarden JA. Potential value of aneurysm sac volume measurements in addition to diameter measurements after endovascular aneurysm repair. *J Endovasc Ther* 2009; 16: 506–13.

33. Ribakove GH, Katz ES, Galloway AC, et al. Surgical implications of transesophageal echocardiography to grade the atheromatous aortic arch. *Ann Thorac Surg* 1992; 53: 758–61.

34. Torres WE, Maurer DE, Steinberg HV, Robbins S, Bernardino ME. CT of aortic aneurysms: the distinction between mural and thrombus calcification. *AJR Am J Roentgenol* 1988; 150: 1317–9.

35. Machida K, Tasaka A. CT patterns of mural thrombus in aortic aneurysms. *J Comput Assist Tomogr* 1980; 4: 840–2.

36. Erbel R. Diseases of the aorta. In: *Diseases of the Heart*, Julian DG, Camm AJ, Fox KM, Hall RJC, Poole-Wilson PA (eds). W B Saunders, London, 1966, 1299–330.

37. Kälsch H, Lehmann N, Möhlenkamp S, et al. Body-surface adjusted aortic reference diameters for improved identification of patients with thoracic aortic aneurysms: results from the population-based Heinz Nixdorf Recall study. *Int J Cardiol* 2013; 163: 72–8.

38. Kuehl H, Eggebrecht H, Boes T, et al. Detection of inflammation in patients with acute aortic syndrome: comparison of FDG-PET/CT imaging and serological markers of inflammation. *Heart* 2008; 94: 1472–7.

39. Webb MR, Ebeler SE. Comparative analysis of topoisomerase IB inhibition and DNA intercalation by flavonoids and similar compounds: structural determinates of activity. *Biochem J* 2004; 384: 527–41.

40. Kobayashi Y, Ishii K, Oda K, et al. Aortic wall inflammation due to Takayasu arteritis imaged with 18F-FDG PET coregistered with enhanced CT. *J Nucl Med* 2005; 46: 917–22.

41. Ben-Haim S, KupzoV E, Tamir A, Israel O. Evaluation of 18F-FDG uptake and arterial wall calcifications using 18F-FDG PET/CT. *J Nucl Med* 2004; 45: 1816–21.

42. Balink H, Spoorenberg A, Houtman PM, Brandenburg A, Verberne HJ. Early recognition of aortitis of the aorta ascendens with (18) F-FDG PET/CT: syphilitic? *Clin Rheumatol* 2013 [Epub ahead of print].

43. Spacek M, Stadler P, Bělohlávek O, Sebesta P. Contribution to FDG-PET/CT diagnostics and post-operative monitoring of patients with mycotic aneurysm of the thoracic aorta. *Acta Chir Belg* 2010; 110: 106–8.

44. Mizoguchi M, Tahara N, Tahara A, et al. Pioglitazone attenuates atherosclerotic plaque inflammation in patients with impaired glucose tolerance or diabetes: a prospective, randomized, comparator-controlled study using serial FDG PET/CT imaging study of carotid artery and ascending aorta. *JACC Cardiovasc Imaging* 2011; 4: 1110–8.

45. Pape LA, Tsai TT, Isselbacher EM, et al.; International Registry of Acute Aortic Dissection (IRAD) Investigators. Aortic diameter >or = 5.5 cm is not a good predictor of type A aortic dissection: observations from the International Registry of Acute Aortic Dissection (IRAD). *Circulation* 2007; 116: 1120–7.

46. Koullias G, Modak R, Tranquilli M, Korkolis DP, Barash P, Elefteriades JA. Mechanical deterioration underlies malignant behavior of aneurysmal human ascending aorta. *J Thorac Cardiovasc Surg* 2005; 130: 677–83.

47. Mohr-Kahaly S, Erbel R, Kearney P, Puth M, Meyer J. Aortic intramural haemorrhage visualized by transesophageal echocardiography: findings and prognostic implications. *J Am Coll Cardiol* 1994; 23: 658–64.

48. Nienaber CA, Fattori R, Lund G, et al. Nonsurgical reconstruction of thoracic aortic dissection by stent-graft placement. *N Engl J Med* 1999; 340: 1539–45.

49. Svensson LG, Kouchoukos NT, Miller DC, et al.; Society of Thoracic Surgeons Endovascular Surgery Task Force. Expert consensus document on the treatment of descending thoracic aortic disease using endovascular stent-grafts. *Ann Thorac Surg* 2008; 85(1 Suppl): S1–41.

50. Eggebrecht H, Baumgart D, Schmermund A, et al. Endovascular stent-graft repair for penetrating atherosclerotic ulcer of the descending aorta. *Am J Cardiol* 2003; 91: 1150–3.

51. Gandini R, Chiocchi M, Maresca L, Pipitone V, Messina M, Simonetti G. Chronic contained rupture of an abdominal aortic aneurysm: from diagnosis to endovascular resolution. *Cardiovasc Intervent Radiol* 2008; 31 Suppl 2: S62–6.

52. Sterpetti AV, Blair EA, Schultz RD, Feldhaus RJ, Cisternino S, Chasan P. Sealed rupture of abdominal aortic aneurysms. *J Vasc Surg* 1990; 11: 430–5.

53. Mosquera VX, Marini M, Lopez-Perez JM, Muñiz-Garcia J, Herrera JM, Cao I, Cuenca JJ. Role of conservative management in traumatic aortic injury: comparison of long-term results of conservative, surgical, and endovascular treatment. *J Thorac Cardiovasc Surg* 2011; 142: 614–21.

54. Berger FH, van Lienden KP, Smithuis R, Nicolaou S, van Delden OM. Acute aortic syndrome and blunt traumatic aortic injury: pictorial review of MDCT imaging. *Eur J Radiol* 2010; 74: 24–39.

55. Mosquera VX, Marini M, Muñiz J, et al. Traumatic aortic injury score (TRAINS): an easy and simple score for early detection of traumatic aortic injuries in major trauma patients with associated blunt chest trauma. *Intensive Care Med* 2012; 38: 1487–96.

56. Malhotra AK, Fabian TC, Croce MA, Weiman DS, Gavant ML, Pate JW. Minimal aortic injury: a lesion associated with advancing diagnostic techniques. *J Trauma* 2001; 51: 1042–8.

57. Lee WA, Matsumura JS, Mitchell RS, et al. Endovascular repair of traumatic thoracic aortic injury: clinical practice guidelines of the Society for Vascular Surgery. *J Vasc Surg* 2011; 53: 187–92.

58. Azizzadeh A, Keyhani K, Miller CC III, Coogan SM, Safi HJ, Estrera AL. Blunt traumatic aortic injury: initial experience with endovascular repair. *J Vasc Surg* 2009; 49: 1403–8.

59. Gharde P, Aggarwal V, Chauhan S, Kiran U, Devagourou V. Iatrogenic acute aortic dissection during cardioplegic cannula insertion detected by transesophageal echocardiography. *J Cardiothorac Vasc Anesth* 2012; 26: e3–5.

60. Timek TA, Hooker R, Patzelt L, Bernath G. Conservative management and resolution of iatrogenic type A aortic dissection in a patient with previous cardiac surgery. *J Thorac Cardiovasc Surg* 2012; 144: e18–21.

61. Stanger O, Pepper J. Should iatrogenic type A aortic dissection in patients with previous cardiac surgery be managed conservatively? *J Thorac Cardiovasc Surg* 2013; 145: 612–3.

62. Rylski B, Hoffmann I, Beyersdorf F, et al. Iatrogenic acute aortic dissection type A: insight from the German Registry for Acute Aortic Dissection Type A (GERAADA). *Eur J Cardiothorac Surg* 2013 [Epub ahead of print].

63. Martins D, Guerra M, Mota JC, Vouga L. [Repair of iatrogenic aortic dissection during Bentall operation in a patient with annulo-aortic ectasia and mitral regurgitation]. *ReV Port Cir Cardiotorac Vasc* 2011; 18: 157–9.

64. Wykrzykowska JJ, Ligthart J, Lopez NG, Schultz C, Garcia-Garcia H, Serruys PW. How should I treat an iatrogenic aortic dissection as a complication of complex PCI? *EuroIntervention* 2012; 7: 1111–7.

65. Noguchi K, Hori D, Nomura Y, Tanaka H. Iatrogenic acute aortic dissection during percutaneous coronary intervention for acute myocardial infarction. *Ann Vasc Dis* 2012; 51: 78–81.

66. LeontyeV S, Borger MA, Legare JF, et al. Iatrogenic type A aortic dissection during cardiac procedures: early and late outcome in 48 patients. *Eur J Cardiothorac Surg* 2012; 41: 641–6.

67. GillinoV AM, Lytle BW, Kaplon RJ, Casselman FP, Blackstone EH, Cosgrove DM. Dissection of the ascending aorta after previous cardiac surgery: differences in presentation and management. *J Thorac Cardiovasc Surg* 1999; 117: 252–60.

68. Januzzi JL, Sabatine MS, Eagle KA, et al.; International Registry of Aortic Dissection Investigators. Iatrogenic aortic dissection. *Am J Cardiol* 2002; 89: 623–6.

69. Welch TD, Foley T, Barsness GW, et al. Iatrogenic aortic dissection or intramural haematoma? *Circulation* 2012; 125: e415–8.

70. Garg P, Buckley O, Rybicki FJ, Resnic FS. Resolution of iatrogenic aortic dissection illustrated by computed tomography. *Circ Cardiovasc Interv* 2009; 2: 261–3.

71. Carstensen S, Ward MR. Iatrogenic aortocoronary dissection: the case for immediate aortoostial stenting. *Heart Lung Circ* 2008; 17: 325–9.

72. Muhs BE, Vincken KL, van Prehn J, et al. Dynamic cine-CT angiography for the evaluation of the thoracic aorta; insight in dynamic changes with implications for thoracic endograft treatment. *Eur J Vasc Endovasc Surg* 2006; 32: 532–6.

73. Schlösser FJ, Mojibian HR, Dardik A, Verhagen HJ, Moll FL, Muhs BE. Simultaneous sizing and preoperative risk stratification for thoracic endovascular aneurysm repair: role of gated computed tomography. *J Vasc Surg* 2008; 48: 561–70.

Index